LEXICON MEDICUM;

OR

MEDICAL DICTIONARY;

CONTAINING AN EXPLANATION OF THE TERMS IN

ANATOMY,
BOTANY,
CHEMISTRY,
MATERIA MEDICA,
MIDWIFERY,
MINERALOGY,
PHARMACY,
PHYSIOLOGY,
PRACTICE OF PHYSIC,
SURGERY,

AND THE VARIOUS BRANCHES OF

NATURAL PHILOSOPHY CONNECTED WITH MEDICINE

SELECTED, ARRANGED, AND COMPILED FROM THE BEST AUTHORS.

" Nec aranearum sane texus ideo melior, quia ex se fila gignunt, nec noster vilior quia ex alienis libamus ut apes."

JUST. LIPS. *Monit. Polit.* Lib. i. cap. i.

By ROBERT HOOPER, M.D. F.L.S.

THIRTEENTH AMERICAN, FROM THE LAST LONDON EDITION,
WITH ADDITIONS FROM AMERICAN AUTHORS ON BOTANY, CHEMISTRY, MATERIA MEDICA, MINERALOGY, &c.

By SAMUEL AKERLY, M.D.

FORMERLY PHYSICIAN TO THE NEW-YORK CITY DISPENSARY, RESIDENT PHYSICIAN TO THE CITY HOSPITAL, LATE HOSPITAL SURGEON UNITED STATES' ARMY, PHYSICIAN TO THE NEW-YORK INSTITUTION FOR THE INSTRUCTION OF THE DEAF AND DUMB, &c. &c.

Volume One: A-J

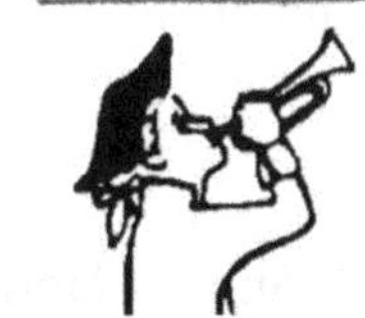

HERITAGE BOOKS
2009

HERITAGE BOOKS
AN IMPRINT OF HERITAGE BOOKS, INC.

Books, CDs, and more—Worldwide

For our listing of thousands of titles see our website
at
www.HeritageBooks.com

A Facsimile Reprint
Published 2009 by
HERITAGE BOOKS, INC.
Publishing Division
100 Railroad Ave. #104
Westminster, Maryland 21157

Originally published
New York:
Harper & Brothers
1843

— Publisher's Notice —
In reprints such as this, it is often not possible to remove blemishes from the original. We feel the contents of this book warrant its reissue despite these blemishes and hope you will agree and read it with pleasure.

International Standard Book Numbers
Paperbound: 978-0-7884-4917-8
Clothbound: 978-0-7884-8080-5

ADVERTISEMENT

TO THE

THIRTEENTH AMERICAN EDITION.

In order to render the Thirteenth American editon of Hooper's Medical Dictionary more acceptable to the Medical public of the United States, considerable additions have been made, selected from American authors, particularly on Materia Medica, Mineralogy, &c. &c. For these additions an acknowledgment is due to Dr. James Thacher, for the extracts we have made from his Medical Biography, to Dr. John W. Webster, of Boston, for the same liberty taken with his Manuel of Chemistry, and to Dr. Jacob Bigelow, for the use of his Treatise on the Materia Medica. Copious extracts have also been made from Professor Cleaveland's Mineralogy, and recourse has been had to the New-York Medical Repository, Barns's Mineralogical Journal, Eaton's Geology, ana other works, for the purpose of introducing new and interesting articles. A number of obsolete terms have been omitted, but lest it might be thought by some to injure the work as a standard of modern as well as of ancient Medical terms, the words omitted have been inserted in the form of an Appendix.

PREFACE.

In the present edition of the Medical Dictionary, the principal additions and improvements are in the introduction of the terms of Botany and those of Mineralogy, and the most modern discoveries in Chemistry and Physiology. The work, therefore, will now be found to contain an account of every article connected with the study of medicine.

In conducting this laborious undertaking, particular attention has been given to,

1 The accentuation, in order that the proper pronunciation of the words may be obtained.

2. The derivation of the terms, and the declension of the words in common use.

3. The definitions, which are from the most approved sources.

4. The introduction of all the modern discoveries in the several branches of medical science

In the selection and arrangement of the most compendious, the most clear, and the most perfect account of the several articles of Anatomy, Biography, Botany, Chemistry, the Materia Medica, Midwifery, Mineralogy, Pathology, Pharmacy, and Physiology; the Compiler has again to acknowledge his obligations to Abernethy, Accum, Aikin, Albinus, Bell, Brande, Bergius, Blanchard, Burns,

Burserius, Callisen, Casselli, Cooper, Cruickshank, Cullen, Davy Denman, Duncan, the Editors of the London and Edinburgh Dispensaries, and of Rees' Cyclopædia, and Motherby's Medical Dictionary, Fourcroy, Good, Haller, Henry, Hoffman, Innis, Latta, Larcy, Lavoisier, Lewis, Linnæus, Majendie, Meyer, Murray, Nicholson, Orfila, Pott, Richerand, Richter, Saunders, Sauvage, Scarpa, Smith, Sœmmering, Swediaur, Symonds, Thomas, Thompson, Turton, Ure (from whose condensed and comprehensive work on chemistry large extracts have been made), Vaughan, Vossius. Willan, Woodville, &c. &c.

It was his original intention to give to each writer the merit of the particular description selected from his work: but having occasion to consult, frequently to abridge, and sometimes to alter, various passages; and finding it difficult, and in many instances impossible, to discover the original writer of several articles; and convinced at the same time that it would be attended with no particular advantage, he has preferred making a general acknowledgment to particularizing the labours of each individual. If he has been so fortunate as to have compressed within the narrow limits of the present publication much general and useful information, his object will be fully answered.

A NEW

MEDICAL DICTIONARY.

A. 1. In composition this letter, the *a* in Greek and *a* in Latin, signifies *without:* thus *aphonia*, without voice, *acaulis*, without stem, *aphyllus*, without a leaf, &c.

2. A. AA. (From *ανα*, which signifies of each.) Abbreviations of *ana*, which word is used in prescriptions after the mention of two or more ingredients, when it implies, that the quantity mentioned of each ingredient should be taken; thus, ℞. *Potassæ nitratis—Sacchari albi* āā ʒj. Take nitrate of potassa and white sugar, of each one drachm.

AA'RON. A physician of Alexandria, author of thirty books in the Syriac tongue, containing the whole practice of physic, chiefly collected from the Greek writings, and supposed to have been written before A. D. 620. He first mentioned, and described, the small-pox and measles, which were probably brought thither by the Arabians. He directed the vein under the tongue to be opened in jaundice, and noticed the white colour of the fæces in that disease. His works are lost, except some fragments, preserved by Rhazes.

AA'VORA. The fruit of a species of palm-tree which grows in the West Indies and Africa. It is of the size of a hen's egg, and included with several more in a large shell. In the middle of the fruit there is a hard nut, about the size of a peach stone, which contains a white almond, very astringent, and useful against a diarrhœa.

ABA'CTUS. *Abigeatus*. Among the ancient physicians, this term was used for a miscarriage, procured by art, or force of medicines, in contradistinction to *abortus*, which meant a natural miscarriage.

A'BACUS. (From a Hebrew word, signifying dust.) A table for preparations, so called from the usage of mathematicians of drawing their figures upon tables sprinkled with dust.

ABAI'SIR. *Abasis*. Ivory black; and also calcareous powder.

ABALIENA'TIO. Abalienation; or a decay of the body, or mind.

ABALIENA'TUS. 1. Corrupted.

2. A part so destroyed as to require immediate extirpation.

3. The total destruction of the senses, whether external or internal, by disease.

ABAPTI'STA. (From *a*, priv. and *βαπτω*, to plunge.) *Abaptiston*. 1. The shoulders of the old trepan.

2. This term is employed by Galen, Fabricius ab Aquapendente, Scultetus, and others, to denote the conical saw with a circular edge, (otherwise called modiolus, or terebra,) which was formerly used by surgeons to perforate the cranium.

ABAPTI'STON. See *Abaptista*.

ABARNAHAS. A chemical term formerly used in the transmutation of metals, signifying *luna plena, magnes*, or *magnesia*.

ABARTICULATION. (From *ab*, and *articulus*, a joint.) A species of articulation which has evident motion. See *Diarthrosis*.

ABA'SIS. See *Abaisir*.

ABBREVIATION. The principal uses of medicinal abbreviations are in prescriptions, in which they are certain marks, or half words, used by physicians for despatch and conveniency when they prescribe; thus:—℞ readily supplies the place of *recipe—h. s.* that of *hora somni—n. m.* that of *nux moschata—elect.* that of *electarium*, &c.; and in general all the names of compound medicines, with the several ingredients, are frequently wrote only up to their first or second syllable, or sometimes to their third or fourth, to make them clear and expressive. Thus *Croc. Anglic.* stands for *Crocus Anglicanus—Conf. Aromat.* for *Confectio Aromatica*, &c. A point being always placed at the end of such syllable, shows the word to be incomplete.

ABBREVIATUS. Abbreviate; shortened. A term often used in botany.

ABDO'MEN. (*Abdomen, inis.* n.; from *abdo*, to hide; because it hides the viscera. It is also derived from *abdere*, to hide, and *omentum*, the caul; by others *omen* is said to be only a termination, as from *lego, legumen*, so from *abdo, abdomen.*) The belly. The largest cavity in the body, bounded superiorly by the diaphragm, by which it is separated from the chest; inferiorly by the bones of the pubes and ischium; on each side by various muscles, the short ribs and ossa ilii; anteriorly by the abdominal muscles, and posteriorly by the vertebræ of the loins, the os sacrum and os coccygis. Internally it is invested by a smooth membrane, called peritoneum, and externally by muscles and common integuments.

In the cavity of the belly are contained,

Anteriorly and *laterally*,

1. The epiploon. 2. The stomach. 3. The large and small intestines. 4. The mesentery. 5. The lacteal vessels. 6. The pancreas. 7. The spleen. 8. The liver and gall-bladder.

Posteriorly, without the peritoneum,

1. The kidneys. 2. The supra-renal glands. 3. The ureters. 4. The receptaculum chyli. 5. The descending aorta. 6. The ascending vena cava.

Inferiorly in the pelvis, and *without the peritoneum*,

In men, 1. The urinary bladder. 2. The spermatic vessels. 3. The rectum.

In women, besides the urinary bladder and intestinum rectum, there are,

1. The uterus. 2. The four ligaments of the uterus. 3. The two ovaria. 4. The two Fallopian tubes. 5. The vagina.

The fore part of this cavity, as has been mentioned, is covered with muscles and common integuments, in the middle of which is the navel. It is this part of the body which is properly called abdomen; it is distinguished, by anatomists, into regions. See *Body*.

The posterior part of the abdomen is called the loins, and the sides the flanks.

ABDOMINALIS. (From *abdomen*, the belly.) Abdominal; pertaining to the belly.

Abdominal hernia. See *Hernia*.

Abdominal muscles. See *Muscles*.

Abdominal regions. See *Body*.

Abdominal ring. See *Annulus Abdominis*.

ABDU'CENS. See *Abducent*.

ABDUCENS LABIORUM. See *Levator anguli oris*.

ABDUCENT. (*Abducens;* from *ab*, from, and *ducere*, to draw.) The name of some muscles which draw parts back in the opposite direction to others. See *Abductor*.

Abducent muscles. See *Abductor*.

Abducent nerves. See *Nervi abducentes*.

ABDUC'TOR. (From *abduco*, to draw away.) *Abducens*. A muscle, the office of which is to pull back or draw the member to which it is affixed from some other. The antagonist is called *adductor*.

ABDUCTOR AURICULARIS. See *Posterior auris*

ABDUCTOR AURIS. See *Posterior auris*.

ABDUCTOR BREVIS ALTER. See *Abductor pollicis manus*.

ABDUCTOR INDICIS MANUS. An internal interosseous muscle of the fore-finger, situated on the hand. *Abductor* of Douglas; *Semi-interosseous indicis* of Winslow; *Abductor indicis* of Cowper. It arises from the superior part of the metacarpal bone, and the os tra pezium, on its inside, by a fleshy beginning, runs towards the metacarpal bone of the fore-finger, adheres to it, and is connected by a broad tendon to the superior part of the first phalanx of the fore-finger. Sometimes it arises by a double tendon. Its use is to draw the fore-finger from the rest, towards the thumb, and to bend it somewhat towards the palm.

ABDUCTOR INDICIS PEDIS. An internal interosseous muscle of the fore-toe, which arises tendinous and fleshy, by two origins, from the root of the inside of the metatarsal bone of the fore-toe, from the outside of the root of the metatarsal bone of the great toe, and from the os cuneiforme internum, and is inserted tendinous into the inside of the root of the first joint of the fore-toe. Its use is to pull the fore-toe inwards, from the rest of the small toes.

ABDUCTOR LONGUS POLLICIS MANUS. See *Extensor ossis metacarpi pollicis manûs.*

ABDUCTOR MEDII DIGITI PEDIS. An interosseous muscle of the foot, which arises tendinous and fleshy, from the inside of the root of the metatarsal bone of the middle toe internally, and is inserted tendinous into the inside of the root of the first joint of the middle toe. Its use is to pull the middle toe inwards.

ABDUCTOR MINIMI DIGITI MANUS. A muscle of the little finger, situated on the hand. *Carpo-phalangien du petit doigt* of Dumas; *Extensor tertii internodii minimi digiti* of Douglas; *Hypothenar minor* of Winslow. It arises fleshy from the pisiform bone, and from that part of the *ligamentum carpi annulare* next it, and is inserted, tendinous, into the inner side of the upper end of the first bone of the little finger. Its use is to draw the little finger from the rest.

ABDUCTOR MINIMI DIGITI PEDIS. A muscle of the little toe. *Calcaneo-phalangien du petit doigt* of Dumas; *Adductor* of Douglas; *Parathenar major* of Winslow, by whom this muscle is divided into two, *Parathenar major* and *metatarseus; Adductor minimi digiti* of Cowper. It arises tendinous and fleshy, from the semicircular edge of a cavity on the inferior part of the protuberance of the os calcis, and from the rest of the metatarsal bone of the little toe, and is inserted into the root of the first joint of the little toe externally. Its use is to bend the little toe, and its metatarsal bone, downwards, and to draw the little toe from the rest.

ABDUCTOR OCULI. See *Rectus externus oculi.*

ABDUCTOR POLLICIS MANUS. A muscle of the thumb, situated on the hand. *Scaphosus-phalangien du pouce* of Dumas; *Adductor pollicis manûs*, and *Adductor brevis alter* of Albinus; *Adductor thenar Riolani* of Douglas (the *adductor brevis alter* of Albinus is the inner portion of this muscle); *Adductor pollicis* of Co[illegible] It arises by a broad tendinous and fleshy beginning, from the ligamentum carpi annulare, and from the os trapezium, and is inserted tendinous into the outer side of the root of the first bone of the thumb. Its use is, to draw the thumb from the fingers.

ABDUCTOR POLLICIS PEDIS. A muscle of the great toe situated on the foot. *Calcaneo-phalangien du pouce* of Dumas; *Abductor* of Douglas; *Thenar* of Winslow; *Abductor pollicis* of Cowper. It arises fleshy, from the inside of the root of the protuberance of the os calcis, where it forms the heel, and tendinous from the same bone, where it joins the os naviculare; and is inserted tendinous into the internal sesamoid bone and root of the first joint of the great toe. Its use is to pull the great toe from the rest.

ABDUCTOR TERTII DIGITI PEDIS. An interosseous muscle of the foot, that arises tendinous and fleshy from the inside and the inferior part of the root of the metatarsal bone of the third toe; and is inserted tendinous into the inside of the root of the first joint of the third toe. Its use is to pull the third toe inwards.

ABEBÆ'OS. (From *a*, neg. and βεβαιος, firm.) *Abebæus.* Weak, infirm, unsteady. A term made use of by Hippocrates, de Signis.

ABEBÆ'US. See *Abebæos.*

ABELMO'SCHUS. (An Arabian word.) See *Hibiscus Abelmoschus.*

Abelmosch. See *Hibiscus Abelmoschus.*

Abelmusk. See *Hibiscus Abelmoschus.*

ABERRA'TIO. (From *ab* and *erro*, to wander from.) Formerly applied to some deviations from what was natural, as a dislocation, and monstrosities.

ABE'SSI. (An Arabian term which means filth.) The alvine excrements.

A'BESUM. Quicklime

ABEVACUA'TIO. (From *ab*, dim, and *evacuo*, to pour out.) A partial or incomplete evacuation of the peccant humours, either naturally or by art.

ABICUM. The thyroid cartilage.

A'BIES. (*Abies, etis.* fem.; from *abeo*, to proceed because it rises to a great height; or from απιος, a wild pear, the fruit of which its cones something resemble.) The fir. See *Pinus.*

ABIES CANADENSIS. See *Pinus Balsamea.*

ABIGEA'TUS. See *Abactus.*

ABIO'TOS. (From *a*, neg. and βιοω, to live.) Deadly. A name given to hemlock, from its deadly qualities. See *Conium maculatum.*

ABLACTA'TIO. (From *ab*, from, and *lac*, milk.) Ablactation, or the weaning of a child from the breast

ABLATION. (*Ablatio;* from *aufero*, to take away. 1. The taking away from the body whatever is hurtful. A term that is seldom used but in its general sense, to clothing, diet, exercise, &c. In some old writings, it expresses the intervals between two fits of a fever, or the time of remission.

2. Formerly chemists employed this term to signify the removal of any thing that is either finished or else no longer necessary in a process.

ABLUE'NT. (*Abluens;* from *abluo*, to wash away.) Abstergent. Medicines which were formerly supposed to purify or cleanse the blood.

ABLUTION. (*Ablutio;* from *abluo*, to wash off.) 1. A washing or cleansing either of the body or the intestines.

2. In chemistry it signifies the purifying of a body, by repeated affusions of a proper liquor.

ABOLI'TIO. (From *aboleo*, to destroy.) The separation or destruction of diseased parts.

ABORSUS. A miscarriage.

ABORTIENS. Miscarrying.

In botany, it is sometimes used synonymously with *sterilis*, sterile or barren.

ABORTION. (*Abortio;* from *aborior*, to be sterile.) *Aborsus; Amblosis; Diaphthora, Ectrosis; Exambloma; Examblosis; Apopallesis; Apopalsis; Apophthora.* Miscarriage, or the expulsion of the fœtus from the uterus, before the seventh month, after which it is called premature labour. It most commonly occurs between the eighth and eleventh weeks of pregnancy, but may happen at a later period. In early gestation, the ovum sometimes comes off entire; sometimes the fœtus is first expelled, and the placenta afterwards. It is preceded by floodings, pains in the back, loins, and lower part of the abdomen, evacuation of the water, shiverings, palpitation of the heart, nausea, anxiety, syncope, subsiding of the breasts and belly, pain in the inside of the thighs, opening and moisture of the os tincæ. The principal causes of miscarriage are blows or falls; great exertion or fatigue; sudden frights and other violent emotions of the mind; a diet too sparing or too nutritious; the abuse of spirituous liquors; other diseases, particularly fevers, and hæmorrhages; likewise excessive bleeding, profuse diarrhœa or cholic, particularly from accumulated fæces; immoderate venery, &c. The spontaneous vomiting so common in pregnancy, rarely occasions this accident: but when induced and kept up by drastic medicines, it may be very likely to have that effect. Abortion often happens without any obvious cause, from some defect in the uterus, or in the fœtus itself, which we cannot satisfactorily explain. Hence it will take place repeatedly in the same female at a particular period of pregnancy; perhaps in some measure from the influence of habit.

The treatment of abortion must vary considerably according to the constitution of the patient, and the causes giving rise to it. If the incipient symptoms should appear in a female of a plethoric habit, it may be proper to take a moderate quantity of blood from the arm, then clear the bowels by some mild cathartic, as the sulphas magnesiæ in the infusum rosæ, afterwards exhibiting small doses of nitrate of potash, directing the patient to remain quiet in a recumbent position, kept as cool as possible, with a low diet, and the antiphlogistic regimen in other respects. Should there be much flooding, cloths wetted with cold water ought to be applied to the region of the uterus, or even introduced into the vagina, to obstruct the escape of the blood mechanically. Where violent forcing pains attend, opium should be given by the mouth, or in the form of glyster, after premising proper evacuations.

Should these means not avail to check the discharge of the forcing pains, and particularly if the water be evacuated, there can be no expectation of preventing the miscarriage; and where there is reason for believing the fœtus dead, from the breasts having previously subsided, the morning sickness gone off, the motion stopped, &c. it will be proper rather to encourage it by manual assistance.

If on the other hand females of a delicate and irritable habit, rather deficient in blood, be subject to abortion, or where this accident is threatened by profuse evacuations and other debilitating causes, it may be more probably prevented by a diet nutritious, yet easy of digestion, with tonic medicines, and the use of the cold bath, attending at the same time to the state of the bowels, giving opium if pain attend, and carefully avoiding the several exciting causes.

[When a female has suffered several abortions, it becomes almost impossible to prevent a repetition at the same period of gestation in a subsequent pregnancy. Nothing, however, will be so successful in preventing a recurrence of a similar misfortune, as in allowing the uterine vessels to recover their tone; for which purpose a sufficient time must intervene before the next conception, otherwise the remedies above recommended will have little or no effect. A.]

ABORTIVE. (*Abortivus*; from *aborior*, to be sterile.) That which is capable of occasioning an abortion, or miscarriage, in pregnant women. It is now generally believed, that the medicines which produce a miscarriage, effect it by their violent operation on the system, and not by any specific action on the womb.

[From the violent operation of the *secale cornutum*, or *spurred rye*, upon the gravid uterus, it has been thought that it would act at any period of gestation as an abortive; but the experiments and trials made with it, have proved it to be inert, having no specific action upon the uterus, except in time of labour. A.]

ABORTUS. A miscarriage.

Abra'sa. (From *abrado*, to shave off.) Ulcers attended with abrasion.

ABRASION. (*Abrasio*; from *abrado*, to tear off.) This word is generally employed to signify the destruction of the natural mucus of any part, as the stomach, intestines, urinary bladder, &c. It is also applied to any part slightly torn away by attrition, as the skin, &c.

A'brathan. Corrupted from abrotanum, southernwood. See *Artemisia abrotanum*.

A'brette. See *Hibiscus Abelmoschus*.

Abro'ma. (From *a*, neg. and βρωμα, food; *i. e.* not fit to be eaten.) A tree of New South Wales, which yields a gum.

ABRO'TANUM. (Αβροτανον; from *a*, neg. and βροτος, mortal; because it never decays: or from αβρος, soft, and τονος, extension; from the delicacy of its texture.) Common southernwood. See *Artemisia*.

Abrotanum mas. See *Artemisia*.

ABROTONI'TES. (From *abrotanum*.) A wine mentioned by Dioscorides, impregnated with *abrotanum*, or southernwood, in the proportion of about one hundred ounces of the dried leaves, to about seven gallons of must.

ABRUPTE'. Abruptly. Applied to pinnate leaves which terminate without an odd leaf or lobe:—*folia abruptè pinnata*.

Abscede'ntia. (From *abscedo*, to separate.) Decayed parts of the body, which, in a morbid state, are separated from the sound.

ABSCESS. (*Abscessus*; from *abscedo*, to depart: because parts, which were before contiguous, become separated, or depart from each other.) *Abscessio*; *Imposthuma*. A collection of pus in the cellular membrane, or in the viscera, or in bones, preceded by inflammation. Abscesses are variously denominated according to their seat: as empyema, when in the cavity of the pleura; vomica, in the lungs; panaris, in any of the fingers; hypopyon, in the anterior chamber of the eye; arthropuosis, in a joint; lumbar abscess, &c.

The formation of an abscess is the result of inflammation terminating in suppuration. This is known by a throbbing pain, which lessens by degrees, as well as the heat, tension, and redness of the inflamed part; and if the pus be near the surface, a cream-like whiteness is soon perceived, with a prominence about the middle, or at the inferior part, then a fluctuation may be felt, which becomes gradually more distinct, till at length the matter makes its way externally. When suppuration occurs to a considerable extent, or in a part of importance to life, there are usually rigours, or sudden attacks of chilliness, followed by flushes of heat; and unless the matter be soon discharged, and the abscess healed, hectic fever generally comes on. When abscesses form in the cellular membrane in persons of a tolerably good constitution, they are usually circumscribed, in consequence of coagulable lymph having been previously effused, and having obliterated the communication with the adjoining cells; but in those of a weakly, and especially a scrophulous constitution, from this not occurring, the pus is very apt to diffuse itself, like the water in anasarca. Another circumstance, which may prevent its readily reaching the surface, is its collecting under an aponeurosis, or other part of dense structure, when the process of ulceration will rather extend in another direction; thus pus accumulating in the loins, may descend to the lower part of the thigh.

When suppuration occurs, if the inflammation have not yet subsided, it may be necessary to employ means calculated to moderate this, in order to limit the extent of the abscess: but evacuations must not be carried too far, or there will not be power in the system to heal it afterwards. If the disease be near the surface, fomentations or warm emollient poultices should be employed, to take off the tension of the skin, and promote the process of ulceration in that direction. As soon as fluctuation is obvious, it will be generally proper to make an opening, lest contiguous parts of importance should be injured; and often at an earlier period, where the matter is prevented from reaching the surface by a fascia, &c., but it is sometimes advisable to wait awhile, especially in large spontaneous abscesses, where the constitution is much debilitated, till by the use of a nutritious diet, with bark and other tonic means, this can be somewhat improved. There are different modes of opening abscesses. 1. By incision or puncture; this is generally the best, as being least painful, and most expeditious, and the extent of the aperture can be better regulated. 2. By caustic; this may be sometimes preferable when suppuration goes on very slowly in glandular parts, (especially in scrophulous and venereal cases,) lessening the subjacent tumour, giving free vent to the matter, and exciting more healthy action in the sore; but it sometimes causes much deformity, it can hardly reach deep seated abscesses, and the delay may be often dangerous. 3. By seton; this is sometimes advantageous in superficial abscesses, (where suppuration is likely to continue,) about the neck and face, leaving generally but a small scar; likewise when near joints, or other important parts liable to be injured by the scalpel or caustic. See *Lumbar Abscess*, and *Ulcer*.

ABSCES'SUS. See *Abscess*.

ABSCISSION. (*Abscissio*; from *ab*, and *scindo*, to cut.) 1. The cutting away some morbid, or other part, by an edged instrument. The abscision of the prepuce makes what we call circumcision.

2. Abscission is sometimes used by medical writers to denote the sudden termination of a disease in death, before it arrives at its decline.

3. Celsus frequently uses the term *abscissa vox* to express a loss of voice.

Absinthites. Absinthiac, or absinthiated. Something tinged or impregnated with the virtues of absinthium or wormwood.

ABSI'NTHIUM. (*Absinthium*, *thii*, n. αψινθιον; from *a*, neg. and ψινθος, pleasant: so called from the disagreeableness of the taste.) Wormwood. See *Artemisia*.

Absinthium commune. Common Wormwood. See *Artemisia Absinthium*.

Absinthium maritimum. Sea Wormwood. See *Artemisia Maritima*.

Absinthium ponticum. Roman Wormwood. See *Artemisia Pontica*.

Absinthium vulgare. Common Wormwood. See *Artemisia Absinthium*.

ABSORBENS. See *Absorbent*.

ABSORBENT. (*Absorbens*; from *absorbeo*, to suck up.) 1. The small, delicate, transparent vessels, which take up substances from the surface of the body, or from any cavity, and carry it to the blood, are termed absorbents or absorbing vessels. They are denominated, according to the liquids which they convey lacteals and lymphatics. See *Lacteal* and *Lymphatic.*

2. Those medicines are so termed, which have no acrimony in themselves, and destroy acidities in the stomach and bowels; such are magnesia, prepared chalk, oyster-shells, crabs' claws, &c.

3. Substances are also so called by chemists, which have the faculty of withdrawing moisture from the atmosphere.

Absorbing vessels. See *Absorbent.*

ABSORPTION. (*Absorptio;* from *absorbeo,* to suck up.) 1. A function in an animated body, arranged by physiologists under the head of natural actions. It signifies the taking up of substances applied to the mouths of absorbing vessels; thus the nutritious part of the food is absorbed from the intestinal canal by the lacteals; thus mercury is taken into the system by the lymphatics of the skin, &c. The principle by which this function takes place, is a power inherent in the mouths of the absorbents, a *vis insita,* dependent on the degree of irritability of their internal membrane by which they contract and propel their contents forwards.

2. By this term chemists understand the conversion of a gaseous fluid into a liquid or solid, on being united with some other substance. It differs from condensation in this being the effect of mechanical pressure.

[*Absorption by plants.*—In 1804, Dr. Foote sent to Dr. Mitchill of New-York, a peach, with the following account of it:—"I present you with a peach by the bearer. You will readily perceive that I could not be induced to this from any thing very promising in its aspect, the richness of its flavour, or the singularity of its species. On tasting, you will find it highly charged with *muriate of soda:* and when I inform you that it has undergone no artificial management, but possessed this property when plucked from the tree, you may find some difficulty in explaining the fact.

"This peach was presented to me by Mr. Solomon Brewer, of Westchester Co., New-York, my former residence. Mr. B. is a respectable man, and the present clerk of the town in which he lives. The history he gives me of this natural *salt-peach* is, that it grew in his neighbourhood, on a tree, around the body and roots of which had been accidentally poured a quantity of pork or beef-brine; that its fruit ripens in the month of September; that the effect of the brine had been, to produce a sickness and decay in the tree; and that at this time (Sept. 1804) it presents the singular fact of a tree hanging tolerably full of *salt peaches.* He was unable to inform me of the precise time of the occurrence, but that it was the fore-part of summer, and after the fruit had obtained its shape and some size. This fact, as respects the vegetable kingdom, is in my mind an isolated one.

"I have felt the more interest in noticing this fact, as it contributes much to strengthen and confirm the opinion you long since advanced, that certain vegetables, as wheat, partake much of the properties of the manure which is used as their aliment, and thence urge with much propriety the importance of the subject to agriculturists."—See *Med. Repos. of New-York,* vol. viii. p. 209. A.]

ABSTEMIOUS. (*Abstemius;* from *abs,* from, and *temetum,* wine.) Refraining absolutely from all use of wine; but the term is applied to a temperate mode of living, with respect to food generally.

ABSTE'NTIO. Cælius Aurelianus uses this word to express a suppression, or retention: thus, *abstentio stercorum,* a retention of the excrements, which he mentions as a symptom very frequent in a satyriasis. In a sense somewhat different, he uses the word *abstenta,* applying it to the pleura, where he seems to mean that the humour of the inflamed pleura is prevented, by the adjacent bones, from extending itself.

ABSTERGENT. (*Abstergens;* from *abstergo,* to cleanse away.) Any application that cleanses or clears away foulness. The term is seldom employed by modern writers.

ABSTRACTION. (From *abstraho,* to draw away.) A term employed by chemists in the process of humid distillation, to signify that the fluid body is again drawn off from the solid, which it had dissolved.

A'BSUS. The Egyptian lotus.

ABVACUA'TIO. (From *abvacuo,* to empty.) A morbid discharge; a large evacuation of any fluid, as of blood from a plethoric person. A term used by some old writers.

ACA'CIA. (*Acacia, æ.* f. ακακια; from ακαζω, to sharpen.) The name of a genus of plants in the Linnæan system. Class, *Polygamia;* Order, *Monœcia.* The Egyptian thorn.

ACACIA CATECHU. This plant affords a drug, formerly supposed to be an earthy substance brought from Japan, and therefore called *terra Japonica,* or Japan earth; afterwards it appeared to be an extract prepared in India, it was supposed till lately, from the juice of the *Mimosa catechu,* by boiling the wood and evaporating the decoction by the heat of the sun. But the shrub is now ascertained to be an acacia, and is termed *Acacia catechu.* It grows in great abundance in the kingdom of Bahar, and catechu comes to us principally from Bengal and Bombay. It has received the following names; *Acachou; Faufel; Cætchu; Caschu; Catechu; Cadtchu; Cashow; Caitchu; Castjoe; Gachu; Cate; Kaath.* The natives call it *Cutt,* the English who reside there *Cutch.* In its purest state, it is a dry pulverable substance, outwardly of a reddish colour, internally of a shining dark brown, tinged with a reddish hue; in the mouth it discovers considerable adstringency, succeeded by a sweetish mucilaginous taste. It may be advantageously employed for most purposes where an adstringent is indicated; and is particularly useful in alvine fluxes, where astringents are required. Besides this, it is employed also in uterine profluvia, in laxity and debility of the viscera in general; and it is an excellent topical adstringent, when suffered to dissolve leisurely in the mouth, for laxities and ulcerations of the gums, aphthous ulcers in the mouth, and similar affections. This extract is the basis of several formulæ in our pharmacopœias, particularly of a tincture: but one of the best forms under which it can be exhibited, is that of simple infusion in warm water with a proportion of cinnamon, for by this means it is at once freed of its impurities and improved by the addition of the aromatic.

Fourcroy says that catechu is prepared from the seeds of a kind of palm, called areca. Sir Humphrey Davy has analyzed catechu, and from his examination it appears, that from Bombay is of uniform texture, red-brown colour, and specific gravity 1.39: that from Bengal is more friable and less consistent, of a chocolate colour externally, but internally chocolate streaked with red-brown, and specific gravity 1.28. The catechu from either place differs little in its properties. Its taste is astringent, leaving behind a sensation of sweetness. It is almost wholly soluble in water. Two hundred grains of picked catechu from Bombay afforded 109 grains of tannin, 66 extractive matter, 13 mucilage, 10 residuum, chiefly sand and calcareous earth. The same quantity from Bengal; tannin 97 grains, extractive matter 73 mucilage 16, residual matter, being sand, with a small quantity of calcareous and aluminous earths, 14. Of the latter, the darkest parts appeared to afford most tannin, the lightest most extractive matter. The Hindoos prefer the lightest coloured, which has probably most sweetness, to chew with the betel-nut.

Of all the astringent substances we know, catechu appears to contain the largest proportion of tannin; and Mr. Purkis found, that one pound was equivalent to seven or eight of oak bark for the purpose of tanning leather.

[The *tinctura Japonica* is a powerful and useful astringent in looseness of the bowels. Many persons take this preparation when they are not aware of it, and when there is no occasion. It is used to colour fictitious and imitation brandies made in the United States, and from the quantity used, these liquors always produce costiveness. A.]

ACACIA GERMANICA. German acacia.

1. The name of the German black-thorn or sloe-tree, the *Prunus spinosa* of Linnæus.

2. The name of the inspissated juice of the fruit, as made in Germany; which, as well as the tree, is there called also *Acacia nostras.* It is now fallen into disuse.

ACACIA INDICA. See *Tamarindus Indica.*

ACACIA NOSTRAS. See *Acacia Germanica.*

ACACIA VERA. 1. The systematic name of the tree which affords gum-arabic, formerly supposed to be a *Mimosa. Acacia:—spinis stipularibus patentibus, foliis bipinnatis, partialibus extimis glandula interstinctis, spicis globosis pedunculatis,* of Wildenow

The Egyptian Thorn. This tree yields the true Acacia Gum, or Gum-Arabic, called also *Gummi acanthinum; Gummi thebaicum; Gummi scorpionis; Gum-lamac; Gummi senega*, or *senica*, or *senegalense.*

Cairo and Alexandria were the principal marts for gum-arabic, till the Dutch introduced the gum from Senegal into Europe, about the beginning of the seventeenth century, and this source now supplies the greater part of the vast consumption of this article. The tree which yields the Senegal gum, grows abundantly on the sands, along the whole of the Barbary coast, and particularly about the river Senegal. There are several species, some of which yield a red astringent juice, but others afford only a pure, nearly colourless, insipid gum, which is the great article of commerce. These trees are from eighteen to twenty feet high, with thorny branches. The gum makes its appearance about the middle of November, when the soil has been thoroughly saturated with periodical rains. The gummy juice is seen to ooze through the trunk and branches, and, in about a fortnight, it hardens into roundish drops, of a yellowish white, which are beautifully brilliant where they are broken off, and entirely so when held in the mouth for a short time, to dissolve the outer surface. No clefts are made, nor any artificial means used by the Moors, to solicit the flow of the gum. The lumps of gum-senegal are usually about the size of partridge eggs, and the harvest continues about six weeks. This gum is a very wholesome and nutritious food; thousands of the Moors support themselves entirely upon it during the time of harvest. About six ounces is sufficient to support a man for a day; and it is, besides, mixed with milk, animal broths, and other victuals.

The gum-arabic, or that which comes directly from Egypt and the Levant, only differs from the gum-senegal in being of a lighter colour, and in smaller lumps; and it is also somewhat more brittle. In other respects, they resemble each other perfectly.

Gum-arabic is neither soluble in spirit nor in oil; but, in twice its quantity of water, it dissolves into a mucilaginous fluid, of the consistence of a thick syrup, and in this state answers many useful pharmaceutical purposes, by rendering oily, resinous, and pinguious substances miscible with water. The glutinous quality of gum-arabic renders it preferable to other gums and mucilages as a demulcent in coughs, hoarsenesses, and other catarrhal affections. It is also very generally employed in ardor urinæ, diarrhœas, and calculous complaints.

2. The name *Acacia vera* has also been used to denote the expressed juice of the immature pods of the tree termed *Acacia veravel.* This inspissated juice is brought from Egypt in roundish masses, wrapped up in thin bladders. It is considered as a mild astringent medicine. The Egyptians give it, in spitting of blood, in the quantity of a drachm, dissolved in any convenient liquor, and repeat this dose occasionally. They likewise employ it in collyria, for strengthening the eyes, and in gargles, for quinsies. It is now seldom used as a medicine, being superseded by the use of catechu, or kino.

Acacia veravel. See *Acacia vera.*

Acacia Zeylonica. See *Hæmatoxylon Campechianum.*

Acacia gum. See *Acacia vera.*

Acacos. The thrush. See *Aphtha.*

ACALYCINUS. (From *a*, priv. and *calyx*, a flower-cup.) Without a calyx.

ACALYCIS. (From *a*, priv. and *calyx*, a flower-cup.) Without a calyx or flower-cup. Applied to plants which have no calyx.

Aca'matos. (From *a*, neg. and καμνω, to grow weary.) A perfect rest of the muscles, or that disposition of a limb which is equally distinct from flexion and extension.

ACA'NTHA. (Ακανθα; from ακη, a point.)

1. A thorn; or any thing pointed.

2. Sometimes applied to the spina dorsi.

Acantha'bolus. (From ακανθα, a thorn; and βαλλω, to cast out.) An instrument, or forceps, for taking out or removing thorns, or whatever may stick in the flesh. —*Paulus Ægineta.*

Aca'nthe. The name of the artichoke in ancient authors.

ACA'NTHINUM. (From ακανθα, a thorn.) Gum-arabic was called *gummi acanthinum*, because it is produced from a thorny tree. See *Acacia Vera.*

Acanticone. See *Epidote.*

ACA'NTHULUS. (From ακανθα, a thorn.) A surgical instrument to draw out thorns or splinters, or to remove any extraneous matter from wounds.

ACA'NTHUS. (*Acanthus, i.* m. ακανθος; from ακανθα, a thorn; so named from being rough and prickly.) The name of a genus of plants in the Linnæan system. Class, *Didynamia;* Order, *Angiospermia.* Bear's-breech.

Acanthus mollis. The systematic name of the bear's-breech, or brank-ursine. *Acanthus:—foliis sinuatis inermibus*, of Linnæus. *Branca ursina* of the shops. The leaves and root abound with a mucilage, which is readily extracted by boiling or infusion. The roots are the most mucilaginous. Where this plant is common, it is employed for the same purposes to which althæa and other vegetables possessing similar qualities are applied among us. It is fallen into disuse. The herb-women too often sell the leaves of bear's-foot, and of cow's parsnip, for the bear's-breech.

Aca'pnon. (From *a*, priv. and καπνος, smoke.) 1. Common wild marjoram.

2. Unsmoked honey.

ACAROIS. The name of a genus of plants, from New South Wales.

Acarois resinifera. The name of a tree which affords the Botany bay gum. See *Botany bay.*

[Gum Acaroides, New Holland resin, or earthy gum-lac. This is the produce of the tree called *Acarois resinifera*, or resin-bearing Acarois. The tree grows abundantly in New Holland, near Botany bay. The substance under consideration is usually found in the ground near the trees from which it has spontaneously exuded. From some resemblance it bears (though by no means a near one) to the article called *gum-lac*, it has been known as the *earthy gum-lac.* It is of yellowish, brownish, or yellowish brown colour, and sometimes contains roots, sticks, and other foreign substances. It has been distinguished in commerce by the term *Botany bay resin.* They refer its importation into England to the year 1799. An account of its chemical properties was published by Lichtenstein in Crell's Journal, and afterwards by Dr. Thompson, in the fourth volume of his Chemistry, p. 138. It was known to the early navigator Tasman, and was brought to New-York and presented to Dr. Mitchill many years ago by some of our navigators. For some time past it has been regarded in Massachusetts as a powerful restorative, or an invigorating medicine in cases of gastric or general debility.

Gum Acaroides is insoluble in water: alcohol or distilled spirits is its proper menstruum. Even in powder its use is improper, as it is not acted upon by the intestinal or alimentary fluids. It is therefore neither administered in substance, infusion, or decoction. It is mostly prescribed in the form of tincture: Tinctura gummi acaroidis. Tincture of New Holland resin.

The proper rule is to make a saturated tincture, of which *a tea-spoon full* may be given once in *three* or *four hours*, according to the circumstances, in milk, jelly, or syrup, water being apt to decompose it. From Kite's essay upon this production, it appears,

1. That dyspepsia has been exceedingly relieved by it, and even wholly removed.

2. That it is an excellent restorative in the debility consequent upon the depletion and exhaustion of acute diseases.

3. It is said to have done good in hysteria

4. Cholera, with cramps of the lower extremities, is reported to have yielded to its powers.

5. The morbid evacuations and commotions of diarrhœa are reported to have yielded to its virtue, after opium had failed.

6. Chronic and atonic catarrhs have been benefitted by its administration.

7. It is alleged to have been remarkably serviceable in incipient dysentery, as well as in that of long duration.

8. In various spasmodic affections, such as stitches in the sides, cramp of the stomach, rheumatic twinges, &c., it has often afforded relief after opiates had failed.

It must be observed, however, that it is not to be prescribed in cases of high action, or phlogistic diathesis, nor during the prevalence of inflammatory symptoms.

From this abstract of the practice with this remedy, no doubt can be entertained of its value, nor of the propriety of considering the discovery of its qualities, as worthy to be considered among the happy events attending the modern Materia Medica.—*Mitchill's MS. Lectures*. A.]

A'CARUS. (From ακαρης, small.) The tick. An insect which breeds in the skin. A very numerous genus of minute insects which infest the skin of animals, and produce various complaints. Those which are found on the human body are

1. The *acarus domesticus*, or domestic tick.
2. The *acarus scabiei*, or itch tick.
3. The *acarus autumnalis*, or harvest-bug.

ACATALE'PSIA. (From *a*, neg. and καταλαμβανω, to apprehend.) Uncertainty in the prognosis or judgment of diseases.

ACA'TALIS. (From *a*, neg. and χατεω, to want.) The juniper tree: so named from the abundance of its seeds.

ACATA'POSIS. (From *a*, neg. and καταπινω, to swallow.) Difficult deglutition.

Aca'statos. (From *a*, neg. and καθιστημι, to determine.) Inconstant.

1. Fevers were so called which are anomalous in their appearance and irregular in their paroxysms.
2. Turbid urine without sediment.

ACAULIS. (From *a*, priv. and *caulis*, a stem.) Without stem. Plants destitute of stem are called *acaules*, stemless; as *Cypripedium acaule*, and *Carduus acaulis*. This term must not be too rigidly understood.

ACCELERA'TOR. (From *accelero*, to hasten or propel.) The name of a muscle of the penis.

Accelerator urinæ. A muscle of the penis. *Ejaculator Seminis; Bulbo-syndesmo-caverneux* of Dumas; *Bulbo-cavernosus* of Winslow. It arises fleshy from the sphincter ani and membranous part of the urethra, and tendinous from the crus, near as far forwards as the beginning of the corpus cavernosum penis; the inferior fibres run more transversely, and the superior descend in an oblique direction. It is inserted into a line in the middle of the bulbous part of the urethra, where each joins with its fellow; by which the bulb is completely closed. The use of these muscles is to drive the urine or semen forward, and by grasping the bulbous part of the urethra, to push the blood towards its corpus cavernosum, and the glans, by which they are distended.

ACCESSION. (*Accesio; from accedo*, to approach.) The commencement of a disease. A term mostly applied to a fever which has paroxysms or exacerbations: thus the accession of fever, means the commencement or approach of the febrile period.

ACCESSO'RIUS. (From *accedo*, to approach: so called from the course it takes.) Connected by contact or approach.

Accessorius lumbalis. A muscle of the loins. See *Sacro-lumbalis*.

Accessorius nervus. The name given by Willis to two nerves which ascend, one on each side, from the second, fourth, and fifth cervical pairs of nerves, through the great foramen of the occipital bone, and pass out again from the cranium through the foramina lacera, with the par vagum, to be distributed on the trapezius muscle.

ACCI'PITER. (From *accipio*, to take.)

1. The hawk; so named from its rapacity.
2. A bandage which was put over the nose: so called from its likeness to the claw of a hawk, or from the tightness of its grasp.

ACCIPITRI'NA. (From *accipiter*, the hawk.) The herb hawk-weed· which Pliny says was so called because hawks are used to scratch it, and apply the juice to their eyes to prevent blindness.

ACCLI'VIS. A muscle of the belly, so named from the oblique ascent of its fibres. See *Obliquus internus abdominis*.

Accouchement. The French word for the act of delivery.

Accoucheur. The French for a midwife.

ACCRETIO. (From *ad*, and *cresco*, to increase.) Accretion.

1. Nutrition; growth.
2. The growing together of parts naturally separate as the fingers or toes.

Accuba'tio. (From *accumbo*, to recline.) Childbed; reclining.

Ace'dia. (From *a*, priv. and κηδος, care.) Carelessness, neglect in the application of medicines. Hippocrâtes sometimes uses this word, in his treatise on the glands, to signify fatigue or trouble.

ACE'PHALUS. (*Acephalus, i.* m. ακεφαλος; from *a*, priv. and κεφαλη, a head.) Without a head. A term applied to a lusus naturæ, or monster, born without a head.

[This term is also applied by modern naturalists to a certain portion of the gelatinous or soft bodied animals, which were formerly classed among the *Vermes* of Linnæus. They are now termed *Acephalous Molluscæ*, or headless molluscæ, having no distinct part corresponding to the head of other animals. A.]

A'CER. (*Acer, eris.* neut.; from *acer*, sharp: because of the sharpness of its juice.) The name of a genus of plants in the Linnæan system. Class *Polygamia*; Order, *Monœcia*.

Acer campestre. The common maple. This tree yields a sweetish, soft, milky sap, which contains a salt with basis of lime, possessed, according to Sherer, of peculiar properties. It is white, semitransparent, not altered by the air, and soluble in one hundred parts of cold, or fifty of boiling water.

Acer pseudoplatanus. The maple-tree, falsely named sycamore. It is also called *Platanus traga*. This tree is common in England, though not much used in medicine. The juice, if drank while fresh, is said to be a good antiscorbutic. All its parts contain a saccharine fluid; and if the root or branches be wounded in the spring, a large quantity of liquor is discharged, which, when inspissated, yields a brown sort of sugar and syrup like molasses.

Acer saccharinum. The sugar maple-tree. Large quantities of sugar are obtained from this tree in New-England and Canada, which is much used in France, where it is commonly known by the name of *Saccharum Canadense* or *Saccharum Acernum*, maple sugar. It has been supposed that all Europe might be supplied from the maple of America, which grows in great quantities in the western counties of all the middle States of the American Union. It is as tall as the oak, and from two to three feet in diameter; puts forth a white blossom in the spring, before any appearance of leaves; its small branches afford sustenance for cattle, and its ashes afford a large quantity of excellent potash. Twenty years are required for it to attain its full growth. Tapping does not injure it; but, on the contrary, it affords more syrup, and of a better quality, the oftener it is tapped. A single tree has not only survived, but flourished, after tapping, for forty years. Five or six pounds of sugar are usually afforded by the sap of one tree; though there are instances of the quantity exceeding twenty pounds. The sugar is separated from the sap either by freezing, by spontaneous evaporation, or by boiling. The latter method is the most used. Dr. Rush describes the process; which is simple, and practised without any difficulty by the farmers.

From frequent trials of this sugar, it does not appear to be in any respect inferior to that of the West Indies It is prepared at a time of the year when neither insect, nor the pollen of plants, exists to vitiate it, as is the case with common sugar. From calculations grounded on facts, it is ascertained, that America is now capable of producing a surplus of one-eighth more than its own consumption.

[The Acer Saccharinum, or sugar-maple tree, abounds in the state of New-York and many other parts of the United States. It furnishes a great amount of rough sugar in the interior of the country and the new settlements, where foreign and refined sugars are but little used. Very little effort has heretofore been made to introduce it into market as an article of commerce. But in 1828 several hundred barrels of this sugar, from the Territory of Michigan, reached the city of New-York by way of the great Western canal. It was sold at auction for six cents per pound; and when refined and converted into loaf sugar, it afforded a reasonable profit to the refiner. A.]

ACERATE. *Aceras*. A salt formed of the acid of the *Acer campestre* with an alkaline, earthy, or metallic base.

ACE'RATOS. From *a*, neg. and κεραω, or κεραννυμι, to mix.) Unmixed; uncorrupted. This term is applied sometimes to the humours of the body by Hippocrates. Paulus Ægineta mentions a plaster of this name.

ACERB. (*Acerbus* from *acer* sharp.) A species

of taste which consists in a degree of acidity, with an addition of roughness; properties common to many immature fruits.

Ace'rbitas. Acerbness.

ACERIC ACID. A peculiar acid, said to exist in the juice of the common maple, *Acer campestre* of Linnæus. It is decomposed by heat, like the other vegetable acids.

ACE'RIDES. (From *α*, priv. and *κερος*, wax.) Soft plasters, made without wax.

ACEROSUS. (From *acus*, a needle.) 1. Acerose: having the shape of a needle. Applied to leaves which are so shaped, as in *Pinus sylvestris* and *Juniperus communis*.

2. (From *acus*, chaff.) Chaffy: applied to coarse bread, &c.

ACESCENT. (*Acescens;* from *aceo*, to be sour or tart.) Turning sour or acid. Substances which readily run into the acid fermentation, are so said to be, as some vegetable and animal juices and infusions. The suddenness with which this change is effected, during a thunder-storm, even in corked bottles, has not been accounted for. In some morbid states of the stomach, also, it proceeds with astonishing rapidity.

ACE'STA. (From *ακεομαι*, to cure.) Distempers which are easily cured.

Ace'stis. Borax.

ACETA'BULUM. (*Acetabulum, i.* n.; from *acetum*, vinegar: so called because it resembles the *acetabulum*, or old saucer in which vinegar was held for the use of the table.) A name given by Latin writers to the cup-like cavity of the os innominatum, which receives the head of the thigh-bone. See *Innominatum os.*

ACETA'RIUM. (From *acetum*, vinegar: because it is mostly made with vinegar.) A sallad or pickle.

ACE'TAS. (*Acetas, tis;* f. from *acetum*, vinegar.) An acetate A salt formed by the union of the acetic acid, with a salifiable base. Those used in medicine are the acetates of ammonia, lead, potassa, and zinc.

Acetas ammoniæ. Acetate of ammonia. See *Ammonia acetatis liquor.*

Acetas plumbi. Acetate of lead. See *Plumbi acetas* and *Plumbi acetatis liquor.*

Acetas potassæ. Acetate of potassa. See *Potassæ acetas.*

Acetas zinci. A metallic salt composed of zinc and acetic acid. It is used by some as an astringent against inflammation of the eyes, urethra, and vagina, diluted in the same proportion as the sulphate of zinc.

Acetate. See *Acetas.*

Acetate of Ammonia. See *Ammoniæ acetatis liquor.*

Acetate of Potassa. See *Potassæ acetas.*

Acetate of Zinc. See *Acetas zinci.*

Acetated vegetable Alcali. See *Potassæ acetas.*

Acetated volatile Alcali. See *Ammoniæ acetatis liquor.*

ACETIC ACID. *Acidum aceticum.* The same acid which, in a very dilute and somewhat impure state, is called vinegar. Acetic acid is found combined with potassa in the juices of a great many plants; particularly the *Sambucus nigra*, *Phœnix dactilifera*, *Galium verum*, and *Rhus typhinus.* "Sweat, urine, and even fresh milk, contain it. It is frequently generated in the stomachs of dyspeptic patients. Almost all dry vegetable substances, and some animal, subjected in close vessels to a red heat, yield it copiously. It is the result likewise of a spontaneous fermentation, to which liquid vegetable and animal matters are liable. Strong acids, as the sulphuric and nitric, develope the acetic by their action on vegetables. It was long supposed, on the authority of Boerhaave, that the fermentation which forms vinegar is uniformly preceded by the vinous. This is a mistake: cabbages sour in water, making sour crout; starch, in starch-makers' sour waters; and dough itself, without any previous production of wine.

"The varieties of acetic acid known in commerce are four: 1. Wine vinegar. 2. Malt vinegar. 3. Sugar vinegar. 4. Wood vinegar.

"We shall describe first the mode of making these commercial articles, and then that of extracting the absolute acetic acid of the chemist, either from these vinegars, or directly from chemical compounds, of which it is a constituent.

"The following is the plan of making vinegar at present practised in Paris. The wine destined for vinegar is mixed in a large tun with a quantity of wine lees, and the whole being transferred into cloth-sacks, placed within a large iron-bound vat, the liquid matter is extruded through the sacks by superincumbent pressure. What passes through is put into large casks, set upright, having a small aperture in their top. In these it is exposed to the heat of the sun in summer, or to that of a stove in winter. Fermentation supervenes in a few days. If the heat should then rise too high, it is lowered by cool air and the addition of fresh wine. In the skilful regulation of the fermentative temperature consists the art of making good wine vinegar. In summer the process is generally completed in a fortnight: in winter, double the time is requisite. The vinegar is then run off into barrels, which contain several chips of birch-wood. In about a fortnight it is found to be clarified, and is then fit for the market. It must be kept in close casks.

"The manufacturers at Orleans prefer wine of a year old for making vinegar. But if by age the wine has lost its extractive matter, it does not readily undergo the acetous fermentation. In this case, acetification, as the French term the process, may be determined by adding slips of vines, bunches of grapes, or green woods.

"Almost all the vinegar of the north of France being prepared at Orleans, the manufactory of that place has acquired such celebrity, as to render their process worthy of a separate consideration. The Orleans' casks contain nearly 400 pints of wine. Those which have been already used are preferred. They are placed in three rows, one over another, and in the top have an aperture of two inches' diameter, kept always open. The wine for acetification is kept in adjoining casks, containing beech shavings, to which the lees adhere. The wine, thus clarified, is drawn off to make vinegar. One hundred pints of good vinegar, boiling hot, are first poured into each cask, and left there for eight days. Ten pints of wine are mixed in, every eight days, till the vessels are full. The vinegar is allowed to remain in this state fifteen days before it is exposed to sale.

"The *used* casks, called *mothers*, are never emptied more than half, but are successively filled again, to acetify new portions of wine. In order to judge if the *mother* works, the vinegar-makers plunge a spatula into the liquid; and according to the quantity of froth which the spatula shows, they add more or less wine. In summer, the atmospheric heat is sufficient. In winter, stoves heated to about 75° Fahr. maintain the requisite temperature in the manufactory.

"In some country districts, the people keep, in a place where the temperature is mild and equable, *a vinegar cask*, into which they pour such wine as they wish to acetify; and it is always preserved full by replacing the vinegar drawn off, by new wine. To establish this household manufacture, it is only necessary to buy at first a small cask of good vinegar.

"At Gand, a vinegar from beer is made, in which the following proportions of grain are found to be most advantageous:—

1880 Paris lbs.	malted barley.
700 —	wheat.
500 —	buckwheat.

These grains are ground, mixed, and boiled, along with twenty-seven casks full of river water, for three hours. Eighteen casks of good beer for vinegar are obtained. By a subsequent decoction, more fermentable liquid is extracted, which is mixed with the former. The whole brewing yields 3000 English quarts.

"In this country, vinegar is usually made from malt. By mashing with hot water, 100 gallons of wort are extracted in less than two hours from 1 boll of malt. When the liquor has fallen to the temperature of 75° Fahr. 4 gallons of the barm of beer are added. After thirty-six hours it is racked off into casks, which are laid on their sides, and exposed, with their bung-holes loosely covered, to the influence of the sun in summer; but in winter they are arranged in a stove-room. In three months this vinegar is ready for the manufacture of sugar of lead. To make vinegar for domestic use, however, the process is somewhat different. The above liquor is racked off into casks placed upright, having a false cover, pierced with holes fixed at about a foot from their bottom. On this a considerable quantity of *rape*, or the refuse from the makers of British wine, or otherwise a quantity of low-priced raisins, is laid. The liquor is turned into another barrel every twenty-four hours, in which time it has begun to grow warm. Sometimes, indeed, the vinegar is fully fermented, as above, without the rape, which is added towards the end, to communicate flavour. Two large casks are in this case worked together, as is described long ago by Boerhaave, as follows:

"'Take two large wooden vats or hogsheads; and in each of these, place a wooden grate or hurdle, at the distance of a foot from the bottom. Set the vessel upright; and on the grate, place a moderately close layer of green twigs, or fresh cuttings of the vine. Then fill up the vessel with the footstalks of grapes, commonly called the rape, to the top of the vessel, which must be left quite open.

"'Having thus prepared the two vessels, pour into them the wine to be converted into vinegar, so as to fill one of them quite up, and the other but half-full. Leave them thus for twenty-four hours, and then fill up the half-filled vessel with liquor from that which is quite full, and which will now in its turn only be left half-full. Four-and-twenty hours afterwards, repeat the same operation; and thus go on, keeping the vessels alternately full and half-full during twenty-four hours, till the vinegar be made. On the second or third day, there will arise in the half-filled vessel a fermentative motion, accompanied with a sensible heat, which will gradually increase from day to day. On the contrary, the fermenting motion is almost imperceptible in the full vessel; and as the two vessels are alternately full and half-full, the fermentation is by this means in some measure interrupted, and is only renewed every other day in each vessel.

"'When this motion appears to have entirely ceased, even in the half-filled vessel, it is a sign that the fermentation is finished; and therefore the vinegar is then to be put into casks close stopped, and kept in a cool place.

"'A greater or less degree of warmth accelerates or checks this, as well as the spirituous fermentation. In France, it is finished in about fifteen days, during the summer; but if the heat of the air be very great, and exceed the twenty-fifth degree of Reaumur's thermometer (88 1-4° Fahr.) the half-filled vessel must be filled up every twelve hours; because, if the fermentation be not so checked in that time, it will become violent, and the liquor will be so heated, that many of the spirituous parts, on which the strength of the vinegar depends, will be dissipated, so that nothing will remain after the fermentation but a vapid liquor, sour indeed, but effete. The better to prevent the dissipation of the spirituous parts, it is a proper and usual precaution to close the mouth of the half-filled vessel in which the liquor ferments, with a cover made of oak wood. As to the full vessel, it is always left open, that the air may act freely on the liquor it contains: for it is not liable to the same inconveniences, because it ferments but very slowly.'

"Good vinegar may be made from a weak syrup, consisting of 18 oz. of sugar to every gallon of water. The yeast and rape are to be here used as above described. Whenever the vinegar (from the taste and flavour) is considered to be complete, it ought to be decanted into tight barrels or bottles, and well secured from access of air. A momentary ebullition before it is bottled is found favourable to its preservation. In a large manufactory of malt vinegar, a considerable revenue is derived from the sale of yeast to the bakers.

"Vinegar obtained by the preceding methods has more or less of a brown colour, and a peculiar but rather grateful smell. By distillation in glass vessels the colouring matter, which resides in a mucilage, is separated, but the fragrant odour is generally replaced by an empyreumatic one. The best French wine vinegars, and also some from malt, contain a little alcohol, which comes over early with the watery part, and renders the first product of distillation scarcely denser, sometimes even less dense, than water. It is accordingly rejected. Towards the end of the distillation the empyreuma increases. Hence only the intermediate portions are retained as distilled vinegar. Its specific gravity varies from 1.005 to 1.015, while that of common vinegar of equal strength varies from 1.010 to 1.025.

"A crude vinegar has been long prepared for the calico printers, by subjecting wood in iron retorts to a strong red heat."

"The acetic acid of the chemist may be prepared in the following modes; 1st. Two parts of fused acetate of potassa with one of the strongest oil of vitriol yield, by slow distillation from a glass retort into a refrigerated receiver, concentrated acetic acid. A small portion of sulphurous acid, which contaminates it, may be removed by re-distillation, from a little acetate of lead. 2d. Or four parts of good sugar of lead, with one part of sulphuric acid treated in the same way, afford a slightly weaker acetic acid. 3d. Gently calcined sulphate of iron, or green vitriol, mixed with sugar of lead in the proportion of 1 of the former to 2 1-2 of the latter, and carefully distilled from a porcelain retort into a cooled receiver, may be also considered a good economical process. Or without distillation, if 100 parts of well-dried acetate of lime be cautiously added to 60 parts of strong sulphuric acid, diluted with 5 parts of water, and digested for 24 hours, and strained, a good acetic acid, sufficiently strong for every ordinary purpose, will be obtained.

"The distillation of acetate of copper, or of lead *per se*, has also been employed for obtaining strong acid. Here, however, the product is mixed with a portion of the fragrant pyro-acetic spirit, which it is troublesome to get rid of. Undoubtedly the best process for the strong acid is that first described, and the cheapest the second or third. When of the utmost possible strength its sp. gravity is 1.062. At the temperature of 50° F. it assumes the solid form, crystallizing in oblong rhomboidal plates. It has an extremely pungent odour, affecting the nostrils and eyes even painfully, when its vapour is incautiously snuffed up. Its taste is eminently acid and acrid. It excoriates and inflames the skin.

"The purified wood vinegar, which is used for pickles and culinary purposes, has commonly a specific gravity of about 1.009; when it is equivalent in acid strength to good wine or malt vinegar of 1.014. It contains about 1-20 of its weight of absolute acetic acid, and 19-20 of water. But the vinegar of fermentation=1.014 will become only 1.023 in acetate, from which, if 0.005 be subtracted for mucilage or extractive, the remainder will agree with the density of the acetate from wood. A glass hydrometer of Fahrenheit's construction is used for finding the specific gravities. It consists of a globe of about 3 inches' diameter, having a little ballast ball drawn out beneath, and a stem above of about 3 inches long, containing a slip of paper with a transverse line in the middle, and surmounted with a little cup for receiving weights or poises. The experiments on which this instrument, called an *Acetometer*, is constructed, have been detailed in the sixth volume of the Journal of Science."

"An acetic acid of very considerable strength may also be prepared by saturating perfectly dry charcoal with common vinegar, and then distilling. The water easily comes off, and is separated at first; but a stronger heat is required to expel the acid. Or by exposing vinegar to very cold air, or to freezing mixtures, its water separates in the state of ice, the interstices of which are occupied by a strong acetic acid, which may be procured by draining. The acetic acid, or radical vinegar of the apothecaries, in which they dissolve a little camphor, or fragrant essential oil, has a specific gravity of about 1.070. It contains fully 1 part of water to 2 of the crystallized acid. The pungent smelling salt consists of sulphate of potash moistened with that acid.

"Acetic acid acts on *tin*, *iron*, *zinc*, *copper*, and *nickel*; and it combines readily with the *oxydes* of many *other metals*, by mixing a solution of their sulphates with that of an acetate of lead."

"Acetic acid dissolves *resins*, *gum-resins*, *camphor*, and *essential oils*."

"Acetic acid and common vinegar are sometimes fraudulently mixed with sulphuric acid to give them strength. This *adulteration* may be detected by the addition of a little chalk, short of their saturation. With pure vinegar the calcareous base forms a limpid solution, but with sulphuric acid a white insoluble gypsum. Muriate of barytes is a still nicer test. British fermented vinegars are allowed by law to contain a little sulphuric acid, but the quantity is frequently exceeded. Copper is discovered in vinegars by supersaturating them with ammonia, when a fine blue colour is produced; and lead by sulphate of soda, hydrosulphurets, sulphuretted hydrogen, and gallic acid. None of these should produce any change on genuine vinegar." See *Lead.*

"Salts consisting of the several bases, united in definite proportions to acetic acid, are called *acetates.* They are characterized by the pungent smell of vinegar, which they exhale on the affusion of sulphuric acid; and by their yielding on distillation in a moderate red heat a very light, odorous, and combustible liquid called pyro-acetate (SPIRIT); which see. They are all soluble in water; many of them so much so as to be uncrystallizable. About 30 different acetates have been formed, of which only a very few have been applied to the uses of life.

"The acetic acid unites with all the *alkalies* and most of the *earths;* and with these bases it forms compounds, some of which are crystallizable, and others have not yet been reduced to a regularity of figure The salts it forms are distinguished by their great solubility; their decomposition by fire, which carbonizes them; the spontaneous alteration of their solution; and their decomposition by a great number of acids, which extricate from them the acetic acid in a concentrated state. It unites likewise with most of the metallic oxides.

"With *barytes* the saline mass formed by the acetic acid does not crystallize; but, when evaporated to dryness, it deliquesces by exposure to air. This mass is not decomposed by acid of arsenic. By spontaneous evaporation, however, it will crystallize in fine transparent prismatic needles, of a bitterish acid taste, which do not deliquesce when exposed to the air, but rather effloresce.

'With *potassa* this acid unites, and forms a deliquescent salt scarcely crystallizable, called formerly *foliated earth of tartar,* and *regenerated tartar.* The solution of this salt, even in closely stopped vessels, is spontaneously decomposed: it deposites a thick, mucous, flocculent sediment, at first gray, and at length black; till at the end of a few months nothing remains in the liquor but carbonate of potassa, rendered impure by a little coaly oil.

"With *soda* it forms a crystallizable salt, which does not deliquesce. This salt has very improperly been called mineral foliated earth. According to the new nomenclature, it is acetate of soda.

'The salt formed by dissolving *chalk* or other calcareous earth in distilled vinegar, formerly called *salt of chalk,* or *fixed vegetable sal ammoniac,* and by Bergman *calx acetata,* has a sharp bitter taste, appears in the form of crystals resembling somewhat ears of corn, which remain dry when exposed to the air, unless the acid has been superabundant, in which case they deliquesce."

Of the *acetate of strontian* little is known, but that it has a sweet taste, is very soluble, and is easily decomposed by a strong heat.

"The salt formed by uniting vinegar with *ammonia,* called by the various names of *spirit of Mindererus, liquid sal ammoniac, acetous sal ammoniac,* and by Bergman *alkali volatile acetatum,* is generally in a liquid state, and is commonly believed not to be crystallizable, as in distillation it passes entirely over into the receiver. It nevertheless may be reduced into the form of small needle-shaped crystals, when this liquor is evaporated to the consistence of a syrup."

"With *magnesia* the acetic acid unites, and after a perfect saturation, forms a viscid saline mass, like a solution of gum-arabic, which does not shoot into crystals, but remains deliquescent, has a taste sweetish at first, and afterwards bitter, and is soluble in spirit of wine. The acid of this saline mass may be separated by distillation without addition.

"*Glucine* is readily dissolved by acetic acid. This solution, Vauquelin informs us, does not crystallize; but is reduced by evaporation to a gummy substance, which slowly becomes dry and brittle; retaining a kind of ductility for a long time. It has a saccharine and pretty strongly astringent taste, in which that of vinegar, however, is distinguishable.

"*Yttria* dissolves readily in acetic acid, and the solution yields by evaporation crystals of acetate of yttria."

"*Alumine,* obtained by boiling alum with alkali, and edulcorated by digesting in an alkaline lixivium, is dissolved by distilled vinegar in a very inconsiderable quantity."

"*Acetate of zircone* may be formed by pouring acetic acid on newly precipitated zircone. It has an astringent taste."

"Vinegar dissolves the true gums, and partly the gum-resins, by means of digestion.

"Boerhaave observes, that vinegar by long boiling dissolves the flesh, cartilages, bones, and ligaments of animals."—*Ure's Chemical Dictionary.*

Moderately rectified pyroligneous acid has been recommended for the preservation of animal food; but the empyreumatic taint it communicates to bodies immersed in it, is not quite removed by their subsequent ebullition in water. See *Acid, Pyrolignous.*

The utility of vinegar as a condiment for preserving and seasoning both animal and vegetable substances in various articles of food is very generally known. It affords an agreeable beverage, when combined with water in the proportion of a table-spoonful of the former to half a pint of the latter. It is often employed as a medicine in inflammatory and putrid diseases, when more active remedies cannot be procured. Relief has likewise been obtained in hypochondriacal and hysteric affections, in vomiting, fainting, and hiccough, by the application of vinegar to the mouth. If this fluid be poured into vessels and placed over the gentle heat of a lamp in the apartments of the sick, it greatly contributes to disperse foul or mephitic vapours, and consequently to purify the air. Its anticontagious powers are now little trusted to, but its odour is employed to relieve nervous headache, fainting fits, or sickness occasioned by crowded rooms.

As an external application, vinegar proves highly efficacious when joined with farinaceous substances, and applied as a cataplasm to sprained joints; it also forms an eligible lotion for inflammations of the surface, when mixed with alcohol and water in about equal proportions. Applied to burns and scalds, it is said to be highly serviceable whether there is a loss of substance or not, and to quicken the exfoliation of carious bone. (Gloucester Infirmary.) Mixed with an infusion of sage, or with water, it forms a popular and excellent gargle for an inflamed throat, also for an injection to moderate the fluor albus. Applied cold to the nose in cases of hæmorrhage, also to the loins and abdomen in menorrhagia, particularly after parturition, it is said to be very serviceable. An imprudent use of vinegar internally is not without considerable inconveniences. Large and frequent doses injure the stomach, coagulate the chyle, and produce not only leanness, but an atrophy. When taken to excess by females, to reduce a corpulent habit, tubercles in the lungs and a consumption have been the consequence.

["When any of the vinous liquors are exposed to the free access of atmospheric air, at a temperature of 80 to 85 degrees, they undergo a second fermentation, terminating in the production of a sour liquid, called vinegar. During this process a portion of the oxygen of the air is converted into carbonic acid; hence, unlike vinous fermentation, the contact of the atmosphere is necessary, and the most obvious phenomenon is the removal of carbon from the beer or wine. Vinegar is usually obtained from malt liquor or cider, while wine is employed as its source in those countries where the grape is abundantly cultivated.—*Webster's Manuel of Chemistry.*

Vinegar for ordinary use may also be made from sugar, molasses, raisins, or other fruits, or from the refuse of fruits, as follows:

"Take the skins of raisins after they have been used in making wine, and pour three times their own quantity of water upon them; stir them well about, and then set the cask in a warm place, also covered, and the liquor in a few weeks' time will become a sound vinegar, which drawn off from its sediments, put into another cask, and well bunged down, will be a good vinegar for the table."—*Beastall's Useful Guide.* A.]

ACETIFICATION (*Acetificatio;* from *acetum,* vinegar, and *fio,* to make.) The action or operation by which vinegar is made.

ACETOMETER. An instrument for estimating the strength of vinegars. See *Acetic Acid.*

ACETO'SA. (From *acesco,* to be sour.) Sorrel. A genus of plants in some systems of botany. See *Rumex.*

ACETOSE'LLA. (From *acetosa,* sorrel: so called from the acidity of its leaves.) Wood-sorrel. See *Oxalis acetosella.*

ACETOUS. (*Acetosus;* from *acetum*, vinegar.) Of or belonging to vinegar.

Acetous Acid. See *Acetum*

Acetous Fermentation. See *Fermentation.*

ACE'TUM. (*Acetum, i.* n.; from *acer*, sour.) Vinegar. A sour liquor obtained from many vegetable substances dissolved in boiling water, and from fermented and spirituous liquors, by exposing them to heat and contact with air; under which circumstances they undergo the acid fermentation, and afford the liquor called vinegar. Common vinegar consists of acetic acid combined with a large portion of water, and with this are in solution portions of gluten, mucilage, sugar, and extractive matter, from which it derives its colour, and frequently some of the vegetable acids, particularly the malic and the tartaric. See *Acetic Acid.*

ACETUM AROMATICUM. Aromatic vinegar. A preparation of the Edinburgh Pharmacopœia, thought to be an improvement of what has been named *thieves' vinegar.*

Take of the dried tops of rosemary, the dried leaves of sage, of each four ounces; dried lavender flowers, two ounces; cloves, two drachms; distilled vinegar, eight pounds. Macerate for seven days, and strain the expressed juice through paper. Its virtues are antiseptic, and it is a useful composition to smell at in crowded courts of justice, hospitals, &c. where the air is offensive.

ACETUM COLCHICI. Vinegar of meadow-saffron. Take of fresh meadow-saffron root sliced, an ounce; acetic acid, a pint; proof spirit, a fluid ounce. Macerate the meadow-saffron root in the acid, in a covered glass vessel, for three days; then press out the liquor and set it by, that the feculencies may subside; lastly, add the spirit to the clear liquor. The dose is from ʒss to ʒiss.

ACETUM DISTILLATUM. See *Acidum aceticum dilutum.*

ACETUM SCILLÆ. Vinegar of squills. Take of squills recently dried, one pound; dilute acetic acid, six pints; proof spirit, half a pint. Macerate the squills with the vinegar in a glass vessel, with a gentle heat for twenty-four hours; then express the liquor and set it aside until the fæces subside. To the decanted liquor add the spirit. This preparation of squills is employed as an attenuant, expectorant, and diuretic. Dose, xv. to lx. drops.

A'CHEIR. (From *a*, neg. and χειρ, hand.) Without hands.

ACHI'COLUM. By this word Cælius Aurelianus, Acut. lib. iii. cap. 17, expresses the sudatorium of the ancient baths, which was a hot room where they used to sweat.

ACHILLE'A. (*Achillea, æ,* f. Αχιλλεια: from Achilles, who is said to have made his tents with it, or to have cured Telephus with it.) 1. The name of a genus of plants in the Linnæan system. Class *Syngenesia;* Order, *Polygamia superflua.*

2. The pharmaceutical name of the milfoil. See *Achillea millefolium.*

ACHILLEA AGERATUM. Maudlin, or maudlin tansy. *Balsamita fœmina; Eupatorium Mesues* This plant, the ageratum of the shops, is described by Linnæus as *Achillea:—foliis lanceolatis, obtusis, acutoserratis.* It is esteemed in some countries as anthelminthic and alterative, and is given in hepatic obstructions. It possesses the virtues of tansy.

ACHILLEA MILLEFOLIUM. The systematic name of the common yarrow, or milfoil. *Achillea; Myriophyllon; Chiliophyllon; Lumbus veneris; Militaris herba; Stratiotes; Carpentaria; Speculum veneris.* The leaves and flowers of this indigenous plant, *Achillea—foliis bipinnatis nudis; laciniis linearibus dentatis; caulibus superne sulcatis* of Linnæus, have an agreeable, weak, aromatic smell, and a bitterish, rough, and somewhat pungent taste. They are both directed for medicinal use in the Edinburgh Pharmacopœia; in the present practice, however, they are almost wholly neglected.

ACHILLEA PTARMICA. The systematic name of the sneeze-wort, or bastard pellitory. *Pseudopyrethrum; Pyrethrum sylvestre; Draco sylvestris; Tarchon sylvestris; Sternutamentoria; Dracunculus pratensis.* The flowers and roots of this plant, *Achillea—foliis lanceolatis, acuminatis, argute serratis,* have a hot biting taste, approaching to that of pyrethrum, with which they also agree in their pharmaceutical properties. Their principal use is as a masticatory and sternutatory.

Achillea foliis pinnatis. See *Genipi verum.*

ACHI'LLES. The son of Peleus and Thetis, one of the most celebrated Grecian heroes. A tendon is named after him, and also a plant with which he is said to have cured Telephus.

ACHILLIS TENDO. The tendon of the gastrocnemii muscles. So called, because, as fable reports, Thetis, the mother of Achilles, held him by that part when she dipped him in the river Styx, to make him invulnerable. Homer describes this tendon, and some writers suppose it was thus named by the ancients, from their custom of calling every thing *Achillean,* that had any extraordinary strength or virtue. Others say it was named from its action in conducing to swiftness of pace, the term importing so much. The tendon of Achilles is the strong and powerful tendon of the heel which is formed by the junction of the gastrocnemius and soleus muscles, and which extends along the posterior part of the tibia from the calf to the heel. See *Gastrocnemius externus,* and *Gastrocnemius internus.*

When this tendon is unfortunately cut or ruptured, as it may be in consequence of a violent exertion, or spasm of the muscles of which it is a continuation, the use of the leg is immediately lost, and unless the part be afterwards successfully united, the patient must remain a cripple for life. When the tendon has been cut, the division of the skin allows the accident to be seen. When the tendon has been ruptured, the patient hears the sound like that of the smack of a whip, at the moment of the occurrence. In whatever way the tendon has been divided, there is a sudden incapacity, or at least an extreme difficulty, either of standing or walking. Hence the patient falls down, and cannot get up again. Besides these symptoms there is a very palpable depression between the ends of the tendon; which depression is increased when the foot is bent, and diminished, or even quite removed when the foot is extended. The patient can spontaneously bend his foot, none of the flexor muscles being interested. The power of extending the foot is still possible, as the peronei muscles, the tibialis posticus, and long flexors, remain perfect, and may perform this motion. The indications are to bring the ends of the divided parts together, and to keep them so, until they have become firmly united. The first object is easily fulfilled by putting the foot in a state of complete extension; the second, namely, that of keeping the ends of the tendon in contact, is more difficult. It seems unnecessary to enumerate the various plans devised to accomplish these ends. The following is Desault's method: After the ends of the tendon had been brought into contact by moderate flection of the knee, and complete extension of the foot, he used to fill up the hollows on each side of the tendon with soft lint and compresses. The roller applied to the limb, made as much pressure on these compresses as on the tendon, and hence this part could not be depressed too much against the adjacent parts. Desault next took a compress about two inches broad, and long enough to reach from the toes to the middle of the thigh, and placed it under the foot, over the back of the leg and lower part of the thigh. He then began to apply a few circles of a roller round the end of the foot, so as to fix the lower extremity of the longitudinal compress; after covering the whole foot with the roller, he used to make the bandage describe the figure of 8, passing it under the foot and across the place where the tendon was ruptured, and the method was finished by encircling the limb upward with the roller as far as the upper end of the longitudinal compress.

A'CHLYS. (Αχλυς.) Darkness; cloudiness. An obsolete term, generally applied to a close, foggy air, or a mist.

1. Hippocrates, de Morbis Mulierum, lib. ii. signifies by this word air, condensed air in the womb.

2. Galen interprets it of those, who, during sickness, lose that lustre and loveliness observed about the pupil of the eye in health.

3. Others express it by an ulcer on the pupil of the eye, or the scar left there by an ulcer.

4. It means also an opacity of the cornea; the same as the caligo cornea of Dr. Cullen.

ACHME'LLA. See *Spilanthus acmella.*

A'CHOLUS. (From *a*, priv. and χολη, bile.) Deficient in bile.

A'CHOR. (*Achor, oris.* m. αχωρ, qu. αχνωο; from αχνη, bran: according to Blanchard it is derived from α, priv. and χωρος, space, as occupying but a small compass.) *Lactumen; Abas; Acores; Cerion; Favus; Crusta lactea* of authors. The scald-head; so called from the branny scales thrown off it. A disease which attacks the hairy scalp of the head, for the most part, of young children, forming soft and scaly eruptions. Dr. Willan, in his description of different kinds of pustules, defines the achor, a pustule of intermediate size between the phlyzacium and psydracium, which contains a straw-coloured fluid, having the appearance and nearly the consistence of strained honey. It appeared most frequently about the head, and is succeeded by a dull white or yellowish scab. Pustules of this kind, when so large as nearly to equal the size of phlyzacia, are termed ceria or favi, being succeeded by a yellow semi-transparent, and sometimes cellular, scab, like a honeycomb. The achor differs from the favus and tinea only in the degree of virulence. It is called favus when the perforations are large; and tinea when they are like those which are made by moths in cloth; but generally by tinea is understood a dry scab on the hairy scalp of children, with thick scales and an offensive smell. When this disorder affects the face, it is called crusta lactea or milk scab. Mr. Bell, in his Treatise on Ulcers, reduces the tinea capitis and crusta lactea to some species of herpes, *viz.* the herpes pustulosus, differing only in situation.

ACHORISTOS. Inseparable. This term was applied by the ancients, to symptoms, or signs, which are inseparable from particular things. Thus, softness is inseparable from humidity; hardness from fragility; and a pungent pain in the side is an inseparable symptom of a pleurisy.

ACHRAS. The name of a genus of plants in the Linnæan system. Class, *Hexandria;* Order, *Monogynia.* The sapota plum-tree.

ACHRAS SAPOTA. The systematic name of the tree which affords the oval-fruited sapota, seeds of which are sometimes given in the form of emulsion in calculous complaints. It is a native of South America, and bears a fruit like an apple, which has, when ripe, a luscious taste, resembling that of the marmalade of quinces, whence it is called natural marmalade. The bark of this, and the *Achras mammosa* is very astringent, and is used medicinally under the name of *Cortex jamaicensis.*

ACHREI'ON. Useless. Applied by Hippocrates to the limbs which, through weakness, become useless.

ACHROI'A. A paleness.

A'CHYRON. Αχυρον. This properly signifies bran, or chaff, or straw. Hippocrates, de Morbis Mulierum, most probably means by this word, bran. Achyron also signifies a straw, hair, or any thing that sticks upon a wall.

A'CIA. (From ακη, a point.) A needle with thread in it for chirurgical operations.

A'CICYS. Weak, infirm, or faint. In this sense it is used by Hippocrates, de Morb. lib. iv.

ACID. (*Acidum, i.* n.) 1. That which impresses upon the organs of taste a sharp or sour sensation. The word *sour*, which is usually employed to denote the simple impression, or lively and sharp sensation produced on the tongue by certain bodies, may be regarded as synonymous to the word *acid.* The only difference which can be established between them, is, that the one denotes a weak sensation, whereas the other comprehends all the degrees of force, from the least perceptible to the greatest degree of causticity: thus we say that verjuice, gooseberries, or lemons, are *sour;* but we use the word acid to express the impression which the nitric, sulphuric, or muriatic acids make upon the tongue.

2. Acids are an important class of chemical compounds. In the generalization of facts presented by Lavoisier and the associated French chemists, it was the leading doctrine that acids resulted from the union of a peculiar combustible base called the *radical,* with a common principle technically called oxygen, or the *acidifier.* This general position was founded chiefly on the phenomena exhibited in the formation and decomposition of sulphuric, carbonic, phosphoric, and nitric acids; and was extended by a plausible analogy to other acids, the radicals of which were unknown.

"I have already shown," says Lavoisier, "that phosphorus is changed by combustion into an extremely light, white, flaky matter. Its properties are likewise entirely altered by this transformation; from being insoluble in water, it becomes not only soluble, but so greedy of moisture as to attract the humidity of the air with astonishing rapidity. By this means it is converted into a liquid, considerably more dense, and of more specific gravity than water. In the state of phosphorus before combustion, it had scarcely any sensible taste; by its union with oxygen it acquires an extremely sharp and sour taste; in a word, from one of the class of combustible bodies, it is changed into an incombustible substance, and becomes one of those bodies called acids.

"This property of a combustible substance, to be converted into an acid by the addition of oxygen, we shall presently find belongs to a great number of bodies. Wherefore strict logic requires that we should adopt a common term for indicating all these operations which produce analogous results. This is the true way to simplify the study of science, as it would be quite impossible to bear all its specific details in the memory if they were not classically arranged. For this reason we shall distinguish the conversion of phosphorus into an acid by its union with oxygen, and in general every combination of oxygen with a combustible substance, by the term *oxygenation;* from this I shall adopt the verb to oxygenate; and of consequence shall say, that in oxygenating phosphorus, we convert it into an acid.

"Sulphur also, in burning, absorbs oxygen gas; the resulting acid is considerably heavier than the sulphur burnt; its weight is equal to the sum of the weights of the sulphur which has been burnt, and of the oxygen absorbed; and, lastly, this acid is weighty, incombustible, and miscible with water in all proportions.

"I might multiply these experiments, and show, by a numerous succession of facts, that all acids are formed by the combustion of certain substances; but I am prevented from doing so in this place by the plan which I have laid down, of proceeding only from facts already ascertained to such as are unknown, and of drawing my examples only from circumstances already explained. In the mean time, however, the examples above cited may suffice for giving a clear and accurate conception of the manner in which acids are formed. By these it may be clearly seen that oxygen is an element common to them all, and which constitutes or produces their acidity; and that they differ from each other according to the several natures of the oxygenated or acidified substances. We must, therefore, in every acid, carefully distinguish between the acidifiable base, which de Morveau calls the radical, and 'the acidifying principle or oxygen.'" *Elements,* p. 115.

"Although we have not yet been able either to compose or to decompound this acid of sea salt, we cannot have the smallest doubt that it, like all other acids, is composed by the union of oxygen with an acidifiable base. We have, therefore, called this unknown substance the muriatic base, or muriatic radical." P. 122. 5th *Edition.*

Berthollet maintains, that Lavoisier had given too much latitude to the idea of oxygen being the universal acidifying principle. "In fact," says he, "it is carrying the limits of analogy too far to infer, that all acidity, even that of the muriatic, fluoric, and boracic acids, arises from oxygen, because it gives acidity to a great number of substances. Sulphuretted hydrogen, which really possesses the properties of an acid, proves directly that acidity is not in all cases owing to oxygen. There is no better foundation for concluding that hydrogen is the principle of alcalinity, not only in the alcalies, properly so called, but also in magnesia, lime, strontian, and barytes, because ammonia appears to owe its alcalinity to hydrogen.

"These considerations prove that oxygen may be regarded as the most usual principle of acidity, but that this species of affinity for the alcalies may belong to substances which do not contain oxygen; that we must not, therefore, always infer, from the acidity of a substance, that it contains oxygen, although this may be an inducement to suspect its existence in it; still less should we conclude, because a substance contains oxygen, that it must have acid properties; on the contrary, the acidity of an oxygenated substance shows that the oxygen has only experienced an incomplete saturation in it, since its properties remain predominant."

This generalization of the French chemists concerning oxygen, was first experimentally combated by Sir Humphry Davy, in a series of dissertations published in the Philosophical Transactions.

"His first train of experiments was instituted with the view of operating by voltaic electricity on muriatic and other acids freed from water. Substances which are now known by the names of chlorides of phosphorus and tin, but which he then supposed to contain dry muriatic acid, led him to imagine that intimately combined water was the real acidifying principle, since acid properties were immediately developed in the above substances by the addition of that fluid, though previously they exhibited no acid powers. In July, 1810, however, he advanced those celebrated views concerning acidification, which, in the opinion of the best judges, display an unrivalled power of scientific research. The conclusions to which these led him, were incompatible with the general hypothesis of Lavoisier. He demonstrated that oxymuriatic acid is, as far as our knowledge extends, a *simple* substance, which may be classed in the same order of natural bodies as oxygen gas, being determined like oxygen to the positive surface in voltaic combinations, and like oxygen combining with inflammable substances, producing heat and light. The combinations of oxymuriatic acid with inflammable bodies were shown to be analogous to oxydes and acids in their properties and powers of combination, but to differ from them in being, for the most part, decomposable by water; and, finally, that oxymuriatic acid has a stronger attraction for most inflammable bodies than oxygen. His preceding decomposition of the alcalies and earths having evinced the absurdity of that nomenclature which gives to the general and essential constituent of alcaline nature, the term oxygen or acidifier; his new discovery of the simplicity of oxymuriatic acid, showed the theoretical system of chemical language to be equally vicious in another respect. Hence this philosopher most judiciously discarded the appellation oxymuriatic acid, and introduced in its place the name chlorine, which merely indicates an obvious and permanent character of the substance, its greenish yellow colour. The more recent investigations of chemists on fluoric, hydriodic, and hydrocyanic acids, have brought powerful analogies in support of the chloridic theory, by showing that hydrogen alone can convert certain undecompounded bases into acids well characterized, without the aid of oxygen."

"After these observations on the nature of acidity, we shall now state the general properties of the acids.

"1. The taste of these bodies is for the most part sour, as their name denotes; and in the stronger species it is acrid and corrosive.

"2. They generally combine with water in every proportion, with a condensation of volume and evolution of heat.

"3. With a few exceptions they are volatilized or decomposed at a moderate heat.

"4. They usually change the purple colours of vegetables to a bright red.

"5. They unite in definite proportions with the alcalies, earths, and metallic oxydes, and form the important class of salts. This may be reckoned their characteristic and indispensable property."

"Thenard has lately succeeded in communicating to many acids *apparently* a surcharge of oxygen, and thus producing a supposed new class of bodies, the *oxygenized acids*, which are, in reality, combinations of the ordinary acids with oxygenized water, or with the deutoxide of hydrogen."

"The class of acids has been distributed into three orders, according as they are derived from the mineral, the vegetable, or the animal kingdom. But a more specific distribution is now requisite. They have also been arranged into those which have a single, and those which have a compound basis or radical. This arrangement is not only vague, but liable in other respects to considerable objections. The chief advantage of a classification is to give general views to beginners in the study, by grouping together such substances as have analogous properties or composition. These objects will be tolerably well attained by the following divisions and subdivisions.

"1st. Acids from inorganic nature, or which are procurable without having recourse to animal or vegetable products.

"2d. Acids elaborated by means of organization.

"The first group is subdivided into three families: 1st. Oxygen acids; 2d. Hydrogen acids; 3d. Acids destitute of both these supposed acidifiers.

Family 1st.—Oxygen acids.
Section 1st, Non-metallic.

1. Boracic.	11. Hypophosphorus.
2. Carbonic.	12. Phosphorus.
3. Chloric.	13. Phosphatic.
4. Perchloric ?	14. Phosphoric.
5. Chloro-Carbonic.	15. Hyposulphurous.
6. Nitrous.	16. Sulphurous.
7. Hyponitric.	17. Hyposulphuric
8. Nitric.	18. Sulphuric
9. Iodic.	19. Cyanic ?
10. Iodo-Sulphuric.	

Section 2d, Oxygen acids.—Metallic.

1. Arsenic.	6. Columbic.
2. Arsenious.	7. Molybdic.
3. Antimonious	8. Molybdous.
4. Antimonic	9. Tungstic.
5. Chromic.	

Family 2d.—Hydrogen acids.

1. Fluoric.	6. Hydroprussic, or Hydro-cyanic.
2. Hydriodic.	
3. Hydrochloric, or Muriatic	7. Hydrosulphurous.
	8. Hydrotellurous.
4. Ferroprussic.	9. Sulphuroprussic.
5. Hydroselenic.	

Family 3d.—Acids without Oxygen or Hydrogen

1. Chloriodic.	3. Fluoboric.
2. Chloroprussic, or Chlorocyanic.	4. Fluosilicic.

Division 2d.—Acids of Organic Origin

1. Aceric.	24. Meconic.
2. Acetic.	25. Menispermic.
3. Amniotic.	26. Margaric.
4. Benzoic.	27. Melassic ?
5. Boletic.	28. Mellitic.
6. Butyric.	29 Moroxylic
7. Camphoric.	30. Mucic.
8. Caseic.	31. Nanceic ?
9. Cevadic.	32. Nitro-leucic.
10. Cholesteric.	33. Nitro-saccharic
11. Citric.	34. Oleic.
12. Delphinic.	35. Oxalic.
13. Ellagic ?	36. Purpuric.
14. Formic.	37. Pyrolithic.
15. Fungic.	38. Pyromalic.
16. Gallic.	39. Pyrotartaric.
17. Igasuric.	40. Rosasic.
18. Kinic.	41. Saclactic.
19. Laccic.	42. Sebacic.
20. Lactic.	43. Suberic.
21. Lampic.	44. Succinic.
22. Lithic, or Uric.	45. Sulphovinic ?
23. Malic.	46. Tartaric.

The acids of the last division are all decomposable at a red heat, and afford generally carbon, hydrogen, oxygen, and, in some few cases, also nitrogen. The mellitic is found like amber in wood coal, and, like it, is undoubtedly of organic origin."

Acid, aceric. See *Aceric acid.*
Acid, acetic. See *Acetum.*
Acid, acetous. See *Acetum.*
Acid, aerial. See *Carbonic acid.*
Acid, ætherial. See *Æthers.*
Acid, aluminous. See *Sulphuric acid.*
Acid, amniotic. See *Amniotic acid.*
Acid, animal. See *Acid.*
Acid, antimonic. See *Antimony.*
Acid, antimonous. See *Antimony.*
Acid of ants. See *Formic acid.*
Acid, arsenical. See *Arsenic.*
Acid, arsenious. See *Arsenic.*
Acid, benzoic. See *Benzoic acid.*
Acid, boletic. See *Boletic acid.*
Acid, boracic. See *Boracic acid.*
Acid, camphoric. See *Camphoric acid.*
Acid, carbonic. See *Carbonic acid.*
Acid, caseic. See *Caseic acid.*
Acid, cetic. See *Cetic acid.*

Acid, chloric See *Chloric acid.*
Acid, chloriodic. See *Chloriodic acid.*
Acid, chlorous. See *Chlorous acid.*
Acid, chloro-carbonic. See *Chloro-carbonous acid* and *Phosgene.*
Acid, chloro-cyanic. See *Chloro-cyanic acid.*
Acid, chloro-prussic. See *Chloro-cyanic acid.*
Acid, chromic. See *Chromic acid.*
Acid, citric. See *Citric acid.*
Acid, columbic. See *Columbic acid.*
Acid, cyanic. See *Prussic acid.*
Acid, dephlogisticated muriatic. See *Chlorine.*
Acid, dulcified. Now called Æther.
Acid, ellegic. See *Ellagic acid.*
Acid, ferro-chyazic. See *Ferro-chyazic acid.*
Acid, ferro-prussic. See *Ferro-prussic acid.*
Acid, ferruretted-chyazic. See *Ferro-prussic acid.*
Acid, fluoboric. See *Fluoboric acid.*
Acid, fluoric. See *Fluoric acid.*
Acid, fluoric, silicated. See *Fluoric acid.*
Acid, fluosilicic. See *Fluoric acid.*
Acid, formic. See *Formic acid.*
Acid, fungic. See *Fungic acid.*
Acid, gallic. See *Gallic acid.*
Acid, hydriodic. See *Hydriodic acid.*
Acid, hydrochloric. See *Muriatic acid.*
Acid, hydrocyanic. See *Prussic acid.*
Acid, hydrofluoric. See *Fluoric acid.*
Acid, hydrophosphorous. See *Phosphorous acid.*
Acid, hydrophtoric. See *Fluoric acid.*
Acid, hydrosulphuric. See *Sulphuretted hydrogen.*
Acid, hydrothionic. See *Sulphuretted hydrogen.*
Acid, hyponitrous. See *Hyponitrous acid.*
Acid, hypophosphorous. See *Hypophosphorous acid.*
Acid, hyposulphuric. See *Hyposulphuric acid.*
Acid, hyposulphurous. See *Hyposulphurous acid.*
Acid, igasuric. See *Igasuric acid.*
Acid, imperfect. These acids are so called in the chemical nomenclature, which are not fully saturated with oxygen. Their names are ended in Latin by *osum*, and in English by *ous:* e. g. *acidum nitrosum*, or nitrous acid.
Acid, iodic. See *Iodic acid.*
Acid, iodosulphuric. See *Iodosulphuric acid.*
Acid, kinic. See *Kinic acid.*
Acid, krameric. See *Krameric acid.*
Acid, laccic. See *Laccic acid.*
Acid, lactic. See *Lactic acid.*
Acid, lampic. See *Lampic acid.*
Acid, lethic. See *Lethic acid.*
Acid, malic. See *Malic acid.*
Acid, manganesic. See *Manganesic acid.*
Acid, margaritic. See *Margaritic acid.*
Acid, meconic. See *Meconic acid.*
Acid, mellitic. See *Mellitic acid.*
Acid, menispermic. See *Menispermic acid.*
Acid of milk. See *Mucic acid.*
Acid, mineral. Those acids which are found to exist in minerals, as the sulphuric, the nitric, &c. See *Acid.*
Acid, molybdic. See *Molybdic acid.*
Acid, molybdous. See *Molybdous acid.*
Acid, moroxylic. See *Moroxylic acid.*
Acid, mucic. See *Mucic acid.*
Acid, mucous. See *Mucic acid.*
Acid, muriatic. See *Muriatic acid.*
Acid, muriatic, dephlogisticated.
Acid, nanceic. See *Nanceic acid.*
Acid of nitre. See *Nitric acid.*
Acid, nitric. See *Nitric acid.*
Acid, nitro-leucic. See *Nitro-leucic acid.*
Acid, nitro-muriatic. See *Nitro-muriatic acid.*
Acid, nitro-saccharine. See *Nitro-saccharic acid.*
Acid, nitro sulphuric. See *Nitro-sulphuric acid*
Acid, nitrous. See *Nitrous acid.*
Acid, Œnothionic. See *Œnothionic acid.*
Acid, oleic. See *Oleic acid.*
Acid, oxalic. See *Oxalic acid.*
Acid, oxiodic. See *Iodic acid.*
Acid, oxychloric. See *Perchloric acid.*
Acid, oxymuriatic. See *Chlorine.*
Acid, perchloric. See *Perchloric acid.*
Acid, perfect. An acid is termed perfect in the chemical nomenclature, when it is completely saturated with oxygen. The names are ended in Latin by *icum*, and in English by *ic:* e. g. *acidum nitricum*, or *nitric acid.*
Acid, perlate. See *Perlate acid.*
Acid, pernitrous. See *Hyponitrous acid*
Acid, phosphatic. See *Phosphatic acid.*
Acid, phosphoric. See *Phosphoric acid.*
Acid, phosphorous. See *Phosphorous acid.*
Acid, prussic. See *Prussic acid.*
Acid, purpuric. See *Purpuric acid.*
Acid, pyro-acetic. See *Pyro-acetic acid.*
Acid, pyrocitric. See *Pyrocitric acid.*
Acid, pyroligneous. See *Pyro-ligneous acid*
Acid, pyromucous. See *Pyro-mucic acid.*
Acid, pyrotartarous. See *Pyrotartaric acid*
Acid, rheumic. See *Rheumic acid.*
Acid, saccho-lactic. See *Mucic acid.*
Acid, saclactic. See *Mucic acid.*
Acid, sebacic. See *Sebacic acid.*
Acid, selenic. See *Selenic acid.*
Acid, silicated fluoric.
Acid, sorbic. See *Sorbic acid.*
Acid, stannic. See *Stannic acid.*
Acid, stibic. See *Stibic acid.*
Acid, stibious. See *Stibious acid.*
Acid, suberic. See *Suberic acid.*
Acid, succinic. See *Succinic acid.*
Acid of sugar. See *Oxalic acid.*
Acid, sulpho-cyanic. See *Sulphuro-prussic acid.*
Acid, sulphovinous. See *Sulphovinic acid.*
Acid, sulphureous. See *Sulphureous acid.*
Acid, sulphuretted chyazic. See *Sulphuro-prussic acid.*
Acid, sulphuric. See *Sulphuric acid.*
Acid of tartar. See *Tartaric acid.*
Acid, tartaric. See *Tartaric acid.*
Acid, telluric. See *Telluric acid.*
Acid, tungstic. See *Tungstic acid.*
Acid, uric. See *Lithic acid.*
Acid, vegetable. Those which are found in the vegetable kingdom, as the citric, malic, acetic, &c. See *Acid.*
Acid of vinegar. See *Acetum.*
Acid of vinegar, concentrated. See *Acetum.*
Acid of vitriol. See *Sulphuric acid.*
Acid, vitriolic. See *Sulphuric acid.*
Acid, zumic. See *Zumic acid.*

ACIDIFIABLE. Capable of being converted into an acid by an acidifying principle. Substances possessing this property are called *radicals* and *acidifiable bases.*

ACIDIFICATION. (*Acidificatio;* from *acidum*, an acid.) The formation of an acid; also the impregnation of any thing with acid properties.

ACIDIFYING. See *Acid.*

ACIDIMETRY. The measurement of the strength of acids. This is effected by saturating a given weight of them with an alkaline base; the quantity of which requisite for the purpose, is the measure of their power.

ACIDITY. *Aciditas.* Sourness.

ACIDULOUS. *Acidula*, Latin; *acidule*, French. Slightly acid: applied to those salts in which the base is combined with such an excess of acid, that they manifestly exhibit acid properties, as the supertartrate and the supersulphate of potassa.

Acidulous waters. Mineral waters, which contain so great a quantity of carbonic acid gas, as to render them acidulous, or gently tart to the taste. See *Mineral waters.*

ACIDULUS. Acidulated. Any thing blended with an acid juice in order to give it a coolness and brisk ness.

A'CIDUM. (*Acidum*, i. n.; from *aceo*, to be sour.) An acid. See *Acid.*

Acidum aceticum. See *Acidum aceticum dilutum.*

Acidum aceticum dilutum. Dilute acetic acid. Take of vinegar, a gallon.

Distil the acetic acid in a sand bath, from a glass retort into a receiver also of glass, and kept cold; throw away the first pint, and keep for use the six succeeding pints, which are distilled over.

In this distillation, the liquor should be kept moderately boiling, and the heat should not be urged too far, otherwise the distilled acid will have an empyreumatic smell and taste, which it ought not to possess. If the acid be prepared correctly, it will be colourless, and of a grateful, pungent, peculiar acid taste. One fluid ounce ought to dissolve at least ten grains of carbonate of lime, or white marble. This liquor is the *acetum distillatum;* the *acidum acetosum* of the London Pharmacopœia of 1787, and the *acidum aceticum* of that of 1822, and the *acidum aceticum dilutum* of the present. The compounds of the acid of vinegar, directed to be used by the new London Pharmacopœia, are *acetum colchici*, *acetum scillæ*, *ceratum plumbi acetatis*, *liquor ammoniæ acetatis*, *liquor plumbi acetatis*, *liquor plumbi acetatis dilutis*, *oxymel*, *oxymel scillæ*, *potassæ acetas*, and the *cataplasma sinapis*.

ACIDUM ACETICUM CONCENTRATUM. When the acid of vinegar is greatly concentrated, that is, deprived of its water, it is called concentrated acid of vinegar, and radical vinegar.

Distilled vinegar may be concentrated by freezing: the congelation takes place at a temperature below 28 degrees, more or less, according to its strength; and the congealed part is merely ice, leaving, of course, a stronger acid. If this be exposed to a very intense cold, it shoots into crystals; which being separated, liquefy, when the temperature rises, and the liquor is limpid as water, extremely strong, and has a highly pungent acetous odour. This is the pure acid of the vinegar; the foreign matter remaining in the uncongealed liquid.

Other methods are likewise employed to obtain the pure and concentrated acid. The process of Westendorf, which has been often followed, is to saturate soda with distilled vinegar; obtain the acetate by crystallization; and pour upon it, in a retort, half its weight of sulphuric acid. By applying heat, the acetic acid is distilled over; and, should there be any reason to suspect the presence of any sulphuric acid, it may be distilled a second time, from a little acetate of soda. According to Lowitz, the best way of obtaining this acid pure, is to mix three parts of the acetate of soda with eight of supersulphate of potassa; both salts being perfectly dry, and in fine powder, and to distil from this mixture in a retort, with a gentle heat.

It may also be obtained by distilling the verdigris of commerce, with a gentle heat. The concentrated acid procured by these processes, was supposed to differ materially from the acetous acids obtained by distilling vinegar; the two acids were regarded as differing in their degree of oxygenizement, and were afterward distinguished by the names of acetous and acetic acids. The acid distilled from verdigris was supposed to derive a quantity of oxygen from the oxyde of copper, from which it was expelled. The experiments of Adet have, however, proved the two acids to be identical; the acetous acid, therefore, only differs from the acetic acid in containing more water, rendering it a weaker acid, and of a less active nature. There exists, therefore, only one of acid vinegar, which is the acetic; its compounds are termed *acetates*.

ACIDUM ACETOSUM. See *Acetum*.

ACIDUM ÆTHEREUM. See *Sulphuric acid*.

ACIDUM ALUMINOSUM. (So called because it exists in alum.) See *Sulphuric acid*.

ACIDUM ARSENICUM. See *Arsenic*.

ACIDUM BENZOICUM. Benzoic acid. The London Pharmacopœia directs it to be made thus:—Take of gum benzoin a pound and a half: fresh lime, four ounces: water, a gallon and a half: muriatic acid, four fluid ounces. Rub together the benzoin and lime; then boil them in a gallon of the water, for half an hour, constantly stirring; and, when it is cold, pour off the liquor. Boil what remains a second time, in four pints of water, and pour off the liquor as before. Mix the liquors, and boil down to half, then strain through paper, and add the muriatic acid gradually, until it ceases to produce a precipitate. Lastly, having poured off the liquor, dry the powder in a gentle heat; put it into a proper vessel, placed in a sand bath; and by a very gentle fire, sublime the benzoic acid. In this process a solution of benzoate of lime is first obtained; the muriatic acid then, abstracting the lime, precipitates the benzoic acid, which is crystallized by sublimation.

The Edinburgh Pharmacopœia forms a benzoate of soda, precipitates the acid by sulphuric acid, and afterward crystallizes it by solution in hot water, which dissolves a larger quantity than cold.

Benzoic acid has a strong, pungent, aromatic, and peculiar odour. Its crystals are ductile, not pulverizable; it sublimes in a moderate heat, forming a white irritating smoke. It is soluble in about twenty-four times its weight of boiling water, which as it cools, precipitates 19-20ths of what it had dissolved. It is soluble in alcohol.

Benzoic acid is very seldom used in the cure of diseases; but now and then it is ordered as a stimulant against convulsive coughs and difficulty of breathing. The dose is from one grain to five.

ACIDUM BORACICUM. See *Boracic acid*.

ACIDUM CARBONICUM. See *Carbonic acid*.

ACIDUM CATHOLICON. See *Sulphuric acid*.

ACIDUM CITRICUM. See *Citric acid*.

ACIDUM MURIATICUM. See *Muriatic acid*.

ACIDUM MURIATICUM OXYGENATUM. See *Oxygenized muriatic acid*.

ACIDUM NITRICUM. See *Nitric acid*.

ACIDUM NITRICUM DILUTUM. Take of nitric acid a fluid ounce; distilled water nine fluid ounces. Mix them.

ACIDUM NITROSUM. See *Nitrous acid*.

ACIDUM PHOSPHORICUM. See *Phosphoric acid*

ACIDUM PRIMIGENIUM. See *Sulphuric acid*.

ACIDUM SUCCINICUM. See *Succinic acid*.

ACIDUM SULPHUREUM. See *Sulphureous acid*.

ACIDUM SULPHURICUM. See *Sulphuric acid*.

ACIDUM SULPHURICUM DILUTUM. *Acidum vitriolicum dilutum*. *Spiritus vitrioli tenuis*. Take of sulphuric acid a fluid ounce and a half; distilled water, fourteen fluid ounces and a half. Add the water gradually to the acid.

ACIDUM TARTARICUM. See *Tartaric acid*.

ACIDUM VITRIOLICUM. See *Sulphuric acid*.

ACIDUM VITRIOLICUM DILUTUM. See *Acidum sulphuricum dilutum*.

A'CIES. Steel.

ACINACIFORMIS. (From *acinaces*, a Persian scimitar, or sabre, and *forma*, resemblance.) Acinaciform; shaped like a sabre, applied to leaves: as those of the *mysembryanthemum acinaciforme*.

ACINE'SIA. (From ακινησια, immobility.) A loss of motion and strength.

ACINIFORMIS. (From *acinus*, a grape, and *forma*, a resemblance.) Aciniform. A name given by the ancients to some parts which resembled the colour and form of an unripe grape, as the uvea of the eye, which was called *tunica acinosa*, and the choroid membrane of the eye, which they named *tunica aciniforma*.

A'CINUS. (*Acinus*, i. m.; a grape.) 1. In anatomy, those glands which grow together in clusters are called by some *acini glandulosi*.

2. In botany, a small berry, which, with several others, composes the fruit of the mulberry, blackberry, &c.

ACINUS BILIOSUS. The small glandiform bodies of the liver, which separate the bile from the blood, were formerly called *acini biliosi*: they are now, however, termed *penicilli*. See *Liver*.

ACMA'STICOS. A species of fever, wherein the heat continues of the same tenor to the end. *Actuarius*.

A'CME. (From ακμη, a point.) The height or crisis. A term applied by physicians to that period or state of a disease in which it is at its height. The ancients distinguished diseases into four stages: 1. The *Arche*, the beginning or first attack. 2. *Anabasis*, the growth. 3. *Acme*, the height. 4. *Paracme*, or the decline of the disease.

ACME'LLA. See *Spilanthus*.

A'CNE. ακνη. *Acna*. A small pimple, or hard tubercle on the face. Foesius says, that it is a small pustule or pimple, which arises usually about the time that the body is in full vigour.

ACNE'STIS. (From α, priv. and κναω, to scratch.) That part of the spine of the back, which reaches from the metaphrenon, which is the part between the shoulder-blades, to the loins. This part seems to have been originally called so in quadrupeds only, because they cannot reach it to scratch.

A'COE. ακοη. The sense of hearing.

ACOE'LIUS. (From α, priv. and κοιλια, the belly.) Without belly. It is applied to those who are so wasted, as to appear as if they had no belly. *Galen*.

ACOE'TUS. Ακοιτος. An epithet for honey, mentioned by Pliny; because it has no sediment, which is called κοιτη.

ACO'NION. Ακονιον. A particular form of medicine among the ancient physicians, made of powders levigated, and probably like collyria for the disorders of the eyes.

ACONITA. (*Aconita*, æ, f.; from *aconitum*, the

name of a plant.) A poisonous vegetable principle, probably alcaline, recently extracted from the *aconitum napellus*, or wolf's bane, by Mons. Brandes The details have not yet reached this country.

ACONITE. See *Aconitum.*

ACONI'TUM. (*Aconitum*, i. m.) Aconite. 1. A genus of plants in the Linnæan system, all the species of which have powerful effects on the human body. Class, *Polyandria*; Order, *Trygynia.*

2. The pharmacopœial name of the common, or blue, wolf's-bane. See *Aconitum napellus.*

Aconitum anthora. The root of this plant *Aconitum—floribus pentagynus, foliorum laciniis linearibus* of Linnæus, is employed medicinally. Its virtues are similar to those of the *aconitum napellus.*

Aconitum napellus. Monk's hood. Aconite. Wolf's-bane. *Camorum. Canicida. Cynoctanum. Actonitum;—foliorum laciniis linearibus, superne latioribus, linea exaratis* of Linnæus. This plant is cultivated in our gardens as an ornament, but is spontaneously produced in Germany, and some other northern parts of Europe. Every part is strongly poisonous, but the root is unquestionably the most powerful; and, when first chewed, imparts a slight sensation of acrimony; but afterward, an insensibility or stupor at the apex of the tongue, and a pungent heat of the lips, gums, palate, and fauces are perceived, followed with a general tremor and sensation of chilliness. The juice applied to a wound seemed to affect the whole nervous system; even by keeping it long in the hand, or on the bosom, we are told unpleasant symptoms have been produced. The fatal symptoms brought on by this poison are, convulsions, giddiness, insanity, violent purgings, both upwards and downwards, faintings, cold sweats, and death itself. Dr. Stoerk appears to be the first who gave the wolf's-bane internally, as a medicine; and since his experiments were published, 1762, it has been generally and successfully employed in Germany and the northern parts of Europe, particularly as a remedy for obstinate rheumatisms; and many cases are related where this disease was of several years' duration, and had withstood the efficacy of other powerful medicines, as mercury, opium, antimony, hemlock, &c. yet, in a short time, was entirely cured by the aconitum. Instances are also given us of its good effects in gout, scrofulous swellings, venereal nodes, amaurosis, intermittent fevers, paralysis, ulceration, and scirrhus. This plant has been generally prepared as an extract or inspissated juice, after the manner directed in the Pharmacopœia: its efficacy is much diminished on being long kept. Like all virulent medicines, it should first be administered in small doses. Stoerk recommends two grains of the extract to be rubbed into a powder, with two drachms of sugar, and to begin with ten grains of this powder, two or three times a day. We find, however, that the extract is oftener given from one grain to ten for a dose; and Stoll, Scherekbecker, and others, increased this quantity considerably. Instead of the extract, a tincture has been made of the dried leaves macerated in six times their weight of spirits of wine, and forty drops given for a dose. Some writers say that the napellus is not poisonous in Sweden, Poland, &c.; but it should be noted that the species which is not poisonous, is the aconitum lycoctonum of Linnæus.

Acopa. Dioscorides's name for the buck-bean or *Menyanthes trifoliata* of Linnæus.

A'COPON. (From *α*, priv. and *κοπος*, weariness.) It signifies originally whatever is a remedy against weariness, and is used in this sense by Hippocrates. Aph. viii. lib. ii. But in time, the word was applied to certain ointments. According to Galen and Paulus Ægineta, the *Acopa pharmaca* are remedies for indispositions of body which are caused by long or vehement motion.

Acopos. The name of a plant in Pliny, supposed to be the buck-bean or *Menyanthes trifoliata* of Linnæus.

A'COR. (*Acor, oris*, m.; from *aceo* to be sour.) Acidity. It is sometimes used to express that sourness in the stomach contracted by indigestion, and from whence flatulencies and acid belching arise.

Acor'dina. Indian tutty.

ACO'RIA. (From *α*, priv. and *κορεω*, to satiate.) Insatiability. In Hippocrates, it means good appetite and digestion.

ACORN. See *Quercus robur.*

A'CORUS. (*Acorus*, i. m.; *ακορον*, from *κορη*, the pupil; because it was esteemed good for the disorders of the eyes.) The name of a genus of plants in the Linnæan system. Class, *Hexandria.* Order, *Digynia.*

Acorus calamus. The systematic name of the plant which is also called *Calamus aromaticus; Acorus verus; Calamus odoratus; Calamus vulgaris; Diringa; Jacerantatinga; Typha aromatica; Clava rugosa.* Sweet-flag, or acorus. *Acorus; Scapi mucrone longissimo foliaceo* of Linnæus. The root has been long employed medicinally. It has a moderately strong aromatic smell; a warm, pungent, bitterish taste; and is deemed useful as a warm stomachic. Powdered, and mixed with some absorbent, it forms a useful and pleasant dentifrice.

Acorus palustris. See *Iris palustris.*

Acorus verus. See *Acorus calamus.*

Acorus vulgaris. See *Iris palustris.*

A'COS. (*Ακος*, from *ακεομαι*, to heal.) A remedy or cure.

ACO'SMIA. (From *α*, neg. and *κοσμος*, beautiful.) Baldness; ill-health: irregularity, particularly of the critical days of fevers.

Aco'ste. (From *ακοστη*, barley.) An ancient food made of barley.

ACOTYLE'DON. (*Acotyledon, onis*, n. from *α*, priv. and *κοτυληδων*. Without a cotyledon; applied in botany to a seed or plant which is not furnished with a cotyledon; *Semen acotyledon.*) All the mosses are *plantæ acotyledones.*

ACOU'STIC. (*Acousticus*: from *ακουω*, to hear.) 1. Belonging to the ear or to sound.

2. That which is employed with a view to restore the sense of hearing, when wanting or diminished. No remedies of this kind, given internally, are known to produce any uniform effect.

Acoustic nerve. See *Portio mollis.*

Acoustic duct. See *Meatus auditorius.*

Acræ'palos. See *Acraipala.*

Acrai'pala. (*Ακραιπαλος*. From *α*, neg. and *κραιπαλη*, surfeit.) Remedies for the effects of a debauch

Acra'sia. (From *α*, and *κεραω*, to mix.) Unhealthiness; intemperance.

Acrati'a. (From *α*, and *κρατος*, strength.) Weakness or intemperance.

Acrati'sma. (From *ακρατον*, unmixed wine. The derivation of this word is the same as *Acrasia*, because the wine used on the occasion was not mixed with water.) A breakfast among the old Greeks, consisting of a morsel of bread, soaked in pure unmixed wine.

Acrato'meli. (From *ακρατον*, pure wine; and *μελι*, honey.) Wine mixed with honey.

A'CRE. (From *ακρος*, extreme.) The extremity of the nose or any other part.

A'CREA. (From *ακρος*, extreme.) *Acroteria.* The extremities; the legs, arms, nose, and ears.

Acribei'a. (From *ακριβης*, accurate.) An exact and accurate description and diagnosis, or distinction, of diseases.

ACRID. *Acris.* A term employed in medicine to express a taste, the characteristic of which is pungency joined with heat.

ACRIMONY. (*Acrimonia*, from *acris*, acrid.) A quality in substances by which they irritate, corrode, or dissolve others. It has been supposed until very lately, there were acid and alkaline acrimonies in the blood, which produced certain diseases; and although the humoral pathology is nearly and improperly exploded, the term venereal acrimony, and some others, are still and must be retained.

A'CRIS. 1. Acrid. See *Acrid.*

2. Any fractured extremity.

Acri'sia. (From *α*, priv. and *κρινω*, to judge or separate.) A turbulent state of a disease, which will scarcely suffer any judgment to be formed thereof.

A'critus. (From *α*, neg. and *κρινω*, to judge.) A disease without a regular crisis, the event of which it is hazardous to judge.

ACROBY'STIA. (From *ακρος*, extreme, and *βυω*, to cover.) The prepuce which covers the extremity of the penis.

ACROCHEIRE'SIS. (From *ακρος*, extreme, and *χειρ*, a hand.) An exercise among the ancients. Probably a species of wrestling, where they only held by the hands.

ACROCHEI'RIS. (From ακρος, extreme, and χειρ, a hand.) Gorræus says, it signifies the arm from the elbow to the ends of the fingers; χειρ signifying the arm, from the scapula to the fingers' end.

ACROCHO'RDON. (From ακρος, extreme, and χορδη, a string.) Galen describes it as a round excrescence on the skin, with a slender base; and that it hath its name because of its situation on the surface of the skin. The Greeks call that excrescence an *achrochordon*, where something hard concretes under the skin, which is rather rough, of the same colour as the skin, slender at the base and broader above. Their size rarely exceeds that of a bean.

ACROCO'LIA. (From ακρος, extreme, and κωλον, a limb.) These are the extremities of animals which are used in food, as the feet of calves, swine, sheep, oxen, or lambs, and of the broths of which jellies are frequently made. Castellus from Budæus adds, that the internal parts of animals are also called by this name.

ACHROLE'NION. Castellus says it is the same as *Olecranon*.

ACROMA'NIA. (From ακρος, extreme, and μανια, madness.) Total or incurable madness.

ACRO'MION. (From ακρον, extremity, and ωμος, the shoulder.) A process of the scapula or shoulder-blade. See *Scapula*.

ACROMPHA'LIUM. (Ακρομφαλον; from ακρος, extreme. and ομφαλος, the navel.) *Acromphalon*. The tip of the navel.

ACRO'MPHALON. See *Acromphalium*.

ACRO'NIA. (From ακρον, the extremity.) The amputation of an extremity, as a finger.

ACRO'PATHOS. (From ακρος, extreme, and παθος, a disease.) *Acropathus*. It signifies literally a disease at the top or superior part. Hippocrates in his treatise De Superfœtatione, applies it to the internal orifice of the uterus; and in Prædict. lib. ii. to cancers which appear on the surface of the body.

ACRO'PATHUS. See *Acropathos*.

A'CROPIS. (From ακρον, the extremity, and οψ, the voice.) Imperfect articulation, from a fault in the tongue.

ACROPO'STHIA. (From ακρος, extreme, and ποσθη, the prepuce.) The extremity of the prepuce; or that part which is cut off in circumcision.

ACRO'PSILON. (From ακρος, extreme, and ψιλος, naked.) The extremity of the denuded glans penis.

ACRO'SPELOS. (From ακρος, extreme, and πελος, black, so called because its ears, or tops, are often of a blackish colour.) *Acrospelus*. The bromus discordis, or wild oat grass.

ACRO'SPELUS. See *Acrospelos*.

ACROTE'RIA. (From ακρος, extreme.) The extreme parts of the body; as the hands, feet, nose, ears, chin, &c.

ACROTERIA'SMUS. (From ακρος, *summus*.) The amputation of an extremity.

ACROTHY'MIA. See *Acrothymion*.

ACROTHY'MION. (From ακρος, extreme, and θυμος, thyme.) *Acrothymia*. *Acrothymium*. A sort of wart, described by Celsus, as hard, rough, with a narrow basis, and broad top; the top of the colour of thyme; it easily splits and bleeds.

ACROTHYMIUM. See *Acrothymion*.

ACROTICUS. (From ακρος, *summus*; whence ἀκρότης, ητος; *summitas*; *cacumen*.) A disease affecting the external surface.

ACROTICA. The name of an order in Good's Nosology.

ACROTISMUS. *Acrotismus*; (From *a*. priv. and κροτος, *pulsus*, defect of pulse.) Acrotism or pulselessness. A term synonymous with asphyxia, and applied to a species of entasia in Good's Nosology.

ACTÆ'A. (From αγω, to break.) *Acte*. The elder-tree, so called from its being easily broken. See *Sambucus nigra*.

A'CTINE. The herb *Bunias*, or *Napus*.

ACTINOBOLI'SMUS. (From ακτιν, a ray, and βαλλω, to cast out.) *Diradiatio*. Irradiation. It is applied to the spirits, conveying the inclinations of the mind to the body.

ACTINOLITE. The name of a mineral which is found in primitive districts.

[" This mineral possesses all the essential characters of hornblende. In fact, common hornblende and actynolite, separated only by slight differences, when viewed in the extremes, do in other cases insensibly pass into each other. The actynolite has usually a greater transparency, a more lively green colour, arising from the chrome which it contains, and differs also in the result of fusion by the blow-pipe.

" The actynolite occurs in prismatic crystals which are commonly long and incomplete, sometimes extremely minute and even fibrous, and variously aggregated into masses more or less large. Its prevailing colour is green, sometimes pure emerald green, but varying from a dark or leek green to a pale green, which is sometimes shaded with gray, yellow, or brown. Its colours are liable to change in consequence of decomposition. It scratches grass, but its prisms are often very brittle in a transverse direction. Its cross fracture is often a little chonchoidal, and more shining than that of common hornblende. Its specific gravity is about 3.30.

" It melts by the blow-pipe into a gray or yellowish-gray enamel. It contains, according to Langier, of

Silex	50.00
Magnesia	19.25
Lime	9.75
Alumine	0.75
Oxide of iron	11.00
Oxide of chrome	5.00
	95.75

Its green colour is derived from the chrome, but is often modified by the large quantity of iron which is present. It presents the following varieties, which pass into each other: 1. common actynolite; 2. glassy; 3. acicular; 4. fibrous.

" Actynolite is found in primitive rocks, or in veins which traverse them; it is sometimes in metallic beds. It is perhaps most common in minerals which contain magnesia. Its more distinct crystals occur in talc, quartz, and limestone.

" It is found in various parts of the United States. In Maryland, near Baltimore, all its varieties occur in granite or gneiss. In Pennsylvania, at Concord in Chester county, in large masses of an emerald-green colour. In Connecticut, near New-Haven, in serpentine; its structure generally radiated. In Maine, at Brunswick, all its varieties occur, sometimes in granite and gneiss, but more frequently in limestone."—*Cleaveland's Mineralogy*. A.]

ACTION. (*Actio*, *nis*. f.; from *ago*, to act.) 1 The operation or exertion of an active power.

2. Any faculty, power, or function. The actions or functions of the body are usually divided by physiologists into vital, natural, or animal. 1. The *vital* functions, or actions, are those which are absolutely necessary to life, and without which animals cannot exist; as the action of the heart, lungs, and arteries. 2. The *natural* functions are those which are instrumental in repairing the several losses which the body sustains: digestion, and the formation of chyle, &c. fall under this head. 3. The *animal* actions are those which we perform at will, as muscular motion, and all the voluntary motions of the body.

Independently of these properties, each part may be said to have an action peculiar to itself—for instance, the liver, by virtue of a power which is peculiar to it, forms continually a liquid which is called bile: the same thing takes place in the kidneys with regard to the urine. The voluntary muscles, in certain states, become hard, change their form, and contract. These are, however, referrible to vitality. It is upon these the attention of the physiologist ought to be particularly fixed. Vital action depends evidently upon nutrition, and reciprocally, nutrition is influenced by vital action.—Thus, an organ that ceases to nourish, loses at the same time its faculty of acting; consequently the organs, the action of which is oftenest repeated, possess a more active nutrition; and, on the contrary, those that act least, possess a much slower nutritive motion.

The mechanism of vital action is unknown. There passes into the organ that acts an insensible molecular motion, which is as little susceptible of description as the nutritive motion. Every vital action, however simple, is the same in this respect.

ACTUAL. This word is applied to any thing endued with a property or virtue which acts by an immediate power inherent in it: it is the reverse of potential: thus, a red-hot iron or fire is called an actual cautery, in contradistinction from caustics, which are called potential cauteries. Boiling water is actually hot; brandy, producing heat in the body, is potentially hot, though of itself cold

Actual cautery. The red-hot iron, or any red-hot substance. See *Actual.*

ACTUA'RIUS. This word was originally a title of dignity given to physicians at the court of Constantinople; but became afterward the proper name of a celebrated Greek physician, John, (the son of Zachary, a Christian writer,) who flourished there about the 12th or 13th century. He is said to be the first Greek author who has treated of mild cathartics, as manna, cassia, &c., though they were long before in use among the Arabians. He appears also to have first noticed distilled waters. His works, however, are chiefly compiled from his predecessors.

ACTUATION. (From *ago*, to act.) That change wrought on a medicine, or any thing taken into the body, by the vital heat, which is necessary, in order to make it act and have its effect.

ACUITAS. Acrimony.

ACUITIO. (From *acuo*, to sharpen.) The sharpening an acid medicine by an addition of something more acid; or, in general, the increasing the force of any medicine, by an addition of something that hath the same sort of operation in a greater degree.

ACULEA'TUS. (From *aculeus*, a prickle.) Prickly; covered with sharp-pointed bodies: applied to stems covered with sharp-pointed bodies, the prickles of which separate with the epidermis, as in *Rosa centifolia.*

ACU'LEUS. (From *acus*, a needle; from ἀκη, or ἀκις; *cuspis*, a point.) A prickle or sharp point. A species of armature with which the stems, branches, and other parts of several plants are furnished; as in the rose, raspberry, gooseberry. The *part* on which it grows is said to be aculeated, thus:—

Caulis aculeatus; as in the *Rosa canina.*

Folia aculeata; as in *Solanum marginatum.*

Calix aculeatus; as in *Solanum aculeatum.*

Stipula aculeata; as in *Rosa cinnamomia.*

Legumen aculeatum; as in *Scorpiurus muricata.*

From the *direction* it has:—

Aculeus rectus, not curved; as in *Rhamnus spina christi*, and *Rosa eglanteria.*

Aculeus incurvus, curved inward; as in *Mimosa cineraria.*

Aculeus recurvus, curved downward; as in *Rubus fruticosus*, and *Rosa rubiginosa.*

From the *number* in one place:—

Aculeus solitarius; as in *Rosa canina.*

Aculeus bifidus, or *geminatus*, in pairs; there being two joined at the basis; as in *Rhamnus spina christi.*

Aculeus trifidus, three in one; as in *Barbaris vulgaris.*

A'CULON. (From *a*, neg. and κυλοω, to roll round;) so called because its fruit is not involved in a cup, or sheath, like others.

Aculos. The fruit or acorn of the ilex.

A'CULOS. See *Aculon.*

ACU'MEN. 1. A point.

2. The extremity of a bone.

ACUMINATUS. (From *acuo*, to point.) Acuminate; or terminated by a point somewhat elongated. Applied by botanists to several parts of plants. An acuminate leaf is seen in the *Syringa vulgaris.* Acuminate leaf-stalk; as that of *Saxifraga stellaris.*

ACUPUNCTU'RA. (From *acus*, a needle, and *punctura*, a prick.) Acupuncture. A bleeding performed by making many small punctures.

[The operation of making small punctures in certain parts of the body with a needle, for the purpose of relieving diseases, is practised in Siam, Japan, and other oriental countries, for the cure of headaches, lethargies, convulsions, colics, &c. The practice of acupuncture is not followed in England nor America. In a modern French work it has been highly commended; but, the author sets so rash an example, and is so wild in his expectations of what may be done by the thrust of a needle, that the tenor of his observations will not meet with many approvers. For instance, in one case, he ventured to pierce the epigastric region so deeply, that the coats of the stomach were supposed to have been perforated: this was done for the cure of an obstinate cough, and is alleged to have effected a cure. But if this be not enough to excite wonder, I am sure the author's suggestion to run a long needle into the right ventricle of the heart, in cases of asphyxia, must create that sensation.—See *Cooper's Surg. Dict.* A.]

A'CURON. (From *a*, neg. and κυρω, to happen.) A name of the *Alisma*, because it produces no effect if taken internally.

ACUSPASTO'RIS. A name of the *Scandix anthriscus*, the shepherd's needle, or Venus's comb.

ACUTANGULARIS. *Acutangulatus.* Acutangular: applied to parts of plants, as *caulis acutangularis.*

ACUTE'. Sharply. Applied in natural history to express form; as *folium acut dentatum; acutè emarginatus*, which means sharply dentate, and with sharp divisions.

ACUTENA'CULUM. (From *acus*, a needle, and *tenaculum*, a handle.) The handle for a needle, to make it penetrate easy when stitching a wound. Heister calls the *portaiguille* by this name.

ACUTUS. Sharp. 1. Used by naturalists to designate form; thus acute-leaved; as in *rumex acutus* &c.

2. In pathology, it is applied to a sharp pungent pain; and to a disease which is attended with violent symptoms, terminates in a few days, and is attended with danger. It is opposed to a chronic disease, which is slow in its progress, and not so generally dangerous.

ACY'ISIS. (From *a*, neg. and κυω, to conceive.) A defect of conception, or barrenness in women.

A'CYRUS. (From *a*, priv. and κυρος, authority; so named from its little note in medicine.) The German leopard's-bane. See *Arnica montana.*

ADÆMO'NIA. (From *a*, priv. and δαιμων, a genius of fortune.) See *Ademonia.*

Adam's Apple. See *Pomum Adami.*

ADAM'S NEEDLE. The roots of this plant, *Yucca gloriosa* of Linnæus, are thick and tuberous, and are used by the Indians instead of bread; being first reduced into a coarse meal. This, however, is only in times of scarcity.

ADAMANTINE SPAR. A stone remarkable for its extreme hardness, which comes from the peninsula of Hither India, and also from China.

[Its colour is dark brown, and its internal lustre usually very strong. It comes from China, and almost always contains grains of magnetic oxide of iron. A specimen was found by chemists to contain,

Alumine	86.50
Silex	5.25
Oxide of iron	6.50
	98.25

The corundum appears to belong to primitive rocks, and particularly to granite, into the composition of which it sometimes enters; hence scales of mica and particles of feldspar sometimes adhere to its surface.

In the United States, it is by some supposed to exist in Maryland, near Baltimore; and in Connecticut, at Haddam, in the same granite, which contains chrysoberyl, &c. It may be employed, like emery, in polishing hard substances.—*Cleav. Min.* A.]

A'DAMAS. (From *a* neg. and δαμαω, to conquer; as not being easily broken.) The adamant or diamond, the most precious of all stones, and which was formerly supposed to possess extraordinary cordial virtues.

ADAMI'TA, or *Adamitum.* A hard stone in the bladder.

[ADAMS, DR. SAMUEL, was the only son of Samuel Adams, late governor of Massachusetts. He was born at Boston, in October, 1751. His preparatory education was at a Latin school in his native town. He entered Harvard University at the age of fourteen years, and was graduated in 1770. His professional education was acquired under the direction of Dr. Joseph Warren, and he practised in Boston. When hostilities commenced with Great Britain, in 1775, Dr. Adams, imbued with the patriotic spirit of his father, engaged as surgeon in the hospital department of the United States' army. Commencing his public services at Cambridge, by attending the soldiers who were wounded at Lexington and Bunker's Hill, he afterward removed to Danbury, and successively to various stations in several of the states, and continued in the service during the revolutionary war; after which he returned to his native town with a broken constitution, and unable to recommence his professional pursuits: he died on the 17th of January, 1788. He possessed a substantial mind, social feelings, and a generous heart; and his greatest pleasure was to do good to his fellow-men.—*Thacher's Med. Biography.* A.]

ADANSO'NIA. (From *Adanson* who first described the Æthiopian sour gourd, a species of this genus.) The name of a genus of plants. Class, *Polyandria;* Order, *Monadelphia.* Monkeys' bread.

ADANSONIA DIGITATA. This is the only species of the genus yet discovered. It is called the Æthiopian sour gourd and monkeys' bread. *Baobab. Bahobab.* It grows mostly on the west coast of Africa, from the Niger to the kingdom of Benin. The bark is called *lalo:* the negroes dry it in the shade; then powder and keep it in little cotton bags; and put two or three pinches into their food. It is mucilaginous, and generally promotes perspiration. The mucilage obtained from this bark is a powerful remedy against the epidemic fevers of the country that produces these trees; so is a decoction of the dried leaves. The fresh fruit is as useful as the leaves, for the same purposes.

ADA'RCES. (From *α*, neg. and *δερκω*, to see.) A saltish concretion found about the reeds and grass in marshy grounds in Galatia, and so called because it hides them. It is used to clear the skin with, in leprosies, tetters, &c. Dr. Plott gives an account of this production in his *Natural History of Oxfordshire.* It was formerly in repute for cleansing the skin from freckles.

Adarticulation. See *Arthrodia.*

ADDEPHA'GIA. (From *αδην*, abundantly, and *φαγω*, to eat.) Insatiability. A voracious appetite. See *Bulimia.*

ADDER. See *Coluber berus.*

ADDITAME'NTUM. (From *addo*, to add.) An addition to any part, which, though not always, is sometimes found. A term formerly employed as synonymous with *epiphysis*, but now only applied to two portions of sutures of the skull. See *Lambdoidal* and *Squamous Sutures.*

ADDITAMENTUM COLI. See *Appendicula cæci vermiformis.*

ADDUCENS. (From *ad*, and *duco*, to draw.) The name of some parts which draw those together to which they are connected.

ADDUCENS OCULI. See *Rectus internus oculi.*

ADDU'CTOR. (From *ad*, and *duco*, to draw.) A drawer or contractor. A name given to several muscles, the office of which is to bring forwards or draw together those parts of the body to which they are annexed.

ADDUCTOR BREVIS FEMORIS. A muscle of the thigh, which, with the *adductor longus* and *magnus femoris*, forms the *triceps adductor femoris. Adductor femoris secundus* of Douglas; *Triceps secundus* of Winslow. It is situated on the posterior part of the thigh, arising tendinous from the os pubis, near its joining with the opposite os pubis below, and behind the adductor longus femoris, and is inserted tendinous and fleshy, into the inner and upper part of the linea aspera, from a little below the trochanter minor, to the beginning of the insertion of the adductor longus femoris. See *Triceps adductor femoris.*

ADDUCTOR FEMORIS PRIMUS. See *Adductor longus femoris.*

ADDUCTOR FEMORIS SECUNDUS. See *Adductor brevis femoris.*

ADDUCTOR FEMORIS TERTIUS. See *Adductor magnus femoris.*

ADDUCTOR FEMORIS QUARTUS. See *Adductor magnus femoris.*

ADDUCTOR INDICIS PEDIS. An external interrosseous muscle of the fore-toe, which arises tendinous and fleshy by two origins, from the root of the inside of the metatarsal bone of the fore-toe, from the outside of the root of the metatarsal bone of the great toe, and from the os cuneiform internum. It is inserted, tendinous, into the inside of the root of the first joint of the fore-toe. Its use is to pull the fore-toe inwards from the rest of the small toes.

ADDUCTOR LONGUS FEMORIS. A muscle situated on the posterior part of the thigh, which, with the *adductor brevis*, and *magnus femoris*, forms the *triceps adductor femoris Adductor femoris primus* of Douglas. *Triceps minus* of Winslow. It arises by a pretty strong roundish tendon, from the upper and interior part of the os pubis, and ligament of its synchondrosis, on the inner side of the pectineus, and is inserted along the middle part of the linea aspera. See *Triceps adductor femoris.*

ADDUCTOR MAGNUS FEMORIS. A muscle which, with the *adductor brevis femoris*, and the *adductor longus femoris*, forms the *Triceps adductor femoris; Adductor femoris tertius et quartus* of Douglas. *Triceps magnus* of Winslow. It arises from the symphysis pubis, and all along the flat edge of the thyroid foramen, from whence it goes to be inserted into the linea aspera throughout its whole length. See *Triceps adductor femoris.*

ADDUCTOR MINIMI DIGITI PEDIS. An internal interrosseous muscle of the foot. It arises, tendinous and fleshy, from the inside of the root of the metatarsal bone of the little toe. It is inserted, tendinous, into the inside of the root of the first joint of the little toe. Its use is to pull the little toe inwards.

ADDUCTOR OCULI. See *Rectus internus oculi.*

ADDUCTOR POLLICIS. See *Adductor pollicis manûs.*

ADDUCTOR POLLICIS MANUS. A muscle of the thumb, situated on the hand. *Adductor pollicis; Adductor ad minimum digitum.* It arises, fleshy, from almost the whole length of the metacarpal bone that sustains the middle finger; from thence its fibres are collected together. It is inserted, tendinous, into the inner part of the root of the first bone of the thumb. Its use is to pull the thumb towards the fingers.

ADDUCTOR POLLICIS PEDIS. A muscle of the great toe, situated on the foot. *Antithenar* of Winslow. It arises, by a long, thin tendon, from the os calcis, from the os cuboides, from the os cuneiforme externum, and from the root of the metatarsal bone of the second toe. It is inserted into the external os sesamoideum, and root of the metatarsal bone of the great toe. Its use is to bring this toe nearer to the rest.

ADDUCTOR PROSTATÆ. A name given by Sanctorini to a muscle, which he also calls *Levator prostatæ*, and which Winslow calls *Prostaticus superior.* Albinus, from its office, had very properly called it *Compressor prostatæ.*

ADDUCTOR TERTII DIGITI PEDIS. An external interosseous muscle of the foot, that arises, tendinous and fleshy, from the roots of the metatarsal bones of the third and little toe. It is inserted, tendinous, into the outside of the root of the first joint of the third toe Its use is to pull the third toe outward.

ADE'LPHIA. (Ἀδελφια, a relation.) Hippocrates calls diseases by this name that resemble each other.

ADEMO'NIA. (From *α*, priv. and *δαιμων*, a genius, or divinity, or fortune.) *Adæmonia.* Hippocrates uses this word for uneasiness, restlessness, or anxiety felt in acute diseases, and some hysteric fits.

A'DEN. (*Aden, enis,* m.; *αδην*, a gland.)

1. A gland. See *Gland.*

2. A bubo. See *Bubo.*

ADENDE'NTES. An epithet applied to ulcers which eat and destroy the glands.

ADE'NIFORMIS. (From *aden*, a gland, and *forma*, resemblance.) Adeniform. 1. Glandiform, or resembling a gland.

2. A term sometimes applied to the prostate gland.

ADENO'GRAPHY. (*Adenographia;* from *αδην*, a gland, and *γραφω*, to write.) A treatise on the glands.

ADENOI'DES. (From *αδην*, a gland, and *ειδος*, resemblance.) Glandiform: resembling a gland. An epithet applied also to the prostate gland.

ADENO'LOGY. (*Adenologia;* from *αδην*, a gland, and *λογος*, a treatise.) The doctrine of the glands.

ADENOUS. (*Adenosus,* from *αδην*, a gland) Gland-like.

ADEPHA'GIA. (From *αδην*, abundantly, and *φαγω*, to eat.) Insatiable appetite. See *Bulimia.*

A'DEPS. (*Adeps, ipis,* m. and f.) Fat. An oily secretion from the blood into the cells of the cellular membrane. See *Fat.*

ADEPS ANSERINUS. Goose-grease.

ADEPS PRÆPARATA. Prepared lard. Cut the lard into small pieces, melt it over a slow fire, and press it through a linen cloth.

ADEPS SUILLA. Hog's lard. This forms the basis of many ointments, and is used extensively for culinary purposes.

ADEPT. (From *Adipiscor*, to obtain.) 1. A skilful alchymist. Such are called so as pretend to some extraordinary skill in chemistry; but these have too often proved either enthusiasts or impostors.

2. The professors of the *Adepta Philosophia*, that philosophy the end of which is the transmutation of metals, and a universal remedy, were also called Adepts.

3. So Paracelsus calls that which treats of the diseases that are contracted by celestial operations, or communicated from heaven.

ADFLA'TUS. A blast; a kind of erysipelas, or St. Anthony's fire.

ADHÆSION. (*Adhesio;* from *adhæro*, to stick to.) The growing together of parts.

ADHÆSIVE. (*Adhæsivus;* from *adhæro*, to stick to.) Having the property of sticking.

ADHÆSIVE INFLAMMATION. That species of inflammation which terminates by an adhesion of the inflamed surfaces.

ADHÆSIVE PLASTER. A plaster made of common litharge plaster and resin, is so called because it is used for its adhesive properties. See *Emplastrum resinæ.*

ADHATO'DA. (A Zeylanic term, signifying expelling a dead fœtus.) See *Justicia adhatoda.*

ADIACHY'TOS. (From *α*, neg. and *διαχύω*, to diffuse, scatter, or be profuse.) Decent in point of dress. Hippocrates thinks the dress of a fop derogatory from the physician, though thereby he hide his ignorance, and obtain the good opinion of his patients.

ADIA'NTHUM. (*Adiantum*, i. n. *αδιαντον*; from *α*, neg. and *διαινω*, to grow wet: so called, because its leaves are not easily made wet.) The name of a genus of plants in the Linnæan system Class, *Cryptogamia;* Order, *Filices.* Maiden-hair.

ADIANTHUM AUREUM The golden maiden-hair. See *Polytrichum.*

ADIANTHUM CAPILLUS VENERIS. Maiden-hair. The leaves of this plant are somewhat sweet and austere to the palate, and possess mucilaginous qualities. A syrup, the *syrop de capillaire* is prepared from them, which is much esteemed in France against catarrhs. Orange-flower water, and a proportion of honey, it is said, are usually added. It acts chiefly as a demulcent, sheathing the inflamed sides of the glottis.

ADIANTHUM PEDATUM. *Adianthum canadense.* This plant is in common use in France for the same purposes as the common adianthum capillus veneris in this country, and appears to be far superior to it.

ADIAPHOROUS. *Adiaphorus.* A term which implies the same with neutral; and is particularly used of some spirits and salts, which are neither of an acid nor alcaline nature.

ADIAPNEU'STIA. (From the privative particle *α*, and *διαπνεω, perspiro.*) A diminution or obstruction of natural perspiration, and that in which the ancients chiefly placed the cause of fevers.

ADIARRHŒ'A. (From *α*, priv. and *διαῤῥεω*, to flow out or through.) A suppression of the necessary evacuations from the bowels.

ADIPOCI'RE. (*Adipocera*, æ. f.; from *adeps*, fat, and *cera*, wax.) A particular spermaceti or fat-like substance formed by the spontaneous conversion of animal matter, under certain conditions. This conversion has long been well known, and is said to have been mentioned in the works of Lord Bacon. "On the occasion of the removal of a very great number of human bodies from the ancient burying-place des Innocens at Paris, facts of this nature were observed in the most striking manner. Fourcroy may be called the scientific discoverer of this peculiar matter, as well as the saponaceous ammoniacal substance contained in bodies abandoned to spontaneous destruction in large masses. This chemist read a memoir on the subject in the year 1789 to the Royal Academy of Sciences, from which the general contents are here abstracted.

"At the time of clearing the before-mentioned burying-place, certain philosophers were specially charged to direct the precautions requisite for securing the health of the workmen. A new and singular object of research presented itself, which had been necessarily unknown to preceding chemists. It was impossible to foretell what might be the contents of a soil overloaded for successive ages with bodies resigned to the putrefactive process. This spot differed from common burying-grounds, where each individual object is surrounded by a portion of the soil. It was the burying-ground of a large district, wherein successive generations of the inhabitants had been deposited for upwards of three centuries. It could not be foreseen that the entire decomposition might be retarded for more than forty years; neither was there any reason to suspect that any remarkable difference would arise from the singularity of situation.

"The remains of the human bodies immersed in this mass of putrescence, were found in three different states, according to the time they had been buried, the place they occupied, and their relative situations with regard to each other. The most ancient were simply portions of bones, irregularly dispersed in the soil, which had been frequently disturbed. A second state, in certain bodies which had always been insulated, exhibited the skin, the muscles, the tendons, and aponeurosis, dry, brittle, hard, more or less gray, and similar to what are called mummies in certain caverns where this change has been observed, as in the catacombs at Rome, and the vault of the Cordeliers at Toulouse.

"The third and most singular state of these soft parts was observed in the bodies which filled the common graves or repositories. By this appellation are understood cavities of thirty feet in depth, and twenty on each side, which were dug in the burying-ground of the Innocents, and were appropriated to contain the bodies of the poor; which were placed in very close rows, each in its proper wooden bier. The necessity for disposing a great number, obliged the men charged with this employment to arrange them so near each other that these cavities might be considered when filled, as an entire mass of human bodies separated only by two planks of about half an inch thick. Each cavity contained between one thousand and fifteen hundred. When one common grave of this magnitude was filled, a covering of about one foot deep of earth was laid upon it, and another excavation of the same sort was made at some distance. Each grave remained open about three years, which was the time required to fill it. According to the urgency of circumstances, the graves were again made on the same spot after an interval of time, not less than fifteen years, nor more than thirty. Experience had taught the workmen, that this time was not sufficient for the entire destruction of the bodies, and had shown them the progressive changes which form the object of Fourcroy's memoir.

"The first of these large graves, opened in the presence of this chemist, had been closed for fifteen years. The coffins were in good preservation, but a little settled, and the wood had a yellow tinge. When the covers of several were taken off, the bodies were observed at the bottom, leaving a considerable distance between their surface and the cover, and flattened as if they had suffered a strong compression. The linen which had covered them was slightly adherent to the bodies; and with the form of the different regions, exhibited on removing the linen, nothing but irregular masses of a soft ductile matter of a gray-white colour These masses environed the bones on all sides, which had no solidity, but broke by any sudden pressure. The appearance of this matter, its obvious composition, and its softness, resembled common white cheese; and the resemblance was more striking from the print which the threads of the linen had made upon its surface. This white substance yielded to the touch, and became soft when rubbed for a time between the fingers.

"No very offensive smell was emitted from these bodies. The novelty and singularity of the spectacle, and the example of the grave-diggers, dispelled every idea either of disgust or apprehension. These men asserted that they never found this matter, by them called *gras* (fat,) in bodies interred alone; but that the accumulated bodies of the common graves only were subject to this change. On a very attentive examination of a number of bodies passed to this state, Fourcroy remarked, that the conversion appeared in different stages of advancement, so that, in various bodies, the fibrous texture and colour, more or less red, were discernible within the fatty matter; that the masses covering the bones were entirely of the same nature, offering indistinctly in all the regions a gray substance, for the most part soft and ductile, sometimes dry, always easy to be separated in porous fragments, penetrated with cavities, and no longer exhibiting any traces of membranes, muscles, tendons, vessels, or nerves. On the first inspection of these white masses, it might have been concluded that they were simply the cellular tissue, the compartments and vesicles of which they very well represented.

"By examining this substance in the different regions of the body, it was found that the skin is particularly disposed to this remarkable alteration. It was afterward perceived that the ligaments and tendons no longer existed, or at least had lost their tenacity; so that the bones were entirely unsupported, and left to the action of their own weight. Whence their relative places were preserved in a certain degree by mere juxtaposition; the least effort being sufficient to separate them. The grave-diggers availed themselves of this circumstance in the removal of the bodies. For they rolled them up from head to feet, and by that means separated from each other the extremities of the bones, which had formerly been articulated. In all those bodies which were changed into the fatty matter, the abdominal cavity had disappeared. The teguments and muscles of this region being converted into the white matter, like the other soft parts, had subsided upon the vertebral column, and were so flattened as to leave no place for the viscera; and accordingly there was scarcely ever any trace observed in the almost obliterated cavity. This observation was for a long time matter of astonishment to the investigators. In vain did they seek in the greater number of bodies, the place and substance of the stomach, the intestines, the bladder, and even the liver, the spleen, the kidneys, and the matrix in females. All these viscera were confounded together, and for the most part no traces of them were left. Sometimes only certain irregular masses were found, of the same nature as the white matter, of different bulks, from that of a nut to two or three inches in diameter, in the regions of the liver or of the spleen.

"The thorax likewise offered an assemblage of facts no less singular and interesting. The external part of this cavity was flattened and compressed like the rest of the organs; the ribs, spontaneously luxated in their articulations with the vertebræ, were settled upon the dorsal column; their arched part left only a small space on each side between them and the vertebræ. The pleura, the mediastinum, the large vessels, the aspera arteria, and even the lungs and the heart, were no longer distinguishable; but for the most part had entirely disappeared, and in their place nothing was seen but some parcels of the fatty substance. In this case, the matter which was the product of decomposition of the viscera charged with blood and various humours, differs from that of the surface of the body, and the long bones, in the red or brown colour possessed by the former. Sometimes the observers found in the thorax a mass irregularly rounded, of the same nature as the latter, which appeared to them to have arisen from the fat and fibrous substance of the heart. They supposed that this mass, not constantly found in all the subjects, owed its existence to a superabundance of fat in this viscus, where it was found. For the general observation presented itself, that, in similar circumstances, the fat parts undergo this conversion more evidently than the others, and afford a larger quantity of the white matter.

"The external region in females exhibited the glandular and adipose mass of the breast converted into the fatty matter, very white and very homogeneous.

"The head was, as has already been remarked, environed with the fatty matter; the face was no longer distinguishable in the greatest number of subjects; the mouth, disorganized, exhibited neither tongue nor palate; and the jaws, luxated and more or less displaced, were environed with irregular layers of the white matter. Some pieces of the same matter usually occupied the place of the parts situated in the mouth; the cartilages of the nose participated in the general alteration of the skin; the orbits, instead of eyes, contained white masses; the ears were equally disorganized; and the hairy scalp, having undergone a similar alteration to that of the other organs, still retained the hair. Fourcroy remarks incidentally, that the hair appears to resist every alteration much longer than any other part of the body. The cranium constantly contained the brain contracted in bulk; blackish at the surface, and absolutely changed like the other organs. In a great number of subjects which were examined, this viscus was never found wanting, and it was always in the above-mentioned state; which proves that the substance of the brain is greatly disposed to be converted into the fat matter.

"Such was the state of the bodies found in the burial-ground des Innocens. Its modifications were also various. Its consistence in bodies lately changed, that is to say, from three to five years, was soft and very ductile, containing a great quantity of water. In other subjects converted into this matter for a long time, such as those which occupied the cavities which had been closed thirty or forty years, this matter is drier, more brittle, and in denser flakes. In several, which were deposited in dry earth, various portions of the fatty matter had become semitransparent. The aspect, the granulated texture, and brittleness of this dried matter, bore a considerable resemblance to wax.

"The period of the formation of this substance had likewise an influence on its properties. In general, all that which had been formed for a long time was white, uniform, and contained no foreign substance, or fibrous remains; such, in particular, was that afforded by the skin of the extremities. On the contrary, in bodies recently changed, the fatty matter was neither so uniform nor so pure as in the former; but it was still found to contain portions of muscles, tendons, and ligaments, the texture of which, though already altered and changed in its colour, was still distinguishable. Accordingly, as the conversion was more or less advanced, these fibrous remains were more or less penetrated with the fatty matter, interposed as it were between the interstices of the fibres. This observation shows, that it is not merely the fat which is thus changed, as was natural enough to think at first sight. Other facts confirm this assertion. The skin, as has been remarked, becomes easily converted into very pure white matter, as does likewise the brain, neither of which has been considered by anatomists to be fat. It is true, nevertheless, that the unctuous parts, and bodies charged with fat, appear more easily and speedily to pass to the state under consideration. This was seen in the marrow, which occupied the cavities of the longer bones. And again, it is not to be supposed but that the greater part of these bodies had been emaciated by the illness which terminated their lives; notwithstanding which, they were all absolutely turned into this fatty substance.

"An experiment made by Poulletier de la Salle, and Fourcroy likewi e, evinced that a conversion does not take place in the fat alone. Poulletier had suspended in his laboratory a small piece of the human liver, to observe what would arise to it by the contact of the air. It partly putrefied, without, however, emitting any very noisome smell. Larvæ of the dermestes and bruchus attacked and penetrated it in various directions; at last it became dry, and after more than ten years' suspension, it was converted into a white friable substance resembling dried agaric, which might have been taken for an earthy substance. In this state it had no perceptible smell. Poulletier was desirous of knowing the state of this animal matter, and experiment soon convinced him and Fourcroy that it was far from being in the state of an earth. It melted by heat, and exhaled in the form of vapour, which had the smell of a very fetid fat; spirit of wine separated a concrescible oil, which appeared to possess all the properties of spermaceti. Each of the three alcalies converted it into soap; and, in a word, it exhibited all the properties of the fatty matter of the burial-ground of the Innocents exposed for several months to the air. Here then was a glandular organ, which in the midst of the atmosphere had undergone a change similar to that of the bodies in the burying-place; and this fact sufficiently shows, that an animal substance which is very far from being of the nature of grease, may be totally converted into this fatty substance.

"Among the modifications of this remarkable substance in the burying-ground before-mentioned, it was observed that the dry, friable, and brittle matter, was most commonly found near the surface of the earth, and the soft, ductile matter at a greater depth. Fourcroy remarks, that this dry matter did not differ from the other merely in containing less water, but likewise by the volatilization of one of its principles."

The grave-diggers assert, that near three years are required to convert a body into this fatty substance. But Dr. Gibbes of Oxford found, that lean beef secured in a running stream, was converted into this fatty matter at the end of a month. He judges from the that running water is most favourable to this process. He took three lean pieces of mutton, and poured on each a quantity of the three common mineral acids. At the end of three days, each was much changed: that in the nitric acid was very soft, and converted into the fatty matter; that in the muriatic acid was not in that time so much altered; the sulphuric acid had turned the other black. Lavoisier thinks that this process may hereafter prove of great use in society. It is not easy to point out what animal substance, or what situation, might be the best adapted for an undertaking of this kind.

The result of Fourcroy's inquiries into the ordinary changes of bodies recently deposited in the earth, was not very extensive. The grave-diggers informed him, that those bodies interred do not perceptibly change colour for the first seven or eight days; that the putrid process disengages elastic fluid, which inflates the abdomen, and at length bursts it; that this event instantly causes vertigo, faintness, and nausea in such persons as unfortunately are within a certain distance of the scene where it takes place; but that when the object of its action is nearer, a sudden privation of sense, and frequently death, is the consequence. These men are taught by experience, that no immediate danger is to be feared from the disgusting business they are engaged in, excepting at this period, which they regard with the utmost terror. They resisted every inducement and persuasion which these philosophers made use of, to prevail on them to assist their researches into the nature of this active and pernicious vapour. Fourcroy takes occasion from these facts, as well as from the pallid and unwholesome appearance of the grave-diggers, to reprobate burials in great towns or their vicinity.

Such bodies as are interred alone, in the midst of a great quantity of humid earth, are totally destroyed by passing through the successive degrees of the ordinary putrefaction; and this destruction is more speedy, the warmer the temperature. But if these insulated bodies be dry and emaciated; if the place of deposition be likewise dry, and the locality and other circumstances such, that the earth, so far from receiving moisture from the atmosphere, becomes still more effectually parched by the solar rays;—the animal juices are volatilized and absorbed, the solids contract and harden, and a peculiar species of mummy is produced. But every circumstance is very different in the common burying-grounds. Heaped together almost in contact, the influence of external bodies affects them scarcely at all, and they become abandoned to a peculiar disorganization, which destroys their texture, and produces the new and most permanent state of combination here described. From various observations, it was found, that this fatty matter was capable of enduring in these burying-places for thirty or forty years, and is at length corroded and carried off by the aqueous putrid humidity which there abounds.

Among other interesting facts afforded by the chemical examination of this substance are the following from experiments by Fourcroy.

1. This substance is fused at a less degree of heat than that of boiling water, and may be purified by pressure through a cloth, which disengages a portion of fibrous and bony matter. 2. The process of destructive distillation by a very graduated heat was begun, but not completed, on account of its tediousness, and the little promise of advantage it afforded. The products which came over were water charged with volatile alcali, a fat oil, concrete volatile alcali, and no elastic fluid during the time the operation was continued. 3. Fragments of the fatty matter exposed to the air during the hot and dry summer of 1786 became dry, brittle, and almost pulverulent at the surface. On a careful examination, certain portions were observed to be semitransparent, and more brittle than the rest. These possessed all the apparent properties of wax, and did not afford volatile alcali by distillation. 4. With water this fatty matter exhibited all the appearances of soap, and afforded a strong lather. The dried substance did not form the saponaceous combination with the same facility or perfection as that which was recent. About two-thirds of this dried matter separated from the water by cooling, and proved to be the semitransparent substance resembling wax. This was taken from the surface of the soapy liquor, which being then passed through the filter, left a white soft shining matter, which was fusible and combustible. 5. Attempts were made to ascertain the quantity of volatile alcali in this substance, by the application of lime, and of the fixed alcalies, but without success: for it was difficult to collect and appreciate the first portions which escaped, and likewise to disengage the last portions. The caustic volatile alcali, with the assistance of a gentle heat, dissolved the fatty matter, and the solution became perfectly clear and transparent at the boiling temperature of the mixture, which was at 185° F. 6. Sulphuric acid, of the specific gravity of 2. 0, was poured upon six times its weight of the fatty matter, and mixed by agitation. Heat was produced, and a gas or effluvium of the most insupportable putrescence was emitted, which infected the air of an extensive laboratory for several days. Fourcroy says, that the smell cannot be described, but that it is one of the most horrid and repulsive that can be imagined. It did not, however, produce any indisposition either in himself or his assistants. By dilution with water, and the ordinary processes of evaporation and cooling, properly repeated, the sulphates of ammonia and of lime were obtained. A substance was separated from the liquor, which appeared to be the waxy matter, somewhat altered by the action of the acid. 7. The nitrous and muriatic acids were also applied, and afforded phenomena worthy of remark, but which for the sake of conciseness are here omitted. 8. Alcohol does not act on this matter at the ordinary temperature of the air. But by boiling it dissolves one-third of its own weight, which is almost totally separable by cooling as low as 55°. The alcohol, after this process, affords by evaporation a portion of that waxy matter which is separable by acids, and is therefore the only portion soluble in cold alcohol. The quantity of fatty matter operated on was 4 ounces, or 2304 grains, of which the boiling spirit took up the whole except 26 grains, which proved to be a mixture of 20 grains of ammoniacal soap, and 6 or 8 grains of the phosphates of soda and of lime. From this experiment, which was three times repeated with similar results, it appears that alcohol is well suited to afford an analysis of the fatty matter. It does not dissolve the neutral salts; when cold, it dissolves that portion of concrete animal oil from which the volatile alcali had flown off; and when heated, it dissolves the whole of the truly saponaceous matter, which is afterward completely separated by cooling. And accordingly it was found, that a thin plate of the fatty matter, which had lost nearly the whole of its volatile alcali, by exposure to the air for three years, was almost dissolved by the cold alcohol.

The concrete oily or waxy substance obtained in these experiments constitutes the leading object of research, as being the peculiar substance with which the other well-known matters are combined. It separates spontaneously by the action of the air, as well as by that of acids. These last separate it in a state of greater purity, the less disposed the acid may be to operate in the way of combustion. It is requisite, therefore, for this purpose, that the fatty matter should be previously diffused in 12 times its weight of hot water; and the muriatic or acetous acid is preferable to the sulphuric or the nitrous. The colour of the waxy matter is grayish; and though exposure to the air, and also the action of the oxygenated muriatic acid did produce an apparent whiteness, it nevertheless disappeared by subsequent fusion. No method was discovered by which it could be permanently bleached.

The nature of this wax or fat is different from that of any other known substance of the like kind. When slowly cooled after fusion, its texture appears crystalline or shivery, like spermaceti; but a speedy cooling gives it a semitransparency resembling wax. Upon the whole, nevertheless, it seems to approach more nearly to the former than to the latter of these bodies. It has less smell than spermaceti, and melts at 127° F.; Dr. Bostock says 92°. Spermaceti requires 6° more of heat to fuse it, (according to Dr. Bostock 20°.) The spermaceti did not so speedily become brittle by cooling as the adipocire. One ounce of alcohol of the strength between 39 and 40 degrees of Baume's aerometer, dissolved when boiling hot 12 gros of this substance, but the same quantity in like circumstances dissolved only 30 or 36 grains of spermaceti. The separation of these matters was also remarkably different, the spermaceti being more speedily deposited, and in a much more regular and crystalline form. Ammonia dissolves with singular facility, and even in the cold, this concrete oil separated from the fatty matter; and by heat it forms a transparent solution, which is a true soap. But no excess of ammonia can produce such an effect with spermaceti.

Fourcroy concludes his memoir with some speculations on the change to which animal substances in peculiar circumstances are subject. In the modern chemistry, soft animal matters are considered as a composition of the oxydes of hydrogen and carbonated azote, more complicated than those of vegetable matters, and therefore more incessantly tending to alteration. If then the carbon be conceived to unite with the oxygen, either of the water which is present, or of the other animal matters, and thus escape in large quantities in the form of carbonic acid gas, we shall perceive the reason why this conversion is attended with so great a loss of weight, namely, about nine-tenths of the whole. The azote, a principle so abundant in animal matters, will form ammonia by combining with the hydrogen; part of this will escape in the vaporous form, and the rest will remain fixed in the fatty matter. The residue of the animal matters deprived of a great part of their carbon, of their oxygen, and the whole of their azote, will consist of a much greater proportion of hydrogen, together with carbon and a minute quantity of oxygen. This, according to the theory of Fourcroy, constitutes the waxy matter, or adipocire, which, in combination with ammonia, forms the animal soap, into which the dead bodies are thus converted.

Muscular fibre, macerated in dilute nitric acid, and afterward well washed in warm water, affords pure adipocire, of a light yellow colour, nearly of the consistence of tallow, of a homogeneous texture, and of course free from ammonia. This is the mode in which it is now commonly procured for chemical experiment.

Ambergris appears to contain adipocire in large quantity, rather more than half of it being of this substance.

Adipocire has been more recently examined by Chevreul. He found it composed of a small quantity of ammonia, potassa, and lime, united to much margarine, and to a very little of another fatty matter different from that. Weak muriatic acid seizes the three alcaline bases. On treating the residue with a solution of potassa, the margarine is precipitated in the form of a pearly substance, while the other fat remains dissolved. Fourcroy being of opinion that the fatty matter of animal carcasses, the substance of biliary calculi, and spermaceti, were nearly identical, gave them the same name of adipocire; but it appears from the researches of Chevreul that these substances are very different from each other.

In the Philosophical Transactions for 1813, there is a very interesting paper on the above subject by Sir E. Home and Mr. Brande. He adduces many curious facts to prove that adipocire is formed by an incipient and incomplete putrefaction. Mary Howard, aged 44, died on the 12th May, 1790, and was buried in a grave ten feet deep at the east end of Shoreditch churchyard, ten feet to the east of the great common sewer, which runs from north to south, and has always a current of water in it, the usual level of which is eight feet below the level of the ground, and two feet above the level of the coffins in the graves. In August, 1811, the body was taken up, with some others buried near it, for the purpose of building a vault, and the flesh in all of them was converted into adipocire or spermaceti. At the full and new moon the tide raises water into the graves, which at other times are dry. To explain the extraordinary quantities of fat or adipocire formed by animals of a certain intestinal construction, Sir E. observes, that the current of water which passes through their colon, while the loculated lateral parts are full of solid matter, places the solid contents in somewhat similar circumstances to dead bodies in the banks of a common sewer.

The circumstance of ambergris, which contains 60 per cent. of fat, being found in immense quantities in the lower intestines of the spermaceti whales, and never higher up than seven feet from the anus, is an undeniable proof of fat being formed in the intestines; and as ambergris is only met with in whales out of health it is most probably collected there from the absorbents, under the influence of disease, not acting so as to take it into the constitution. In the human colon, solid masses of fat are sometimes met with in a diseased state of that canal. A description and analysis by Doctor Ure of a mass of ambergris, extracted in Perthshire from the rectum of a living woman, were published in a London Medical Journal in September, 1817. There is a case communicated by Dr. Babington, of fat formed in the intestines of a girl four and a half years old, and passing off by stool. Mr. Brande found, on the suggestion of Sir E. Home, that muscle digested in bile, is convertible into fat, at the temperature of about 100°. If the substance, however, pass rapidly into putrefaction, no fat is formed. Fæces voided by a gouty gentleman after six days' constipation, yielded, on infusion in water, a fatty film. This process of forming fat in the lower intestines by means of bile, throws considerable light upon the nourishment derived from clysters, a fact well ascertained, but which could not be explained. It also accounts for the wasting of the body, which so invariably attends all complaints of the lower bowels. It accounts too for all the varieties in the turns of the colon, which we meet with in so great a degree in different animals. This property of the bile explains likewise the formation of fatty concretions in the gall bladder so commonly met with, and which, from these experiments, appear to be produced by the action of the bile on the mucus secreted in the gall bladder; and it enables us to understand how want of the gall bladder in children, from mal-formation, is attended with excessive leanness, notwithstanding a great appetite, and leads to an early death. Fat thus appears to be formed in the intestines, and from thence received into the circulation, and deposited in almost every part of the body. And as there appears to be no direct channel by which any superabundance of it can be thrown out of the body, whenever its supply exceeds the consumption, its accumulation becomes a disease, and often a very distressing one.

[In the New-York Medical Repository, vol. ii. p. 325, is related the case of a person who was drowned, and whose body was converted into this substance after lying in the mud of a river for a year. We have seen a piece of meat raised out of a well by pumping, into which it had fallen, and where it was completely changed into adipocire. A barrel of meat, which had undergone a change and become adipocire, was raised from the British frigate Hussar, sunk near Hell-Gate during the revolutionary war, where it had remained in eight or ten fathoms of salt water near fifty years. A single body of a female, consisting of a solid mass of adipocire, was dug up in dry ground, near the City Hall in New-York. A box of candles, taken from a sunken wreck on the coast of Brazil, was changed in appearance and consistence, and had become a mass of adipocire. The bones of a huge cetaceous animal were dug up in the low grounds about New-Orleans: when they were exhibited as a show in New-York, in 1828, adipocire was discovered in the cells of the spongy part of the jaw-bone. A.]

ADI'POSE. (*Adiposus;* from *adeps*, fat.) Fatty; as adipose membrane, &c.

ADIPOSE MEMBRANE. *Membrana adiposa.* The fat collected in the cells of the cellular membrane.

ADI'PSA. (From *a*, neg. and διψα, thirst.) 1. So the Greeks called medicines, &c. which abate thirst.

2. Hippocrates applied this word to oxymel.

ADI'PSIA. (From *a*, neg. and διψα, thirst.) A want of thirst. A genus of disease in the class *locales*, and order *dysorexiæ* of Cullen's Nosology. It is mostly symptomatic of some disease of the brain.

ADI'PSOS. So called because it allays thirst.) 1. The Egyptian palm-tree, the fruit of which is said to be the *Myrobalans*, which quench thirst.

2. Also a name for liquorice.

ADJUTO'RIUM. (From *ad* and *juvo*, to help.) A name of the *humerus*, from its usefulness in lifting up the fore-arm.

ADJUVA'NTIA. Whatever assists in preventing or curing disease.

ADNATA TUNICA. *Albuginea oculi; Tunica albuginea oculi.* A membrane of the eye mostly confounded with the *conjunctiva*. It is, however, thus formed: five of the muscles which move the eye, take their origin from the bottom of the orbit, and the sixth arises from the edge of it; they are all inserted by a tendinous expansion, into the anterior part of the *tunica sclerotica*, which expansion forms the adnata, and gives the whiteness peculiar to the fore-part of the eye. It lies between the *sclerotica* and *conjunctiva*.

ADNA'TUS. (From *adnescor*, to grow to.) A term applied to some parts which appear to grow to others: as *tunica adnata, stipulæ adnatæ, folium adnatum*.

ADOLESCE'NTIA. See *Age*.

Ado'nion. (From Αδωνις, the youth from whose blood it was feigned to have sprung.) *Adonium*. See *Artemisia abrotanum*.

Adonium. See *Adonion*.

ADO'PTER. *Tubus intermedius*. A chemical vessel with two necks, used to combine retorts to the cucurbits or matrasses in distillation, with retorts instead of receivers.

A'dor. A sort of corn, called also spelta.

A'dos. Forge water, or water in which red-hot iron is extinguished.

AD PONDUS OMNIUM. The weight of the whole. These words are inserted in pharmaceutical preparations, or prescriptions, when the last ingredient ought to weigh as much as all the others put together.

ADPRESSUS. Approximated. A term in botany, applied to branches of leaves when they rise in a direction nearly parallel to the stem, and are closely applied to them, as in the branches of the *Genista tinctoria* and leaves of the *Thlaspi campestris*.

Adra Rhi'za. Blancard says the root of the Aristolochia is thus named.

Adra'chne. The strawberry bay-tree. A species of *Arbutus*.

Adrara'gi. An Indian name for our garden-saffron.

ADROBO'LON. (From αδρος, large, and βωλος, a globe, bole, or mass.) Indian bdellium, which is coarser than the Arabian. See *Bdellium*.

ADSCENDENS. See *Ascendens*.

ADSTRICTION. Costiveness.

ADSTRINGENT. See *Astringent*.

[ADULARIA. This is the most perfect variety of feldspar, and bears to common feldspar, in many respects, the relation of rock crystal to common quartz. Adularia is more or less translucent, and sometimes transparent and limpid. Its colour is white, either a little milky, or with a tinge of green, yellow, or red. But it is chiefly distinguished by presenting, when in certain positions, whitish reflections, which are often slightly tinged with blue or green, and exhibit a pearly or silver lustre. These reflections, which are often confined to certain spots, proceed in most cases from the interior of the crystal.

Adularia is sometimes cut into plates and polished. The *fish's eye, moonstone*, and *argentine*, of lapidaries, come chiefly from Persia, Arabia, and Ceylon, and belong to adularia, as do also the *water opal* and *girasole* of the Italians.—*Cleavl. Min.*

It has been found in the states of Maryland, Pennsylvania, New-York, and Massachusetts. A.]

ADUSTION. *Adustio*. 1. An inflammation about the brain, and its membranes, with a hollowness of the eyes, a pale colour, and a dry body; obsolete.

2. In surgery, adustion signifies the same as cauterization, and means the application of any substance to the animal body, which acts like fire. The ancient surgeons, especially the Arabians, were remarkably fond of having recourse to adustion in local diseases; but the use of actual heat is very rarely admitted by the moderns.

ADVENTITIOUS. (*Adventitius*; from *advenio*, to come to.) Any thing that accidentally, and not in the common course of natural causes, happens to make a part of another. Something accruing or befalling a person or thing from without. It is used in medicine in opposition to hereditary; as when diseases may be transmitted from the parent and also acquired, as is the case with gout and scrofula. They are sometimes hereditary, and very often adventitious.

ADVERSIFO'LIA. (From *adversus*, opposite, and *folium*, a leaf.) A plant with alternate leaves.

Adversifo'liæ plantæ. 1. Plants the leaves of which stand opposite to each other on the same stem or branch.

2. The name of a class in Sauvages' *Methodus Foliorum*. Valerian, teasel, honey-suckle, &c. are examples.

ADVERSUS. Opposite. Applied in natural history to parts which stand opposite to each other; as *plantæ adversifoliæ*, the leaves standing opposite to each other on the same stem, as in valerian, teasel, honeysuckle, &c.

ADYNA'MIA. (*Adynamia, æ*, f.; Αδυναμια, from α, priv. and δυναμις, power.) A defect of vital power.

Adyna'miæ. (The plural of *Adynamia*.) The second order of the class *neuroses* of Cullen's Nosology; it comprehends *syncope, dyspepsia, hypochondriasis*, and *chlorosis*.

Ady'namon. (From α, neg. and δυναμις, strength.) *Adynamum*. Among ancient physicians, it signified a kind of weak factitious wine, prepared from must, boiled down with water; to be given to patients to whom pure or genuine wine might be hurtful.

Adynamum. See *Adynamon*.

[ÆDELITE. A mineral described by Kirwan, containing, according to Bergman, silex from 62 to 69 parts, alumine from 18 to 20, lime from 8 to 16, water 3 to 4.—*Cleav. Min.* A.]

ÆDOI'A. (From αιδως, modesty; or from α, neg. and ειδεω, to see; as not being decent to the sight.) The pudenda, or parts of generation.

ÆDOPSO'PHIA. (From αιδοια, *pudenda*; and ψοφεω, to break wind.) A term used by Sauvages and Sagar, to signify a flatus from the bladder, or from the womb, making its escape through the vagina.

ÆDOPTO'SIS. (*Ædoptosis*; from αιδοῖον, the groin; pl. αιδοια, *pudenda*; and πτωσις, a falling down.) Genital prolapsi. The name of a genus of diseases in Good's Nosology.

ÆGAGRO'PILUS (From αιγαγρος, a wild goat, and *pila*, a ball.) *Ægagropila*.

1. A ball found in the stomach of deer, goats, hogs, horned cattle, as cows, &c. It consists of hairs which they have swallowed from licking themselves. They are of different degrees of hardness, but have no medicinal virtues. Some rank these balls among the *Bezoars*. Hieronymus Velschius wrote a treatise on the virtues of this.

2. A species of conferva found in Wallenfenmoor, from its resembling these concretions, is also so named.

Æ'GIAS. A white speck on the pupil of the eye, which occasions a dimness of sight.

ÆGI'DES. *Aglia*. A disorder of the eyes mentioned by Hippocrates. Foësius thinks the disease consists of small cicatrices in the eye, caused by an afflux of corrosive humours upon the part. But in one passage of Hippocrates, Foësius says it signifies small white concretions of humours which stick upon the pupil, and obscure the sight.

ÆGI'DION. A collyrium or ointment for inflammations and defluxions of the eyes.

Æ'GILOPS. 1. The same as *Ægylops*.

2. Wild fescue grass, so called from its supposed virtue in curing the disorder named Ægylops. It is a species of *Bromus* in the Linnæan system.

ÆGINE'TA, Paulus. A celebrated surgeon of the island of Ægina, from which he derived his name. He is placed by Le Clerc in the fourth century; by others in the seventh. He was eminently skilled in his profession, and his works are frequently cited by Fabricius ab Aquapendente. He is the first author that notices the cathartic quality of rhubarb. He begins his book with the description of the diseases of women; and is said to be the first that deserves the appellation of a man midwife.

Ægine'tia. Malabrian broom rape. A species of *Orobancha*.

Æ'GIS. A film on the eye.

ÆGO'CERAS. (From αιξ, a goat, and κερας, a horn; so called, because the pods were supposed to resemble the horns of a goat.) Fœnugreek. See *Trigonella Fœnumgræcum*.

ÆGO'LETHRON. (From αιξ, a goat, and ολεθρος, destruction: so named from the opinion of its being poisonous to goats.) Tournefort says it is the *Chamærododendron*, now the *Azalæa pontica* of Linnæus.

ÆGO'NYCHON. (From αιξ, a goat, and ονυξ, a hoof: because of the hardness of the seed.) See *Lithospermum officinale*.

ÆGOPO'DIUM. (*Ægopodium, i*. n.; from αιξ, a goat, and πους, a foot: from its supposed resemblance to a goat's foot.) A genus of plants in the Linnæan system. Class, *Pentandria*; Order, *Digynia*. Goatweed. The following species was formerly much esteemed.

Ægopodium podagraria. Goatweed. This plant is sedative, and was formerly applied to mitigate pains of gout, and to relieve piles, but not now employed. In its earlier state it is tender and esculent.

ÆGOPROSO'PON. (From αιξ, a goat, and προσωπον, a face: so called because goats are subject to defects in the eyes, or from having in it some ingredients named after the goat.) A name of a lotion for the eyes, when inflamed.

Æ'GYLOPS. (*Ægylops*, *opis*, m.; from αιξ, a goat, and ωψ, an eye.) *Anchilops.* A disease so named from the supposition that goats were very subject to it. The term means a sore just under the inner angle of the eye. The best modern surgeons seem to consider the ægylops only as a stage of the fistula lachrymalis. Paulus Ægineta calls it anchilops, before it bursts, and ægylops after. When the skin covering the lachrymal sac has been for some time inflamed, or subject to frequent returning inflammations, it most commonly happens that the puncta lachrymalia are affected by it; and the fluid, not having an opportunity of passing off by them, distends the inflamed skin, so that at last it becomes sloughy, and bursts externally. This is that state of the disease which is called perfect *aigylops*, or *ægylops*.

ÆGY'PTIA MUSCATA. See *Hibiscus abelmoschus.*

ÆGYPTI'ACUM. A name given to different unguents of the detergent or corrosive kind. We meet with a black, a red, a white, a simple, a compound, and a magistral ægyptiacum. The simple ægyptiacum, which is that usually found in our shops, is a composition of verdigris, vinegar, and honey, boiled to a consistence. It is usually supposed to take its name from its dark colour, wherein it resembles that of the natives of Egypt. It is improperly called an unguent, as there is no oil, or rather fat in it.

ÆGY'PTIUM PHARMACUM AD AURES. Aëtius speaks of this as excellent for deterging fœtid ulcers of the ears, which he says it cures, though the patient were born with them.

AEIPATHEI'A. (From αει, always, and παθος, a disease.) Diseases of long duration.

ÆNEA. (From æs, brass, so called because it was formerly made of brass.) A catheter.

ÆO'NION. The common house leek. See *Sempervivum tectorum.*

ÆO'RA. (From αιωρεω, to lift up, to suspend on high.) Exercise without muscular action; as swinging. A species of exercise used by the ancients, and of which Aëtius gives the following account. Gestation, while it exercises the body, the body seems to be at rest. Of this motion there are several kinds. First, swinging in a hammock, which, at the decline of a fever, is beneficial. Secondly, being carried in a litter, in which the patient either sits or lies along. It is useful when the gout, stone, or such other disorder attends, as does not admit of violent motions. Thirdly, riding in a chariot, which is of service in most chronical disorders; especially before the more violent exercises can be admitted. Fourthly, sailing in a ship or boat. This produces various effects, according to the different agitation of the waters, and, in many tedious chronical disorders, is efficacious beyond what is observed from the most skilful administration of drugs. These are instances of a passive exercise.

ÆQUA'LIS. Equal. Applied by botanists to distinguish length; as *filimenta æqualia; pedunculi æquales*, &c.

Æ'QUE. Equally. The same as *ana.*

ÆQUIVALVIS. *Æquivalve.* A botanical term, implying, composed of equal valves.

A'ER. (*Aer*, *eris*, m.; from αηρ.) The fluid which surrounds the globe. See *Air* and *Atmosphere.*

Æ'RA. Darnel, or lolium.

Ærated alkaline water. An alkaline water impregnated with carbonic acid.

ÆRIAL. Belonging to air.

Ærial Acid. See *Carbonic acid.*

Ærial plants. Those plants are so called which, after a certain time, do not require that their roots should be fixed to any spot in order to maintain their life, which they do by absorption from the atmosphere. Such are a curious tropical tribe of plants called *cacti*, the epidendrum, flos æris, and the ficus australis.

ÆRI'TIS. The *Anagallis*, or pimpernell.

ÆROLITE. A meteoric stone.

AEROLO'GICE. See *Aerology.*

AEROLO'GY. (*Aerologia*, *æ*, f.; from αηρ, the air, and λογος, a discourse.) *Aerologice.* That part of medicine which treats of the nature and proper ties of air.

AERO'MELI. Honey dew; also a name for manna.

ÆROMETER. An instrument for making the necessary corrections in pneumatic experiments to ascertain the mean bulk of the gases.

AEROPHO'BIA. Fear of air or wind.

1. Said to be a symptom of phrenitis and hydrophobia.

2. A name of *Hydrophobia.*

AERO'PHOBUS. (From αηρ, air, and φοβος, fear.) According to Cœlius Aurelianus, some phrenetic patients are afraid of a lucid, and others of an obscure air: and these he calls *aerophobi.*

AERO'SIS. The aerial vital spirit of the ancients.

ÆROSTATION. *Ærostatio.* A name commonly, but not very correctly, given to the art of raising heavy bodies into the atmosphere, by buoyancy of heated air, or gases of small specific gravity, enclosed in a bag, which from being usually of a spherical form, is called a balloon.

ÆRO'SUS LAPIS. So Pliny calls the *Lapis calaminaris*, upon the supposition that it was a copper ore.

ÆRU'CA. Verdigris.

ÆRU'GO. (*Ærugo*, *ginis*, f., from *æs*, copper.)
1. The rust of any metal, particularly of copper.

2. Verdigris. See *Verdigris.*

ÆRUGO ÆRIS. Rusts of copper or verdigris. See *Verdigris.*

ÆRUGO PRÆPARA'TA. See *Verdigris.*

ÆS. Brass.

ÆSCULA'PIUS, said to be the son of Apollo, by the nymph Coronis, born at Epidaurus, and educated by Chiron, who taught him to cure the most dangerous diseases, and even raise the dead; worshipped by the ancients as the god of medicine. His history is so involved in fable, that it is useless to trace it minutely His two sons, Machaon and Podalirius, who ruled over a small city in Thessaly, after his death accompanied the Greeks to the siege of Troy: but Homer speaks merely of their skill in the treatment of wounds; and divine honours were not paid to their father till a latter period. In the temples raised to him, votive tablets were hung up, on which were recorded the diseases cured, as they imagined, by his assistance.

Æ'SCULUS. (*Æsculus*, *i*, m.; from *esca*, food.) The name of a genus of plants in the Linnæan system Class, *Heptandria;* Order, *Monogynia.* Horse-chesnut.

ÆSCULUS HIPPOCASTANUM. The systematic name for the common horse-chesnut tree. *Castanea equina, pavina. Æsculus—foliolis septenis* of Linnæus. The fruit of this tree, when dried and powdered, is recommended as an errhine. The bark is highly esteemed on the continent as a febrifuge; and is, by some, considered as being superior in quality to the Peruvian bark. The bark intended for medical use is to be taken from those branches which are neither very young nor very old, and to be exhibited under similar forms and doses, as directed with respect to the Peruvian bark. It rarely disagrees with the stomach; but its astringent effects generally require the occasional administration of a laxative. During the late scarcity of grain, some attempts were made to obtain starch from the horse-chesnut, and not without success.

ÆSTHE'TICA. (From αισθάνομαι, to feel, or perceive.) Diseases affecting the sensation. The name of an order of diseases in Good's Nosology. See *Nosology.*

ÆSTIV'ALIS. (From *æstas*, summer.) Æstival; belonging to summer. Diseases of animals and plants which appear in the summer.

ÆSTIVALES PLANTÆ. Plants which flower in summer. A division according to the seasons of the year.

ÆSTIVA'TIO. Æstivation; the action of the summer, or its influence on things.

ÆSTPHARA. Incineration, or burning of the flesh, or any other part of the body.

ÆSTUA'RIUM. A stove for conveying heat to all parts of the body at once. A kind of vapour bath. Ambrose Paré calls an instrument thus, which he describes for conveying heat to any particular part. Palmarius, De Morbis Contagiosis, gives a contrivance under this name, for sweating the whole body.

ÆSTUA'TIO. The boiling up, or rather the fermenting of liquors when mixed.

Æ'STUS. *Æstus*, *ûs*, m.; from the Hebrew *esh*,

heat. Heat; applied to the feeling merely of heat, and sometimes to that of inflammation in which there is heat and redness.

ÆSTUS VOLATICUS. 1. Sudden heat, or scorching, which soon goes off, but which for a time reddens the part.

2. According to Vogel, synonymous with phlogosis.

3. *Erythema volaticum* of Sauvages.

ÆTAS. See *Age*.

Æ'THER. (*Æther, eris*, m.; from αιθηρ: a supposed fine subtile fluid.) Æther. A volatile liquor, obtained by distillation, from a mixture of alcohol and a concentrated acid.

The medical properties of æther, when taken internally, are antispasmodic, cordial, and stimulant. Against nervous and typhoid fever, all nervous diseases, but especially tetanic affections, soporose diseases from debility, asthma, palsy, spasmopic colic, hysteria, &c. it always enjoys some share of reputation. Regular practitioners seldom give so much as empirics, who sometimes venture upon large quantities, with incredible benefit. Applied externally, it is of service in the headache, toothache, and other painful affections. Thus employed, it is capable of producing two very opposite effects, according to its management; for, if it be prevented from evaporating, by covering the place to which it is applied closely with the hand, it proves a powerful stimulant and rubefacient, and excites a sensation of burning heat, as is the case with solutions of camphor in alcohol, or turpentine. In this way it is frequently used for removing pains in the head or teeth. On the contrary, if it be dropped on any part of the body, exposed freely to the air, its rapid evaporation produces an intense degree of cold; and, as this is attended with a proportional diminution of bulk in the part, applied in this way, it has frequently contributed to the reduction of the intestine, in cases of strangulated hernia.

ÆTHER RECTIFICATUS. *Æther vitriolicus.* Rectified æther. Take of sulphuric æther, fourteen fluid ounces. Fused potash, half an ounce. Distilled water, eleven fluid ounces.

First dissolve the potash in two ounces of the water, and add thereto the æther, shaking them well together, until they are mixed. Next, at a temperature of about 200 degrees, distil over twelve fluid ounces of rectified æther, from a large retort into a cooled receiver. Then shake the distilled æther well with nine fluid ounces of water, and set the liquor by, so that the water may subside. Lastly, pour off the supernatant rectified æther, and keep it in a well-stopped bottle.

Sulphuric æther is impregnated with some sulphureous acid, as is evident in the smell, and with some ætherial oil: and these require a second process to separate them. Potash unites to the acid, and requires to be added in a state of solution, and in sufficient quantities, for the purpose of neutralizing it; and it also forms a soap with the oil. It is advantageous also to use a less quantity of water than exists in the ordinary solution of potash; and therefore the above directions are adopted in the last London Pharmacopœia. For its virtues, see *Æther*.

ÆTHER SULPHURICUS. *Naphtha vitrioli; Æther vitriolicus.* Sulphuric æther. Take of rectified spirit, sulphuric acid, of each, by weight, a pound and a half. Pour the spirit into a glass retort, then gradually add to it the acid, shaking it after each addition, and taking care that their temperature, during the mixture, may not exceed 120 degrees. Place the retort very cautiously into a sand bath, previously heated to 200 degrees, so that the liquor may boil as speedily as possible, and the æther may pass over into a tubulated receiver, to the tubulure of which another receiver is applied, and kept cold by immersion in ice, or water. Continue the distillation until a heavier part also begins to pass over, and appear under the æther in the bottom of the receiver. To the liquor which remains in the retort, pour twelve fluid ounces more of rectified spirit, and repeat the distillation in the same manner.

It is mostly employed as an excitant, nervine, antispasmodic, and diuretic, in cases of spasms, cardialgia, enteralgia, fevers, hysteria, cephalalgia, and spasmodic asthma. The dose is from min. xx to ʒij. Externally, it cures toothache, and violent pains in the head. See *Æther*.

ÆTHER VITRIOLICUS. See *Æther sulphuricus* and *Æther rectificatus*.

ÆTHE'REA HERBA. The plant formerly so called is supposed to be the Eryngium.

ÆTHERIAL OIL. See *Oleum Ætherium*.

Æ'THIOPS. A term applied formerly to several preparations, because of a black colour, like the skin of an Æthiopian.

ÆTHIOPS ANTIMONIA'LIS. A preparation of antimony and mercury, once in high repute, and still employed by some practitioners in cutaneous diseases A few grains are to be given at first, and the quantity increased as the stomach can bear it.

ÆTHIOPS MARTIALIS. A preparation of iron, formerly in repute, but now neglected.

Æthiops mineral. The substance heretofore known by this name, is called by the London College, *Hydrargyri sulphuretum nigrum.*

ÆTHMOID. See *Ethmoid*.

Æthmoid Artery. See *Ethmoid Artery*.

Æthmoid Bone. See *Ethmoid Bone*.

ÆTHU'SA. (*Æthusa, æ*, f.; from αιθουσα, beggarly.) The name of a genus of plants of the Linnæan system. Class, *Pentandria;* Order, *Digynia*.

ÆTHUSA MEUM. The systematic name of the *meum* of the Pharmacopœias. Called also *Meum athamanticum; Meu; Spignel; Baldmoney*. The root of this plant is recommended as a carminative, stomachic. and for attenuating viscid humours, and appears to be nearly of the same nature as lovage, differing in its smell, being rather more agreeable, somewhat like that of parsnips, but stronger, and being in its taste less sweet, and more warm, or acrid.

ÆTIOLOGY. (*Ætiologia, æ*, f.; αιτιολογια: from αιτια, a cause, and λογος, a discourse.) The doctrine of the causes of diseases.

ÆTITES. Eagle stone. A stone formed of oxyde of iron, containing in its cavity some concretion which rattles on shaking the stone. Eagles were said to carry them to their nest, whence their name: and superstition formerly ascribed wonderful virtues to them.

[This is now arranged among the ores of iron by the name of the *nodular argillaceous oxide of iron.* See *Cleav. Min.* A.]

AE'TIUS. A physician, called also *Amidenus*, from the place of his birth. He flourished at Alexandria, about the end of the fifth century, and left sixteen books, divided into four *tetrabiblia*, on the practice of physic and surgery, principally collected from Galen and other early writers, but with some original observations. He appears very partial to the use of the cautery, both actual and potential, especially in palsy; which plan of treatment Mr. Pott revived in paraphlegia; and it has since often been adopted with success. Aëtius is the earliest writer who ascribed medical efficacy to the external use of the magnet, particularly in gout and convulsions; but rather on the report of others, than as what he had personally experienced.

ÆTO'CION. *Ætolium*. The granum cnidium. See *Daphne mezereon*.

ÆTO'NYCHUM. See *Lithospermum*.

AFFECTION. (*Affectio, onis*, f. This is expressed in Greek by παθος: hence *pathema, passio.*) Any existing disorder of the whole body, or a part of it; as hysterics, leprosy, &c. Thus, by adding a descriptive epithet to the term affection, most distempers may be expressed. And hence we say febrile affection, cutaneous affection, &c., using the word affection synonymously with disease.

AFFINITY. (*Affinitas, atis*, f.; a proximity of relationship.) The term affinity is used indifferently with attraction. See *Attraction*.

AFFINITY OF AGGREGATION. See *Attraction*.

AFFINITY, APPROPRIATE. See *Affinity, intermediate.*

AFFINITY OF COMPOSITION. See *Attraction*.

AFFINITY, COMPOUND. When three or more bodes, on account of their mutual affinity, unite and form one homogeneous body, then the affinity is termed compound affinity or attraction: thus, if to a solution of sugar and water be added spirits of wine, these three bodies will form a homogeneous liquid by compound affinity.

AFFINITY, DIVELLENT. See *Affinity, quiescent.*

AFFINITY, DOUBLE. *Double elective attraction.* When two bodies, each consisting of two elementary parts, come into contact, and are decomposed, so that their elements become reciprocally united, and produce two new compound bodies, the decomposition is then termed decomposition by double affinity: thus, if we add common salt, which consists of muriatic acid and soda, to nitrate of silver, which is composed of nitric acid and oxyde of silver, these two bodies will be decompounded; for the nitric acid unites with the soda, and the oxyde of silver with the muriatic acid, and thus may be obtained two new bodies. The common salt and nitrate of silver therefore mutually decompose each other by what is called double affinity.

Affinity, intermediate. *Appropriate affinity.* Affinity of an intermedium is, when two substances of different kinds, that show to one another no component affinity, do, by the assistance of a third, combine, and unite into a homogeneous whole: thus, oil and water are substances of different kinds, which, by means of alcali, combine and unite into a homogeneous substance: hence the theory of lixiviums, of washing, &c. See *Attraction.*

Affinity, quiescent. Mr. Kirwan employs the term *Quiescent affinity* to mark that, by virtue of which, the principle of each compound, decomposed by double affinity, adhere to each other; and *Divellent affinity*, to distinguish that by which the principles of one body unite and change order with those of the other: thus, sulphate of potash is not completely decomposed by the nitric acid or by lime, when either of these principles is separately presented; but if the nitric acid be combined with lime, this nitrate of lime will decompose the sulphate of potash. In this last case, the affinity of the sulphuric acid with the alcali is weakened by its affinity to the lime. This acid, therefore, is subject to two affinities, the one which retains it to the alcali, called *quiescent*, and the other which attracts it toward the lime, called *divellent* affinity.

Affinity, reciprocal. When a compound of two bodies is decomposed by a third, the separated principle being in its turn capable of decomposing the new combination: thus ammonia and magnesia will separate each other from muriatic acid.

Affinity, simple. *Single elective attraction.* If a body, consisting of two component parts, be decomposed on the approach of a third, which has a greater affinity with one of those component parts than they have for each other, then the decomposition is termed decomposition by *simple* affinity: for instance, if pure potash be added to a combination of nitric acid and lime, the union which existed between these two bodies will cease, because the potash combines with the nitric acid, and the lime, being disengaged, is precipitated. The reason is, that the nitric acid has a greater affinity for the pure potash than for the lime, therefore it deserts the lime, to combine with the potash. When two bodies only enter into chemical union, the affinity, which was the cause of it, is also termed *simple* or *single elective* attraction; thus the solution of sugar and water is produced by simple affinity, because there are but two bodies.

AFFLA'TUS. (From *ad* and *flare*, to blow.) A vapour or blast. A species of erysipelas, which attacks people suddenly, so named upon the erroneous supposition that it was produced by some unwholesome wind blowing on the part.

AFFUSION. (*Affusio;* from *ad*, and *fundo*, to pour upon.) Pouring a liquor upon something. The affusion of cold water, or pouring two or three quarts on the patient's head and body, is sometimes practised by physicians, but lately introduced by Dr. Currie, of Liverpool, in the treatment of typhus fever, and which appears to possess a uniformity of success, which we look for in vain in almost any other branch of medical practice. The remedy consists merely in placing the patient in a bathing-tub, or other convenient vessel, and pouring a pailful of cold water upon his body; after which he is wiped dry, and again put to bed. It should be noted,

First, That it is the *low contagious fever* in which the cold affusion is to be employed: the first symptoms of which are a dull headache, with restlessness and shivering; pains in the back, and all over the body, the tongue foul, with great prostration of strength; the headache becoming more acute, the heat of the body, by the thermometer, 102° to 105°, or more; general restlessness, increasing to delirium, particularly in the night.

Secondly, That it is *in the early stage of the disease* we must employ the remedy; and generally *in the state of the greatest heat and exacerbation.*

Thirdly, It is *affusion*, not *immersion*, that must be employed.

Since the first publication of Dr. Currie's work, the practice of affusion has been extended throughout England; and its efficacy has been established in some stages of the disease, from which the author had originally proscribed the practice of it. One of the cautionary injunctions which had been given for the affusion of cold water in fever, was *never to employ it in cases where the patient had a sense of chilliness upon him*, even if the thermometer, applied to the trunk of the body, indicated a preternatural degree of heat. In his last edition of Reports, however, Dr. Currie has given the particulars of a case of this kind, in which the cold affusion was so managed as to produce a successful event.

In fevers *arising from*, or *accompanied by*, *topical inflammation*, his experience does not justify the use of cold affusion; though, in a great variety of these cases, the warm affusion may be used with advantage "And," says he, "though I have used the cold affusion in some instances, so late as the twelfth or fourteenth day of contagious fever, with safety and success, yet it can only be employed, at this advanced period, in the instances in which the heat keeps up steadily above the natural standard, and the respiration continues free. In such cases, I have seen it appease agitation and restlessness, dissipate delirium, and, as it were, snatch the patient from impending dissolution. But it is in the *early stages* of fever (let me again repeat) that it ought always to be employed, if possible; and where, without any regard to the heat of the patient, it is had recourse to in the last stage of fever, after every other remedy has failed, and the case appears desperate, (of which I have heard several instances,) can it appear surprising that the issue should sometimes be unfavourable?"

Numerous communications from various practitioners, in the West and East Indies, in Egypt and America, also show the efficacy of affusion in the raging fevers of hot countries.

AFORA. (From *a*, priv. and *fores*, a door.) Having a door or valve: applied to plants, the seed vessel of which is not furnished with a valvule.

AFTER-BIRTH. See *Placenta.*

A'ga cretensium. The small Spanish milk-thistle.

AGALACTA'TIO. See *Agalactia.*

AGALA'CTIA. (Αγαλακτια; from *a*, priv. and γαλα, milk.) *Agalaxis; Agalactio; Agalactatio.* A defect of milk in childbirth.

AGALA'CTOS. (From *a*, priv. and γαλα, milk.) An epithet given to women who have no milk when they lie in.

AGALA'XIS. See *Agalactia.*

Agallochum. See *Lignum aloes.*

Agallochum verum. See *Lignum aloes.*

Aga'lluge. See *Lignum aloes.*

Agallugum. See *Lignum aloes.*

AGALMATOLITE. See *Figurestone.*

AGARIC. See *Agaricus.*

Agaricoi'des. (From αγαρικος, the agaric, and ειλος, resemblance.) A species of fungus like the agaric.

AGA'RICUS. Agaric. The name of a genus of plants in the Linnæan system. Class, *Cryptogamia;* Order, *Fungi.* The plants of this genus appear to approach nearer to the nature of animal matter than any other productions of the vegetable kingdom, as, beside hydrogen, oxygen, and carbon, they contain a considerable portion of nitrogen, and yield ammonia by distillation. Prof. Proust has likewise discovered in them the benzoic acid, and phosphate of lime.

The mushrooms, remarkable for the quickness of their growth and decay, as well as for the fœtor attending their spontaneous decomposition, were unaccountably neglected by analytical chemists, though capable of rewarding their trouble, as is evinced by the recent investigations and discoveries of Messrs. Vauquelin and Braconnot. The insoluble fungous portion of the mushroom, though it resembles woody fibre in some respects, yet being less soluble than it in alcalies, and yielding a nutritive food, is evidently a peculiar product, to which accordingly the name of *fungin* has been given. Two new vegetable acids, the boletic and fungic, were also fruits of these researches.

The six following species have been submitted to chemical analysis; the results are affixed to each. 1.

Agaricus campestris, an ordinary article of foo analyzed by Vauquelin, gave the following constituents: 1. Adipocire. On expressing the juice of the agaric, and subjecting the remainder to the action of boiling alkohol, a fatty matter is extracted, which falls down in white flakes as the alkohol cools. It has a dirty white colour; a fatty feel, like spermaceti; and, exposed to heat, soon melts, and then exhales the odour of grease. 2. An oily matter. 3. Vegetable albumen. 4. The sugar of mushrooms. 5. An animal matter soluble in water and alkohol: on being heated, it evolves the odour of roasting meat, like osmazome. 6. An animal matter not soluble in alkohol. 7. Fungin. 8. Acetate of potash.

2. *Agaricus volvaceus* afforded Braconnot fungin, gelatin, vegetable albumen, much phosphate of potash, some acetate of potash, sugar of mushrooms, a brown oil, adipocire, wax, a very fugacious deleterious matter, uncombined acid, supposed to be the acetic, benzoic acid, muriate of potash, and a deal of water; in all 14 ingredients.

3. *Agaricus acris*, or *piperatus*, was found by Braconnot, after a minute analysis, to contain nearly the same ingredients as the preceding, without the wax and benzoic acid, but with more adipocire.

4. *Agaricus stypticus.* From twenty parts of this Braconnot obtained of resin and adipocire 1.8, fungin 16.7, of an unknown gelatinous substance, a potash salt, and a fugacious acrid principle, 1.5.

5. *Agaricus bulbosus*, was examined by Vauquelin, who found the following constituents: an animal matter insoluble in alkohol; osmazome; a soft fatty matter of a yellow colour and acrid taste; an acid salt, (not a phosphate.) The insoluble substance of the agaric yielded an acid by distillation.

6. *Agaricus theogolus.* In this, Vauquelin found sugar of mushrooms; osmazome; a bitter acrid fatty matter; an animal matter not soluble in alkohol; a salt containing a vegetable acid.

Agaricus albus. See *Boletus laricis.*

Agaricus campestris. There are several species of the agaric, which go by the term mushroom; as the *Agaricus chantarellus, deliciosus, violaceus*, &c.; but that which is eaten in this country is the *Agaricus campestris* of Linnæus. Similar to it in quality is the champignon, or *Agaricus pratensis.* Broiled with salt and pepper, or stewed with cream and some aromatic, they are extremely delicious, and, if not eaten to excess, salubrious. Great care should be taken to ascertain that they are the true fungus, and not those of a poisonous nature. Catchup is made by throwing salt on mushrooms, which causes them to part with their juice.

Agaricus chantarellus. A species of fungus, esteemed a delicacy by the French. Broiled with salt and pepper, it has much the flavour of a roasted cockle.

Agaricus chirurgorum. See *Boletus igniarius.*

Agaricus cinnamomeus. Brown mushroom. This species of agaric is of a pleasant smell. When broiled, it gives a good flavour.

Agaricus deliciosus. This fungus, well seasoned, and then broiled, has the exact flavour of a roasted muscle. It is in season in September.

Agaricus mineralis. A mineral; the mountain milk, or mountain meal, of the Germans It is one of the purest of the native carbonates of lime, found chiefly in the clefts of rocks, and at the bottom of some lakes, in a loose or semi-indurated form. It has been used internally in hæmorrhages, strangury, gravel, and dysenterics; and externally as an application to old ulcers, and weak and watery eyes.

[It is composed of very minute particles, feebly cohering, fine or soft to the touch, and soiling the fingers. Its texture is spongy, and hence it usually swims for a moment when placed on water. Its colour is white, either pure, or tinged with yellow, &c. It is a very pure carbonate of lime.

Agaric mineral undoubtedly proceeds from the gradual disintegration of other varieties of carbonate of lime, and is deposited from water in the cavities or fissures of other calcareous rocks.

Var. 1. Fossil Farina. This variety differs but little from that just described, and has probably a similar origin. It appears in thin, white crusts, light as cotton, and very easily reducible to powder. These crusts are attached to the lateral or lower surfaces of beds of shell, limestone, &c.—*Cleav. Min.* A.]

Agaricus muscarius. Bug agaric; so called from its known virtue in destroying bugs. This reddish fungus is the *Agaricus—stipitatus, lamellis dimidiatis solitarus, stipite volvato, apice dilatato, basi ovato*, of Linnæus. It is not much known in this country. Haller relates that six persons of Lithuania perished at one time, by eating this kind of mushroom; and that in others it has caused delirium. The following account from Orfila, of the effects of this species in the animal economy, is interesting. Several French soldiers ate, at two leagues from Polosck, in Russia, mushrooms of the above kind. Four of them, of a robust constitution, who conceived themselves proof against the consequences under which their feebler companions were beginning to suffer, refused obstinately to take an emetic. In the evening, the following symptoms appeared. Anxiety, sense of suffocation, ardent thirst, intense griping pains, a small and irregular pulse, universal cold sweats, changed expression of countenance, violet tint of the nose and lips, general trembling, fœtid stools. These symptoms becoming worse, they were carried to the hospital. Coldness and livid colour of the limbs, a dreadful delirium, and acute pains, accompanied them to the last moment. One of them sunk a few hours after his admission into the hospital; the three others had the same fate in the course of the night. On opening their dead bodies, the stomach and intestines displayed large spots of inflammation and gangrene; and putrefaction seemed advancing very rapidly. It is employed externally to strumous phagedenic, and fistulous ulcers, as an escharotic.

Agaricus piperatus. The plant thus named by Linnæus, is the pepper mushroom; also called pepper agaric. It is the *Fungus piperatus albus, lacteo-succo turgens* of Ray. *Fungus albus acris.* When freely taken, fatal consequences are related by several writers to have been the result. When this vegetable has even lost its acrid juice by drying, its caustic quality still remains.

Agaricus pratensis. The champignon of Hudson's Flora Anglica. This plant has but little smell, and is rather dry, yet when broiled and stewed, communicates a good flavour.

Agaricus violaceus. Violet mushroom. This fungus requires much broiling, but when sufficiently done and seasoned, it is as delicious as an oyster. Hudson's *bulbosus* is only a variety of this.

AGATE. A mineral found chiefly in Siberia and Saxony, which consists of chalcedony blended with variable proportions of jasper, amethyst, quartz, opal, heliotrope, and carnelion.

[This name is usually applied to an aggregate of certain quartzy or siliceous substances, intimately combined, possessing a great degree of hardness, a compact and fine texture, agreeable colours, variously arranged and intermixed, and susceptible of a good polish. The minerals which most frequently enter into the composition of agates, are common chalcedony, carnelion, and jasper, to which are sometimes added flint, hornstone, common quartz, amethyst, heliotrope, and opal. The *chalcedony*, however, is the most common and abundant ingredient, and may frequently be considered the *base* of the agate; in fact, some agates are composed entirely of chalcedony differently coloured. In most cases, only two or three of the aforementioned ingredients occur in the same agate; but, though variously intermixed, each ingredient usually remains perfectly distinct.

Agates exhibit the colours already mentioned, while describing the simple minerals which compose them. But these colours are often so arranged, as to present the resemblance of some well-known object. Hence arises much of the beauty of agates; and hence also most of the distinctive names they have received in the arts. Of these a few will be mentioned. 1. Onyx agate. 2. Eyed agate. 3. Dotted agate. 4. Moss agate. 5. Dendritic agate. 6. Spotted or figured agate. 7. Breccia agate. 8. Fortification agate. 9. Ribband agate, &c. *Cleav. Min.* A.]

[Agatized wood. This substance appears to have been produced by the process common y called the petrifaction of wood. It is essentially composed of siliceous earth, which it is highly probable has been gradually deposited, as the vegetable matter was decomposed and removed. Both its form and texture indicate its origin. Thus it presents more or less distinctly, the form of the trunk, branches, roots, or knots, which once belonged to the vegetable. The surface is rough or longitudinally striated. Its texture is fibrous, and the fibres often intertwined like those of wood. Its longitudinal fracture is usually fibrous or splintery, and its cross fracture imperfectly conchoidal, with little or no lustre.—*Cleav. Min.*

Agatized wood has been found in various parts of the United States. We have seen in the possession of Dr. Mitchill some remarkable specimens of siliceous petrifactions or agatized madrepores, echini, &c. from the West-Indian islands. A.]

AGE. *Ætas.* The ancients reckoned six stages of life.

1. *Pueritia*, childhood, which is to the fifth year of our *age*.

2. *Adolescentia*, youth, reckoned to the eighteenth, and youth properly so called, to the twenty-fifth year.

3. *Juventus*, reckoned from the twenty-fifth to the thirty-fifth year.

4. *Virilis ætas*, manhood, from the thirty-fifth to the fiftieth year.

5. *Senectus*, old *age*, from fifty to sixty.

6. *Crepita ætas*, decrepit age, which ends in death.

AGENE'SIA. (Αγενησια; from α, neg. γενναω, or γινομαι, to beget.) Male sterility, or impotency in man. A term employed by Vogel and Good. See *Nosology*.

A'GER. (*Ager*, *gri.* m.; from αγρος.) The common earth or soil.

Ager naturæ. The womb.

AGE'RATUM. (Αγηρατον; from α, priv. and γηρας, *senectus:* never old, evergreen; because its flowers preserve their beauty a long time.) See *Achillæa ageratum*.

AGEU'STIA. (From α, neg. and γευομαι, *gusto*, to taste.) *Agheustia; Apogeustia; Apogeusis.* A defect or loss of taste. A genus of disease in the class *locales*, and order *dysæsthesiæ* of Cullen. The causes are fever or palsy, whence he forms two species: the latter he calls *organic*, arising from some affection in the membrane of the tongue, by which relishing things, or those which have some taste, are prevented from coming into contact with the nerves; the other *atonic*, arising without any affection of the tongue.

AGGLUTINA'NTIA. Adhesive medicines which heal by causing the parts to stick together.

AGGLUTINA'TION. (*Agglutinatio; from ad* and *glutino*, to glue together.) The adhesive union or sticking together of substances.

Agglut'tio. Obstruction in the œsophagus, or a difficulty in swallowing.

AGGREGATE. (*Aggregatus; from aggrego*, to assemble together.) Aggregated or added together. 1. When bodies of the same kind are united, the only consequence is, that one larger body is produced. In this case, the united mass is called an aggregate, and does not differ in its chemical properties from the bodies from which it was originally made. Elementary writers call the smallest parts into which an aggregate can be divided without destroying its chemical properties, integrant parts. Thus the integrant parts of common salt are the smallest parts which can be conceived to remain without change; and beyond these, any further subdivision cannot be made without developing the component parts, namely, the alcali and the acid; which are still further resolvable into their constituent principles.

2. A term applied to glands, flowers, gems, &c. An aggregate flower is one which consists of a number of smaller flowers or fructifications, collected into a head by means of some part common to them all. In this view aggregate flowers are opposed to simple flowers which have a single fructification, complete in its parts, nine of which are common to many flowers.

Aggregate gem. A term applied in botany when two, three, or even more gems appear at the same time.

Aggregate glands. (From *aggrego*, to assemble together.) *Glandulæ aggregatæ.* An assemblage of glands, as those on some parts of the internal surface of the intestines.

Aggregate peduncle. Clustered flower stalks, so called when several grow together, as in *verbascum nigrum.*

Aggregation, affinity of. See *Attraction.*

Aggregation, attraction of. See *Attraction.*

AGGREGATUS. See *Aggregate.*

AGHEU'STIA. See *Ageustia.*

AGITATO'RIA. Convulsive diseases.

AGLACTA'TIO. Defect of milk.

AGLA'XIS. Defect of milk.

Aglium. 1. A shining tubercle or pustule on the face.

2. A white speck on the eye. See *Ægides.*

A'gnacal. A tree, which, according to Ray, grows about the isthmus of Darien, and resembles a pear tree, the fruit of which is a great provocative to venery.

Agna'ta. See *Adnata tunica.*

AGNI'NA. (*Agnina;* from *agnus*, a lamb.) Aëtius calls one of the membranes which involve the fœtus by the name of *membrana agnina*, which he derives from its tenderness. See *Amnios.*

AGNOI'A. (From α, priv. and γινωσκω, to know.) Forgetfulness.

A'GNUS. A lamb.

Agnus castus. (Called *agnus*, from the down upon its surface, which resembles that upon a lamb's skin; and *castus*, because the chaste matrons, at the feasts of Ceres, strewed them upon their beds and lay upon them.) See *Vitex agnus castus.*

[Agnus tartaricus. This is a vegetable production, and belongs to the ferns. It is the root of the Polypodium Barometz, belonging to the class Cryptogamia, and order Felices of Linnæus. The root of this plant is covered with a sort of orange-coloured wool among the radicals, and has a peculiar oblong figure, which, when put in a proper position, has a remote resemblance to a sheep. When pulled up by the roots, the stipes of the leaves, except four, are cut away, and those left behind are trimmed to resemble legs, and this Chinese juggle has had great sway in the world, and has deceived even Dr. Darwin, who has figured and noticed it in his Botanic Garden as a plant growing in the form of an animal.—*Notes from Mitchill's Lectures.* A.]

Agomphi'asis. A looseness of the teeth.

A'gone. (Αγονη; from α, neg. and γονος, offspring: so called because it was supposed to cause barrenness.) Henbane. See *Hyosciamus niger.*

AGO'NIA. Sterility, impotence, agony.

Agoni'sticum. (Αγωνιστικον; from αγωνιαω, to struggle.) A term used by ancient physicians to signify water extremely cold, which was directed to be given in large quantities, in acute erysipelatous fevers, with a view of overpowering or struggling with the febrile heat of the blood.

A'GONOS. (From α, priv. and γονος, or γονη, an offspring.) Barren. Hippocrates calls those women so who have no children, though they might have if the impediment were removed.

AGRE'STIS. 1. Pertaining to the field; the trivial name of many plants.

2. In the works of some old writers, it expresses an ungovernable malignity in a disease.

A'GRIA. 1. A name of the *Ilex aquifolium*, or common holly.

2. A malignant pustule, of which the ancient surgeons, and particularly Celsus, describe two sorts; one which has been so called, is small, and casts a roughness or redness over the skin, slightly corroding it; smooth about its centre; spreads slowly; and is of a round figure. The second ulcerates, with a violent redness and corrosion, so as to make the hair fall off; it is of an unequal form, and turns leprous.

AGRIA'MPELOS. (From αγριος, wild, and αμπελος, a vine.) The wild vine, or white bryony. See *Bryonia.*

AGRIELÆ'A. (From αγριος, wild, and ελαια, the oilve-tree.) The oleaster, or wild olive.

AGRI'FOLIUM. (From ακις, a prickle, and φυλλον, a leaf.) The holly-tree. Which should rather be called *acifolium*, from its prickly leaves.

AGRIMO'NIA. (*Agrimonia, æ*, f.; from αγρος, a field, and μονος, alone: so named from its being the chief of all wild herbs.) Agrimony.

1. The name of a genus of plants in the Linnæan system. Class, *Dodecandria;* Order, *Digynia.*

2. The pharmacopœial name of the common agrimony. See *Agrimonia eupatoria.*

Agrimonia eupatoria. The systematic name of the common agrimony. *Agrimonai* of the pharmacopœias; *Agrimonia—foliis caulinis pinnatis, foliolis undique serratis, omnibus minutis interstinctis, fruc tibus hispidis* of Linnæus. It is common in fields about hedges and shady places, flowering in June and July. It has been principally regarded in the character of a mild astringent and corroborant, and many authors recommend it as a deobstruent, especially in hepatic and other visceral obstructions. Chomel relates two instances of its successful use in cases where the liver was much enlarged and indurated. It has been used with advantage in hæmorrhagic affections, and to give tone to a lax and weak state of the solids. In cutaneous disorders, particularly in scabies, we have been told that it manifests great efficacy. For this purpose it was given infused with liquorice in the form of tea; but, according to Alston, it should be always exhibited in the state of powder. It is best used while fresh, and the tops, before the flowers are formed, possess the most virtue. Cullen observes that the agrimony has some astringent powers, but they are feeble; and pays little attention to what has been said in its favour.

AGRIMONY. See *Agrimonia.*

Agrimony hemp. See *Bidens tripartita.*

AGRIOCA'RDAMUM. (From αγριος, wild, and καρδαμον, the nasturtium.) Sciatica cresses, or wild garden cress.

AGRIOCA'STANUM. (From αγριος, wild, and καςανον, the chestnut.) Earth of pig-nut. See *Bunium bulbo-castanum.*

AGRIOCI'NARA. (From αγριος, wild, and κιναρα, artichoke.) Wild artichoke; not so good as the cultivated for any purpose. See *Cinara scolymus.*

AGRIOCOCCIME'LA. (From αγριος, wild, κοκκυς, a berry, and μηλεα, an apple-tree.) The *Prunus spinosa* of Linnæus.

AGRIOME'LA. The crab-apple.

A'GRION. *Agriophyllon.* The *peucedanum silaus,* or hog's fennel.

AGRIOPASTINA'CA. (From αγριος, wild, and *pastinaca,* a carrot.) Wild carrot, or parsnip.

AGRIOPHY'LLON. See *Agrion.*

AGRIORI'GANUM. (From αγριος, wild, and οριγανον, marjoram.) Wild marjoram. See *Origanum vulgare.*

AGRIOSELI'NUM. (From αγριος, wild, and σελινον, parsley.) Wild parsley. Lee *Smyrnium olusatrum.*

AGRIOSTA'RI. (From αγριος, wild, and ςαις, wheat.) Field-corn, a species of Triticum.

AGRIPA'LMA. (From αγριος, wild, and παλμα, a palm-tree.) *Agripalma gallis.* The herb motherwort, or wild-palm.

AGRIPA'LMA GALLIS. See *Agripalma.*

AGRI'PPÆ. Those children which are born with their feet foremost are so called, because that was said to be the case with Agrippa the Roman, who was named *ab ægro partu,* from his difficult birth.

A'GRIUM. An impure sort of natron. The purer sort was called *halmyrhaga.*

AGROSTEMMA. (Αγρου ςεμμα, the garland of the field.) The name of a genus of plants. Class *Decandria;* Order, *Pentagynia.* Cockle.

AGROSTEMMA GITHAGO. This plant has been called *Nigellastrum; Pseudo melanthium; Lychnis segetum major; Githago; Nigella officinarum; Lychnoides segetum.* Cockle. It has no particular virtues, and is fallen into disuse.

AGROSTIS. (From αγρος, a field.) The name of a genus of plants. Class, *Triandria;* Order, *Digynia.* Bentgrass.

AGRU'MINA. Leeks; wild onions.

AGRY'PNIA. (From α, priv. and υπνος, sleep.) Watchfulness; sleeplessness. The name of a genus in Good's Nosology. See *Nosology.*

AGRYPNOCO'MA. (From αγρυπνος, without sleep, and κωμα, a lethargy.) A lethargic kind of watchfulness, in which the patient is stupidly drowsy, and yet cannot sleep.

AGUE. See *Febris Intermittens.*

Ague cake. The popular name for a hard tumour, most probably the spleen on the left side of the belly, lower than the false ribs in the region of the spleen, said to be the effect of intermittent fevers. However frequent it might have been formerly, it is now very rare, and although then said to be owing to the use of bark, it is now less frequent since the bark has been generally employed.

Ague drop. A medicine sold for the cure of agues, composed of arsenite of potassa in solution in water. The regular substitute for the quack medicine called the tasteless ague drop, which has cured thousands of that complaint, is the liquor arsenicalis, or Fowler's arsenical solution.

Ague-free. A name given by some to sassafras, on account of its supposed febrifuge virtue.

AGUSTINE. (From α, priv. and γευςια, taste, that is tasteless.) *Augustina.* A new earth discovered in the Saxon beryl, or beryl of Georgien Stadt, (a stone greatly resembling the beryl of Siberia) by Professor Tromsdorff, of Erfurth, in Germany, to which he has given the name of *agustine,* on account of the property of forming salts which are nearly destitute of taste. This earth is white and insipid: when moistened with water, it is somewhat ductile, but is not soluble in that fluid. Exposed to a violent heat, it becomes extremely hard, but acquires no taste. It combines with acids, forming salts which have little or no taste. It does not combine either in the humid or dry way with alcalies, or with their carbonates. It retains carbonic acid but feebly. It dissolves in acids equally well after having been hardened by exposure to heat, as when newly precipitated. With sulphuric acid it forms a salt which is insipid, and scarcely soluble, but an excess of acid renders it soluble, and capable of crystallizing in stars. With an excess of phosphoric acid it forms a very soluble salt. With nitrous acid it forms a salt scarcely soluble.

AGUTIGUEPOO'BI BRAZILIENSIS. An Indian name of the arrow-root. See *Maranta.*

[AIGUE MARINE, called by some *aqua marina;* one of the precious stones which has been found in various parts of the United States. It is a name sometimes employed to designate the beryl. A.]

AIMATEI'A. A black bilious and blood-like discharge from the bowels.

AIMORRHŒ'A. See *Hæmorrhagia.*

AIMO'RRHOIS. See *Hæmorrhois.*

AIPATHEI'A. (From αει, always, and παθος, a disease.) Diseases of long continuance.

AI'PI. *Aipima coxera. Aipipoca.* Indian words for Cassada. See *Jatropha manihot.*

AIR. This term was, till lately, used as the generic name for such invisible and exceedingly rare fluids as possess a very high degree of elasticity, and are not condensible into the liquid state by any degree of cold hitherto produced; but as this term is commonly employed to signify that compound of aëriform fluids which constitutes our atmosphere, it has been deemed advisable to restrict it to this signification, and to employ as the generic term the word GAS, for the different kinds of air, except what relates to our atmospheric compound.

AIR, ATMOSPHERIC. "The immense mass of permanently elastic fluid which surrounds the globe we inhabit," says Dr. Ure, "must consist of a general assemblage of every kind of air which can be formed by the various bodies that compose its surface. Most of these, however, are absorbed by water; a number of them are decomposed by combination with each other; and some of them are seldom disengaged in considerable quantities by the processes of nature. Hence it is that the lower atmosphere consists chiefly of oxygen and nitrogen, together with moisture and the occasional vapours or exhalations of bodies. The upper atmosphere seems to be composed of a large proportion of hydrogen, a fluid of so much less specific gravity than any other, that it must naturally ascend to the highest place, where, being occasionally set on fire by electricity, it appears to be the cause of the aurora borealis and fire-balls. It may easily be understood, that this will only happen on the confines of the respective masses of common atmospherical air, and of the inflammable air; that the combustion will extend progressively, though rapidly, in flashings from the place where it commences; and that when by any means a stream of inflammable air, in its progress toward the upper atmosphere, is set on fire at one end, its ignition may be much more rapid than what happens higher up, where oxygen is wanting, and at the same time more definite in its figure and progression, so as to form the appearance of a fire-ball.

That the air of the atmosphere is so transparent as to be invisible except by the blue colour it reflects when in very large masses, as is seen in the sky or region above us, or in viewing extensive landscapes; that it is without smell, except that of electricity, which it sometimes very manifestly exhibits; altogether without taste, and impalpable; not condensible by any degree of cold into the dense fluid state, though easily changing its dimensions with its temperature; that it gravitates and is highly elastic; are among the numerous observations and discoveries which do honour to the sagacity of the philosophers of the seventeenth century. They likewise knew that this fluid is indispensably necessary to combustion, but no one, except the great, though neglected, John Mayow, appears to have formed any proper notion of its manner of acting in that process.

The air of the atmosphere, like other fluids, appears to be capable of holding bodies in solution. It takes up water in considerable quantities, with a diminution of its own specific gravity: from which circumstance, as well as from the consideration that water rises very plentifully in the vaporous state *in vocuo*, it seems probable, that the air suspends vapour, not so much by a real solution, as by keeping its particles asunder, and preventing their condensation. Water likewise dissolves or absorbs air.

Mere heating or cooling does not affect the chemical properties of atmospherical air; but actual combustion, or any process of the same nature, combines its oxygen, and leaves its nitrogen separate. Whenever a process of this kind is carried on in a vessel containing atmospherical air, which is enclosed either by inverting the vessel over mercury, or by stopping its aperture in a proper manner, it is found that the process ceases after a certain time; and that the remaining air (if a combustible body capable of solidifying the oxygen, such as phosphorus, have been employed,) has lost about a fifth part of its volume, and is of such a nature as to be incapable of maintaining any combustion for a second time, or of supporting the life of animals. From these experiments it is clear, that one of the following deductions must be true:—1. The combustible body has emitted some principle, which, by combining with the air, has rendered it unfit for the purpose of further combustion; or, 2. It has absorbed part of the air which was fit for that purpose, and has left a residue of a different nature; or, 3. Both events have happened; namely, that the pure part of the air has been absorbed, and a principal has been emitted, which has changed the original properties of the remainder.

The facts must clear up these theories. The first induction cannot be true, because the residual air is not only of less bulk, but of less specific gravity, than before. The air cannot therefore have received so much as it has lost. The second is the doctrine of the philosophers who deny the existence of phlogiston, or a principle of inflammability; and the third must be adopted by those who maintain that such a principle escapes from bodies during combustion. This residue was called phlogisticated air, in consequence of such an opinion.

In the opinion that inflammable air is the phlogiston, it is not necessary to reject the second inference that the air has been no otherwise changed than by the mere subtraction of one of its principles; for the pure or vital part of the air may unite with inflammable air supposed to exist in a fixed state in the combustible body; and if the product of this union still continues fixed, it is evident, that the residue of the air, after combustion, will be the same as it would have been if the vital part had been absorbed by any other fixed body. Or, if the vital air be absorbed while inflammable air or phlogiston is disengaged, and unites with the aëriform residue, his residue will not be heavier than before, unless the inflammable air it has gained exceeds in weight the vital air it has lost; and if the inflammable air falls short of that weight, the residue will be lighter.

These theories it was necessary to mention; but it has been sufficiently proved by various experiments, that combustible bodies take oxygen from the atmosphere, and leave nitrogen; and that when these two fluids are again mixed in due proportions, they compose a mixture not differing from atmospherical air.

The respiration of animals produces the same effect on atmospherical air as combustion does, and their constant heat appears to be an effect of the same nature. When an animal is included in a limited quantity of atmospherical air, it dies as soon as the oxygen is consumed; and no other air will maintain animal life but oxygen, or a mixture which contains it. Pure oxygen maintains the life of animals much longer than atmospherical air, bulk for bulk.

It is to be particularly observed, however, that, in many cases of combustion, the oxygen of the air, in combining with the combustible body, produces a compound, not solid, or liquid, but aëriform. The residual air will therefore be a mixture of the nitrogen of the atmosphere with the consumed oxygen, converted into another gas. Thus, in burning charcoal, the carbonic acid gas generated, mixes with the residual nitrogen, and makes up exactly, when the effect of heat ceases, the bulk of the original air. The breathing of animals, in like manner, changes the oxygen into carbonic acid gas, without altering the atmospherical volume.

There are many provisions in nature by which the proportion of oxygen in the atmosphere, which is continually consumed in respiration and combustion, is again restored to that fluid. In fact there appears, as far as an estimate can be formed of the great and general operations of nature, to be at least as great an emission of oxygen as is sufficient to keep the general mass of the atmosphere at the same degree of purity. Thus, in volcanic eruptions, there seems to be at least as much oxygen emitted or extricated by fire from various minerals, as is sufficient to maintain the combustion, and perhaps even to meliorate the atmosphere And in the bodies of plants and animals, which appear in a great measure to derive their sustenance and augmentation from the atmosphere and its contents, it is found that a large proportion of nitrogen exists. Most plants emit oxygen in the sunshine, from which it is highly probable that they imbibe and decompose the air of the atmosphere, retaining carbon, and emitting the vital part. Lastly, if to this we add the decomposition of water, there will be numerous occasions in which this fluid will supply us with disengaged oxygen; while, by a very rational supposition, its hydrogen may be considered as having entered into the bodies of plants for the formation of oils, sugars, mucilages, &c., from which it may be again extricated.

To determine the respirability or purity of air, it is evident that recourse must be had to its comparative efficacy in maintaining combustion, or some other equivalent process.

From the latest and most accurate experiments, the proportion of oxygen in atmospheric air is by measure about 21 per cent.; and it appears to be very nearly the same, whether it be in this country or on the coast of Guinea, on low plains or lofty mountains, or even at the height of 7250 yards above the level of the sea, as ascertained by Gay Lussac, in his aërial voyage in September, 1805. The remainder of the air is nitrogen, with a small portion of aqueous vapour, amounting to about one per cent. in the driest weather, and a still less portion of carbonic acid, not exceeding a thousandth part of the whole.

As oxygen and nitrogen differ in specific gravity in the proportion of 135 to 121, according to Kirwan, and of 139 to 120, according to Davy, it has been presumed, that the oxygen would be more abundant in the lower regions, and the nitrogen in the higher, if they constituted a mere mechanical mixture, which appears contrary to the fact. On the other hand, it has been urged, that they cannot be in the state of chemical combination, because they both retain their distinct properties unaltered, and no change of temperature or density takes place on their union. But perhaps it may be said, that, as they have no repugnance to mix with each other, as oil and water have, the continual agitation to which the atmosphere is exposed, may be sufficient to prevent two fluids, differing not more than oxygen and nitrogen in gravity, from separating by subsidence, though simply mixed. On the contrary, it may be argued, that to say chemical combination cannot take place without producing new properties, which did not exist before in the component parts, is merely begging the question; for though this generally appears to be the case, and often in a very striking manner, yet combination does not always produce a change of properties, as appears in M. Biot's experiments with various substances; of which we may instance water, the refraction of which is precisely the mean of that of the oxygen and hydrogen, which are indisputably combined in it.

To get rid of the difficulty, Mr. Dalton of Manchester

framed an ingenious hypothesis, that the particles of different gases neither attract nor repel each other; so that one gas expands by the repulsion of its own particles, without any more interruption from the presence of another gas, than if it were in a vacuum. This would account for the state of atmospheric air, it is true; but it does not agree with certain facts. In the case of the carbonic acid gas in the Grotto del Cano, and over the surface of brewers' vats, why does not this gas expand itself freely upward, if the superincumbent gases do not press upon it? Mr. Dalton himself, too, instances as an argument for his hypothesis, that oxygen and hydrogen gases, when mixed by agitation, do not separate on standing. But why should either oxygen or hydrogen require agitation, to diffuse it through a vacuum, in which, according to Mr. Dalton, it is placed?

The theory of Berthollet appears consistent with all the facts, and sufficient to account for the phenomenon. If two bodies be capable of chemical combination, their particles must have a mutual attraction for each other. This attraction, however, may be so opposed by concomitant circumstances, that it may be diminished in any degree. Thus we know, that the affinity of aggregation may occasion a body to combine slowly with a substance for which it has a powerful affinity, or even entirely prevent its combining with it; the presence of a third substance may equally prevent the combination; and so may the absence of a certain quantity of caloric. But in all these cases the attraction of the particles must subsist, though diminished or counteracted by opposing circumstances. Now we know that oxygen and nitrogen are capable of combination; their particles, therefore, must attract each other; but in the circumstances in which they are placed in our atmosphere, that attraction is prevented from exerting itself, to such a degree as to form them into a chemical compound, though it operates with sufficient force to prevent their separating by their difference of specific gravity. Thus the state of the atmosphere is accounted for, and every difficulty obviated, without any new hypothesis.

The exact specific gravity of atmospherical air, compared to that of water, is a very nice and important problem. By reducing to 60° Fahr. and to 30 inches of the barometer, the results obtained with great care by Biot and Arago, the specific gravity of atmospherical air, appears to be 0.001220, water being represented by 1.000000. This relation expressed fractionally is 1-820, or water is 820 times denser than atmospherical air. Mr. Rice, in the 77th and 78th numbers of the Annals of Philosophy, deduces from Sir George Shuckburgh's experiments 0.00120855 for the specific gravity of air. This number gives water to air as 827.437 to 1. If with Mr. Rice we take the cubic inch of water=252.525 gr., then 100 cubic inches of air by Biot's experiments will weigh 30.808 grains, and by Mr. Rice's estimate 30.519. He considers with Dr. Prout the atmosphere to be a compound of 4 volumes of nitrogen, and 1 of oxygen; the specific gravity of the first being to that of the second as 1.1111 to 0.9722. Hence

0.8 vol. nitr. sp. gr.	0.001166	=0.000933
0.2 oxy.	0.001340	=0.000268
		0.001201

The numbers are transposed in the Annals of Philosophy by some mistake.

Biot and Arago found the specific gravity of oxygen to be 1.10359
and that of nitrogen 0.96913
air being reckoned, ... 1.00000
Or compared to water as unity,—

Nitrogen is	0.001182338
Oxygen,	0.001346379
And 0.8 nitrogen	=0.00094587
0.2 oxygen	=0.00026927
	0.00121514
And 0.79 nitrogen	=0.000934
0.21 oxygen	=0.000283
	0.001217

A number which approaches very nearly to the result of experiment. Many analogies, it must be confessed, favour Dr. Prout's proportions; but the greater number of experiments on the composition and density of the atmosphere agree with Biot's results. Nothing can decide these fundamental chemical proportions, except a new, elaborate, and most minutely accurate series of experiments. We shall then know whether the atmosphere contains in volume 20 or 21 per cent. of oxygen."—*Ure's Chem. Dict.*

Air, alcaline. See *Ammonia.*
Air, azotic. See *Nitrogen.*
Air, fixed. See *Carbonic acid.*
Air, fluoric. See *Fluoric acid.*
Air, hepatic. See *Hydrogen sulphuretted.*
Air, heavy inflammable. See *Carburetted hydrogen.*
Air, inflammable. See *Hydrogen.*
Air, marine. See *Muriatic acid.*
Air, nitrous. See *Nitrous.*
Air, phlogisticated. See *Nitrogen.*
Air, phosphoric. See *Hydrogen phosphuretted.*
Air, sulphureous. See *Sulphureous acid.*
Air, vital. See *Oxygen.*

AISTHETE'RIUM. (From αισθανομαι, to perceive.) The sensorium commune, or common sensory, or seat, or origin of sensation.

AIX LA CHAPE'LLE. Called Aken by the Germans. A town in the south of France, where there is a sulphureous water, Thermæ Aquis-granensis, the most striking feature of which, and what is almost peculiar to it, is the unusual quantity of sulphur it contains: the whole, however, is so far united to a gaseous basis, as to be entirely volatilized by heat; so that none is left in the residuum after evaporation. In colour it is pellucid, in smell sulphureous, and in taste saline, bitterish, and rather alcaline. The temperature of these waters varies considerably, according to the distance from the source and the spring itself. In the well of the hottest bath, it is, according to Lucas, 136° Monet, 146°; at the fountain where it is drank, it is 112°. This thermal water is much resorted to on the Continent for a variety of complaints. It is found essentially serviceable in the numerous symptoms of disorders in the stomach and biliary organs, that follow a life of high indulgence in the luxuries of the table; in nephritic cases, which produce pain in the loins, and thick mucous urine with difficult micturition. As the heating qualities of this water are as decided as in any of the mineral springs, it should be avoided in cases of a general inflammatory tendency, in hectic fever and ulceration of the lungs; and in a disposition to active hæmorrhagy. As a hot bath, this water is even more valuable and more extensively employed than as an internal remedy. The baths of Aix la Chapelle may be said to be more particularly medicated than any other that we are acquainted with. They possess both temperature of any degree that can be borne; and a strong impregnation with sulphur in its most active forms; and a quantity of alcali, which is sufficient to give it a very soft soapy feel, and to render it more detergent than common water. From these circumstances, these baths will be found of particular service in stiffness and rigidity of the joints and ligaments, which is left by the inflammation of gout and rheumatism, and in the debility of palsy, where the highest degree of heat which the skin can bear is required. The sulphureous ingredient renders it highly active in almost every cutaneous eruption, and in general in every foulness of the skin; and here the internal use of the water should attend that of the bath These waters are also much employed in the distressing debility which follows a long course of mercury and excessive salivation. Aken water is one of the few natural springs that are hot enough to be employed as a vapour bath, without the addition of artificial heat. It is employed in cases in which the hot bath is used; and is found to be a remarkably powerful auxiliary in curing some of the worst species of cutaneous disorders. With regard to the dose of this water to be begun with, or the degree of heat to bathe in, it is in all cases best to begin with small quantities and low degrees of heat, and gradually increase them, agreeably to the effects and constitution of the patient. The usual time of the year for drinking these waters is from the beginning of May to the middle of June, or from the middle of August to the latter end of September.

AIZO'ON. (From αει, always, and ζω, to live.) *Aizoum.* 1. An evergreen aquatic plant, like the aloe, said to possess antiscorbutic virtues.

2. The house leek. See *Sempervivum tectorum*.

AIZOUM. See *Aizoon*.

AJA'VA. An ancient name of a seed used in the East as a remedy for the colic.

AJUGA. (From *a*, priv. and ζυγον, a yoke.) 1. The name of a genus of plants in the Linnæan system.

2. The pharmacopœial name of the creeping bugloss. See *Ajuga pyramidalis*.

AJUGA PYRAMIDALIS. *Consolida media. Bugula.* Upright bugloss. Middle consound. This plant, *Ajuga—caule tetragono foliis radicalibus maximis*, of Linnæus, possesses subadstringent and bitter qualities: and has been recommended in *phthisis*, *aphthæ*, and *cynanche*.

[AKANTICONE. The name of a mineral synonymous with the *epidote* of Haüy, *pistazit* of Werner, *glassy actynolite* of Kirwan, &c. A.]

A'KENSIDE, MARK. An English physician, born at Newcastle-upon-Tyne, in 1721; but more distinguished as a poet, especially for his "Pleasures of the Imagination." After studying at Edinburgh, and graduating at Leyden, he settled in practice; but though appointed physician to the queen, as well as to St. Thomas's Hospital, he is said not to have been very successful. He died of a putrid fever, in his 49th year. He has left a Dissertation on Dysentery in Latin, admired for its elegance; and several small Tracts in the Philosophical and London Medical Transactions.

AL. The Arabian article, which signifies *the;* it is applied to a word by way of eminence, as the Greek *o* is. The Easterns express the superlative by adding *God* thereto, as *the mountain of God*, for the highest mountain; and it is probable that *Al* relates to the word *Alla*, God: so *Alchemy*, may be *the chemistry of God*, or the most exalted perfection of chemical science.

A'LA. 1. The wing of a bird.

2. The arm-pit, so called because it answers to the pit under the wing of a bird.

3. An accidental part of the seed of a plant; consisting of a membraneous prolongation from the side of the seed, and distinguished by the number into

Semina monoterygia: one-winged, as in *Bignonia*.
Dipterygia: two-winged, as in *Betula*.
Tripterygia: three-winged.
Tetrapterygia: four-winged.
Polypterigia: many-winged, or *Molendinacea:* windmill-winged, for so the many-winged seeds of some umbelliferous plants are termed.

4. The two lateral or side petals of a papilionaceous or butterfly-shaped flower.

ALA AURIS. The upper part of the external ear.

ALA INTERNA MINOR. See *Nymphæ*.

ALA NASI. 1. The cartilage of the nose which forms the outer part of the nostrils.

2. The sides of the nose are called *alæ nasi*.

ALA VESPERTILIONIS. That part of the ligament of the womb, which lies between the tubes and the ovarium; so called from its resemblance to the wing of a bat.

ALABASTER. Among the stones which are known by the name of marble, and have been distinguished by a considerable variety of denominations by statuaries and others, whose attention is more directed to their external character and appearance than their component parts, alabasters are those which have a greater or less degree of imperfect transparency, a granular texture, are softer, take a duller polish than marble, and are usually of a white colour. Some stones, however, of a veined and coloured appearance, have been considered as alabasters, from their possessing the first-mentioned criterion; and some transparent and yellow sparry stones have also received this appellation.

[Alabaster is a variety of compact gypsum. It is found in compact masses of a fine grain, whose fracture is even, or splintery, and nearly or quite dull, or sometimes a little foliated. It is nearly opaque, and its colours are commonly white or gray, sometimes shaded with yellow, red, &c. or variously mingled. Its specific gravity is sometimes only 1.87. It is sometimes in concretions.

Compact gypsum, and some varieties of granular gypsum, are employed in sculpture and architecture, under the name of *alabaster*. The same name is also given to certain varieties of carbonate of lime. It may be well to employ the term gypseous and calcareous alabaster.—*Cleav. Min.*

The cabinet of the New-York Lyceum of Natural History contains some very fine specimens of gypseous alabaster, from various parts of the United States. A.]

ALÆFO'RMIS. (*Alæformis;* from *Ala*, a wing, and *forma*, resemblance.) Wing-like. Any thing like a wing.

ALAI'A PHTHI'SIS. (From αλαιος, blind, and φθισις, a wasting.) A consumption from a flux of humours from the head.

[ALALITE. A rare mineral, consisting principally of silex, magnesia, and lime, found in the form of prismatic crystals, otherwise called diopside. A.]

ALANDAHLA. The Arabian for bitter. The bitter apple. See *Cucumis colocynthis*.

ALANFU'TA. An Arabian name of a vein between the chin and lower lip, which was formerly opened to prevent fœtid breath.

ALARIA OSSA. The wing-like processes of the sphenoid bone.

ALA'RIS. (*Alaris;* from *ala*, a wing.) Formed like, or belonging to a wing.

ALARIS EXTERNUS. *Musculus alaris externus.* A name of the external pterygoid muscle; so called because it takes its rise from the wing-like process of the sphenoid bone.

ALARIS VENA. The innermost of the three veins in the bend of the arm.

ALATE'RNUS. A species of rhamnus.

ALA'TUS. (From *ala*, a wing.) Winged. 1 Applied to stems and leaf-stalks, when the edges or angles are longitudinally expanded into leaf-like borders; as in *Ænopordium acanthium; Lathyrus latifolius*, &c. and the leaf-stalk of the orange tribe, citrus, &c

2. One who has prominent scapulæ like the wings of birds.

ALBAGRAS NIGRA. So Avicenna names the *Lepra ichthyosis*, or *Lepra Græcorum*.

ALBAME'NTUM. (From *albus*, white.) The white of an egg.

ALBA'NUM. Urinous salt.

ALBA'TIO. (From *albus*, white.) *Albificati*. The calcination or whitening of metals.

A'LBICANS. (From *albico*, to grow white.) Inclining to white. Whitish.

ALBICA'NTIA CO'RPORA. *Corpora albicantia Willisii.* Two small round bodies or projections from the base of the brain, of a white colour.

ALBIN. A mineral found in Bohemia; so called from its white colour.

ALBI'NUM. See *Gnaphalium dioicum*.

ALBI'NUS BERNARD SIEGFRED, son of a physician, and professor at Leyden of the same name, was born near the end of the 17th century, and prosecuted his studies with so much zeal and success, that he was appointed, on the recommendation of Boerhaave, professor of anatomy and surgery, when only 20 years old. This office he filled for half a century, and acquired a greater reputation than any of his predecessors. He has left several valuable anatomical works; and particularly very accurate descriptions, and plates of the muscles and bones, which are still highly esteemed.

A'LBORA. A sort of itch; or rather of leprosy Paracelsus says, it is a complication of the morphew, serpigo, and leprosy. When cicatrices appear in the face like the serpigo, and then turn to small blisters of the nature of the morphew, it is the albora. It terminates without ulceration, but by fœtid evacuations in the mouth and nostrils; it is also seated in the root of the tongue.

ALBUCA'SIS, an Arabian physician and surgeon of considerable merit, who lived about the beginning of the twelfth century. He has copied much from preceding writers, but added also many original observations; and his works may be still perused with pleasure. He insisted on the necessity of a surgeon being skilled in anatomy to enable him to operate with success, as well as acquainted with the materia medica, that he may apply his remedies with propriety. He appears to have extracted polypi from the nose, and performed the operation of bronchotomy. He is the first who left distinct descriptions and delineations of the instruments used in surgery, and of the manner of employing them.

ALBUGI'NEA. (*Albuginia;* from *albus*, white: so

called on account of its white colour.) The name of a membrane of the eye and of the testicle.

ALBUGINEA OCULI. See *Adnata tunica*.

ALBUGINEA TESTIS. *Tunica albuginea testis*. The innermost coat of the testicle. A strong, white, and dense membrane, immediately covering the body or substance of the testicle. On its outer surface it is smooth, but rough and uneven on the inner. See *Testicle*.

ALBU'GO. A white opacity of the cornea of the eye. The Greeks named it *leucoma;* the Latins, *albugo*, *nebula*, and *nubecula*. Some ancient writers have called it *pterygium*, *janua oculi*, *onyx*, *unguis*, and *ægides*. It is a variety of Cullen's *Caligo corneæ*.

[Albugo, (from *albus*, white.) It is a white opacity of the cornea, not of a superficial kind, but affecting the very substance of this membrane. A.]

ALBUM BALSAMUM. The balsam of copaiba. See *Copaiba*.

ALBUM GRÆCUM. The white dung of dogs. It was formerly applied as a discutient, to the inside of the throat, in quinsies, being first mixed with honey; medicines of this kind have long since justly sunk into disuse.

ALBUM OLUS. See *Valeriana locusta*.

ALBU'MEN. *Albumine*. 1. Coagulable lymph. This substance, which derives its name from the Latin for the white of an egg, in which it exists abundantly, and in its purest natural state, is one of the chief constituent principles of all the animal solids. Beside the white of egg, it abounds in the serum of blood, the vitreous and crystalline humours of the eye, and the fluid of dropsy. Fourcroy claims to himself the honour of having discovered it in the green feculæ of plants in general, particularly in those of the cruciform order, in very young ones, and in the fresh shoots of trees, though Rouelle appears to have detected it there long before. Vauquelin says it exists also in the mineral water of Plombieres.

Seguin has found it in remarkable quantity in such vegetables as ferment without yest, and afford a vinous liquor; and from a series of experiments, he infers, that albumen is the true principle of fermentation, and that its action is more powerful in proportion to its solubility, three different degrees of which he found it to possess.

The chief characteristic of albumen is its coagulability by the action of heat. If the white of an egg be exposed to a heat of about 134° F. white fibres begin to appear in it, and at 160° it coagulates into a solid mass In a heat not exceeding 212 it dries, shrinks, and assumes the appearance of horn. It is soluble in cold water before it has been coagulated, but not after; and when diluted with a very large portion, it does not coagulate easily. Pure alcalies dissolve it, even after coagulation. It is precipitated by muriate of mercury, nitro-muriate of tin, acetate of lead, nitrate of silver, muriate of gold, infusion of galls and tannin. The acids and metallic oxydes coagulate albumen. On the addition of concentrated sulphuric acid, it becomes black, and exhales a nauseous smell. Strong muriatic acid gives a violet tinge to the coagulum, and at length becomes saturated with ammonia. Nitric acid, at 70° F. disengages from it abundance of azotic gas; and if the heat be increased, prussic acid is formed; after which carbonic acid and carburetted hydrogen are evolved, and the residue consists of water containing a little oxalic acid, and covered with a lemon-coloured fat oil. If dry potassa or soda be triturated with albumen, either liquid or solid, ammoniacal gas is evolved, and the calcination of the residuum yields an alcaline prussiate.

On exposure to the atmosphere in a moist state, albumen passes at once to the state of putrefaction.

Solid albumen may be obtained by agitating white of egg with ten or twelve times its weight of alcohol. This seizes the water which held the albumen in solution; and this substance is precipitated under the form of white flocks or filaments, which cohesive attraction renders insoluble, and which consequently may be freely washed with water. Albumen thus obtained is like fibrine, solid, white, insipid, inodorous, denser than water, and without action or vegetable colours. It dissolves in potassa and soda more easily than fibrine; but in acetic acid and ammonia, with more difficulty. When these two animal principles are separately dissolved in potassa, muriatic acid added to the albuminous, does not disturb the solution, but it produces a cloud in the other.

Fourcroy and several other chemists have ascribed the characteristic coagulation of albumen by heat to its oxygenation. But cohesive attraction is the real cause of the phenomenon. In proportion as the temperature rises, the particles of water and albumen recede from each other, their affinity diminishes, and then the albumen precipitates. However, by uniting albumen with a large quantity of water, we diminish its coagulating property to such a degree, that heat renders the solution merely opalescent. A new-laid egg yields a soft coagulum by boiling; but when, by keeping, a portion of the water has transuded so as to leave a void space within the shell, the concentrated albumen affords a firm coagulum.

An *analogous phenomenon* is exhibited by acetate of alumina, a solution of which, being heated, gives a precipitate in flakes, which re-dissolve as the caloric which separated the particles of acid and base escapes, or as the temperature falls. A solution containing 1-10 of dry albumen forms by heat a solid *coagulum;* but when it contains only 1-15, it gives a glary liquid. One-thousandth part, however, on applying heat, occasions opalescence. Putrid white of egg, and the *pus* of ulcers, have a similar smell. According to Dr. Bostock, a drop of a saturated solution of corrosive sublimate let fall into water containing 1-2000 of albumen, occasions a milkiness and curdy precipitate. On adding a slight excess of the mercurial solution to the albuminous liquid, and applying heat, the precipitate which falls, being dried, contains in every 7 parts 5 of albumen. Hence that salt is the most delicate test of this animal product. The yellow pitchy precipitate occasioned by tannin, is brittle when dried, and not liable to putrefaction. But tannin, or infusion of galls, is a much nicer test of gelatin than of albumen.

The cohesive attraction of coagulated albumen makes it resist putrefaction. In this state it may be kept for weeks under water without suffering change. By long digestion in weak nitric acid, albumen seems convertible into gelatin. By the analysis of Gay Lussac and Thénard, 100 parts of albumen are formed of 52.883 carbon, 23.872 oxygen, 7.540 hydrogen, 15.705 nitrogen; or, in other terms, of 52.883 carbon, 27.127 oxygen and hydrogen. in the proportion for constituting water, 15.705 nitrogen, and, 4.285 hydrogen in excess. The negative pole of a voltaic pile in high activity coagulates albumen; but if the pile be feeble, coagulation goes on only at the positive surface. Albumen, in such a state of concentration as it exists in serum of blood, can dissolve some metallic oxydes, particularly the protoxide of iron. Orfila has found white of egg to be the best antidote to the poisonous effects of corrosive sublimate on the human stomach. As albumen occasions precipitates with the solutions of almost every metallic salt, probably it may act beneficially against other species of mineral poison.

From its coagulability albumen is of great use in clarifying liquids.

It is likewise remarkable for the property of rendering leather supple, for which purpose a solution of whites of eggs in water is used by leather-dressers.—*Ure's Chem. Dict.*

2. In botany, the term *albumen* is applied to a farinaceous, fleshy, or horny substance, which makes up the chief bulk of some seeds, as grapes, corn, palms, lilies, never rising out of the ground, nor assuming the office of leaves, being destined solely to nourish the germinating embryo, till its roots perform their office. In the date palm, this part is nearly as hard as stone, in *mirabilis* it is like wheat-flour. It is wanting in several tribes of plants, as those with compound or with cruciform flowers, and the cucumber or gourd kind, according to Gardner. Some few leguminous plants have it, and a great number of others, which, like them, have cotyledons besides. We are not, however, to suppose, that so important an organ is altogether wanting, even in the above-mentioned plants. The farinaceous matter destined to nourish their embryos, is unquestionably lodged in their cotyledons, the sweet taste of which, as they begin to germinate, often evinces its presence, and that it has undergone the same change as in barley. The albumen of the nutmeg is remarkable for its eroded variegated appearance, and aromatic quality; the cotyledons of this plant are very small.—*Smith.*

Albumen ovi. *Albugo ovi; Albumen albor ovi; Ovi albus liquor; Ovi candidum albumentum; Clareta.* The white of an egg.

ALBURNUM. (From *albus*, white.) The soft white substance, which, in trees, is found between the liber, or inner bark, and the wood. In process of time it acquires solidity, becoming itself the wood. While soft, it performs a very important part of the functions of growth, which ceases when it becomes hard. A new circle of alburnum is annually formed over the old, so that a transverse section of the trunk presents a pretty correct register of the tree's age, each zone marking one year. From its colour and comparative softness, it has been called by some writers, the *adeps arborum.* The alburnum is found in largest quantities in trees that are vigorous. In an oak six inches in diameter, this substance is nearly equal in bulk to the wood.

A'LBUS, White. This term is applied to many parts, from their white colour; as *linea alba, lepra alba, macula alba*, &c.

A'LCAHEST. An Arabic word to express a universal dissolvent, which was pretended to by Paracelsus and Van Helmont. Some say that Paracelsus first used this word, and that it is derived from the German words *al* and *geest*, i. e. *all spirit:* and that Van Helmont borrowed the word, and applied it to his invention, which he called the universal dissolvent.

A'LCALI. (Arabian.) This word is spelt indifferently with a *c* or a *k*. See *Alkali.*

ALCALIZATION. The impregnating any spirituous fluid with an alcali.

ALCANNA. (Indian word.) See *Anchusa.*

A'lcaol. The solvent for the preparation of the philosopher's stone.

ALCARRAZES. A species of porous pottery made in Spain.

A'LCEA. (*Alcea, æ.* f.; from αλκη, strength.) The name of a genus of plants in the Linnæan system. Class, *Monadelphia;* Order, *Polyandria.* Hollyhock.

Alcea Ægyptiaca villosa. See *Hibiscus Abelmoschus.*

Alcea Indica. See *Hibiscus Abelmoschus.*

Alcea rosea. Common hollyhock. The flowers of this beautiful tree are said to possess adstringent and mucilaginous virtues. They are seldom used medicinally.

Alchemia. See *Alchemy.*

ALCHEMI'LLA. (*Alchemilla, æ.* f. So called because it was celebrated by the old alchemists.)

1. The name of a genus of plants in the Linnæan system. Class, *Tetrandria;* Order, *Monogynia.* Ladies' mantle.

2. The pharmacopœial name of the plant called ladies' mantle. Sea *Alchemilla vulgaris.*

Alchemilla vulgaris. Ladies' mantle. This plant, *Alchemilla:—Foliis lobatis* of Linnæus, was formerly esteemed as an adstringent in hæmorrhages, fluor albus, &c. given internally. It is fallen into disuse.

ALCHEMIST. One who practises the mystical art of alchemy.

A'LCHEMY. *Alchemia; Alchimia; Alkima.* That branch of chemistry which relates to the transmutation of metals into gold;—the forming a panacea or universal remedy,—an alcahest, or universal menstruum,—a universal ferment, and many other absurdities.

Alchimia. See *Alchemy.*

ALCHIMI'LLA. See *Alchemilla.*

A'lchitron. 1. Oil of Juniper.

2. Also the name of a dentifrice of Messue.

A'LCHYMY. Alchemy.

A'LCOHOL. See *Alkohol.*

ALCYO'NIUM. It is difficult to say what the Greeks called by this name. Dioscorides speaks of five sorts of it. It is a spongy plant-like substance, met with on the sea-shore, of different shapes and colours. This bastard sponge is calcined with a little salt, as a dentifrice, and is used to remove spots on the skin.

ALDER. See *Betula alnus.*

Alder, berry-bearing. See *Rhamnus frangula.*

Alder wine. See *Betula alnus.*

Aldrum. See *Alzum.*

Aldum. See *Alzum.*

ALE. *Cerevisia; Liquor cereris; Vinum hordeaceum.* A fermented liquor made from malt and hops, and chiefly distinguished from beer, made from the same ingredients, by the quantity of hops used therein, which is greater in beer, and therefore renders the liquor more bitter, and fitter for keeping. Ale, when well fermented, is a wholesome beverage, but seems to disagree with those subject to asthma, or any disorder of the respiration, or irregularity in the digestive organs. The old dispensatories enumerate several medicated ales, such as *cerevisia oxydorica*, for the eyes; *cerevisia antiarthritica*, against the gout; *cephalica, epileptica*, &c. See *Beer.*

ALEI'ON. (Αλειον, copious.) Hippocrates uses this word as an epithet for water.

ALEI'PHA. (From αλειφω, to anoint.) Any medicated oil.

ALELAI'ON. (From αλς, salt, and ελαιον, oil.) Oil beat up with salt, to apply to tumours. Galen frequently used it.

ALE'MA. (From α. priv. and λιμος, hunger.) Meat, food, or any thing that satisfies the appetite.

ALE'MBIC. (*Alembicus.* Some derive it from the Arabian particle *al*, and αμβιξ; from αμβαινω, to ascend. Avicenna declares it to be Arabian.) Moorshead. A chemical utensil made of glass, metal, or earthenware, and adapted to receive volatile products from retorts. It consists of a body to which is fitted a conical head, and out of this head descends laterally a beak to be inserted into the receiver.

ALE'MBROTH. (A Chaldee word, importing the key of art.) 1. Some explain it as the name of a salt, *sal mercurii*, or *sal philosophorum & artis;* others say it is named *alembrot* and *sal fusionis* or *sal fixionis* *Alembroth desiccatum* is said to be the *sal tartari*, hence this word seems to signify alkaline salt, which opens the bodies of metals by destroying their sulphurs, and promoting their separation from the ores. From analogy, it is supposed to have the same effect in conquering obstructions and attenuating viscid fluids in the human body.

2. A peculiar earth, probably containing a fixed alkali, found in the island of Cyprus, has also this appellation.

3. A solution of the corrosive sublimate, to which the muriate of ammonia has been added, is called sal alembroth.

Alepe'nsis. A species of ash-tree, which produces manna.

A'les. (From αλς, salt.) A compound salt.

Aleu'ron. (From αλεω, to grind.) Meal.

ALEXANDERS See *Smyrnium olusatrum.*

Alexanders, round-leaved. See *Smyrnium perfoliatum.*

ALEXA'NDRIA. (*Alexandria.*) *Alexandrina.* The bay-tree, or laurel, of Alexandria.

Alexa'ndrium. *Emplastrum viride.* A plaster described by Celsus, made with wax, alum, &c.

ALEXICA'CUM. (From αλεξω, to drive away, and κακον, evil.) An antidote or amulet, to resist poison.

ALEXIPHA'RMIC. (*Alexipharmicum;* from αλεξω, to expel, and φαρμακον, a poison.) *Antipharmicum; Caco-alexiteria.* A medicine supposed to preserve the body against the power of poisons, or to correct or expel those taken. The ancients attributed this property to some vegetables and even waters distilled from them. The term, however, is now very seldom used.

ALEXIPYRE'TICUM. (From αλεξω, to drive away, and πυρετος, fever.) A febrifuge.

ALEXIPY'RETOS. *Alexipyretum.* A remedy for a fever.

Ale'xir. An elixir.

ALEXITE'RIUM. (*Alexiterium, i.* n.; from αλεξω, to expel, and τηρεω, to preserve.) A preservative medicine against poison, or contagion.

ALGA. A sea-weed.

Algæ. 1. The name of an *order* or division of the class *Cryptogamia* in the Linnæan system of plants. The name of one of the seven *families* or natural tribes into which the whole vegetable kingdom is divided by Linnæus in his Philosophia Botanica. He defines them plants, the roots, leaves, and stems of which are all in one. Under this description are comprehended all the sea-weeds and some other aquatic plants.

2. In the sexual system of plants *Algæ* constitute the third *order* of the class, Cryptogamia. From their admitting of little distinction of root, leaf, or stem, and

the parts of their flowers being equally incapable of description, the genera are distinguished by the situation of what is supposed to be the flowers or seeds, or by the resemblance which the whole plant bears to some other substance.

The parts of fructification of the algæ are in *calycules* of which there are three varieties:—

1. *Pelta*, target; a flat, oblong fruit, seen in the *Lichen caninus*.

2. *Scutella*, the saucer; a round, hollow, or flat fruit, as in *Lichen stellaris*.

3 *Tuberculum*, the tubercle; a hemispherical fruit, observable in *Lichen geographicus*.

In the fuci, the parts of fructification are sometimes in hollow bladders; and in some of the ulvæ, it is dispersed through the whole substance of the plant.

A'LGAROTH. (So called from Victorius Algaroth, a physician of Verona, and its inventor.) *Algarot; Algaroth; Mercurius vitæ; Pulvis Algarothi; Pulvis angelicus· Mercurius mortis.* The antimonial part of the butter of antimony, separated from some of its acid by washing it in water. It is violently emetic in doses of two or three grains, and is preferred by many for making the emetic tartar.

ALGE'DO. (From αλγος, pain.) A violent pain about the anus, perinæum, testes, urethra, and bladder, arising from the sudden stoppage of a virulent gonorrhœa. A term very seldom used.

ALGE'MA. (From αλγεω, to be in pain.) *Algemodes; Algematodes.* Uneasiness; pain of any kind.

A'LGOR. A sudden chilliness or rigour.

ALGOSAREL. The Arabian term for the wild carrot. See *Daucus sylvestris*.

ALHA'GI. (Arabian.) A species of *Hedysarum.* The leaves are hot and pungent, the flowers purgative.

ALHA'NDALA. An Arabian name for the colocynth, or bitter apple.

ALHA'SEF. (Arabian.) *Alhasaf.* A sort of fœtid pustule, called also *Hydroa*.

A'LIA SQUILLA. (From αλιος, belonging to the sea, and σκιλλα, a shrimp.) The prawn. A species of the genus *cancer*.

A'LICA. (From *alo*, to nourish) In general signification, a grain, a sort of food admired by the ancients. It is not certain whether it is a grain or a preparation of some kind thereof.

ALICASTRUM. (From *alica*, as *siliquastrum* from *siliqua*.) A kind of bread mentioned by Celsus.

A'LICES. (From αλιζω, to sprinkle.) Little red spots in the skin, which precede the eruption of pustules in the small-pox.

ALIENA'TIO MENTIS. Estrangement of the mind.

ALIENA'TION. (*Alienatio;* from *alieno*, to estrange.) A term applied to any wandering of the mind.

ALIENA'TUS. Alienated. A leaf is so termed when the first leaves give way to others totally different from them, and the natural habit of the genus, as is the case in many of the *mimosæ* from New Holland.

ALIFO'RMIS. Alæform, or wing-like. A name given by anatomists and naturalists to some parts from their supposed resemblance, as aliform muscles, &c. See *Alæformis*.

ALIMENT. (*Alimentum;* from *alo*, to nourish.) The name of aliment is given generally to every substance, which being subjected to the action of the organs of digestion, is capable by itself of affording nourishment. In this sense an aliment is extracted necessarily from vegetables or animals: for only those bodies that have possessed life are capable of serving usefully in the nutrition of animals during a certain time. This manner of regarding aliments appears rather too confined. Why refuse the name of aliments to substances which, in reality, cannot of themselves afford nourishment, but which contribute efficaciously to nutrition, since they enter into the composition of the organs, and of the animal fluids? Such are the muriate of soda, the oxyde of iron, silicia, and particularly water, which is found in such abundance in the bodies of animals, and is so necessary to them. It appears preferable to consider as an aliment every substance which can serve in nutrition; establishing, however, the important distinction between substances which can nourish of themselves, and those which are useful to nutrition only in concert with the former.

In respect to their nature, aliments are different from each other, by the proximate principles which predominate in their composition. They may be distinguished into nine classes:—

1st, Farinaceous aliments: wheat, barley, oats, rice, rye, maize, potato, sago, salep, peas, haricots, lentils, &c.

2d, Mucilaginous aliments: carrots, salsafy, (goats-beard) beet-root, turnip, asparagus, cabbage, lettuce, artichoke, cardoons, pompions, melons, &c.

3d, Sweet aliments: the different sorts of sugar figs, dates, dried grapes, apricots, &c.

4th, Acidulous aliments: oranges, gooseberries, cherries, peaches, strawberries, raspberries, mulberries, grapes, prunes, pears, apples, sorrel, &c.

5th, Fatty and oily aliments: cocoa, olives, sweet almonds, nuts, walnuts, the animal fats, the oils, butter, &c.

6th, Caseous aliments: the different sorts of milk, cheese, &c.

7th, Gelatinous aliments: the tendons, the aponeurosis, the chorion, the cellular membrane, young animals, &c.

8th, Albuminous aliments: the brain, the nerves, eggs, &c.

9th, Fibrinous aliments: the flesh and the blood of different animals.

We might add to this list a great number of substances that are employed as medicines, but which doubtless are nutritive, at least in some of their immediate principles; such are manna, tamarinds, the *pulp of cassia*, the extracts and saps of vegetables, the animal or vegetable decoctions.

Among aliments there are few employed such as nature presents them; they are generally prepared, and disposed in such a manner as to be suitable to the action of the digestive organs. The preparations which they undergo are infinitely various, according to the sort of aliment, the people, the climates, customs, the degree of civilization: even fashion is not without its influence on the art of preparing aliments.

In the hand of the skilful cook, alimentary substances almost entirely change their nature:—form, consistence, odour, taste, colour, composition, &c., every thing is so modified that it is impossible for the most delicate tastes to recognise the original substance of certain dishes.

The useful object of cookery is to render aliments agreeable to the senses, and of easy digestion; but it rarely stops here: frequently with people advanced in civilization its object is to excite delicate palates, or difficult tastes, or to please vanity. Then, far from being a useful art, it becomes a real scourge, which occasions a great number of diseases, and has frequently brought on premature death.

We understand by *drink*, a liquid which, being introduced into the digestive organs, quenches thirst, and so by this repairs the habitual losses of our fluid humours: the drinks ought to be considered as real aliments.

The drinks are distinguished by their chemical composition:—

1st, Water of different sorts, spring water, river water, water of wells, &c.

2d, The juices and infusions of vegetables and animals, juices of lemon, of gooseberries, whey, tea, coffee, &c.

3d, Fermented liquors: the different sorts of wine, beer, cider, perry, &c.

4th, The alcoholic liquors: brandy, alcohol, ether, rum, sack, ratafia.

ALIMENTARY *Alimentarius.* Nourishing or belonging to food.

ALIMENTARY CANAL. *Canalis alimentarius.* Alimentary duct. A name given to the whole of those passages which the food passes through from the mouth to the anus. This duct may be said to be the true characteristic of an animal; there being no animal without it, and whatever has it, being properly ranged under the class of animals. Plants receive their nourishment by the numerous fibres of their roots, but have no common receptacle for digesting the food received, or for carrying off the excrements. But in all, even the lowest degree of animal life, we may observe a stomach, if not also intestines, even where we cannot perceive the least formation of any organs of the senses, unless that common one of feeling, as in oysters.

Alimentary duct. 1. The alimentary canal. See *Alimentary canal.*

2. The thoracic duct is sometimes so called. See *Thoracic duct.*

Alimos. Common liquorice.

A'limum. A species of arum.

Alipa'sma. (From αλειφω, to anoint.) An ointment rubbed upon the body to prevent sweating.

Alipow. A species of turbith, found near Mount Ceti, in Languedoc. It is a powerful purgative, used instead of senna, but is much more active.

ALI'PTÆ. (From αλειφω, to anoint.) Those who anointed persons after bathing.

Alisanders. The same as alexanders.

ALI'SMA. (*Alisma;* from αλς, the sea.) The name of a genus of plants in the Linnæan system. Class, *Hexandria;* Order, *Polygynia.* Water-plantain.

Alisma plantago aquatica. The systematic name of the water-plantain, now fallen into disuse.

A'lit. *Alith.* Asafœtida.

A'lkahat glaube'ri. An alkaline salt.

A'lkahest. An imaginary universal menstruum, or solvent. See *Alcahest.*

A'lkahest glaube'ri. An alkaline salt.

ALKALESCENT. *Alkalescens.* Any substance in which alkaline properties are beginning to be developed, or to predominate, is so termed.

A'LKALI. (*Alcali,* in Arabic, signifies burnt; or from *al* and *kali,* i. e. the essence, or the whole of kali, the plant from which it was originally prepared, though now derived from plants of every kind. *Alcali; alifi; alafor; alafort; calcadis.*

Alkalies may be defined, those bodies which combine with acids, so as to neutralize or impair their activity, and produce salts. Acidity and alkalinity are therefore two correlative terms of one species of combination. When Lavoisier introduced oxygen as the acidifying principle, Morveau proposed hydrogen as the alkalifying principle, from its being a constituent of volatile alcali or ammonia. But the splendid discovery by Sir H. Davy, of the metallic basis of potassa and soda, and of their conversion into alkalies, by combination with oxygen, has banished for ever that hypothetical conceit. It is the mode in which the constituents are combined, rather than the nature of the constituents themselves, which gives rise to the acid or alkaline condition. Some metals combined with oxygen in one proportion, produce a body possessed of alkaline properties; in another proportion, of acid properties. And on the other hand, ammonia and prussic acid prove that both the alkaline and acid conditions can exist independent of oxygen. These observations, by generalizing our notions of acids and alkalies, have rendered the definitions of them very imperfect. The difficulty of tracing a limit between the acids and alkalies is still increased, when we find a body sometimes performing the functions of an acid, sometimes of an alkali. Nor can we diminish this difficulty by having recourse to the beautiful law discovered by Sir H. Davy, that oxygen and acids go to the positive pole, and hydrogen alkalies, and inflammable bases to the negative pole. We cannot in fact give the name of acid to all the bodies which go to the first of these poles, and that of alkali to those that go to the second; and if we wished to define the alkalies by bringing into view their electric energy, it would be necessary to compare them with the electric energy which is opposite to them. Thus we are always reduced to define alkalinity by the property which it has of saturating acidity, because alkalinity and acidity are two correlative and inseparable terms. M. Gay Lussac conceives the alkalinity which the metallic oxides enjoy, to be the result of two opposite properties, the alkalifying property of the metal, and the acidifying of oxygen, modified both by the combination and by the proportions.

The alkalies may be arranged into three classes: 1st, Those which consist of a metallic basis combined with oxygen. These are three in number, potassa, soda, and lithia. 2d, That which contains no oxygen, viz. ammonia. 3d, Those containing oxygen, hydrogen, and carbon. In this class we have aconita, atropia, brucia, cicuta, datura, delphia, hyosciama, morphia, strychnia, and perhaps some other *truly vegetable* alkalies. The order of vegetable alkalies may be as numerous as that of vegetable acids. The earths, lime, barytes, and strontites, were enrolled among the alkalies by Fourcroy, but they have been kept apart by other systematic writers, and are called alkaline earths.

Besides neutralizing acidity, and thereby giving birth to salts, the first four alkalies having the following properties:—

1st, They change the purple colour of many vegeta bles to a green, the reds to a purple, and the yellows to a brown. If the purple have been reddened by acid, alkalies restore the purple.

2d, They possess this power on vegetable colours *after* being saturated with carbonic acid, by which criterion they are distinguishable from the akaline earths.

3d, They have an acrid and urinous taste.

4th, They are powerful solvents or corrosives of animal matter; with which, as well as with oils in general, they combine, so as to produce neutrality.

5th, They are decomposed, or volatilized, at a strong red heat.

6th, They combine with water in every proportion, and also largely with alcohol.

7th, They continue to be soluble in water when neu tralized with carbonic acid; while the alkaline earths thus become insoluble.

It is needless to detail at length Dr. Murray's specu lations on alkalinity. They seem to flow from a pa. tial view of chemical phenomena. According to him either oxygen or hydrogen may generate alkalinity, but the combination of both principles is necessary to give this condition its utmost energy. "Thus the class of alkalies will exhibit the same relations as the class of acids. Some are compounds of a base with oxygen; such are the greater number of the metallic oxydes, and probably of the earths. Ammonia is a compound of a base with hydrogen. Potassa, soda, barytes, strontites, and probably lime, are compounds of bases with oxygen and hydrogen; and these last, like the analogous order among the acids, possess the highest power." Now, perfectly dry and caustic ba rytes, lime, and strontites, as well as the dry potassa and soda obtained by Gay Lussac and Thenard, are not inferior in alkaline power to the same bodies after they are slacked or combined with water. 100 parts of lime destitute of hydrogen, that is, pure oxyde of calcium, neutralize 78 parts of carbonic acid. But 132 parts of Dr. Murray's *strongest* lime, that is, the hydrate, are required to produce the same alkaline effect. If we ignite nitrate of barytes, we obtain, as is well known, a perfectly dry barytes, or protoxide of barium; but if we ignite crystallized barytes, we obtain the same alkaline earth combined with a prime equivalent of water. These two different states of barytes were demonstrated by M. Berthollet in an excellent paper published in the 2d volume of the Memoirs D'Arcueil, so far back as 1809. "The first barytes," (that from crystallized barytes) says he, "presents all the characters of a combination; it is engaged with a substance which *diminishes* its action on other bodies, which renders it more fusible, and which gives it by fusion the appearance of glass. This substance is nothing else but water; but in fact, by adding a little water to the second barytes (that from ignited nitrate) and by urging it at the fire, we give it the properties of the first." Page 47. 100 parts of barytes void of hydrogen, or dry barytes, neutralize 28 1-2 of dry carbonic acid. Whereas 111 2-3 parts of the hydrate, or what Dr. Murray has styled the most energetic, are required to produce the same effect. In fact, it is not hydrogen which combines with the pure barytic earth, but hydrogen and oxygen in the state of water. The proof of this is, that when carbonic acid and that hydrate unite, the exact quantity of water is disengaged. The protoxide of barium, or pure barytes, has never been combined with hydrogen by any chemist.—*Ure's Chem. Dict.*

Alkali causticum. Caustic alkali. An alkali is so called when deprived of the carbonic acid it usually contains, for it then becomes more caustic, and more violent in its action.

Alkali, caustic volatile. See *Ammonia.*

Alkali, phlogisticated. Prussian alkali. When a fixed alkali is ignited with bullock's blood, or other animal substances, and lixiviated, it is found to be in a great measure saturated with prussic acid: from the theories formerly adopted respecting this combination, it was called phlogisticated alkali.

Alkali fixum. Fixed alkali. Those alkalies are

so called that emit no characteristic smell, and cannot be volatilized, but with the greatest difficulty. Two kinds of fixed alkalies have only hitherto been made known, namely potassa and soda. See *Potassa* and *Soda*.

Alkali, fossile. See *Soda.*

Alkali, mineral. See *Soda.*

Alkali, Prussian. See *Alkali, phlogisticated.*

Alkali, vegetable. See *Potassa.*

Alkali, volatile. See *Ammonia.*

ALKALI'NA. Alkalines. A class of substances described by Cullen as comprehending the substances otherwise termed *antacida.* They consist of alkalies, and other substances which neutralize acids. The principal alkalines in use, are the carbonates and subcarbonates of soda and potassa, the subcarbonate of ammonia, lime-water, chalk, magnesia and its carbonate.

ALKALIZATION. *Alkalizatio.* The impregnating any thing with an alkaline salt, as spirit of wine, &c.

ALKALOMETER. The name of an instrument for determining the quantity of alkali in commercial potassa and soda.

A'LKANET. (*Alkanah*, a reed, Arabian.) See *Anchusa tinctoria.*

ALKA'NNA. See *Anchusa.*

ALKA'NNA VE'RA. See *Lawsonia inermis.*

ALKEKE'NGI. (Arabian.) The winter-cherry. See *Physalis alkekengi.*

ALKE'RMES. A term borrowed from the Arabs, denoting a celebrated remedy, of the form and consistence of a confection, whereof the kermes is the basis. See *Kermes.*

ALKIMA. See *Alchemy.*

A'LKOHOL. (An Arabian word, which signifies antimony: so called from the usage of the Eastern ladies to paint their eyebrows with antimony, reduced to a most subtile powder; whence it at last came to signify any thing exalted to its highest perfection.) *Alcohol; Alkol; Spiritus vinosus rectificatus; Spiritus vini rectificatus; spiritus vini concentratus; Spiritus vini rectificatissimus.*

1. This term is applied in strictness only to the pure spirit obtainable by distillation and subsequent rectification from all liquids that have undergone vinous fermentation, and from none but such as are susceptible of it. But it is commonly used to signify this *spirit* more or less imperfectly freed from water, in the state in which it is usually met with in the shops, and in which, as it was first obtained from the juice of the grape, it was long distinguished by the name of spirit of wine. At present it is extracted chiefly from grain or molasses in Europe, and from the juice of the sugar cane in the West Indies; and in the diluted state in which it commonly occurs in trade, constitutes the basis of the several spirituous liquors called brandy, rum, gin, whiskey, and cordials, however variously denominated or disguised.

As we are not able to compound alkohol immediately from its ultimate constituents, we have recourse to the process of fermentation, by which its principles are first extricated from the substances in which they were combined, and then united into a new compound; to distillation, by which this new compound, the alkohol, is separated in a state of dilution with water, and contaminated with essential oil; and to rectification, by which it is ultimately freed from these.

It appears to be essential to the fermentation of alkohol, that the fermenting fluid should contain saccharine matter, which is indispensable to that species of fermentation called vinous. In France, where a great deal of wine is made, particularly at the commencement of the vintage, that is too weak to be a saleable commodity, it is a common practice to subject this wine to distillation, in order to draw off the spirit; and as the essential oil that rises in this process is of a more pleasant flavour than that of malt or molasses, the French brandies are preferred to any other; though even in the flavour of these there is a difference, according to the wine from which they are produced. In the West Indies a spirit is obtained from the juice of the sugar-cane, which is highly impregnated with its essential oil, and well known by the name of *rum.* The distillers in this country use grain, or molasses, whence they distinguish the products by the name of *malt spirits*, and *molasses spirits.* It is said that a very good spirit may be extracted from the husks of gooseberries or currants, after wine has been made from them.

As the process of malting developes the saccharine principle of grain, it would appear to render it fitter for the purpose; though it is the common practice to use about three parts of raw grain with one of malt. For this two reasons may be assigned: by using raw grain, the expense of malting is saved, as well as the duty on malt; and the process of malting requires some nicety of attention, since, if it be carried too far, part of the saccharine matter is lost, and if it be stopped too soon, this matter will not be wholly developed. Besides, if the malt be dried too quickly, or by any unequal heat, the spirit it yields will be less in quantity, and more unpleasant in flavour. Another object of economical consideration is, what grain will afford the most spirit in proportion to its price, as well as the best in quality. Barley appears to produce less spirit than wheat; and if three parts of raw wheat be mixed with one of malted barley, the produce is said to be particularly fine. This is the practice of the distillers in Holland for producing a spirit of the finest quality; but in England they are expressly prohibited from using more than one part of wheat to two of other grain. Rye, however, affords still more spirit than wheat.

Other articles have been employed, though not generally, for the fabrication of spirit, as carrots and potatoes; and we are lately informed by Professor Proust, that from the fruit of the carob tree he has obtained good brandy in the proportion of a pint from five pounds of the dried fruit.

To obtain pure alkohol, different processes have been recommended; but the purest rectified spirit obtained as above described, being that which is least contaminated with foreign matter, should be employed. Rouelle recommends to draw off half the spirit in a water bath; to rectify this twice more, drawing off two-thirds each time; to add water to this alkohol, which will turn it milky by separating the essential oil remaining in it; to distil the spirit from this water; and finally rectify it by one more distillation.

Baumé sets apart the first running, when about a fourth is come over, and continues the distillation till he has drawn off about as much more, or till the liquor runs off milky. The last running he puts into the still again, and mixes the first half of what comes over with the preceding first product. This process is again repeated, and all the first products being mixed together, are distilled afresh. When about half the liquor is come over, this is to be set apart as pure alkohol.

Alkohol in this state, however, is not so pure as when, to use the language of the old chemists, it has been *dephlegmated*, or still further freed from water, by means of some alkaline salt. Boerhaave recommended, for this purpose, the muriate of soda, deprived of its water of crystallization by heat, and added hot to the spirit. But the subcarbonate of potassa is preferable. About a third of the weight of the alkohol should be added to it in a glass vessel, well shaken, and then suffered to subside. The salt will be moistened by the water absorbed from the alkohol; which being decanted, more of the salt is to be added, and this is to be continued till the salt falls dry to the bottom of the vessel. The alkohol in this state will be reddened by a portion of the pure potassa, which it will hold in solution, from which it must be freed by distillation in a water bath. Dry muriate of lime may be substituted advantageously for the alkali.

As alkohol is much lighter than water, its specific gravity is adopted as the test of its purity. Fourcroy considers it as rectified to the highest point when its specific gravity is 829, that of water being 1000; and perhaps this is nearly as far as it can be carried by the process of Rouelle or Baumé simply. Bories found the first measure that came over from twenty of spirit at 836 to be 820, at the temperature of 71° F. Sir Charles Blagden, by the addition of alkali, brought it to 813, at 60° F. Chaussier professes to have reduced it to 798; but he gives 998.35 as the specific gravity of water. Lowitz asserts that he has obtained it at 791, by adding as much alkali as nearly to absorb the spirit; but the temperature is not indicated. In the shops, it is about 835 or 840: according to the London College it should be 815.

It is by no means an easy undertaking to determine

the strength or relative value of spirits, even with sufficient accuracy for commercial purposes. The following requisites must be obtained before this can be well done: the specific gravity of a certain number of mixtures of alcohol and water must be taken so near each other, as that the intermediate specific gravities may not perceptibly differ from those deduced from the supposition of a mere mixture of the fluids; the expansions or variations of specific gravity in these mixtures must be determined at different temperatures; some easy method must be contrived of determining the presence and quantity of saccharine or oleaginous matter which the spirit may hold in solution, and the effect of such solution on the specific gravity; and lastly, the specific gravity of the fluid must be ascertained by a proper floating instrument with a graduated stem or set of weights; or, which may be more convenient, with both.

The most remarkable characteristic property of alkohol, is its solubility or combination in all proportions with water; a property possessed by no other combustible substance, except the acetic spirit obtained by distilling the dry acetates. When it is burned in a chimney which communicates with the worm-pipe of a distilling apparatus, the product, which is condensed, is found to consist of water, which exceeds the spirit in weight about one-eighth part; or more accurately, 100 parts of alkohol, by combustion, yield 136 of water. If alkohol be burned in closed vessels with vital air, the product is found to be water and carbonic acid. Whence it is inferred that alkohol consists of hydrogen, united either to carbonic acid, or its acidifiable base; and that the oxygen uniting on the one part with the hydrogen, forms water; and on the other with the base of the carbonic acid, forms that acid.

The most exact experiments on this subject are those recently made by De Saussure. The alkohol he used had, at 62.8°, a specific gravity or 0.8302; and by Richter's proportions, it consists of 13.8 water, and 86.2 of absolute alkohol. The vapour of alkohol was made to traverse a narrow porcelain tube ignited; from which the products passed along a glass tube about six feet in length, refrigerated by ice. A little charcoal was deposited in the porcelain, and a trace of oil in the glass tube. The resulting gas being analyzed in an exploding eudiometer, with oxygen, was found to resolve itself into carbonic acid and water. Three volumes of oxygen disappeared for every two volumes of carbonic acid produced; a proportion which obtains in the analysis by oxygenation of olefiant gas. Now, as nothing resulted but a combustible gas of this peculiar constitution, and condensed water equal to 1000-4064 of the original weight of the alkohol, we may conclude that vapour of water and olefiant gas are the sole constituents of alkohol. Subtracting the 13.8 per cent. of water in the alkohol at the beginning of the experiment, the absolute alcohol of Richter will consist of 13.7 hydrogen, 51.98 carbon, and 34.32 oxygen. Hence Gay Lussac infers, that alkohol, in vapour, is composed of one volume olefiant gas, and one volume of the vapour of water, condensed by chemical affinity into one volume.

The sp. gr. of olefiant gas is................	0.97804
of aqueous vapour is............	0.62500
Sum=	1.60304
And alkoholic vapour is=	1.6133

These numbers approach nearly to those which would result from two prime equivalents of olefiant gas, combined with one of water; or ultimately, three of hydrogen, two of carbon, and one of oxygen.

The mutual action between alkohol and acids produces a light, volatile, and inflammable substance, called æther. Pure alkalies unite with spirit of wine, and form alkaline tinctures. Few of the neutral salts unite with this fluid, except such as contain ammonia. The carbonated fixed alkalies are not soluble in it. From the strong attraction which exists between alkohol and water, it unites with this last in saline solutions, and in most cases precipitates the salt. This is a pleasing experiment, which never fails to surprise those who are unacquainted with chemical effects. If, for example, a saturated solution of nitre in water be taken, and an equal quantity of strong spirit of wine be poured upon it, the mixture will constitute a weaker spirit, which is incapable of holding the nitre in solution; it therefore falls to the bottom instantly, in the form of minute crystals.

The degree of solubility of many neutral salts in alkohol have been ascertained by experiments made by Macquer, of which an account is published in the Memoirs of the Turin Academy.

All deliquescent salts are soluble in alkohol. Alkohol holding the strontitic salts in solution, gives a flame of a rich purple. The cupreous salts and boracic acid give a green; the soluble calcareous, a reddish; the barytic, a yellowish.

The alkohol of 0.825 has been subjected to a cold of −91° without congealing.

When potassium and sodium are put in contact with the strongest alkohol, hydrogen is evolved. When chlorine is made to pass through alkohol in a Woolfe's apparatus, there is a mutual action. Water, an oily-looking substance, muriatic acid, a little carbonic acid and carbonaceous matter, are the products. This oily substance does not redden turnsole, though its analysis by heat shows it to contain muriatic acid. It is white, denser than water, has a cooling taste analogous to mint, and a peculiar, but not æthereous odour. It is very soluble in alkohol, but scarcely in water. The strongest alkalies hardly operate on it.

It was at one time maintained, that alkohol did not exist in wines, but was generated and evolved by the heat of distillation. On this subject Gay Lussac made some decisive experiments. He agitated wine with litharge in fine powder, till the liquid became as limpid as water, and then saturated it with subcarbonate of potassa. The alkohol immediately separated and floated on the top. He distilled another portion of wine *in vacuo*, at 59° Fahr., a temperature considerably below that of fermentation. Alkohol came over. Mr. Brande proved the same position by saturating wine with subacetate of lead, and adding potassa.

Adem and Duportal have substituted for the redistillations used in converting wine or beer into alkohol, a single process of great elegance. From the capital of the still a tube is led into a large copper recipient. This is joined by a second tube to a second recipient, and so on through a series of four vessels, arranged like a Woolfe's apparatus. The last vessel communicates with the worm of the first refrigeratory. This, the body of the still, and the two recipients nearest it, are charged with the wine or fermented liquor. When ebullition takes place in the still, the vapour issuing from it communicates soon the boiling temperature to the liquor in the two recipients. From these the volatilized alkohol will rise and pass into the third vessel, which is empty. After communicating a certain heat to it, a portion of the finer or less condensible spirit will pass into the fourth, and thence, in a little, into the worm of the first refrigeratory. The wine round the worm will likewise acquire heat, but more slowly. The vapour that in that event may pass uncondensed through the first worm, is conducted into a second, surrounded with cold water. Whenever the still is worked off, it is replenished by a stop-cock from the nearest recipient, which, in its turn, is filled from the second, and the second from the first worm tub. It is evident, from this arrangement, that by keeping the third and fourth recipients at a certain temperature, we may cause alkohol, of any degree of lightness, to form directly at the remote extremity of the apparatus. The utmost economy of fuel and time is also secured, and a better flavoured spirit is obtained. The *arrière gout* of bad spirit can scarcely be destroyed by infusion with charcoal and redistillation. In this mode of operating, the taste and smell are excellent, from the first. Several stills on the above principle have been constructed at Glasgow for the West India distillers, and have been found extremely advantageous. The excise laws do not permit their employment in the home trade.

If sulphur in sublimation meet with the vapour of alkohol, a very small portion combines with it, which communicates a hydrosulphurous smell to the fluid. The increased surface of the two substances appears to favour the combination. It had been supposed, that this was the only way in which they could be united; but Favre has lately asserted, that having digested two drachms of flowers of sulphur in an ounce of alkohol, over a gentle fire not sufficient to make it boil, for twelve hours, he obtained a solution that gave twenty-three grains of precipitate. A similar mixture left to stand for a month in a place exposed to the solar rays, afforded sixteen grains of precipitate; and another from which the light was excluded, gave thirteen grains. If alkohol be boiled with one-fourth of its weight of sulphur for an hour, and filtered hot, a small quantity of minute crystals will be deposited on cooling; and the clear fluid will assume an opaline hue on being diluted with an equal quantity of water, in which state it will pass the filter, nor will any sediment be deposited for several hours. The alkohol used in the last-mentioned experiment did not exceed 840.

Phosphorus is sparingly soluble in alkohol, but in greater quantity by heat than in cold. The addition of water to this solution affords an opaque milky fluid, which becomes clear by the subsidence of the phosphorus.

Earths seem to have scarcely any action upon alkohol. Quicklime, however, produces some alteration in this fluid, by changing its flavour, and rendering it of a yellow colour. A portion is probably taken up.

Soaps are dissolved with great facility in alkohol, with which they combine more readily than with water. None of the metals, or their oxydes, are acted upon by this fluid. Resins, essential oils, camphor, bitumen, and various other substances, are dissolved with great facility in alkohol, from which they may be precipitated by the addition of water. From its property of dissolving resins, it becomes the menstruum of some varnishes.

Camphor is not only extremely soluble in alkohol, but assists the solution of resins in it. Fixed oils, when rendered drying by metallic oxydes, are soluble in it, as well as when combined with alkalies.

Wax, spermaceti, biliary calculi, urea, and all the animal substances of a resinous nature, are soluble in alkohol; but it curdles milk, coagulates albumen, and hardens the muscular fibre and coagulum of the blood.

The uses of alkohol are various. As a solvent of resinous substances and essential oils, it is employed both in pharmacy and by the perfumer. When diluted with an equal quantity of water, constituting what is called proof spirit, it is used for extracting tinctures from vegetable and other substances, the alkohol dissolving the resinous parts, and the water the gummy. From giving a steady heat without smoke when burnt in a lamp, it was formerly much employed to keep water boiling on the tea-table. In thermometers, for measuring great degrees of cold, it is preferable to mercury, as we cannot bring it to freeze. It is in common use for preserving many anatomical preparations, and certain subjects of natural history; but to some it is injurious, the molluscæ for instance, the calcareous covering of which it in time corrodes. It is of considerable use, too, in chemical analysis, as appears under the different articles to which it is applicable.

From the great expansive power of alkohol, it has been made a question, whether it might not be applied with advantage in the working of steam engines. From a series of experiments made by Betancourt, it appears, that the steam of alkohol has, in all cases of equal temperature, more than double the force of that of water; and that the steam of alkohol at 174° F. is equal to that of water 212°; thus there is a considerable diminution of the consumption of fuel, and where this is so expensive as to be an object of great importance, by contriving the machinery so as to prevent the alkohol from being lost, it may possibly at some future time be used with advantage, if some other fluid of great expansive power, and inferior price, be not found more economical.

Alkohol may be decomposed by transmission through a red-hot tube: it is also decomposable by the strong acids, and thus affords that remarkable product, ETHER, and OLEUM VINI.—*Ure's Chem. Dict.*

2. The alkohol of the London Pharmacopœia is directed to be made thus:—Take of rectified spirit, a gallon; subcarbonate of potassa, three pounds. Add a pound of the subcarbonate of potassa, previously heated to 300°, to the spirit, and macerate for twenty-four hours, frequently stirring them; then pour off the spirit, and add to it the rest of the subcarbonate of potassa heated to the same degree; lastly, with the aid of a warm bath, let the alkohol distil over, keep it in a well-stopped bottle. The specific gravity of alkohol is to the specific gravity of distilled water, as 815 to 1,000.

ALLAGITE. A carbosilicate of manganese.

ALLANITE. A mineral, first recognised as a distinct species by Mr. Allan of Edinburgh. It is massive and of a brownish black colour.

[Before the blowpipe it froths, and is converted into scoria. In nitric acid it forms a jelly. It contains silex 35.4, lime 9.2, oxide of cerium 33.9, alumine 4.1, oxide of iron 25.4, volatile matter 4.0. It is found in Greenland, and associated with mica and feldspar. A.]

ALLANTOI'DES. (From αλλας, a hog's pudding, and ειδος, likeness: because in some brutal animals it is long and thick.) *Membrana allantoides.* A membrane of the fœtus, peculiar to brutes, which contains the urine discharged from the bladder.

ALLELUI'A. (Hebrew. *Praise the Lord.*) So named from its many virtues. See *Oxalis acetosella.*

ALL-GOOD. See *Chenopodium bonushenricus.*

ALL-HEAL. See *Heraclium* and *Stachys.*

ALLIA'CEOUS. (*Alliaceus;* from *allium,* garlick.) Pertaining to garlick.

ALLIA'RIA. (From *allium,* garlick: from its smell resembling garlick.) See *Erysimum alliaria.*

A'LLIUM. (*Allium, i. n.*; from *oleo,* to smell; because it stinks: or from αλεω, to avoid; as being unpleasant to most people.) Garlick.

1. The name of a genus of plants in the Linnæan system. Class, *Hexandria;* Order, *Monogynia.*

2. The pharmacopœial name of garlick. See *Allium sativum.*

ALLIUM CEPA. *Cepa. Allium:—scapo nudo inferne ventricoso longiore, foliis teretibus,* of Linnæus. The Onion. Dr. Cullen says, onions are acrid and stimulating, and possess very little nutriment. With bilious constitutions they generally produce flatulency, thirst, headache, and febrile symptoms: but where the temperament is phlegmatic, they are of infinite service, by stimulating the habit and promoting the natural secretions, particularly expectoration and urine. They are recommended in scorbutic cases, as possessing antiscorbutic properties. Externally, onions are employed in suppurating poultices, and suppression of urine in children is said to be relieved by applying them, roasted, to the pubes.

ALLIUM PORRUM. The Leek or Porret. *Porrum* Every part of this plant, but more particularly the root, abounds with a peculiar odour. The expressed juice possesses diuretic qualities, and is given in the cure of dropsical diseases, and calculous complaints, asthma, and scurvy. The fresh root is much employed for culinary purposes.

ALLIUM SATIVUM. *Allium; Theriaca rusticorum* Garlick. *Allium:—caule planifolio bulbifero, bulbo composito, staminibus tricuspidatis,* of Linnæus. This species of Garlick, according to Linnæus, grows spontaneously in Sicily; but, as it is much employed for culinary and medicinal purposes, it has been long very generally cultivated in gardens. Every part of the plant, but more especially the root, has a pungent acrimonious taste, and a peculiarly offensive strong smell. This odour is extremely penetrating and diffusive; for, on the root being taken into the stomach, the alliaceous scent impregnates the whole system, and is discoverable in the various excretions, as in the urine, perspiration, milk, &c. Garlick is generally allied to the onion, from which it seems only to differ in being more powerful in its effects, and in its active matter, being in a more fixed state. By stimulating the stomach, they both favour digestion, and, as a stimulus, are readily diffused over the system. They may, therefore, be considered as useful condiments with the food of phlegmatic people, or those whose circulation is languid, and secretions interrupted; but with those subject to inflammatory complaints, or where great irritability prevails, these roots, in their acrid state, may prove very hurtful. The medicinal uses of garlick are various; it has been long in estimation as an expectorant in pituitous asthmas, and other pulmonary affections, *unattended* with inflammation. In hot bilious constitutions, therefore, garlick is improper: for it frequently produces flatulence, headache, thirst, heat, and other inflammatory symptoms. A free use of it is said to promote the piles in habits disposed to this complaint. Its utility as a diuretic in dropsies is attested by unquestionable authorities; and its febrifuge power has not only been experienced in preventing the paroxysms of intermittents, but even in subduing the plague. Bergius says quartans have been cured by it; and he begins by giving one bulb, or clove, morning and evening, addi every day one more, till four or five cloves be taken at a dose: if the fever then vanishes, the dose is to be diminished, and it will be sufficient to take one or two cloves, twice a day, for some weeks. Another virtue of garlick is that of an anthelminthic. It has likewise been found of great advantage in scorbutic cases, and in calculous disorders, acting in these not only as a diuretic, but, in several instances, manifesting a lithontriptic power. That the juice of alliaceous plants, in general, has considerable effects upon human calculi, is to be inferred from the experiments of Lobb; and we are abundantly warranted in asserting that a decoction of the beards of leeks, taken, liberally, and its use persevered in for a length of time, has been found remarkably successful in calculous and gravelly complaints. The penetrating and diffusive acrimony of garlick, renders its external application useful in many disorders, as a rubefacient, and more especially as applied to the soles of the feet, to cause a revulsion from the head or breast, as was successfully practised and recommended by Sydenham. As soon as an inflammation appears, the garlick cataplasm should be removed, and one of bread and milk be applied, to obviate excessive pain. Garlick has also been variously employed externally, to tumours and cutaneous diseases: and, in certain cases of deafness, a clove, or small bulb of this root, wrapt in gauze or muslin, and introduced into the meatus auditorius, has been found an efficacious remedy. Garlick may be administered in different forms; swallowing the clove entire, after being dipped in oil, is recommended as most effectual; where this cannot be done, cutting it into pieces without bruising it, and swallowing these may be found to answer equally well, producing thereby no uneasiness in the fauces. On being beaten up and formed into pills, the active parts of this medicine soon evaporate: this Dr. Woodville, in his Medical Botany, notices, on the authority of Cullen, who thinks that Lewis has fallen into a gross error, in supposing dry garlick more active than fresh. The syrup and oxymel of garlick, which formerly had a place in the British Pharmacopœias, are now expunged. The cloves of garlick are by some bruised, and applied to the wrists, to cure agues, and to the bend of the arm to cure the toothache: when held in the hand, they are said to relieve hiccough; when beat with common oil into a poultice, they resolve sluggish humours; and, if laid on the navels of children, they are supposed to destroy worms in the intestines.

Allium victoriale. *Victorialis longa.* The root, which when dried loses its alliaceous smell and taste, is said to be efficacious in allaying the abdominal spasms of gravid females.

ALLOCHROITE. A massive opaque mineral of a grayish, yellowish, or reddish colour.

[This mineral resembles certain varieties of the garnet in some of its physical characters, but more particularly in composition. It contains silex 37.0, lime 30.0, alumine 5.0, oxide of iron 18.5, oxide of manganese 6.25;=96.75. *Cleav. Min.* A.]

ALLOEO'SIS. (From αλλος, another.) Alteration in the state of a disease.

Alloeo'tica. (From αλλος, another.) Alteratives. Medicines which change the appearance of the disease.

ALLOGNO'SIS. (From αλλος, another, and γινωσκω, to know.) Delirium; perversion of the judgment; incapability of distinguishing persons.

ALLOPHANE. A mineral of a blue, and sometimes a green or brown colour.

ALLO'PHASIS. (From αλλος, another, and φαω, to speak.) According to Hippocrates, a delirium, where the patient is not able to distinguish one thing from another.

ALLOTRIOPHA'GIA. (From αλλοτριος, foreign, and φαγω, to eat.) In Vogel's Nosology, it signifies the greedily eating unusual things for food. See *Pica.*

ALLOY. Allay. 1. Where any precious metal is mixed with another of less value, the assayers call the latter the alloy, and do not in general consider it in any other point of view than as debasing or diminishing the value of the precious metal.

2. Philosophical chemists have availed themselves of this term to distinguish all metallic compounds in general. Thus brass is called an alloy of copper and zinc; bell metal an alloy of copper and tin.

Every alloy is distinguished by the metal which predominates in its composition, or which gives it its value. Thus English jewellery trinkets are ranked under alloys of gold, though most of them deserve to be placed under the head of copper. When mercury is one of the component metals, the alloy is called *amalgam.* Thus we have an amalgam of gold, silver, tin, &c. Since there are about thirty different permanent metals, independent of those evanescent ones that constitute the bases of the alkalies and earths, there ought to be about 870 different species of binary alloy. But only 132 species have been hitherto made and examined. Some metals have so little affinity for others, that as yet no compound of them has been effected, whatever pains have been taken. Most of these obstacles to alloying, arise from the difference in fusibility and volatility. Yet a few metals, the melting point of which is nearly the same, refuse to unite. It is obvious that two bodies will not combine, unless their affinity or reciprocal attraction be stronger than the cohesive attraction of their individual particles. To overcome this cohesion of the solid bodies, and render affinity predominant, they must be penetrated by caloric. If one be very difficult of fusion, and the other very volatile, they will not unite unless the reciprocal attraction be exceedingly strong. But if their degree of fusibility be almost the same, they are easily placed in the circumstances most favourable for making an alloy. If we are therefore far from knowing all the binary alloys which are possible, we are still further removed from knowing all the triple, quadruple, &c. which may exist. It must be confessed, moreover, that this department of chemistry has been imperfectly cultivated.

Besides, alloys are not, as far as we know, definitely regulated like oxydes in the proportions of their component parts. 100 parts of mercury will combine with 4 or 8 parts of oxygen, to form two distinct oxydes, the black and the red; but with no greater, less, or intermediate proportions. But 100 parts of mercury will unite with 1, 2, 3, or with any quantity up to 100 or 1000, of tin or lead. The alloys have the closest relations in their physical properties with the metals. They are all solid at the temperature of the atmosphere, except some amalgams; they possess metallic lustre, even when reduced to a coarse powder: are completely opaque, and more or less dense, according to the metals which compose them; are excellent conductors of electricity; crystallize more or less perfectly; some are brittle, others ductile and malleable; some have a peculiar odour; several are very sonorous and elastic. When an alloy consists of metals differently fusible, it is usually malleable while cold, but brittle while hot; as is exemplified in brass.

The density of an alloy is sometimes greater, sometimes less than the mean density of its components, showing that, at the instant of their union, a diminution or augmentation of volume takes place. The relation between the expansion of the separate metals and that of their alloys, has been investigated only in a very few cases. Alloys containing a volatile metal are decomposed, in whole or in part, at a strong heat. This happens with those of arsenic, mercury, tellurium, and zinc. Those that consist of two differently fusible metals, may often be decomposed by exposing them to a temperature capable of melting only one of them. This operation is called eliquation. It is practised on the great scale to extract silver from copper. The argentiferous copper is melted with 3 1-2 times its weight of lead; and the triple alloy is exposed to a sufficient heat. The lead carries off the silver in its fusion, and leaves the copper under the form of a spongy lump The silver is afterward recovered from the lead by another operation.

Some alloys oxydize more readily by heat and air, than when the metals are separately treated. Thus 3 of lead and 1 of tin, at a dull red, burn visibly, and are almost instantly oxydized. Each by itself in the same circumstances, would oxydize slowly, and with out the disengagement of light.

The formation of an alloy must be regulated by the nature of the particular metals.

The degree of affinity between metals may be in some measure estimated by the greater or less facility with which, when of different degrees of fusibility or volatility, they unite, or with which they can after union be separated by heat. The greater or less tendency to separate into different proportional alloys, by long-con tinued fusion, may also give some information on this subject. Mr. Hatchett remarked, in his admirable researches on metallic alloys, that gold made standard with the usual precautions by silver, copper, lead, antimony, &c. and then cast into vertical bars, was by no means a uniform compound; but that the top of the bar, corresponding to the metal at the bottom of the crucible, contained the larger proportion of gold. Hence, for thorough combination, two red-hot crucibles should be employed; and the liquified metals should be alternately poured from the one into the other. And to prevent unnecessary oxydizement by exposure to air, the crucibles should contain, besides the metal, a mixture of common salt and pounded charcoal. The melted alloy should also be occasionally stirred up with a rod of pottery.

The most direct evidence of a chemical change having taken place in the two metals by combination, is when the alloy melts at a much lower temperature than the fusing points of its components. Iron, which is nearly infusible, when alloyed with gold acquires almost the fusibility of this metal. Tin and lead form solder, an alloy more fusible than either of its components; but the triple compound of tin, lead, and bismuth, is most remarkable on this account. The analogy is here strong, with the increase of solubility which salts acquire by mixture, as is exemplified in the uncrystallizable residue of saline solutions, or mother waters, as they are called. Sometimes two metals will not directly unite, which yet, by the intervention of a third, are made to combine. This happens with mercury and iron, as has been shown by Messrs. Aiken, who effected this difficult amalgamation by previously uniting the iron to tin or zinc.

The tenacity of alloys is generally, though not always, inferior to the mean of the separate metals. One part of lead will destroy the compactness and tenacity of a thousand of gold. Brass made with a small proportion of zinc, is more ductile than copper itself; but when one-third of zinc enters into its composition, it becomes brittle.

In common cases, the specific gravity affords a good criterion whereby to judge of the proportion in an alloy, consisting of two metals of different densities.—*Ure.*

ALLSPICE. See *Myrtes Pimenta.*

ALLUVIAL. That which is deposited in valleys, or in plains, from neighbouring mountains, or the overflowing of rivers. Gravel, loam, clay, sand, brown coal, wood coal, bog iron ore, and calc tuff, compose the alluvial deposites.

A'LMA. The first motion of a fœtus to free itself from its confinement.

2. Water.—*Rulandus.*

ALMABRI. A stone like amber.

ALMA'NDA CATHARTICA. A plant growing on the shores of Cayenne and Surinam, used by the inhabitants as a remedy for the colic; supposed to be cathartic.

ALME'NE. Rock salt.

ALMOND. See *Amygdalus.*

Almond, bitter. See *Amygdalus.*

Almond, sweet. See *Amygdalus.*

Almond paste. This cosmetic for softening the skin and preventing chops, is made of four ounces of blanched bitter almonds, the white of an egg, rose water and rectified spirits, equal parts, as much as is sufficient.

Almonds of the ears. A popular name for the tonsils, which have been so called from their resemblance to an almond in shape. See *Tonsils.*

Almonds of the throat. A vulgar name for the tonsils. See *Tonsils.*

ALNABATI. In Avicenna and Serapion, this word means the *siliqua dulcis*, a gentle laxative. See *Ceratonia siliqua.*

A'LNUS. (*Alno*, Italian.) The alder. The pharmacopœial name of two plants, sometimes used in medicine, though rarely employed in the present practice.

1. *Alnus rotundifolia; glutinosa; viridis.* The common alder-tree. See *Betula alnus.*

2. *Alnus nigra.* The black or berry-bearing alder. See *Rhamnus Frangula.*

A'LOE. (*Aloë, ës.* fr. from *ahlah*, a Hebrew word, signifying growing near the sea.) The name of a genus of plants of the Linnæan system. Class *Hexandria.* Order, *Monogynia.* The Aloe.

Aloë Caballina. See *Aloë perfoliata.*

Aloë Guineensis. See *Aloë perfoliata.*

ALOE PERFOLIATA. *Aloë Succotorina; Aloë Zocotorina.* Succotorine aloes is obtained from a variety of the *Aloë perfoliata* of Linnæus:—*foliis caulinis dentatis, amplexicaulibus vaginantibus, floribus corymbosis cernuis, pedunculatis subcylindricis.* It is brought over wrapped in skins, from the Island of Socotora, in the Indian Ocean; it is of a bright surface, and in some degree pellucid; in the lump of a yellowish red colour, with a purplish cast; when reduced into powder, it is of a golden colour. It is hard and friable in very cold weather; but in summer it softens very easily between the fingers. It is extremely bitter, and also accompanied with an aromatic flavour, but not so much as to cover its disagreeable taste. Its scent is rather agreeable, being somewhat similar to that of myrrh. Of late this sort has been very scarce, and its place in a great measure supplied by another variety, brought from the Cape of Good Hope, which is said to be obtained from the *Aloë spicata* of Linnæus, by inspissating the expressed juice of the leaves, whence it is termed in the London Pharmacopœia *Extractum aloës spicatæ.*

The *Aloë hepatica, vel Barbadensis*, the common or Barbadoes or hepatic aloes, was thought to come from a variety of the *Aloë perfoliata* described:—*floribus pedunculatis, cernuis corymbosis, subcylindricis, foliis spinosis, confertis, dentatis, vaginantibus, planis, maculatis;* but Dr. Smith has announced, that it will be shown in Sibthorp's Flora Græca, to be from a distinct species, the *Aloë vulgaris*, or true αλοη of Dioscorides; and it is therefore termed in the London Pharmacopœia, *Aloës vulgaris extractum.* The best is brought from Barbadoes in large gourd-shells; an inferior sort in pots, and the worst in casks. It is darker coloured than the Socotorine, and not so bright; it is also drier and more compact, though sometimes the sort in casks is soft and clammy. To the taste it is intensely bitter and nauseous, being almost wholly without that aroma which is observed in the Socotorine. To the smell it is strong and disagreeable.

The *Aloë caballina, vel Guineensis*, or horse-aloes, is easily distinguished from both the foregoing, by its strong rank smell; in other respects it agrees pretty much with the hepatic, and is now not unfrequently sold in its place. Sometimes it is prepared so pure and bright as scarcely to be distinguishable by the eye, even from the Socotorine, but its offensive smell betrays it; and if this also should be dissipated by art, its wanting the aromatic flavour of the finer aloes will be a sufficient criterion. This aloe is not admitted into the materia medica, and is employed chiefly by farriers.

The general nature of these three kinds is nearly the same. Their particular differences only consist in the different proportions of gum to their resin, and in their flavour. The smell and taste reside principally in the gum, as do the principal virtues of the aloes. Twelve ounces of Barbadoes aloes yield nearly 4 ounces of resin, and 8 of gummy extract. The same quantity of Socotorine aloes yields 3 ounces of resin and 9 of gummy extract.

Aloes is a well-known stimulating purgative, a property which it possesses not only when taken internally, but also by external application. The cathartic quality of aloes does not reside in the resinous part of the drug, but in the gum, for the pure resin has little or no purgative power. Its medium dose is from 5 to 15 grains, nor does a larger quantity operate more effectually. Its operation is exerted on the large intestines; principally on the rectum. In small doses long continued, it often produces much heat and irritation, particularly about the anus, from which it sometimes occasions a bloody discharge; therefore, to those who were subject to piles, or of an hæmorrhagic diathesis, or even in a state of pregnancy, its exhibition has been productive of considerable mischief; but on the contrary, by those of a phlegmatic constitution, or those suffering from uterine obstructions (for the stimulant action of aloes, it has been supposed, may be extended to the uterus) and in some cases of dyspepsia, palsy, gout, and worms, aloes may be employed as a laxative with peculiar advantage. In all diseases of the bilious tribe, aloes is the strongest purge, and the best preparations for this purpose are the pilula ex aloe cum myrrha, the tinctura aloës, or the extractum colocynthidis compositum. Its efficacy in jaundice is very considerable, as it proves a succedaneum to the bile, of which in that disease there is a defective supply to the intestine either in quantity or quality. Aloes therefore may be considered as injurious where inflammation or irritation exists in the bowels or neighbouring parts, in pregnancy, or in habits disposed to piles; but highly serviceable in all hypochondriac affections, cachectic habits, and persons labouring under oppression of the stomach caused by irregularity. Aromatics correct the offensive qualities of aloes the most perfectly. The canella alba answers tolerably, and without any inconvenience; but some rather prefer the essential oils for this purpose. Dr. Cullen says, "If any medicine be entitled to the appellation of a *stomach purge*, it is certainly aloes. It is remarkable with regard to it, that it operates almost to as good a purpose in a small as in a large dose; that one or two grains will produce one considerable dejection, and 20 grains will do no more, except it be that in the last dose the operation will be attended with gripes, &c. Its chief use is to render the peristaltic motion regular, and it is one of the best cures in habitual costiveness. There is a difficulty we meet with in the exhibition of purgatives, viz. that they will not act but in their full dose, and will not produce half their effect if given in half the dose. For this purpose we are chiefly confined to aloes. Neutral salts in half their dose will not have half their effect; although even from these, by large dilution, we may obtain this property; but besides them and our present medicine, I know no other which has any title to it except sulphur. Aloes sometimes cannot be employed. It has the effect of stimulating the rectum more than other purges, and with justice has been accused of exciting hæmorrhoidal swellings, so that we ought to abstain from it in such cases, except when we want to promote them. Aloes has the effect of rarifying the blood and disposing to hæmorrhagy, and hence it is not recommended in uterine fluxes. Fœtid gums are of the same nature in producing hæmorrhagy, and perhaps this is the foundation of their emmenagogue power." Aloes is administered either simply in powders, which is too nauseous, or else in composition;—1. With purgatives, as soap, scammony, colocynth, or rhubarb. 2. With aromatics, as canella, ginger, or essential oils. 3. With bitters, as gentian. 4. With emmenagogues, as iron, myrrh, wine, &c. It may be exhibited in pills as the most convenient form, or else dissolved in wine, or diluted alkohol. The officinal preparations of aloes are the following:—

1. Pilulæ Aloës.
2. Pilula Aloës Composita
3. Pilulæ Aloës cum Assafœtidâ.
4. Pilula Aloës cum Colocynthide.
5. Pilula Aloës cum Myrrha.
6. Tinctura Aloës.
7. Tinctura Aloës Ætherialis.
8. Tinctura Aloës et Myrrha.
9. Vinum Aloës.
10. Extractum Aloës.
11. Decoctum Aloës Compositum.
12. Pulvis Aloës Compositus.
13. Pulvis Aloës cum Canella.
14. Pulvis Aloës cum Guaiaco.
15. Tinctura Aloës Composita.
16. Extractum Colocynthidis Compositum.
17. Tinctura Benzoini Composita.

Aloë Socotorina. See *Aloë perfoliata.*

Aloë Zocotorina. See *Aloë perfoliata.*

ALOEDA'RIA. (From αλοη, the aloe.) Compound purging medicines: so called from having aloes as the chief ingredient.

ALOEPHANGINA. Medicines formed by a combination of aloes and aromatics.

ALOES. *Fel naturæ.* The inspissated juice of the aloe plant. Aloes is distinguished into three species, *socotorine*, *hepatic*, and *caballine*; of which the two first are directed for officinal use in our pharmacopœias. See *Aloë perfoliata.*

ALOES LIGNUM. See *Lignum Aloës.*

ALOE'TIC. A medicine wherein aloes is the chief or fundamental ingredient.

ALOGOTRO'PHIA. (From αλογος, disproportionate, and τρεφω, to nourish.) Unequal nourishment, as in the rickets.

ALO'PECES. (From αλωπηξ, the fox.) The psoæ muscles are so called by Fallopius and Vesalius because in the fox they are particularly strong.

ALOPE'CIA. (From αλωπηξ, a fox: because the fox is subject to a distemper that resembles it; or, as some say, because the fox's urine will occasion baldness.) Baldness, or the falling off of the hair. A genus of disease in Sauvages' Nosology.

ALOPECUROIDEA. (From *alopecurus*, the fox-tail grass.) Resembling the alopecurus. The name of a division of grasses.

ALO'SA. (From αλισκω, to take: because it is ravenous.) See *Clupea alosa.*

ALOSA'NTHI. (From αλς, salt, and ανθος, a flower.) *Alosanthum.* Flowers of salt.

A'LOSAT. Quicksilver.

ALOSOHOC. Quicksilver.

A'LPHITA. (*Alphita*, the plural of αλφιτον, the meal of barley in general.) By Hippocrates this term is applied to barley-meal either toasted or fried. Galen says that κριμνα is coarse meal, αλευρον is fine meal, and αλφιτα is a middling sort.

ALPHI'TIDON. *Alphitedum.* It is when a bone is broken into small fragments like *alphite* or bran.

ALPHO'NSIN. The name of an instrument for extracting balls. It is so called from the name of its inventor, Alphonso Ferrier, a Neapolitan physician. It consists of three branches, which separate from each other by their elasticity, but are capable of being closed by means of a tube in which they are included.

ALPHOSIS. The specific name of a disease in the genus *Epichrosis* of Good's Nosology.

A'LPHUS. (Αλφος; from αλφαινω, to change: because it changes the colour of the skin.) A species of leprosy, called by the ancients *vitilago*, and which they divided into *alphus*, *melas*, and *leuce*. See *Lepra*

A'LPINI BALSAMUM. Balm of Gilead.

ALPI'NUS, PROSPER, a Venetian, born in 1553, celebrated for his skill in medicine and botany. After graduating at Padua, he went to Egypt, and during three years carefully studied the plants of that country, and the modes of treating diseases there; of which he afterward published a very learned account. He has left also some other less important works. He was appointed physician to the celebrated Andrew Doria; and subsequently botanical professor at Padua, which office he retained till his death in 1616.

A'LSINE. (*Alsine, es.* f.; from αλσος, a grove: so called because it grows in great abundance in woods and shady places.) The name of a genus of plants in the Linnæan system. Class, *Pentandria;* Order, *Trigynia.* Chickweed.

ALSINE MEDIA. *Morsus gallinæ centunculus.* The systematic name for the plant called chickweed, which, if boiled tender, may be eaten like spinach, and forms also an excellent emollient poultice.

ALSTON, CHARLES, born in Scotland in 1683, was early attached to the study of botany, and distinguished himself by opposing the sexual system of Linnæus. He afterward studied under Boerhaave at Leyden; then returning to his native country, was materially instrumental, in conjunction with the celebrated Alexander Monro, in establishing the medical school at Edinburgh, where he was appointed professor of botany and materia medica. He died in 1760. His "Lectures on the Materia Medica," a posthumous work, abound in curious and useful facts, which will long preserve their reputation.

A'LTERATIVE. (*Alterans;* from *altero*, to change.) Alterative medicines are those remedies which are given with a view to re-establish the healthy functions of the animal economy, without producing any sensible evacuation.

ALTERNÆ PLANTÆ. Alternate leaved plants. The name of a class of plants in Sauvages' Methodus foliorum.

ALTERNANS. Alternate; placed alternately. A term applied by botanists to leaves, gems, &c.

ALTERNUS. Alternate. In botany, this term is applied to branches and leaves when they stand singly on each side, in such a manner that between every two on one side there is but one on the opposite side, as on the branches of the *Althæá officinalis*, *Rhamnus catharticus*, and leaves of the *Malva rotundifolia.*

ALTHÆ'A. (*Althæa, æ.* f.; from αλθεω, to heal so called from its supposed qualities in healing.) 1 The name of a genus of plants of the Linnæan system

Class, *Monadelphia;* Order, *Polyandria.* Marsh-mallow.

2. The pharmacopœial name of the marsh-mallow. See *Althea Officinalis.*

ALTHÆA OFFICINALIS. The systematic name of the marsh-mallow. *Malvaviscus*; *Aristalthæa. Althæa:—foliis simplicibus tomentosis.* The mucilaginous matter with which this plant abounds, is the medicinal part of the plant; it is commonly employed for its emollient and demulcent qualities in tickling coughs, hoarseness, and catarrhs, in dysentery, and difficulty and heat of urine. The leaves and root are generally selected for use. They relax the passages in nephritic complaints, in which last case a decoction is the best preparation. Two or three ounces of the fresh roots may be boiled in a sufficient quantity of water to a quart, to which one ounce of gum-arabic may be added. The following is given where it is required that large quantities should be used. An ounce of the dried roots is to be boiled in water, enough to leave two or three pints to be poured off for use: if more of the root be used, the liquor will be disagreeably slimy. If sweetened, by adding a little more of the root of liquorice, it will be very palatable. The root had formerly a place in many of the compounds in the pharmacopœias, but now it is only directed in the form of syrup.

ALTHE'XIS. (From αλθειν, to cure, or heal.) Hippocrates often uses this word to signify the cure of a distemper.

ALUDEL. A hollow sphere of stone, glass, or earthenware, with a short neck projecting at each end, by means of which one globe might be set upon the other. The uppermost has no opening at the top. They were used in former times for the sublimation of several substances.

ALUM. See *Alumen.*

ALUM EARTH. A massive mineral of a blackish brown colour, a dull lustre, an earthy and somewhat slaty fracture, sectile and rather soft, containing charcoal silica, alumina, oxyde of iron, sulphur, sulphates of lime, potassa, and iron, magnesia, muriate of potassa, and water.

ALUM SLATE. A massive mineral of a bluish black colour, or slate containing alum.

ALU'MEN. (*Alum*, an Arabian word.) *Assos; Azub; Aseb; Elanula; Sulphas aluminæ acidulus cum potassâ; Super-sulphas aluminæ et potassæ; Argilla vitriolata.* Alum. This important salt has been the object of innumerable researches both with regard to its fabrication and composition. It is produced, but in a very small quantity, in the native state; and this is mixed with heterogeneous matters. It effloresces in various forms upon ores during calcination, but it seldom occurs crystallized. The greater part of this salt is factitious, being extracted from minerals called alum ores, such as,

1. Sulphuretted clay. This constitutes the purest of all aluminous ores, namely, that of La Tolfa, near Civita Vecchia, in Italy. It is white, compact, and as hard as indurated clay, whence it is called *petra aluminaris.* It is tasteless and mealy; one hundred parts of this ore contain above forty of sulphur and fifty of clay, a small quantity of potassa, and a little iron. Bergman says it contains forty-three of sulphur in one hundred, thirty-five of clay, and twenty-two of siliceous earth. This ore is first torrefied to acidify the sulphur, which then acts on the clay, and forms the alum.

2. The pyritaceous clay, which is found at Schwemsal, in Saxony, at the depth of ten or twelve feet. It is a black and hard, but brittle substance, consisting of clay, pyrites, and bitumen. It is exposed to the air for two years, by which means the pyrites are decomposed, and the alum is formed. The alum ores of Hesse and Liege are of this kind; but they are first torrefied, which is said to be a disadvantageous method.

3. The schistus aluminaris contains a variable proportion of petroleum and pyrites intimately mixed with it. When the last are in a very large quantity, this ore is rejected as containing too much iron. Professor Bergman very properly suggested, that by adding a proportion of clay, this ore may turn out advantageously for producing alum. But if the petrol be considerable, it must be torrefied. The mines of Becket in Normandy, and those of Whitby, in Yorkshire, are of this species.

4. Volcanic aluminous ore. Such is that of Salfaterra near Naples. It is in the form of a white saline earth, after it has effloresced in the air · or else it is in a stony form.

5. Bituminous alum ore is called shale, and is in the form of a schistus, impregnated with so much oily matter, or bitumen, as to be inflammable. It is found in Sweden, and also in the coal mines at Whitehaven, and elsewhere.

Chaptal has fabricated alum on a large scale from its component parts. For this purpose he constructed a chamber 91 feet long, 48 wide, and 31 high in the middle. The walls are of common masonry, lined with a pretty thick coating of plaster. The floor is paved with bricks, bedded in a mixture of raw and burnt clay; and this pavement is covered with another, the joints of which overlap those of the first, and instead of mortar, the bricks are joined with a cement of equal parts of pitch, turpentine, and wax, which, after having been boiled till it ceases to swell, is used hot. The roof is of wood, but the beams are very close together, and grooved lengthwise, the intermediate space being filled up by planks fitted into the grooves, so that the whole is put together without a nail. Lastly, the whole of the inside is covered with three or four successive coatings of the cement above-mentioned, the first being laid on as hot as possible; and the outside of the wooden roof was varnished in the same manner. The purest and whitest clay being made into a paste with water, and formed into balls half a foot in diameter, these are calcined in a furnace, broken to pieces, and a stratum of the fragments laid on the floor. A due proportion of sulphur is then ignited in the chamber, in the same manner as for the fabrication of sulphuric acid; and the fragments of burnt clay, imbibing this as it forms, begin after a few days to crack and open, and exhibit an efflorescence of sulphate of alumina. When the earth has completely effloresced, it is taken out of the chamber, exposed for some time in an open shed, that it may be the more intimately penetrated by the acid, and is then lixiviated and crystallized in the usual manner. The cement answers the purpose of lead on this occasion very effectually, and, according to Chaptal, costs no more than lead would at three farthings a pound.

Curaudau has lately recommended a process for making alum without evaporation. One hundred parts of clay and five of muriate of soda are kneaded into a paste with water, and formed into loaves. With these a reverberatory furnace is filled, and a brisk fire is kept up for two hours. Being powdered, and put into a sound cask, one-fourth of their weight of sulphuric acid is poured over them by degrees, stirring the mixture well at each addition. As soon as the muriatic gas is dissipated, a quantity of water equal to the acid is added, and the mixture stirred as before. When the heat is abated, a little more water is poured in; and this is repeated till eight or ten times as much water as there was acid is added. When the whole has settled, the clear liquor is drawn off into leaden vessels, and a quantity of water equal to this liquor is poured on the sediment. The two liquors being mixed, a solution of potassa is added to them, the alkali in which is equal to one-fourth of the weight of the sulphuric acid. Sulphate of potassa may be used, but twice as much of this as of the alkali is necessary. After a certain time, the liquor, by cooling, affords crystals of alum equal to three times the weight of the acid used. It is refined by dissolving it in the smallest possible quantity of boiling water. The residue may be washed with more water, to be employed in lixiviating a fresh portion of the ingredients.

Its sp. gravity is about 1.71. It reddens the vegetable blues. It is soluble in 16 parts of water at 60°, and in 3-4 of its weight at 212°. It effloresces superficially on exposure to air, but the interior remains long unchanged. Its water of crystallization is sufficient at a gentle heat to fuse it. If the heat be increased it froths up, and loses fully 45 per cent. of its weight in water. The spongy residue is called *burnt* or calcined *alum*, and is used by surgeons as a mild escharotic. A violent heat separates a great portion of its acid.

Alum was thus analyzed by Berzelius: 1*st*, 20 parts (grammes) of pure alum lost, by the heat of a spirit lamp, 9 parts, which gives 45 per cent. of water. The dry salt was dissolved in water, and its acid precipitated by muriate of barytes; the sulphate of which, obtained after ignition, weighed 20 parts; indicating in 100 parts 34.3 of dry sulphuric acid. 2*d*, Ten parts of alum were dissolved in water, and digested with an excess of ammonia. Alumina, well washed and burned, equivalent to 10.67 per cent. was obtained. In another experiment, 10.86 per cent. resulted. 3*d*, Ten parts of alum dissolved in water, were digested with carbonate of strontites, till the earth was completely separated. The sulphate of potassa, after ignition, weighed 1.815, corresponding to 0.981 potassa, or in 100 parts to 9.81.

Alum, therefore, consists of

Sulphuric acid	34.33
Alumina	10.86
Potassa	9.81
Water	45.00
	100.00

or, Sulphate of alumina	36.85
Sulphate of potassa	18.15
Water	45.00
	100.00

Thenard's analysis, Ann. de Chimie, vol. 59, or Nicholson's Journal, vol. 18, coincides perfectly with that of Berzelius in the product of sulphate of barytes. From 400 parts of alum, he obtained 490 of the ignited barytic salt; but the alumina was in greater proportion, equal to 12.54 per cent. and the sulphate of potassa less, or 15.7 in 100 parts.

Vauquelin, in his last analysis, found 48.58 water; and by Thenard's statement there are indicated

34.23	dry acid,
7.14	potassa,
12.54	alumina,
46.09	water.
100.00	

If we rectify Vauquelin's erroneous estimate of the sulphate of barytes, his analysis will also coincide with the above. Alum, therefore, differs from the simple sulphate of alumina previously described, which consisted of 3 prime equivalents of acid and 2 of earth, merely by its assumption of a prime of sulphate of potassa. It is probable that all the aluminous salts have a similar constitution. It is to be observed, moreover, that the number 34.36 resulting from the theoretic proportions, is, according to Gilbert's remarks on the Essay of Berzelius, the just representation of the dry acid in 100 of sulphate of barytes, by a corrected analysis, which makes the prime of barytes 9.57.

Should ammonia be suspected in alum, it may be detected, and its quantity estimated, by mixing quicklime with the saline solution, and exposing the mixture to heat in a retort, connected with a Woolfe's apparatus. The water of ammonia being afterward saturated with an acid, and evaporated to a dry salt, will indicate the quantity of pure ammonia in the alum. A variety of alum, containing both potassa and ammonia, may also be found. This will occur where urine has been used, as well as muriate of potassa, in its fabrication. If any of these bisulphates of allumina and potassa be acted on in a watery solution, by gelatinous alumina, a neutral triple salt is formed, which precipitates in a nearly insoluble state.

When alum in powder is mixed with flour or sugar, and calcined, it forms the *pyrophorus* of Homberg.

Mr. Winter first mentioned, that another variety of alum can be made with *soda*, instead of potassa. This salt, which crystallizes in octahedrons, has been also made with pure muriate of soda, and bisulphate of alumina, at the laboratory of Hurlett, by Mr. W. Wilson. It is extremely difficult to form, and effloresces like the sulphate of soda.

On the subject of soda-alum, Dr. Ure published a short paper in the Journal of Science for July, 1822. The form and taste of this salt are exactly the same as those of common alum; but it is less hard, being easily crushed between the fingers, to which it imparts an appearance of moisture. Its specific gravity is 1.6. 100 parts of water at 60° F. dissolve 110 of it; forming a solution, whose sp. gravity is 1.296. In this respect, potassa alum is very different. For 100 parts of water dissolve only from 8 to 9 parts, forming a saturated solution, the specific gravity of which is no more than 1.0465. Its constituents are, by Dr. Ure's analysis,—

Sulphuric acid	34.00	4 primes,		33.96
Alumina	10.75	3	—	10.82
Soda	6.48	1	—	6.79
Water	49.00	25	—	48.43
	100.23			100.00

Or it consists of 3 primes sulphate of alumina+1 sulphate of soda. To each of the former, 5 primes of water may be assigned, and to the latter 10, as in Glauber's salts.

The only injurious *contamination* of alum is sulphate of iron. It is detected by ferro-prussiate of potassa.

Oxymuriate of alumina, or the chloride, has been proposed by Mr. Wilson of Dublin, as preferable to solution of chlorine, for discharging the turkey-red die.

Alum is used in large quantities in many manufactories. When added to tallow, it renders it harder. Printer's cushions, and the blocks used in the calico manufactory, are rubbed with burnt alum to remove any greasiness, which might prevent the ink or colour from sticking. Wood sufficiently soaked in a solution of alum does not easily take fire; and the same is true of paper impregnated with it, which is fitter to keep gunpowder, as it also excludes moisture. Paper impregnated with alum is useful in whitening silver, and in silvering brass without heat. Alum mixed in milk helps the separation of its butter. If added in a very small quantity to turbid water, in a few minutes it renders it perfectly limpid, without any bad taste or quality; while the sulphuric acid imparts to it a very sensible acidity, and does not precipitate as soon, or so well, the opaque earthy mixtures that render it turbid. It is used in making pyrophorus, in tanning, and in many other manufactories, particularly in the art of dying, in which it is of the greatest and most important use, by cleansing and opening the pores on the surface of the substance to be died, rendering it fit for receiving the colouring particles, (by which the alum is generally decomposed,) and at the same time making the colour fixed. Crayons generally consist of the earth of alum, powdered and tinged for the purpose.—*Ure's Chem. Dict.*

In medicine it is employed internally as a powerful astringent in cases of passive hæmorrhages from the womb, intestines, nose, and sometimes lungs. In bleedings of an active nature, i. e. attended with fever, and a plethoric state of the system, it is highly improper. Dr. Percival recommends it in the *colica pictonum* and other chronic disorders of the bowels, attended with obstinate constipation. (See Percival's Essays.) The dose advised in these cases is from 5 to 20 grains, to be repeated every four, eight, or twelve hours. When duly persisted in, this remedy proves gently laxative, and mitigates the pain.

Alum is also powerfully tonic, and is given with this view in the dose of 10 grains made into a bolus three times a day, in such cases as require powerful tonic and astringent remedies. Another mode of administering it is in the form of whey made by boiling a drachm of powdered alum in a pint of milk for a few minutes, and to be taken in the quantity of a tea-cup full three times a day. Dr. Cullen thinks it ought to be employed with other astringents in diarrhœas. In active hæmorrhages, as was observed, it is not useful, though a powerful medicine in those which are passive. It should be given in small doses, and gradually increased. It has been tried in the diabetes without success; though, joined with nutmeg, it has been more successful in intermittents, given in a large dose, an hour or a little longer, before the approach of the paroxysm. In gargles, in relaxation of the uvula, and other swellings of the mucous membrane of the fauces, divested of acute inflammation, it has been used with advantage.

Externally, alum is much employed by surgeons as a lotion for the eyes, and is said to be preferable to sulphate of zinc or acetate of lead in the ophthalmia membranarum. From two to five grains dissolved in an ounce of rose-water, forms a proper collyrium. It is also applied as a styptic to bleeding vessels, and to ulcers, where there is too copious a secretion of pus. It has proved successful in inflammation of the eyes, in the form of cataplasm, which is made by stirring or shaking a lump of alum in the whites of two eggs, till they form a coagulum, which is applied to the eye between two pieces of thin linen rag. Alum is also employed as an injection in cases of gleet or fluor albus.

When deprived of its humidity, by placing it in an earthen pan over a gentle fire, it is termed burnt alum, *alumen exsiccatum*, and is sometimes employed by surgeons to destroy fungous flesh, and is a principal ingredient in most styptic powders.

Alum is also applied to many purposes of life; in this country, bakers mix a quantity with the bread, to render it white; this mixture makes the bread better adapted for weak and relaxed bowels; but in opposite states of the alimentary canal, this practice is highly pernicious.

The officinal preparations of alum are:

1. Alumen exsiccatum.
2. Solutio sulphatis cupri ammoniati.
3. Liquor aluminis compositus.
4. Pulvis sulphatis aluminis compositus.

ALUMEN CATINUM. A name of potassa.

ALUMEN COMMUNE. See *Alumen*.

ALUMEN CRYSTALLINUM. See *Alumen*.

ALUMEN EXSICCATUM. Dried Alum. Expose alum in an earthen vessel to the fire, so that it may dissolve and boil, and let the heat be continued and increased until the boiling ceases. See *Alumen*.

ALUMEN FACTITIUM. See *Alumen*.

ALUMEN ROMANUM. See *Alumen*.

ALUMEN RUBRUM. See *Alumen*.

ALUMEN RUPEUM. See *Alumen*.

ALUMEN RUTILUM. See *Alumen*.

ALUMEN USTUM. See *Alumen*.

ALU'MINA. Alumine. *Terra Alumina*. Earth of alum. Pure clay. One of the primitive earths, which, as constituting the plastic principle of all clays, loams, and boles, was called argil or the argillaceous earth, but now, as being obtained in greatest purity from alum, is styled alumina. It was deemed elementary matter till Sir H. Davy's celebrated electro-chemical researches led to the belief of its being, like barytes and lime, a metallic oxyde.

The purest native alumina is found in the oriental gems, the sapphire and ruby. They consist of nothing but this earth, and a small portion of colouring matter. The native porcelain clays or kaolins, however white and soft, can never be regarded as pure alumina. They usually contain fully half their weight of silica, and frequently other earths. To obtain pure alumina we dissolve alum in 20 times its weight of water, and add to it a little of the solution of carbonate of soda, to throw down any iron which may be present. We then drop the supernatant liquid into a quantity of the water of ammonia, taking care not to add so much of the aluminous solution as will saturate the ammonia. The volatile alkali unites with the sulphuric acid of the alum, and the earthy basis of the latter is separated in a white spongy precipitate. This must be thrown on a filter, washed, or edulcorated, as the old chemists expressed it, by repeated affusions of water, and then dried. Or if an alum, made with ammonia instead of potassa, as is the case with some French alums, can be got, simple ignition dissipates its acid and alkaline constituents, leaving pure alumina.

Alumina prepared by the first process is white, pulverulent, soft to the touch, adheres to the tongue, forms a smooth paste without grittiness in the mouth, insipid, inodorous, produces no change in vegetable colours, insoluble in water, but mixes with it readily in every proportion, and retains a small quantity with considerable force; is infusible in the strongest heat of a furnace, experiencing merely a condensation of volume and consequent hardness, but is in small quantities melted by the oxyhydrogen blowpipe. Its specific gravity is 2.000 in the state of powder, but by ignition it is augmented.

Every analogy leads to the belief that alumina contains a peculiar metal, which may be called *aluminum*. The first evidences obtained of this position are presented in Sir H. Davy's researches. Iron negatively electrified by a very high power being fused in contact with pure alumina, formed a globule whiter than pure iron which effervesced slowly in water, becoming covered with a white powder. The solution of this in muriatic acid, decomposed by an alkali, afforded alumina and oxyde of iron. By passing potassium in vapour through alumina heated to whiteness, the greatest part of the potassium became converted into potassa, which formed a coherent mass with that part of the alumina not decompounded; and in this mass there were numerous gray particles, having the metallic lustre, and which became white when heated in the air, and which slowly effervesced in water. In a similar experiment made by the same illustrious chemist, a strong red heat only being applied to the alumina, a mass was obtained, which took fire spontaneously by exposure to air, and which effervesced violently in water. This mass was probably an alloy of aluminum and potassium. The conversion of potassium into its deutoxyde, dry potassa, by alumina, proves the presence of oxygen in the latter. When regarded as an oxyde, Sir H. Davy estimates its oxygen and basis to be to one another as 15 to 33; or as 10 to 22. The prime equivalent of alumina would thus appear to be $1.0+2.2=3.2$. But Berzelius's analysis of sulphate of alumina seems to indicate 2.136 as the quantity of the earth which combines with five of the acid. Hence aluminum will come to be represented by $2.136-1=1.136$.

Alumina which has lost its plasticity by ignition, recovers it by being dissolved in an acid or alkaline menstruum, and then precipitated. In this state it is called a hydrate, for when dried in a steam heat it retains much water; and therefore resembles in composition wavellite, a beautiful mineral, consisting almost entirely of alumina, with about 28 per cent. of water.

Alumina is widely diffused in nature. It is a constituent of every soil, and of almost every rock. It is the basis of porcelain, pottery, bricks, and crucibles. Its affinity for vegetable colouring matter, is made use of in the preparation of lakes, and in the arts of dying and calico printing. Native combinations of alumina, constitute the fullers' earth, ochres, boles, pipeclays, &c.

The salts of alumina have the following general characters:

1. Most of them are very soluble in water, and their solutions have a sweetish acerb taste.
2. Ammonia throws down their earthy base, even though they have been previously acidulated with muriatic acid.
3. At a strong red heat they give out a portion of their acid.
4. Phosphate of ammonia gives a white precipitate.
5. Hydriodate of potassa produces a flocculent precipitate of a white colour, passing into a permanent yellow.
6. They are not affected by oxalate of ammonia, tartaric acid, ferroprussiate of potassa, or tincture of galls: by the first two tests they are distinguishable from yttria; and by the last two, from that earth and glucina.
7. If bisulphate of potassa be added to a solution of an aluminous salt moderately concentrated, octahedral crystals of alum will form.

ALUMINITE. A mineral of a snow white colour, dull, opaque, and having a fine earthy fracture. It consists of sulphuric acid, alumina, water, silica, lime, and oxyde of iron.

ALUMINOUS. Pertaining to alum.

Aluminous waters. Waters impregnated with particles of alum.

ALUMINUM. See *Alumina*.

ALUSIA. (From αλυσις, a wandering.) *Alysis*; Illusion; Hallucination. A term used by Good to a species of his genus *Empathemata*. See *Nosology*.

ALVEAR'IUM. (From *alveare*, a bee-hive.) That part of the meatus auditorius externus is so called, which contains the wax of the ear.

ALVE'OLUS. (A diminutive of *alveus*, a cavity.) The socket of a tooth.

A'LVEUS. (*Alveus*, *i.* m., a cavity.) A cavity.

ALVEUS AMPULLESCENS. That part of the duct conveying the chyle to the subclavian vein, which swells out.

ALVEUS COMMUNIS. The common duct, or communication of the ampullæ of the membranaceous semicircular canals in the internal ear, is so termed by Scarpa.

ALVIDU'CA. (From *alvus*, the belly, and *duco*, to draw.) Purging medicines.

ALVIFLUXUS. (From *alvus*, and *fluo*, to flow.) A diarrhœa, or purging.

ALVUS. (*Alvus*, *i.* f. and sometimes m. *ab alluendo, quâ sordes alluuntur*.) The belly, stomach, and entrails.

A'LYCE. (From $\alpha\lambda\upsilon\omega$, to be anxious.) That anxiety which attends low fevers.

ALY'PIA. (From α, neg. and $\lambda\upsilon\pi\eta$, pain.) Without pain; applied to a purgation of the humours, without pain.

ALY'PIAS. *Alypum.* A species of turbith, the *globularia alypum;* so called because it purges without pain.

ALYSIS. See *Alusia.*

ALY'SMUS. (From $\alpha\lambda\upsilon\omega$, to be restless.) Restlessness.

ALY'SSUM. (From α, neg. and $\lambda\upsilon\sigma\sigma\alpha$, the bite of a mad dog; so called because it was foolishly thought to be a specific in the cure of the bite of a mad-dog.) Mad-wort. See *Marrubium alyssum.*

ALYSSUM GALENI. See *Marrubium verticillatum.*

ALYSSUM PLINII. See *Galium album.*

ALYSSUM VERTICILLATUM. The *Marrubium verticillatum.*

A'LZUM. *Aldum; Aldrum.* The name of the tree which produces gum bdellium, according to some ancient authors.

A'MA. ($\mathrm{A}\mu\alpha$, together.) A word used in composition.

AMADINE. A substance, the properties of which are intermediate between those of starch and gum. See *Starch.*

AMADOU. A variety of the *boletus igniarius,* found on old ash and other trees. It is boiled in water to extract its soluble parts, then dried and beat with a mallet to loosen its texture. It has now the appearance of very spongy doe-skin leather. It is lastly impregnated with a solution of nitre, and dried, when it is called spunk, or German tinder; a substance much used on the continent for lighting fires, either from the collision of flint and steel, or from the sudden condensation of air in the atmospheric pyrophorus.

AMA'LGAM. (*Amalgama;* from $\alpha\mu\alpha$ and $\gamma\alpha\mu\epsilon\iota\nu$, to marry.) A substance produced by mixing mercury with a metal, the two being thereby incorporated. See *Alloy.*

AMAME'LIS. (From $\alpha\mu\alpha$, and $\mu\eta\lambda\epsilon\alpha$, an apple.) The bastard medlar of Hippocrates.

AMANI'TÆ. (From α, priv. and $\mu\alpha\nu\iota\alpha$, madness; so called, because they are eatable and not poisonous, like some others.) A tribe of fungous productions, called mushrooms, truffles, and morells, and by the French, champignons.

AMARA DULCIS. See *Solanum dulcamara.*

AMA'RACUS. (From α, neg. and $\mu\alpha\rho\alpha\iota\nu\omega$, to decay: because it keeps its virtues a long time.) Marjoram.

Amaranth, esculent. See *Amaranthus oleraceus.*

AMARA'NTHUS. (*Amaranthus, i.* m.; from α, neg. and $\mu\alpha\rho\alpha\iota\nu\omega$, to decay: because the flower, when cut, does not soon decay.) The name of a genus of plants in the Linnæan system. Class, *Monœcia;* Order, *Pentandria.*

AMARANTHUS OLERACEUS. *Esculent amaranth.* The leaves of this, and several other species, are eaten in India the same as cabbage is here.

AMA'RUS. Bitter. See *Bitter.* The principal bitters used medicinally are,

1. The *pure bitters;* gentiana lutea, humulus lupulus, and quassia amara.
2. *Styptic bitters;* cinchona officinalis, croton cascarilla, quassia simarouba.
3. *Aromatic bitters;* artemisia absinthium, anthemis nobilis, hyssopus, &c.

AMATORIA FEBRIS. (From *amo,* to love.) See *Chlorosis.*

AMATORIA VENEFICIA. (From *amo,* to love, and *veneficium,* witchcraft.) Philters. Love powders.

AMATO'RIUS. A term given to a muscle of the eye, by which that organ is moved in ogling. See *Rectus inferior oculi.*

AMATZQUI'TI. An Indian term. See *Arbutus unedo.*

AMAURO'SIS. (*Amauroses, is.* f. $\mathrm{A}\mu\alpha\upsilon\rho\omega\sigma\iota\varsigma$; from $\alpha\mu\alpha\upsilon\rho\omega$, to darken or obscure.) *Gutta serena; Amblyopia.* A disease of the eye attended with a diminution or total loss of sight, without any visible injury to the organ, and arising from a paralytic affection of the retina and optic nerve. A genus of disease in the class *locales,* and order *dysæsthesiæ* of Cullen. It arises generally from compression of the optic nerves; *amaurosis compressionis;* from debility, *amaurosis atonica;* from spasm, *amaurosis spasmodica;* or from poisons, *amaurosis venenata.*

The symptoms of amaurosis are noted for being very irregular. In many cases, the pupil is very much dilated, immoveable, and of its natural black colour. Sometimes, however, in the most complete and incurable cases, the pupil is of its natural size, and the iris capable of free motion. In some cases, the pupil has a dull, glassy, or horny appearance. Sometimes its colour is greenish, occasionally whitish and opaque, so as to be liable to be mistaken for an incipient cataract. Richter mentions a degree of strabismus, as the only symptom, except the loss of sight, as invariably attendant on amaurosis.

The blindness produced by amaurosis, is generally preceded by an imaginary appearance of numerous insects, or substances, like cobwebs, interposing themselves between objects and the eye. The origin of a cataract on the other hand, is usually attended with a simple cloudiness of vision.

Violent contusions of the head, apoplectic fits, flashes of lightning, frequent exposure to the rays of the sun, severe exercise, strong passions, drunkenness, and other causes of paralytic affections, are enumerated as producing this complaint. Sometimes tumours within the cranium, bony projections, &c. have been found compressing the optic nerves: but in many instances no morbid appearance could be traced, to account for the blindness.

The disorder is generally difficult to be removed: but is sometimes much benefited by general and local stimulants, persevered in for a considerable time. If there are marks of congestion in the head, local bleeding, active purging, and other evacuations, would be proper in the first instance. Blisters and issues behind the ear or neck should also be tried. Richter speaks of much success from the use of medicines acting steadily on the bowels, after premising an emetic. Mr. Ware observes, that in some cases the pupil is contracted, indicating probably, internal inflammation; and then the internal use of mercury, especially the oxymuriate, will be most beneficial. Electricity has been sometimes serviceable, taking the aura or sparks, or even gentle shocks: but galvanism is certainly preferable. Errhines are often useful, as the compound powder of asarabacca; Mr. Ware particularly recommends the hydrargyrus vitriolatus of the former London Pharmacopœia. Stimulants have been sometimes usefully applied to the eye itself, as the vapour of oil of turpentine, an infusion of capsicum, &c. Where the intention of a blister is to stimulate, it is best applied to the temple on the affected side.

AMBER. *Succinum.* A beautiful bituminous substance, which takes a good polish, and, after a slight rubbing, becomes so electric, as to attract straws and small bodies; it was called $\eta\lambda\epsilon\kappa\tau\rho o\nu$, *electrum,* by the ancients, and hence the word electricity. "Amber is a hard, brittle, tasteless substance, sometimes perfectly transparent, but mostly semitransparent or opaque, and of a glossy surface: it is found of all colours, but chiefly yellow or orange, and often contains leaves or insects; its specific gravity is from 1.065 to 1.100; its fracture is even, smooth, and glossy; it is capable of a fine polish, and becomes electric by friction; when rubbed or heated, it gives a peculiar agreeable smell, particularly when it melts, that is at 550° of Fahrenheit, but it then loses its transparency: projected on burning coals, it burns with a whitish flame, and a whitish-yellow smoke, but gives very little soot, and leaves brownish ashes; it is insoluble in water and alcohol, though the latter, when highly rectified, extracts a reddish colour from it; but it is soluble in the sulphuric acid, which then acquires a reddish-purple colour, and is precipitable from it by water. No other acid dissolves it, nor is it soluble in essential or expressed oils, without some decomposition and long digestion; but pure alkali dissolves it. By distillation it affords a small quantity of water, with a little acetous acid, an oil, and a peculiar acid. The oil rises at first colourless: but, as the heat increases, becomes brown, thick, and empyreumatic. The oil may be rectified by successive distillations, or it may be obtained very light and limpid at once, if it be put into a glass alembic with water, as the elder Rouelle directs, and distilled at a heat not greater than 212° Fahr. It requires to be kept in stone bottles, however, to retain this state; for in glass vessels it becomes brown by the action of light.

Amber is met with plentifully in regular mines in

some parts of Prussia. The upper surface is composed of sand, under which is a stratum of loam, and under this a bed of wood, partly entire, but chiefly mouldered or changed into a bituminous substance. Under the wood is a stratum of sulphuric or rather aluminous mineral, in which the amber is found. Strong sulphureous exhalations are often perceived in the pits.

Detached pieces are also found occasionally on the sea-coast in various countries. It has been found in gravel beds near London. In the Royal Cabinet at Berlin there is a mass of 18lbs. weight, supposed to be the largest ever found. Jussieu asserts, that the delicate insects in amber, which prove the tranquillity of its formation, are not European. Haüy has pointed out the following distinctions between mellite and copal, the bodies which most closely resemble amber. Mellite is infusible by heat. A bit of copal heated at the end of a knife takes fire, melting into drops, which flatten as they fall; whereas amber burns with spitting and frothing; and when its liquefied particles drop, they rebound from the plane which receives them. The origin of amber is at present involved in perfect obscurity, though the rapid progress of vegetable chemistry promises soon to throw light on it. Various frauds are practised with this substance. Neumann states as the common practices of workmen, the two following: The one consists in surrounding the amber with sand in an iron pot, and cementing it with a gradual fire for forty hours, some small pieces placed near the sides of the vessel being occasionally taken out for judging of the effect of the operation: the second method, which he says is that most generally practised, is by digesting and boiling the amber about twenty hours with rapeseed oil, by which it is rendered both clear and hard.

Werner has divided it into two sub-species, the white and the yellow: but there is little advantage in the distinction. Its ultimate constituents are the same with those of vegetable bodies in general; viz. carbon, hydrogen, and oxygen.

In the second volume of the Edinburgh Philosophical Journal, Dr. Brewster has given an account of some optical properties of amber, from which he considers it established beyond a doubt that amber is an *indurated vegetable juice;* and that the traces of a regular structure, indicated by its action upon polarized light, are not the effect of the ordinary laws of crystallization by which *mellite* has been formed, but are produced by the same causes which influence the mechanical condition of gum-arabic, and other gums, which are known to be formed by the successive deposition and induration of vegetable fluids."—*Ure's Chem. Dict.* See *Oleum Succini*, and *Succinic Acid.*

[Amber has heretofore been chiefly obtained from the shores of the Baltic in Prussia. It has however been found in other countries.

In the state of New-Jersey, on Crosswick's creek, four miles from Trenton, it occurs in alluvial soil. The amber is both yellow and whitish, and occurs in grains or small masses, seldom exceeding an inch in length. It rests on lignite or carbonated wood, or even penetrates it, and is sometimes connected with pyrites. The stratum of lignite, which contains the amber, rests on a coarse, ferruginous sand, and is covered by a soft bluish clay, embracing masses of pyrites. Above the clay is a bed of sand. Amber exists also near Woodbury, in the same state, in large plates in a bed of marl; also at Camden, opposite Philadelphia, where a transparent specimen, almost white, and several inches in diameter, has been found in a stratum of gravel.

Most naturalists are induced to believe that amber is a resinous juice, which once proceeded from certain trees, but has since been gradually mineralized in the interior of the earth. It occurs in masses, whose weight usually varies from a fraction of an ounce to a few pounds; and its largest masses, which are extremely rare, do not much exceed 20lbs.—*Cleav. Min.*

The largest mass perhaps ever seen, was recently found between Memel and Koningsberg, measuring 14 inches in length, by 9 1-4 in breadth, and weighing 21lbs.—*Month. Mag. Oct.* 1811. A.]

AMBER SEED. See *Hibiscus abelmoschus.*

AMBERGRIS. (*Ambragrisea, æ.* f.) A concrete, found in very irregular masses, floating on the sea near the Molucca islands, Madagascar, Sumatra, on the coast of Coromandel, Brazil, America, China, and Japan. It has also been taken out of the intestines of the *Physeter macrocephalus*, the spermaceti whale. As it has not been found in any whales but such as are dead or sick, its production is generally supposed to be owing to disease, though some have a little too peremptorily affirmed it to be the cause of the morbid affection. As no large piece has ever been found without a greater or less quantity of the beaks of the *Sepia octopodia*, the common food of the spermaceti whale, interspersed throughout its substance, there can be little doubt of its originating in the intestines of the whale; for if it were occasionally swallowed by it only, and then caused disease, it would be frequently found without these, when it is met with floating or thrown upon the shore.

Ambergris is found of various sizes, generally in small fragments, but sometimes so large as to weigh near two hundred pounds. When taken from the whale it is not so hard as it becomes afterward on exposure to the air. Its specific gravity ranges from 780 to 926. If good, it adheres like wax to the edge of a knife with which it is scraped, retains the impression of the teeth or nails, and emits a fat odoriferous liquid on being penetrated with a hot needle. It is generally brittle; but, on rubbing it with the nail, it becomes smooth like hard soap. Its colour is either white, black, ash-coloured, yellow, or blackish; or it is variegated, namely, gray with black specks, or gray with yellow specks. Its smell is peculiar, and not easy to be counterfeited. At 144° it melts, and at 212° is volatilized in the form of a white vapour. But, on a red-hot coal, it burns, and is entirely dissipated. Water has no action on it; acids, except nitric, act feebly on it; alkalies combine with it, and form a soap; æther and the volatile oils dissolve it; so do the fixed oils, and also ammonia, when assisted by heat; alkohol dissolves a portion of it, and is of great use in analyzing it, by separating its constituent parts. According to Boillon la Grange, who has given the latest analysis of it, 3820 parts of ambergris consist of adipocire 2016 parts, a resinous substance 1167, benzoic acid 425, and coal 212. But Bucholtz could find no benzoic acid in it. Dr. Ure examined two different specimens with considerable attention. The one yielded benzoic acid, the other, equally genuine to all appearance, afforded none.

An alkoholic solution of ambergris, added in minute quantity to lavender water, tooth powder, hair powder, wash balls, &c. communicates its peculiar fragrance. Its retail price being in London so high as a guinea per oz. leads to many adulterations. These consist of various mixtures of benzoin, labdanum, meal, &c. scented with musk. The greasy appearance and smell which heated ambergris exhibits, afford good *criteria*, joined to its solubility in hot æther and alkohol.

It has occasionally been employed in medicine, but its use is mostly confined to the perfumer. Dr. Swediaur took thirty grains of it without perceiving any sensible effect. A sailor, who took half an ounce of it, found it a good purgative.—*Ure's Chem. Dict.*

[Ambergris, which is a concretion from the intestines of the spermaceti whale, also contains a considerable portion of fatty matter, amounting in some specimens to 60 per cent. It is only found in the unhealthy animal. Its chief constituent is a substance very analogous to cholesterine, and to which Peltier and Caventou have given the name of *ambreine.* By digestion in nitric acid, ambreine is converted into a peculiar acid called the *ambreic acid. Webster's Manual of Chem. Boston*, 1828. A.]

The medical qualities of ambergris are stomachic, cordial, and antispasmodic. It is very seldom used in this country.

AMBLO'SIS. (Αμβλωσις; from αμβλοω, to cause abortion.) A miscarriage.

AMBLO'TICA. (Αμβλωτικα; from αμβλοω, to cause abortion.) Medicines which were supposed to occasion abortion.

AMBLYGONITE. A greenish-coloured mineral that occurs in granite, along with green topaz and tourmaline, near Pinig, in Saxony. It seems to be a species of spodumine.

AMBLYO'PIA. (*Amblyopia, æ.* f.; from αμβλος, dull, and ωψ, the eye.) *Amblyosmus; Amblytes.* Hippocrates means by this word, dimness of sight to which old people are subject. Paulus Actuarius, and the best modern writers, seem to think that amblyopia means the same thing as the incomplete amaurosis. See *Amaurosis*.

AMBLYO'SMUS. See *Amblyopia*.

AMBLYTES. See *Amblyopia*.

A'MBO. An Indian name of the mango.

A'MBON. (From αμβαινω, to ascend.) Celsus uses this term to signify the margin or tip of the sockets in which the heads of the large bones are lodged.

A'MBONE. The same as ambe.

A'MBRA. Amber. Also an aromatic gum.

AMBRA CINERACEA. Ambergris and gray amber.

AMBRA GRISEA. Ambergris.

A'MBRAM. Amber.

AMBREINE. See *Ambergris*.

AMBREIC ACID. See *Ambergris*. A.]

AMBRE'TTE. See *Hibiscus abelmoschus*.

AMBULATI'VA. (From *ambulo*, to walk.) A species of herpes; so called because it walks or creeps, as it were, about the body.

AMBU'STIO. (*Ambustio*, *onis*. f.; from *amburo*, to burn.) See *Burn*.

AMBUSTUM. A burn or scald.

AME'LLA. The same as achmella.

AMENORRHŒA. (*Amenorrhœa*, *æ*. f.; from *a*, priv. μην, a month, and ῥεω, to flow.) A partial or total obstruction of the menses in women from other causes than pregnancy and old age. The menses should be regular as to quantity and quality; and that this discharge should observe the monthly period, is essential to health. When it is obstructed, nature makes her efforts to obtain for it some other outlet. When these efforts of nature fail, the consequence may be, pyrexia, pulmonic diseases, spasmodic affections, hysteria, epilepsia, mania, apoplexia, chlorosis, according to the general habit and disposition of the patient. Dr. Cullen places this genus in the class *locales*, and order *epischeses*. His species are, 1. *Emansio mensium;* that is, when the menses do not appear so early as is usually expected. See *Chlorosis*. 2. *Suppressio mensium*, when, after the menses appearing and continuing as usual for some time, they cease without pregnancy occurring. 3. *Amenorrhœa difficilis, vel Menorrhagia difficilis*, when this flux is too small in quantity, and attended with great pain, &c.

The causes of a suppression of the menses appear mostly to operate by inducing a constriction of the extreme vessels; such as cold, fear, and other depressing passions, an indolent life, the abuse of acids, &c. It is sometimes symptomatic of other diseases, in which considerable debility occurs, as phthisis pulmonalis. When the discharge has been some time interrupted, particularly in persons previously healthy, hæmorrhages will often happen from other outlets, the nose, stomach, lungs, &c. even in some instances a periodical discharge of blood from an ulcer has occurred. The patient generally becomes obstinately costive, often dyspeptic; colicky pains, and various hysterical symptoms likewise are apt to attend. The means of chief efficacy in restoring the uterine function are those calculated to relax spasm, assisted sometimes by such as increase arterial action, particularly in protracted cases. The former will be employed with most probability of success, when symptoms of a menstrual effort appear. They are, especially the hip-bath, fomentations to the hypogastrium, sitting over a vessel of hot water, so that the vapour may be applied to the pudenda; with antispasmodic medicines, as the compound galbanum pill, castor, &c. but especially opium. If the patient be plethoric, venæsection should be premised. In cases of long standing, the object will be to bring about a determination of blood to the uterus. This may be accomplished by emmenagogues, of which savine and cantharis are most to be relied upon; though the latter would be improper, if hæmaturia had occurred. Certain cathartics are also very useful, particularly aloes, which appear to operate especially on the rectum, and thus sympathetically influence the uterus. Electric shocks passed through the hypogastric region, may likewise contribute to the cure.

In cases of scanty and painful menstruation, the means pointed out above as calculated to take off constriction of the uterine vessels, should be resorted to; especially the hip-bath, and the free use of opium.

AMENTACEÆ PLANTÆ. Amentaceous plants. A division of plants in natural arrangements of botanists.

AMENTA'CEUS. Having an amentum or catkin, as the willow, birch, beech, poplar, &c.

AME'NTIA. (*Amentia*, *æ*. f.; from *a*, priv. and *mens*, the mind.) Imbecility of intellect, by which the relations of things are either not perceived, or not recollected. A disease in the class *neuroses*, and order *vesaniæ* of Cullen. When it originates at birth, it is called *amentia congenita*, natural stupidity; when from the infirmities of age, *amentia senilis*, dotage or childishness; and when from some accidental cause, *amentia acquisita*.

AME'NTUM. (Derived from its fancied resemblance to a cat's-tail, and by Festus, from the Greek ἁμμα, a bond or thong.) *Julus; Nucamentum; Catulus.* Catkin. A species of inflorescence, considered by some as a species of calyx. It is a simple peduncle covered with numerous chaffy scales, under which are the flowers or parts of fructification. The distinctions of catkins are into,

1. *Cylindrical:* as in *Corylus avellana; Beta alba; Alnus*.
2. *Globose:* as in *Fagus sylvatica; Platanus orientalis; Urtica pilulifera*.
3. *Ovate:* as in the Female *Pinus sylvestris*.
4. *Filiform:* seen in *Fagus pumila* and *Castanea pumila*.
5. *Attenuate*, slender towards the end: as in *Fagus castanea*.
6. *Thick:* in *Juglans regia*.
7. *Imbrecate*, scaly. as in *Juniperus communis*, and *Salix fusca*.
8. *Paleaceous*, chaffy: as in *Pinus sylvestris*.
9. *Naked:* the scales being so small or wanting, that the parts of fructification appear naked, as in *Excoccaria*.

American balsam. See *Myroxylum Peruiferum*.

[AMERICAN CENTAURY. This is the *Chironia angularis* of Linnæus. It is a native of damp, rich soils, in the middle and southern parts of the United States, where it is commonly known by the name of *centaury*. Every part of the plant is a pure, strong bitter, and communicates its qualities to both water and alkohol. It appears to be a remedy in considerable use at the south for intermittent fever. On the stomach it exerts an invigorating influence, and promotes appetite and digestion. It may be given in powder, in doses of ten or twenty grains, or in infusion, which is the more common mode.—*Bigelow's Sequel*, &c. A.]

[AMERICAN COLUMBO. This is the *Frasera Walteri* of Michaux. It is a tall, rank, perennial plant, growing spontaneously in the southern and western parts of the United States. It is the *Swertia frazera* of Smith, in Rees's Cyclopedia. The root, which is large and fleshy, has a considerable degree of bitterness, and when cut in slices and dried, has some resemblance to the imported columbo. Owing to its comparative cheapness, it has been substituted in druggists' shops for columbo, to which it is incomparably inferior in bitterness. It is however an article of considerable tonic powers, and, when fresh, is said to be emetic and cathartic.—*Big. Seq.* A.]

[AMERICAN HELLEBORE. Veratrum viride. The plant bearing this name grows on wet meadows, and on the banks of brooks throughout the United States. It sends up a tuft of large plaited leaves early in the spring, and in June produces a panicle of green flowers It is often designated by the name of *poke-root*, though a very different plant from the *Phytolacca*.

Its properties resemble those of the *Veratrum Album* of Europe, to which plant it is so closely allied in appearance, that many botanists have considered them the same species. The root has a bitter taste, accompanied with acrimony, and leaves a permanent impression on the mouth and fauces. It abounds with a resinous juice, which adheres closely to a knife with which it has been cut. This is taken up by alkohol, and precipitated by water. The decoction has an intensely bitter taste, probably owing to an extractive principle. The distilled water has a slightly unpleasant taste, without bitterness or pungency. *Veratrine* probably exists in this root.

Like the white Hellebore, it is an acrid emetic, and a powerful stimulant, followed by sedative effects. From the sum of my observations respecting it, I am satisfied that the root, when not impaired by long keeping or exposure, is, in sufficient doses, a strong emetic, commencing its operation tardily, but continuing it in many instances for a long time; in large doses affecting the functions of the brain and nervous system, in a powerful manner, producing giddiness, impaired vision, prostration of strength, and diminution of the vital powers.

From three to six grains in powder will commonly occasion vomiting, the activity being in some degree proportionate to the freshness of the article. Dr. Ware found, that doses somewhat larger did not act with undue violence, in the case of some alms-house patients. A *wine*, prepared like that of white hellebore, has produced relief in gout and rheumatism, in doses of less than a fluid drachm.—*Big. Mat. Med.* A.]

[AMERICAN SENNA. Cassia Marilandica. This is a tall plant, with yellow flowers, growing in most parts of the United States. Its botanical affinity to the Cassia Senna, probably first led to a suspicion of its cathartic powers. Its leaves abound with resin, and have also some extractive and volatile matter. An ounce of the dried leaves, infused in water, proves cathartic, and the plant, being easy of acquisition, is not unfrequently used for this purpose by country practitioners.—*Big. Seq.* A.]

AMERICA'NUM TUBEROSUM. The potatoe. See *Solanum toberosum.*

AMETHY'STA PHARMACA. (From *a*, neg. and *μεθυ*, wine.) Medicines which were said either to prevent or remove the effects of wine.—*Galen.*

AMETHY'STUS. (From *a*, neg. and *μεθυσκω*, to be inebriated: so called, because in former times, according to Plutarch, it was thought to prevent drunkenness. —*Ruland. in Lex. Chem.*) The amethyst. "A gem of a violet colour, and great brilliancy, said to be as hard as the ruby or sapphire, from which it only differs in colour. This is called the oriental amethyst, and is very rare. When it inclines to the purple or rosy colour, it is more esteemed than when it is nearer to the blue. These amethysts have the same figure, hardness, specific gravity, and other qualities, as the best sapphires or rubies, and come from the same places, particularly from Persia, Arabia, Armenia, and the West Indies. The occidental amethysts are merely coloured crystals or quartz."

AMIANTHUS. See *Asbestos.*

AMI'CULUM. A little short cloak. It is the same as the amnios, but anciently meant a covering for the pubes of boys, when they exercised in the gymnasium. —*Rhodius.*

AMIDINE. A substance produced, according to Saussure, when we abandon the paste of starch to itself, at the ordinary temperature, with or without the contact of air.

A'MIDUM. See *Amylum.*

AMINÆ'UM. A wine produced in Aminæa, formerly a province of Italy; called also Salernum. Also a strong wine vinegar. Galen mentions *Aminæum Neapolitanum*, and *Aminæum Siculum.*

A'MMI. (*Ammium, i.* n. Αμμι; from *αμμος*, sand, from its likeness to little gravel-stones.) 1. The name of a genus of plants in the Linnean system.

2. The pharmacopœial name of the herb bishop's weed, of which there are two sorts. See *Sison ammi* and *ammi majus.*

AMMI MAJUS. The systematic name for the *ammi vulgare* of the shops. The seeds of this plant, *Ammi—foliis inferioribus pinnatis, lanceolatis serratis; superioribus, multifidis, linearibus*, of Linnæus; are less powerful than those of the *Sison ammi*, but were exhibited with the same views.

AMMI VE'RUM. See *Sison Ammi.*

AMMI VULGARE. See *Ammi majus.*

AMMION. *Ammium.* Cinnabar.

AMMOCHO'SIA. (From *αμμος*, sand, and *χεω*, to pour.) A remedy for drying the body by sprinkling it with hot sand.—*Oribasius.*

AMMO'NIA. (*Ammonia, æ.* f; so called because it is obtained from sal ammoniac, which received its name from being dug out of the earth near the temple of Jupiter Ammon.) Ammonia gas. The substance so called is an aëriform or alkaline air. "There is a saline body, formerly brought from Egypt, where it was separated from soot by sublimation, but which is now made abundantly in Europe, called sal ammoniac. From this salt pure ammonia can be readily obtained by the following process: Mix unslacked quicklime with its own weight of sal ammoniac, each in fine powder, and introduce them into a glass retort. Join to the beak of the retort, by a collar of caoutchouc, (a neck of an Indian rubber bottle answers well,) a glass tube about 18 inches long, containing pieces of ignited muriate of lime. This tube should lie in a horizontal position, and its free end, previously bent obliquely by the blowpipe, should dip into dry mercury in a pneumatic trough. A slip of porous paper, as an additional precaution, may be tied round the tube, and kept moist with æther. If a gentle heat from a charcoal chaffer or lamp be now applied to the bottom of the retort, a gaseous body will bubble up through the mercury. Fill a little glass tube, sealed at one end, with the gas, and transfer it, closely stopped at the other end, into a basin containing water. If the water rise instantly and fill the whole tube, the gas is pure, and may be received for examination.

Ammonia is a transparent, colourless, and consequently invisible gas, possessed of elasticity, and the other mechanical properties of the atmospherical air. Its specific gravity is an important datum in chemical researches, and has been rather differently stated. Now as no aëriform body is more easily obtained in a pure state than ammonia, this diversity, among accurate experimentalists, shows the nicety of this statical operation. Biot and Arago make it = 0.59669 by experiment, and by calculation from its elementary gases, they make it = 0.59438. Kirwan says that 100 cubic inches weigh 18.16 gr. at 30 inches of bar. and 61° F., which compared to air reckoned 30.519, gives 0.59540. Sir H. Davy determines its density to be = 0.590, with which estimate the theoretic calculations of Dr. Prout, in the sixth volume of the Annals of Philosophy, agree.

This gas has an exceedingly pungent smell, well known by the old name of spirits of hartshorn. An animal plunged into it speedily dies. It extinguishes combustion, but being itself to a certain degree combustible, the flame of a taper immersed in it is enlarged before going out. It has a very acrid taste. Water condenses it very rapidly.

Water is capable of dissolving easily about one-third of its weight of ammoniacal gas, or 460 times its bulk. Hence, when placed in contact with a tube filled with this gas, water rushes into it with explosive velocity.

Ammoniacal gas, perfectly dry, when mixed with oxygen, explodes with the electric spark, and is converted into water and nitrogen, as has been shown in an ingenious paper by Dr. Henry. But the simplest, and perhaps most accurate mode of resolving ammonia into its elementary constituents, is that first practised by Berthollet, the celebrated discoverer of its composition. This consists in making the pure gas traverse very slowly an ignited porcelain tube of a small diameter.

The alkaline nature of ammonia is demonstrated, not only by its neutralizing acidity, and changing the vegetable reds to purple or green, but also by its being attracted to the negative pole of a voltaic arrangement. When a pretty strong electric power is applied to ammonia in its liquid or solid combinations, simple decomposition is effected; but in contact with mercury, very mysterious phenomena occur. If a globule of mercury be surrounded with a little water of ammonia, or placed in a little cavity in a piece of sal ammoniac, and then subjected to the voltaic power by two wires, the negative touching the mercury, and the positive the ammoniacal compound, the globule is instantly covered with a circulating film, a white smoke rises from it, and its volume enlarges, while it shoots out ramifications of a semi-solid consistence over the salt. The amalgam has the consistence of soft butter, and may be cut with a knife. Whenever the electrization is suspended, the crab-like fibres retract towards the central mass, which soon, by the constant formation of white saline films, resumes its pristine globular shape and size. The enlargement of volume seems to amount occasionally to ten times that of the mercury, when a small globule is employed. Sir H. Davy, Berzelius, and Gay Lussac and Thenard, have studied this singular phenomenon with great care. They produced the very same substance by putting an amalgam of mercury and potassium into the moistened cupel of sal ammoniac. It becomes five or six times larger, assumes the consistence of butter, while it retains its metallic lustre.

What takes place in these experiments? In the second case, the substance of metallic aspect which we obtain is an ammoniacal hydruret of mercury and potassium. There is formed, besides, muriate of potassa. Consequently a portion of the potassium of the amalgam decomposes the water, becomes potassa, which itself decomposes the muriate of ammonia. Thence result hydrogen and ammonia, which, in the nascent state, unite to the undecomposed amalgam. In the first experiment, the substance which, as in the second, presents the metallic aspect, is only an ammoniacal hydruret of mercury; its formation is accompanied by the perceptible evolution of a certain quantity of chlorine at the positive pole. It is obvious, therefore, that the salt is decomposed by the electricity. The hydrogen of the muriatic acid, and the ammonia, both combine with the mercury.

Ammonia is not affected by a cherry-red heat. According to Guyton de Morveau, it becomes a liquid at about 40°—0°, or at 0° the freezing point of mercury; but it is uncertain whether the appearances he observed may not have been owing to hygrometric water, as happens with chlorine gas. The ammoniacal liquid loses its pungent smell as its temperature sinks, till at —50° it gelatinizes, if suddenly cooled; but if slowly cooled it crystallizes.

Oxygen, by means of electricity, or a mere red heat, resolves ammonia into water and nitrogen. When there is a considerable excess of oxygen, it acidifies a portion of the nitrogen into nitrous acid, whence many fallacies in analysis have arisen. Chlorine and ammonia exercise so powerful an action on each other, that when mixed suddenly, a sheet of white flame pervades them. The simplest way of making this fine experiment, is to invert a matress, with a wide mouth and conical neck, over another with a taper neck, containing a mixture of sal ammoniac and lime, heated by a lamp. As soon as the upper vessel seems to be full of ammonia, by the overflow of the pungent gas, it is to be cautiously lifted up, and inserted, in a perpendicular direction, into a wide-mouthed glass decanter or flask, filled with chlorine. On seizing the two vessels thus joined with the two hands covered with gloves, and suddenly inverting them, like a sand-glass, the heavy chlorine and light ammonia, rushing in opposite directions, unite, with the evolution of flame. As one volume of ammonia contains, in a condensed state, one and a half of hydrogen, which requires for its saturation just one and a half of chlorine, this quantity should resolve the mixture into muriatic acid and nitrogen, and thereby give a ready analysis of the alkaline gas. If the proportion of chlorine be less, sal ammoniac and nitrogen are the results. The same thing happens on mixing the aqueous solutions of ammonia and chlorine. But if large bubbles of chlorine be let up in ammoniacal water of moderate strength, luminous streaks are seen in the dark to pervade the liquid, and the same reciprocal change of the ingredients is effected.

Gay Lussac and Thenard state, that when 3 parts of ammoniacal gas and 1 of chlorine are mixed together, they condense into sal ammoniac, and azote, equal to 1-10 the whole volume, is given out.

Iodine has an analogous action on ammonia; seizing a portion of its hydrogen to form hydriodic acid, whence hydriodate of ammonia results; while another portion of iodine unites with the liberated nitrogen to form the explosive pulverulent iodine.

Cyanogen and ammoniacal gas begin to act upon each other whenever they come into contact, but some hours are requisite to render the effect complete. They unite in the proportion nearly of 1 to 1 1-2, forming a compound which gives a dark orange-brown colour to water, but dissolves in only a very small quantity of water. The solution does not produce prussian blue with the salts of iron.

By transmitting ammoniacal gas through charcoal ignited in a tube, prussic or hydrocyanic acid is formed.

The action of the alkaline metals on gaseous ammonia, is very curious. When potassium is fused in that gas, a very fusible olive-green substance, consisting of potassium, nitrogen, and ammonia is formed; and a volume of hydrogen remains exactly equal to what would result from the action on water of the quantity of potassium employed. Hence, according to Thenard, the ammonia is divided into two portions. One is decomposed, so that its nitrogen combines with the potassium, and its hydrogen remains free, while the other is absorbed in whole or in part by the nitroguret of potassium. Sodium acts in the same manner. The olive substance is opaque, and it is only when in plates of extreme thinness that it appears semitransparent; it has nothing of the metallic appearance; it is heavier than water; and, on minute inspection, seems imperfectly crystallized. When it is exposed to a heat progressively increased, it melts, disengages ammonia, and hydrogen, and nitrogen, in the proportions constituting ammonia; then it becomes solid, still preserving its green colour, and is converted into a nitroguret of potassium or sodium. Exposed to the air at the ordinary temperature, it attracts only its humidity, but not its oxygen, and is slowly transformed into ammoniacal gas, and potassa or soda. It burns vividly when projected into a hot crucible, or when heated in a vessel containing oxygen. Water and acids produce also sudden decomposition, with the extrication of heat. Alkalies or alkaline salts are produced. Alkohol likewise decomposes it with similar results. The preceding description of the compound of ammonia with potassium, as prepared by Gay Lussac and Thenard, was controverted by Sir H. Davy.

The experiments of this accurate chemist led to the conclusion, that the presence of moisture had modified their results. In proportion as more precautions are taken to keep every thing absolutely dry, so in proportion is less ammonia regenerated. He seldom obtained as much as 1-10 of the quantity absorbed; and he never could procure hydrogen and nitrogen in the proportions constituting ammonia; there was always an excess of nitrogen. The following experiment was conducted with the utmost nicety. 3 1-2 gr. of potassium were heated in 12 cubic inches of ammoniacal gas; 7.5 were absorbed, and 3.2 of hydrogen evolved. On distilling the olive-coloured solid in a tube of platina, 9 cubical inches of gas were given off, and half a cubical inch remained in the tube and adapters. Of the nine cubical inches, one-fifth of a cubical inch only was ammonia; 10 measures of the permanent gas mixed with 7.5 of oxygen, and acted upon by the electrical spark, left a residuum of 7.5. He infers that the results of the analysis of ammonia, by electricity and potassium, are the same.

On the whole we may legitimately infer, that there is something yet unexplained in these phenomena. The potassium separates from ammonia as much hydrogen, as an equal weight of it would from water. If two volumes of hydrogen be thus detached from the alkaline gas, the remaining volume, with the volume of nitrogen, will be left to combine with the potassium, forming a triple compound, somewhat analogous to the cyanides, a compound capable of condensing ammonia.

When ammoniacal gas is transmitted over ignited wires of iron, copper, platina, &c. it is decomposed completely, and though the metals are not increased in weight, they have become extremely brittle. Iron, at the same temperature, decomposes the ammonia, with double the rapidity that platinum does. At a high temperature, the protoxyde of nitrogen decomposes ammonia.

Of the ordinary metals, zinc is the only one which liquid ammonia oxydizes and then dissolves. But it acts on many of the metallic oxydes. At a high temperature the gas deoxydizes all those which are reducible by hydrogen. The oxydes soluble in liquid ammonia, are the oxyde of zinc; the protoxyde and peroxyde of copper; the oxyde of silver; the third and fourth oxydes of antimony; the oxyde of tellurium; the protoxides of nickel, cobalt, and iron, the peroxyde of tin, mercury, gold, and platinum. The first five are very soluble, the rest less so. These combinations can be obtained by evaporation, in the dry state, only with copper, antimony, mercury, gold, platinum, and silver; the four last of which are very remarkable for their detonating property. See the particular metals.

All the acids are susceptible of combining with ammonia, and they almost all form with it neutral compounds. Gay Lussac made the important discovery, that whenever the acid is gaseous, its combination with ammoniacal gas takes place in a simple ratio of determinate volumes, whether a neutral or a subsalt be formed.

Ammoniacal salts have the following general characters:—

1st, When treated with a caustic fixed alkali or earth, they exhale the peculiar smell of ammonia

2d, They are generally soluble in water, and crystallizable.

3d, They are all decomposed at a moderate red heat; and if the acid be fixed, as the phosphoric or boracic, the ammonia comes away pure.

4th, When they are dropped into a solution of muriate of platina, a yellow precipitate falls."—*Ure's Chem. Dict.*

The preparations of ammonia in use are,

1. Liquor ammoniæ. See *Ammoniæ liquor*.
2. The sub-carbonate of ammonia. See *Ammoniæ subcarbonas*, and *ammoniæ subcarbonatis liquor*.
3. The acetate of ammonia. See *Ammoniæ acetatis liquor*.
4. The muriate of ammonia. See *Sal ammoniac.*
5. Ferrum ammoniatum.
6. Several tinctures and spirits, holding ammonia in solution.

Ammonia, argentate of. Fulminating silver.

Ammonia acetata. See *Liquor ammoniæ acetatis.*

Ammonia muriata. See *Sal ammoniac.*

Ammonia præparata. See *Ammonia subcarbonas.*

Ammoniac, sal. See *Sal Ammoniac.*

AMMONI'ACUM. (Αμμονιακον; so called from *Ammonia*, whence it was brought.) *Gum-ammoniac.* A concrete gummy resinous juice, composed of little lumps, or tears, of a strong and somewhat ungrateful smell, and nauseous taste, followed by a bitterness. There has, hitherto, been no information had concerning the plant which affords this drug; but Wildenow considers it to be the *Heracleum gummiferum*, having raised that plant from the seeds, which are sometimes found in the drug. It is imported here from Turkey, and from the East Indies. It consists, according to Braconnot, of 70 resin, 18.4 gum. 4.4 glutinous matter, 6 water, and 1.2 loss in 100 parts. Gum ammoniacum is principally employed as an expectorant, and is frequently prescribed in asthma and chronic catarrh. Its dose is from 10 to 30 grains. It is given in the form of pill or diffused in water, and is frequently combined with squill, or tartarized antimony. In large doses it proves purgative. Externally, it is applied as a discutient, under the form of plaster, to white swellings of the knee, and to indolent tumours. The officinal preparations are ammoniacum purificatum. Emplastrum ammoniaci; Empl. ammoniaci cum hydrargyro; Mistura ammoniaci.

Ammoniæ acetatis liquor. A solution of acetate of ammonia; formerly called *Aqua ammoniæ acetatæ.* Take of sub-carbonate of ammonia, two ounces; dilute acetic acid, four pints. Add the acid to the salt, until bubbles of gas shall no longer arise, and mix. The effervescence is occasioned by the escape of carbonic acid gas, which the acetic acid expels, and neutralizes the ammonia.

If the acid rather predominate, the solution is more grateful to the taste: and provided that acid be correctly prepared, the proportions here given will be found sufficient; where the acid cannot be depended on, it will be right to be regulated rather by the cessation of effervescence than by quantity.

This preparation was formerly known in the shops under the name of *spirit of Mindererus.* When assisted by a warm regimen, it proves an excellent and powerful sudorific; and, as it operates without quickening the circulation, or increasing the heat of the body, it is admissible in febrile and inflammatory diseases, in which the use of stimulating sudorifics are attended with danger. Its action may likewise be determined to the kidneys, by walking about in the cool air. The common dose is half an ounce, either by itself, or along with other medicines, adapted to the same intention.

Ammoniæ carbonas. See *Ammoniæ subcarbonas.*

Ammoniæ liquor. *Liquor of Ammonia.* Take of muriate of ammonia eight ounces; lime newly prepared, six ounces; water, four pints. Pour on the lime a pint of the water, then cover the vessel, and set them by for an hour; then add the muriate of ammonia, and the remaining water previously made boiling hot, and cover the vessel again; strain the liquor when it has cooled; then distil from it twelve fluid ounces of the solution of ammonia into a receiver cooled to the temperature of 50°. The specific gravity of this solution should be to that of distilled water, as 4.960 to 1000.

Lime is capable of decomposing muriate of ammonia at a temperature much below that of boiling water; so that when the materials are mixed, a solution of ammonia and of muriate of lime is obtained. This being submitted to distillation, the ammonia passes over with a certain portion of the water, leaving behind the muriate of lime dissolved in the rest. The proportion of water directed seems, however, unnecessarily great, which obliges the operator to employ larger vessels than would otherwise suffice. But the process now directed is certainly much easier, more economical, and more uniform in its results, than that of former pharmacopœias.

This preparation is colourless and transparent with a strong peculiar smell; it parts with the ammonia in the form of gas, if heated to 130 degrees, and requires to be kept, with a cautious exclusion of atmospherical air, with the carbonic acid of which it readily unites on this latter account, the propriety of keeping it in small bottles instead of a large one, has been suggested.

This is the *aqua ammoniæ puræ* of the shops, and the *alcali volatile causticum.*

Water of ammonia is very rarely given internally, although it may be used in doses of ten or twenty drops, largely diluted, as a powerful stimulant in asphyxia and similar diseases. Externally it is applied to the skin as a rubefacient, and in the form of gas to the nostrils, and to the eyes as a stimulant: in cases of torpor, paralysis, rheumatism, syncope, hysteria, and chronic ophthalmia.

Ammoniæ murias. See *Sal ammoniacæ.*

Ammoniæ nitras. *Alcali volatile nitratum; Sal ammoniacus nitrosus; Ammonia nitrata.* A salt composed of the nitric acid and ammonia, the virtues of which are internally diuretic and deobstruent, and externally resolvent and sialogogue.

Ammoniæ subcarbonas. Subcarbonate of ammonia. This preparation was formerly called *ammonia præparata,* and *sal volatilis salis ammoniaci,* and *sal volatilis.* It is made thus:—Take of muriate of ammonia, a pound: of prepared chalk, dried, a pound and a half. Reduce them separately to powder; then mix them together, and sublime in a heat gradually raised, till the retort becomes red. In this preparation a double decomposition takes place, the carbonic acid of the chalk uniting with the ammonia, and forming subcarbonate of ammonia, which is volatilized while muriate of lime remains in the vessel.

This salt possesses nervine and stimulating powers, and is highly beneficial in the dose of from two to eight grains, in nervous affections, debilities, flatulency, and acidity from dyspepsia.

Ammoniæ subcarbonatis liquor. *Liquor ammoniæ carbonatis.* Solution of subcarbonate of ammonia. Take of subcarbonate of ammonia, four ounces; distilled water a pint. Dissolve the subcarbonate of ammonia in the water, and filter the solution through paper. This preparation possesses the properties of ammonia in its action on the human body See *Ammoniæ subcarbonas.*

Ammonicated copper, liquor of. See *Cupri ammoniati liquor.*

Ammo'nion. (From αμμος, sand.) Aëtius uses this term to denote a collyrium of great virtue in many diseases of the eye, which was said to remove sand or gravel from the eyes.

AMMONI'TES. Petrifactions, which have likewise been distinguished by the name of *cornua ammonis,* and are called *snake-stones* by the vulgar, consist chiefly of lime-stone. They are found of all sizes, from the breadth of half an inch to more than two feet in diameter; some of them rounded, others greatly compressed, and lodged in different strata of stones and clays. They appear to owe their origin to shells of the nautilus kind.

AMMO'NIUM. Berzelius first gave this name to a supposed metal which with oxygen he conceives to form the alkali called ammonia. It is now generally used by all chemists. See *Ammonia.*

AMNE'SIA. (From α, priv. and μνησις, memory.) *Amnestia.* Forgetfulness; mostly a symptomatic affection.

Amne'stia. See *Amnesia.*

A'MNIOS. (From αμνος, a lamb, or lamb's skin.) *Amnion.* The soft internal membrane which surrounds the fœtus. It is very thin and pellucid in the early stage of pregnancy, but acquires considerable thickness and strength in the latter months. The amnios contains a thin watery fluid, in which the fœtus is suspended. See *Liquor amnii.*

AMNIO'TIC. (*Amnioticus;* from *amnios:* so called because it is obtained from the membrane of that name.) Of or belonging to the amnios.

Amniotic acid. *Acidum amnioticum.* A peculiar acid found in the liquor of the amnios of the cow. It exists in the form of a white pulverulent powder. It is slightly acid to the taste, but sensibly reddens vegetable blues. It is with difficulty soluble in cold, but readily soluble in boiling water, and in alkohol. When exposed to a strong heat, it exhales an odour of ammonia and of prussic acid. Assisted by heat, it decomposes carbonate of potassa, soda, and ammonia. It produces no change in the solutions of silver, lead, or mercury, in nitric acid. Amniotic acid may be obtained by evaporating the liquor of the amnios of the cow to a fourth part, and suffering it to cool; crystals of amniotic acid will be obtained in considerable quantity. Whether this acid exists in the liquor of the amnios of other animals, is not yet known.

AMO'MUM. (*Amomum, i.* n.; from an Arabian word, signifying a pigeon, the foot of which it was thought to resemble.) The name of a genus of plants in the Linnæan system. Class *Monanaria;* Order, *Monogynia.*

Amomum cardamomum. The former systematic name for the *cardamomum minus.* See *Elettaria cardamomum.*

Amomum granum paradisi. The systematic name of the plant which affords the grains of paradise. *Cardamomum majus; Meleguetta; Maniguetta; Cardamomum piperatium.* Grains of paradise, or the greater cardamom seeds, are contained in a large brown, somewhat triangular flask, the thickness of one's thumb, and pyramidal. The seeds are angular, and of a reddish brown colour, smaller than pepper, and resemble very much the seeds of the *cardamomum minus.* They are extremely hot, and similar in virtue to pepper.

Amomum verum. True stone parsley. The fruit is about the size of a grape, of a strong and grateful aromatic taste, and penetrating smell. The seeds have been given as a carminative.

Amomum zingiber. The former systematic name of the plant which affords ginger. See *Zingiber officinale.*

Amo'rge. See *Amurca.*

AMPELITE. The aluminous ampelite, is the alum slate; and the graphic, the graphic slate.

AMPELOSA'GRIA. (From αμπελος, a vine, and αγριος, wild.) See *Bryonia alba.*

AMPHEMERI'NA. See *Amphemerinos.*

AMPHEMERI'NOS. (Fom αμφι, about and ημερα, a day.) *Amphemerina.* A fever of one day's duration.

AMPHIARTHRO'SIS. Αμφιαρθρωσις; from αμφι, both, and αρθρωσις, an articulation: so called from its partaking both of diarthrosis and synarthrosis.) A mixed species of connexion of bones, which admits of an obscure motion, as is observed in the metacarpal and metatarsal bones, and the vertebræ.

AMPHIBIUM. (From αμφι, *ambo,* and βιος, vita.) An amphibious animal, or one that lives both on land and in the water. The *amphibious* animals, according to Linnæus, are a class, the heart of which is furnished with one ventricle and one auricle, in which respiration is in a considerable degree voluntary.

AMPHIBLESTROI'DES. (From αμφιβλεςρον, a net, and ειδος, a resemblance.) Reteform or net-like; a term which has been applied to the retina.

Amphibole. Some species of actionlite and hornblende have this name.

[This is the name given by Haüy, to a mineral, the synonyms of which are:—

Tremolith of Werner,
La Tremolithe of Brochant,
Grammatite of Brogniart,
Tremolite of Cleaveland. A.]

Amphibolites. Trap rocks are so called in geology, the basis of which is hornblende.

AMPHIBRA'NCHIA. (From αμφι, about, and βραγχια, the jaws.) The fauces or parts about the tonsils, according to Hippocrates and Foësius.

Amphicau'stis. (From αμφι, about, and καυςις, ripe corn.) A sort of wild barley.

2. Eustachius says, it was also to express the private parts of a woman.

AMPHIDEON. (From αμφι, on both sides, and δαιω, to divide.) *Amphidæum; Amphidium.* The os tincæ, or mouth of the womb, which opens both ways, was so called by the ancients.

AMPHIDIARTHRO'SIS. The same as *Amphiarthrosis.*

Amphigene. A name of Vesuvian.

[This name is given by Haüy to that crystalline substance, frequently found among volcanic productions, and which other mineralogists have called *Leucite.* A.]

AMPHIMERI'NA. (From αμφι, about, and ημερα, a day.) A fever of one day's continuance.

AMPHIME'TRION. (From αμφι, about, and μητρα, the womb.) *Amphimetrium.* The parts about the womb. *Hippocrates.*

A'mphiplex. (From αμφι, about, and πλεκτω, to connect.) According to Rufus Ephesius, the part situated between the scrotum and anus, and which is connected with the thighs.

Amphipneuma. (From αμφι, about, and πνευμα, breath.) A difficulty of breathing.—*Hippocrates.*

AMPHI'POLIS. (From αμφι, about, and πολεω, to attend.) *Amphipolus.* One who attends the bed of a sick person, and administers to him.—*Hippocrates.*

Amphismi'la. (From αμφι, on both sides, and σμιλη, an incision-knife.) A dissecting knife, with an edge on both sides. *Galen.*

AMPLECTENS. Embracing, clasping.

AMPLEXICAULIS. (From *amplector,* to surround, and *caulis,* a stem.) Embracing or clasping the stem. *Folium amplexicaule* is a leaf, the base of which surrounds the stem, as in *Papaver somniferum* and *Carduus marianus;* and the *Senesio hirsutus,* has a leafstalk which embraces the stem as its base.

AMPU'LLA. (Αμβολλα; from αναβαλλω, to swell out.) A bottle.

1. All bellied vessels are so called in chemistry, as bolt-heads, receivers, cucurbits, &c.

2. In anatomy this term is applied by Scarpa to the dilated portions of the membranaceous semicircular canals, just within the vestibulum of the ear.

3. In botany; it is a small membranaceous bag attached to the roots and the emersed leaves of some aquatic plants, rendering them buoyant.—*Thompson.*

AMPULLE'SCENS. (From *ampulla,* a bottle.) The most tumid part of the thoracic duct is called *alveus ampullescens.*

AMPUTA'TIO. (From *amputo,* to cut off.) *Ectome.* Amputation; a surgical operation, which consists in the removal of a limb or viscus: thus we say, a leg, a finger, the penis, &c. when cut off, are amputated; but when speaking of a tumour or excrescence, it is said to be removed, or dissected out.

AMULE'TUM. (From αμμα, a bond; because it was tied round the person's neck; or rather from αμυνω, to defend.) An amulet, or charm; by wearing which the person was supposed to be defended from the admission of all evil: in particular, an antidote against the plague.

Amu'rca. (From αμεργω, to press out.) *Amorge.*
1. A small herb, whose expressed juice is used in dying.

2. The sediment of the olive, after the oil has been pressed from it; recommended by Hippocrates and Galen as an application to ulcers.

Amu'tica. (From αμυτ7ω, to scratch.) Medicines that, by vellicating or scratching, as it were, the bronchia, stimulate it to the discharge of whatever is to be thrown off the lungs.

A'myche. (From αμυσσω, to scratch.)

1. A superficial laceration or exulceration of the skin: a slight wound.—*Hippocrates.*

2. Scarification.—*Galen.*

AMY'GDALA. (*Amygdala, æ.* f.; Αμυγδαλη; from αμυσσω, to lancinate: so called, because after the green husk is removed from the fruit, there appear upon the shell certain fissures, as it were lacerations.)

1. The fruit called the almond. See *Amygdalis communis.*

2. The tonsil glands of the throat are sometimes termed, from their resemblance, *Amygdalæ.*

Amygdala amara. The bitter almond. See *Amygdalus communis.*

AMYGDALA DULCIS. The sweet almond. See *Amygdalus communis.*

AMYGDALÆ OLEUM. See *Amygdalus communis.*

AMYGDALOID. (*Amygdaloides;* from *amygdalus*, an almond, and εἰδος, resemblance.) Almond-like.

1. A name given to some parts of the body and to parts of vegetables and minerals, which resemble almonds.

2. A compound mineral consisting of spheroidal particles or vesicles of lithomarge, green earth, calc spar, steatite imbedded in a basis of fine-grained greenstone or wacke, containing sometimes, also, crystals of hornblende.

[Amygdaloid is a compound rock, composed of a basis, in which are imbedded various simple minerals. But these imbedded minerals are not crystals and grains, apparently of cotemporaneous origin with the basis itself, *as in the case of porphyry.* On the contrary, their form, though sometimes irregular, is usually spheroidal or oval, like that of an *almond;* and hence the name of this rock, (from *Amygdala*, an almond.) —*Cleav. Min.* A.]

AMY'GDALUS. (*Amygdalus*, *i.* m.; from *amygdala*, the derivation of which look to.) The name of a genus of plants in the Linnæan system. Class *Icosandria;* Order, *Monogynia.* The almond-tree.

AMYGDALUS COMMUNIS. The systematic name of the plant which affords the common almond. *Amygdalus—foliis serratis infimis glandulosis, floribus sessilibus geminis* of Linnæus.

The almond is a native of Barbary. The same tree produces either bitter or sweet. Sweet almonds are more in use as food than medicine; but they are said to be difficult of digestion, unless extremely well comminuted. Their medicinal qualities depend upon the oil which they contain in the farinaceous matter, and which they afford on expression, nearly in the proportion of half their weight. It is very similar to olive oil; perhaps rather purer, and is used for the same purposes. The oil thus obtained is more agreeable to the palate than most of the other expressed oils, and is therefore preferred for internal use, being generally employed with a view to obtund acrid juices, and to soften and relax the solids, in tickling coughs, hoarseness, costiveness, nephritic pains, &c. Externally, it is applied against tension and rigidity of particular parts. The milky solutions of almonds in watery liquors, usually called emulsions, possess, in a certain degree, the emollient qualities of the oil, and have this advantage over pure oil, that they may be given in acute or inflammatory disorders, without danger of the ill effects which the oil might sometimes produce by turning rancid. The officinal preparations of almonds are the expressed oil, the confection, and the emulsion; to the latter, the addition of gum-arabic is sometimes directed, which renders it a still more useful demulcent in catarrhal affections, stranguries, &c.

Bitter almonds yield a large quantity of oil, perfectly similar to that obtained from sweet almonds, but the matter remaining after the expression of the oil, is more powerfully bitter than the almond in its entire state. Great part of the bitter matter dissolves by the assistance of heat, both in water and rectified spirit; and a part arises also with both menstrua in distillation. Bitter almonds have been long known to be poisonous to various brute animals; and some authors have alleged that they are also deleterious to the human species; but the facts recorded upon this point appear to want further proof. However, as the noxious quality seems to reside in that matter which gives it the bitterness and flavour, it is very probable, that when this is separated by distillation, and taken in a sufficiently concentrated state, it may prove a poison to man, as is the case with the common laurel, to which it appears extremely analogous. Bergius tells us, that bitter almonds, in the form of emulsion, cured obstinate intermittents, after the bark had failed. A simple water is distilled from bitter almonds, after the oil is pressed out, which possesses the same qualities, and in the same degree, as that drawn from cherry-stones. These afforded, formerly, the now-exploded *aqua cerasorum nigrorum*, or black cherry-water.

AMYGDALUS PERSICA. The systematic name of the common peach-tree. The fruit is known to be grateful and wholesome, seldom disagreeing with the stomach, unless this organ is not in a healthy state, or the fruit has been eaten to excess, when effects similar to those of the other dulco-acid summer fruits may be produced. The flowers, including the calyx as well as the corolla, are the parts of the persica used for medicinal purposes. These have an agreeable but weak smell, and a bitterish taste. Boulduc observes, "that when distilled, without addition, by the heat of a water-bath, they yield one-sixth their weight, or more, of a whitish liquid, which communicates to a considerable quantity of other liquids a flavour like that of the kernels of fruits. These flowers have a cathartic effect, and especially to children, have been successfully given in the character of a vermifuge; for this purpose, an infusion of a drachm of flowers dried, or half an ounce in their recent state, is the requisite dose. The leaves of the peach are also found to possess anthelmintic power, and from a great number of experiments appear to have been given with invariable success both to children and adults. However, as the leaves and flowers of this plant manifest, in some degree, the quality of those of the laurocerasus, they ought to be used with caution."

A'MYLA. (From *amylum*, starch.) This term has been applied to some chemical fæcula, or highly pulverized residuum. Obsolete.

AMY'LEON. *Amylion.* Starch.

A'MYLUM. (*Amylum*, *i.* n. Αμυλον; from *a*, priv. and μυλη, a mill; because it was formerly made from wheat, without the assistance of a mill.) *Amyleon; Amylion.* See *Starch.*

AMY'RIS. (From *a*, intensive, and μυρον, ointment, or balm; so called from its use, or smell.) The name of a genus of plants in the Linnæan system. Class, *Octandria;* Order, *Monogynia*, of which two species are used in medicine.

AMYRIS ELEMIFERA. The systematic name of the plant from which it is supposed we obtain the resin called *gum-elemi.* The plant is described by Linnæus: *Amyris:—foliis ternis quinato pinnatisque subtus tomentosis.* Elemi is brought here from the Spanish West Indies: it is most esteemed when softish, somewhat transparent, of a pale whitish colour, inclining a little to green, and of a strong, though not unpleasant smell. It is only used in ointments and plasters, and is a powerful digestive.

AMYRIS GILEADENSIS. The systematic name of the plant from which the *opobalsamum* is obtained. It has been called by a variety of names, as *Balsamum genuinum antiquorum; Balsamelæon; Ægyptiacum balsamum; Balsamum Asiaticum; Balsamum Judaicum, Balsamum Syriacum; Balsamum e Mecca; Balsamum Alpini; Oleum balsami; Carpobalsamum; Xylobalsamum.* Balsam, or balm of Gilead; Balsam of Mecca. A resinous juice, obtained by making incisions into the bark of the *Amyris:—foliis ternatis integerrimis, pedunculis unifloris lateralibus* of Linnæus. This tree grows spontaneously, particularly near to Mecca, on the Asiatic side of the Red Sea. The juice of the fruit is termed *carpobalsamum* in the pharmacopœias, and that of the wood and branches *xylobalsamum.* The best sort is a spontaneous exudation from the tree, and is held in so high estimation by the Turks, that it is rarely, if ever, to be met with genuine among us. The medicinal virtues of the genuine balsam of Gilead, have been highly rated, undoubtedly with much exaggeration. The common balsam of Mecca is scarcely used; but its qualities seem to be very similar to those of the balsam of Tolu, with perhaps more acrimony. The dose is from 15 to 50 drops.

A'MYUM. (From *a*, priv. and μυς, muscle.) A limb so emaciated that the muscles scarcely appear.

ANA. In medical prescriptions it means "of each." See *A.*

ANA'BASIS. (From αναβαινω, to ascend.)

1. An ascension, augmentation, or increase of a disease, or paroxysm. It is usually meant of fevers.—*Galen.*

2. A species of the *equisetum*, or horse-tail plant.

ANABA'TICA. (From αναβαινω, to ascend.) An epithet formerly applied to a continual fever, when it increases in malignity.

ANABE'XIS. (From αναβηττω, to cough up.) An expectoration of matter by coughing.

ANABLE'PSIS. (From ανα and βλεπω, to see again.) The recovery of sight after it has been lost.

ANABLYSIS. (From ανα and βλυζω, to gush out again.) Ebullition or effervescence.

ANA'BOLE. (From αναβαλλω, to cast up.) The

discharge of any thing by vomit; also dilatation, or extension.—*Galen.*

ANABROCHE'SIS. (From ανα and βροχεω, to reabsorb.) The reabsorption of matter.

ANABROCHI'SMOS. (From αναβροχεω, to reabsorb.) *Anabrochismus.* The taking up and removing the hair on the eyelids, when they become troublesome.—*Galen, Ægineta,* and others.

ANABRO'SIS. (From αναβροσκω, to devour.) A corrosion of the solid parts, by sharp and biting humours.—*Galen.*

ANACA'RDIUM. (From ανα, without, and καρδια, a heart.) Without heart; because the pulp of the fruit, instead of having the seed enclosed, as is usually the case, has the nut growing out of the end of it. The name of a genus of plants. Class, *Enneandria;* Order, *Monogynia.*

ANACARDIUM OCCIDENTALE. The cashewnut. The oil of this nut is an active caustic, and employed as such in its native country: but neither it, nor any part of the fruit, is used medicinally in this country. It is a useful marking ink, as any thing written on linen or cotton with it, is of a brown colour, which gradually grows blacker, and is very durable.

ANACARDIUM ORIENTALE. The Malacca bean. See *Avicennia tomentosa.*

ANACATHA'RSIS. (From ανα, and καθαιρομαι, to purge up.) An expectoration of pus, or a purgation by spitting, contra-distinguished from catharsis, or evacuation downwards. In this sense the word is used by Hippocrates and Galen. Blanchard denotes, by this word, medicines which operate upwards, as vomiting, &c.

ANACATHA'RTIC. (*Anacatharticus;* from ανακαθαιρομαι, to purge upwards.) Promoting expectoration, or vomiting.

ANA'CHRON. Mineral alkali.

ANA'CLASIS. (From ανακλαω, to bend back.) A reflection or recurvature of any of the members, according to Hippocrates.

ANA'CLISIS. (From ανακλενω, to recline.) A couch, or sick-bed.—*Hippocrates.*

ANACO'CHE. (From ανακωχεω, to retard.) Delay in the administration of medicines; also slowness in the progress of a disease.—*Hippocrates.*

ANACŒLIA'SMUS. (From ανα, and κοιλια, the bowels.) A gentle purge, which was sometimes used to relieve the lungs.

ANACOLLE'MA. (From ανα, and κολλαω, to glue together.) A collyrium made of agglutinant substances, and stuck on the forehead.—*Galen.*

ANACONCHOLI'SMOS. (From ανακογχολιζω, to sound as a shell.) A gargarism: so called, because the noise made in the throat is like the sound of a shell.—*Galen.*

ANACTE'SIS. (From ανακταομαι, to recover.) Restoration of strength; recovery from sickness.—*Hippocrates.*

ANACUPHI'SMA. (From ανακουφιζω, to lift up.) A kind of exercise mentioned by Hippocrates, which consists in lifting the body up and down, like our weigh jolt, and dumb bells.

ANACYCE'SIS. (From ανακυκαω, to mix.) The mixture of substances, or medicines, by pouring one upon another.

ANACY'CLEON. (From ανακυκλοω, to wander about.) *Anacycleus.* A mountebank, or wandering quack.

ANACYRI'OSIS. (From ανα, and κυρος, authority.) By this word, Hippocrates means that gravity and authority which physicians should preserve among sick people and their attendants.

ANADIPLO'SIS. (From αναδιπλοω, to reduplicate.) A reduplication or frequent return of a paroxysm, or disease.—*Galen.*

ANA'DOSIS. (From ανω, upwards, and διδωμι, to give.) 1. A vomit.

2. The distribution of aliment all over the body.

3. Digestion.

ANA'DROME. (From ανω, upwards, and δρεμω, to run.) A pain which runs from the lower extremities to the upper parts of the body.—*Hippocrates.*

ANÆ'DES. (From α, priv. and αιδως, a shame.) Shameless. Hippocrates uses this word metaphorically for without restraint; and applies it to water rushing into the aspera arteria.

ANÆSTHE'SIA. (*Anæsthesia, æ.* f. Αναισθησια; from α, priv. and αισθανομαι, to feel.) Loss of the sense of touch. A genus of disease in the class *Locales,* and order *Dysæsthesiæ* of Cullen.

ANAGA'LLIS. (From αναγελαω, to laugh; because, by curing the spleen, it disposes persons to be cheerful.) 1. The name of a genus of plants in the Linnæan system.

2. The pharmacopœial name of the *anagallis arvensis.*

ANAGALLIS ARVENSIS. The systematic name for the *Anagallis—foliis indivisis, caule procumbente* of Linnæus. A small and delicately formed plant, which does not appear to possess any particular properties.

ANAGARGALI'CTUM. (From ανα, and γαργαρεων, the throat.) A gargarism, or wash for the throat.

ANAGARGARI'STUM. A gargle.

ANAGLY'PHE. (From αναγλυφω, to engrave.) A part of the fourth ventricle of the brain was formerly thus called, from its resemblance to a pen, or style.

ANAGNO'SIS. (From αναγινωσκω, to know.) The persuasion, or certainty, by which medical men judge of a disease from its symptoms.—*Hippocrates.*

ANA'GRAPHE. (From αναγραφω, to write.) A prescription or receipt.

ANALCINE. Cubic zeolite. A mineral found in granite, gneiss, trap rocks, and lavas, at Calton Hill, Edinburgh, in Bohemia, and Ferroe islands. From its becoming *feebly* electrical by heat, it has got this name. [Derived from Αναλκις. Weak.]

ANALE'NTIA. A fictitious term used by Paracelsus for epilepsy.

ANALE'PSIA. (From ανα, and λαμβανω, to take again.) A species of epilepsy, which proceeds from a disorder of the stomach, and with which the patient is apt to be seized very often and suddenly.

ANALE'PSIS. (From αναλαμβανω, to restore.) A recovery of strength after sickness.

ANALE'PTIC. (*Analepticus;* from αναλαμβανω, to recruit or recover.) That which recovers the strength which has been lost by sickness.

ANALO'SIS. (From αναλισκω, to consume.) A consumption, or wasting.

ANA'LYSIS. (Αναλυσις; from αναλυω, to resolve.) The resolution by chemistry, of any matter into its primary and constituent parts. The processes and experiments which chemists have recourse to, are extremely numerous and diversified, yet they may be reduced to two species, which comprehend the whole art of chemistry. The first is, *analysis,* or decomposition; the second, *synthesis,* or composition. In *analysis,* the parts of which bodies are composed, are separated from each other: thus, if we reduce cinnabar, which is composed of sulphur and mercury, and exhibit these two bodies in a separate state, we say we have decomposed or analyzed cinnabar. But if, on the contrary, several bodies be mixed together, and a new substance be produced, the process is then termed chemical composition, or *synthesis:* thus, if by fusion and sublimation, we combine mercury with sulphur, and produce cinnabar, the operation is termed chemical composition, or composition by synthesis. Chemical analysis consists of a great variety of operations. In these operations the most extensive knowledge of such properties of bodies as are already discovered must be applied, in order to produce simplicity of effect, and certainty in the results. Chemical analysis can hardly be executed with success, by one who is not in possession of a considerable number of simple substances in a state of great purity, many of which, from their effects, are called reagents. The word analysis is often applied by chemists to denote that series of operations, by which the component parts of bodies are determined, whether they be merely separated, or exhibited apart from each other; or whether these distinctive properties be exhibited by causing them to enter into new combinations, without the perceptible intervention of a separate state; and, in the chemical examination of bodies, analysis or separation can scarcely ever be effected, without synthesis taking place at the same time.

ANAMNE'SIS. (From αναμιμνησκω, to remember.) Remembrance, or recollection of what has been done.—*Galen.*

ANAMNE'STIC. (From the same.) A remedy for bad memory, or whatever strengthens the memory.

ANA'NAS. The egg-shaped pine-apple. See *Bromelia Ananas.*

ANA'NCE. (From αναγκαζω, to compel.) Necessity. It is applied to any desperate operation.—*Hippocrates.*

Anaphalanti'asis. (From αναφαλαντος, bald.) A thinness of hair upon the eyebrows.—*Gorræus.*

Ana'phora. (From αναφερω, to bring up.) It is applied to a person who spits blood.—*Gorræus.*

ANAPHORY'XIS. (From αναφορυσσω, to grind down.) The reducing of any thing to dust, or a very fine powder.

ANAPHRODI'SIA. (*Anaphrodisia*, æ. f.; from α, priv. and αφροδισια, the feast of Venus.) Impotence. A genus of disease in the class *Locales*, and order *Dysorexiæ* of Cullen. It either arises from paralysis, *anaphrodisia paralytica;* or from gonorrhœa, *anaphrodisia gonorrhoica.*

Anaphro'meli. (From α, neg. αφρος, froth, and μελι, honey.) Clarified honey.

ANAPLA'SIS. (From αναπλασσω, to restore again.) A restoration of flesh where it has been lost; also the reuniting a fractured bone.—*Hippocrates.*

ANAPLERO'SIS. (From αναπληροω, to fill again.) The restitution or filling up of wasted parts.—*Galen.*

Anaplero'tica. (From the same.) Medicines renewing flesh: incarnatives, or such medicines as fill up a wound so as to restore it to its original shape.—*Galen.*

Anapleu'sis. (From αναπλευω, to float upon.) The rotting of a bone, so that it drops off, and lies upon the flesh. Exfoliation, or separation of a bone.—*Hippocrates, Ægineta*, &c.

ANAPNEU'SIS. (From αναπνευω, to respire.) Respiration.

ANA'PNOE. Respiration.

ANAPTO'SIS. (From αναπιπτω, to fall back.) A relapse.

Ana'ptysis. The same as *Anacatharsis.*

Anarrhegni'mia. (From ανα, and ῥηγνυμι, to break again.) *Anarrhexis.* A fracture; the fresh opening of a wound.

ANARRHŒ'A. (From ανα, upwards, and ῥεω, to flow.) A flux of humours from below upwards.—*Schneider de Catarrho.*

Anarrho'pia. (From ανα, upwards, and ῥεπω, to creep.) A flux of humours, from below upwards.—*Hippocrates.*

A'NAS. (*Anas, tis.* f.; from νεω, to swim, *a nando.*) A genus of birds in the Linnæan system.

Anas cygnus. The swan. The flesh of the young swan or cygnet is tender, and a great delicacy.

Anas domestica. The tame duck. The flesh of this bird is difficult of digestion, and requires that warm and stimulating condiments be taken with it to enable the stomach to digest it.

ANASA'RCA. (*Anasarca*, æ. f.; from ανα, through, and σαρξ, flesh.) *Sarcites.* A species of dropsy from a serous humour, spread between the skin and flesh, or rather a general accumulation of lymph in the cellular system. Dr. Cullen ranks this genus of disease in the class *Cachexiæ*, and the order *Intumescentiæ.* He enumerates the following species, viz. 1. *Anasarca serosa:* as when the due discharge of serum is suppressed, &c. 2. *Anasarca oppilata:* as when the blood-vessels are considerably pressed, which happens to many pregnant women, &c. 3. *Anasarca exanthematica:* this happens after ulcers, various eruptive disorders, and particularly after the *erysipelas.* 4. *Anasarca anæmia* happens when the blood is rendered extremely poor from considerable losses of it. 5. *Anasarca debilium:* as when feebleness is induced by long illness, &c.

This species of dropsy shows itself at first with a swelling of the feet and ancles towards the evening, which, for a time, disappears again in the morning. The tumefaction is soft and inelastic, and when pressed upon by the finger, retains its mark for some time, the skin becoming much paler than usual. By degrees the swelling ascends upwards, and occupies the trunk of the body; and at last, even the face and eyelids appear full and bloated; the breathing then becomes difficult, the urine is small in quantity, high coloured, and deposites a reddish sediment; the belly is costive, the perspiration much obstructed, the countenance yellow, and a considerable degree of thirst, with emaciation of the whole body, prevails. To these symptoms succeed torpor, heaviness, a troublesome cough, and a slow fever. In some cases the water oozes out, through the pores of the cuticle; in others, being too gross to pass by these, it raises the cuticle in small blisters; and sometimes the skin, not allowing the water to escape through it, is compressed and hardened, and is at the same time so much distended as to give the tumour a considerable degree of firmness. For the causes of this disease, see *Hydrops.*

In those who have died of anasarca, the whole of the cellular membrane has been distended with a fluid, mostly of a serous character. Various organic diseases have occurred; and the blood is said to be altered in consistence, according to the degree of the disease. In general a cure can be more readily effected when it arises from topical or general debility, than when occasioned by visceral obstruction; and in recent cases, than in those of long continuance. The skin becoming somewhat moist, with a diminution of thirst, and increased flow of urine, are very favourable. In some few cases the disease goes off by a spontaneous crisis by vomiting, purging, &c. The indications of treatment in anasarca are, 1. To evacuate the fluid already collected. 2. To prevent its returning again. The first object may be attained mechanically by an operation; or by the use of those means, which increase the action of the absorbents: the second by removing any exciting causes, which may still continue to operate; and at the same time endeavouring to invigorate the system. Where the quantity of fluid collected is such as to disturb the more important functions, the best mode of relieving the patient is to make a few small incisions with a lancet, not too near each other, through the integuments on the fore and upper part of each thigh; the discharge may be assisted by pressure, and when a sufficient quantity has been evacuated, it is better to heal them by the first intention. In the use of issues or blisters, there is some risk of inducing gangrene, especially if applied to the legs: and the same has happened from scarifications with the cupping instrument. Absorption may be promoted by friction, and bandaging the parts, which will at the same time obviate farther effusion; but most powerfully by the use of different evacuating remedies, especially those which occasion a sudden considerable discharge of fluids. Emetics have been often employed with advantage; but it is necessary to guard against weakening the stomach by the frequent repetition of those which produce much nausea; and perhaps the benefit results not so much from the evacuation produced by the mouth, as from their promoting other excretions; antimonials in particular inducing perspiration, and squill increasing the flow of urine, &c.; for which purpose they may be more safely given in smaller doses: in very torpid habits, mustard may claim the preference. Cathartics are of much greater and more general utility; where the bowels are not particularly irritable, the more drastic purgatives should be employed and repeated as often as the strength will allow; giving, for example, every second or third morning, jalap, scammony, colocynth, or gamboge, joined with calomel or the supertartrate of potassa and some aromatic, to obviate their griping. Elaterium is perhaps the most powerful, generally vomiting as well as purging the patient, but precarious in its strength and therefore better given in divided doses, till a sufficient effect is produced. Diuretics are universally proper, and may be given in the intervals, where purgatives can be borne, otherwise constantly persevered in; but unfortunately the effects of most of them are uncertain. Saline substances in general appear to stimulate the kidneys, whether acid, alkaline, or neutral; but the acetate, and supertartrate of potassa, are chiefly resorted to in dropsy. Dr. Ferriar, of Manchester, has made an important remark of the latter salt, that its diuretic power is much promoted by a previous operation on the bowels, which encourages the more liberal use of it; indeed, if much relied upon, a drachm or two should be given three times or oftener in the day. It is obviously, therefore, best adapted to those cases, in which the strength is not greatly impaired; and the same holds with the nauseating diuretics, squill, colchicum, and tobacco. The latter has been strongly recommended by Dr. Fowler of York, in the form of tincture; the colchicum, as an oxymel by some German physicians; but the squill is most in use, though certainly very precarious if given alone. In languid and debilitated habits, we prefer the more stimulant diuretics, as juniper, horseradish, mustard, garlic, the spiritus ætheris nitrici, &c.; even turpentine, or the tinctura cantharidis, may be proper, where milder means have failed. Digitalis is often a very powerful remedy, from the utility of which in inflammatory diseases we might expect it to answer best in persons of great natural strength, and not much exhausted by the disorder; but Dr. Withering expressly states that its diuretic effects appear most certainly and beneficially, where the pulse is feeble or intermitting, the countenance pale, the skin cold, and the tumours readily pitting on pressure; which has been since confirmed by other practitioners: it should be begun with in small doses two or three times a day, and progressively increased till the desired operation on the kidneys ensues, unless alarming symptoms appear in the mean time. Opium and some other narcotics have been occasionally useful as diuretics in dropsy, but should be only regarded as adjuvants, from their uncertain effects. In the use of diuretics, a very important rule is, not to restrict the patient from drinking freely. This was formerly thought necessary on theoretical grounds; whereby the thirst was aggravated to a distressing degree, and the operation of remedies often prevented, especially on the kidneys. Sir Francis Milman first taught the impropriety of this practice, which is now generally abandoned; at least so long as the flow of urine is increased in proportion to the drink taken, it is considered proper to indulge the patient with it. Another evacuation, which it is very desirable to promote in anasarca, is that by the skin, but this is with difficulty accomplished: nauseating emetics are the most powerful means, but transient in their effect, and their frequent use cannot be borne. If a gentle diaphoresis can be excited, it is as much as we could expect; and perhaps on the whole most beneficial to the patient. For this purpose the compound powder of ipecacuanha, saline substances, and antimonials in small doses, assisted by tepid drink, and warmth applied to the surface, may be had recourse to. Sometimes much relief is obtained by promoting perspiration locally by means of the vapour-bath. Mercury has been much employed in dropsy, and certainly appears often materially to promote the operation of other evacuants, particularly squill and digitalis; but its chief utility is where there are obstructions of the viscera, especially the liver, of which, however, ascites is usually the first result: its power of increasing absorption hardly appears, unless it is carried so far as to affect the mouth, when it is apt to weaken the system so much as greatly to limit its use. The other indication of invigorating the constitution, and particularly the exhalant arteries, may be accomplished by tonic medicines, as the several vegetable bitters, chalybeates in those who are remarkably pale, and, if there be a languid circulation, stimulants may be joined with them: a similar modification will be proper in the diet, which should be always as nutritious as the patient can well digest; directing also in torpid habits pungent articles, as garlic, onions, mustard, horseradish, &c. to be freely taken, which will be farther useful by promoting the urine. Rhenish wine, or punch made with hollands and supertartrate of potassa, may be allowed for the drink. Regular exercise, such as the patient can bear, (the limbs being properly supported, especially by a well-contrived laced stocking) ought to be enjoined, or diligent friction of the skin, particularly of the affected parts, employed when the tumefaction is usually least, namely, in the morning. The cold bath, duly regulated, may also, when the patient is convalescent, materially contribute to obviate a relapse.

ANASPA'SIS. (From *ανα*, and *σπαω*, to draw together.) Hippocrates uses this word to signify a contraction of the stomach.

ANA'SSYTOS. (From *ανα*, upwards, and *σευομαι*, to agitate.) *Anassytus.* Driven forcibly upwards. Hippocrates applies this epithet to air rushing violently upwards, as in hysteric fits.

ANASTA'LTICA. (From *ανασελλω*, to contract.) Styptic or refrigerating medicines.

ANA'STASIS. (From *ανασημι*, to cause to rise.) 1. A recovery from sickness; a restoration of health.

2. It likewise signifies a migration of humours, when expelled from one place and obliged to remove to another.—*Hippocrates.*

ANASTOMO'SIS. (From *ανα*, through, and *σομα*, a mouth.) The communication of vessels with one another.

ANASTOMO'TIC (*Anastomoticus;* from *ανα*, through, and *σομα*, the mouth.) That which opens the pores and mouths of the vessels, as cathartics, diuretics, deobstruents, and sudorifics.

ANATASE. A mineral found only in Dauphiny and Norway.

[This name is given by Haüy and Brogniart, to the octahedral oxide of Titanium, which has been found in various parts of the United States, in the forms of

The oxide of titanium,
The ferruginous oxide,
The silico-calcareous oxide.

See Bruce's Mineralogical Journal, in which numerous specimens are figured and described by him. A.]

ANA'TES. (From *nates*, the buttocks.) A disease of the anus. *Festus*, &c.

ANATO'MIA. See *Anatomy.*

ANA'TOMY. (*Ανατομια*, or *ανατομη*, *Anatomia*, *æ.* f. and *Anatome, es;* from *ανα*, and *τεμνω*, to cut up.) *Androtomy.* The dissection or dividing of organized substances to expose the structure, situation, and uses of parts. Anatomy is divided into that of animals strictly so called, also, denominated *zootomy*, and that of vegetables or *phytotomy.*

The anatomy of brute animals and vegetables is comprised under the term comparative anatomy, because their dissection was instituted to illustrate or compare by analogy their structure and functions with those of the human body.

ANATOMY, COMPARATIVE. Zootomy. The dissection of brutes, fishes, polypi, plants, &c. to illustrate or compare them with the structure and functions of the human body.

ANATRE'SIS. (From *ανα*, and *τιτραω*, to perforate.) A perforation like that which is made upon the skull by trepanning.

ANATRI'BE. (From *ανατριβω*, to rub.) Friction all over the body.

ANATRI'PSIS. Friction all over the body.—*Moschion de Morb. Mulieb.* and *Galen.*

ANA'TRON. (Arabian.) The name of a lake in Egypt, where it was produced. See *Soda.*

ANA'TROPE. (From *ανατρεπω*, to subvert.) *Anatrophe; Anatropha.* A relaxation or subversion of the stomach, with loss of appetite and nausea. Vomiting; indigestion.—*Galen.*

ANA'TRUM. Soda.

ANAU'DIA. (From *α*, priv. and *αυδη*, the speech.) Dumbness; privation of voice; catalepsy.—*Hippocrates.*

ANA'XYRIS. (From *αναξυρις*, the sole.) The herb sorrel; so called because its leaf is shaped like the sole of the shoe.

ANCEPS. (*Anceps, ipitis.* adjective.) Two-edged; that is, compressed, having the edges sharp like a two-edged sword; applied to stems and leaves of plants, as in the *Sisyrinchium striatum, Iris graminea*, and leaves of the *Typha latifolia.*

A'NCHA. (Arabian, to press upon, as being the support of the body.) The thigh.—*Avicenna, Forestius*, &c.

A'NCHILOPS. (From *αγχι*, near, and *ωψ*, the eye.) A disease in the inward corner of the eye. See *Ægilops.*

ANCHORA'LIS. (From *αγκων*, the elbow.) The projecting part of the elbow on which we lean, called generally the olecranon. See *Ulna.*

ANCHORALIS PROCESSUS. The olecranon, a process of the ulna.

ANCHOVY. See *Clupea encrasicolus.*

Anchovy Pear. See *Grias cauliflora.*

ANCHU'SA. (*Anchusa, æ.* f.; from *αγχειν*, to strangle: from its supposed constringent quality; or, as others say, because it strangles serpents.) 1. The name of a genus of plants in the Linnæan system. Class, *Pentandria;* Order, *Monogynia.*

2. The name in some pharmacopœias for the alkanet root and bugloss. See *Anchusa officinalis*, and *Anchusa tinctoria.*

ANCHUSA OFFICINALIS. The officinal bugloss. In some pharmacopœias it is called *Buglossa; Buglossum angustifolium majus; Buglossum vulgare majus; Buglossum sylvestre; Buglossum sativum. Anchusa—foliis lanceolatis strigosis, spicis secundis imbricatis, calycibus quinque partitis*, of Linnæus; it was formerly esteemed as a cordial in melancholic and hypochondriacal diseases. It is seldom used in modern practice, and then only as an aperient and refrigerant.

Anchusa tinctoria. The systematic name for the anchusa or alkanna of the pharmacopœias. This plant grows wild in France, but is cultivated in our gardens. The root is externally of a deep purple colour. To oil, wax, turpentine, and alkohol, it imparts a beautiful deep red colour, for which purpose it is used. Its medicinal properties are scarcely perceptible.

A'nchyle. See *Ancyle.*

ANCHYLOMERI'SMA. (From αγχυλομαι, to bend.) Sagar uses this term to express a concretion, or growing together of the soft parts.

ANCHYLO'SIS. (From αγχυλομαι, to bend.) A stiff joint. It is divided into the *true* and *spurious*, according as the motion is entirely or but partly lost. This state may arise from various causes, as tumefaction of the ends of the bones, caries, fracture, dislocation, &c. also dropsy of the joint, fleshy excrescences, aneurisms, and other tumours. It may also be owing to the morbid contraction of the flexor muscles, induced by the limb being long kept in a particular position, as a relief to pain, after burns, mechanical injuries, &c. The rickets, white swellings, gout, rheumatism, palsy, from lead particularly, and some other disorders, often lay the foundation for anchylosis: and the joints are very apt to become stiff in advanced life. Where the joint is perfectly immoveable, little can be done for the patient; but in the spurious form of complaint, we must first endeavour to remove any cause mechanically obstructing the motion of the joint, and then to get rid of the morbid contraction of the muscles. If inflammation exist, this must be first subdued by proper means. Where extraneous matters have been deposited, the absorbents must be excited to remove them: and where the parts are preternaturally rigid, emollient applications will be serviceable. Fomentations, gentle friction of the joint and of the muscles, which appear rigid, with the camphor linament, &c. continued for half an hour or more two or three times a day; and frequent attempts to move the joint to a greater extent, especially by the patient exerting the proper muscles, not with violence, but steadily for some time, are the most successful means: but no rapid improvement is to be expected in general. Sometimes, in obstinate cases, rubbing the part with warm brine occasionally, or applying stimulant plasters of ammoniacum, &c. may expedite the cure; and in some instances, particularly as following rheumatism, pumping cold water on the part every morning has proved remarkably beneficial. Where there is a great tendency to contraction of the muscles, it will be useful to obviate this by some mechanical contrivance. It is proper to bear in mind, where, from the nature of the case, complete anchylosis cannot be prevented, that the patient may be much less inconvenienced by its being made to occur in a particular position; that is in the upper extremities generally a bent, but in the hip or knee an extended one.

A'nci. A term formerly applied to those who have a distorted elbow.

A'ncinar. Borax.

ANCIPITIUS. (From *Anceps.*) Two-edged: applied to a leaf which is compressed and sharp at both edges, as that of the *Typha latifolia.*

Ancirome'le. See *Ancylomele.*

A'NCON. (From αγκαζομαι, to embrace; *απο του αγκεισθαι ετερω οςεω το οςεον*: because the bones meeting and there uniting, are folded one into another.) The elbow.

ANCONE'US. (From αγκων, the elbow.) A small triangular muscle, situated on the back part of the elbow. *Anconeus minor* of Winslow; *Anconeus vel cubitalis Riolani* of Douglas. It arises from the ridge, and from the external condyle of the humerus, by a thick, strong, and short tendon: from this it becomes fleshy, and, after running about three inches obliquely backward, it is inserted by its oblique fleshy fibres into the back part or ridge of the ulna. Its use is to extend the fore-arm.

Anconeus externus. See *Triceps extensor cubiti.*

Anconeus internus. See *Triceps extensor cubiti.*

Anconeus major. See *Triceps extensor cubiti.*

Anconeus minor. See *Anconeus.*

ANCONOID. (*Anconoideus*; from αγκων, the elbow.) Belonging to the elbow.

Anconoid process. See *Ulna.*

A'NCTER. (Αγκτηρ, a bond, or button.) A fibula or button, by which the lips of wounds are held together.—*Gorræus.*

ANCTERIA'SMUS. (From αγκτηρ, a button.) The operation of closing the lips of wounds together by loops, or buttons.—*Galen.*

Ancu'bitus. A disease of the eyes with a sensation as if sand were in them.—*Joh. Anglic. Ros. Ang.*

A'NCYLE. (From αγκυλος, crooked.) *Anchyle.* A species of contraction, called a stiff joint.—*Galen*

Ancylion. See *Ancyloglossum.*

ANCYLOBLE'PHARON. (*Ancyloblepharum, i.* n.; from αγκυλη, a hook, and βλεφαρον, an eyelid.) A disease of the eye, by which the eylids are closed together.—*Aëtius.*

ANCYLOGLO'SSUM. (*Ancyloglossum, i.* n.; from αγκυλη, a hook, and γλωσσα, the tongue.) *Ancylion* of Ægineta. Tongue-tied. A contraction of the frænulum of the tongue.

ANCYLOME'LE. (From αγκυλος, crooked, and μηλη, a probe.) *Ancyromele: Ancirómele.* A crooked probe, or a probe with a hook, with which surgeons search wounds.—*Galen,* &c.

ANCYLO'SIS. See *Anchylosis.*

Ancylo'tomus. (From αγκυλη, a hook, and τεμνω, to cut.) A crooked chirurgical knife, or bistoury. A knife for loosening the tongue, not now used.

A'ncyra. (Αγκυρα, an anchor.) A chirurgical hook. Epicharmus uses this word for the membrum virile, according to Gorræus.

ANCYROI'DES. (*Ancyroides processus;* from αγκυρα, an anchor, and ειδος, a likeness.) A process of the scapula was so called, from its likeness to the beak of an anchor. The coracoid process of the scapula. See *Scapula.*

Ancyrome'le. See *Ancylomele.*

ANDALUSITE. A massive mineral, of a flesh, and sometimes rose-red colour, belonging to primitive countries, and first found in Andalusia in Spain.

[It has been found also in the United States. The hardness of this mineral is nearly equal to that of corundum. Its specific gravity is 3.16. Its structure is more or less distinctly crystalline. It is perfectly infusible by the blow-pipe. It contains alumine 52, silex 38, potash 8, iron 2.

It differs from feldspar by its greater hardness and its infusibility; and from corundum, by its structure and less specific gravity. Some mineralogists, however, are inclined to believe this mineral to be feldspar intimately mixed with corundum; and hence its hardness.—*Cleav. Min.* A.]

Anderson's pills. These consist of Barbadoes aloes, with a proportion of jalap, and oil of aniseed.

[ANDERSON, ALEXANDER, M.D. Dr. Anderson, of the city of New-York, received his degree of Doctor in Medicine from the Medical faculty of Columbia College. He afterward turned his attention to the subject of engraving in wood, and finally abandoned his profession of a physician for the employment of an engraver, in which he now stands pre-eminent, being a self-taught artist. His wood engravings are excellent, and many of them equal copperplate. He has made this art subservient to his first profession, by engravings illustrating the intestines, blood-vessels, &c., as well as subjects of botany and natural history. He is a modest, unassuming man, and is now (1829) in the height of his reputation and usefulness. A.]

[ANDERSON, JAMES, M.D. Having successfully terminated his academical pursuits at an early age, Dr. Anderson commenced the study of medicine under the direction of his father, a very respectable physician from Scotland. He attended a course of lectures, by Professors Shippen and Morgan, in the school of Philadelphia, then in its infancy; and next sailed for Edinburgh, at that time the focus of medical literature. Circumstances, which it is unnecessary to mention, not permitting him to remain long enough to obtain a degree, he returned to this country with an ample certificate, signed by his preceptors, Cullen, the elder Munro, and the whole board of professors. Immediately on his return, he commenced the practice of physic in conjunction with his father. Deeply versed in general, and particularly in medical science, and devoted almost beyond example to the performance of his professional duties, he soon obtained a reputation, unenjoyed by any of his competitors. For a period of upwards of thirty years, he retained a practice of an extent certainly without a parallel in this section of the country. Advancing rapidly toward his sixtieth year, and feeling the infirmities consequent on a life so laborious, he retired to his seat near Chestertown. In this situation, however, he was not allowed the repose which he anticipated. Though the native vigour of his constitution was broken down by the invasion of disease, and by those accidents to which his course of life subjected him, he attended almost to the close of it, to the calls of his patients. He died December 8th, 1820, at his seat in the vicinity of Chestertown, Maryland, in the 69th year of his age.—*Thacher's Med. Biog.* A.]

ANDI'RA. A tree of Brazil, the fruit of which is bitter and astringent, and used as a vermifuge.

ANDRANATO'MIA. (From ανηρ, a man, and τεμνω, to cut.) *Andranatome.* The dissection of the human body, particularly of the male.—*M. Aur. Severinus, Zootome Democrit.*

ANDRAPODOCAPE'LUS. (From ανδροποδον, a slave, and καπηλος, a dealer.) A crimp. Galen calls by this name the person whose office it was to anoint and slightly to wipe the body, to cleanse the skin from foulness.

ANDREOLITE. A species of crop-stone.

ANDROCŒTE'SIS. (From ανερ, a man, and κοιτεω, to cohabit with.) 1. The venereal act.

2. The infamous act of sodomy.—*Moschion*, &c.

ANDRO'GYNUS. (From ανερ, a man, and γυνη, a woman.) 1. An hermaphrodite.

2. An effeminate person.—*Hippocrates.*

3. A plant is said to be androgenous, which produces both male and female flowers from the same root, as the walnut, beech, horn-beam, nettle, &c.

ANDRO'MACHUS, of *Crete*, was physician to the emperor Nero. He invented a composition, supposed to be an antidote against poison, called after him, *Theriaca Andromachi*, which he dedicated to that emperor in a copy of Greek verses still preserved. This complicated preparation long retained its reputation, but is now deservedly abandoned.

ANDRO'NION. *Andronium.* A kind of plaster used by Ægineta for carbuncles, invented by Andron.

ANDROPO'GON. (From ανηρ, a man, and πωγων, a beard.) The name of a genus of plants in the Linnæan system. Class, *Polygamia:* Order, *Monœcia.*

ANDROPOGON NARDUS. The systematic name of Indian nard or spikenard. *Spica nardi; Spica Indica.* The root of this plant is an ingredient in the mithridate and theriaca; it is moderately warm and pungent, accompanied with a flavour not disagreeable. It is said to be used by the Orientals as a spice.

ANDROPOGON SCHÆNANTHUS. The systematic name of the camel-hay, or Sweet-rush. *Juncus odoratus; Fœnum camelorum; Juncus aromaticus.* The dried plant is imported into this country from Turkey and Arabia. It has an agreeable smell, and a warm, bitterish, not unpleasant taste. It was formerly employed as a stomachic and deobstruent.

ANDRO'TOMIA. *Androtome.* Human dissection, particularly of the male.

ANDRY, NICHOLAS, a physician, born at Lyons in 1658. He was made professor of medicine at Paris in 1701, and lived to the age of 84. Besides a Treatise on Worms, and other minor publications, and contributions in the Medical and Philosophical Journals, he was author of a work, still esteemed, called "Orthopedie," or the art of preventing and removing deformities in children; which he proposed to effect by regimen, exercise, and various mechanical contrivances.

ANE'BIUM. (From αναβαινω, to ascend.) The herb alkanet, so called from its quick growth. See *Anchusa.*

ANELE'SIS. (From ανειλεω, to roll up.) *Aneilema.* An involution of the guts, such as is caused by flatulence and gripes.—*Hippocrates.*

ANE'MIA. (From ανεμος, wind.) Flatulence.

ANE'MONE. (From ανεμος, wind; so named, because it does not open its flowers till blown upon by the wind.) The name of a genus of plants in the Linnæan system. Class, *Polyandria;* Order, *Polyginia.* The wind flower.

ANEMONE HEPATICA. The systematic name for the *hepatica nobilis* of the pharmacopœias. *Herba trinitatis.* Hepatica, or herb trinity. This plant possesses mildly adstringent and corroborant virtues, with which intentions infusions of it have been drunk as tea, or the powder of the dry leaves given to the quantity of half a spoonful at a time.

ANEMONE NEMOROSA. The systematic name of the *ranunculus albus* of the pharmacopœias. The bruised leaves and flowers are said to cure tinea capitis applied to the part. The inhabitants of Kamskatka, it is believed, poison their arrows with the root of this plant.

ANEMONE PRATENSIS. The systematic name for the *Pulsatilla nigricans* of the pharmacopœias. This plant, *Anemone—pedunculo involucrato, petalis apice reflexis, foliis bipinnatis*, of Linnæus, has been received into the Edinburgh pharmacopœia upon the authority of Baron Stoerck, who recommended it as an effectual remedy for most of the chronic diseases affecting the eye, particularly amaurosis, cataract, and opacity of the cornea, proceeding from various causes. He likewise found it of great service in venereal nodes, nocturnal pains, ulcers, caries, indurated glands, suppressed menses, serpiginous eruptions, melancholy, and palsy. The plant, in its recent state, has scarcely any smell; but its taste is extremely acrid, and, when chewed, it corrodes the tongue and fauces.

ANENCE'PHALUS. (From α. priv. and εγκεφαλος, the brain.) A monster without brains. Foolish.—*Galen de Hippocrate.*

A'NEOS. A loss of voice and reason.

ANEPITHY'MIA. (From α. priv. and επιθυμια, desire.) Loss of appetite.

A'NESIS. (From ανιημι, to relax.) A remission, or relaxation, of a disease, or symptom. *Aëtius*, &c.

ANE'SUM. See *Anisum.*

ANE'THUM (*Anethum, i. n.* Ανεθον; from ανευ, afar, and θεω, to run: so called because its roots run out a great way.)

1. The name of a genus of plants in the Linnæan system. Class, *Pentandria;* Order, *Digynia.*

2. The pharmacopœial name of the common dill. See *Anethum graveolens.*

ANETHUM FŒNICULUM. The systematic name for the *fœniculum* of the shops. Sweet fennel, *Anethum—fructibus ovatis* of Linnæus. The seeds and roots of this indigenous plant are directed by the colleges of London and Edinburgh. The seeds have an aromatic smell, and a warm sweetish taste, and contain a large proportion of essential oil. They are stomachic and carminative. The root has a sweet taste, but very little aromatic warmth, and is said to be pectoral and diuretic.

ANETHUM GRAVEOLENS. The systematic name of the *Anethum* of the shops. *Anethum—fructibus compressis*, of Linnæus.—*Dill. Anet.* This plant is a native of Spain, but cultivated in several parts of England. The seeds are directed for use by the London and Edinburgh Pharmacopœias: they have a moderately warm, pungent taste, and an aromatic, but sickly smell. There is an essential oil, and a distilled water prepared from them, which are given in flatulent colics and dyspepsia. They are also said to promote the secretion of milk.

ANE'TICA. (*Aneticus;* from ανιημαι, to relax.) Medicines which assuage pain, according to Andr Tiraquell.

ANETUS. (From ανιημι, *remitto.*) A name given by Good, in his Study of Medicine, to a genus of diseases which embraces intermittent fevers. See *Nosology.*

ANEURI'SMA. (*Aneurisma, matis*, neut. Ανευρυσμα; from ανευρυνω, to dilate.) An aneurism; a preternatural tumour formed by the dilatation of an artery. A genus of disease ranked by Cullen in the class *Locales*, and order *Tumores.* There are three species of aneurism: 1. The *true aneurism, aneurisma verum*, which is known by the presence of a pulsating tumour. The artery either seems only enlarged at a small part of its tract, and the tumour has a determinate border, or it seems dilated for a considerable length, in which circumstance the swelling is oblong, and loses itself so gradually in the surrounding parts, that its margin cannot be exactly ascertained. The first, which is the most common, is termed *circumscribed true aneurism;* the last, the *diffused true aneurism.* The symptoms of the circumscribed true aneurism, take place as follows: the first thing the patient perceives is an extraordinary throbbing in some particular situation, and, on paying a little more attention, he discovers there a small pulsating tumour, which entirely disappears when compressed, but returns again as soon as the pressure is removed. It is commonly unattended with pain or change in the colour of the skin. When once the tumour has originated, it continually grows larger, and at length attains a very considerable size. In proportion as it becomes larger, its pulsation becomes weaker, and, indeed, it is almost quite lost, when the disease has acquired much magnitude. The diminution of the pulsation has been ascribed to the coats of the artery, losing their dilatable and elastic quality, in proportion as they are distended and indurated; and, consequently, the aneurismal sac being no longer capable of an alternate diastole and systole from the action of the heart. The fact is also imputed to the coagulated blood, deposited on the inner surface of the sac, particularly in large aneurisms, in which some of the blood is always interrupted in its motion. In true aneurisms, however, the blood does not coagulate so soon, nor so often, as in false ones. Whenever such coagulated blood lodges in the sac, pressure can only produce a partial disappearance of the swelling. In proportion as the aneurismal sac grows larger, the communication into the artery beyond the tumours is lessened. Hence, in this state, the pulse below the swelling becomes weak and small, and the limb frequently cold and œdematous. On dissection, the lower continuation of the artery is found preternaturally small, and contracted. The pressure of the tumour on the adjacent parts also produces a variety of symptoms, ulcerations, caries, &c. Sometimes an accidental contusion, or concussion, may detach a piece of coagulum from the inner surface of the cyst, and the circulation through the sack be obstructed by it. The coagulum may possibly be impelled quite into the artery below, so as to induce important changes. The danger of an aneurism arrives when it is on the point of bursting, by which occurrence the patient usually bleeds to death; and this sometimes happens in a few seconds. The fatal event may generally be foreseen, as the part about to give way becomes particularly tense, elevated, thin, soft, and of a dark purple colour. 2. The *false* or *spurious aneurism, aneurisma spurium*, is always owing to an aperture in the artery, from which the blood gushes into the cellular substance. It may arise from an artery being lacerated in violent exertions; but the most common occasional cause is a wound. This is particularly apt to occur at the bend of the arm, where the artery is exposed to be injured in attempting to bleed. When this happens, as soon as the puncture has been made, the blood gushes out with unusual force, of a bright scarlet colour and in an irregular stream, corresponding to the pulsation of the artery. It flows out, however, in an even and less rapid stream when pressure is employed higher up than the wound. These last are the most decisive marks of the artery being opened; for blood often flows from a vein with great rapidity, and in a broken current, when the vessel is very turgid and situated immediately over the artery, which imparts its motion to it. The surgeon endeavours precipitately to stop the hæmorrhage by pressure; and he commonly occasions a *diffused false aneurism*. The external wound in the skin is closed, so that the blood cannot escape from it; but insinuates itself into the cellular substance. The swelling thus produced is uneven, often knotty, and extends upwards and downwards, along the tract of the vessel. The skin is also usually of a dark purple colour. Its size increases as long as the internal hæmorrhage continues, and, if this should proceed above a certain pitch, mortification of the limb ensues. 3. The *varicose aneurism, aneurisma varicosum:* this was first described by Dr. W. Hunter. It happens when the brachial artery is punctured in opening a vein: the blood then rushes into the vein, which becomes varicose. Aneurisms may happen in any part of the body, except the latter species, which can only take place where a vein runs over an artery. When an artery has been punctured, the tourniquet should be applied, so as to stop the flow of blood by compressing the vessel above; then the most likely plan of obviating the production of spurious aneurism appears to be applying a firm compress immediately over the wound, and securing it by a bandage, or in any other way, so as effectually to close the orifice, yet not prevent the circulation through other vessels: afterward keeping the limb as quiet as possible, enjoining the antiphlogistic regimen, and examining daily that no extravasation has happened, which would require the compress being fixed more securely, previously applying the tourniquet, and pressing the effused blood as much as possible into the vessel. If there should be much coldness or swelling of the limb below, it will be proper to rub it frequently with some spirituous or other stimulant embrocation. It is only by trial that it can be certainly determined when the wound is closed; but always better not to discontinue the pressure prematurely. The same plan may answer, when the disease has already come on, if the blood can be entirely, or even mostly, pressed into the artery again; at any rate, by determining the circulation on collateral branches, it will give greater chance of success to a subsequent operation. There is another mode, stated to have sometimes succeeded, even when there was much coagulated blood; namely, making strong pressure over the whole limb, by a bandage applied uniformly, and moistened to make it sit closer, as well as to obviate inflammation; but this does not appear so good a plan, at least in slighter cases. If however the tumour be very large, and threatens to burst, or continues spreading, the operation should not be delayed. The tourniquet being applied, a free incision is to be made into the tumour, the extravasated blood removed, and the artery tied both above and below the wound, as near to it as may be safe; and if any branch be given off between, this must be also secured. It is better not to make the ligatures tighter, than may be necessary to stop the flow of blood; and to avoid including any nerve if possible. Sometimes, where extensive suppuration or caries has occurred, or gangrene is to be apprehended, amputation will be necessary: but this must not be prematurely resolved upon, for often after several weeks the pulse has returned in the limb below. In the true aneurism, when small and recent, cold and astringent applications are sometimes useful; or making pressure on the tumour, or on the artery above, may succeed; otherwise an operation becomes necessary to save the patient's life; though unfortunately it oftener fails in this than in the spurious kind; gangrene ensuing, or hæmorrhage; this chiefly arises from the arteries being often extensively diseased, so that they are more likely to give way, and there is less vital power in the limb. A great improvement has been made in the mode of operating in these cases by Mr. John Hunter, and other modern surgeons, namely, instead of proceeding as already explained in the spurious aneurism, securing the artery some way above, and leaving the rest in a great measure to the powers of nature. It has been now proved by many instances, that when the current of the blood is thus interrupted, the tumour will cease to enlarge, and often be considerably diminished by absorption. There is reason for believing too, that the cures effected spontaneously, or by pressure, have been usually owing to the trunk above being obliterated. There are many obvious advantages in this mode of proceeding; it is more easy, sooner performed, and disorders the system less, particularly as you avoid having a large unhealthy sore to be healed; besides there is less probability of the vessel being diseased at some distance from the tumour. In the popliteal aneurism, for example, the artery may be secured rather below the middle of the thigh, where it is easily come at. The tourniquet therefore being applied, and the vessel exposed, a strong ligature is to be passed round it; or, which is perhaps preferable, two ligatures a little distant, subsequently cutting through the artery between them, when the two portions contract among the surrounding flesh. It is proper to avoid including the nerve or vein, but not unnecessarily detach the vessel from its attachments. For greater security one end of each ligature, after being tied, may be passed through the intercepted portion of artery, that they may not be forced off. Then the wound is to be closed by adhesive plaster, merely leaving the ends of the ligatures hanging out, which will after some time come away. However it must be remembered that hæmorrhage is liable to occur, when this happens, even three or four weeks after the operation; so that proper precautions are required, to check it as soon as possible; likewise the system should be lowered previously, and kept so during the cure. When a true aneurism changes into the spurious form, which is known by the tumour spreading, becoming harder, and with a less distinct pulsation, the operation becomes immediately necessary. When an aneurism is out of the reach of an operation, life may be prolonged by occasional bleeding, a spare diet, &c.; and when the tumour becomes apparent externally, carefully guarding it from injury. In the varicose aneurism an operation will be very seldom if ever required, the growth of the tumour being limited.

Aneurisma spurium. See *Aneurisma.*

Aneurisma varicosum. See *Aneurisma.*

Aneurisma verum. See *Aneurisma.*

ANE'XIS. (From ανεχω, to project.) A swelling, or protuberance.

ANGEIOLO'GY. (*Angeiologia*, *æ*. f.; from αγγειον, a vessel, and λογος, a discourse.) A dissertation, or reasoning, upon the vessels of the body.

ANGEIOTI'SMUS. (From αγγειον, a vessel, and τεμνω, to cut.) An angeiotomist, or skilful dissector of the vessels.

ANGEIO'TOMY. (*Angeiotomia;* from αγγειον, a vessel, and τεμνω, to cut.) The dissection of the blood-vessels of an animal body; also the opening of a vein, or an artery.

ANGE'LICA. (So called from its supposed angelic virtues.) 1. The name of a genus of plants in the Linnæan system. Class *Pentandria;* Order, *Digynia.* Angelica.

2. The pharmacopœial name of the garden angelica. See *Angelica archangelica.*

Angelica archangelica. The systematic name for the *angelica* of the shops. *Milzadella Angelica—foliorum impari lobato* of Linnæus. A plant, a native of Lapland, but cultivated in our gardens. The roots of angelica have a fragrant, agreeable smell, and a bitterish, pungent taste. The stalk, leaves, and seeds, which are also directed in the pharmacopœias, possess the same qualities, though in an inferior degree. Their virtues are aromatic and carminative. A sweatmeat is made, by the confectioners, of this root, which is extremely agreeable to the stomach, and is surpassed only by that of ginger.

Angelica, garden. See *Angelica archangelica.*

Angelica pilula. Anderson's Scots pill.

Angelica sativa. See *Angelica sylvestris.*

Angelica sylvestris. *Angelica sativa.* Wild angelica. *Angelica—foliis æqualibus ovato-lanceolatis serratis,* of Linnæus. This species of angelica possesses similar properties to the garden species, but in a much inferior degree. It is only used when the latter cannot be obtained. The seeds, powdered and put in the hair, kill lice.

Angelica, wild. See *Angelica sylvestris.*

ANGELICUS. (From *angelus*, an angel.) Some plants, &c. are so called, from their supposed superior virtues.

Angelicus pulvis. Submuriate of mercury.

ANGELI'NA. *Angelina zanoni acostæ.* A tree of vast size, sometimes above sixteen feet thick, growing in rocky and sandy places in Malabar in the East Indies. It bears ripe fruit in December. The dried leaves heated are said to alleviate pain and stiffness of the joints, and dismiss swelling of the testes caused by external violence; and are also said to be useful in the cure of venereal complaints.

Angelinæ cortex. The name of the tree from which the *Cortex Angelinæ* is procured. It is a native of Grenada. This bark has been recommended as an anthelmintic for children.

Angeloca'cos. The purging Indian plum. See *Myrobalanus.*

A'ngi. (From *angor*, anguish; because of their pain.) Buboes in the groin.—*Fallopius de Morbo Gallico.*

ANGIGLO'SSUS. (From αγκυλη, a hook, and γλωσσα, the tongue.) A person who stammers.

ANGI'NA. (*Angina*, *æ*. f.; from αγχω, to strangle; because it is often attended with a sense of strangulation.) A sore throat. See *Cynanche.*

Angina lini. A name used by some of the later Greeks writers to express what the more ancient writers of this nation called *linozostres*, and the Latins *epilinum*. which is the *cuscuta* or dodder, growing on the *linum* or flax, as that on the thyme was called *epithymum.* See *Cuscuta.*

Angina maligna. Malignant or putrid sore throat. See *Cynanche maligna.*

Angina parotidea. The mumps. See *Cynanche parotidea.*

Angina pectoris. *Syncope ang nosa* of Dr. Parry. An acute constrictory pain at the lower end of the sternum, inclining rather to the left side, and extending up into the left arm, accompanied with great anxiety Violent palpitations of the heart, laborious breathings, and a sense of suffocation, are the characteristic symptoms of this disease. It is found to attack men much more frequently than women, particularly those who have short necks, who are inclinable to corpulency, and who, at the same time, lead an inactive and sedentary life. Although it is sometimes met with in persons under the age of twenty, still it more frequently occurs in those who are between forty and fifty In slight cases, and in the first stage of the disorder, the fit comes on by going up hill, up stairs, or by walking at a quick pace after a hearty meal; but as the disease advances, or becomes more violent, the paroxysms are apt to be excited by certain passions of the mind; by slow walking, by riding on horseback, or in a carriage; or by sneezing, coughing, speaking, or straining at stool. In some cases, they attack the patient from two to four in the morning, or whilst sitting or standing, without any previous exertion or obvious cause. On a sudden, he is seized with an acute pain in the breast, or rather at the extremity of the sternum, inclining to the left side, and extending up into the arm, as far as the insertion of the deltoid muscle, accompanied by a sense of suffocation, great anxiety, and an idea that its continuance or increase, would certainly be fatal. In the first stage of the disease, the uneasy sensation at the end of the sternum, with the other unpleasant symptoms, which seemed to threaten a suspension of life by a perseverance in exertion, usually go off upon the person's standing still, or turning from the wind; but, in a more advanced stage, they do not so readily recede, and the paroxysms are much more violent. During the fit, the pulse sinks, in a greater or less degree, and becomes irregular; the face and extremities are pale, and bathed in a cold sweat, and, for a while, the patient is perhaps deprived of the powers of sense and voluntary motion. The disease having recurred more or less frequently during the space of some years, a violent attack at last puts a sudden period to his existence. Angina pectoris is attended with a considerable degree of danger; and it usually happens that the person is carried off suddenly. It mostly depends upon an ossification of the coronary arteries, and then we can never expect to effect a radical cure. During the paroxysms, considerable relief is to be obtained from fomentations, and administering powerful antispasmodics, such as opium and æther combined together. The application of a blister to the breast is likewise attended sometimes with a good effect. As the painful sensation at the extremity of the sternum often admits of a temporary relief, from an evacuation of wind by the mouth, it may be proper to give frequent doses of carminatives, such as peppermint, carraway, or cinnamon water. Where these fail in the desired effect, a few drops of ol. anisi, on a little sugar, may be substituted.

With the view of preventing the recurrence of the disorder, the patient should carefully guard against passion, or other emotions of the mind: he should use a light, generous diet, avoiding every thing of a heating nature; and he should take care never to overload the stomach, or to use any kind of exercise immediately after eating. Besides these precautions, he should endeavour to counteract obesity, which has been considered as a predisposing cause; and this is to be effected most safely by a vegetable diet, moderate exercise at proper times, early rising, and keeping the body perfectly open. It has been observed that angina pectoris is a disease always attended with considerable danger, and, in most instances, has proved fatal under every mode of treatment. We are given, however, to understand, by Dr. Macbride, that of late, several cases of it have been treated with great success, and the disease radically removed, by inserting a large issue on each thigh. These, therefore, should never be neglected. In one case, with a view of correcting, or draining off the irritating fluid, he ordered, instead of issues, a mixture of lime water with a little of the spirituous juniperi comp., and an alterative proportion of Huxham's antimonial wine, together with a plain, light, perspirable diet. From this course the patient was soon apparently mended; but it was not until after the insertion of a large issue in each thigh, that he was restored to perfect health.

ANGINI TONSILLARIS. See *Cynanche tonsillaris.*

ANGINA TRACHEALIS. See *Cynanche trachealis.*

ANGIOCARPI. The name given by Persoon to a division of funguses which bear their seeds internally. They are either hard or membranous tough and leathery.

ANGIOLO'GY. (*Angiologia;* from αγγειον, a vessel, and λογος, a discourse) The doctrine of the vessels of the human body.

ANGIOSPERMIA. (From αγγος, a vessel, and σπερμα, a seed.) The name of an order of plants in the class *Didynamia* of the sexual system of Linnæus, the seeds of which are lodged in a pericarpium or seed-vessel.

ANGIOSPERMÆ HERBÆ. Those plants, the seeds of which are enclosed in a covering or vessel.

A'NGLICUS. (From *Anglia*, England.) The sweating sickness, which was so endemic and fatal in England, was called Sudor Anglicanus. See *Sudor Anglicus.*

ANGO'LAM. A very tall tree of Malabar, possessing vermifuge powers.

ANGO'NE. (From αγχω, to strangle.) A nervous sort of quinsy, or hysteric suffocation, where the fauces are contracted and stopped up without inflammation.

A'NGOR. (*Angor, oris.* m.: from *Ango.*) Agony or intense bodily pain.—*Galen.*

A'NGOS. (Αγγος, a vessel.) A vessel. A collection of humours.

ANGULATUS. Angled.—A term used to designate stem, leaves, petioles, &c. which present several acute angles in their circumference. There are several varieties of angular stems.

1. *Triangulatus*, three-angled; as in *Cactus triangularis.*

2. *Quadrangulatus*, four-angled; as in *Cactus tetragonus.*

3. *Quinqueangulatus*, five-angled; as in *Cactus pentagonus.*

4. *Hexangulatus*, six-angled; as in *Cactus hexagonus.*

5. *Multiangulatus*, many-angled; as in *Cactus cereus.*

6. *Obtusangularis*, obtuse-angled; as in *Scrofularia nodosa.*

7. *Acutangulatus*, acute-angled; as in *Scrofularia aquatica.*

8. *Caulis triqueter*, three-sided, but with flat sides; as in *Hedysarum triquetrum*, *Viola mirabilis*, *Carex acuta.*

9. *Caulis tetaquetrus*, quadrangular with flat sides; as in *Hypericum quadrangulare*, *Mentha officinalis.*

For angular leaves, See *Leaf*, *Petiole*, &c.

ANGULOSUS. Angular.

ANGUSTU'RÆ CORTEX. A bark imported from Angustura. See *Cusparia.*

ANHELA'TION. (*Anhelatio;* from *anhelo*, to breathe with difficulty.) *Anhelitus.* Shortness of breathing.

ANHYDRITE. Anhydrous gypsum. There are six varieties of this mineral su hate of lime. 1. The compact.—2. The granular. 3. The fibrous. 4. The radiated. 5. The sparry or cube spar. 6. The siliciferous or vulpinite.

ANHYDROS. A name given by the ancient Greeks, to express one of those kinds of *Strychna* or nightshades, which, when taken internally, caused madness.

ANHYDROUS. (From *a*, neg. and υδωρ, water. Without water.

ANICE'TON. (From *a*, priv. and νικη, victory.) A name of a plaster invented by Crito, and so called because it was thought an infallible or invincible remedy for achores, or scald-head. It was composed of litharge, alum, and turpentine, and is described by Galen.

Anil. The name of the Indigo plant.

A'NIMA. A soul: whether rational, sensitive, or vegetative. The word is pure Latin, formed of ανεμος, breath. It is sometimes used by physicians to denote the principle of life in the body, in which sense Willis calls the blood *anima brutalis.* By chemists it was used figuratively for the volatile principle in bodies, whereby they were capable of being raised by the fire; and by the old writers on botany, materia medica, and pharmacy, it was frequently employed to denote its great efficacy: hence *anima, hepates, aloes, rhabarbari*, &c.

ANIMA ALOES. Refined aloes.

ANIMA ARTICULORUM. A name of the Hermodactyles. See *Hermodactylus.*

ANIMA HEPATIS. Sal martis.

ANIMA PULMONUM. The soul of the lungs. A name given to saffron, on account of its use in asthmas.

ANIMA RHABARBAR The best rhubarb.

ANIMA SATURNI. A preparation of lead.

ANIMA VENERIS. A preparation of copper.

ANIMAL. An organized body endowed with life and voluntary motion. The elements which enter into the composition of the bodies of animals are solid, liquid, gaseous, and inconfinable.

Solid Elements. Phosphorus, sulphur, carbon, iron, manganese, potassium, lime, soda, magnesia, silica, and alumina.

Liquid Elements. Muriatic acid; water, which in this case may be considered as an element, enters into the organization, and constitutes three-fourths of the bodies of animals.

Gaseous Elements. Oxygen, hydrogen, azote.

Inconfinable Elements. Caloric, light, electric, and magnetic fluids.

These diverse elements, united with each other, three and three, four and four, &c. according to laws still unexplained, form what we name the proximate principles of animals.

Proximate Materials, or Principles. These are divided into azotized, and non-azotized.

The azotized principles are: albumen, fibrin, gelatin, mucus, cheese-curd principle, urea, uric acid, osmazome, colouring matter of the blood.

The non-azotized principles are: the acetic, benzoic, lactic, formic, oxalic, rosacic, acids; sugar of milk, sugar of diabetic urine, picromel, yellow colouring matter of bile, and of other liquids or solids which become yellow accidentally, the blistering principle of cantharides, spermaceti, biliary calculus, the odoriferous principles of ambergris, musk, castor, civet, &c which are scarcely known, except for their faculty of acting on the organ of smell.

Animal fats are not immediate, simple, proximate principles. It is proved that human fat, that of the pig, of the sheep, &c. are principally formed by two fatty bodies, *stearin*, and *elain*, which present very different characters that may be easily separated.

Neither is the butter of the cow a simple body; it contains acetic acid, a yellow colouring principle, an odorous principle, which is very manifest in fermented cheese.

We must not reckon among these substances, adipocire, a matter which is seen in bodies long buried in the earth; it is composed of *margarine*, of a fluid acic fat, of an orange colouring principle, and of a peculiar odorous substance. Nor must this substance be confounded with spermaceti, and the biliary calculus, which are themselves very different from each other. It does not contain a single principle analogous to them.

Organic Elements. The materials or principles above mentioned combine among themselves, and from their combination arise the organic elements, which are solid or liquid. The laws or forces that govern these combinations are entirely unknown.

Organic Solids. The solids have sometimes the form of canals, sometimes that of large or small plates, at other times they assume that of membranes. In man the total weight of solids is generally eight or nine times less than that of liquids. This proportion is nevertheless variable according to many circumstances.

The ancients believed that all the organic solids might be reduced by ultimate analysis to simple fibres, which they supposed were formed of earth, oil, and iron. Haller, who admitted this idea of the ancients, owns that this fibre is visible only to the eye of the mind. *Invisibilis est ea fibra sola; mentis acie distinguimus.* This is just the same as if he had said that it does not exist at all, which nobody at present doubts.

The ancients also admitted secondary fibres, which they supposed to be formed by particular modifications of the simple fibre. Thence, the nervous, muscular, parenchymatous, osseous fibre.

Chaussier has lately proposed to admit four sorts of fibres, which he calls *luminary*, *nerval*, *muscular*, and *albuginous*.

Science was nearly in this state when Pinel conceived the idea of distinguishing the organic solids, not by fibres, but by tissues or systems. Bichât applied it to all the solid parts of the bodies of animals: the classification of Bichât has been perfected by Dupuytren and Richerand.

Classification of the Tissues.

	Tissue	Varieties	
1.	Cellular		System.
2.	Vascular	Arterial. Venous. Lymphatic.	
3.	Nervous	Cerebral. Ganglaic.	
4.	Osseous		
5.	Fibrous	Fibrous. Fibro-cartilaginous. Dermoid.	
6.	Muscular	Voluntary. Involuntary.	
7.	Erectile		
8.	Mucous		
9.	Serous		
10.	Horny or Epidemic	Hairy. Epidermoid.	
11.	Parenchymatous, Glandular.		

These systems, associated with each other and with the fluids, compose the *organs* or instruments of life. When many organs tend by their action toward a common end, we name them, collectively considered, an *apparatus*. The number of apparatus, and their disposition, constitute the differences of animals.—*Magendie*.

Animal actions. *Actiones animales*. Those actions, or functions, are so termed, which are performed through the means of the mind. To this class belong the external and internal senses, the voluntary action of muscles, voice, speech, watching, and sleep. See *Action*.

Animal Heat. See *Heat, animal*.

Animal Œconomy. See *Œconomy, animal*.

Animal Oil. *Oleum animale*. *Oleum animale Dippolii*. An empyreumatic oil, obtained from the bones of animals, recommended as an anodyne and antispasmodic.

A'nimé gummi. The substance which bears this name in the shops is a resin. See *Hymenæa courbaril*.

A'nimi deliquium. (From *animus*, the mind, and *delinquo*, to leave.) Fainting. See *Syncope*.

A'NIMUS. This word is to be distinguished from *anima*; which generally expresses the faculty of reasoning, and *animus*, the being in which that faculty resides.

Anin'ga. A root which grows in the Antilles islands, and is used by sugar-bakers for refining their sugar.

ANISCA'LPTOR. (From *anus*, the breech, and *scalpo*, to scratch.) The latissimus dorsi is so called, because it is the muscle chiefly instrumental in performing this office.—*Bartholin*.

Anisotachys. (From ανισος, unequal, and ταχυς, quick.) A quick and unequal pulse.—*Gorræus*.

ANI'SUM. (From *a*. neg. and ισος, equal.) See *Pimpinella anisum*.

Anisum sinense. See *Illicium anisatum*.

Anisum stellatum. See *Illicium*.

Anisum vulgare. See *Pimpinella anisum*.

ANNEAL. We know too little of the arrangement of particles to determine what it is that constitutes or produces brittleness in any substance. In a considerable number of instances of bodies which are capable of undergoing ignition, it is found that sudden cooling renders them hard and brittle. This is a real inconvenience in glass, and also in steel, when this metalic substance is required to be soft and flexible. The inconveniences are avoided by cooling them very gradually, and this process is called annealing. Glass vessels, or other articles, are carried into an oven or apartment near the great furnace, called the leer, where they are permitted to cool, in a greater or less time, according to their thickness and bulk. The annealing of steel, or other metallic bodies, consists simply in heating them and suffering them to cool again, either upon the hearth of the furnace, or in any other situation where the heat is moderate, or at least the temperature is not very cold.

Annoto. See *Bixa orleana*.

ANNUAL. (*Annuus*, yearly.) A term applied in botany to plants and roots, which are produced from the seed, grow to their full extent, and die in one year or season, as *Papaver somniferum*, *Helianthus annuus*, *Hordeum triticum*, &c.

Annue'ntes. (From *annuo*, to nod.) Some muscles of the head were formerly so called, because they perform the office of nodding, or bending the head downwards.—*Cowper*, &c.

ANNULAR. (*Annularis*; from *Annulus*, a ring, because it is ring-like, or the ring is worn on it, or it surrounds any thing like a ring; thus, annular bone, &c

Annular bone. *Circulus osseus*. A ring-like bone placed before the cavity of the tympanum in the fœtus.

Annular cartilage. See *Trachæa*.

ANNULA'RIS. *Annularis digitus*. The ring-finger. The one between the little and middle fingers.

Annularis processus. See *Pons varolii*.

A'NNULUS. (*Annulus*, *i*. m., a ring.) A ring. In botany applied to the slender membrane surrounding the stem of the fungi.

Annulus abdominis. The abdominal ring. An oblong separation of tendinous fibres, called an opening, in each groin, through which the spermatic chord in men, and the round ligament of the uterus in women, pass. It is through this part that the abdominal viscera fall in that species of hernia, which is called bubonocele. See *Obliquus externus abdominis*.

A'NO. (Ανω, upwards; in opposition to κατω, downwards.) Upwards.

ANOCATHA'RTIC. (From ανω, upwards, and καθαιρω, to purge.) Emetic, or that which purges upwards.

ANOCHEI'LON. (From ανω, upwards, and χειλος the lip.) The upper lip.

Ano'dia. (From *a*, neg. and οδος, the way.) Hippocrates uses this word for inaccuracy and irregularity in the description and treatment of a disease.

ANO'DYNA. See *Anodyne*.

ANODYNE. (*Anodynus*; from *a*, priv. and ωδυνη, pain.) Those medicines are termed *Anodynes*, which ease pain and procure sleep. They are divided into three sorts; paregorics, or such as assuage pain; hypnotics, or such as relieve by procuring sleep; and narcotics, or such as ease the patient by stupifying him.

Ano'dynum martiale. Ferrum ammoniatum precipitated from water by potassa.

Ano'dynum minerale. Sal prunella.

ANOMALOUS. (From *a*. priv. and νομος, a law.) This term is often applied to those diseases, the symptoms of which do not appear with that regularity which is generally observed in diseases. A disease is also said to be anomalous, when the symptoms are so varied as not to bring it under the description of any known affection.

ANO'MPHALOS. (From *a*, priv. and ομφαλος, the navel.) *Anomphalus*. Without a navel.

ANO'NYMUS. (*Anonymus*, from *a*, priv. and ονομα, name.) Nameless; some eminences of the brain are called *columnæ anonymæ*; and it was formerly applied to one of the cricoid muscles.

ANO'RCHIDES. (From *a*, priv. and ορχις, the testicle.) Children are so termed which come into the world without testicles. This is a very common occurrence. The testicles of many male infants at the time of birth are within the abdomen. The time of their descent is very uncertain, and instances have occurred where they have not reached the scrotum at the age of ten or fifteen.

ANORE'XIA. (*Anorexia*, *æ*, f.; from *a*, priv. and ορεξις, appetite.) A want of appetite, without loathing of food. Cullen ranks this genus of disease in the class *Locales*, and order *Dysorexiæ*. He believes it to be generally symptomatic, but enumerates two species, viz. the *Anorexia humoralis*, and the *Anorexia atonica*. See *Dyspepsia*.

ANO'SMIA. (*Anosmia*, *æ*, f.; from *a*, neg. and οζω, to smell.) A loss of the sense of smelling. This genus of disease is arranged by Cullen in the order *Locales*, and order *Dysæsthæsiæ*. When it arises from a disease of the Schneiderian membrane, it is termed *Anosmia organica*; and when from no manifest cause *Anosmia atonica*.

ANSER. (*Anser, eris.* m.; a goose or gander.) The name of a genus of birds.

ANSER DOME'STICUS. The tame goose. The flesh of this bird is somewhat similar to that of the duck, and requires the assistance of spirituous and stimulating substances, to enable the stomach to digest it. Both are very improper for weak stomachs.

ANSERI'NA. (From *anser*, a goose; so called because geese eat it.) See *Potentilla anserina.*

ANT. See *Formica rufa.*

Ant, acid of. See *Formic acid.*

ANTACID. (*Antacidus;* from αντι, against, and *acidus*, acid.) That which destroys acidity. The action of antacids in the human stomach, is purely chemical, as they merely combine with the acid present, and neutralize it. They are only palliatives, the generation of acidity being to be prevented by restoring the tone of the stomach and its vessels. Dyspepsia and diarrhœa are the diseases in which they are employed. The principal antacids in use are the alkalies; *e. g.* Liquoris potassæ, gutt. xv. or from 5 to 15 gr. of subcarbonate of potassa, or soda dissolved in water. The solution of soda called double soda-water, or that of potassa supersaturated with carbonic acid, is more frequently used, as being more pleasant. Ammonia has been recommended as preferable to every other antacid, from 10 to 20 drops of the liquor ammoniæ in a cupful of water. The liquor calcis, or lime water, is likewise used to correct acidity, two or three ounces being taken occasionally. Creta præparata alone, or with the addition of a small quantity of any aromatic —chelæ cancrorum præparatæ; magnesia also and its carbonate, are used for the same purpose.

ANTAGONIST. (*Antagonistus*, counteracting.) A term applied to those muscles which have opposite functions. Such are the flexor and extensor of any limb, the one of which contracts it, the other stretches it out; and also the abductors and adductors. Solitary muscles are those without any antagonist, as the heart, &c.

ANTA'LGIC. (*Antalgicus;* from αντι, against, and αλγος, pain.) That which relieves pain.

ANTA'LKALINE. (*Antalkalinus;* from αντι, against, and *alkali*, an alcali.) That which possesses the power of neutralizing alkalies. All the acids are of this class.

ANTAPHRODISI'AC. *Antaphrodisiacus;* from αντι, against, and Αφροδιτη, Venus. Antivenereal, or whatever extinguishes amorous desires.

ANTAPHRODI'TIC. The same.

ANTAPO'DOSIS. (From ανταποδιδωμι, to reciprocate.) A vicissitude, or return of the paroxysm of fevers.—*Hippocrates.* Called by Galen *eipidosis.*

ANTARTHRI'TIC. See *Antiarthritic.*

ANTASTHMA'TIC. See *Antiasthmatic.*

ANTATRO'PHIC. See *Antiatrophic.*

ANTECHE'SIS. (From αντεχομαι, to resist.) A violent stoppage in the bowels, which resists all efforts to remove it.—*Hippocrates.*

ANTELA'BIUM. (From *ante*, before, and *labium*, a lip.) The extremity of the lip.

ANTE'MBASIS. (From αντι, mutually, and εμβαινω, to enter.) A coalescence, or union of bone.—*Galen.*

ANTEME'TIC. See *Antiemetic.*

ANTENEA'SMUS. (From αντι, against, and τεινεσμος, implacable.) That species of madness in which the patient endeavours to destroy himself.

ANTEPHIA'LTIC. See *Antiphialtic.*

ANTEPILE'PTIC. See *Antiepileptic.*

ANTE'RIOR. Before. A term applied to what may be situated before another of the same kind, as a muscle, a projection, eminence, lobe, artery, &c.

ANTERIOR AURIS. *Musculus anterior auris.* One of the common muscles of the ear, situated before the external ear. It arises thin and membranous, near the posterior part of the *zygoma*, and is inserted into a small eminence on the back of the helix, opposite to the concha, which it draws a little forwards and upwards.

ANTERIOR INTERCOSTAL. *Nervus intercostalis anterior. Splanchnic nerve.* A branch of the great intercostal that is given off in the thorax.

ANTERIOR MALLEI. See *Laxator tympani.*

ANTHE'LIX. See *Antihelix.*

ANTHE'LMIA. (From αντι, against, and ελμινς, a worm; so called, because it was thought of great virtue in expelling worms.) See *Spigelia anthelmia*, and *Marilandica.*

ANTHELMINTIC. (*Anthelminticus;* from αντι, against, and ελμινς, a worm.) Whatever procures the evacuation of worms from the stomach and intestines. The greater number of anthelmintics act mechanically, dislodging the worms, by the sharpness or roughness of their particles, or by their cathartic operation. Some seem to have no other qualities than those of powerful bitters by which they either prove noxious to these animals, or remove that debility of the digestive organs, by which the food is not properly assimilated, or the secreted fluids poured into the intestines are not properly prepared; circumstances from which it has been supposed the generation of worms may arise. The principal medicines belonging to this class, are, mercury, gamboge, Geoffræa inermis, tanacetum, polypodium filix mas, spigelia marilandica, artemisia santonica, olea Europæa, stannum pulverisatum, ferri limaturæ, and dolichos pruriens; which see under their respective heads.

A'NTHEMIS. (*Anthemis, midis.* fœm.; from ανθεω, *floreo;* because it bears an abundance of flowers.) 1. The name of a genus of plants in the Linnæan system. Class, *Syngenesia;* Order, *Polygamia superflua.*

2. The name in the London Pharmacopœia for chamomile. See *Anthemis nobilis.*

ANTHEMIS COTULA. The systematic name of the plant called *Cotula fœtida: Chamæmelum fœtidum*, in the pharmacopœias. Mayweed. Stinking chamomile. This plant, *Anthemis:—receptaculis conicis paleis setaceis, seminibus nudis*, of Linnæus, has a very disagreeable smell; the leaves, a strong, acrid, bitterish taste; the flowers, however, are almost insipid. It is said to have been useful in hysterical affections, but is very seldom employed.

ANTHEMIS NOBILIS. The systematic name for the *Chamæmelum; Chamæmelum nobile; Chamomilla romana; Euanthemon* of Galen. *Anthemis* of the last London pharmacopœia. Common chamomile. *Anthemis—foliis pinnato-compositis linearibus acutis subvillosis*, of Linnæus. Both the leaves and flowers of this indigenous plant have a strong though not ungrateful smell, and a very bitter, nauseous taste; but the latter are the bitterer, and considerably more aromatic. They possess tonic and stomachic qualities, and are much employed to restore tone to the stomach and intestines, and as a pleasant and cheap bitter. They have been long successfully used for the cure of intermittents, as well as of fevers of the irregular nervous kind, accompanied with visceral obstructions. The flowers have been found useful in hysterical affections, flatulent or spasmodic colics, and dysentery; but, from their laxative quality, Dr. Cullen tells us they proved hurtful in diarrhœas. A simple infusion is frequently taken to excite vomiting, or for promoting the operation of emetics. Externally they are used in the *decoctum pro fomento*, and are an ingredient in the *decoctum malvæ compositum.*

ANTHEMIS PYRETHRUM. The plant from which we obtain the pyrethrum of the pharmacopœias; *Asterantium; Buphthalmum creticum; Bellis montana putescens acris; Dentaria; Herba salivaris; Pes Alexandrinus.* Spanish Chamomile; pellitory of Spain. *Anthemis:—caulibus simplicibus unifloris decumbentibus—foliis pinnato-multifidis*, of Linnæus. This root, though cultivated in this country, is generally imported from Spain. Its taste is hot and acrid, its acrimony residing in a resinous principle. The ancient Romans, it is said, employed the root of this plant as a pickle. In its recent state, it is not so pungent as when dried, and yet, if applied to the skin, it produces inflammation. Its qualities are stimulant; but it is never used, except as a masticatory, for relieving toothaches, rheumatic affections of the face, and paralysis of the tongue, in which it affords relief by stimulating the excretory ducts of the salival glands.

ANTHERA. (From ανθος, a flower.)

1. A compound medicine used by the ancients; so called from its florid colour.—*Galen. Ægineta.*

2. The male part of the fructification of plants:—so called by Linnæus, by way of eminence. The male genital organ of plants consists of three parts, the filament, anther, and pollen. The anthera is the little head or extremity which rests on the filament.

Different terms are applied to the anthers from their figure:

1. *Oblong;* as in *Lilium candidum.*

2. *Globose*, as in *Mercurialis annua*.
3. *Semilunar;* as in *Fragaria vesca*.
4. *Angular;* as in *Tulipa gesneriana*.
5. *Linear;* as in the grasses and *Protea*.
6. *Didymous;* as in *Digitalis purpurea*.
7. *Arrow shaped;* as in *Crocus sativus*.
8 *Bifid*, parted half way down in two; as in the grasses and *Erica*.
9. *Shield like*, or *peltate*, of a round shape; as in *Taxus baccata*.
10. *Dentate*, with a tooth-like margin; as in *Taxus baccata*.
11. *Hairy;* as in *Lamium album*.
12. *Bicorn*, with two divisions like horns; as in *Arbutus uva ursi* and *Vaccinium myrtillus*.
13. *Cristate*, having cartilaginous points.
14. *Crucial;* as in *Mellitis*.
15. *Double* or *twin-like;* as in *Callisia* and *Hura*.
16. *Rostrate;* as in *Osbeckia*.
17. *Subulate*, or awl-shaped; as in the genus *Rolla*.
18. *Cordate;* as in *Cupraria*.
19. *Reniform*, kidney-shaped; as in *Tradescantia* and *Ginora*.
20. *Trigonal*, or three-cornered; as in the *Rose*.
21. *Tetragonal*, or four-cornered, as in *Cannabis* and *Dictamnus*.

From their situation:

22. *Erect*, with its base upon the apex of the filament; as in *Tulipa gesneriana*.
23. *Incumbent*, lying horizontally upon the filament, as in *Amaryllis formossima*.
24. *Versatile* when the incumbent anther adheres so loosely to the filament, that the least agitation of the plant puts it in motion; as in *Secale cereale*.
25. *Lateral*, adhering laterally to the filament; as in *Dianthera*.
26. *Sessile*, the filament almost wanting; as in *Aristolochia clematitis*.
27. *Free*, not united to any other anther.
28. *Connate*, united together; as in *Viola odorata*.

ANTHODIUM. A species of calyx, which contains many flowers being common to them all.

It is distinguished from its structure into,

1. *Monophyllous*, consisting of one leaflet perfect at its base, but cut at its limb or margin; as in *Tragopogon*.
2. *Polyphyllous*, consisting of several leaflets; as in *Carduus* and *Centaurea*.
3. *Simple*, consisting of one series of leaflets; as in *Cacalia porophyllum*.
4. *Equal*, when all the leaves of the *Anthodium simplex* are of the same length, as in *Ethulia*.
5. *Imbrecate* or *squamose*, as in *Centaurea cyanus*.
6. *Squarrose*, the leaflets bent backward at their extremities.
7. *Scabrous*, rough, consisting of dry leaflets; as in *Centaurea glastifolia* and *jacea*.
8. *Spinous*, the leaflets having thorns; as in *Cynaa scolymus* and *Centaurea sonchifolia*.
9. *Turbinate;* as in *Tarconanthus camphoratus*.
10. *Globose;* as in *Centaurea calcitrapa*.
11. *Hemispherical*, round below and flat above; as in *Anthemis* and *Chrysocoma*.
12. *Cylindrical*, long and round; as with *Eupatorium*.
13. *Calcyculate*, the basis surrounded by another small leafy anthodium; as in *Leontodon taraxacum*, *Senecio*, and *Crepis*.

ANTHOPHYLLITE. A massive mineral, of a brown colour, found at Konigsberg, in Norway.

[This substance has been observed only in amorphous masses, whose longitudinal fracture is foliated, or radiated, and whose cross fracture is uneven. The lustre of the most perfect laminæ is somewhat metallic. Its natural joints, of which two are much more perfect than the others, are parallel to the faces of a rectangular four-sided prism. It is rather difficult to break, and strongly scratches fluate of lime, but produces little or no effect on glass. It is feebly translucent at the edges, and its colour is brown, tinged with violet. Its powder is whitish, and rough to the touch. Its specific gravity varies from 3.11, to 3.29. Before the blow-pipe it is infusible. It contains silex 62.66, alumine 13.33, magnesia 4.0, lime 3.33, oxide of iron 12.00, manganese 3.25, water 1.43. It is softer, lighter, and has less lustre, than Labrador stone.—*Cleav. Min.* A.]

ANTHOPHY'LLUS. (From ανθος, a flower, and φυλλον, a leaf; so called from the fragance of the flowers and the beauty of the leaves.) The clove is so termed when it has been suffered to grow to maturity.—*Bauhin.*

ANTHOPHY'LLUS. (From ανθος, a flower, and φιλεω, to love.) A florist.

A'NTHORA. (*Quasi antithora.* Αντιθορα; from αντι, against, and θορα, monkshood: so called, because it is said to counteract the effects of the thorn or monkshood.) A species of Wolfsbane. See *Aconitum anthora.*

A'NTHOS FLORES. The flowers of the *rosmarinus* are so termed in some pharmacopœias. See *Rosmarinus officinalis.*

ANTHRA'CIA. 1. The name of a genus of diseases in Good's Nosology. See *Nosology.*

2. A name of the carbuncle. See *Anthrax.*

ANTHRACITE. Blind coal, Kilkenny coal, or glance coal. There are three varieties, conchoidal, slaty, and columnar.

[When pulverized and heated, it becomes red, and slowly consumes with a very light lambent flame, without smoke, and when pure emits no sulphureous or bituminous odour; it leaves a variable proportion of reddish ashes. Slaty glance coal consists of carbon, with from 3 to 30 per cent. of earth and iron. This mineral occurs in imbedded masses, beds, or veins, in primitive, transition, and floetz rocks. It is found in gneiss, in micaceous shistus, in mineral veins, with calcareous spar, native silver, mineral pitch, and red iron ore; and has been discovered by Jameson in the independent coal formation in the Isle of Arran.—*Phillips's Min.*

The coal of Rhode-Island is mingled with quartz, and occasionally with fibrous asbestos; yet it has but little hydrogen, and less bitumen. It is overlaid by coarse shale, containing numerous and strong impressions of ferns.

In Pennsylvania there are two great coal formations; one situated S. E. of the mountains, and the other N. W. The former is the Anthracite or glance coal, extending almost from Delaware along the head waters of the Lehigh and Schuylkill, and to Wilkesbarre on the Susquehannah, and along the Juniata.—*Mitchill's Notes to Phil. Min.*

This formation of Anthracite has been traced for ninety or a hundred miles in the state of Pennsylvania, and mines have been opened in many places on the branches of the Susquehannah, Schuylkill, and Delaware rivers, and some of them bordering on the states of New-Jersey and New-York. In many places it is near the surface, and appears to be inexhaustible. It is now extensively used as fuel, and its consumption is increasing. A.]

ANTHRACO'SIS OCULI. A red, livid, burning, sloughy, very painful tumour, occurring on the eyelids.—*Ægineta.*

ANTHRAX. (*Anthrax, acis.* m.; from ανθραξ, a burning coal.) *Anthracia; Anthrocosia; Anthrocoma; Carbunculus; Carbo; Rubinus versus; Codisella; Granatristum; Pruna; Persicus ignus* of Avicenna. A hard and circumscribed inflammatory tubercle like a boil, which sometimes forms on the cheek, neck, or back, and in a few days becomes highly gangrenous. It then discharges an extremely fœtid sanies from under the black core, which, like a burning coal, continues destroying the surrounding parts It is supposed to arise from a peculiar miasma, is most common in warm climates, and often attends the plague.

ANTHROPOGRA'PHY. (*Anthropographia;* from ανθρωπος, a man, and γραφω, to write.) Description of the structure of man.

ANTHROPOLO'GY. (*Anthpopologia;* from ανθρωπος, a man, and λογος, a discourse.) The description of man.

ANTHYPNO'TIC. (*Anthypnoticus;* from αντι, against, and υπνος, sleep.) That which prevents sleep or drowsiness.

ANTHYPOCHONDRI'AC. (*Anthypochondriacus*, from αντι, against, and ὑποχονδρια, the hypochondria.) That which is adapted to cure low-spiritedness or disorders of the hypochondria.

ANTHYSTE'RIC. (*Anthystericus;* from αντι, against, and υστερα, the womb.) That which relieves the hysteric passion

A'NTI (Αν7ι, against.) There are many names compounded with this word, as *Antiasthmatic; Antihysteric; Antidysenteric*, &c.; which signify medicines against the asthma, hysterics, dysentery, &c.

ANTIA'GRA. (From αν7ιας, a tonsil, and αγρα, a prey.) *Antiagri.* A tumour of the tonsils.—*Ulpian, Roland*, &c.

ANTIARTHRI'TIC. (*Antiarthriticus;* from αν7ι, against, and αρθρι7ις, the gout.) Antiarthritic. Against the gout.

ANTIASTHMATIC. (*Antiasthmaticus;* from αν7ι, against, and ασθμα, an asthma.) Antasthmatic. Against the asthma.

ANTIATROPHIC. (*Antiatrophicus;* from αν7ι, against, and α7ροφια, an atrophy.) Against an atrophy or wasting away.

ANTICACHE'CTIC (*Anticachecticus;* from αν7ι, against, and καχεξια, a cachexy.) Medicines against a cachexy, or bad habit of body.

ANTICA'RDIUM. (From αν7ι, against, or opposite, and καρδια, the heart.) The hollow at the bottom of the breast, commonly called scrobiculus cordis, or the pit of the stomach.

ANTICATARRHA'L. (*Anticatarrhalis;* from αν7ι, against, and κα7αρρος, a catarrh.) That which relieves a catarrh.

ANTICAUSO'TIC. (From αν7ι, against, and καυσος, a burning fever.) Remedies against burning fevers. We read, in Corp. Pharm. of Junken, of a *syrupus anticausoticus.*

A'NTICHEIR. (From αν7ι, against, and χειρ, the hand.) The thumb.—*Galen.*

ANTICNE'MION. (From αντι, against, or opposite, and κνημη, the calf of the leg.) That part of the tibia which is bare of flesh, and opposite the calf of the leg. The shin-bone.—*Galen.*

ANTICO'LIC. (From αντι, against, and κωλικη, the colic.) Remedies against the colic.

ANTIDIA'STOLE. (From αντι, against, and διαςελλω, to distinguish.) An exact and accurate distinction of one disease, or symptom, from another.

ANTIDI'NIC. (From αντι, against, and δινος, circumgyration.) Medicines against a vertigo, or giddiness.—*Blanchard.*

ANTIDOTARIUM. (*Antidotarium, i.* n.; from αντιδοτος, an antidote.) A term used by former writers for what we now call a dispensatory; a place where antidotes are prescribed and prepared. There are antidotaries extant of several authors, as those of *Nicholaus, Mesue, Myrepsus*, &c.

ANTI'DOTUS. From αντι, against, and διδωμι, to give.) 1. An antidote.

2. A preservative against sickness.

3. A remedy.—*Galen.*

ANTIDYSENTE'RIC. (*Antidysentericus;* from αντι, against, and δυσεντερια, a flux.) Medicines against a dysentery.

ANTIEMETIC. (*Antiemeticus;* from αντι, against, and εμεω, to vomit.) Antemetic. That which prevents or stops vomiting.

ANTIEPHIALTIC. (*Antiephialticus;* from αντι, against, and εφιαλτης, the nightmare.) Antephialtic. Against the nightmare.

ANTIEPILEPTIC. (*Antiepilepticus;* from αντι, against, and επιληψις, the epilepsy.) Antepileptic. Against epilepsy.

ANTIFEBRI'LE. (*Antifebrilis;* from αντι, against, and *febris*, a fever.) A febrifuge, a remedy against fever.

ANTIHE'CTIC. (*Antihecticus;* from αντι, against, and ἑκτικος, a hectic fever.) A remedy against a hectic fever

ANTIHE'CTICUM POTERII. *Antimonium diaphoreticum Joviale.* A medicine invented by Poterius, formerly extolled as effectual in hectic fevers, but now disregarded. It is an oxyde of tin and chalybeated regulus of antimony, in consequence of their deflagration with nitre.

ANTIHE'LIX. (*Antihelix, licis.* m.; from αντι, against, and ελιξ, the helix.) The inner circle of the external ear, so called from its opposition to the outer circuit, called the helix.

ANTIHELMINTIC. See *Anthelmintic.*

ANTIHYSTER'IC. (*Antihystericus;* from αντι, against, and ὑςερικα, hysterics.) Medicines which prevent or relieve hysterics.

ANTILE'PSIS. (From αντιλαμβανω, to take hold of.) The securing of bandages or ligatures from slipping. —*Hippocrates.*

ANTILO'BIUM. (From αντι, opposite, and λοβος, the bottom of the ear.) The tragus or that part of the ear which is opposite the lobe.

ANTILOI'MIC. (*Antiloimicus;* from αντι, against, and λοιμος, the plague.) Remedies or preventives against the plague.

ANTI'LOPUS. The antelope. An African beast resembling a deer, the hoofs and horns of which were formerly given in hysteric and epilectic cases.

ANTILY'SSUS. (From αντι, against, and λυσσα, the bite of a mad dog.) A medicine or remedy against the bite of a mad dog.

ANTIMONIA'L. (*Antimonialis;* from *antimonium*, antimony.) An antimonial or composition in which antimony is a chief ingredient. A preparation of antimony.

Antimonial powder. See *Antimonialis pulvis.*

ANTIMONIA'LIS PULVIS. Antimonial powder. Take of sulphuret of antimony, powdered, a pound; hartshorn shavings, two pounds. Mix and throw them into a broad iron pot heated to a white heat, and stir the mixture constantly until it acquires an ash colour. Having taken it out, reduce it to powder, and put it into a coated crucible, upon which another inverted crucible, having a small hole in its bottom, is to be luted. Then raise the fire by degrees to a white heat, and keep it so for two hours. Reduce the residuary mass to a very fine powder. The dose is from five to ten grains. It is in high esteem as a febrifuge, sudorific, and antispasmodic. The diseases in which it is mostly exhibited are, most species of asthenic and exanthematous fevers, acute rheumatism, gout, diseases arising from obstructed perspiration, dysuria, nervous affections, and spasms.

This preparation was introduced into the former London pharmacopœia as a substitute for a medicine of extensive celebrity, Dr. James's powder; to which, however, the present form more nearly assimilates in its dose, and it is more manageable in its administration, by the reduction of the proportion of antimony to one-half.

Antimonic acid. See *Antimony.*

Antimonious acid. See *Antimony.*

ANTIMONII OXYDUM. *Oxyde of Antimony.* This preparation is now directed to be made by dissolving an ounce of tartarized antimony, and two drams of subcarbonate of ammonia, separately in distilled water, mixing the solutions and boiling, till the oxyde of antimony is precipitated, which is to be washed with water, and dried. This must not be confounded with the old calcined or diaphoretic antimony, being a much more active preparation. See *Antimony.*

In its effects, it will be found to agree pretty much with the antimonium tartarizatum; but it is very little employed.

ANTIMONII SULPHURETUM PRÆCIPITATUM. *Sulphur antimonii præcipitatum.* Precipitated sulphuret of antimony. This preparation of antimony appears to have rendered that called kermes mineral unnecessary. It is made thus:—Take of sulphuret of antimony, in powder, two pounds;—of the solution of potassa, four pints:—of distilled water, three pints.

Mix; and boil the mixture over a slow fire for three hours, stirring it well, and occasionally adding distilled water, so that the same measure may be preserved. Strain the solution quickly through a double linen cloth, and while it is yet hot, drop in gradually, as much sulphuric acid as may be required to precipitate the powder; then wash away the sulphate of potassa by hot water; dry the precipitated sulphuret of antimony, and reduce it to powder. In this process part of the water is decomposed, and its oxygen unites partly with the antimony; the oxyde of antimony, as well as the potassa, combines with sulphur and hydrogen, forming hydrosulphuret of antimony and hydroguretted sulphuret of potassa: if the solution be allowed to cool, the former of these partly precipitates, constituting the kermes mineral; but the addition of the sulphuric acid throws down the whole of it at once, mixed with some sulphur, furnished with the decomposition of the hydroguretted sulphuret of potassa.

As an alterative and sudorific, it is in high estimation, and given in diseases of the skin and glands; and, joined with calomel, it is one of the most powerful and penetrating alteratives we are in possession of

Antimonii tartarizati vinum. Wine of tartarized antimony. Take of tartarized antimony, one scruple; boiling distilled water, eight fluid ounces; rectified spirit, two fluid ounces. Dissolve the tartarized antimony in the boiling distilled water, and add the spirit to the filtered liquor. Four fluid drachms of this contain one grain of tartarized antimony.

ANTIMONITE. A salt formed by the combination of the antimonous acid with alkaline and other bases. See *Antimony.*

ANTIMO'NIUM. See *Antimony*

Antimonium calcinatum. An oxyde of antimony.

Antimonium diaphoreticum. An old name for an oxyde of antimony.

Antimonium tartarizatum. *Tartarus emeticus; Tartarum emeticum; Tartarus antimonialus; Tartris antimonii cum potassa; Tartarum stibiatum.* Tartar emetic. It is obtained by boiling the fusible oxyde of antimony with supertartrate of potassa, the excess of tartaric acid dissolves the oxyde, and a triple salt is obtained by crystallization. The London Pharmacopœia directs thus Take of glass of antimony finely legivated, supertartrate of potassa in powder, of each a pound; boiling distilled water a gallon; mix the glass of antimony and the supertartrate of potassa well together, and then add them by degrees to the distilled water, which is to be kept boiling and constantly stirred; boil the whole for a quarter of an hour, and then set it by. Filter it when cold, and evaporate the filtered liquor so that crystals may form in it. A solution of this salt in dilute wine is ordered in the Pharmacopœia. See *Antimonii tartarizati vinum.*

Tartar emetic is the most useful of all the antimonial preparations. Its action is not dependent on the state of the stomach, and, being soluble in water, its dose is easily managed, while it also acts more speedily. In doses of from one to three, four, or five grains, it generally acts powerfully as an emetic, and is employed whenever we wish to obtain the effects which result from full vomiting. As patients are differently affected by this medicine, the safest mode of exhibiting it is: ℞. *Antimonii tartarazati,* gr. iii. *Aquæ distillatæ,* ℥ iv. Misce et cola. Dosis ℥ ss. omni horæ quadrante, donec supervenerit vomitus.

For children, emetic tartar is not so safe for an emetic as ipecacuanha powder: when great debility of the system is present, even a small dose has been known to prove fatal. Sometimes it proves cathartic. In smaller doses it excites nausea, and proves a powerful diaphoretic and expectorant. As an emetic it is chiefly given in the beginning of fevers and febrile diseases; when great debility is present, and in the advanced stages of typhoid fever, its use is improper, and even sometimes fatal. As a diaphoretic, it is given in small doses, of from an eighth to a quarter of a grain; and as an expectorant, in doses still smaller. Emetic tartar, in small doses, combined with calomel, has been found a powerful yet safe alterative in obstinate eruptions of the skin. ℞. *Antimonii tartarizati,* gr iv. *Hydrargyri submuriatis,* gr. xvi. *Confectionis rosæ gallicæ,* q. s. Divide in pil. xxiv. Capiat i. mane nocteque ex thea sassafras.

In the form of powder, or dissolved in water, it is applied by a pencil to warts and obstinate ulcers: it is also given in the form of clyster, with a view to produce irritation in soporose diseases, apoplexy, ileus, and strangulated hernia. The powder mixed with any fluid, and rubbed on the scorbiculus cordis, excites vomiting. Another property which tartar emetic has, when rubbed on the skin, is that of producing a crop of pustules very like to the small-pox, and with this view it is used against rheumatic pains, white, and other obstinate swellings. The best antidote against the bad effects of too large a quantity of this and other antimonial preparations, is a decoction of the bark of cinchona; in defect of which, tea and other astringents may be used. In a larger dose, this salt is capable of acting as a violent poison. The best antidotes are demulcent drinks, infusions of bark, tea, and sulphuretted hydrogen water, which instantly converts the energetic salt into a relatively mild sulphuret: anodynes are useful afterward.

Antimonium vitrifactum. Glass of antimony. An oxyde of antimony, with a little sulphuret.

ANTIMONY. (*Antimonium, i. n.* Αντιμονιον. The origin of this word is very obscure. The most received etymology is, from αντι, against, and μονος, a monk; because Valentine, by an injudicious administration of it, poisoned his brother monks.) *Stibium.* A metal found *native,* but very rarely; it has in that state, a metallic lustre, and is found in masses of different shapes; its colour is white, between those of tin and silver. It generally contains a small portion of arsenic. It is likewise met with in the state of an oxyde, *antimonial ochre.* The most abundant ore of it is that in which it is combined with sulphur, *the gray ore of antimony,* or *sulphuret of antimony* The colour of this ore is bluish, or steel-gray, of a metallic lustre, and is often extremely beautifully variegated. Its texture is either compact, foliated, or striated. The striated is found both crystallized, massive, and disseminated: there are many varieties of this ore.

Properties of Antimony.—Antimony is a metal of a grayish white, having a slight bluish shade, and very brilliant. Its texture is lamellated, and exhibits plates crossing each other in every direction. Its surface is covered with herbarisations and foliage. Its specific gravity is 6.702. It is sufficiently hard to scratch all the soft metals. It is very brittle, easily broken, and pulverizable. It fuses at 810° Fahr. It can be volatilized, and burns by a strong heat. When perfectly fused, and suffered to cool gradually, it crystallizes in octahedra. It unites with sulphur and phosphorus. It decomposes water strongly at a red heat. It is soluble in alkaline sulphurets. Sulphuric acid, boiled upon antimony, is feebly decomposed Nitric acid dissolves it in the cold. Muriatic acid scarcely acts upon it. The oxygenated muriatic acid gas inflames it, and the liquid acid dissolves it with facility. Arsenic acid dissolves it by heat with difficulty. It unites, by fusion, with gold, and renders it pale and brittle. Platina, silver, lead, bismuth, nickel, copper, arsenic, iron, cobalt, tin, and zinc, unite with antimony by fusion, and form with it compounds, more or less brittle. Mercury does not alloy with it easily unless very pure. We are little acquainted with the action of alkalies upon it. Nitrate of potassa is decomposed by it. It fulminates by percussion with oxygenated muriate of potassa. Antimony forms three, probably four, distinct combinations with oxygen:

1. The *protoxyde,* a blackish gray powder obtained from a mixture of powder of antimony and water at the positive pole of a voltaic circuit.

2. The *deutoxyde,* obtained by digesting the metal in powder, in muriatic acid, and pouring the solution in water of potassa. Wash and dry the precipitate. It is a powder of a dirty white colour which melts in a moderate red heat, and crystallizes as it cools.

3. The *tritoxyde,* or *antimonious acid,* which as immediately produced by the combustion of the metal, called formerly, from its fine white colour, the argentine flowers of antimony. It forms the salts called *antimonites* with the different bases.

4. The *peroxyde,* or *antimonic acid.* This is formed when the metal in powder is ignited along with six times its weight of nitre in a silver crucible. The excess of potassa and nitre being afterward separated by hot water, the antimoniate of potassa is then to be decomposed by muriatic acid, when the insoluble antimonic acid of a straw colour will be obtained.

Methods of obtaining antimony. 1. To obtain antimony, heat 32 parts of filings of iron to redness, and project on them, by degrees, 100 parts of antimony; when the whole is in fusion, throw on it, by degrees, 20 parts of nitrate of potassa, and after a few minutes quiet fusion, pour it into an iron melting cone, previously heated and greased.

2. It may also be obtained by melting eight parts of the ore mixed with six of nitrate of potassa, and three of supertartrate of potassa, gradually projected into a red-hot crucible, and fused.

To obtain perfectly pure antimony, Margraaf melted some pounds of the sulphuret in a luted crucible, and thus scorified any metals it might contain. Of the antimony thus purified, which lay at the bottom, he took sixteen ounces, which he oxydized cautiously first with a slow, and afterward with a strong heat, until it ceased to smell of sulphur, and acquired a grayish-white colour. Of this gray powder he took four ounces, mixed them with six drachms of supertartrate of potassa, and three of charcoal, and kept them in fusion in a well-covered and luted crucible, for one nour, and thus obtained a metallic button that weighed one ounce, seven drachms, and twenty grains.

The metal, thus obtained, he mixed with half its weight of desiccated subcarbonate of soda, and covered the mixture with the same quantity of the subcarbonate. He then melted it in a well-covered and luted crucible, in a very strong heat, for half an hour, and thus obtained a button which weighed one ounce, six drachms, and seven grains, much whiter and more beautiful than the former. This he again treated with one and a half ounce of subcarbonate of soda, and obtained a button, weighing one ounce, five drachms, and six grains. This button was still purer than the foregoing. Repeating these fusions with equal weights of subcarbonate of soda three times more, and an hour and a half each time, he at last obtained a button so pure as to amalgamate with mercury with ease, very hard, and in some degree malleable; the scoriæ formed in the last fusion were transparent, which indicated that they contained no sulphur, and hence it is the obstinate adherence of the sulphur that renders the purification of this metal so difficult.

"Chlorine gas and antimony combine with combustion, and a *bichloride* results. This was formerly prepared by distilling a mixture of two parts of corrosive sublimate with one of antimony. The substance which came over having a fatty consistence, was called *butter of antimony*. It is frequently crystallized in four-sided prisms. It is fusible and volatile at a moderate heat; and is resolved by water alone into the white oxyde and muriatic acid. Being a bichloride, it is eminently corrosive, like the bichloride of mercury, from which it is formed. It consists of 45.7 chlorine + 54.3 antimony, according to Dr. John Davy's analysis, when the composition of the sulphuret is corrected by its recent exact analysis by Berzelius. But 11 antimony + 2 primes chlorine = 9.0, give the proportion per cent. of 44.1 + 55.5; a good coincidence, if we consider the circuitous process by which Dr. Davy's analysis was performed. Three parts of corrosive sublimate, and one of metallic antimony, are the equivalent proportions for making butter of antimony.

Iodine and antimony combine by the aid of heat into a solid *iodine*, of a dark red colour.

The *phosphuret* of this metal is obtained by fusing it with solid phosphoric acid. It is a white semicrystalline substance. The sulphuret of antimony exists abundantly in nature. It consists, according to Berzelius, of 100 antimony + 37.25 sulphur. The proportion given by the equivalent ratio is 100 + 36.5. The only important alloys of antimony are those of lead and tin; the former constitutes type-metal, and contains about one-sixteenth of antimony; the latter alloy is employed for making the plates on which music is engraved.

The salts of antimony are of two different orders; in the first, the deutoxyde acts the part of a salifiable base; in the second, the tritoxide and peroxide act the part of acids, neutralizing the alkaline and other bases, to constitute the antimonites and antimoniates.

The only distinct combination of the first order entitled to our attention, is the triple salt called *tartrate of potassa and antimony*, or tartar emetic, and which, by Gay Lussac's new views, would be styled cream-tartrate of antimony. This constitutes a valuable and powerful medicine, and therefore the mode of preparing it should be correctly and clearly defined. As the dull white deutoxyde of antimony is the true basis of this compound salt, and as that oxyde readily passes by mismanagement into the tritoxide or antimonious acid, which is altogether unfit for the purpose, adequate pains should be taken to guard against so capital an error. In the British pharmacopœias, the glass of antimony is now directed as the basis of tartar emetic. More complex and precarious formulæ were formerly introduced. The new edition of the Pharmacopée Française has given a recipe, which appears, with a slight change of proportions, to be unexceptionable. Take of the sulphuretted vitreous oxide of antimony, levigated and acidulous tartrate of potassa, equal parts. From a powder, which is to be put into an earthen or silver vessel, with a sufficient quantity of pure water. Boil the mixture for half an hour, adding boiling water from time to time; filter the hot liquor, and evaporate to dryness in a porcelain capsule; dissolve in boiling water the result of the evaporation, evaporate till the solution acquires the spec. grav 1.161, and then let it repose, that crystals be obtained which, by this process, will be pure. By another recipe, copied, with some alteration, from Mr. Phillips's prescription, into the appendix of the French Pharmacopœia, a subsulphate of antimony is formed first of all, by digesting two parts of sulphuret of antimony in a moderate heat, with three parts of oil of vitriol. This insoluble subsulphate being well washed, is then digested in a quantity of boiling water, with its own weight of cream of tartar, and evaporated at the density 1.161, after which it is filtered hot. On cooling, crystals of the triple tartrate are obtained. One might imagine, that there is a chance of obtaining by this process a mixture of sulphate of potassa, and perhaps of a triple sulphate of antimony, along with the tartar emetic. Probably this does not happen, for it is said to yield crystals, very pure, very white, and without any mixture whatever.

Pure tartar emetic is in colourless and transparent tetrahedrons or octohedrons. It reddens litmus. Its taste is nauseous and caustic. Exposed to the air, it effloresces slowly. Boiling water dissolves half its weight, and cold water a fifteenth part. Sulphuric, nitric, and muriatic acids, when poured into a solution of this salt, precipitate its cream of tartar; and soda, potassa, ammonia, or their carbonates, throw down its oxyde of antimony. Barytes, strontites, and lime waters occasion not only a precipitate of oxyde of antimony, like the alkalies, but also insoluble tartrates of these earths. That produced by the alkaline hydrosulphurets is wholly formed of kermes; while that caused by sulphuretted hydrogen, contains both kermes and cream of tartar. The decoctions of several varieties of cinchona, and of several bitter and astringent plants, equally decompose tartar emetic; and the precipitate then always consists of the oxyde of antimony, combined with the vegetable matter and cream of tartar. Physicians ought, therefore, to beware of such incompatible mixtures. When tartar emetic is exposed to a red heat, it first blackens, like all organic compounds, and afterward leaves a residuum of metallic antimony and subcarbonate of potassa. From this circumstance, and the deep brownish red precipitate, by hydrosulphurets, this antimonial combination may readily be recognised. The precipitate may further be dried on a philter, and ignited with black flux, when a globule of metallic antimony will be obtained. Infusion of galls is an active precipitant of tartar emetic.

The composition of this salt, according to M. Thenard, is 35.4 acid, 39.6 oxyde, 16.7 potassa, and 8.2 water. The presence of the latter ingredient is obvious, from the undisputed phenomenon of efflorescence. If we adopt the new views of M. Gay Lussac, this salt may be a compound of a prime equivalent of tartar = 23.825, with a prime equivalent of deutoxide of antimony = 13. On this hypothesis, we would have the following proportions:

2 primes acid,	= 16.75	45.4
1 prime potassa,	= 5.95	16.2
1 prime water,	= 1.125	3.1
4 oxyde of antimony,	= 13.00	35.3
	36.825	100.0

But very little confidence can be reposed in such atomical representations.

The deutoxyde seems to have the property of combining with sulphur in various proportions. To this species of compound must be referred the liver of antimony, glass of antimony, and *crocus metallorum* of the ancient apothecaries. Sulphuretted hydrogen forms, with the deutoxide of antimony, a compound which possessed at one time great celebrity in medicine, and of which a modification has lately been introduced into the art of calico printing. By dropping hydrosulphuret of potassa, or of ammonia, into the cream tartrate, or into mild muriate of antimony, the hydrosulphuric of the metallic oxyde precipitates of a beautiful deep orange colour. This is *kermes mineral.* Cluzel's process for obtaining a fine *kermes*, light, velvety, and of a deep purple-brown, is the following: one part of pulverized sulphuret of antimony, 22 1-2 parts of crystallized subcarbonate of soda, and 200 parts of water, are to be boiled together in an iron pot. Filter the hot liquor into warm earthen pans, and allow them to cool very slowly. At the end of 24 hours, the kermes is deposited. Throw it on a filter, wash it with water which had been boiled and then cooled out of contact with air. Dry the kermes at a temperature of 85°, and preserve in corked phials. Whatever may be the process employed, by boiling the liquor, after cooling and filtration, on new sulphuret of antimony, or upon that which was left in the former operation, this new liquid will deposite, on cooling, a new quantity of kermes. Besides the hydrosulphuretted oxyde of antimony, there is formed a sulphuretted hydrosulphuret of potassa or soda. Consequently the alkali seizes a portion of the sulphur from the antimonial sulphuret, water is decomposed; and, while a a portion of its hydrogen unites to the alkaline sulphuret, its oxygen, and the other portion of its hydrogen, combine with the sulphuretted antimony. It seems, that the resulting kermes remains dissolved in the sulphuretted hydrosulphuret of potassa or soda; but as it is less soluble in the cold than the hot, it is partially precipitated by refrigeration. If we pour into the supernatant liquid, after the kermes is deposited and removed, any acid, as the dilute nitric, sulphuric, or muriatic, we decompose the sulphuretted hydrosulphuret of potassa or soda. The alkaline base being laid hold of, the sulphuretted hydrogen and sulphur to which they were united are set at liberty; the sulphur and kermes fall together, combine with it, and form an orange-coloured compound, called the golden sulphuret of antimony. It is a hydroguretted sulphuret of antimony. Hence, when it is digested with warm muriatic acid, a large residuum of sulphur is obtained, amounting sometimes to 12 per cent. Kermes is composed, by Thenard, of 20.3 sulphuretted hydrogen, 4.15 sulphur, 72.76 oxyde of antimony, 2.79 water and loss; and the golden sulphuret consists of 17.87 sulphuretted hydrogen, 68.3 oxyde of antimony, and 12 sulphur.

By evaporating the supernatant kermes liquid, and cooling, crystals form, which have been lately employed by the calico printer to give a topical orange. These crystals are dissolved in water, and the solution, being thickened with paste or gum, is applied to cloth in the usual way. When the cloth is dried, it is passed through a dilute acid, when the orange precipitate is deposited and fixed on the vegetable fibres.

An empirical antimonial medicine, called James's powder, has been much used in this country. The inventor called it his *fever powder*, and was so successful in his practice with it, that it obtained very great reputation, which it still in some measure retains. Probably, the success of Dr. James was in a great measure owing to his free use of the bark, which he always gave as largely as the stomach would bear, as soon as he had completely evacuated the primæ viæ by the use of his antimonial preparation, with which at first he used to combine some mercurial. His specification, lodged in chancery, is as follows: "Take antimony, calcine it with a continued protracted heat, in a flat, unglazed, earthen vessel, adding to it from time to time a sufficient quantity of any animal oil and salt, well dephlegmated; then boil it in melted nitre for a considerable time, and separate the powder from the nitre by dissolving it in water." The real recipe has been studiously concealed, and a false one published in its stead. Different formulæ have been offered for imitating it. That of Dr. Pearson furnishes a mere mixture of an oxyde of antimony, with phosphate of lime. The real powder of James, according to this chemist, consists of 57 oxyde of antimony, with 43 phosphate of lime. It seems highly probable that superphosphate of lime would act on oxyde of antimony in a way somewhat similar to cream of tartar, and produce a more chemical combination than what can be derived from a precarious ustulation, and calcination of hartshorn shavings and sulphuret of antimony, in ordinary hands. The antimonial medicines are powerful deobstruents, promoting particularly the cuticular discharge. The union of this metallic oxyde with sulphuretted hydrogen, ought undoubtedly to favour its medicinal agency in chronic diseases of the skin. The kermes deserves more credit than it has hitherto received from British physicians.

The compounds, formed by the antimonious and antimonic acids with the bases, have not been applied to any use. Muriate of barytes may be employed as a test for tartar emetic. It will show, by a precipitate insoluble in nitric acid, if sulphate of potassa be present. If the crystals be regularly formed, more tartar need not be suspected."—*Ure's Chem. Dict.*

The preparations of antimony formerly in use were very many: those now directed to be kept are;—

1. *Sulphuretum antimonii.*
2. *Oxydum antimonii.*
3. *Sulphuretum antimonii præcipitatum.*
4. *Antimonium tartarizatum.*
5. *Vinum antimonii tartarizati.*
6. *Pulvis antimonialis.*

ANTI'MORIS. (From αντι, against, and μορος, death, or disease.) A medicine to prolong life.

ANTINEPHRI'TIC. (*Antinephriticus;* from αντι, against, and νεφριτις, a disease of the kidneys.) A remedy against disorders of the kidneys.

ANTIODONTALGIC. (*Antiodontalgicus;* from αντι, against, and οδονταλγια, the toothache.) Against the toothache.

ANTIODONTA'LGICUS. An insect described by Germi in a small work published at Florence 1794, so called from its property of allaying the toothache. It is a kind of curculio found on a species of thistle, *Carduus spinosissimus.* If twelve or fifteen of these insects, in the state of larva, or when come to perfection, be bruised and rubbed slowly between the fore-finger and thumb until they have lost their moisture, and if the painful tooth, where it is hollow, be touched with that finger, the pain ceases sometimes instantaneously A piece of shamoy leather will answer the same purpose with the finger. If the gums are inflamed, the remedy is of no avail. Other insects possess the property of curing the toothache; such as the *Scarabeus ferrugineus* of Fabricius; the *Coccinella septempunctata,* or lady-bird; the *Chrysomela populi,* and the *Chrysomela sanguinolenta.* This property belongs to several kinds of the *Coleoptera.*

ANTIPARALY'TIC. (*Antiparalyticus;* from αντι, against, and παραλυσις, the palsy.) Against the palsy.

ANTIPATHY. (*Antipathia, æ.* f. Αντιπαθης, from αντιπαθεω, to have a natural repugnance or dislike; from αντι, against, and παθος, an affection.) 1. An aversion to particular objects.

2. The name of a genus of diseases in some classifications.

ANTIPERISTA'LTIC. (*Antiperistalticus;* from αντι, against, and περιςελλω, to contract.) Whatsoever obstructs the peristaltic motion of the intestines.

ANTIPERI'STATIS. (From αντι, against, and περιςημι, to press.) A compression on all sides. *Theophrastus de igne.*

ANTIPHA'RMIC. (*Antipharmicus;* from αντι, against, and φαρμακον, a poison.) The same as alexipharmic. Remedies or preservatives against poison.—*Dioscorides.*

ANTIPHLOGI'STIC. (*Antiphlogisticus;* from αντι, against, and φλεγω, to burn.) A term applied to those medicines, plans of diet, and other circumstances, which tend to oppose inflammation, or which, in other words, weaken the system by diminishing the activity of the vital power.

ANTIPHTHI'SIC. (*Antiphthisicus;* from αντι, against, and φθισις, consumption.) Against a consumption.

ANTI'PHTHORA. (From αντι, against, and φθορα, corruption.) A species of wolfsbane which resists corruption. See *Aconitum anthora.*

ANTIPHY'SIC. (*Antiphysicus;* from αντι, against, and φυσαω, to blow.) A carminative or remedy against wind.

ANTIPLEURI'TIC. (*Antipleuriticus;* from αντι, against, and πλευριτις, pleurisy.) Against a pleurisy.

ANTIPODA'GRIC. (*Antipodagricus;* from αντι, against, and ποδαγρα, the gout.) That which relieves or removes the gout.

ANTIPRAXIA. (From αντι against. and πρασσω, to work.) A contrariety of functions and temperaments in divers parts. Contrariety of symptoms.

ANTIPYRE'TIC. (*Antipyreticus;* from αντι, against, and πυρετος, fever.) Against a fever.

ANTIQUARTANA'RIA. (From αντι, against, and *quartana,* a quartan fever.) Remedies against quartan agues.

ANTIQUA'RTICUM. The same as Antiquartanaria.

ANTIRRHI'NUM. (Αντιῤῥινον; from αντι against, and ῥις, the nose: so called because it represents the nose of a calf.) The name of a genus of plants in the

Linnæan system. Class, *Didynamia;* Order, *Angiospermia.*

Antirrhinum elatine. The systematic name of the plant we call fluellin, or female speedwell. *Elatine* of the shops. The leaves of this plant have a roughish bitter taste, but no smell. It was formerly much used against scurvy and old ulcerations, but now wholly forgotten.

Antirrhinum linaria. The systematic name for the *linaria* of the pharmacopœias. *Osyris; Urinaria; Antirrhinum—foliis lanceolatis linearibus confertis, caule erecto, spicis terminalibus sessilibus, floribus imbricatis* of Linnæus. Common toad-flax. A perennial indigenous plant, common in barren pastures, hedges, and the sides of roads, flowering from July to September. The leaves have a bitterish and somewhat saline taste, and when rubbed between the fingers, have a faint smell, resembling that of elder. They are said to be diuretic and cathartic, and in both characters to act powerfully, especially in the first; hence the name *urinaria.* They have been recommended in dropsies and other disorders requiring powerful evacuations. The linaria has also been used as a resolvent in jaundice, and such diseases as were supposed to arise from visceral obstructions. But the plant has been chiefly valued for its effects when externally applied, especially in hæmorrhoidal affections, for which both the leaves and flowers have been employed in various forms of ointment, fomentation, and poultice. Dr. Wolph first invented an ointment of this plant for the piles. The Landgrave of Hesse, to whom he was physician, constantly interrogated him, to discover its composition; but Wolph obstinately refused, till the prince promised to give him a fat ox annually for the discovery: hence, to the following verse, which was made to distinguish the linaria from the escula, viz.

" *Escula lactescit, sine lacte linaria crescit.*" The hereditary Marshal of Hesse added,

" *Escula nil nobis, sed dat linaria taurum.*"

ANTISCO'LIC. (*Antiscolicus;* from αντι, against, and σκωληξ, a worm.) Remedies against worms. See *Anthelmintic.*

ANTISCORBU'TIC. (*Antiscorbuticus,* from αντι, against, and *scorbutus,* the scurvy.) Medicines which cure the scurvy.

ANTISEPTIC. (*Antisepticus,* from αντι, against, and σηπω, to putrefy.) Whatever possesses a power of preventing animal substances from passing into a state of putrefaction, and of obviating putrefaction when already begun. This class of medicines comprehends four orders:

1. *Tonic antiseptics;* as cinchona, cusparia, chamæmelum, &c. which are suited for every condition of body, and are, in general, preferable to other antiseptics, for those with relaxed habits.

2. *Refrigerating antiseptics;* as acids, which are principally adapted for the young, vigorous, and plethoric.

3. *Stimulating antiseptics;* as wine and alkohol, best adapted for the old and debilitated.

4. *Antispasmodic antiseptics;* as camphor and asafœtida, which are to be selected for irritable and hysterical habits.

[" The presence of air, though not necessary to putrefaction, materially accelerates it, and those gases which contain no oxygen, are very efficient in checking or altogether preventing the process. Carbonic acid also remarkably retards putrefaction; and if boiled meat be carefully confined in vessels containing that gas, it remains for a very long time unchanged, as seen in Mr. Appert's method of preserving meat."

" There are several substances which, by forming new combinations with animal matter, retard or prevent putrefaction; such as chlorine, and many of the saline and metallic compounds; sugar, alkohol, volatile oils, acetic acids, and many other vegetable substances, also stand in the list of antiputrefactives, though their mode of operating is by no means understood."—*Webster's Man. of Chem.*

The alkaline earths and salts are antiseptics, and act by absorbing the acids formed in the process of putrefaction. Carbon or charcoal of wood is one of the most powerful antiseptics. It will restore tainted meat, and purify offensive water. Casks are now charred to contain water on long sea voyages, and it will continue pure and sweet in these for a long time. Charcoal in powder is successfully used in the cure of looseness of the bowels, and it has been known to cure intermittent fevers. A.]

Anti'spasis. (From αντι, against, and σπαω, to draw.) A revulsion. The turning the course of the humours, while they are actually in motion.—*Galen.*

ANTISPASMODIC. (*Antispasmodicus;* from αντι, against, and σπασμος, a spasm.) Possessing the power of allaying, or removing, inordinate motions in the system, particularly those involuntary contractions which take place in muscles, naturally subject to the command of the will. Spasm may arise from various causes. One of the most frequent is a strong irritation, continually applied; such as dentition, or worms. In these cases, narcotics prove useful, by diminishing irritability and sensibility. Sometimes spasm arises from mere debility; and the obvious means of removing this is by the use of tonics. Both narcotics and tonics, therefore, are occasionally useful as antispasmodics, such as opium, camphor, and æther, in the one class, and zinc, mercury, and Peruvian bark, in the other. But there are, farther, several other substances, which cannot be with propriety referred to either of these classes; and to these, the title of antispasmodics is more exclusively appropriated. The principal antispasmodics, properly so called, are moschus, castoreum, oleum animale empyreumaticum, petroleum, ammonia, asafœtida, sagapenum, galbanum, valeriana, crocus, melaleuca leucadendron. The narcotics, used as antispasmodics, are æther, opium, camphor. The tonics, used as antispasmodics, are cuprum, zincum, hydrargyrum, cinchona.

ANTI'THENAR. (From αντι, against, and θεναρ, the palm of the hand or foot.) A muscle of the foot. See *Adductor pollicis pedis.*

ANTITRA'GICUS. *Antitragus.* One of the proper muscles of the ear, the use of which is to turn up the tip of the antitragus a little outwards, and to depress the extremity of the antihelix towards it.

ANTITRAGUS. (*Antitragus, i.* m. from αντι, and τραγος, the tragus.) An eminence of the outer ear, opposite to the tragus.

ANTIVENE'REAL. (From αντι, against, and *venereus,* venereal.) Against the venereal disease.

ANTO'NII SANCTI IGNIS. (So called because St. Anthony was supposed to cure it miraculously. In the Roman missal, St. Anthony is implored as being the preserver from all sorts of fire.) St. Anthony's fire. See *Erysipelas.*

Antophy'llon. (From αντι, against, and φυλλον a leaf; so called because its leaves are opposite.) The male caryophyllus.

A'NTRUM. (*Antrum, i.* n. a den or cave.) 1 A cavity which has a small opening into it.

2. The cochlea of the ear.

Antrum buccinosum. The cochlea of the ear

Antrum genæ. See *Antrum of Highmore.*

Antrum highmorianum. See *Antrum of Highmore.*

Antrum of highmore. (From the name of an anatomist, who gave the first accurate description of it.) *Antrum Highmorianum; Antrum genæ; Sinus maxillaris pituitarius; Antrum maxillæ superioris.* Maxillary sinus. A large cavity in the middle of each superior maxillary bone, between the eye and the roof of the mouth, lined by the mucous membrane of the nose. See *Maxillare superius, os.*

One or both antra are liable to several morbid affections. Sometimes their membranous lining inflames and secretes pus. At other times, in consequence of inflammation, or other causes, various excrescences and fungi are produced in them. Their bony parietes are occasionally affected with exostosis, or caries Extraneous bodies may be lodged on them, and it is even asserted that insects may be generated in them, and cause, for many years, afflicting pains. Abscesses in the antrum are by far the most common. Violent blows on the cheek, inflammatory affections of the adjacent parts, and especially of the pituitary membrane lining the nostrils, exposure to cold and damp and, above all things, bad teeth, may induce inflammation and suppuration in the antrum. The first symptom is a pain, at first imagined to be a toothache, particularly if there should be a carious tooth at this part of the jaw. This pain, however, extends more into the nose than that usually does which arises from a decayed tooth; it also affects, more or less, the eye, the orbit, and the situation of the frontal sinuses. But even such symptoms are insufficient to characterize the disease, the nature of which is not unequivocally evinced, till a much later period. The complaint is, in general, of much longer duration than one entirely dependent on a caries of the tooth, and its violence increases more and more, until at last a hard tumour becomes perceptible below the cheek-bone. The swelling by degrees extends over the whole cheek; but it afterward rises to a point, and forms a very circumscribed hardness, which may be felt above the back grinders. This symptom is accompanied by redness, and sometimes by inflammation and suppuration of the external parts. It is not uncommon also, for the outward abscess to communicate with that within the antrum. The circumscribed elevation of the tumour, however, does not occur in all cases. There are instances in which the matter makes its way towards the palate, causing the bones of the part to swell, and at length rendering them carious, unless timely assistance be given. There are other cases, in which the matter escapes between the fangs and sockets of the teeth. Lastly, there are other examples, in which matter, formed in the antrum, makes its exit at the nostril of the same side when the patient is lying with his head on the opposite one, in a low position. If this mode of evacuation should be frequently repeated, it prevents the tumour both from pointing externally, and bursting, as it would do if the purulent matter could find no other vent. This evacuation of the pus from the nostril is not very common. The method of cure consists in extracting one of the dentes molares from the affected side; and then perforating through the socket into the bony cavity. A mild injection may afterward be employed to cleanse the sinus occasionally.

Antrum maxillæ. See *Antrum of Highmore.*

Antrum maxillare. See *Antrum of Highmore.*

Antrum pylori. A concavity of the stomach approaching the pylorus.

Anty'lion. (From *Antyllus*, its inventor.) An astringent application, recommended by Paulus Ægineta.

A'NUS. (*Anus*, *i.* masc. *quasi onus;* as carrying the burden of the bowels.)

1. The fundament; the lower extremity of the great intestine, named the rectum, is so called; and its office is to form an outlet for the fæces. The anus is furnished with muscles which are peculiar to it, viz. the *sphincter*, which forms a broad circular band of fibres, and keeps it habitually closed, and the *levatores ani*, which serve to dilate and draw it up to its natural situation, after the expulsion of the fæces. It is also surrounded, as well as the whole of the neighbouring intestine, with muscular fibres, and a very loose sort of cellular substance. The anus is subject to various diseases, especially piles, ulceration, abscesses, excrescences, prolapsus; and imperforation in new-born infants.

2. The term *anus* is also applied to a small opening of the third ventricle of the brain, which leads into the fourth.

[*Fissure of the anus.* In the New-York Medical and Physical Journal, a very interesting case of this malady is related by the patient himself. He was successfully operated upon by Professor Alexander H. Stevens, M.D., of the College of Physicians and Surgeons of New-York. The fissure was on one side, and the incision was made directly upon it and through the sphincter. The relief from the most agonizing pain was immediate and permanent. We find a note on the subject of this disease in the Philadelphia edition of *Cooper's First Lines of the Practice of Surgery*, which we quote.

"Baron Boyer has recently called the attention of Surgeons to what he has denominated *fissure of the anus.* Though this disease was noticed by Ætius, it passed unobserved by modern surgeons until the time of Sabatier, who imperfectly described it. Baron Boyer has met with many cases of it, and it is now understood by all the surgeons of Paris, where it is said to be not uncommon. It has been generally confounded with ulcerated piles, blind fistula, or other diseases of the rectum. The symptoms it occasions have been considered inexplicable by the surgeon, though exceedingly distressing to the patient. Fissure of the anus is an oblong ulceration of the extremity of the rectum, just where the mucous membrane joins the skin. The ulceration is generally a little above the anus, so that it is not easily discovered, unless the sides of the rectum are drawn outwards, and the gut partially everted. Moreover, the fissure is superficial, and presents nothing striking to the eye, and is, therefore, more likely to pass unobserved. The mucous membrane is more red than natural at the edges of the ulcerated portion, which is entirely absorbed; but there is nothing unnatural to be felt with the fingers, except a very remarkable constriction, which accompanies, or rather precedes, this disease. It would appear, that this constriction is, indeed, the cause of the malady, which results from the efforts to expel hardened fæces through the contracted passage. The introduction of the finger causes exquisite pain."

"The first symptom of the disease, is pain felt in evacuating the rectum, greatly aggravated by costiveness, and rendered most excruciating by the hardness of the fæces. Hence the sufferer is led to use injections and mild laxative medicines. In the commencement, the pain subsides at the expiration of about half an hour; in its progress, the paroxysms lengthen to several hours' duration, and the patients writhe in agony, not knowing what position to put themselves in. They suffer least in bed, and remain there several days without leaving it. The pain has accessions without any known cause, and often ceases in the same manner."

"The pain appears to be owing to a retention of excrementitious matter near the extremity of the rectum, the expulsion of which is prevented by the constriction of the sphincter ani. The fæces are, sometimes, streaked with a line of blood, especially if they be hard; but this is not always the case: sometimes there is a discharge per anum of a white liquid matter, in small quantities; this is what would be expected from an inflamed or ulcerated mucous membrane, but occasionally the ulceration extends to the muscular coat of the intestine."

"These symptoms vary in different patients. In delicate and nervous women, a variety of remote symptoms occur, and often conceal the origin of the primary complaint, which is mistaken for cancer of the rectum, ulceration of the womb, &c."

"In this disease there are two distinct occurrences: viz. constriction of the anus, and ulceration or fissure. The former is the cause of the latter. Ulceration without constriction, as we every day see in fistula in ano, does not occasion so severe pain as is felt in this complaint. With respect to the treatment of this complaint, if it be slight, it will sometimes yield to laxative medicines and the application of leeches to the peri næum. But these means are not generally sufficient It is then necessary to divide with the knife the whole of the sphincter ani, and that if possible, immediately at the seat of the fissure. The incision should be at least one-third of an inch deep, especially near the verge of the anus, and an inch long. After the operation, or at any rate, before cicatrization begins, a tent is to be introduced and kept in the rectum, without which the operation would be unsuccessful When the fissure is in the anterior part of the anus, as the sphincter could not be safely divided in that direction, it is best to cut towards the coccyx. After the cure the rectum is found more ample than before." A.]

Anus, artificial. An accidental opening in the parietes of the abdomen, to which opening some part of the intestinal canal leads, and through which the fæces are either wholly or in part discharged. When strangulated hernia occurs, in which the intestine is simply pinched, and this event is unknown; when it has not been relieved by the usual means; or when the necessary operation has not been practised in time; the protruded part becomes gangrenous, and the fæces escape. But if the patient should be at last operated upon, his fæces are discharged through the wound, and the intestines are more easily emptied. In both cases the excrement continues to be discharged from the artificial opening. In this way an artificial anus is formed, through which the excrement is evacuated during life.

Any'drion. (From *α*, priv. and *υδωρ*, water; so called, because they who eat of it become thirsty.) A species of night-shade, according to Blancard.

Anypeu'thynus. (From *α*, neg. and *υπευθυνος*, blameable.) Hippocrates, in his Precepts, uses this word to signify an accidental event, which cannot be charged on the physician, and for which he is not accountable.

AO'RTA. (*Aorta, æ.* f.; from αηρ, air, and τηρεω, to keep: so called because the ancients supposed that only air was contained in it.) The great artery of the body, which arises from the left ventricle of the heart, forms a curvature in the chest, and descends into the abdomen. See *Artery*.

APALACHI'NE GALLIS. (From απαλακω, to repel; because it is supposed to repel infection.) See *Ilex cassine*.

APARI'NE. (From ρινη, a file; because its bark is rough, and rasps like a file.) Goose-grass. See *Galium aparine*.

APARTHRO'SIS. (From απο and αρθρον, a joint.) Articulation.

APATITE. A phosphate of lime mineral, of a white wine, yellow, green and red colour, found in primitive rocks in Cornwall and Devonshire.

[There are several varieties of the phosphate of lime. The first variety (apatite) yielded Klaproth, lime 55.00, phosphoric acid, 45.00.

Its solubility in acids, and inferior hardness, may serve to distinguish it from the chrysoberil, tourmaline, topaz, chrysolite, beryl, emerald, and some varieties of quartz; all of which it more or less resembles, especially the *emerald*, *beryl*, and *chrysolite*. From carbonate of lime it differs by its greater hardness, and want of effervescence in acids; and it does not, like the fluate of lime, when its powder is thrown into warm sulphuric acid, yield a gas capable of corroding glass, unless from the accidental presence of a small quantity of that salt. The variety of phosphate of lime, called apatite, usually in crystals, sometimes presents a low six-sided prism, the primitive form.

The same gangure, which contains the crystals, often embraces grains or small granular masses, having a crystalline structure, but nearly or quite destitute of a regular form. The apatite occurs in veins, or is disseminated in granite, gneiss, or other primitive rocks. It is associated with quartz, feldspar, fluate of lime, garnets, the oxydes of iron, tin, &c.

Apatite has been found in Maryland, Pennsylvania, and New-York; also in the States of Connecticut and Maine.—*Cl. Min.* A.]

APE'LLA. (From α, priv. and *pellis*, skin.) Shortness of the prepuce. Galen gives this name to all whose prepuce, either through disease, section, or otherwise, will not cover the glans.

APE'PSIA. (*Apepsia, æ* f. Απεψια; from α, priv. and πεπτω, to digest.) Indigestion. See *Dyspepsia*.

APE'RIENS PALPEBRARUM RECTUS. See *Levator palpebræ superioris*.

APERIENT. (*Aperiens;* from *aperio*, to open.) 1. That which gently opens the bowels.

2. Applied also to muscles, the office of which is to open parts; as the levator palpebræ superioris, which is called, in some anatomical works, aperiens palpebræ.

APERI'STATON. See *Aperistatus*.

APERI'STATUS. (From α, neg. and περιϛημι, to surround.) *Aperistaton*. An epithet used by Galen, of an ulcer which is not dangerous, nor surrounded by inflammation.

APE'RTOR OCULI. See *Levator palpebræ superioris*.

APETALUS. (From α, priv. and *petalum*, a petal.) Without a petal or corol.

APETALÆ PLANTÆ. Plants without petals. The name of a division of plants in most systems of botany.

APEUTHY'SMENUS. (From απο and ευθυς, straight.) A name formerly given to the intestinum rectum, or straight gut.

A'PEX. 1. The extremity of a part; as the apex of the tongue, apex of the nose, &c.

2. The extremity of a leaf, *apex folii*.

3. The *anthera* of a flower of Tournefort, Rivinus, and Ray.

APHANI'SMUS. (From αφανιζω, to remove from the sight.) The removal, or gradual decay, of a disorder.

APHANITE. The name given by Haüy to a rock apparently homogeneous, but really compound, in which amphibole is the predominant principle.

APHÆ'RESIS. (From αφαιρεω, to remove.) This term was formerly much used in the schools of surgery, to signify that part of the art which consists in taking off any diseased or preternatural part of the body.

APHELXIA. (*Aphelxia, æ.* f.; from αφελκω, *abstraho* to separate or abstract.) Revery. A genus of diseases in Good's classification constituted by absence or abstraction of mind. See *Nosology*.

APHEPSE'MA. (From απο, and εψω, to boil.) A decoction.

A'PHESIS. (From αφιημι, to remit.) The remission or termination of a disorder.

APHISTE'SIS. (From αφιϛημι, to draw from.) An abscess.

Aphlogistic lamp. One which burns without flame.

A'PHODOS. (From απο, and οδος, departure.) Excrement. The dejection of the body.

APHO'NIA. (Αφωνια; from α, priv. and φωνη, the voice.) A suppression of the voice, without either syncope or coma. A genus of disease in the class *Locales*, and order *Dyscinesiæ*, of Cullen.

1. When it takes place from a tumour of the fauces, or about the glottis, it is termed *aphonia gutturalis*.

2. When from a disease of the trachea, *aphonia trachealis*.

3. And when from a paralysis, or want of nervous energy, *aphonia atonica*.

APHORIA. (*Aphoria, æ.* f.; from α, negative, and φερω, *fero, paris*.) Barrenness. The name of a genus of diseases in Good's new classification. See *Nosology*.

A'PHORISM. (*Aphorismus;* from αφοριζω, to distinguish.) A maxim, or principle, comprehended in a short sentence.

APHRITE. Earth foam. A carbonate of lime usually found in calcareous veins at Gera in Misnia and Thuringia.

[APHRIZITE. A variety of schorl, sometimes in nine-sided prisms, terminated at one extremity by three faces, and at the other by six, of which three are larger than the others, and stand on those three lateral edges of the prism, each of which contains an angle of 120°.—*Cl. Min.* A.]

APHRODI'SIA. (From Αφροδιτη, Venus.) An immoderate desire of venery.

APHRODISIAC (*Aphrodisiacus;* from αφροδισια, venery.) That which excites a desire for venery.

APHRODISIA'STICON. (From αφρος, froth.) A troch so called by Galen, because it was given in dysenteries, where the stools were frothy.

APHRODI'SIUS MORBUS. (From Αφροδιτη, Venus.) The venereal disease.

APHTHA. (*Aphtha, æ.* f. Αφθαι; from απτω, to inflame.) The thrush. Frog, or sore mouth. *Aphtha lactucimen* of Sauvages. *Ulcera serpentia oris*, or spreading ulcers in the mouth, of Celsus. *Pustula oris. Alcola. Vesiculæ gingivarum. Acacos. Aphtha infantum*. A disease ranked by Cullen in the class *Pyrexiæ*, order *Exanthemata*. Children are very subject to it. It appears in small, white ulcers upon the tongue, gums, and around the mouth and palate, resembling small particles of curdled milk. When the disease is mild, it is confined to these parts; but when it is violent and of long standing, it is apt to extend through the whole course of the alimentary canal, from the mouth down to the anus; and so to excite severe purgings, flatulencies, and other disagreeable symptoms. The disease when recent and confined to the mouth, may in general be easily removed; but when of long standing, and extending down to the stomach and intestines, it very frequently proves fatal.

The thrush sometimes occurs as a chronic disease, both in warm climates and in those northern countries where the cold is combined with a considerable degree of moisture, or where the soil is of a very marshy nature. It may, in some cases, be considered as an idiopathic affection; but it is more usually symptomatic. It shows itself, at first, by an uneasy sensation, or burning heat in the stomach, which comes on by slow degrees, and increases gradually in violence. After some time, small pimples, of about the size of a pin's head, show themselves on the tip and edges of the tongue; and these, at length, spread over the whole inside of the mouth, and occasion such a tenderness and rawness, that the patient cannot take any food of a solid nature; neither can he receive any vinous or spirituous liquor into his mouth, without great pungency and pain being excited; little febrile heat attends but there is a dry skin, pale countenance, small pulse, and cold extremities. These symptoms will probably continue for some weeks, the general health being sometimes better and sometimes worse, and then the patient will be attacked with acrid eructations, or severe purgings, which greatly exhaust his strength, and produce considerable emaciation of the whole body. After a little time, these symptoms cease, and he again enjoys better health; but, sooner or later, the acrid matter shows itself once more in the mouth, with greater virulence than before, and makes frequent translations to the stomach and intestines, and so from these to the mouth again, until, at last, the patient is reduced to a perfect skeleton. Elderly people, and persons with a shattered constitution, are most liable to its attacks. The treatment of the thrush in children is generally to be begun with the exhibition of a gentle emetic: then clear the bowels, if confined, by rhubarb and magnesia, castor oil, or other mild aperients; or sometimes in gross, torpid habits by a dose of calomel. In general the prevalence of acid in the primæ viæ appears to lead to the complaint; whence antacid remedies prove beneficial in its progress: when the patient is costive, giving the preference to magnesia; when relaxed, to chalk, which may be sometimes joined with aromatics, the mild vegetable astringents, or even a little opium, if the diarrhœa be urgent. Where the child is very weak, and the aphthæ of a dark colour, the decoction of bark or other tonics must be had recourse to. The separation of the sloughs and healing of the ulcers may be promoted by washing the mouth occasionally with the honey of borax, diluted with two or three parts of rose water; or where they are of a dark colour, by the decoction of bark, acidulated with sulphuric acid. The diet should be light and nutritious, especially where there is much debility. As the complaint is subsiding, particular attention is required to obviate the bowels becoming confined. In the chronic aphthæ affecting grown persons, pretty much the same plan of treatment is to be pursued: besides which, the compound powder of ipecacuanha and other diaphoretics, assisted by the occasional use of the warm bath, wearing flannel next the skin, particularly in a damp cold climate, &c. appear to be beneficial.

APHYLLUS. (From *α*, priv. and *φυλλον*, a leaf.) Leafless. A term applied to parts of plants which are so conditioned when similar parts of other plants have leaves. Thus a stem is said to be aphyllous when it is altogether void of leaves. Linnæus uses the term *nudus*. Examples are found in *Cuscuta Europæa*, dodder; *Asphodelus fistulosus*, &c.

Aphyllæ plantæ. Aphyllous plants, or plants without leaves. Some plants being entirely devoid of leaves, are naturally arranged under one head, to which this name is given.

A'PIS. The name of a genus of insects in the Linnæan system. The bee.

Apis mellifica. The systematic name of the honey-bee. It was formerly dried and powdered, and thus given internally as a diuretic. It is to the industry of this little animal that we are indebted for honey and wax. See *Mel* and *Cera*. The venom of the bee, according to Fontana, bears a close resemblance to that of the viper. It is contained in a small vesicle, and has a hot acrid taste like that of the scorpion.

A'PIUM. (*Apium*, *i.* n.; from *ηπιος*, *Doricè*, *απιος*, mild: or from *apes*, bees; because they are fond of it.) 1. The name of a genus of plants in the Linnæan system. Class, *Pentandria*; Order, *Digynia*.

2. The pharmacopœial name of the herb smallage. See *Apium graveolens*.

Apium graveolens. The systematic name for the *apium* of the pharmacopœias. *Apium—foliolis caulinis, cuneiformibus, umbellis, sessilibus*, of Linnæus. Smallage The root, seeds, and fresh plant, are aperient and carminative.

Apium hortense. See *Apium petroselinum*.

Apium petroselinum. The systematic name for the *petroselinum* of the pharmacopœias. *Petroselinum vulgare. Apium hortense.* Common parsley. *Apium—foliis caulinis linearibus, involucellis minutis*, of Linnæus. Both the roots and seeds of this plant were formerly directed by the London College for medicinal use, and the root is still retained in the Edinburgh Pharmacopœia; the former have a sweetish taste, accompanied with a slight warmth or flavour, somewhat resembling that of carrot; the latter are in taste warmer and more aromatic than any other part of the plant, and manifest considerable bitterness. The roots are said to be aperient and diuretic, and have been employed in nephritic pains and obstructions of urine. The seeds possess aromatic and carminative powers but are seldom prescribed.

[APLOME of Haüy, Brochant, Brogniart. This very rare mineral has been observed only in dodecaedrons with rhombic faces, marked by striæ, parallel to the shorter diagonals. This dodecaedron is supposed to be derived from a cube by one of the most simple laws of decrement: viz. that of a single range of particles parallel to all the edges of a cube. Hence its name from the Greek Απλοος, simple.

The Aplome gives fire with steel, and feebly scratches quartz. Its specific gravity is 3.44. Its fracture in some parts is uneven and nearly dull; while in others it is shining and slightly conchoidal. Its colour is usually a deep brown, sometimes yellowish green. It is usually opaque, but the small crystals often transmit an orange-coloured light.

It is fusible by the blow-pipe into a blackish glass. It is composed of silex, 40.0, alumine 20.0, lime 14.5, oxyde of iron 14.5, manganese 2.0, ferruginous silex 2.0; = 93.00.

It differs from the garnet in the direction of its striæ and its inferior specific gravity. It has been found in Siberia and Saxony.—*Cl. Min.* A.]

APLONÆ. A deep orange-brown mineral, mostly considered to be a variety of the garnet.

APNEU'STIA. (From *α*, and *πνεω*, to breathe.) A defect or difficulty of respiration, such as happens in a cold, &c. *Foesius.*

Apnœa'. The same.—*Galen.*

Apocapni'smus. (From *απο*, and *καπνος*, smoke.) A fumigation.

Apocalha'rsis. (From *απο*, and *καθαιρω*, to purge.) An evacuation of humours. A discharge downwards, and sometimes applied, with little discrimination, to vomiting.

Apocaulize'sis. (From *αποκαυλιζω*, to break transversely.) A transverse fracture.—*Hippocrates.*

APOCENO'SIS. (From *απο*, and *κενοω*, to evacuate.) 1. A flow or evacuation of any humour.

2. The name of an order in the class *Locales* of Cullen, which embraces diseases characterized by a superabundant flux of blood, or other fluid, without pyrexia.

Apo'cope. (From *απο*, and *κοπτω*, to cut from.) Abscission, or the removal of a part by cutting it off.

Apo'crisis. (From *απο*, and *κρινω*, to secrete from.) A secretion of superabundant humours.—*Hippocrates.*

Apocru'sticon. See *Apocrustinum.*

Apocru'stinum. (From *αποκρουω*, to repel.) *Apocrusticon.* An astringent or repellent medicine.—*Galen.*

Apocye'sis. (From *απο*, and *κυω*, to bring forth.) Parturition, or the bringing forth of a child.—*Galen.*

Apodacry'tica. (From *απο*, and *δακρυ*, a tear) Medicines which, by exciting tears, remove superfluous humours from the eyes, as onions, &c.—*Pliny.*

Apogeu'sis. See *Ageustia.*

Apogeu'stia. See *Ageustia.*

Apoginome'sis. (From *απογινομαι*, to be absent.) The remission or absence of a disease.—*Hippocrates.*

Apoglauco'sis. (From *απο*, and *γλαυκος*, sky-coloured; so called because of its bluish appearance.) See *Glaucoma.*

Apo'gonum. (From *απο*, and *γινομαι*, to beget.) A living fœtus in the womb.—*Hippocrates.*

Apolep'sis. (From *απο*, and *λαμβανω*, to take from.) An interception, suppression, or retention of urine, or any other natural evacuation.—*Hippocrates.*

Apolino'sis. (From *απο*, and *λινον*, flax.) The method of curing a fistula, according to Ægineta, by the application of raw flax.

Apo'lysis. (From *απο*, and *λυω*, to release.) The solution or termination of a disease. The removal of a bandage.—*Erotianus.*

APOMA'GMA. (From *απο*, and *ματτω*, to cleanse from.) Any thing used to cleanse and wipe away filth from sores, as sponge, &c.—*Hippocrates.*

Apomathe'ma. (From *απο*, neg. and *μανθανω*, to learn.) Hippocrates expresses, by this term, a forgetfulness of all that has been learnt.

Apo'meli. (From *απο*, from, and *μελι*, honey.) An oxymel, or decoction, made with honey.

APONEURO'SIS. (From *απο*, and *νευρον*, a nerve from an erroneous supposition of the ancients, that it was formed by the expansion of a nerve.) A tendinous expansion. See *Muscle*.

APO'NIA. (From *a*, priv. and πονος, pain.) Freedom from pain.

APONITRO'SIS. (From απο, and νιτρον, nitre.) The sprinkling an ulcer over with nitre.

APOPALLE'SIS. (From αποπαλλω, to throw off hastily.) An abortion, or premature expulsion of a fœtus.—*Hippocrates*.

APOPALSIS. See *Apopallesis*.

APOPEDA'SIS. (From απο, and πηδαω, to jump from.) A luxation.

APOPHLEGMA'SIA. (From απο, and φλεγμα, phlegm.) A discharge of phlegm or mucus.

APOPHLEGMA'TIC. (*Apophlegmaticus*; from απο, and φλεγμα, phlegm.) *Apophlegmatizantia*; *Apophlegmatizonta*. 1. Medicines which excite the secretion of mucus from the mouth and nose.

2. Masticatories.

3. Errhines.

APOPHLEGMATIZANTIA. See *Apophlegmatic*.

APOPHLEGMATIZONTA. See *Apophlegmatic*.

APOPHRA'XIS. (From απο, and φρασσω, to interrupt.) A suppression of the menstrual discharge.

APOPHTHA'RMA. (From απο, and φθειρω, to corrupt.) A medicine to procure abortion.

APOPHTHE'GMA. (From αποφθεγγομαι, to speak eloquently.) A short maxim, or axiom; a rule.

APO'PHTHORA. (From αποφθειρω, to be abortive.) An abortion.

APOPHY'ADES. The ramifications of the veins and arteries.—*Hippocrates*.

APO'PHYAS. (From αποφυω, to proceed from.) Any thing which grows or adheres to another, as a wart to the finger.

APOPHYLLITE. *Ichthyophthalmite*. Fish-eye stone. A mineral composed of silex, potassa, and water, found in the iron mine of Utoe, in Sweden.

[This mineral occurs in laminated masses, or in regular crystals, having a strong, and *peculiar* external lustre, which is intermediate between vitreous and pearly. When exposed to the flame of a lamp it exfoliates. Before the blow-pipe it melts with some difficulty into a white enamel. Its fragments, placed in cold nitric acid, are gradually converted into a whitish, flaky substance. Its powder forms a jelly in nitric or muriatic acid. It contains silex 51, lime 28, potash 4, water 17. It is lighter and harder than sulphate of barytes, but much less hard than adularia, both of which it may resemble.—*Cl. Min.* A.]

APO'PHYSIS. (From αποφυω, to proceed from.) 1. In anatomy. *Appendix*; *Probole*, *Ecphysis*; *Processus*; *Productio*; *Projectura*; *Protuberantia*. A process, projection, or protuberance of a bone beyond a plain surface; as the nasal apophysis of the frontal bone, &c.

2. In botany, this word is applied to a fleshy tubercle under the basis of the capsule or dry fruit adhering to the frondose mosses.

APOPLE'CTA VENA. A name formerly applied to the internal jugular vein; so called because in apoplexies it appears full and turgid.—*Bartholin*.

APOPLE'CTIC. (From αποπληξια, an apoplexy.) Belonging to an apoplexy.

APOPLE'XY. (*Apoplexy*, æ. f.; from απο, and πλησσω, to strike or knock down; because persons, when seized with this disease, fall down suddenly.) A sudden abolition, in some degree, of the powers of sense and motion, the patient lying in a sleep-like state; the action of the heart remaining, as well as the respiration, often with a stertorous noise. Cullen arranges it in the class *Neuroses*, and order *Comata*:

1. When it takes place from a congestion of blood, it is termed *Apoplexia sanguinea*.

2. When there is an abundance of serum, as in persons of a cold phlegmatic temperament, *Apoplexia serosa*.

3. If it arise from water in the ventricles of the brain, it is called *Apoplexia hydrocephalica*. See *Hydrocephalus*.

4. If from a wound, *Apoplexia traumatica*.

5. If from poisons, *Apoplexia venenata*.

6. If from the action of suffocating exhalations, *Apoplexia suffocata*.

7. If from passions of the mind, *Apoplexia mentalis*.

8. And when it is joined with catalepsy, *Apoplexia cataleptica*.

Apoplexy makes its attack chiefly at an advanced period of life; and most usually on those who are of a corpulent habit, with a short neck, and large head; and who lead an inactive life, make use of a full diet, or drink to excess. The immediate cause of apoplexy, is a compression of the brain, produced either by an accumulation of blood in the vessels of the head, and distending th m to such a degree, as to compress the medullary portion of the brain; or by an effusion of blood from the red vessels, or of serum from the exhalants; which fluids are accumulated in such a quantity as to occasion compression. These states, of overdistension and of effusion, may be brought on by whatever increases the afflux, and impetus of the blood in the arteries of the head; such as violent fits of passion, great exertions of muscular strength, severe exercise, excess in venery, stooping down for any length of time, wearing any thing too tight about the neck, overloading the stomach, long exposure to excessive cold, or a vertical sun, the sudden suppression of any long-accustomed evacuation, the application of the fumes of certain narcotic and metallic substances, such as opium, alkohol, charcoal, mercury, &c. and by blows, wounds, and other external injuries: in short, apoplexy may be produced by whatever determines too great a flow of blood to the brain, or prevents its free return from that organ.

The young, and those of a full plethoric habit, are most liable to attacks of the sanguineous apoplexy; and those of a phlegmatic constitution, or who are much advanced in life, to the serous. Apoplexy is sometimes preceded by headache, giddiness, dimness of sight, loss of memory, faltering of the tongue in speaking, numbness in the extremities, drowsiness, stupor, and nightmare, all denoting an affection of the brain; but it more usually happens that, without much previous indisposition, the person falls down suddenly, the countenance becomes florid, the face appears swelled and puffed up, the vessels of the head, particularly of the neck and temples, seem turgid and distended with blood; the eyes are prominent and fixed, the breathing is difficult and performed with a snorting noise, and the pulse is strong and full Although the whole body is affected with the loss of sense and motion, it nevertheless takes place often more upon one side than the other, which is called hemiplegia, and in this case, the side least affected with palsy is somewhat convulsed.

In forming an opinion as to the event, we must be guided by the violence of the symptoms. If the fit is of long duration, the respiration laborious and stertorous, and the person much advanced in years, the disease, in all probability, will terminate fatally. In some cases, it goes off entirely; but it more frequently leaves a state of mental imbecility behind it, or terminates in a hemiplegia, or in death. Even when an attack is recovered from, it most frequently returns again, after a short period of time, and in the end proves fatal. In dissections of apoplexy, blood is often found effused on the surface and in the cavities of the brain; and in other instances, a turgidity and distention of the blood-vessels are to be observed. In some cases, tumours have been found attached to different parts of the substance of the brain, and in others, no traces of any real affection of it could be observed.

On an attack of sanguineous apoplexy, all compression should be removed from the neck, the patient laid with his head a good deal raised, and a free admission of cool air allowed. Then blood should be taken freely from the arm or the temporal artery, or the jugular vein; which it may be sometimes necessary to repeat, if the symptoms continue, and the patient is still plethoric; or if blood can less be spared, cupping or leeches may lessen the congestion in the brain. The next object should be thoroughly to evacuate the bowels by some active purgative, as calomel joined with jalap, or with extract of colocynth, or followed by infusion of senna and some neutral salt, with a lit tle tartarized antimony or tincture of jalap repeated every two hours till it operates; or a draught of tincture of senna and wine of aloes, where the bowels are very torpid, may answer the purpose. Stimulant clysters will also be proper, particularly if the patient cannot swallow, as common salt and syrup of buckthorn, with a proper quantity of gruel, infusion of senna or infusion of colocynth; or a turpentine clyster in elderly torpid habits. Cold should then be applied assiduously to the scalp, the hair being previously shaved, and a blister to the back of the neck; and diaphoretic medicines may be exhibited, avoiding, however, those which contain opium. Sinapisms to the feet may also be useful, particularly if these are cold. If under these means, the sensibility does not gradually return, some of the gentle diffusible stimulants will be proper, as ammonia, mustard, æther, camphor, &c.: and at this period, a blister to the scalp may come in aid. By some practitioners emetics are recommended, but their use is hazardous, especially if sufficient evacuations be not premised: and the same may be observed of sternutatories. In the serous form of the disease, general bleeding is inadmissible, and even the local abstraction of blood should be very sparingly made; the bowels should be kept open, especially by aloetic or mercurial formulæ, but not procuring profuse discharges; and the other secretions maintained, especially by the use of the diffusible stimulants already mentioned; blisters to the head, and errhines may be here also useful. When apoplectic symptoms have been occasioned by opium, or other narcotics, the timely discharge of this by an active emetic will be the most important measure; but in a plethoric habit, bleeding should be premised; subsequently various stimulants may be employed, as ammonia, vinegar, &c. endeavouring to procure a determination to the surface, and rousing the patient from his torpid state. The prevention of the sanguineous form of the disease will be best attempted by abstemiousness, regular moderate exercise, and keeping up the evacuations; an issue or seton may also be useful; but under urgent circumstances, bleeding, especially topical, must be resorted to. In leucophlegmatic habits, a more nutritious diet will be proper.

APOPNI'XIS. (From αποπνιγω, to suffocate.) A suffocation.—*Moschion.*

APOPSOPHE'SIS. (From απο, and ψοφεω, to emit wind.) The emission of wind by the anus or uterus, according to Hippocrates.

APOPSY'CHIA. (From απο, from, and ψυχη, the mind.) The highest degree of deliquium, or fainting, according to Galen.

APO'PTOSIS. (From αποπιπτω, to fall down.) A prolapsus, or falling down of any part through relaxation.—*Erotian.*

Apore'xis. (From απο, and ορεγω, to stretch out.) A play with balls, in the gymnastic exercises.

Apo'ria. (From α, priv. and πορος, a duct.) Restlessness, uneasiness, occasioned by the interruption of perspiration, or any stoppage of the natural secretions.

Aporrhi'psis. (From αποῤῥιπτω, to cast off.) Hippocrates used this word to signify that kind of insanity where the patient tears off his clothes, and casts them from him.

Aposceparni'smus. (From απο, from, and σκεπαρνιζω, to strike with a hatchet.) *Deasciatio.* A species of fracture, when part of a bone is chipped off.—*Gorræus.*

Aposcha'sis. (From απο, and σχαζω, to scarify.) *Aposchasmus.* A scarification. Venesection.—*Hippocrates.*

[APOSEPEDINE. The products of the fermentation of cheese have been examined by M. Bracconnot, who has shown that the substance, called by Proust *caseous oxide*, has no claim to such a title, and proposes to call it *Aposepedine*, from απο, and σηπεδων, (result of putrefaction). To obtain this substance, the curd of skim-milk, spontaneously coagulated, is to be mixed with water, and exposed in an open vessel until the putrefaction has fully obtained its height. By filtration, a liquor is obtained which, on being concentrated by evaporation, yields a product of a very fœtid odour, owing apparently to the presence of an oily substance. Towards the close of the evaporation, vapours of acetic acid pass over, and a liquid of the consistence of syrup remains; which, on cooling, concretes into a granulated, reddish mass like honey, and of a saline bitter taste. Treated by alkohol, it is separated into a soluble and insoluble portion. The latter is the *Aposepedine* of M. Bracconnot; the former is the *caseate of ammonia* of Proust.—*Webster's Man. Chem.* A.]

Aposi'tia. (From απο, from, and σιτος, food.) *Apositios.* A loathing of food.—*Galen.*

Apospa'sma. (From αποσπαω, to tear off.) A violent, irregular fracture of a tendon, ligament, &c. *Galen.*

Aposphaceli'sis. (From απο, and σφακελος, a mortification.) Hippocrates uses this word to denote a mortification of the flesh in wounds, or fractures, caused by too tight a bandage.

APO'STASIS. (From απο, and ιςημι, to recede from.) 1. An abscess, or collection of matter.

2. The coming away of a fragment of bone by fracture.

3. When a distemper passes away by some outlet, Hippocrates calls it an *apostasis by excretion.*

4. When the morbific matter, by its own weight, falls and settles on any part, an *apostasis by settlement.*

5. When one disease turns to another, an *apostasis by metastasis.*

APOSTA'XIS. (From αποςαζω, to distil from.) Hippocrates uses this word to express the defluxion or distillation of any humour, or fluid: as blood from the nose.

APOSTELUS. An apostle. An ointment and other things were formerly so designated from some famous inventer; as unguentum apostelorum, because it has twelve ingredients in it.

APOSTEMA. (*Apostema, atis.* n.; from αφιςημι, to recede.) The term given by the ancients to abscesses in general. See *Abscess.*

APOSTEMA'TIAI. Those who, from an inward abscess, void pus downward, are thus called by Aretæus.

Aposteri'gma. (From αποςηριγω, *fulcio.*) Galen uses this word to denote a rest of a diseased part, a cushion.

Apo'strophe. (From απο, and ςρεφω, to turn from.) Thus Paulus Ægineta expresses an aversion for food.

APOSYRINGE'SIS. (From απο, and συριγξ, a fistula.) The degeneracy of a sore into a fistula.—*Hippocrates.*

APOSY'RMA. (From απο, and συρω, to rub off.) An abrasion or disquamation of the bones or skin.—*Hippocrates.*

APOTANEUSIS. (From απο, and τεινω, to extend.) An extension, or elongation, of any member or substance.

Apotelme'sis. (From απο, and τελμα, a bog.) An expurgation of filth, or fæces.

APOTHE'CA. (Αποθηκη; from αποτιθημι, to reposit.) A shop, or vessel, where medicines are sold, or deposited.

APOTHECA'RY. (*Apothecarius;* from απο, and τιθημι, *pono,* to put: so called from his employ being to prepare, and keep in readiness, the various articles in the *Materia Medica*, and to compound them for the physician's use; or from αποθηκη, a shop.) In every European country, except Great Britain, the *apothecary* is the same as we name in England the *druggist* and *chemist.*

APOTHERAPEI'A. (From απο, and θεραπευω, to cure.) A perfect cure, according to Hippocrates.

Apotherapeu'tica. (From αποθεραπευω, to heal.) Therapeutics. That part of medicine which teaches the art of curing disorders.

Apothe'rmum. (From απο, and θερμη, heat.) An acrimonious pickle, with mustard, vinegar, and oil.—*Galen.*

APO'THESIS. (From απο, and τιθημι, to replace.) The reduction of a dislocated bone, according to Hippocrates.

APOTHLI'MMA. (From απο, and θλιβω, to press from.) The dregs or expressed juice of a plant.

Apothrau'sis. (From απο, and θραυω, to break.) The taking away the splinters of a broken bone.

Apo'tocus. (From απο, and τικτω, to bring forth.) Abortive; premature.—*Hippocrates.*

Apotre'psis. (From απο, and τρεπω, to turn from.) A resolution or reversion of a suppurating tumour.

Apotropæ'a. (From αποτρεπω, to avert.) An amulet, or charm, to avert diseases.—*Foësius.*

A'POZEM. (*Apozema.* From απο, and ζεω, to boil.) A decoction.

Apozeu'xis. (From απο, and ζευγνυμι, to separate.) The separation or removal of morbid parts.—*Hippocrates.*

Apo'zymos (From απο, and ζυμη, ferment.) Fermented.

APPARA'TUS. (From *apparco*, to appear, or be ready at hand.) This term is applied to the instruments and the preparation and arrangement of every thing necessary in the performance of any operation, medical, surgical, or chemical.

APPARATUS ALTUS. See *Lithotomy*.

APPARATUS MAJOR. See *Lithotomy*.

APPARATUS MINOR. See *Lithotomy*.

APPARATUS, PNEUMATIC. The discovery of aëriform fluids has, in modern chemistry, occasioned the necessity of some peculiar instruments, by means of which those substances may, in distillations, solutions, or other operations, be caught, collected, and properly managed. The proper instruments for this are styled the pneumatic apparatus. Any kind of air is specifically lighter then any liquid; and, therefore, if not decomposed by it, rises through it in bubbles. On this principle rests the essential part of the apparatus, adapted to such operations. Its principal part is the pneumatic trough, which is a kind of reservoir for the liquid, through which the gas is conveyed and caused to rise, and is filled either with water or with quicksilver. Some inches below its brim a horizontal shelf is fastened, in dimension about half or the third part of the trough, and in the water-trough this is provided on its foremost edge with a row of holes, into which, from underneath, short-necked funnels are fixed. The trough is filled with water sufficient to cover the shelf, to support the receivers, which being previously filled with water are placed invertedly, their open end turned down upon the above-mentioned holes, through which afterward the gases, conveyed there and directed by means of the funnels, rise in the form of air bubbles.

In some cases the trough must be filled with quicksilver, because water absorbs or decomposes some kinds of air. The price and specific gravity of that metal make it necessary to give to the quicksilver trough smaller dimensions. It is either cut in marble, or made of wood well joined. The late Karsto has contrived an apparatus, which, to the advantage of saving room, adds that of great conveniency.

To disengage gases, retorts of glass, either common or tubulated, are employed, and placed in a sand-bath, or heated by a lamp. Earthen, or coated glass retorts, are put in the naked fire. If necessary, they are joined with a metallic or glass conveying pipe. When, besides the aëriform, other fluids are to be collected, the middle or intermediate bottle finds its use; and to prevent, after cooling, the rising of the water from the trough into the disengaging vessel, the tube of safety is employed. For the extrication of gases taking place in solutions, for which no external heat is required, the bottle called disengaging bottle, or proof, may be used. For receivers, to collect disengaged airs, various cylinders of glass are used, whether graduated or not, either closed at one end or open at both; and in this last case, they are made air-tight by a stopper fitted by grinding. Besides these, glass bells and common bottles are employed.

To combine with water, in a commodious way, some gases that are only gradually and slowly absorbed by it, the glass apparatus of Parker is serviceable.

APPENDI'CULA. A little appendage.

APPENDICULA CÆCI VERMIFORMIS. A vermicular process, about four inches in length, and the size of a goose-quill, which hangs to the intestinum cæcum of the human body.

APEPNDICULÆ EPPILOICÆ. *Appendicces coli adiposæ.* The small appendices of the colon and rectum, which are filled with adipose substance. See *Omentum*.

APPENDICULA'TUS. Applied to leaves, leafstalks, &c. that are furnished with an additional organ for some particular purpose not essential to it; as the *Dionæa muscipula*, the leaves of which terminate each in a pair of toothed irritable lobes, that close over and imprison insects; as also the leaf of the *Nepentha distillatorea*, which bears a covered pitcher full of water; the leaves of our *Utriculum*, which have numerous bladders attached to them which seem to secrete air and float them; and the petiolus of the *Dipsacus pilosus*, which has little leaves at its base.

APPENDIX. 1. An appendage; that which belongeth to any thing.

2. See *Apophysis*.

APPLE. See *Pyrus*

Apple, acid of. See *Malic acid.*

Apple, pine. See *Bromelia ananus.*

Apple, thorn. See *Datura stramonium.*

Appropriate affinity. See *Affinity intermediate*

APRICOT. See *Prunus armeniaca.*

APYRE'XIA. (From α, priv. and πυρεξια, a fever. Apyrexia. Without fever.—The intermission of feverish heat.

APYRI'NUS. (From α, priv. and πυρην, *nucleus*, a kernel.) Without a kernel.

APYRINÆ PLANTÆ. Plants without kernels. The name in Gerard's arrangement of a class of plants.

APYROUS. Bodies which sustain the action of a strong heat for a considerable time, without change of figure or other properties, have been called apyrous; but the word is now very seldom used. It is synonymous with *refractory*.

A'QUA. See *Water*.

AQUÆ AERIS FIXI. Water impregnated with fixed air. This is liquid carbonic acid, or water impregnated with carbonic acid. It sparkles in the glass, has a pleasant acidulous taste, and forms an excellent beverage. It diminishes thirst, lessens the morbid heat of the body, and acts as a powerful diuretic. It is also an excellent remedy in increasing irritability of the stomach, as in advanced pregnancy, and it is one of the best anti-emetics which we possess.

AQUA ALUMINIS COMPOSITA. Compound solution of alum, formerly called aqua aluminosa bateana. See *Liquor aluminis compositus*.

AQUA AMMONIÆ ACETATÆ. See *Ammonia acetatis liquor*.

AQUA AMMONIÆ PURÆ. See *Ammonia.*

AQUA ANETI. See *Anethum graveolens.*

AQUA CALCIS. See *Calcis liquor.*

AQUA CARUI. See *Carum carui.*

AQUA CINNAMOMI. See *Laurus cinnamomum.*

AQUA CŒLESTIS. A preparation of copper.

AQUA CUPRI AMMONIATI. See *Cupri ammoniati liquor.*

AQUA CUPRI VITRIOLATI COMPOSITA. This preparation of the Edinburgh Pharmacopœia is used externally, to stop hæmorrhages of the nose, and other parts. It is made thus: ℞ *Cupri vitriolati, Aluminis, sing.* ℥ss. *Aquæ puræ,* ℥iv. *Acidi vitriolici,* ʒij. Boil the salts in water until they are dissolved; then filter the liquor and add the acid.

AQUA DISTILLATA. Distilled water. This is made by distilling water in clean vessels, until about two-thirds have come over. In nature, no water is found perfectly pure. Spring or river water always contains a portion of saline matter, principally sulphate of lime; and, from this impregnation, is unfit for a number of pharmaceutic preparations. By distillation, a perfectly pure water is obtained. The London College directs ten gallons of common water; of which, first distil four pints, which are to be thrown away; then distil four gallons. This distilled water is to be kept in glass vessels. See *Water*

AQUA FŒNICULI. See *Anethum fœniculum.*

AQUA FORTIS. This name is given to a weak and impure nitric acid, commonly used in the arts. It is distinguished by the terms *double* and *single*, the single being only half the strength of the other. The artists who use these acids call the more concentrated acid, which is much stronger even than the double aqua fortis, *spirit of nitre*. This distinction appears to be of some utility, and is therefore not improperly retained by chemical writers. See *Nitric acid.*

AQUA KALI PRÆPARATI. See *Potassæ subcarbonatis liquor.*

AQUA KALI PURI. See *Potassæ liquor.*

AQUA LITHARGYRI ACETATI. See *Plumbi acetatis liquor.*

AQUA LITHARGYRI ACETATI COMPOSITA. See *Plumbi acetatis liquor dilutus.*

AQUA MARINE. See *Beryl.*

AQUA MENTHÆ PIPERITÆ. See *Mentha piperita.*

AQUA MENTHÆ SATIVÆ. See *Mentha viridis.*

AQUA MENTHÆ VIRIDIS. See *Mentha viridis*

AQUA DE NAPOLI. See *Aquetta.*

AQUA PIMENTÆ. See *Myrtus pimenta.*

AQUA PULEGII. See *Mentha Pulegium.*

AQUA REGIA. *Aqua regalis.* This acid, which is a mixture of the nitric and muriatic acids, lately called nitro-muriatic, and now chlorine, was formerly called aqua regalis, because it was, at that time, the only acid that was known to be able to dissolve gold. See *Chlorine.*

Aqua rosæ. See *Rosa centifolia.*

Aqua styptica. A name formerly given to a combination of powerful astringents, viz. sulphate of copper, sulphate of alum, and sulphuric acid. It has been applied topically to check hæmorrhage, and, largely diluted with water, as a wash in purulent ophthalmia. See *Aqua cupri vitriolati composita.*

Aqua Toffania. See *Aquetta.*

Aqua vitæ. Ardent spirit of the first distillation has been distinguished in commerce by this name.

Aqua zinci vitriolati cum camphora. *Aqua vitriolia camphorata.* This is made by dissolving half an ounce of sulphate of zinc in a quart of boiling water, adding half an ounce of camphorated spirit, and filtering. This, when properly diluted, is a useful collyrium for inflammations of the eyes, in which there is a weakness of the parts. Externally, it is applied by surgeons to scorbutic and phagedenic ulcerations.

Aquæ distillatæ. Distilled waters. These are made by introducing vegetables, as mint, penny-royal, &c. into a still with water; and drawing off as much as is found to possess the properties of the plants. The London College orders the waters to be distilled from dried herbs, because fresh are not ready at all times of the year. Whenever the fresh are used, the weights are to be increased. But whether the fresh or dried herbs are employed, the operator may vary the weight according to the season in which they have been produced and collected. Herbs and seeds, kept beyond the space of a year, are improper for the distillation of waters. To every gallon of these waters, five ounces, by measure, of proof spirit are to be added.

Aquæ minerales. See *Mineral waters.*

Aqua stillatitiæ simplices. Simple distilled waters.

Aquæ stillatitiæ spirituosæ. Spirituous distilled waters, now called only spiritus; as spiritus pulegii.

AQUÆDUCT. *Aquæductus;* a canal or duct, so named because it was supposed to carry a watery fluid.

Aquæduct of Fallopius. A canal in the petrous portion of the temporal bone, first accurately described by Fallopius.

Aquatic nut. See *Trapa natans.*

Aquaticæ plantæ. Aquatic plants, or such as grow in or near water. A natural order of plants.

AQUATICUS. (From *aqua*, water.) Aquatic; or belonging to the water.

AQUEOUS. (*Aquosus*, watery.) Of the nature of, or resembling water.

Aqueous humour. *Humor Aquosus.* The very limpid watery fluid, which fills both chambers of the eye. See *Eye.*

AQUE'TTA. The name of a liquid poison, made use of by the Roman women, under the Pontificate of Alexander VII. It was prepared and sold in drops, by Tophania, or Toffania, an infamous woman who resided at Palermo, and afterward at Naples. From her, these drops obtained the name of *Aqua Toffania, Aqua della Toffana;* and also *Aqua di Napoli.* This poison is said by some to be a composition of arsenic, and by others of opium and cantharides.

AQUIFO'LIUM. (From *acus*, a needle, and *folium*, a leaf; so called on account of its prickly leaf.) See *Ilex aquifolium.*

A'QUILA. (Αετος, the eagle.) 1. A species of the extensive genus *Falco* of ornithologists.

2. Aquila, among the ancients, had many other epithets joined with it, as rubra, salutifera, volans, &c.

3. A chemical name formerly used for sal-ammoniac, mercurius præcipitatus, arsenic, sulphur, and the philosopher's stone.

Aquila alba. One of the names given to calomel by the ancients. See *Hydrargyri submurias.*

Aquila alba philosophorum. *Aqua alba ganymodis.* Sublimated sal-ammoniac.

Aquila cœlestis. A panacea, or cure for all diseases; a preparation of mercury.

Aquila veneris. A preparation of the ancients, made with verdigris and sublimed sal-ammoniac.

Aquilæ lignum. Eagle-wood. It is generally sold for the agallochum. See *Lignum aloes.*

Aquilæ venæ. Branches of the jugular veins, which are particularly prominent in the eagle.

AQUILE'GIA. (From *aqua*, water, and *lego*, to gather; so called from the shape of its leaves, which retain water.) The herb columbine.

1. The name of a genus of plants in the Linnæan system. Class, *Polyandria;* Order, *Pentagynia.*

2. The name in the pharmacopœias, for the columbine. See *Aquilegia vulgaris.*

Aquilegia vulgaris. The systematic name of the columbine. The seeds, flowers, and the whole plant, have been used medicinally, the first in exanthematous diseases, the latter chiefly as an antiscorbutic. Though retained in several foreign pharmacopœias, their utility seems to be not allowed in this country.

Aquili'na. (From *Aquila*, an eagle; so called from the resemblance of its leaves to eagle's wings.) The trivial name of a species of pteris. See *Pteris.*

AQUU'LA. (Diminutive of *aqua.*) A small quantity of very fine and limpid water. This term is applied to the pellucid water, which distends the capsule of the crystalline lens, and the lens itself. Paulus Ægineta uses it to denote a tumour consisting of a fatty substance under the skin of the eyelid.

Arabic gum. See *Acaciæ gummi.*

A'racalan. An amulet.

A'raca mira. (Indian.) A shrub growing in the Brazils, the roots of which are diuretic and antidysenteric.

ARA'CHNE. (From *arag*, Hebrew, to weave; or from αραχνη, a spider.) The spider.

ARACHNOID. (*Arachnoides;* from αραχνη, a spider, and ειδος, likeness; so named from its resemblance to a spider's web.) Web-like.

Arachnoid membrane. *Membrana arachnoides.* 1. A thin membrane of the brain, without vessels and nerves, situated between the dura and pia mater, and surrounding the cerebrum, cerebellum, medulla oblongata, and medulla spinalis.

2. The term is also applied by some writers to the tunic of the crystalline lens and vitreous humour of the eye.

ARACK. (Indian.) An Indian spirituous liquor, prepared in many ways, often from rice; sometimes from sugar, fermented with the juice of cocoa-nuts; frequently from toddy, the juice of which flows from the cocoa-nut tree by incision, and from other substances.

A'rados. (From αραδεω, to be turbulent.) Hippocrates uses this term to signify a commotion in the stomach, occasioned by the fermentation of its contents

Aræo'tica. (From αραιοω, to rarefy.) Things which rarefy the fluids of the body.

ARA'LIA. (From *ara*, a bank in the sea; so called because it grows upon the banks near the sea.) The name of a genus of plants in the Linnæan system. Class, *Pentandria;* Order, *Pentagynia.* The berry-bearing angelica. Of the several species of this tree, the roots of the nudicaulis, or naked-stalked, were brought over from North America, where it grows, and sold here for sarsaparilla.

Ara'nea. (From αραω, to knit together.)

1. The name of a genus of insects.

2. The spider.

ARA'NTIUS, Ju'lius Cæsar, a celebrated anatomist and physician, born at Bologna, about the year 1530. After studying under Vesalius, and others, he graduated and became professor there, and died in 1589. In his first work, "On the Human Fœtus," he described the foramen ovale, and ductus arteriosus, and corrected several errors in the anatomy of the gravid uterus, which had been generally derived from the examination of brutes. He afterward showed that the blood, after birth, could only pass from the right to the left side by the heart through the vessels of the lungs, thus preparing for the discovery of the circulation of Harvey. A Treatise on Tumours, and a Commentary on part of Hippocrates, were also written by him.

ARA'TRUM. The plough. A plant has this for a trivial name, because its roots are found to hinder the plough: hence *remora aratri.* See *Ononis spinosa.*

ARBOR. A tree. 1. In botany, a plant, consisting of one trunk which rises to a great height, is very durable, woody, and divided at its top into branches which do not perish in the winter; as the oak, elm, ash, &c.

2. In anatomy, it is applied to parts which ramify like a tree, as the *Arbor vitæ* of the cerebellum.

3. In chemistry, applied to crystallizations which ramify like branches.

ARBOR DIANÆ. See *Silver.*

ARBOR VITÆ. The tree of life.

1. The cortical substance of the cerebellum is so disposed, that, when cut transversely, it appears ramified like a tree, from which circumstance it is termed *arbor vitæ.*

2. The name of a tree formerly in high estimation in medicine. See *Thuya occidentalis.*

ARBORES. One of the natural divisions or families of plants. Trees consist of a single and durable woody trunk, bearing branches, which do not perish in the winter, as *Tilia, Fraxinus, Pyrus,* &c.

ARBUSTIVA. (From *arbustum*, a copse of shrubs or trees.) The name of an order of plants in Linnæus's natural method.

ARBUTHNOT, JOHN, a physician, born in Scotland soon after the restoration, celebrated for his wit and learning. He graduated at Aberdeen, and settling in this metropolis, had the good fortune to be at Epsom, when Prince George of Denmark was taken ill there; whom, having restored to health, he was appointed physician to Queen Anne, but never got into very extensive practice. His chief medical publications were "On the Choice of Aliments," and "On the Effects of Air upon Human Bodies." He died in 1735.

A'RBUTUS. The name of a genus of plants in the Linnæan system. Class, *Decandria;* Order, *Monogynia.*

Arbutus, trailing. See *Arbutus uva ursi.*

ARBUTUS UNEDO. *Amatzquitl; Unedo papyracea.* A decoction of the bark of the root of this plant is recommended in fevers.

ARBUTUS UVA URSI The systematic name for the officinal trailing Arbutus; Bear's berry; Bear's whortle-berry; Bear's whorts; or Bear's bilberries; called also *Vaccaria. Arbutus—caulibus procumbentibus, foliis integerrimis,* of Linnæus. This plant, though employed by the ancients in several diseases, requiring adstringent medicines, had almost entirely fallen into disuse until the middle of the present century, when it first drew the attention of physicians, as a useful remedy in calculous and nephritic complaints, which diseases it appears to relieve by its adstringent qualities.

A'RCA ARCANORUM. The mercury of the philosophers.

A'RCA CORDIS. The pericardium.

ARCA'NUM. A secret. A medicine, the preparation or efficacy of which is kept from the world, to enhance its value. With the chemists, it is a thing secret and incorporeal; it can only be known by experience, for it is the virtue of every thing, which operates a thousand times more than the thing itself.

ARCANUM CATHOLICUM. Bezoar, plantain, and colchicum.

ARCANUM DUPLEX. *Arcanum duplicatum.* A name formerly given to the combination of potassa and sulphuric acid, more commonly called vitriolated tartar, and now sulphate of potassa.

ARCANUM TARTARI. The acetate of potassa.

ARCE'RTHOS. Juniper.

ARCHÆ'US. 1. The universal archæus, or principle of Van Helmont, was the active principle of the material world. See *Vis vitæ.*

2. Good health.

A'RCHE. (From αρχη, the beginning.) The earliest stage of a disease.

ARCHE'NDA. (Arabian.) A powder made of the leaves of the ligustrum, to check the fœtid odour of the feet.

ARCHEO'STIS. White briony.

[ARCHER, JOHN, M. D. of the state of Maryland, a celebrated practitioner of medicine. Many contributions of his, on various subjects of medical science, are to be found in the New-York Medical Repository. He was the first who introduced the Seneca snake-root (polygala senega) as a remedy in Croup. He died in 1814. A.]

Archil. See *Lichen rocella.*

[There are several lichens which abound in colouring matter; of these the most remarkable is the *lichen rocella*, which grows in the south of France, and in the Canary Islands; and which affords the beautiful, but perishable blue, called *litmus, archil,* or *turnsole.* The moss is dried, powdered, mixed with pearlash and urine, and allowed to ferment, during which it becomes red and then blue; in this state it is mixed with carbonate of potassa and chalk, and dried. It is used for dying silk and ribands; and by the chemists as a most delicate test of acids, which it indicates by passing from blue to red; the blue colour is restored by alkalies, which do not render it green. *Cudbear* appears to be a similar preparation of the *lichen tartareus.—Webster's Man. Chem.* A.]

Archilla. See *Lichen rocella.*

ARCHI'THOLOS. (From αρχη, the chief, and θολος, a chamber.) The sudatorium, or principal room of the ancient baths.

ARCHOPTO'MA (From αρχος, the anus, and πιπτω, to fall down.) A bearing down of the rectum, or prolapsus ani.

A'RCHOS. (From αρχος, an arch.) The anus; so called from its shape.

ARCTA'TIO. (From *arcto*, to make narrow.) *Arctitudo.* Narrowness.

1 A constipation of the intestines, from inflammation.

2. A preternatural straitness of the pudendum muliebre.

A'RCTIUM. (From αρκτος, a bear; so called from its roughness.) The name of a genus of plants in the Linnæan system. Class, *Syngenesia;* Order, *Polygamia æqualis.* The burdock.

ARCTIUM LAPPA. The systematic name for the herb clot-bur, or burdock. *Bardana; Arctium; Britannica; Ilaphis.* The plant so called in the pharmacopœias, is the *Arctium—foliis cordatis, inermibus, petiolatis,* of Linnæus. It grows wild in uncultivated grounds. The seeds have a bitterish subacrid taste: they are recommended as very efficacious diuretics, given either in the form of emulsion, or in powder, to the quantity of a drachm. The roots taste sweetish, with a slight austerity and bitterness: they are esteemed aperient, diuretic, and sudorific; and are said to act without irritation, so as to be safely ventured upon in acute disorders. Decoctions of them have been used in rheumatic, gouty, venereal, and other disorders; and are preferred by some to those of sarsaparilla. Two ounces of the roots are to be boiled in three pints of water, to a quart; to this, two drachms of sulphate of potassa have been usually added. Of this decoction, a pint should be taken every day in scorbutic and rheumatic cases, and when intended as a diuretic, in a shorter period.

ARCTIZITE. The foliated species of scapolite. See *Scapolite.*

ARCTU'RA. (From *arcto*, to straiten.) An inflammation of the finger, or toe, from a curvature of the nail.—*Linnæus.*

ARCUA'LIA. (From *arcus*, a bow.) *Arcualis.* The sutura coronalis is so named, from its bow-like shape; and, for the same reason, the bones of the sinciput are called *arcualia ossa.—Bartholin.*

ARCUA'TIO. (From *arcus*, a bow.) A gibbosity of the fore-parts, with a curvation of the sternum, of the tibia, or dorsal vertebræ.—*Avicenna.*

A'RCULÆ. (A dim. of *arca*, a chest.) The orbits or sockets of the eyes.

A'RDAS. (From αρδυω, to defile.) Filth, excrement, or refuse.—*Hippocrates.*

ARDENT. (*Ardens;* from *ardeo*, to burn.) Burning hot. Applied to fevers, alkohol, &c.

ARDOR. (*Ardor, oris.* m.; from *ardeo*, to burn.) A burning heat.

ARDOR FEBRILIS. Feverish heat.

ARDOR URINÆ. Scalding of the urine, or a sense of heat in the urethra.

ARDOR VENTRICULI. Heartburn.

A'REA. 1. An empty space.

2. That kind of baldness where the crown of the head is left naked, like the tonsure of a monk.

ARE'CA. The name of a genus of plants of the class *Palmæ.*

ARECA INDICA. An inferior kind of nutmeg.

ARE'GON. (From αρηγω, to help; so called from its valuable qualities.) A resolvent ointment.

AREMA'ROS. Cinnabar.

ARE'NA. Sand, or gravel.

ARENA'MEL. (From *arena*, sand; so called because it was said to be procured from sandy places.) *Arenamen.* Bole-armenic.

ARENA'TIO. (From *arena*, sand.) Saburation, or the sprinkling of hot sand upon the bodies of patients.—*Baccius de Thermis.*

[ARENDALITE. The same as Arendate; both of which are synonymous with Epidote. A.]

ARENDATE. See *Epidote.*

ARE'NTES. (From *areo*, to dry up.) A sort of ancient cupping-glasses, used without scarifying.

ARE'OLA. (A diminutive of *area*, a void space.) A small red or brown circle, which surrounds the nipples of females. During and after pregnancy, it becomes considerably larger.

AREOMETER. See *Hydrometer.*

ARETÆNOI'DES. See *Arytænoides.*

ARETÆ'US, of Cappadocia; a physician, who practised at Rome, but at what period is uncertain, though the most probable opinion places him between the reigns of Vespasian and Adrian. Eight books of his remain "On the Causes, Signs, and Method of treating acute and chronic Diseases," written in the Greek language, and admired for their pure style, and luminous descriptions, as well as the judicious practice generally recommended. He was partial to the use of hellebore and other drastic medicines; and appears to have been among the first to recommend cantharides for blistering the skin.

A'RETE. (Αρετη, virtue.) Hippocrates uses this word to mean corporeal or mental vigour.

ARE'US. A pessary, invented by Ægineta.

A'RGAL. Argol. Crude tartar, in the state in which it is taken from the inside of wine-vessels, is known in the shops by this name.

ARGASY'LLIS. (From αργος, a serpent; which it is said to resemble.) The plant which was supposed to produce gum-ammoniac. See *Heracleum gummiferum.*

A'RGEMA. (From αργος, white.) *Argemon.* A small white ulcer of the globe of the eye.—*Erotianus. Galen, &c.*

Argentate of ammonia. Fulminating silver.

[This mineral has a laminated or rather slaty structure. Its laminæ or layers, often curved or undulated, are seldom perfectly parallel; but their surface has almost always a pearly lustre, somewhat shining. According to Bournon, these laminæ are composed of minute rhombs, whose summits are so deeply truncated perpendicularly to the axis, that only a very thin portion of the rhomb remains. Indeed this mineral sometimes presents the primitive rhomb. It is translucent, at least at the edges; and its colour is white, shaded with gray, green, or red. It is easily broken; and its spec. grav. is 2.64.

It is nearly a pure carbonate of lime, often containing a little oxide of iron or manganese. Hence at a red heat it often becomes reddish brown.—*Cl. Min.* A.]

ARGENTI NITRAS. *Argentum nitratum; Causticum lunare.* Nitrate of silver. Take of silver an ounce; nitric acid, a fluid ounce; distilled water, two fluid ounces. Mix the nitric acid and water, and dissolve the silver therein on a sand bath; then increase the heat gradually that the nitrate of silver may be dried. Melt the salt in a crucible over a slow fire until the water being evaporated, it shall cease to boil; then pour it quickly into moulds of convenient shape. Its virtues are corrosive and astringent. Internally it is exhibited in very small quantities, in epilepsy, chorea, and other nervous affections, and externally it is employed to destroy fungous excrescences, callous ulcers, fistulas, &c. In the latter disease, it is used as an injection; from two grains to three being dissolved in an ounce of distilled water.

ARGE'NTUM. (*Argentum, i.* m.; from αργος, white, because it is of a white colour.) Silver. See *Silver.*

ARGENTUM FUSUM. Crude mercury.

ARGENTUM MOBILE. Crude mercury.

ARGENTUM NITRATUM. See *Argenti nitras.*

ARGENTUM VIVUM. See *Mercury.*

A'RGES. (From αργος, white.) A serpent, with a whitish skin, deemed by Hippocrates exceedingly venomous.

ARGI'LLA. (*Argilla, æ.* f.; from αργος, white.) Argil. White clay. See *Alumina.*

ARGILLA VITRIOLATA. Alum.

ARGILLACEOUS. Of or belonging to argilla, or aluminous earth. See *Alumina.*

Argillaceous earth. See *Alumina.*

Argillaceous schistus. See *Clay-slate.*

ARGILLITE. See *Clay-slate.*

[ARGILLOLITE. This mineral often strongly resembles certain varieties of compact limestone, or calcareous marl. Its texture is sometimes porous, and sometimes compact, or even slaty. Its fracture is dull and earthy, sometimes splintery or conchoidal. In hardness, also, it differs little from indurated marl, or the softer varieties of compact limestone, and is some times nearly friable. Its particles are sufficiently hard to scratch iron, although its masses may be cut by a knife.

It adheres but slightly to the tongue, and yields an argillaceous odour when moistened. In water it gradually crumbles, but never forms a ductile paste. It is opaque; and its colour is gray, often tinged with yellow or blue; also rose, or pale red, brown, or brownish red, and sometimes greenish. It very often presents white, brown, or greenish spots, nearly round, and is sometimes striped.

It hardens by exposure to heat, but is generally in fusible by the blow-pipe: some varieties melt at their surface. It does not effervesce with acids, by which it is distinguished from those minerals which it most resembles.

Claystone seems to approach very near to jasper, or petrosilex, in a state of decomposition, and sometimes to tripoli.—*Cl. Min.* A.]

ARGYRI'TIS. (From αργυρος, silver.) Litharge, or spume of silver. A kind of earth was formerly so named, which is taken from silver mines, and is bespangled with many particles of silver.

ARGYRO'COME. (From αργυρος, silver, and κομη, hair.) A species of *gnaphalium* or cudweed was so named from its white silvery floscules.

ARGYROLI'BANOS. The white olibanum.

ARGYRO'PHORA. An antidote, in the composition of which there is silver.

ARGYROTROPHE'MA. (From αργος, white, and τροφημα, food.) A white cooling food, made with milk. Milk diet.—*Galen.*

ARHEUMATI'STOS. (From α, neg. and ῥευματιζω to be afflicted with rheums.) Not being afflicted with gouty rheums.

ARICY'MON. (From αρι and κυω, to be quickly impregnated.) A woman who conceives quickly and often.

ARILLUS. (From *arère*, to be dry or parched.) The seed-coat or tunic of the permanent husk that invests a seed, which drying falls off spontaneously. It is a peculiar membrane, thick, and loosely surrounds the seed.

The varieties of arilli are,

1. The *succulent*, pulpy; like a berry in *Evonymus europeus* and *Lætia.*
2. *Cartilaginous;* in *Coffea Arabica.*
3. *Dimidiate*, half round; as in *Taxus baccata.*
4. *Lacerate*, cut-like; as in the mace of the *Myristica moschata.*
5. *Reticulate*, net-like, surrounding the seed like a net; as in the *Orchis* tribe.
6. *Tricuspid;* as in *Malva coromandiliana.*
7. *Hirsute*, hairy; as in *Geranium incanum.*
8. *Villous;* in *Geranium dissectum.*

ARISTA. (From *areo*, to dry.) The awn; a sharp beard, or point, or bristle-like filament, which proceeds from the husk or glume of grasses. Its distinctions are into,

1. *Naked*, without villi; as in *Stipa arguens* and *juncea.*
2. *Plumose*, having white villi; as in *Stipa pennata.*
3. *Straight*, as in *Bromus secalinus*, and *mollis.*
4. *Geniculate*, having a knee-like bend; as with *Avena sativa.*
5. *Recurved*, bent back; as in *Holcus lanatus*, and *Agrostis canina.*
6. *Tortile*, twisted like a rope; as in *Agrostis rubra*, and *Aira montana.*
7. *Terminal*, fixed to the apex of the husk: it is so in *Agrostis miliacea.*
8. *Dorsal*, fixed to the back or outward part of the husk; as in *Agrostis canina; Bromus; Alopecurus.*
9. *Uncinate*, hooked; as in *Panicum hirtellum.*

ARISTALTHÆ'A. (From αριϛος, best, and αλθαια, the althæa.) The common marsh-mallow. See *Althæa officinalis.*

ARISTATUS. (From *arista*, the awn.) Awned. Applied to leaves, leaf-stalks, &c. when terminated by a long rigid spine, which in a leaf does not appear as a contraction. In *Galium aristatum*, the leaf-stalk is awned.

ARISTOLO'CHIA. (*Aristolochia*, *æ*. f.; from αριστος, good, and λοχια or λοχεια, parturition; so called because it was supposed to be of sovereign use in disorders incident to child-birth.) 1. The name of a genus of plants in the Linnæan system. Class, *Gynandria*; Order, *Hexandria*.

2. The pharmacopœial name of the long-rooted birthwort See *Aristolochia longa*.

ARISTOLOCHIA ANGUICIDA. Snake-killing birthwort. *Aristolochia—foliis cordatis, acuminatis; caule volubili, fructicoso; pedunculis solitariis; stipulis cordatis*, of Linnæus. The juice of the root of this plant has the property of so stupifying serpents, that they may be handled with impunity. One or two drops are sufficient; and if more be dropped into the mouth, they become convulsed. So ungrateful is the smell of the root to those reptiles, that it is said they immediately turn from it. The juice is also esteemed as a preventive against the effects usually produced by the bite of venomous serpents.

ARISTOLOCHIA CLEMATITIS. *Aristolochia tenuis*. The systematic name of the *Aristolochia vulgaris* of some pharmacopœias. An extract is ordered by the Wirtemberg Pharmacopœia, and the plant is retained in that of Edinburgh. It is esteemed as possessing antipodagric virtues.

ARISTOLOCHIA FABACEA. See *Fumaria bulbosa*.

ARISTOLOCHIA LONGA. The systematic name for the aristolochia of our pharmacopœias. *Aristolochia —foliis cordatis, petiolatis, integerrimis, obtusiusculis; caule infirmo, floribus solitariis*. The root of this plant only is in use; it possesses a somewhat aromatic smell, and a warm bitterish taste, accompanied with a slight degree of pungency. The virtues ascribed to this root by the ancients were very considerable; and it was frequently employed in various diseases, but particularly in promoting the discharge of the *lochia*; hence its name. It is now very rarely used, except in gouty affections, as an aromatic stimulant.

ARISTOLOCHIA ROTUNDA. The root of this species of birthwort, *Aristolochia—foliis cordatis, subsessilibus, obtusis; caule infirmo; floribus solitariis*, of Linnæus; is used indiscriminately with that of the *aristolochia longa*. See *Aristolochia longa*.

ARISTOLOCHIA SERPENTARIA. The systematic name for the *Serpentaria virginiana* of the pharmacopœias. *Aristolochia; Colubrina virginiana; Viperina; Viperina virginiana; Pestilochia; Contrayerva virginiana*. Virginian snake-root. The plant which affords this root is the *Aristolochia—foliis cordato oblongis planis; caulibus infirmis flexuosis teretibus; floribus solitariis. Caulus geniculata valde nodosa. Flores ad radicem* of Linnæus. Snake-root has an aromatic smell, approaching to that of valerian, but more agreeable; and a warm, bitterish, pungent taste. It was first recommended as a medicine of extraordinary power, in counteracting the poisonous effects of the bites of serpents; this, however, is now wholly disregarded: but as it possesses tonic and antiseptic virtues, and is generally admitted as a powerful stimulant and diaphoretic, it is employed, in the present day, in some fevers where these effects are required. A tinctura is directed both by the London and Edinburgh Pharmacopœias.

ARISTOLOCHIA TENUIS. See *Aristolochia clematitis*.

ARISTOLOCHIA TRILOBATA. Three-lobed birthwort The root, and every part of this plant, *Aristolochia—foliis trilobis, caule volubili, floribus maximis* of Linnæus, is diuretic, and is employed in America against the bite of serpents.

ARISTOLOCHIA VULGARIS. See *Aristolochia clematitis*.

ARISTOPHANEI'ON. (From *Aristophanes*, its inventor.) The name of an ancient emollient plaster, composed of wax, or pitch.—*Gorræus*.

[ARKTIZIT. This mineral is otherwise called *Wernerite*, after the celebrated German mineralogist Werner.

The Wernerite, a rare mineral, occurs in eight-sided prisms, terminated by four-sided summits, whose faces form, with the alternate lateral planes on which they stand, an angle of about 121°. Or it may be called a four sided prism, truncated on its lateral edges. The primitive form appears to be a quadrangular prism, with square bases. It also occurs in irregular grains.

The Wernerite strikes fire with steel, but is scratched by feldspar. Its fracture is both imperfectly foliated and uneven, with a moderate lustre, a little pearly or resinous. Its specific gravity is 3.60.

It is usually more or less translucent; and its colour is greenish gray, or olive green, and sometimes white. The surface of the crystals sometimes has the lustre and aspect of an enamel.

Before the blow-pipe, it froths and melts into an opaque, white enamel. A mean of two analyses, by John, gives silex 45.5, alumine 33.5, lime 13.22, oxide of iron 5.75, oxide of manganese 1.47=99.44.

Its mode of fusion by the blow-pipe, and its imperfectly foliated structure, may serve to distinguish it from most minerals which it resembles.

This mineral is sometimes in tabular masses, but most commonly in crystals which are easily recognised. The general form of these crystals, (certain small faces being neglected,) is a very oblique rhomb, or rather four-sided prism, so flattened that some of its edges become thin and sharp, like the edge of an axe. The primitive form is a four-sided prism, the bases of which are parallelograms, with angles of 101° 30′, and 78° 30′. The integrant particles are oblique, triangular prisms. M. Haüy has described five secondary forms.—*Cl. Min.* A.]

ARMA. (*Arma*, *orum. pl.* n. Arms.) In botany, applied to a species of armature or offensive weapons. They are one of the seven kinds of *fulcra*, or props of plants enumerated by Linnæus in his *Delineatio plantæ*. They are pungent points in some part of a plant. In the present day, arma is used as a generic term embracing the *aculeus*, *furca*, *spina*, and *stimulus*.

ARMATU'RA. 1. See *Arma*.

2. The amnios or internal membrane which surrounds the fœtus.

ARMATURE. See *Arma*.

A'RME. (From αρω, to adapt.) 1. A junction of the lips of wounds.

2. The joining of the sutures of the head.

[ARMINIAN STONE. Quartzy or calcareous substances, penetrated by the azure carbonate of copper, have been called by this name, the copper giving a most beautiful blue colour. A.]

ARMI'LLA. (Diminutive of *armus*, the arm.) The round ligament which confines the tendons of the carpus.

ARMORA'CIA. (From *Armorica*, the country whence it was brought.) See *Cochlearia Armoracia*.

ARMSTRONG, JOHN, a Scotch physician, born in 1709, who, after graduating at Edinburgh, settled in London, but met with little success, having distinguished himself less in his profession than as a poet, particularly by his "Essay on the Art of Preserving Health," in blank verse. He afterward attended the army in Germany, which brought him more into notice as a physician. He attained the age of seventy, and died in pretty good circumstances. His professional publications are not of much note; the principal one is entitled "Medical Essays." He is supposed, however, to have contributed materially to a useful Treatise on the Diseases of Children, published by his brother George, who, after practising many years as an apothecary, obtained a diploma in medicine.

A'RNICA. (*Arnica*, *æ*. f. Αρνικη; from αρς, a lamb; because of the likeness of the leaf of this plant to the coat of the lamb.) Arnica. 1. The name of a genus of plants in the Linnæan system Class, *Syngenesia*; Order, *Polygamia superflua*.

2. The pharmacopœial name of the Mountain arnica See *Arnica montana*.

ARNICA MONTANA. The systematic name for the *arnica* of the pharmacopœias. *Arnica foliis ovatis integris; caulinis geminis oppositis*, of Linnæus. *Doronicum Germanicum. Acyrus*. The flowers of this plant are very generally employed on the Continent. Of the advantages derived from their use, in paralytic and other affections, depending upon a want of nervous energy, there are several proofs; and their extraordinary virtues, as a febrifuge and antiseptic, have been highly extolled by Dr. Collin, of Vienna. Much caution is necessary in regulating the dose, as it is a medicine very apt to produce vomiting, and much uneasiness of the stomach. See *Arnica*.

ARNICA SUEDENSIS. See *Inula dysenterica*.

ARNO'TTO. A Spanish name for a shrub. See *Bixa orleana*.

ARO'MA. (*Aroma, matis*, neut.; from αρι, intensely, and οζω, to smell.) *Spiritis rector*. The odorous principle of plants, and other substances, which have their characteristic smell. This is called by the moderns, *aroma*. Water charged with aroma, is called the distilled water of the substance made use of: thus lavender and peppermint waters are water impregnated with the aroma of the lavender and peppermint.

AROMATA. (Αρωματα, sweet spices, herbs, &c.) Aromatics.

AROMA'TIC. (*Aromaticus;* from αρωμα, an odour.) A term applied to a grateful spicy scent, and an agreeable pungent taste, as cinnamon bark, cardamoms, &c.

Aromatic vinegar. See *Acetum aromaticum*.

AROMATICÆ PLANTÆ. Odoriferous or strong and agreeable smelling plants. The name of a class of plants in some natural arrangements.

AROMA'TICUS CORTEX. A name for canella alba. *Cortex winteranus*.

AROMATOPO'LA. (From αρωμα, an odour, and πωλεω, to sell.) A druggist; a vender of drugs and spiceries.

ARQUEBUSA'DE. (A French word, implying *good for a gun-shot wound*.) *Aqua sclopetaria; Aqua vulneraria; Aqua catapultarum*. The name of a spirituous water, distilled from a farrago of aromatic plants.

ARRA'CK. A spirituous liquor distilled from rice, and drunk, in the rice countries, as brandy is in this island. Its effects on the animal economy are the same.

ARRAGONITE. A mineral of a greenish and pearly gray colour, found at Arragon in Spain, England, and Scotland.

[Although this mineral is composed chiefly of lime and carbonic acid, yet there is reason to believe, that other ingredients are essential to its true composition. It differs from pure carbonate of lime in hardness, specific gravity, and crystalline structure.

In nitric acid it dissolves with effervescence. The analysis of no mineral has ever so much exercised the talents, exhausted the resources, and disappointed the expectations of the most distinguished chemists of Europe, as that of arragonite. Vauquelin and Fourcroy obtained lime 58.5, carbonic acid 41.5; and the analysis of Biot and Thenard, conducted with much ingenuity, scarcely differs from this, except in giving a little water. With these, both Chevenix and Klaproth agree, in finding the arragonite to contain lime and carbonic acid in nearly the same proportions as in the common carbonate of lime. Kirwan in his mineralogy, published in 1794, conjectured that the arragonite might contain *strontian;* and very recently Professor Stromeyer of Gottingen has discovered in this mineral between three and four per cent. of the carbonate of strontian. This discovery will very probably lead to a solution of the preceding difficulty; but it is important that the analysis should be repeated by different chemists.—*Cl. Min.* A.]

A'RRAPHUS. (From α, priv. and ραφη, a suture.) Without suture. It is applied to the cranium when naturally without sutures.

Arrangement of Minerals. See *Minerals, arrangement of*.

ARRHÆ'A. (From α, neg. and ρεω, to flow.) The suppression of any natural flux, as the menses, &c.

ARRHIZUS. (From α, priv. and ριζα, a root: without root.) Applied to paraatical plants, which have no roots, but adhere and imbibe their nourishment by ainastomosing of the vessels; as *Viscum album*, and *Loranthus europeus*.

ARROWHEAD. The *Sagittaria sagittifolia* of Linnæus. The roots of this plant are said to be esculent, but it must be in times of very great scarcity.

Arrow-root. See *Maranta*.

Arrow-shaped. See *Leaf*.

ARSE'NIATE. (*Arsenias, atis*. m.; from *arsenicum*, arsenic.) A salt formed by a combination of arsenic acid with salifiable bases; as arseniate of ammonia, which is produced by the union of ammonia with arsenic acid. The only one used in medicine is the superarseniate of potassa, which is in solution in the liquor arsenicalis. See *Arsenicalis liquor*.

A'RSENIC. (*Arsenicum, i.* n.; from the Arabic term *Arsanek*, or from αρσηυ, for αρρηυ, *masculus;* from its strong and deadly powers.) The name of a metal scattered, in great abundance, over the mineral kingdom. It is found in black, heavy masses of little brilliancy, called *native arsenic* or testaceous arsenic. This exists in different parts of Germany. Mineralized by sulphur, it forms *sulphurized arsenic*. This mineral is met with in Italy, about Mount Vesuvius. There are two varieties of this ore, which differ from each other in colour, occasioned by the different proportions of their component parts. The one is called *yellow sulphurized arsenic*, or *orpiment;* the other, *red sulphurized arsenic*, or *realgar*, or *ruby arsenic;* both are met with in Hungary and different parts of Germany. The colour of the first ore is a lemon-yellow, inclining sometimes to a green; the colour of the latter is a ruby-red; it is more transparent than the former, and found in compact and solid masses, sometimes crystallized in bright needles. Arsenic united to oxygen, constitutes the ore called *native oxyde of arsenic*. This ore is scarce; it is generally found of an earthy appearance, or as an efflorescence, coating native, or metallic arsenic; its colour is a whitish gray; it is rarely met with crystallized. Arsenic exists likewise alloyed with cobalt, antimony, tin, copper, lead, and various other metals.

Method of obtaining Arsenic. In order to obtain metallic arsenic, mix two parts of the white oxyde of arsenic of commerce, with one of black flux (obtained by detonating one part of nitrate of potassa with two of supertartrate of potassa), and put the mixture into a crucible, or melting pot. Invert over this another crucible, lute the two together with a little clay and sand, and apply gradually a red heat to the lower one. The oxyde of arsenic will be reduced, and be found lining the upper crucible in small crystals of a metallic brilliancy.

The charcoal of the black flux takes in this process the oxygen from the white oxyde, and forms carbonic acid gas; which flies off during the process, and the oxyde becomes reduced to the metallic state. This reduction of the oxyde is greatly facilitated by the alkali of the flux.

Remark.—In order to obtain arsenic in a state of absolute purity, the metal thus obtained must be reduced to a powder, dissolved by heat in nitro-muriatic acid, and then precipitated by immersing into the solution a plate of zinc. The arsenic is thus precipitated in a fine powder, and may be reduced to a mass, by exposing it in a covered crucible to a moderate heat.

"It is among the most combustible of the metals, burns with a blue flame, and garlic smell, and sublimes in the state of arsenious acid.

Concentrated sulphuric acid does not attack arsenic when cold; but if it be boiled upon this metal, sulphurous acid gas is emitted, a small quantity of sulphur sublimes, and the arsenic is reduced to an oxyde.

Nitrous acid readily attacks arsenic, and converts it into arsenious acid, or, if much be employed, into arsenic acid.

Boiling muriatic acid dissolves arsenic, but affects it very little when cold. This solution affords precipitates upon the addition of alkalies. The addition of a little nitric acid expedites the solution; and this solution, first heated and condensed in a close vessel, is wholly sublimed into a thick liquid, formerly termed *butter of arsenic*. Thrown in powder into chlorine gas, it burns with a bright white flame, and is converted into a chloride.

None of the earths or alkalies act upon it, unless it be boiled a long while in fine powder, in a large proportion of alkaline solution.

Nitrates detonate with arsenic, convert it into arsenic acid, and this, combining with the base of the nitrate, forms an arseniate, that remains at the bottom of the vessel.

Muriates have no action upon it; but if three parts of chlorate of potassa be mixed with one part of arsenic in fine powder, which must be done with great precaution, and a very light hand, a very small quantity of this mixture placed on an anvil, and struck with a hammer, will explode with flame and a considerable report; if touched with fire, it will burn with considerable rapidity; and if thrown into concentrated sulphuric acid, at the instant of contact a flame rises into the air like a flash of lightning, which is so bright as to dazzle the eye.

Arsenic readily combines with sulphur by fusion and sublimation, and forms a yellow compound called *orpiment*, or a red called *realgar*. The nature of these, and their difference, are not accurately known; but Fourcroy considers the first as a combination of sulphur with the oxyde, and the second as a combination of sulphur with the metal itself, as he found the red sulphuret converted into the yellow by the action of acids.

Arsenic is soluble in fat oils in a boiling heat; the solution is black, and has the consistence of an ointment when cold. Most metals unite with arsenic; which exists in the metallic state in such alloys as possess the metallic brilliancy.

Iodine and arsenic unite, forming an iodide, of a dark, purple-red colour, possessing the properties of an acid. It is soluble in water, and its solution forms a soluble compound with potassa.

Arsenic combines with hydrogen into a very noxious compound, called arsenuretted hydrogen gas. To prepare it, fuse in a covered crucible 3 parts of granulated tin, and 1 of metallic arsenic in powder; and submit this alloy, broken in pieces, to the action of muriatic acid in a glass retort. On applying a moderate heat, the arsenuretted hydrogen comes over, and may be received in a mercurial or water pneumatic trough. Protomuriate of tin remains in the retort.

A prime equivalent of hydrogen is to one of arsenic as 1 to 76; and 2 consequently as 1 to 38. Gehlen fell a victim to his researches on this gas; and therefore the new experiments requisite to elucidate its constitution must be conducted with circumspection. It extinguishes flame, and instantly destroys animal life. Water has no effect upon it. From the experiments of Sir H. Davy, and Gay Lussac and Thenard, there appears to be a solid compound of hydrogen and arsenic, or a hydruret. It is formed by acting with the negative pole of a voltaic battery on arsenic plunged in water. It is reddish brown, without lustre, taste, and smell. It is not decomposed at a heat approaching to cherry-red; but at this temperature it absorbs oxygen; while water and arsenious acid are formed, with the evoluton of heat and light. The proportion of the two constituents is not known.

Arsenic is used in a variety of arts. It enters into metallic combinations, wherein a white colour is required. Glass manufacturers use it; but its effect in the composition of glass does not seem to be clearly explained. Orpiment and realgar are used as pigments."

Arsenic and its various preparations are the most active of all poisons. That which is mostly taken, is the white oxyde, or arsenious acid. See *Arsenious acid.*

[Arsenical pyrites, or arsenical iron, is found in the Highlands of New-York, on the west side of the Hudson. In the town of Warwick, in Orange county, of this state, there is a huge vein of it in a mountain range, sufficient, as is said by a traveller, to poison the whole world. A.]

ARSENIC ACID. *Acidum arsenicum; Acidum arsenicale.* "We are indebted to the illustrious Scheele for the discovery of this acid, though Macquer had before noticed its combinations. It may be obtained by various methods. If six parts of nitric acid be poured on one of the concrete arsenious acids, or white arsenic of the shops, in the pneumato-chemical apparatus, and heat be applied, nitrous gas will be evolved, and a white concrete substance, differing in its properties from the arsenious acid, will remain in the retort. This is the arsenic acid. It may equally be procured by means of aqueous chlorine, or by heating concentrated nitric acid with twice its weight of the solution of the arsenious acid in muriatic acid. The concrete acid should be exposed to a dull red heat for a few minutes. In either case an acid is obtained, that does not crystallize, but attracts the moisture of the air, has a sharp, caustic taste, reddens blue vegetable colours, is fixed in the fire, and of the specific gravity of 3 391.

If the arsenic acid be exposed to a red heat in a glass retort, it melts and becomes transparent, but assumes a milky hue on cooling. If the heat be increased, so that the retort begins to melt, the acid boils, and sublimes into the neck of the retort. If a covered crucible be used instead of the glass retort, and a violent heat applied, the acid boils strongly, and in a quarter of an hour begins to emit fumes. These, on being received in a glass bell, are found to be arsenious acid; and a small quantity of a transparent glass, difficult to fuse, will be found lining the sides of the crucible. This is arseniate of alumina.

Combustible substances decompose this acid. If two parts of arsenic acid be mixed with about one of charcoal, the mixture introduced into a glass retort, coated, and a matrass adapted to it; and the retort then gradually heated in a reverberatory furnace, till the bottom is red; the mass will be inflamed violently, and the acid reduced, and rise to the neck of the retort in the metallic state, mixed with a little oxyde and charcoal powder. A few drops of water, devoid of acidity, will be found in the receiver.

With sulphur the phenomena are different. If a mixture of six parts of arsenic acid, and one of powdered sulphur, be digested together, no change will take place: but on evaporating to dryness, and distilling in a glass retort, fitted with a receiver, a violent combination will ensue, as soon as the mixture is sufficiently heated to melt the sulphur. The whole mass rises almost at once, forming a red sublimate, and sulphurous acid passes over into the receiver.

If pure arsenic acid be diluted with a small quantity of water, and hydrogen gas, as it is evolved by the action of sulphuric acid on iron, be received into this transparent solution, the liquor grows turbid, and a blackish precipitate is formed, which, being well washed with distilled water, exhibits all the phenomena of arsenic. Sometimes, too, a blackish-gray oxyde of arsenic is found in this process.

If sulphuretted hydrogen gas be employed instead of simple hydrogen gas, water and a sulphuret of arsenic are obtained.

With phosphorus, phosphoric acid is obtained, and a phosphuret of arsenic, which sublimes.

The arsenic acid is much more soluble than the arsenious. According to Lagrange, two parts of water are sufficient for this purpose. It cannot be crystallized by any means; but, on evaporation, assumes a thick honey-like consistence.

No acid has any action upon it: if some of them dissolve it by means of the water that renders them fluid, they do not produce any alteration in it. The boracic and phosphoric are vitrifiable with it by means of heat, but without any material alteration in their natures. If phosphorus acid be heated upon it for some time, it saturates itself with oxygen, and becomes phosphoric acid.

The arsenic acid combines with the earthy and alkaline bases, and forms salts very different from those furnished by the arsenious acid.

All these *arseniates* are decomposable by charcoal, which separates arsenic from them by means of heat.

All its *salts*, with the exception of those of potassa, soda, and ammonia, are insoluble in water; but except arseniate of bismuth, and one or two more, very soluble in an excess of arsenic acid. Hence, after barytes or oxyde of lead has been precipitated by this acid, its farther addition re-dissolves the precipitate. This is a useful criterion of the acid, joined to its reduction to the metallic state by charcoal, and the other characters already detailed. Sulphuric acid decomposes the arseniates at a low temperature, but the sulphates are decomposed by arsenic acid at a red heat, owing to the greater fixity of the latter. Phosphoric, nitric, muriatic, and fluoric acids, dissolve, and probably convert into subsalts all the arseniates. The whole of them, as well as arsenic acid itself when decomposed at a red heat by charcoal, yield the characteristic garlic smell of the metallic vapour. Nitrate of silver gives a pulverulent brick-coloured precipitate, with arsenic acid. The acid itself does not disturb the transparency of a solution of sulphate of copper; but a neutral arseniate gives with it a bluish green precipitate; with sulphate of cobalt, a dirty red; and with sulphate of nickel, an apple-green precipitate. These precipitates redissolve, on adding a small quantity of the acid which previously held them in solution. Orfila says, that arsenic acid gives, with acetate of copper, a bluish-white precipitate, but that it exercises no action either on the muriate or acetate of cobalt; but with the ammonio-muriate, it gives a rose-coloured precipitate. Arsenic acid ought to be accounted a more violent poison than even the arsenious.

The *arseniate of barytes* is insoluble, uncrystallizable, soluble in an excess of its acid, and decomposable by sulphuric acid, which precipitates a sulphate of barytes.

The *bin-arseniate of potassa* is made on the great scale in Saxony, by fusing together equal parts of nitre and arsenious acid; dissolving the melted mass, and crystallizing the salt.

Of the *arseniate of strontian* nothing is known, but no doubt it resembles that of barytes.

With *lime-water* this acid forms a precipitate of *arseniate of lime*, soluble in an excess of its base, or in an excess of its acid, though insoluble alone. The acidulous arseniate of lime affords on evaporation little crystals, decomposable by sulphuric acid. The same salt may be formed by adding carbonate of lime to the solution of arsenic acid. This acid does not decompose the nitrate or muriate of lime: but the saturated alkaline arseniates decompose them by double affinity, precipitating the insoluble calcareous arseniate.

If arsenic acid be saturated with *magnesia*, a thick substance is formed near the point of saturation. This *arseniate of magnesia* is soluble in an excess of acid; and on being evaporated takes the form of a jelly, without crystallizing. Neither the sulphate, nitrate, nor muriate of magnesia is decomposed by arsenic acid, though they are by the saturated alkaline arseniates.

Arsenic acid, saturated with *potassa*, does not easily crystallize. This *arseniate*, being evaporated to dryness, attracts the humidity of the air, and turns the syrup of violets green, without altering the solution of litmus. It fuses into a white glass, and with a strong fire is converted into an acidule, part of the alkali being abstracted by the silex and alumina of the crucible. If exposed to a red heat with charcoal in close vessels, it swells up very much, and arsenic is sublimed. It is decomposed by sulphuric acid; but in the humid way the decomposition is not obvious, as the arsenic acid remains in solution. On evaporation, however, this acid and sulphate of potassa are obtained.

If arsenic acid be added to the preceding salt, till it ceases to have any effect on the syrup of violets, it will redden the solution of litmus; and in this state it affords very regular and very transparent crystals, of the figure of quadrangular prisms, terminated by two tetraëdral pyramids, the angles of which answer to those of the prisms. These crystals are the arsenical neutral salt of Macquer. As this salt differs from the preceding arseniate by its crystallizability, its reddening solution of litmus, its not decomposing the calcareous and magnesian salts like it, and its capability of absorbing an additional portion of potassa, so as to become neutral, it ought to be distinguished from it by the term of *acidulous arseniate of potassa.*

With *soda* in sufficient quantity to saturate it, arsenic acid forms a salt crystallizable like the acidulous arseniate of potassa. To form the neutral arseniate, carbonate of soda should be added to the acid, till the mixture be decidedly alkaline. This salt crystallizes from the concentrated solution. It is much more soluble in hot than in cold water. Pelletier says, that the crystals are hexaëdral prisms, terminated by planes perpendicular to their axis. This neutral arseniate of soda, however, while it differs completely from that of potassa in this respect, and in becoming deliquescent instead of crystallizable on the addition of a surplus portion of arsenic acid, resembles the arseniate of potassa in its decomposition by charcoal, by acids, and by the earths.

Combined with *ammonia*, arsenic acid forms a salt affording rhomboidal crystals analogous to those of the nitrate of soda.

The *arseniate of soda* and *ammonia* is formed by mixing the two separate arseniates; and the compound salt gives crystals with brilliant faces. If we redissolve the crystals, and then recrystallize, we should add a little ammonia, otherwise the salt will be acidulous from the escape of some ammonia.

Arsenic acid saturated with *alumina* forms a thick solution, which, being evaporated to dryness, yields a salt insoluble in water, and decomposable by the sulphuric, nitric, and muriatic acids, as well as by all the other earthy and alkaline bases. The arsenic acid readily dissolves the alumina of the crucibles in which it is reduced to a state of fusion; and thus it attacks silex also, on which it has no effect in the humid way.

By the assistance of a strong fire, as Fourcroy asserts, arsenic acid decomposes the alkaline and earthy sulphates, even that of barytes; the sulphuric acid flying off in vapour, and the arseniate remaining in the retort. It acts in the same manner on the nitrate, from which it expels the pure acid. It likewise decomposes the muriates at a high temperature, the muriatic acid being evolved in the form of gas, and the arsenic acid combining with their bases, which it saturates; while the arsenious acid is too volatile to have this effect. It acts in the same manner on the fluates, and still more easily on the carbonates, with which, by the assistance of heat, it excites a brisk effervescence. Lagrange, however, denies that it acts on any of the neutral salts, except the sulphate of potassa and soda, the nitrate of potassa, and the muriates of soda and ammonia, and this by means of heat. It does not act on the phosphates, but precipitates the boracic acids from solutions of borates when heated.

Arsenic acid does not act on gold or platina; neither does it on mercury or silver, without the aid of a strong heat; but it oxydizes copper, iron, lead, tin, zinc, bismuth, antimony, cobalt, nickel, manganese, and arsenic.

This acid is not used in the arts, at least directly, though indirectly it forms a part of some compositions used in dying. It is likewise one of the mineralizing acids combined by nature with some of the metallic oxydes."—*Ure's Chem. Dict.*

Arsenic, oxyde of. See *Arsenious acid.*

Arsenic, white. See *Arsenious acid.*

ARSE'NICAL CAUSTIC. A species of caustic said to possess useful properties, independent of those of destroying morbid parts to which it is applied. It is composed of two parts of levigated antimony to one of white arsenic. This is the caustic so extensively employed under the name of arsenical caustic, by the late Mr Justamond, in his treatment of cancers.

[Arsenic is a powerful, a dangerous, and yet a valuable caustic. Small tumours, excrescences, warts, &c., may be easily and safely removed by it. Alone, it gives much pain; and in large quantities, and applied to an extensive surface, is extremely dangerous. Its painful action may be modified and more safely applied by mixing one part of white arsenic with one of powdered opium, and two of lapis calaminaris. A.]

ARSENICA'LIS LIQUOR. Arsenical solution. Take of sublimed oxyde of arsenic, in very fine powder, sub carbonate of potassa from tartar, of each 64 grains; distilled water a pint. Boil them together in a glass vessel, until the arsenic be entirely dissolved. When the solution is cold, add compound spirit of lavender, four fluid drachms. Then add as much distilled water as may exactly fill a pint measure. This preparation accords with the formula of Dr. Fowler, of Stafford, who first introduced it in imitation of a celebrated popular remedy for intermittents, sold under the name of the tasteless ague-drop. The compound spirit of lavender is only intended to give some colour and taste, without which it would be more liable to mistakes. Where the dose is small, and the effects so powerful, the most minute attention to its proportion and preparation becomes necessary. Each ounce contains four grains of the oxyde, and each drachm half a grain; but it will rarely be proper to go beyond one-sixteenth of a grain as a dose.

Arsenical solution. See *Arsenicalis liquor.*

Arsenici oxydum præparatum. See *Arsenici oxydum sublimatum.*

ARSENICUM ALBUM. *Arsenici oxydum sublimatum; Arsenici oxydum præparatum.* Reduce white arsenic into powder, then put it into a crucible and expose it to the fire, so as to sublime it into another crucible inverted over the former. This is intended to render the arsenic more pure.

Arsenicum album. White arsenic. See *Arsenious acid.*

ARSENICUM CRYSTALLINUM. See *Arsenious acid.*

ARSE'NIOUS ACID. White arsenic. Oxyde of arsenic. *Arsenicum crystallinum, risigallum, aquala, arfar, aquila, zarnick, artaneck.* Rat's bane. The earliest chemists were embarrassed in the determination of the nature of the poisonous white substance known in commerce by the name of *white arsenic* "Fourcroy was the first who distinguished by this name the white arsenic of the shops, which Scheele had proved to be a compound of the metal arsenic with oxygen, and which the authors of the new chemical nomenclature had consequently termed oxyde of arsenic. As, however, it manifestly exhibits the properties of an acid, it has a fair claim to the title; for many oxydes and acids are similar in this, that both consist of a base united with oxygen, and the only difference between them is, that the compound in which the acid properties are manifest is termed an acid, and that in which they are not is called an oxyde.

This acid, which is one of the most virulent poisons known, frequently occurs in a native state, if not very abundantly; and it is obtained in roasting several ores, particularly those of cobalt. In the chimneys of the furnaces where this operation is conducted, it generally condenses in thick semitransparent masses; though sometimes it assumes the form of a powder, or of little needles, in which state it was formerly called flowers of arsenic.

The arsenious acid reddens the most sensible blue vegetable colours, though it turns the syrup of violets green On exposure to the air it becomes opaque, and covered with a slight efflorescence. Thrown on incandescent coals, it evaporates in white fumes, with a strong smell of garlic. In close vessels it is volatilized; and, if the heat be strong, vitrified. The result of this vitrification is a transparent glass, capable of crystallizing in tetraëdra, the angles of which are truncated. It is easily altered by hydrogen and carbon, which deprive it of its oxygen at a red heat, and reduce the metal, the one forming water, the other carbonic acid with the oxygen taken from it; as it is by phosphorus, and by sulphur, which are in part converted into acids by its oxygen, and in part form an arsenical phosphuret or sulphuret with the arsenic reduced to the metallic state. Hence Margraaf and Pelletier, who particularly examined the phosphurets of metals, assert they might be formed with arsenious acid. Its specific gravity is 3.7.

It is soluble in thirteen times its weight of boiling water, but requires eighty times its weight of cold. The solution crystallizes, and the acid assumes the form of regular tetraëdrons, according to Fourcroy; but, according to Lagrange, of octaëdrons, and these frequently varying in figure by different laws of decrement. It crystallizes much better by slow evaporation than by simple cooling.

The solution is very acrid, reddens blue colours, unites with the earthy bases, and decomposes the alkaline sulphurets. Arsenious acid is also soluble in oils, spirits, and alkohol; the last taking up from 1 to 2 per cent. It is composed of 9.5 of metal = 3 oxygen; and its prime equivalent is therefore 12.5. Dr. Wollaston first observed, that when a mixture of it with quicklime is heated in a glass tube, at a certain temperature, ignition suddenly pervades the mass, and metallic arsenic sublimes. As arseniate of lime is found at the bottom of the tube, we perceive that a portion of the arsenious acid is robbed of its oxygen, to complete the acidification of the rest.

There are even some metals, which act upon the solution, and have a tendency to decompose the acid so as to form a blackish precipitate, in which the arsenic is very slightly oxydized.

The action of the other acids upon the arsenious is very different from that which they exert on the metal arsenic. By boiling, sulphuric acid dissolves a small portion of it, which is precipitated as the solution cools. The nitric acid does not dissolve it, but by the help of heat converts it into arsenic acid. Neither the phosphoric nor the carbonic acid acts upon it; yet it enters into a vitreous combination with the phosphoric and boracic acids. The muriatic acid dissolves it by means of heat, and forms with it a volatile compound, which water precipitates; and aqueous chlorine acidifies it completely, so as to convert it into arsenic acid.

The arsenious acid combines with the *earthy* and *alkaline* bases, forming *Arsenites*. The earthy arseniates possess little solubility; and hence the solutions of barytes, strontian, and lime, form precipitates with that of arsenious acid.

This acid enters into another kind of combination with the earths, that formed by *vitrification*. Though a part of this volatile acid sublimes before the glass enters into fusion, part remains fixed in the vitrified substance, to which it imparts transparency, a homogeneous density, and considerable gravity. The arsenical glasses appear to contain a kind of triple salt, since the salt and alkalies enter into an intimate combination at the instant of fusion, and remain afterward perfectly mixed. All of them have the inconvenience of quickly growing dull by exposure to the air.

With the *fixed alkalies* the arsenious acid forms thick arsenites, which do not crystallize; which are decomposable by fire, the arsenious acid being volatilized by the heat; and from which all the other acids precipitate this in powder. These saline compounds were formerly termed livers, because they were supposed to be analogous to the combinations of sulphur with the alkalies.

With *ammonia* it forms a salt capable of crystallization. If this be heated a little, the ammonia is decomposed, the nitrogen is evolved, while the hydrogen, uniting with part of the oxygen of the acid, forms water.

Neither the earthy nor alkaline arsenites have yet been much examined; what is known of them being only sufficient to distinguish them from the arseniates.

The arsenious acid is used in numerous instances in the arts, under the name of *white arsenic*, or of arsenic simply. In many cases it is reduced, and acts in its metallic state.

Many attempts have been made to introduce it into medicine; but as it is known to be one of the most violent poisons, it is probable that the fear of its bad effects may deprive society of the advantages it might afford in this way. An arseniate of potassa was extensively used by the late Dr. Fowler, of York, who published a treatise on it, in intermittent and remittent fevers. He likewise assured the writer, that he had found it extremely efficacious in periodical headache, and as a tonic in nervous and other disorders; and that he never saw the least ill effect from its use, due precaution being employed in preparing and administering it. Externally it has been employed as a caustic to extirpate cancer, combined with sulphur, with bole, with antimony, and with the leaves of crowfoot; but it always gives great pain, and is not unattended with danger. Febvre's remedy was water one pint, extract of hemlock ℥j. Goulard's extract ℥iij. tincture of opium ʒj. arsenious acid gr. x. With this the cancer was wetted morning and evening; and at the same time a small quantity of a weak solution was administered internally. A still milder application of this kind has been made from a solution of one grain in a quart of water, formed into a poultice with crumb of bread.

It has been more lately used as an alterative with advantage in chronic rheumatism. The symptoms which show the system to be *arsenified* are thickness, redness, and stiffness of the *palpebræ*, soreness of the gums, ptyalism, itching over the surface of the body, restlessness, cough, pain at stomach, and headache. When the latter symptoms supervene, the administration of the medicine ought to be immediately suspended. It has also been recommended against chincough; and has been used in considerable doses with success, to counteract the poison of venomous serpents.

Since it acts on the animal economy as a deadly poison in quantities so minute as to be insensible to the taste when diffused in water or other vehicles, it has been often given with criminal intentions and fatal effects. It becomes therefore a matter of the utmost importance to present a systematic view of the phenomena characteristic of the poison, its operation, and consequences.

It is a dense substance, subsiding speedily after agitation in water. Dr. Ure found its sp. gr. to vary from 3.728 to 3.730, which is a little higher than the number given above: 72 parts dissolve in 1000 of boiling water, of which 30 remain in it, after it cools. Cold water dissolves, however, only 3-1000 or 1-10 of the preceding quantity. This water makes the syrup of violets green, and reddens litmus paper. Lime water gives a fine white precipitate with it of arsenite of lime, soluble in an excess of the arsenious solution; sulphuretted hydrogen gas, and hydrosulphuretted water, precipitate a golden yellow sulphuret of arsenic. By this means, 1-100000 of arsenious acid may be detected in water. This sulphuret dried on a filter, and heated in a glass tube with a bit of caustic potassa, is decomposed in a few minutes, and converted into sulphuret of potassa, which remains at the bot tom, and metallic arsenic of a bright steel lustre, which sublimes, coating the sides of the tube. The hydrosulphurets of alkalies do not affect the arsenious solution, unless a drop or two of nitric or muriatic acid be poured in, when the characteristic golden yellow precipitate falls. Nitrate of silver is decomposed by the arsenious acid, and a very peculiar yellow arsenite of silver precipitates; which, however, is apt to be redissolved by nitric acid, and therefore a very minute addition of ammonia is requisite. Even this, however, also, if in much excess, redissolves the silver precipitate.

As the nitrate of silver is justly regarded as one of the best precipitant tests of arsenic, the mode of using it has been a subject of much discussion. This excellent test was first proposed by Mr. Hume of Long Acre, in May 1809. *Phil. Mag.* xxxiii. 401. The presence of muriate of soda indeed, in the arsenical solution, obstructs, to a certain degree, the operation of this reagent. But that salt is almost always present in the *primæ viæ*, and is a usual ingredient in soups, and other vehicles of the poison. If, after the water of ammonia has been added, (by plunging the end of a glass rod dipped in it into the supposed poisonous liquid,) we dip another rod into a solution of pure nitrate of silver, and transfer it into the arsenious solution, either a fine yellow cloud will be formed, or at first merely a white curdy precipitate. But at the second or third immersion of the nitrate rod, a central spot of yellow will be perceived surrounded with the white muriate of silver. At the next immersion, this yellow cloud on the surface will become very conspicuous. Sulphate of soda does not interfere in the least with the silver test.

The ammoniaco-sulphate, or rather ammoniaco-acetate of copper, added in a somewhat dilute state to an arsenious solution, gives a fine grass-green and a very characteristic precipitate. This green arseniate of copper, well washed, being acted on by an excess of sulphuretted hydrogen water, changes its colour, and becomes of a brownish-red. Ferro-prussiate of potassa changes it into a blood-red. Nitrate of silver converts it into the yellow arsenite of silver.

Lastly, if the precipitate be dried on a filter, and placed on a bit of burning coal, it will diffuse a garlic odour. The cupreous test will detect 1-110000 of the weight of the arsenic in water.

The Voltaic battery, made to act by two wires on a little arsenious solution placed on a bit of window-glass, developes metallic arsenic at the negative pole, and if this wire be copper, it will be whitened like tombac.

We may here remark, however, that the most elegant mode of using all these precipitation reagents is upon a plane of glass; a mode practised by Dr. Wollaston in general chemical research, to an extent, and with a success, which would be incredible in other hands than his. Concentrate by heat in a capsule the suspected poisonous solution, having previously filtered it if necessary. Indeed, if it be very much disguised with animal or vegetable matters, it is better first of all to evaporate to dryness, and by a few drops of nitric acid to dissipate the organic products. The clear liquid being now placed in the middle of the bit of glass, lines are to be drawn out from it in different directions. To one of these a particle of weak ammoniacal water being applied, the weak nitrate of silver may then be brushed over it with a hair pencil. By placing the glass in different lights, either over white paper or obliquely before the eye, the slightest change of tint will be perceived. The ammoniaco-acetate should be applied to another filament of the drop, deutacetate of iron to a third, weak ammoniaco-acetate of cobalt to a fourth, sulphuretted water to a fifth, lime water to a sixth, a drop of violet-syrup to a seventh, and the two galvanic wires at the opposite edges of the whole. Thus with one single drop of solution many exact experiments may be made.

But the chief, the decisive trial or *experimentum crucis* remains, which is to take a little of the dry matter, mix it with a small pinch of dry black flux, put it into a narrow glass tube sealed at one end, and after cleansing its sides with a feather, urge its bottom with a blow-pipe till it be distinctly red-hot for a minute. Then garlic fumes will be smelt, and the steel-lustred coating of metallic arsenic will be seen in the tube about one-fourth of an inch above its bottom. Cut the tube across at that point by means of a fine file, detach the scale of arsenic with the point of a penknife; put a fragment of it into the bottom of a small wine-glass along with a few drops of ammoniaco-acetate of copper, and triturate them well together for a few minutes with a round-headed glass rod. The mazarine blue colour will soon be transmuted into a lively grass-green, while the metallic scale will vanish. Thus we distinguish perfectly between a particle of metallic arsenic and one of animalized charcoal. Another particle of the scale may be placed between two smooth and bright surfaces of copper, with a touch of fine oil; and while they are firmly pressed together, exposed to a red-heat. The tombac alloy will appear as a white stain. A third particle may be placed on a bit of heated metal, and held a little under the nostrils, when the garlic odour will be recognised. No danger can be apprehended, as the fragment need not exceed the tenth of a grain.

It is to be observed, that one or two of the precipitation tests may be equivocal from admixtures of various substances. Thus tincture of ginger gives with the cupreous reagent a green precipitate;—and the writer of this article was at first led to suspect from that appearance, that an empirical tincture, put into his hands for examination, did contain arsenic. But a careful analysis satisfied him of its genuineness. Tea covers arsenic from the cupreous test. Such poisoned tea becomes, by its addition, of an obscure olive or violet red, but yields scarcely any precipitate. Sulphuretted hydrogen, however, throws down a fine yellow sulphuret of arsenic.

The true way of obviating all these sources of fallacy, is to evaporate carefully to dryness, and expose the residue to heat in a glass tube. The arsenic sublimes, and may be afterward operated on without ambiguity. M. Orfila has gone into ample details on the modifications produced by wine, coffee, tea, broth, &c. on arsenical tests, of which a good tabular abstract is given in Mr. Thomson's London Dispensatory. But it is evident that the differences in these menstrua, as also in beers, are so great as to render precipitations and changes of colour by reagents very unsatisfactory witnesses, in a case of life and death. Hence the method of evaporation above described should never be neglected. Should the arsenic be combined with oil, the mixture ought to be boiled with water, and the oil then separated by the capillary action of wick-threads. If with resinous substances, these may be removed by oil of turpentine, not by alkohol, (as directed by Dr. Black,) which is a good solvent of arsenious acid. It may moreover be observed, that both tea and coffee should be freed from their tannin by gelatin, which does not act on the arsenic, previous to the use of reagent for the poison. When one part of the arsenious acid in watery solution is added to ten parts of milk, the sulphuretted hydrogen present in the latter, occasions the white colour to pass into a canary yellow; the cupreous test gives it a slight green tint, and the nitrate of silver produces no visible change, though even more arsenic be added; but the hydrosulphurets throw down a golden yellow, with the aid of a few drops of an acid. The liquid contained in the stomach of a rabbit poisoned with a solution of three grains of arsenious acid, afforded a white precipitate with nitrate of silver, grayish-white with lime water, green with the ammoniaco-sulphate, and deep yellow with sulphuretted hydrogen water.

The preceding copious description of the habitudes of arsenious acid in different circumstances, is equally applicable to the soluble arsenites. Their poisonous operation, as well as that of the arsenic acid, has been satisfactorily referred by Mr. Brodie to the suspension of the functions of the heart and brain, occasioned by the absorption of these substances into the circulation, and their constant determination to the nervous system and the alimentary canal. This proposition was established by numerous experiments on rabbits and dogs. Wounds were inflicted, and arsenic being applied to them, it was found that in a short time death supervened with the same symptoms of inflammation of the stomach and bowels, as if the poison had been swallowed.

He divides the morbid affections into three classes: 1*st*, Those depending on the nervous system, as palsy at first of the posterior extremities, and then of the rest of the body, convulsions, dilatation of the pupils and general insensibility: 2*d*, Those which indicate disturbance in the organs of circulation; for example, the feeble, slow, and intermitting pulse, weak contractions of the heart immediately after death, and the impossibility of prolonging them, as may be done in sudden deaths from other causes, by artificial respiration: 3*d*, Lastly, those which depend on lesion of the alimentary canal, as the pains of the abdomen, nauseas, and vomitings, in those animals which were suffered to vomit. At one time it is the nervous system that is most remarkably affected, and at another the organs of circulation. Hence inflammation of the stomach and intestines, ought not to be considered as the immediate cause of death, by the greater number of cases of poisoning by arsenic. However, should an animal not sink under the first violence of the poison, if the inflammation has had time to be developed, there is no doubt that it may destroy life. Mr. Earl states, that a woman who had taken arsenic resisted the alarming symptoms which at first appeared, but died on the fourth day. On opening her body the mucous membrane of the stomach and intestines was ulcerated to a great extent. Authentic cases of poison are recorded, where no trace of inflammation was perceptible in the *primæ viæ*.

The effects of arsenic have been graphically represented by Dr. Black: 'The symptoms produced by a dangerous dose of arsenic begin to appear in a quarter by an hour, or not much longer, after it is taken. First sickness, and great distress at stomach, soon followed by thirst, and burning heat in the bowels. Then come on violent vomiting and severe colic pains, and excessive and painful purging. This brings on faintings, with cold sweats, and other signs of great debility. To this succeed painful cramps, and contractions of the legs and thighs, and extreme weakness, and death.' Similar results have followed the incautious sprinkling of schirrous ulcers with powdered arsenic, or the application of arsenical pastes. The following more minute specification of symptoms is given by Orfila: 'An austere taste in the mouth; frequent ptyalism; continual spitting; constriction of the *pharynx* and *œsophagus;* teeth set on edge; hiccups; nausea; vomiting of brown or bloody matter; anxiety; frequent fainting fits; burning heat at the *precordia;* inflammation of the lips, tongue, palate, throat, stomach; acute pain of stomach, rendering the mildest drinks intolerable; black stools of an indescribable fœtor; pulse frequent, oppressed, and irregular, sometimes slow and unequal; palpitation of the heart; *syncope;* unextinguishable thirst; burning sensation over the whole body, resembling a consuming fire; at times an icy coldness; difficult respiration; cold sweats; scanty urine, of a red or bloody appearance; altered expression of countenance; a livid circle round the eyelids; swelling and itching of the whole body, which becomes covered with livid spots, or with a miliary eruption; prostration of strength; loss of feeling, especially in the feet and hands; delirium, convulsions, sometimes accompanied with an insupportable priapism; loss of the hair; separation of the epidermis; horrible convulsions; and death.'

It is uncommon to observe all these frightful symptoms combined in one individual; sometimes they are altogether wanting, as is shown by the following case, related by M. Chaussier:—A robust man of middle age swallowed arsenious acid in large fragments, and died without experiencing other symptoms than slight *syncopes.* On opening his stomach, it was found to contain the arsenious acid in the very same state in which he had swallowed it. There was no appearance whatever of erosion or inflammation in the intestinal canal. Etmuller mentions a young girl's being poisoned by arsenic, and whose stomach and bowels were sound to all appearance, though the arsenic was found in them. In general, however, inflammation does extend along the whole canal, from the mouth to the *rectum.* The stomach and *duodenum* present frequently gangrenous points, eschars, perforations of all their coats; the villous coat in particular, by this and all other corrosive poisons, is commonly detached, as if it were scraped off or reduced into a paste of a reddish-brown colour. From these considerations we may conclude, that from the existence or non-existence of intestinal lesions, from the extent or seat of the symptoms alone, the physician should not venture to pronounce definitively on the fact of poisoning.

The result of Mr. Brodie's experiments on brutes teaches, that the inflammations of the intestines and stomach are more severe when the poison has been applied to an external wound, than when it has been thrown into the stomach itself.

The best remedies against this poison in the stomach, are copious draughts of bland liquids of a mucilaginous consistence, to inviscate the powder, so as to procure its complete ejection by vomiting. Sulphuretted hydrogen condensed in water, is the only direct antidote to its virulence; Orfila having found, that when dogs were made to swallow that liquid, after getting a poisonous dose of arsenic, they recovered, though their œsophagus was tied to prevent vomiting; but when the same dose of poison was administered in the same circumstances, without the sulphuretted water, that it proved fatal.

When the *viscera* are to be subjected after death to chemical investigation, a ligature ought to be thrown round the œsophagus and the beginning of the colon, and the intermediate stomach and intestines removed. Their liquid contents should be emptied into a basin; and thereafter a portion of hot water introduced into the stomach, and worked thoroughly up and down this *viscus*, as well as the intestines.

After filtration, a portion of the liquid should be concentrated by evaporation in a porcelain capsule, and then submitted to the proper reagents above described. We may also endeavour to extract from the stomach by digestion in boiling water, with a little ammonia, the arsenical impregnation, which has been sometimes known to adhere in minute particles with wonderful obstinacy. This precaution ought, therefore, to be attended to. The heat will dissipate the excess of ammonia in the above operation; whereas, by adding potassa or soda, as prescribed by the German chemists, we introduce animal matter in alkaline solution, which complicates the investigation.

The matters rejected from the patient's bowels before death, should not be neglected. These, generally speaking, are best treated by cautious evaporations to dryness; but we must beware of heating the residuum to 400°, since at that temperature, and perhaps a little under it, the arsenious acid itself sublimes.

Vinegar, hydroguretted alkaline sulphurets, and oils, are of no use as counterpoisons. Indeed, when the arsenic exists in substance in the stomach, even sulphuretted hydrogen water is of no avail, however effectually it neutralize an arsenious solution. Syrups, linseed tea, decoction of mallows, or tragacanth, and warm milk, should be administered as copiously as possible, and vomiting provoked by tickling the fauces with a feather. Clysters of a similar nature may be also employed. Many persons have escaped death by having taken the poison mixed with rich soups; and it is well known, that when it is prescribed as a medicine, it acts most beneficially when given soon after a meal. These facts have led to the prescription of butter and oils; the use of which is, however, not adviseable, as they screen the arsenical particles from more proper menstrua, and even appear to aggravate its virulence. Morgagni, in his great work on the seats and causes of disease, states, that at an Italian feast the dessert was purposely sprinkled over with arsenic instead of flour. Those of the guests who had previously ate and drank little, speedily perished; those who had their stomachs well filled, were saved by vomiting. He also mentions the case of three children who ate a vegetable soup poisoned with arsenic. One of them who took only two spoonfuls, had no vomiting, and died; the other two, who had eaten the rest, vomited, and got well. Should the poisoned patient be incapable of vomiting, a tube of caoutchouc, capable of being attached to a syringe, may be had recourse to The tube first serves to introduce the drink, and to withdraw it after a few instants.

The following tests of arsenic and corrosive sublimate have been lately proposed by Brugnatelli: Take the starch of wheat boiled in water until it is of a proper consistence, and recently prepared; to this add a sufficient quantity of iodine to make it of a blue colour; it is afterward to be diluted with pure water until it becomes of a beautiful azure. If to this, some drops of a watery solution of arsenic be added, the colour changes to a reddish hue, and finally vanishes. The solution of corrosive sublimate poured into iodine and starch, produces almost the same change as arsenic; but if to the fluid acted on by the arsenic we add some drops of sulphuric acid, the original blue colour is restored with more than its original brilliancy, while it does not restore the colour to the corrosive sublimate mixture.—*Ure's Chem. Dict.*

ARTEMISIA. (From a queen of that name, who first used it; or from Αρτεμις, Diana; because it was formerly used in the diseases of women, over whom she presided.) The name of a genus of plants in the Linnæan system. Class, *Syngenesia;* Order, *Polygamia superflua.*

Artemisia abrotanum. The systematic name for the *Abrotanum* of the pharmacopœias. *Abrotanum mas; Adonion; Adonium; Abrathan.* Common southernwood. *Artemisia—foliis setaceis ramosissimis* of Linnæus. A plant possessed of a strong, and, to most people, an agreeable smell; a pungent, bitter, and somewhat nauseous taste. It is supposed to stimulate the whole system, but more particularly the uterus. It is very rarely used unless by way of fomentation, with which intention the leaves are directed.

Artemisia absinthium. The systematic name for the *Absinthium vulgare* of the pharmacopœias. Common wormwood. Falsely called in our markets *Absinthium Romanum,* or Roman wormwood. *Absinthium Ponticum* of Dioscorides and Pliny, according to *Murray. Artemisia—foliis compositis multifidis floribus subglobosis pendulis; receptaculo villoso* of Linnæus. This plant is a native of Britain, and grows about rubbish, rocks, and sides of roads. The leaves of wormwood have a strong disagreeable smell: their taste is nauseous, and so intensely bitter as to be proverbial. The flowers are more aromatic and less bitter than the leaves, and the roots discover an aromatic warmth without bitterness. This species of wormwood may be considered the principal of the herbaceous bitters. Its *virtus,* (in the words of Bergius,) is antiputredinosa, antacida, anthelmintica, resolvens, tonica, spasmodica. And although it is now chiefly employed with a view to the two last-mentioned qualities, yet we are told of its good effects in a great variety of diseases, as intermittent fevers, hypochondriasis, obstructions of the liver and spleen, gout, calculi, scurvy, dropsy, worms, &c. Cullen thinks it is possessed of a narcotic power, and that there is in every bitter, when largely employed, a power of destroying the sensibility and irritability of the nervous system.

Externally, wormwood is used in discutient and antiseptic fomentations. This plant may be taken in powder, but it is more commonly preferred in infusion. The Edinburgh Pharmacopœia directs a tincture of the flowers, which is, in the opinion of Dr. Cullen, a light and agreeable bitter, and, at the same time, a strong impregnation of the wormwood.

Artemisia chinensis. Mugwort of China. *Moxa Japonica; Musia pattræ.* A soft lanuginous substance, called *Moxa,* is prepared in Japan, from the young leaves of this species of mugwort, by beating them when thoroughly dried, and rubbing them between the hands, till only the fine fibres are left. Moxa is celebrated in the eastern countries for preventing and curing many disorders, by being burnt on the skin; a little cone of it laid upon the part, previously moistened, and set on fire on the top, burns down with a temperate and glowing heat, and produces a dark-coloured spot, the ulceration of which is promoted by putting a little garlic, and the ulcer is either healed up when the eschar separates, or kept running for a length of time, as different circumstances may require.

Artemisia glacialis. Mountain wormwood. This is found on Alpine situations, and has similar virtues to common wormwood.

Artemisia judaica. The systematic name for the *Santonicum* of the pharmacopœias, according to some botanists. See *Artemisia santonica.*

Artemisia maritima. The systematic name for the *Absinthium maritimum* of the pharmacopœias. Sea wormwood. Falsely called in our markets, Roman wormwood. *Artemisia—foliis multipartitis, tomentosis; racemis cernuis; flosculis fœmineis ternis* of Linnæus. This plant grows plentifully about the sea-shore, and in salt marshes. The specific differences between it and the common wormwood, *artemisia absinthium,* are very evident. Its taste and smell are considerably less unpleasant than those of the common wormwood, and even the essential oil, which contains the whole of its flavour concentrated, is somewhat less ungrateful, and the watery extract somewhat less bitter than those of the common wormwood. Hence it is preferred, in those cases where the *Artemisia absinthium* is supposed to be too unpleasant for the stomach. A conserve of the tops of this plant was directed by the London pharmacopœia.

Artemisia pontica. The systematic name for the *Absinthium ponticum,* or Roman wormwood, not now used medicinally.

Artemisia rupestris. The systematic name for the *Genipi album* of the pharmacopœias. *Artemisia—foliis pinnatis; caulibus adscendentibus; floribus globosis, cermuis; receptaculo papposo.* It has a grateful smell, and is used in some countries in the cure of intermittents and obstructed catamenia.

Artemisia santonica. *Absinthium santonicum Alexandrinum; Sementina; Absinthium seriphium Ægyptium; Scheba Arabum; Zedoariæ semen; Xantolina; Lumbricorum semina; Cina; Semen contra, Semen sanctum; Artemisia Judaica.* The Tartarian southernwood or wormseed. *Artemisia—foliis caulinis linearibus, pinnato-multifidis; ramis indivisis, spicis secundis reflexis; floribus quinquefloris* of Linnæus. The seeds are small, light, and oval, composed of a number of thin membraneous coats of a yellowish-green colour, with a cast of brown, easily friable, upon being rubbed between the fingers, into a fine chaffy kind of substance. They are brought from the Levant; have a moderately strong and not agreeable smell, somewhat of the wormwood kind, and a very bitter subacrid taste. Their virtues are extracted both by watery and spirituous menstrua. They are esteemed to be stomachic, emmenagogue, and anthelmintic; but it is especially for the last-mentioned powers that they are now administered, and from their efficacy in this way they have obtained the name of wormseed. To adults the dose in substance is from one to two drachms, twice a day. Lewis thinks that the spirituous extract is the most eligible preparation of the santonicum, for the purposes of an anthelmintic.

Artemisia vulgaris. Mugwort. This plant, *Artemisia—foliis pinnatifidis, planis, incisis, subtus tomentosis; racemis simplicibus, recurvatis; floribus radio quinquefloro* of Linnæus, is slightly bitter, and, although in high esteem in former days, is now almost wholly forgotten.

Artemo'nium. (From *Artemon,* its inventor.) A collyrium, or wash for the eyes.

ARTE'RIA. (*Arteria, æ.* f.; from αηρ, air, and τηρεω, to keep; so called because the ancients believed they contained air only.) See *Artery.*

Arteri'aca. (From αρτηρια, an artery.) Medicines formerly used against disorders of the aspera arteria, or trachea.

Arteriæ adiposæ. The arteries which secrete the fat about the kidneys are so called. They are branches of the capsula and diaphragmatic, renal, and spermatic arteries.

Arteriæ venosæ. The four pulmonary veins were so called by the ancients.

Arterio'sus ductus. See *Ductus arteriosus.*

ARTERIO'TOMY. (*Arteriotomia, æ.* f.; from αρτηρια, an artery, and τεμνω, to cut.) The opening of an artery. This operation is frequently performed on the temporal artery.

A'RTERY. *Arteria.* A membraneous pulsating canal, that arises from the heart and gradually becomes less as it proceeds from it. Arteries are composed of three membranes; a common, or external; a muscular; and an internal one, which is very smooth. They are only two in number, the pulmonary artery, and the aorta, and these originate from the heart; the pulmonary artery from the right ventricle, and the aorta from the left: the other arteries are all branches of the aorta. Their termination is either in the veins, or in capillary exhaling vessels, or they anastomose with one another. It is by their means that the blood is carried from the heart to every part of the body, for nutrition, preservation of life, generation of heat, and the secretion of the different fluids. The action of the arteries, called the pulse, corresponds with that of the heart, and is effected by the contraction of their muscular, and great elasticity of their outermost coat.

A table of the Arteries.

All the arteries originate from the pulmonary artery and the aorta.

The *pulmonary artery* emerges from the right ventricle of the heart, soon divides into a right and left branch, which are distributed by innumerable ramifications through the lungs.

The *aorta* arises from the left ventricle of the heart, and supplies every part of the body with blood, in the following order.

a. It forms an *arch*.
b. It then descends along the spine; and,
c. It divides into the two *iliacs*.

a. The ARCH OF THE AORTA gives off three branches.
1. The *arteria innominata*, which divides into the *right carotid* and *right subclavian*.
2. The *left carotid*.
3. The *left subclavian*.

I The *carotids* are divided into *external* and *internal*.

The *external carotids* give off
1. The *thyroid*,
2. The *lingual*,
3. The *labial*,
4. The *inferior pharyngeal*,
5. The *occipital*,
6. The *posterior auris*,
7. The *internal maxillary*, from which the *spinous artery of the dura mater*, the *lower maxillary*, and *several branches about the palate and orbit* arise,
8. The *temporal*.

The *internal carotid* affords,
1. The *ophthalmic*,
2. The *middle cerebral*,
3. The *communicans*, which inosculates with the *vertebral*.

II. The *subclavians* give off the following branches.
1. The *internal mammary*, from which the *thymic*, *comes phrenici*, *pericardiac*, and *phrenico-pericardiac arteries* arise,
2. The *inferior thyroid*, which gives off the *tracheal*, *ascending thyroid*, and *transversalis humeri*,
3. The *vertebral*, which proceeds within the vertebræ, and forms within the cranium the *basilary artery*, from which the *anterior cerebelli*, the *posterior cerebri*, and *many branches about the brain*, are given off,
4. The *cervicalis profunda*,
5. The *cervicalis superficialis*,
6. The *superior intercostal*,
7. The *supra-scapular*.

As soon as the subclavian arrives at the arm-pit, it is called the *axillary artery;* and when the latter reaches the arm, it is called the *brachial*.

The *axillary artery* gives off,
1. *Four mammary arteries*,
2. The *sub-scapular*,
3. The *posterior circumflex*,
4. The *anterior circumflex*, which ramify about the shoulder-joint.

The *brachial artery* gives off,
1. *Many lateral branches*,
2. The *profunda humeri superior*,
3. The *profunda humeri inferior*,
4. The *great anastomosing artery*, which ramifies about the elbow-joint.

The *brachial artery* then divides, about the bend of the arm, into the *ulnar* and *radial arteries*, which are ramified to the ends of the fingers.

The *ulnar artery* gives off,
1. *Several recurrent branches*,
2. The *common interosseal*, of which the *dorsal ulnar*, the *palmaris profunda*, the *palmary arch*, and the *digitals*, are branches.

The *radial artery* gives off,
1. The *radial recurrent*,
2. The *superficialis volæ*, and then divides into the *palmaris profunda*, and the *digitals*.

b. The DESCENDING AORTA gives off,

In the breast,
1. The *bronchial*,
2. The *œsophageal*,
3. The *intercostals*,
4. The *inferior diaphragmatic*.

Within the abdomen,
1. The *cœliac*, which divides into three branches:
 1. The *hepatic*, from which are given off, before it reaches the liver,
  α. The *duodeno-gastric*, which sends off the *right gastro-epiploic* and the *pancreatico-duodenal*,
  β. The *pylorica superior hepatica;*
 2. The *coronaria ventriculi*,
 3. The *splenic*, which emits the *great* and *small pancreatics*, the *posterior gastric*, the *left gastro-epiploic*, and the *vasa brevia;*
2. The *superior mesenteric*,
3. The *emulgents*,
4. The *spermatics*,
5. The *inferior mesenteric*,
6. The *lumbar arteries*,
7. The *middle sacral*.

c. The aorta then bifurcates into the ILIACS, each of which divide into *external* and *internal*.

The *internal iliac*, called also *hypogastric*, gives off,
1. The *lateral sacrals*,
2. The *gluteal*,
3. The *ischiatic*,
4. The *pudica*, from which the *external hæmorrhoidal*, the *perineal*, and the *arteriæ penis* arise,
5. The *obturatory*.

The *external iliac* gives off, in the groin,
1. The *epigastric*,
2. The *circumflexia iliaca;*

It then passes under Poupart's ligament, and is called the *femoral artery;* and sends off,
1. The *profunda*,
2. The *ramus anastomoticus magnus*, which runs about the knee joint;

Having reached the ham, where it gives off some small branches, it is termed the *popliteal*. It then divides into the *anterior* and *posterior tibial*.

The *tibialis antica* gives off,
1. The *recurrent*,
2. The *internal malleolar*,
3. The *external malleolar*,
4. The *tarsal*,
5. The *metatarsal*,
6. The *dorsalis externa halicis*.

The *posterior tibial* sends off,
1. The *nutritia tibiæ*,
2. *Many small branches*,
3. The *internal plantar*,
4. The *external plantar*, from which an *arch* is formed, that gives off the *digitals of the toes*.

ARTHANI'TA. (From αρτος, bread; because it is the food of swine.) The herb sow-bread. See *Cyclamen Europeum*.

ARTHRE'MBOLUS. (From αρθρον, a joint, and εμβαλλω, to impel.) An instrument for reducing luxated bones.

ARTHRI'TIC. (*Arthriticus;* from αρθριτις, the gout.) Pertaining to the gout.

ARTHRITICA HERBA. The *Ægopodium podagraria*. and several other plants, were so called.

ARTHRI'TIS. (*Arthritis, tidis*, fœm.; from αρθρον, a joint: because it is commonly confined to the joints.) The gout. Dr. Cullen, in his Nosology, gives it the name of *podagra*, because he considers the foot to be the seat of idiophatic gout. It is arranged in the class *Pyrexiæ*, and order *phlegmasiæ*, and is divided into four species, the regular, atonic, retrocedent, and misplaced. See *Podagra*.

ARTHROCA'CE. (From αρθρον, a joint, and κακη, a disease.) An ulcer of the cavity of the bone.

ARTHRO'DIA. (*Arthrodia, æ.* f.; from αρθροω, to articulate.) A species of *diarthrosis*, or moveable connexion of bones, in which the head of one bone is received into the superficial cavity of another, so as to admit of motion in every direction, as the head of the humerus with the glenoid cavity of the scapula.

ARTHRODY'NIA. (*Arthrodynia, æ.* f.; from αρθρον, a joint, and οδυνη, pain.) Pain in a joint. It is one of the terminations of acute rheumatism. See *Rheumatismus*.

ARTHROPUO'SIS. (*Arthropuosis, is.* f.; from αρθρον, a joint, and πυον, pus.) *Arthropyosis*. A collection of pus in a joint. It is however frequently applied to other affections. See *Lumbar abscess*.

ARTHROSIA. (*Arthrosiæ;* from αρθροω, to articulate: whence *arthrosis*, *arthrites*.) The name of a genus of disease in Good's new classification, which embraces rheumatism, gout, and white swelling. See *Nosology*.

ARTHRO'SIS. (From αρθροω, to articulate, or join together.) Articulation.

ARTICHOKE. See *Cinara scolymus*.

Artichoke, French. See *Cinara scolymus*.

Artichoke, Jerusalem. See *Helianthus tuberosus.*

ARTICULA'R. (*Articularis;* from *articulus,* a joint.) Belonging to a joint.

ARTICULARIS MORBUS. A name given to a disease which more immediately infests the *articuli,* or joints. The morbus articularis is synonymous with the Greek word arthritis, and our gout.

ARTICULARIS VENA. A branch of the basilic vein is so called because it passes under the joint of the shoulder.

ARTICULATION. (*Articulatio;* from *articulus,* a joint.) The skeleton is composed of a great number of bones, which are all so admirably constructed, and with so much affinity to each other, that the extremity of every bone is perfectly adjusted to the end of the bone with which it is connected: and this connexion is termed their articulation. Anatomists distinguish three kinds of articulation; the first they name *Diarthrosis;* the second, *Synarthrosis;* and the third, *Amphiarthrosis;* which see, under their respective heads.

ARTICULA'TUS. Articulate; jointed. A term applied to roots, stems, leaves, &c., when they are apparently formed of distinct pieces united as if one piece grew out of another, so as to form a jointed, but connected whole: in the *Radix articulata,* radicals shoot out from each joint, as in the *Oxalis acetocella,* wood sorrel. The *Caulis articulata* is exemplified in the *Cactus flagelliformis* and *Lathyrus sylvestris;* the *Cactus opuntia* and *Cactus ficus indica* have articulate leaves. The *Oxalis acetosella* articulate leafstalks.

ARTICULUS. (From *artus,* a joint; from αρθρον.) 1. A joint. See *Articulation.*

2. Botanists apply this term to that part of the stalk of grasses which is intercepted, or lies between two knots; and also to the knot itself.

ARTI'SCUS. (From αρτος, bread.) A troch; so called because it is made like a little loaf.

ARTO'CREAS. (From αρτος, bread, and κρεας, flesh.) A nourishing food, made of bread and various meats, boiled together.—*Galen.*

ARTO'GALA. (From αρτος, bread, and γαλα, milk.) A cooling food made of bread and milk. A poultice.

ARTO'MELI. (From αρτος, bread, and μελι, honey.) A cataplasm made of bread and honey.—*Galen.*

A'RUM. (*Arum, i.* n.; from the Hebrew word *jaron,* which signifies a dart; so named because its leaves are shaped like a dart; or αρα, injury.) 1. The name of a genus of plants in the Linnæan system. Class, *Gynandria;* Order, *Polyandria.*

2. The pharmacopœial name of the common arum. See *Arum maculatum.*

ARUM DRACUNCULUS. The systematic name of the plant called, in English, dragon's wort, and many-leaved arum; *Dracunculus polyphyllus; Colubrina dracontia; Serpentaria gallorum; Erva de Sancta Maria; Gigarus serpentaria; Arum polyphyllum.* The roots and leaves of this plant are extremely acrimonious, more so than the *Arum maculatum,* with which it agrees in medicinal virtues.

ARUM MACULATUM. The systematic name for common arum, or wake-robin; the *arum* of the pharmacopœias. *Arum—acaule; foliis hastatis, integerrimis; spadice clavato* of Linnæus. Common arum or wake-robin. The root is the medicinal part of this plant, which, when recent, is very acrimonious; and, upon being chewed, excites an intolerable sensation of burning and prickling in the tongue, which continues for several hours. When cut in slices and applied to the skin, it has been known to produce blisters. This acrimony, however, is gradually lost by drying, and may be so far dissipated by the application of heat, as to leave the root a bland farinaceous aliment. In this state it has been made into a wholesome bread. It has also been prepared as starch. Its medicinal quality, therefore, resides wholly in the active volatile matter, and consequently the powdered root must lose much of its power, on being long kept. Arum is certainly a powerful stimulant, and, by promoting the secretions, may be advantageously employed in cachectic and chlorotic cases in rheumatic affections, and in various other complaints of phlegmatic and torpid constitutions; but more especially in a weakened or relaxed state of the stomach, occasioned by the prevalence of viscid mucus. If this root is given in powder, great care should be taken that it be young and newly dried, when it may be used in the dose of a scruple, or more, twice a day, but in rheumatisms, and other disorders requiring the full effect of this medicine, the root should be given in a recent state; and, to cover the insupportable pungency it discovers on the tongue, Dr. Lewis advises us to administer it in the form of emulsion, with gum-arabic and spermaceti, increasing the dose from ten grains to upwards of a scruple, three or four times a day. In this way, it generally occasioned a sensation of slight warmth about the stomach, and afterward, in the remoter parts, manifestly promoted perspiration, and frequently produced a plentiful sweat. Several obstinate rheumatic pains were removed by this medicine. The root answers quite as well as garlic for cataplasms, to be applied on the feet in deliriums. The London College, in their Pharmacopœia, 1788, ordered a conserve, in the proportion of half a pound of the fresh root to a pound and a half of double refined sugar, beat together in a mortar, which appears to be one of the best forms of exhibiting arum, as its virtues are destroyed by drying, and are not extracted by any menstruum. It may be given to adults in doses of a drachm.

ARUNDINACEUS. (From *arundo,* a reed.) Arundinaceous or reed-like.

ARUNDINACEÆ PLANTÆ. Arundinaceous plants. A name given to a class of plants by Ray, from their appearance.

ARUNDO. (*Arundo, inis,* f.; supposed to be derived from *areo,* because it soon becomes dry.) The name of a genus of plants in the Linnæan system. Class *Triandria;* Order, *Digynia.*

ARUNDO BAMBOS. The bamboo plant. The young shoots of this plant are prepared by the natives of both Indies with vinegar, garlic, pepper, &c. into excellent pickles, which promote the appetite and assist digestion. A substance called *Tabasheer* or *Tabachir,* which is a concretion of the liquor in the cavities of the cane, and extracted at certain seasons, is much esteemed as a medicine by the orientalists.

ARUNDO SACCHARIFERA. The name of the sugar-cane. See *Saccharum officinale.*

ARYTÆ'NO. Belonging to the arytænoid cartilage. Some muscles are so named because they are connected with this cartilage: they have also the terminal name of the part they go to; as *arytæno-epiglottideus.*

ARYTÆNO-EPIGLOTTIDEUS. A muscle of the epiglottis *Arytæno-Epiglottici* of Winslow. It is composed of a number of fibres running between the arytænoid cartilage and epiglottis. It pulls the side of the epiglottis towards the external opening of the glottis, and when both act, they pull it close upon the glottis.

ARYTÆNOI'D. (*Arytænoideus* and *Arytænoides;* from αρυταινα, a funnel, and ειδος, shape.) The name of some parts, from their being funnel-shapped.

ARYTÆNOID CARTILAGE. *Cartilago arytænoidea* The name of two cartilages of the larynx. See *Larynx.*

ARYTÆNOIDE'US. Applied to some muscles, vessels, nerves, &c.

ARYTÆNOIDEUS MAJOR. See *Arytænoideus transversus.*

ARYTÆNOIDEUS MINOR. See *Arytænoideus obliquus.*

ARYTÆNOIDEUS OBLIQUUS. A muscle of the glottis *Arytænoideus minor* of Douglas. It arises from the base of one arytænoid cartilage, and crossing its fellow, is inserted near the tip of the other arytænoid cartilage. This muscle is occasionally wanting; but when present, and both muscles act, their use is to pull the arytænoid cartilages towards each other.

ARYTÆNOIDEUS TRANSVERSUS. An azygos or single muscle of the glottis. *Arytænoideus major* of Douglas. It arises from the side of one arytænoid cartilage from near its articulation with the cricoid to near its tip. The fibres run across, and are inserted in the same manner into the other arytænoid cartilage Its use is to shut the glottis, by bringing the two arytænoid cartilages, with their ligaments, nearer to each other.

ASAFŒ'TIDA. (*Asafœtida, æ,* f.; from the Hebrew word *asa,* to heal.) See *Ferula.*

ASA'PHATUM. (From *a,* neg. and σαφης, clear, so called by reason of their minuteness.) An intercuta neous disorder, generated in the pores, like worms with black heads

Asa'phia. (From *a*, neg. and σαφης, clear.) A defect in utterance or pronunciation

ASARABACCA. See *Asarum Europæum.*

A'SARUM. (*Asarum*, *i.* n.; from *a*, neg. and σαιρω, to adorn; because it was not admitted into the ancient coronal wreaths.) 1. The name of a genus of plants in the Linnæan system. Class, *Dodecandria;* Order, *Monogynia.*

2. The pharmacopœial name of the asarabacca. See *Asarum Europæum.*

Asarum europæum. The systematic name of the asarabacca of the shops. *Nardus montana; Nardus rustica; Asarum—foliis reniformibus, obtusis, binis* of Linnæus. This plant is a native of England, but not very common. Its leaves are extremely acrid, and are occasionally used, when powdered, as a sternutatory. For this purpose, the leaves, as being less acrid than the roots, are preferred, and in moderate doses, not exceeding a few grains, snuffed up the nose, for several evenings, produce a pretty large watery discharge, which continues for several days together, by which headache, toothache, ophthalmia, and some paralytic and soporific complaints have been effectually relieved.

Prior to the introduction of ipecacuanha, the leaves and root of this plant were frequently employed on account of their emetic power: the dose of the dried leaves was 20 grains; of the dried roots 10 grains. As they were occasionally violent in their operation, they have fallen into disuse.

Asarum hypocistis. A parasitical plant which grows in warm climates, from the roots of the *Cistus.* The juice, *succus hypocistidis*, is a mild astringent, of no particular smell nor flavour. It has fallen into disuse.

ASBESTOS. *Asbestus.* A mineral of which there are five varieties, all more or less flexible and fibrous. 1. *Amianthus* occurs in very long, fine, flexible, elastic fibres, of a white, greenish, or reddish colour. It is somewhat unctuous to the touch, has a silky or pearly lustre, and is slightly translucent. Sectile; tough; sp. grav. from 1 to 2.3.

The ancients manufactured cloth out of the fibres of asbestos, for the purpose, it is said, of wrapping up the bodies of the dead, when exposed on the funeral pile. Several moderns have likewise succeeded in making this cloth, the chief artifice of which seems to consist in the admixture of flax and a liberal use of oil; both which substances are afterward consumed by exposing the cloth for a certain time to a red heat. Although the cloth of asbestos, when soiled, is restored to its primitive whiteness by heating in the fire, it is found, nevertheless, by several authentic experiments, that its weight diminishes by such treatment. The fibres of asbestos, exposed to the violent heat of the blow-pipe, exhibit slight indications of fusion; though the parts, instead of running together, moulder away, and part fall down, while the rest seem to disappear before the current of air. Ignition impairs the flexibility of asbestos in a slight degree.

2. *Common asbestos* occurs in masses of fibres of a dull greenish colour, and of a somewhat pearly lustre. Fragments splintery. It is scarcely flexible, and greatly denser than amianthus. It is more abundant than amianthus, and is found usually in serpentine, as at Portsoy, the Isle of Anglesea, and the Lizard in Cornwall. It was found in the limestone of Glentilt, by Dr. M'Culloch, in a pasty state, but it soon hardened by exposure to air.

3. *Mountain Leather* consists not of parallel fibres like the preceding, but interwoven and interlaced so as to become tough. When in very thin pieces it is called *mountain paper.* Its colour is yellowish-white, and its touch meagre. It is found at Wanlockhead, in Lanarkshire. Its specific gravity is uncertain.

4. *Mountain Cork*, or *Elastic Asbestos*, is, like the preceding, of an interlaced fibrous texture; is opaque, has a meagre feel and appearance, not unlike common cork, and like it, too, is somewhat elastic. It swims on water. Its colours are white, gray, and yellowish-brown; receives an impression from the nail; very tough; cracks when handled, and melts with difficulty before the blow-pipe.

5. *Mountain Wood*, or *Ligniform asbestos*, is usually massive, of a brown colour, and having the aspect of wood. Internal lustre glimmering Soft, sectile, and tough; opaque; feels meagre; fusible into a black slag. Sp. grav. 2.0. It is found in the Tyrol; Dauphiny; and in Scotland, at Glentilt, Portsoy, and Kildrumie.

Ascaloni'tes. A species of onion.

ASCA'RIDES. The plural of *ascaris.*

A'SCARIS. (*Ascaris, idis;* from ασκεω, to move about; so called from its continued troublesome motion.) The name of a genus of intestinal worms. There are several species of this genus. Those which belong to the human body are:—

1. *Ascaris vermicularis*, the thread or maw worm which is very small and slender, not exceeding half an inch in length; it inhabits the rectum.

2. *Ascaris bumbricoides*, the long and round worm which is a foot in length, and about the breadth of goose-quill.

ASCE'NDENS. (From *ad* and *scando*, to ascend. *Adscendens.* Ascending. Applied to muscles, leaves stalks, &c. from their direction; as *musculus obliquus ascendens*, *folium ascendens*, *caulis ascendens*, the leaves of the *geranium vitifolium* and stems of the *hedysarum onobrychis*, &c.

Ascendens obliquus See *Obliquus internus abdominus.*

A'scia. An axe or chisel. A simple bandage; so called from its shape in position.—*Galen.*

ASCIDIATUS. (From *ascidium*,) Ascidiate or pitcherform: a term applied to a leaf and other parts of plants which are so formed; the *folium ascidiatum* is seen in the *Nepenthes Distillatoria*, and in *Saracenia.*

ASCIDIUM. (From ασκιδιον, a small bottle.) The pitcher. A term introduced by Willdenow into botany to express a hollow foliaceous appendage, resembling a small pitcher. It is of rare occurrence, but has been found as a *caulinar*, *foliar*, and a *peduncular* or floral appendage.

1. The *caulinar* belongs to the Austalasian plant *Cephalotus follicularis.*.

2. The *foliar* is peculiar to the genus *Nepenthes.*

3. The *peduncular* on the *Surubea quianensis.*

ASCI'TES. (*Ascites*, *æ.* m.; from ασκος, a sack, or bottle; so called from its bottle-like protuberancy.) Dropsy of the belly. A tense, but scarcely elastic, swelling of the abdomen from accumulation of water Cullen ranks this genus of disease in the class *Cachexiæ*, and order, *Intumescentiæ.* He enumerates two species:

1. *Ascites abdominalis*, when the water is in the cavity of the peritonæum, which is known by the equal swelling of the parietes of the abdomen.

2. *Ascites saccatus*, or encysted dropsy, in which the water is encysted, as in the ovarium: the fluctuation is here less evident, and the swelling is at first partial.

Ascites is often preceded by loss of appetite, sluggishness, dryness of the skin, oppression at the chest, cough, diminution of the natural discharge of urine, and costiveness. Shortly after the appearance of these symptoms, a protuberance is perceived in the hypogastrium, which extends gradually, and keeps on increasing, until the whole abdomen becomes at length uniformly swelled and tense. The distension and sense of weight, although considerable, vary somewhat according to the posture of the body, the weight being felt the most on that side on which the patient lies, while, at the same time, the distention becomes somewhat less on the opposite side. In general, the practitioner may be sensible of the fluctuation of the water, by applying his left hand on one side of the abdomen, and then striking on the other side with his right. In some cases, it will be obvious to the ear. As the collection of water becomes more considerable, the difficulty of breathing is much increased, the countenance exhibits a pale and bloated appearance, an immoderate thirst, the skin is dry and parched, and the urine is very scanty, thick, high coloured, and deposits a lateritious sediment. With respect to the pulse, it is variable, being sometimes considerably quickened, and, at other times, slower than natural. The principal difficulty, which prevails in ascites, is the being able to distinguish, with certainty, when the water is in the cavity of the abdomen, or when it is in the different states of encysted dropsy. To form a just judgment, we should attend to the following circumstances:—When the preceding symptoms gave suspicion of a general hydropic diathesis; when, at the same time, some degree of dropsy appears in other parts of the body; and when, from its first appearance, the swelling has been equally diffused over the whole belly, we may generally presume that the water is in the cavity of the abdomen. But when an ascites has not been preceded by any remarkable cachectic state of the system, and when, at its beginning, the tumour and tension had appeared in one part of the belly more than another, there is reason to suspect an encysted dropsy. Even when the tension and tumour of the belly have become general, yet, if the system or the body in general appear to be little affected; if the patient's strength be little impaired; if the appetite continue pretty entire, and the natural sleep be little interrupted; if the menses in females continue to flow as usual: if there be yet no anasarca, or, though it may have already taken place, if it be still confined to the lower extremities, and there be no leucophlegmatic paleness or sallow colour in the countenance; if there be no fever, nor so much thirst and scarcity of urine as occur in a more general affection: then according as more of these different circumstances take place, there will be the stronger grounds for supposing the ascites to be of the encysted kind. The encysted form of the disease scarcely admits of a perfect cure, though its progress to a fatal termination is generally very slow; and the peritonæal dropsy is mostly very obstinate, depending usually on organic disease in the liver, or other abdominal viscera. The plan of treatment agrees very much with that of *anasarca*; which see. The operation of paracentesis should only be performed where the distension is very great, and the respiration or other important functions impeded; and it will often be better not to draw off the whole of the fluid at once; great care must be taken, too, to keep up sufficient pressure by a broad bandage over the abdomen; for even fatal syncope has arisen from the neglect of this. The contraction of the muscles will be promoted by friction. Cathartics are found more decidedly beneficial than in anasarca, where the bowels will bear their liberal use. Diuretics too, are of great importance in the treatment; and, among other means of increasing the flow of urine, long-continued gentle friction of the abdomen with oil has been sometimes very successful, probably by promoting absorption in the first instance; the only use of the oil seems to be that the friction is thereby better borne. In cases where visceral obstructions have led to the effusion, these must be removed, before a cure can be accomplished: and for this purpose mercury is the remedy most to be depended upon, besides that in combination with squill, or digitalis, it will often prove powerfully diuretic. Tonic medicines, a nutritious diet, and, if the complaint appears giving way, such exercise as the patient can take, without fatigue, with other means of improving the general health, ought not to be neglected.

ASCLEPI'ADES, a celebrated physician, born at Prusa, in Bithynia, who flourished somewhat before the time of Pompey. He originally taught rhetoric, but not meeting with success, applied himself to the study of medicine, in which he soon became famous from the novelty of his theory and practice. He supposes disease to arise from the motion of the particles of the blood and other fluids being obstructed by the straitness of the vessels, whence pain, fever, &c. ensued. He deprecated the use of violent remedies, as emetics and purgatives, but frequently employed clysters, when costiveness attended. In fevers, he chiefly relied on a complete abstinence from food or drink for three days or more; but when their violence abated, allowed animal food and wine. In pleurisies, and other complaints attended with violent pain, he prescribed bleeding; but in those of a chronic nature, depended principally on abstinence, exercise, baths, and frictions. None of his works remain at present. He is said to have pledged his reputation on the preservation of his own health, which he retained to a great age, and died at length from a fall.

ASCLE'PIAS. (From *Asclepias, adis.* f.; so named after its discoverer; or from *Æsculapius*, the god of medicine.) The name of a genus of plants in the Linnæan system. Class, *Pentandria;* Order, *Digynia.*

Asclepias syriaca. Syrian dog's bane. This plant is particularly poisonous to dogs, and also to the human species. Boiling appears to destroy the poison in the young shoots, which are then said to be esculent, and flavoured like asparagus.

Asclepias vincetoxicum. The systematic name for the *vincetoxicum* of the pharmacopœias. *Hermidinaria; Asclepias.* Swallow-wort; Tame poison The root of this plant smells, when fresh, somewhat of valerian; chewed, it imparts at first a considerable sweetness, which is soon succeeded by an unpleasant subacrid bitterness. It is given in some countries in the cure of glandular obstructions.

Ascle'pios. (From *Asclepias*, its inventor.) A dried smegna and collyrium described by Galen.

Asco'ma. (From ασκος, a bottle.) The eminence of the pubes at the years of maturity, so called from its shape.

ASCYROIDEÆ. A name given by Scoipoli to a class of plants which resemble the *Ascyrum*, St. Peter's worth.

A'sef. A pustule like a millet seed.

A'segon. *Asegen; Asogen.* Dragon's blood. See *Calamus rotang.*

ASE'LLIUS, Gaspar, of Cremona, born about the year 1580, taught anatomy at Paris with great reputation. In 1622, he discovered the lacteals in a dog opened soon after a meal, and noticed their valves, but supposed they went to the liver. These vessels, he candidly observes, had been mentioned by some of the earliest medical writers, but not described, nor their function stated; and not being noticed by any modern anatomist previously, the discovery is properly attributed to him. His death took place four years after, subsequent to which his dissertation on the subject was published by his friends.

ASH. See *Fraxinus excelsior.*

[Ashes. The residuum, after the incineration of wood. It is also applied to the alkali extracted by lixiviation, under the names of *Pot-ash*, and *Pearl-ash*, both of which are included in the mercantile title *Ashes.* A.]

Asiaticum balsamum. Balm of Gilead.

A'SINUS. The ass. A species of the genus *Equus.* Its milk is preferred to cow's and other kinds of milk, in phthisical cases, and where the stomach is weak; as containing less oleaginous particles, and being more easily converted into chyle. See *Milk, Asses.*

Asini'num lac. Asses' milk.

Asi'ti. (From α, neg. and σιτος, food.) *Asitia* Those are so called who take no food, for want of appetite.

A'sjogam. (Indian.) A tree growing in Malabar and the East Indies, the juice of which is used against the colic.

Aso'des. (Frem αδω, to nauseate.) A nausea or loathing, or a fever with much sense of heat and nausea.—*Aretæus.*

Aspadia'lis. A suppression of urine from an imperforated urethra.

Aspalathum. See *Lignum aloes.*

ASPALATHUS. (From α, and σπαω, because the thorns were not easily drawn out of the wounds they made.) The name of a genus of plants in the Linnæan system. Class, *Diadelphia;* Order, *Decandria.*

Aspalathus canariensis. The systematic name of the rose-wood tree, or *lignum rhodium* of the ancients. An essential oil is obtained from the roots, which is used principally as a perfume; but is an excellent cordial and carminative given internally. The best preparation is a tincture, made by macerating four ounces of the wood in a pint of rectified spirit.

ASPARAGIN. White transparent crystals, of a peculiar vegetable principle, which spontaneously form in asparagus juice which has been evaporated to the consistence of syrup. They are in the form of rhomboidal prisms, hard and brittle, having a cool and slightly nauseous taste. They dissolve in hot water, but sparingly in cold water, and not at all in alkohol. On being heated, they swell and emit penetrating vapours, which affect the eyes and nose like wood-smoke. Their solution does not change vegetable blues; nor is it affected by hydrosulphuret of potassa, oxalate of ammonia, acetate of lead, or infusion of galls. Lime disengages ammonia from it; though none is evolved by triturating it with potassa. The asparagus juice should be first heated to coagulate the albumen, then filtered and left to spontaneous evaporation for 15 or 20 days. Along with the asparagin crystals, others in needles of little consistency appear, analogous to *mannite*, from which the first can be easily picked out.—*Vauquelin and Robiquet. Annales de Chimie*, vol. lv. and *Nicholson's Journal*, 15.

ASPA'RAGUS. (*Asparagus*, *i.* m. Ασπαραγος, a young shoot before it unfolds its leaves.) 1. The name of a genus of plants in the Linnæan system. Class, *Hexandria*; Order, *Monogynia*. Asparagus.

2. The pharmacopœial name of the sparage. See *Asparagus officinalis*.

ASPARAGUS OFFICINALIS. The systematic name of the asparagus, the root of which has been esteemed as a diuretic. It is mostly employed as a food, but it contains very little nourishment. A peculiar vegetable principle, called asparagin, has been found in this plant. See *Asparagin*.

[ASPARAGUS STONE. This is one of the varieties of the phosphate of lime. Vauquelin found it to contain lime 54.28, phosphoric acid 45.72; by which analysis it appears to differ but little from Apatite, the other variety, which see. A.]

ASPA'SIA. (From α, for αμα, together, and σπαω, to draw.) A constrictive medicine for the pudendum muliebre. *Capivac.*

ASPER. Rough. Applied to parts which are rough, as *linea aspera*, &c.

In the language of botany, *scaber* and *asper* are used synonymously.

ASPER CAULIS. *Caulis scaber*. Scabrous stem; is when it is thickly covered with papillæ which are not visible, but can be felt when running the finger along it; as in *Galium aperine*, *Lithospermum arvense*, *Centaurea nigra*, &c.

ASPERA ARTERIA. (So called from the inequality of its cartilages.) See *Trachea*.

ASPERIFOLIÆ. (From *asper*, rough.) Rough-leaved plants. The name of a class and of an order of plants given by Boerhaave, Ray, Linnæus, &c.

ASPE'RULA. (A diminutive of *asper*, the seeds being rough.) The name of a genus of plants in the Linnæan system. Class, *Tetrandria*; Order, *Monogynia*.

ASPERULA ODORATA. The systematic name for the officinal *matrisylva*. Woodruff. It is a low umbelliferous plant, growing wild in woods and copses, and flowering in May. It hath an agreeable odour, which is much improved by moderate drying; the taste is a little austere. It imparts its flavour to vinous liquors; and is commended as a cordial and deobstruent remedy.

ASPHALTI'TIS. 1. A kind of trefoil.

2. The last vertebra of the loins.

ASPHALTUM. *Asphaltus*. This substance, likewise called *Bitumen Judaicum*, or Jews' Pitch, is a smooth, hard, brittle, black or brown substance, which breaks with a polish, melts easily when heated, and when pure burns without leaving any ashes. It is found in a soft or liquid state on the surface of the Dead sea, but by age grows dry and hard. The same kind of bitumen is likewise found in the earth in other parts of the world; in China; America, particularly in the island of Trinidad; and some parts of Europe, as the Carpathian hills, France, Neufchatel, &c.

According to Neumann, the asphaltum of the shops is a very different compound from the native bitumen; and varies, of course, in its properties, according to the nature of the ingredients made use of in forming it. On this account, and probably from other reasons, the use of asphaltum, as an article of the materia medica, is totally laid aside.

The Egyptians used asphaltum in embalming, under the name of mumia mineralis, for which it is well adapted. It was used for mortar at Babylon.

[This bitumen is dry and solid, and usually very brittle, but often too hard to receive an impression from the finger nail. In some varieties its fracture is more or less conchoidal, and shining with a resinous lustre; in others, it is earthy, or uneven, or nearly dull. The earthy variety is less hard than the others, and seems to be intermediate between Maltha and the harder kinds of Asphaltum.—*Cl. Min.*

The ancient bricks of Babylon, several of which I have had the best opportunities to examine, have a portion of bitumen adhering to them. This is black, and emits, by burning, a somewhat aromatic vapour. It appears to have lost none of its peculiar qualities, during the term of 3000 or 4000 years, since it was first incorporated as a cement, in the walls and towers constructed by the ancient inhabitants of Shinaar. The specimens I possess of modern bitumen from Bosrah, or its vicinity, are substantially the same with that used of old.

Asphaltum of St. Antonio, at the western extremity of Cuba, is compact, deep black, and capable of supporting a flame when heated and set on fire. That from Trinidad island is not so pure; but is stated to be much more abundant. Specimens from St. Stephens, near the Alabama river, were sent me by Mr Magoffin.—*Mitchill's Notes to Philips's Min.* A.]

ASPHO'DELUS. (*Asphodelus*, *i.* m. from ασπις, a serpent, and δειλος, fearful; because it destroys the venom of serpents: or from σποδελος, ashes, because it was formerly sown upon the graves of the dead. 1. The name of a genus of plants in the Linnæan system. Class, *Hexandria*; Order, *Monogynia*.

2. The pharmacopœial name of the daffodil. See *Asphodelus ramosus*.

ASPHODELUS RAMOSUS. The systematic name for the officinal, or branched asphodel. *Asphodelus*:—*caulenudo; foliis enciformibus, carinatis, lævibus*, of Linnæus. The plant was formerly supposed to be efficacious in the cure of sordid ulcers. It is now wholly laid aside.

ASPHY'XIA. (*Asphyxia*, *æ.* f.; from α, priv. and σφυξις, a pulse.) The state of the body, during life, in which the pulsation of the heart and arteries cannot be perceived. There are several species of asphyxia enumerated by different authors. See *Syncope*.

ASPIDI'SCUS. (From ασπις, a buckler.) The sphincter muscle of the anus was formerly so called from its shape.—*Cælius Aurelianus*.

[ASPINWALL, WILLIAM, M. D. was born in Brookline, Mass., on the 23d of May, (old style,) 1743. His ancestors emigrated from England about the year 1630. He was fitted for College by the Rev. Amos Adams, minister of Roxbury, and was graduated at Harvard University, in 1764. It was the personal interest which he took in the revolutionary contest, acting upon a mind deeply imbued with a sense of his country's wrongs, that gave strength and tone to his sentiments in after life. Dr. Aspinwall's language on political subjects was bold and strong, his creed being that of a democratic republican. In the unhappy scenes of party excitement, he unwaveringly adhered to what he deemed original and fundamental principles; but he aimed to preserve a good conscience, and to do justice to the honest opinions, the pure motives, and undoubted integrity of his opponents. He was not a political persecutor; and, when he was in the councils of the State, resolutely declined acting with his coadjutors, who were disposed to drive from office incumbents, whose only fault was what they deemed political heresy.

After the death of the eminent and distinguished Dr. Zabdiel Boylston, the first inoculator of small-pox in America, Dr. Aspinwall established himself in that undertaking, and erected hospitals for that purpose in Brookline. Perhaps no practitioner in the United States ever inoculated so many persons, or acquired such skill and celebrity in treating this malignant disease, as Dr. Aspinwall. Besides his practice in this disorder when it generally spread, he was allowed, after the year 1788, to keep a hospital open at all times, to which great numbers resorted, and from which they returned with warm expressions of satisfaction. He continued in the successful treatment of this disease, till the general introduction of vaccine inoculation. He had made ample accommodation for enlarged practice, and established what might have been justly deemed a sure foundation for prosperity, when vaccine inoculation was first introduced. He well knew that if vaccination possessed the virtues ascribed to it, his schemes of fortune and usefulness arising from inoculation at his hospital, were ruined; that he should be involved in loss, and his anticipations of fortune would be blasted. But as an honest man and faithful physician, he deemed it his duty to inquire into the efficacy of the novel substitute. With the utmost alacrity, therefore, he gave the experiment a fair trial, promptly acknowledged its efficacy, and relinquished his own establishment. The foregoing is corroborated by the following statement, recently made by Dr. Waterhouse, in the Medical Intelligencer

"The late Dr. Aspinwall, a man of great sagacity, and uncommonly well grounded in the principles of his profession, gave evidence of it on the first sight of a vaccine pustule. I had invited all the elder physicians of Boston, and the vicinity of Cambridge, to see the first vaccine pustules ever raised in the new world. They gave them the ordinary inspection on the skin; all but Dr. Aspinwall, whose attention was rivetted on the pustule, its areola, and efflorescence. He came a second time, and viewed the inoculated part in every light, and reviewed it, and seemed loath to leave the sight of it. He seemed wrapped in serious thought, and said repeatedly—'This pustule is so like small-pox, and yet it is not small-pox, that should it, on scabbing, take out a portion of the true skin, so as to leave an indelible mark or pit behind, I shall be ready to conclude that it is a mild species of small-pox, hitherto unknown here.' He had been in the habit of examining the small-pox pimple and pustule through glasses, to know if it '*had taken;*' and he remarked, that they were peculiar, *unique*, and unlike any other eruption he ever saw; but that this *kine-pock* came the nearest to it. Some time after, I gave him a portion of the virus to make his own experiments, and observe the progress of its inoculation, and coincidence of the constitutional symptoms; when he observed, that its progress, febrile affection, and mode of scabbing, were *very like* small-pox, and so of the indelible mark left on the arm; yet, throughout the whole visible affection, *different*. To crown the whole of his honourable conduct, he some time after took all those of my family whom I had vaccinated, into his small-pox hospital, the only licensed one in the state, and there tested them to his satisfaction, and one to the very verge of rigid experiment: and then he said to me and others—'*This new inoculation of yours is no sham. As a man of humanity, I rejoice in it; although it will take from me a handsome annual income.*' His conduct throughout was so strongly marked with superior intelligence, generosity, and honour, as to excite my esteem and respect; and I accordingly dedicate this effusion of gratitude to the memory of the Hon. William Aspinwall, M. D.; a gentleman respectable in public life as a counsellor, and an honour to his profession as a physician."—*Thach. Med. Biog.* A.]

ASPLE'NIUM. (*Asplenium, ii.* n.; from *α*, priv. σπλην, the spleen; because it was supposed to remove disorders of the spleen.) The name of a genus of plants in the Linnæan system. Class, *Cryptogamia;* Order, *Filices.*

ASPLENIUM CETERACH. The systematic name of the herb spleenwort. Miltwaste. *Scolopendria vera; Dorodilla.* This small bushy plant, *Asplenium—frondibus pinnatifidis, lobis alternis confluentibus obtusis* of Linnæus, grows upon old walls and rocks. It has an herbaceous, mucilaginous, roughish taste, and is recommended as a pectoral. In Spain it is given, with great success, in nephritic and calculous diseases.

ASPLENIUM RUTA MURARIA. The systematic name for the *ruta muraria* of the pharmacopœias. It is supposed by some to possess specific virtues in the cure of ulcers of the lungs, and is exhibited in the form of decoction.

ASPLENIUM SCOLOPENDRIUM. The systematic name for the *scolopendrium* of the pharmacopœias. *Phillitis; Lingua cervina.* Harts-tongue. This indigenous plant, *Asplenium—frondibus simplicibus, cordato lingulatis, integerrimis; stipitibus hirsutis* of Linnæus: grows on most shady banks, walls, &c. It has a slightly astringent and mucilaginous sweetish taste. When fresh and rubbed, it imparts a disagreeable smell. Harts-tongue, which is one of the *five capillary* herbs, was formerly much used to strengthen the viscera, restrain hæmorrhages and alvine fluxes, and to open obstructions of the liver and spleen, and for the general purposes of demulcents and pectorals.

ASPLENIUM TRICHOMANES. The systematic name for the *trichomanes* of the pharmacopœias. Common maiden-hair or spleenwort. *Asplenium—frondibus pinnatis, pinnis subrotundis, crenatis* of Linnæus. This plant is admitted into the Edinburgh Pharmacopœia: the leaves have a mucilaginous, sweetish, subastringent taste, without any particular flavour: they are esteemed useful in disorders of the breast, being supposed to promote the expectoration of tough phlegm, and to open obstructions of the viscera.

ASS. See *Asinus*

Ass's milk. See *Asinus.*

ASSABA. A shrub found on the coast of Guinea, the leaves of which are supposed to disperse buboes.

ASSAFŒ'TIDA. See *Ferula assafœtida.*

ASSARABA'CCA. See *Asarum Europeum.*

ASSA'RIUM. A Roman measure of twelve ounces.

ASSARTHRO'SIS. Articulation.

ASSAY. Essay. This operation consists in determining the quantity of valuable or precious metal contained in any mineral or metallic mixture, by analyzing a small part thereof. The practical difference between the analysis and the assay of an ore, consists in this: The analysis, if properly made, determines the nature and quantities of all the parts of the compound; whereas the object of the assay consists in ascertaining how much of the particular metal in question may be contained in a certain determinate quantity of the material under examination. Thus, in the assay of gold or silver, the baser metals are considered as of no value or consequence; and the problem to be resolved is simply, how much of each is contained in the ingot or piece of metal intended to be assayed.

ASSIMULA'TION. (*Assimilatio*, from *ad*, and *similis*, to make like to.) The conversion of the food into nutriment.

ASSISTE'NTES. (From *ad*, and *sisto*, to stand near.) A name of the prostate glands, so called because they lie near the bladder.

ARSO'DES. (From ασαομαι, to nauseate, or from *assare*, to burn.) *Asodes.* A continual fever, attended with a loathing of food.

A'STACUS. (*Astacus, i.* m.; from *α*, neg. and ςαζω, to distil; so called from the hardness and dryness of its shell.) The name of a genus of shell-fish.

ASTACUS FLUVIATILIS. The officinal crevis, or cray-fish. See *Cancer astacus.*

ASTACUS MARINUS. The lobster. See *Cancer gammarus.*

A'STAPSIS. (From ςαφις, uva passa.) A raisin.

ASTERA'NTIUM. (From αςηρ, a star.) The pellitory; so called from its star-like form. See *Anthemis pyrethrum.*

ASTERICUM. (From the star-like appearance of the flowers.) The pellitory. See *Anthemis pyrethrum.*

ASTHE'NIA. (From *α*, priv. and σθενος, strength.) Extreme debility. The asthenic diseases form one great branch of the Brunonian arrangement.

ASTHENOLOGY. (*Asthenologia, æ.* f.; from *α*, priv. and σθενος, strength, and λογος, a treatise.) The doctrine of diseases arising from debility. The disciples of the Brunonian school, as they denominate themselves, maintain peculiar opinions on this subject

A'STHMA. (*Asthma, matis*, neut.: from ασθμαζω to breathe with difficulty.) Difficult respiration returning at intervals, with a sense of stricture across the breast, and in the lungs; a wheezing hard cough, at first, but more free towards the close of each paroxysm, with a discharge of mucus, followed by a remission. It is ranked by Cullen in the class *Neurosis*, and order *Spasmi.* There are, according to him, three species of asthma:—

1. *Asthma spontaneum*, when without any manifest cause.

2. *Asthma plethoricum*, when it arises from plethora

3. *Asthma exanthematicum*, originating from the repulsion of some acrid humour.

Asthma rarely appears before the age of puberty, and seems to attack men more frequently than women, particularly those of a full habit, in whom it never fails, by frequent repetition, to occasion some degree of emaciation. In some instances, it arises from an hereditary predisposition, and in many others, it seems to depend upon a particular constitution of the lungs. Dyspepsia always prevails, and appears to be a very prominent feature in the predisposition. Its attacks are most frequent during the heats of summer, in the dog-days, and in general commence about midnight. On the evening preceding an attack of asthma, the spirits are often much affected, and the person experiences a sense of fulness about the stomach, with lassitude, drowsiness, and a pain in the head. On the approach of the succeeding evening, he perceives a sense of tightness and stricture across the breast, and a sense of straitness in the lungs, impeding respiration. The difficulty of breathing continuing to increase for some length of time, both inspiration and expiration are performed slowly, and with a wheezing noise; the speech becomes difficult and uneasy, a propensity to coughing succeeds, and the patient can no longer remain in a horizontal position, being as it were threatened with immediate suffocation. These symptoms usually continue till towards the approach of morning, and then a remission commonly takes place; the breathing becomes less laborious and more full, and the person speaks and coughs with greater ease. If the cough is attended with an expectoration of mucus, he experiences much relief, and soon falls asleep. When he awakes in the morning, he still feels some degree of tightness across his breast, although his breathing is probably more free and easy, and he cannot bear the least motion, without rendering this more difficult and uneasy; neither can he continue in bed, unless his head and shoulders are raised to a considerable height. Towards evening, he again becomes drowsy, is much troubled with flatulency in the stomach, and perceives a return of the difficulty of breathing, which continues to increase gradually, till it becomes as violent as on the night before. After some nights passed in this way, the fits at length moderate, and suffer more considerable remissions, particularly when they are attended by a copious expectoration in the mornings, and this continues from time to time throughout the day; and the disease going off at last, the patient enjoys his usual rest by night, without further disturbance. The pulse is not necessarily affected in this disease, though often quickened by the difficulty of breathing; and sometimes slight pyrexia attends. In plethoric habits, the countenance is flushed and turgid during the fit; but in others rather pale and shrunk: in the former, too, some difficulty of breathing and wheezing usually remain in the interval; in others the recovery is more complete. On this is founded the common distinction of asthma into the humid, pituitous, or catarrhal, and the dry, spasmodic, or nervous forms. The exciting causes are various:—accumulation of blood, or viscid mucus in the lungs, noxious vapours, a cold and foggy atmosphere, or a close hot air, the repulsion of eruptions, or other metastatic diseases, flatulence, accumulated fæces, violent passions, organic diseases in the thoracic viscera, &c. Sometimes the fits return at pretty regular periods; and it is generally difficult to obviate future attacks, when it has once occurred: but it often continues to recur for many years, and seldom proves fatal, except as inducing hydrothorax, phthisis, &c. The treatment must vary according to the form of the disease. In young persons of a plethoric habit, with great dyspnœa, a flushed countenance, accelerated pulse, &c. the abstraction of blood will be found to afford marked relief; but under opposite circumstances, it might be highly injurious, and we should always avoid repeating it unnecessarily. In ambiguous cases, cupping may be preferred, or leeches to the chest, with blisters. Mild cathartics should also be employed; or where costiveness appears to induce the fits, those of a more active nature. Nauseating emetics are of considerable service, especially where the patient is distressed with viscid mucus, not only by promoting perspiration and expectoration, but also by their antispasmodic power, the return of a paroxysm may often be prevented by their timely use. Squill combined with ipecacuanha is one of the best forms. Where the disease is of the purely spasmodic character, opium will be found the most powerful palliative remedy, especially if combined with æther, though it unfortunately loses some of its power by repetition; the fœtid gum resins are also useful, particularly where the bowels are torpid; and other antispasmodics may be occasionally employed. The practice of smoking, or chewing tobacco, has sometimes appeared extremely beneficial; and a cup of strong coffee has often afforded speedy relief. Means should also be employed for strengthening the system; and where there appears a tendency to serous effusion, digitalis may be very useful. But by far the most important part of the treatment consists in obviating or removing the several exciting causes, whether operating on the lungs immediately, or through the medium of the primæ viæ, &c. Individual experience can alone ascertain what state of the atmosphere as to temperature, dryness, purity, &c. shall be most beneficial to asthmatics, though a good deal depends on habit in this respect: but a due regulation of this, as well as of the diet, and other parts of regimen, will usually afford more permanent relief than any medicines we can employ.

A'STITES. (From *ad*, and *sto*, to stand near.) A name given by the ancients to the prostate glands, because they are situated near the bladder.

ASTRA'GALUS. (*Astragalus*, *i*. m.; Αςραγαλος, a cockle, or die; because it is shaped like the die used in ancient games.) 1. The ankle-bone; a bone of the *tarsus*, upon which the tibia moves. Also called the sling-bone, or first bone of the foot. *Ballistæ os; aristrios; talus; quatrio; tetroros; cavicula; cavilla; diabebos; peza.* It is placed posteriorly and superiorly in the tarsus, and is formed of two parts, one large, which is called its body, the other small, like a process. The part where these two unite is termed the neck.

2. The name of a genus of plants in the Linnæan system. Class, *Diadelphia;* Order, *Decandria.*

ASTRAGALUS EXCAPUS. Stemless milk-vetch. The root of this plant, *Astragalus acaulis excapus;—leguminibus lunatis; foliis villosis* of Linnæus, is said to cure confirmed syphilis, especially when in the form of nodes and nocturnal pains.

ASTRAGALUS TRAGACANTHA. The former systematic name for the plant which affords the gum tragacanth. See *Astragalus verus.*

ASTRAGALUS VERUS. Goat's thorn. Milk-vetch. *Spina hirci; Astragalus tragacantha; Astragalus aculeatus.* We are indebted to a French traveller, of the name of Olivier, for the discovery that the gum tragacanth of commerce, is the produce of a species of astragalus not before known. He describes it under the name of *astragalus verus*, being different both from *A. tragacantha* of Linnæus, and from the *A. gummifera* of Labillardiere. It grows in the North of Persia. Gum-tragacanth, or gum dragant, or dragon, (which is forced from this plant by the intensity of the solar rays, is concreted into irregular lumps or vermicular pieces, bent into a variety of shapes, and larger or smaller proportions, according to the size of the wound from which it issues,) is brought chiefly from Turkey, in irregular lumps, or long vermicular pieces bent into a variety of shapes: the best sort is white, semi-transparent, dry, yet somewhat soft to the touch.

Gum-tragacanth differs from all the other known gums, in giving a thick consistence to a much larger quantity of water; and in being much more difficultly soluble, or rather dissolving only imperfectly. Put into water, it slowly imbibes a great quantity of the liquid, swells into a large volume, and forms a soft but not fluid mucilage; if more water be added, a fluid solution may be obtained by agitation but the liquor looks turbid and wheyish, and on standing, the mucilage subsides, the limpid water on the surface retaining little of the gum. Nor does the admixture of the preceding more soluble gums promote its union with the water, or render its dissolution more durable: when gum-tragacanth and gum-arabic are dissolved together in water, the tragacanth separates from the mixture more speedily than when dissolved by itself.

Tragacanth is usually preferred to the other gums for making up troches, and other like purposes, and is supposed likewise to be the most effectual as a medicine; but on account of its imperfect solubility, is unfit for liquid forms. It is commonly given in powder, with the addition of other materials of similar intention; thus, to one part of gum-tragacanth are added one of gum-arabic, one of starch, and six of sugar.

According to Bucholtz, gum-tragacanth is composed of 57 parts of a matter similar to gum-arabic, and 43 parts of a peculiar substance, capable of swelling in cold water without dissolving, and assuming the appearance of a thick jelly. It is soluble in boiling water, and then forms a mucilaginous solution.

The demulcent qualities of this gum are to be considered as similar to those of gum-arabic. It is seldom given alone, but frequently in combination with more powerful medicines, especially in the form of troches, for which it is peculiarly well adapted: it gives name to an officinal compound powder, and was an ingredient in the compound powder of cerusse.

ASTRA'NTIA. (From αστρον, *astrum*, a star; so called from the star-like shape of its flowers.) The name of a genus of plants in the Linnæan system. Class, *Pentandria;* Order, *Dyginia.*

Astrantia major. *Astrantia vulgaris.*

Astrantia nigra. The herb sanicle master-wort. A rustic purge in the time of Gerard.

A'strape. (From ἀστράπτω, to corruscate.) Lightning. Galen reckons it among the remote causes of epilepsy.

ASTRI'CTUS. (From *astringo*, to bind.) When applied to the belly, it signifies costiveness; thus, *alvus astricta.*

ASTRI'NGENT. (*Astringens;* from *astringo*, to constringe.) Adstringent. That which, when applied to the body, renders the solids denser and firmer, by contracting their fibres, independently of their living, or muscular power. Astringents thus serve to diminish excessive discharges; and by causing greater compression of the nervous fibrillæ, may lessen morbid sensibility or irritability. Hence they may tend indirectly to restore the strength, when impaired by these causes. The chief articles of this class are the acids, alum, lime-water, chalk, certain preparations of copper, zinc, iron, and lead; the gallic acid, which is commonly found united with the true astringent principle, was long mistaken for it. Seguin first distinguished them, and, from the use of this principle in tanning skins, has given it the name of *tannin.* Their characteristic differences are, the gallic acid forms a black precipitate with iron; the astringent principle forms an insoluble compound with albumen.

ASTRONO'MY. (*Astronomia;* from ἄστρον, a star, and νόμος, a law.) The knowledge of the heavenly bodies. Hippocrates ranks this and astrology among the necessary studies of a physician.

ASTRUC, John, a learned physician, born in France, 1684. He studied and took his degrees at Montpelier, and became afterward a professor there. In 1729, he was appointed physician to the king of Poland, but soon returned to his native country, was made consulting physician to the French king, and professor of medicine at Paris, where he attained great celebrity. He was author of numerous medical and philosophical works, but especially one "on Venereal Diseases," which deservedly became extremely popular, and was translated into various modern languages. He lived to the advanced age of 82.

ATA'XIA. (From α, neg. and τάσσω, to order.) Want of regularity in the symptoms of a disease, or of the functions of an animal body.

ATE'CNIA. (From α, neg. and τίκτω, to bring forth.) Venereal impotency: inability to procreate children.

ATHAMANTA. (*Athamanta, æ.* fœm; so named from Athamas in Thessaly.) The name of a genus of plants in the Linnæan system. Class, *Pentandria;* Order, *Digynia.*

Athamanta cretensis. The systematic name for the *daucus creticus* of the pharmacopœias. *Myrrhus annua.* Candy carrot. The seeds of this plant, *Athamanta—foliolis linearibus planis, hirsutis; petalis bipartitis; seminibus oblongis hirsutis*, of Linnæus, are brought from the isle of Candy: they have an aromatic smell, and a slightly-biting taste; and are occasionally employed as carminatives, and diuretics in diseases of the primæ viæ and urinary passages.

Athamanta oreoselinum. The systematic name for the officinal *oreoselinum.* Black mountain parsley. The root and seed of this plant, *Athamanta--foliolis divaricatis* of Linnæus, as well as the whole herb, were formerly used medicinally Though formerly in so high estimation as to obtain the epithet of *polychresta*, this plant is seldom used in the practice of the present day. An extract and tincture prepared from the root were said to be attendant, aperient, deobstruent, and lithontriptic. The oil obtained by distillation from the seed was esteemed to allay the toothache; and the whole was recommended as an antiscorbutic and corroborant.

ATHAMANTICUM. See *Æthusa meum.*

ATHANA'SIA. (From α, priv. and θάνατος, death; so called because its flowers do not wither easily.) 1. The immortal plant. A name given to tansy; because when stuffed up the nose of a dead corpse, it is said to prevent putrefaction. See *Tanacetum vulgare.*

2. It means also immortality.

3. The name of an antidote of Galen, and another of Oribasius.

4. It is the name also of a collyrium described by Aëtius, and of many other compositions.

A'thara. (From ἀθήρ, corn.) A panada, or pap for children, made of bruised corn.

ATHERO'MA. (*Atheroma, atis,* n. Ἀθήρωμα, pulse pap.) An encysted tumour that contains a soft substance of the consistence of a poultice.

ATHRIX. (Ἀθριξ, *debilis*, weak.)

1. Weakness.

2. (From α, *priv.* and θρίξ, a pair.) Baldness.

ATHY'MIA. (From α, neg. and θυμός, courage.)

1. Pusillanimity.

2. Despondency or melancholy.

A'TLAS. (*Atlas, antis,* m.; from Ἀτλάω, to sustain, because it sustains the head; or from the fable of Atlas, who was supposed to support the world upon his shoulders.) The name of the first vertebra This vertebra differs very much from the others. See *Vertebræ.* It has no spinous process which would prevent the neck from being bent backwards, but in its place it has a small eminence. The great foramen of this is much larger than that of any other vertebra Its body, which is small and thin, is, nevertheless, firm and hard. It is somewhat like a ring, and is distinguished into its *great arch*, which serves in the place of its body, and its *small posterior arch.* The atlas is joined superiorly to the head by ginglymus; and inferiorly, to the second cervical vertebra, by means of the inferior oblique processes, and the odontoid process by trochoides.

ATMOMETER. The name of an instrument to measure the quantity of exhalation from a humid surface in a given time.

A'TMOSPHERE. (*Atmosphera, æ.* f.; from ἀτμός vapour, and σφαῖρα, a globe.) The elastic invisible fluid which surrounds the earth to an unknown height, and encloses it on all sides. Neither the properties nor the composition of the atmosphere, seem to have occupied much the attention of the ancients. Aristotle considered it as one of the four elements, situated between the regions of *water* and *fire*, and mingled with two *exhalations*, the *dry* and the *moist;* the first of which occasioned thunder, lightning, and wind; while the second produced rain, snow, and hail.

The opinions of the ancients were vague conjectures, until the matter was explained by the sagacity of Hales, and of those philosophers who followed his career.

Boyle proved beyond a doubt, that the atmosphere contained two distinct substances:—

1. An elastic fluid distinguished by the name of *air.*
2. Water in a state of vapour.

Besides these two bodies, it was supposed that the atmosphere contained a great variety of other substances which were continually mixing with it from the earth, and which often altered its properties, and rendered it noxious or fatal. Since the discovery of carbonic acid gas by Dr. Black, it has been ascertained that this elastic fluid always constitutes a part of the atmosphere.

The constituent parts of the atmosphere, therefore, are:—

1. Air. 2. Water. 3. Carbonic acid gas. 4. Unknown bodies.

1. For the properties, composition, and account of the first, see *Air.*

2. *Water.*—That the atmosphere contains water, has been always known. The rain and dew which so often precipitate from it, the clouds and fogs with which it is often obscured, and which deposite moisture on all bodies exposed to them, have demonstrated its existence in every age. Even when the atmosphere is perfectly transparent, water may be extracted from it in abundance by certain substances. Thus, if concentrated sulphuric acid be exposed to air, it gradually attracts so much moisture, that its weight is increased more than three times: it is converted into diluted acid, from which the water may be separated by distillation. Substances which have the property of abstracting water from the atmosphere, have received the epithet of *hygroscopic*, because they point out the presence of that water. Sulphuric acid, the fixed alkalies, muriate of lime, nitrate of lime, and, in general, all deliquescent salts, possess this property. The greater number of animal and vegetable bodies likewise possess it. Many of them take water from moist air, but give it out again to the air when dry. These bodies

augment in bulk when they receive moisture, and diminish again when they part with it. Hence some of them have been employed as *hygrometers*, or measures of the quantity of moisture contained in the air around them. This they do by means of the increase or diminution of their length, occasioned by the addition or abstraction of moisture. This change of length is precisely marked by means of an index. The most ingenious and accurate hygrometers are those of Saussure and Deluc. In the first, the substance employed to mark the moisture is a human hair, which by its contractions and dilatations is made to turn round an index. In the second, instead of a hair, a very fine thin slip of whalebone is employed. The scale is divided into 100°. The beginning of the scale indicates extreme dryness, the end of it indicates extreme moisture. It is graduated by placing it first in air made as dry as possible by means of salts, and afterward in air saturated with moisture. This gives the extremes of the scale, and the interval between them is divided into 100 equal parts.

The water, which constitutes a component part of the atmosphere, appears to be in the state of vapour, and chemically combined with air in the same manner as one gas is combined with another. As the quantity of the water contained in the atmosphere varies considerably, it is impossible to ascertain its amount with any degree of accuracy.

3. *Carbonic acid gas.*—The existence of carbonic gas as a constituent part of the atmosphere, was observed by Dr. Black immediately after he had ascertained the nature of that peculiar fluid. If we expose a pure alkali or alkaline earth to the atmosphere, it is gradually converted into a carbonate by the absorption of carbonic acid gas. This fact, which had been long known, rendered the inference that carbonic acid gas existed in the atmosphere unavoidable, as soon as the difference between a pure alkali and its carbonate had been ascertained to depend upon that acid. Not only alkalies and alkaline earths absorb carbonic acid when exposed to the air, but several of the metallic oxydes also.

Carbonic acid gas not only forms a constituent part of the atmosphere near the surface of the earth, but at the greatest heights which the industry of man has been able to penetrate. Saussure found it at the top of Mount Blanc, the highest point of the old continent; a point covered with eternal snow, and not exposed to the influence of vegetables or animals. Lime-water, diluted with its own weight of distilled water, formed a pellicle on its surface after an hour and three-quarters exposure to the open air on that mountain; and slips of paper moistened with pure potash, acquired the property of effervescing with acids after being exposed an hour and a half in the same place. This was at a height no less than 15,668 feet above the level of the sea. Humboldt has more lately ascertained the existence of this gas in air, brought by Mr. Garnerin from a height not less than 4280 feet above the surface of the earth, to which height he had risen in an air-balloon. This fact is a sufficient proof that the presence of carbonic acid in air does not depend upon the vicinity of the earth.

Now, as carbonic acid gas is considerably heavier than air, it could not rise to great heights in the atmosphere unless it entered into combination with the air. We are warranted, therefore, to conclude, that carbonic acid is not merely mechanically mixed, but that it is chemically combined with the other constituent parts of the atmosphere. It is to the affinity which exists between carbonic acid and air that we are to ascribe the rapidity with which it disperses itself through the atmosphere, notwithstanding its great specific gravity. Fontana mixed 20,000 cubic inches of carbonic acid gas with the air of a close room, and yet half an hour after he could not discover the traces of carbonic acid in that air. Water impregnated with carbonic acid, when exposed to the air, very soon loses the whole of the combined gas. And when a phial full of carbonic acid gas is left uncorked, the gas, as Bergman first ascertained, very soon disappears, and the phial is found filled with common air.

The difficulty of separating this gas from air, has hitherto prevented the possibility of determining with accuracy the relative quantity of it in a given bulk of air; but from the experiments which have been made, we may conclude with some degree of confidence, that it is not very different from 0.01. From the experiments of Humboldt, it appears to vary from 0.005 to 0.01. This variation will by no means appear improbable, if we consider that immense quantities of carbonic acid gas must be constantly mixing with the atmosphere, as it is formed by the respiration of animals, by combustion, and several other processes which are going on continually. The quantity, indeed, which is daily formed by these processes is so great, that at first sight it appears astonishing that it does not increase rapidly. The consequence of such an increase would be fatal, as air containing 0.1 of carbonic acid extinguishes light, and is destructive to animals. But there is reason to conclude, that this gas is decomposed by vegetables as rapidly as it forms.

4. *Bodies found in the atmosphere.*—From what has been advanced, it appears that the atmosphere consists chiefly of three distinct elastic fluids united together by chemical affinity; namely, air, vapour, and carbonic acid gas; differing in their proportions at different times and in different places; the average proportion of each is,

98.6 air
1.0 carbonic acid
0.4 water

100.0

But besides these bodies, which may be considered as the constituent parts of the atmosphere, the existence of several other bodies has been suspected in it. It is not meant in this place to include among those bodies electric matter, or the substance of clouds and fogs, and those other bodies which are considered as the active agents in the phenomena of meteorology, but merely those foreign bodies which have been occasionally found or suspected in air. Concerning these bodies, however, very little satisfactory is known at present, as we are not in the possession of instruments sufficiently delicate to ascertain their presence. We can indeed detect several of them actually mixing with air, but what becomes of them afterward we are unable to say.

1. Hydrogen gas is said to have been found in air situated near the crater of volcanoes, and it is very possible that it may exist always in a very small proportion in the atmosphere, but this cannot be ascertained till some method of detecting the presence of hydrogen combined with a great proportion of air be discovered.

2. Carburetted hydrogen gas is often emitted by marshes in considerable quantities during hot weather. But its presence has never been detected in air; so that in all probability it is again decomposed by some unknown process.

3. Oxygen gas is emitted abundantly by plants during the day. There is some reason to conclude that this is in consequence of the property which plants have of absorbing and decomposing carbonic acid gas. Now as this carbonic acid gas is formed at the expense of the oxygen of the atmosphere, as this oxygen is again restored to the air by the decomposition of the acid, and as the nature of atmospheric air remains unaltered, it is clear that there must be an equilibrium between these two processes; that is to say, all the carbonic acid formed by combustion must be again decomposed, and all the oxygen abstracted must be again restored. The oxygen gas which is thus continually returning to the air, by combining with it, makes its component parts always to continue in the same ratio.

4. The smoke and other bodies which are continually carried into the air by evaporation, &c. are probably soon deposited again, and cannot therefore be considered with propriety as forming part of the atmosphere.

5. There is another set of bodies, which are occasionally combined with air, and which, on account of the powerful action which they produce on the human body, have attracted a great deal of attention. These are known by the name of *contagions*.

That there is a difference between the atmosphere in different places, as far as respects its effects upon the human body, has been considered as an established point in all ages. Hence some places have been celebrated as healthy, and others avoided as pernicious, to the human constitution. It is well known that in pits and mines the air is often in such a state as to suffocate almost instantaneously those who attempt to breathe it. Some places are frequented by peculiar diseases. It is known that those who are much in the apartments of persons ill of certain maladies, are extremely apt to catch the infection; and in prisons and other places, where crowds of people are confined together, when diseases once commence they are wont to make dreadful havoc. In all these cases, it has been supposed that a certain noxious matter is dissolved by the air, and that it is the action of this matter which produces the mischief.

This noxious matter is, in many cases, readily distinguished by the peculiarly disagreeable smell which it communicates to the air. No doubt this matter differs according to the diseases which it communicates, and the substance from which it has originated. Morveau lately attempted to ascertain its nature; but he soon found the chemical tests hitherto discovered altogether insufficient for that purpose. He has put it beyond a doubt, however, that this contagious matter is of a compound nature, and that it is destroyed altogether by certain agents. He exposed infected air to the action of various bodies, and he judged of the result by the effect which these bodies had in destroying the fœtid smell of the air. The following is the result of his experiments:

1. Odorous bodies, such as benzoin, aromatic plants, &c. have no effect whatever. 2. Neither have the solutions of myrrh, benzoin, &c. in alkohol, though agitated in infected air. 3. Pyroligneous acid is equally inert. 4. Gunpowder, when fired in infected air, displaces a portion of it; but what remains, still retains its fœtid odour. 5. Sulphuric acid has no effect; sulphurous acid weakens the odour, but does not destroy it. Distilled vinegar diminishes the odour, but its action is slow and incomplete. 7. Strong acetic acid acts instantly, and destroys the fœtid odour of infected air completely. 8. The fumes of nitric acid, first employed by Dr. Carmichael Smith, are equally efficacious. 9. Muriatic acid gas, first pointed out as a proper agent by Morveau himself, is equally ineffectual. 10. But the most powerful agent is oxymuriatic acid gas, first proposed by Mr. Cruickshanks, and now employed with the greatest success in the British navy and military hospitals.

Thus there are four substances which have the property of destroying contagious matter, and of purifying the air; but acetic acid cannot easily be obtained in sufficient quantity, and in a state of sufficient concentration to be employed with advantage. Nitric acid is attended with inconvenience, because it is almost always contaminated with nitrous gas. Muriatic acid and oxymuriatic acid are not attended with these inconveniences; the last deserves the preference, because it acts with greater energy and rapidity. All that is necessary is to mix together two parts of salt with one part of the black oxyde of manganese, to place the mixture in an open vessel in the infected chamber, and to pour upon it two parts of sulphuric acid. The fumes of oxymuriatic acid are immediately exhaled, fill the chamber, and destroy the contagion.

Ato'chia. (From α, neg. and τοκος, offspring; from τικτω, to bring forth.) 1. Inability to bring forth children. 2. Difficult labour.

ATOMIC THEORY. In the chemical combination of bodies with each other, it is observed that some unite in all proportions; others in all proportions as far as a certain point, beyond which combination no longer takes place; there are also many examples, in which bodies unite in one proportion only, and others in several proportions; and these proportions are definite, and in the intermediate ones no combination ensues. And it is remarkable, that when one body enters into combination with another, in several different proportions, the numbers indicating the greater proportions are exact simple multiples of that denoting the smallest proportion. In other words, if the smallest portion in which B combines with A, be denoted by 10 A may combine with twice 10 of B, or with three times 10, and so on; but with no intermediate quantities. Examples of this kind have of late so much increased in number, that the law of simple multiples bids fair to become universal with respect at least to chemical compounds, the proportions of which are definite. Mr. Dalton has founded what may be termed the atomic theory of the chemical constitution of bodies. Till this theory was proposed, we had no adequate explanation of the uniformity of the proportions of chemical compounds; or of the nature of the cause which renders combination in other proportions impossible. The following is a brief illustration of the theory: Though we appear, when we effect the chemical union of bodies, to operate on masses, yet it is consistent with the most rational view of the constitution of bodies, to believe, that it is only between their ultimate particles, or atoms, that combination takes place. By the term atoms, it has been already stated we are to understand the smallest parts of which bodies are composed. An atom, therefore, must be mechanically indivisible, and of course a fraction of an atom cannot exist, and is a contradiction in terms Whether the atoms of different bodies be of the same size, or of different sizes, we have no sufficient evidence. The probability is, that the atoms of different bodies are of unequal sizes; but it cannot be determined whether their sizes bear any regular proportion to their relative weights. We are equally ignorant of their shape; but it is probable, though not essential to the theory, that they are spherical. This, however, requires a little qualification. The atoms of all bodies, probably consist of a solid corpuscle, forming a nucleus, and of an atmosphere of heat, by which that corpuscle is surrounded, for absolute contact is never supposed to take place between the atoms of bodies. The figure of a single atom may therefore be supposed to be spherical. But in compound atoms, consisting of a single central atom surrounded by other atoms of a different kind, it is obvious that the figure (contemplating the solid corpuscles only) cannot be spherical; yet if we include the atmosphere of heat, the figure of a compound atom may be spherical, or some shape approaching to a sphere. Taking for granted that combination takes place between the atoms of bodies only, Mr. Dalton has deduced from the relative weights in which bodies unite, the relative weights of their ultimate particles or atoms. When only one combination of any two elementary bodies exists, he assumes, unless the contrary can be proved, that its elements are united atom to atom; single combinations of this sort he calls binary. But if several compounds can be obtained from the same elements, they combine, he supposes, in proportions expressed by some simple multiple of the number of atoms. The following table exhibits a view of these combinations:

1 Atom of A+1 atom of B=1 atom of C, binary.
1 Atom of A+2 atoms of B=1 atom of D, ternary.
2 Atoms of A+1 atom of B=1 atom of E, ternary.
1 Atom of A+3 atoms of B=1 atom of F, quaternary
3 Atoms of A+1 atom of B=1 atom of G, quaternary.

A different classification of atoms has been proposed by Berzelius, viz. into 1. Elementary atoms. 2. Compound atoms. The compound atoms he divides again into three different species; namely; 1st, Atoms formed of only two elementary substances, united or compound atoms of the first order. 2dly, Atoms composed of more than two elementary substances, and these, as they are only found in organic bodies, or bodies obtained by the destruction of organic matter, he calls organic atoms. 3dly, Atoms formed by the union of two or more compound atoms; as, for example, the salts. These he calls compound atoms of the second order. If elementary atoms of different kinds were of the same size, the greatest number of atoms of it that could be combined with an atom of B would be 12; for this is the greatest number of spherical bodies that can be arranged in contact with a sphere of the same diameter. But this equality of size, though adopted by Berzelius, is not necessary to the hypothesis of Mr. Dalton, and is, indeed, supposed by him not to exist.

As an illustration of the mode in which the weight of the atoms of bodies is determined, let us suppose that any two elementary substances, A and B, form a binary compound, and that they have been proved experimentally to unite in the proportion by weight, of five to the former, to four of the latter, then since (according to the hypothesis) they unite particle to particle, those numbers will express the relative weight of their atoms. But besides combining atom to atom singly, 1 atom of A may combine with 2 of B, or with 3, 4, &c. or one atom of B may combine with 2 of A, or with 3, 4, &c. When such a series of compounds exists, the relative proportion of their elements ought necessarily on analysis to be proved to be 5 of A to 4 of B, or 5 to (4+4=) 8 or 5 to (4+4+4=) 12, &c., or contrariwise, 4 of B to 5 of A, or 4 to (5+5=) 10 or 4 to (5+5+5=) 15. Between these there ought to be no intermediate compounds, and the existence of any such (as 5 of A to 6 of B, or 4 of B to 7½ of A) would, if clearly established, militate against the hypothesis. To verify these numbers, it may be proper to examine the combinations of A and B with some third substance, for example, with C. Let us suppose that A and C form a binary compound, in which analysis discovers 5 parts of A, and 3 of C. Then if C and B are also capable of forming a binary compound, the relative proportion of its elements ought to be 4 of B to 3 of C, for these numbers denote the relative weights of their atoms. Now this is precisely the method by which Mr. Dalton has deduced the relative weights of oxygen, hydrogen, and nitrogen, the first two from the known composition of water, and the last two from the proportion of the elements of ammonia. Extending the comparison to a variety of other bodies, he has obtained a scale of the relative weights of their atoms. In several instances additional evidence is acquired of the accuracy of the weight assigned to an element, by our obtaining the same number from an investigation of several of its compounds. For example,

1. In water, the hydrogen is to the oxygen as 1 to 8.
2. In olefiant gas, the hydrogen is to the carbon as 1 to 8.
3. In carbonic acid, the oxygen is to the carbon as 8 to 6.

Whether, therefore, we determine the weight of the atom of carbon from the proportion in which it combines with hydrogen, or with oxygen, we arrive at the same number 6, an agreement which, as it occurs in various other instances, can scarcely be an accidental coincidence. In similar manner, 8 is deducible, as representing the atom of oxygen, both from the combination of that base with hydrogen, and with carbon, and 1 is referred to be the relative weight of the atom of hydrogen, from the two principal compounds into which it enters. In selecting the body which should be assumed as unity, Mr. Dalton has been induced to fix on hydrogen, because it is that body which unites with others in the smallest proportion. Thus in water, we have 1 of hydrogen, by weight, to 8 of oxygen; in ammonia, 1 of hydrogen to 14 of nitrogen; in carburetted hydrogen, 1 of hydrogen to 6 of carbon; and in sulphuretted hydrogen, 1 of hydrogen to 16 of sulphur. Taking for granted that all these bodies are binary compounds, we have the following scale of numbers expressive of the relative weights of the atoms of their elements:

Hydrogen	1
Oxygen	8
Nitrogen	14
Carbon	6
Sulphur	16

Drs. Wollaston and Thomas, and Professor Berzelius, on the other hand, have assumed oxygen as the decimal unit, (the first making it 10, the second 1, and the third 100,) chiefly with a view to facilitate the estimation of its numerous compounds with other bodies. This perhaps is to be regretted, even though the change may be in some respects eligible, because it is extremely desirable that chemical writers should employ a universal standard of comparison for the weights of the atoms of bodies. It is easy, however, to reduce the number to Mr. Dalton's by the rule of proportion. Thus, as 8, Mr. Dalton's number for oxygen, corrected by the latest experiments, is to 1, his number for hydrogen, so is 10, Dr. Wallaston's number for oxygen, 1.25 the number for hydrogen. Sir H. Davy has assumed with Mr. Dalton, the atom of hydrogen as unity; but that philosopher and Berzelius also have modified the theory, by taking for granted that water is a compound of one proportion (atom) of oxygen and two proportions (atoms) of hydrogen. This is founded on the fact that two measures of hydrogen gas and one of oxygen gas are necessary to form water; and on the supposition that equal measures of different gases contain equal numbers of atoms. And as in water the hydrogen is to the oxygen by weight as 1 to 8, two atoms or volumes of hydrogen must, on this hypothesis, weigh 1, and 1 atom or volume of hydrogen 8; or if we denote a single atom of hydrogen by 1, we must express an atom of oxygen by 16. It is objectionable, however, to this modification of the atomic theory, that it contradicts a fundamental proposition of Mr. Dalton, the consistency of which with mechanical principles he has fully shown; namely, that that compound of any two elements which is with most difficulty decomposed, must be presumed, unless the contrary can be proved, to be a binary one. It is easy to determine, in the manner already explained, the relative weights of the atoms of two elementary bodies which unite only in one proportion; but when one body unites in different proportions with another, it is necessary in order to ascertain the weight of its atom, that we should know the smallest proportion in which the former combines with the latter. Thus if we have a body A, 100 parts of which by weight combine with not less than 32 of oxygen, the relative weight of its atom will be to that of oxygen as 100 to 32; or reducing these numbers to their lowest terms, as 25 to 8; and the number 25 will therefore express the relative weight of the atom of A. But if, in the progress of science, it should be found that 100 parts of A are capable of uniting with 16 parts of oxygen, then the relative weight of the atom of A must be doubled; for as 100 is to 16, so is 50 to 8. This example will serve to explain the changes that have been sometimes made in assigning the weights of the atoms of certain bodies, changes which it must be observed always consist either in a multiplication or division of the original weight by some simple number. There are, it must be acknowledged, a few cases in which one body combines with another in different proportions; and yet the greater proportions are not multiples of the less by any entire number. For example, we have two oxydes of iron, the first of which consists of 100 iron and about 30 oxygen; the second of 100 iron and about 45 oxygen. But the numbers 30 and 45 are to each other as 1 to 1½. It will, however, render these numbers 1 and 1½ consistent with the law of simple multiples; if we multiply each of them by 2, it will change them to 2 and 3; and if we suppose that there is an oxyde of iron, though it has not yet been obtained experimentally, consisting of 100 iron and 15 oxygen; for the multiplication of this last number by 2 and 3 will then give us the known oxydes of iron. In some cases where we have the apparent anomaly of one atom of one substance united with 1½ of another, it has been proposed by Dr. Thomson to remove the difficulty by multiplying both numbers by 2, and by assuming that in such compounds we have two atoms of the one combined with 3 atoms of the other. Such combinations, it is true, are exceptions to a law deduced by Berzelius, that in all inorganic compounds one of the constituents is in the state of a single atom: but they are in no respect inconsistent with the views of Mr Dalton, and are indeed expressly admitted by him to be compatible with this hypothesis, as well as confirmed by experience. Thus, it will appear in the sequel, that some of the compounds of oxygen with nitrogen are constituted in this way. Several objections have been proposed to the theory of Mr. Dalton; of these it is only necessary to notice the most important. It has been contended that we have no evidence when one combination only of two elements exists, that it must be a binary one, and that we might equally well suppose it to be a compound of 2 atoms of the one body with one atom of the other. In answer to this objection, we may urge the probability, that when two elementary bodies A and B unite, the most energetic combination will be that in which one atom of A is combined with one atom of B; for an additional atom of B will introduce a new force, diminishing the attraction of these elements for each other, namely, the mutual repulsion of the atoms of B; and this repulsion will be greater in proportion as we increase the number of the atoms of B. 2dly, It has been said, that when more than one compound of two elements exists, we have no proof which of them is the binary compound, and which the ternary. For example, that we might suppose carbonic acid to be a compound of an atom of charcoal, and an atom of oxygen; and carbonic oxyde of an atom of oxygen, with two atoms of charcoal. To this objection, however, it is a satisfactory answer that such a constitution of carbonic acid and carbonic oxyde would be directly contradictory of a law of chemical combination; namely, that it is attended, in most cases, with an increase of specific gravity. It would be absurd, therefore, to suppose carbonic acid, which is the heavier body, to be only once compounded, and carbonic oxyde, which is the lighter, to be twice compounded. Moreover, it is universally observed, that of chemical compounds, the most simple are the most difficult to be decomposed; and this being the case with carbonic oxyde, we may naturally suppose it to be more simple than carbonic acid. 3dly, It has been remarked, that instead of supposing water to consist of an atom of oxygen united with an atom of hydrogen, and that the atom of the former is 7½ times heavier than that of the latter, we might with equal probability conclude, that in water we have 7½ times more atoms in number of oxygen than of hydrogen. But this, if admitted, would involve the absurdity that in a mixture of hydrogen and oxygen gases so contrived that the ultimate atoms of each should be equal in number, 7 atoms of oxygen would desert all the proximate atoms of hydrogen in order to unite with one at a distance, for which they must have naturally a less affinity.

ATONIC. *Atonicus.* Having a diminution of strength.

A'TONY. (*Atonia*, from *a*, neg. and τεινω, to extend.) Weakness, or a defect of muscular power.

ATRABI'LIS. (*Atrabilis*, from *atra*, black, and *bilis*, bile.) 1. Black bile.

2. Melancholy.

Atrabiliaræ capsulæ. (From *atra*, black, and *bilis*.) See *Renal glands*.

ATRACHE'LUS. (From *a*, priv. and τραχηλος, the neck.) Short-necked.

Atrage'ne. See *Clematis vitalba*.

Atra'sia. (From *a*, neg. and τιτραω, to perforate.) *Atresia*. 1. Imperforate.

2. A disease where the natural openings, as the anus or vagina, have not their usual orifice.

Atreta'rum. (From *a*, neg. and τραω, to perforate.) A suppression of urine from the menses being retained in the vagina.

A'TRICES. (From *a*, priv. and θριξ, hair.) Small tubercles about the anus upon which hairs will not grow.—*Vaselius.*

A'trici. Small sinuses in the rectum, which do not reach so far up as to perforate into its cavity.

A'TRIPLEX. (*Atriplex, icis.* f.; said to be named from its dark colour, whence it was called *Atrum olus.*) The name of a genus of plants in the Linnæan system. Class, *Polygamia;* Order, *Monœcia.*

Atriplex fœtida. See *Chenopodium vulvaria.*

Atriplex hortensis. See *Atriplex sativa.*

Atriplex sativa. The systematic name for the *atriplex hortensis* of the pharmacopœias. Orache, the herb and seed of this plant, *Atriplex—caule erecto herbaceo, foliis triangularibus*, of Linnæus, have been exhibited medicinally as antiscorbutics, but the practice of the present day appears to have totally rejected them.

ATROPA. (*Atropa, æ.* f., from Ατροπος, the goddess of destiny: so called from its fatal effects.) The name of a genus of plants in the Linnæan system. Class, *Pentandria;* Order, *Monogynia.*

Atropa belladonna. The systematic name for the *belladonna* of the pharmacopœias. *Solanum melonocerasus; Solanum lethale.* Deadly nightshade or dwale. *Atropa—caule herbaceo; foliis ovatis integris* of Linnæus. This plant has been long known as a strong poison of the narcotic kind, and the berries have furnished many instances of their fatal effects, particularly upon children that have been tempted to eat them. The activity of this plant depends on a principle *sui generis* called *Atropia.* (See *Atropia.*) The leaves were first used internally, to discuss scirrhous and cancerous tumours; and from the good effects attending their use, physicians were induced to employ them internally, for the same disorders; and there are a considerable number of well-authenticated facts, which prove them a very serviceable and important remedy. The dose, at first, should be small; and gradually and cautiously increased. Five grains are considered a powerful dose, and apt to promote dimness of sight, vertigo, &c.

Atropa mandragora. The systematic name for the plant which affords the *radix mandragoræ* of the pharmacopœias. Mandrake. The boiled root is employed in the form of poultice, to discuss indolent tumours.

ATRO'PHIA. (*Atrophia, æ* f.; from *a*, neg. and τρεφω, to nourish.) *Marasmus.* Atrophy. Nervous consumption. This disease is marked by a gradual wasting of the body, unaccompanied either by a difficulty of breathing, cough, or any evident fever, but usually attended with a loss of appetite and impaired digestion. It is arranged by Cullen in the class *Cachexiæ*, and order *Marcores.* There are four species:—

1. When it takes place from too copious evacuations, it is termed *atrophia inanitorum;* and *tabes nutricum;—sudatoria;—à sanguifluxu*, &c.

2. When from famine, *atrophia famelicorum.*

3. When from corrupted nutriment, *atrophia cacachymica.*

4. And when from an interruption in the digestive organs, *atrophia debilium.*

The atrophy of children is called *paidatrophia.* The causes which commonly give rise to atrophy, are a poor diet, unwholesome air, excess in venery, fluor albus, severe evacuations, continuing to give suck too long, a free use of spirituous liquors, mental uneasiness, and worms; but it frequently comes on without any evident cause. Along with the loss of appetite and impaired digestion, there is a diminution of strength, the face is pale and bloated, the natural heat of the body is somewhat diminished, and the lower extremities are œdematous. Atrophy, arise from whatever cause it may, is usually very difficult to cure, and not unfrequently terminates in dropsy.

A'TROPHY. See *Atrophia.*

ATROPIA. A poisonous vegetable principle, probably alkaline, recently extracted from the *Atropa belladonna*, or deadly nightshade, by Brandes. He boiled two pounds of dried leaves of *atropa belladonna* in a sufficient quantity of water, pressed the decoction out, and boiled the remaining leaves again in water. The decoctions were mixed, and some sulphuric acid was added, in order to throw down the albumen and similar bodies; the solution is thus rendered thinner, and passes more readily through the filter. The decoction was then supersaturated with potassa, by which he obtained a precipitate that, when washed with pure water and dried, weighed 89 grains. It consisted of small crystals, from which by solution in acids, and precipitation by alkalies, the new alkaline substance, atropia, was obtained in a state of purity.

The external appearance of atropia varies considerably, according to the different methods by which it is obtained. When precipitated from the decoction of the herb by solution of potassa, it appears in the form of very small short crystals, constituting a sandy powder. When thrown down by ammonia from an aqueous solution of its salts, it appears in flakes like wax, if the solution is much diluted; if concentrated, it is gelatinous like precipitated alumina: when obtained by the cooling of a hot solution in alkohol, it crystallizes in long, acicular, transparent, brilliant crystals, often exceeding one inch in length, which are sometimes feathery, at other times star-like in appearance, and sometimes they are single crystals. Atropia, however, is obtained in such a crystalline state only when rendered perfectly pure by repeated solution in muriatic acid, and precipitation by ammonia. When pure, it has no taste. Cold water has hardly any effect upon dried atropia, but it dissolves a small quantity when it is recently precipitated; and boiling water dissolves still more. Cold alkohol dissolves but a minute portion of atropia; but when boiling, it readily dissolves it. Ether and oil of turpentine, even when boiling, have little effect on atropia.

Sulphate of atropia crystallizes in rhomboidal tables and prisms with square bases. It is soluble in four or five parts of cold water. It seems to effloresce in the air, when freed as much as possible from adhering sulphuric acid, by pressure between the folds of blotting paper. Its composition by Brandes seems to be,

Atropia,	38.93
Sulphuric acid,	36.52
Water,	24.55
	100.00

This analysis would make the prime equivalent of atropia so low as 5.3, oxygen being 1. Muriate of atropia appears in beautiful white brilliant crystals, which are either cubes or square plates similar to the muriate of *daturia.* He makes the composition of this salt to be,

Atropia,	39.19
Muriatic acid,	25.40
Water,	35.41
	100.00

This analysis was so conducted as to be entitled to little attention. Nitric, acetic, and oxalic acids dissolve atropia, and form acicular salts, all soluble in water and alkohol. Mr. Brandes was obliged to discontinue his experiments on the properties of this alkali. The violent headaches, pains in the back, and giddiness, with frequent nausea, which the vapour of atropia occasioned while he was working on it, had such a bad effect on his weak health, that he has entirely abstained from any further experiments.

He once tasted a small quantity of sulphate of atropia. The taste was not bitter, but merely saline; but there soon followed violent headache, shaking in the limbs, alternate sensations of heat and cold, oppression of the chest, and difficulty in breathing, and diminished circulation of the blood. The violence of these symptoms ceased in half an hour. Even the vapour of the different salts of atropia produces giddiness. When exposed for a long time to the vapours of a solution of nitrate, phosphate, or sulphate of atropia, the pupil of the eye is dilated. This happened frequently to him, and when he tasted the salt of atropia, it occurred to such a degree, that it remained so for twelve hours, and the different degrees of light had no influence.—*Schweigger's Journal*, xxviii. 1.

We may observe on the above, that it is highly improbable that atropia should have a saturating power, intermediate between potassa and soda.

ATTE'NUANT. (*Attenuans;* from *attenuo*, to make thin.) An attenuant or diluent is that which possesses the power of imparting to the blood a more thin and more fluid consistence than it had, previous to its exhibition; such are, water, whey, and all aqueous fluids.

ATTO'LLENS. (*Attollens;* from *attollo*, to lift up. Lifting up: a term applied to some muscles, the office of which is to lift up the parts they are affixed to.

Attollens aurem. A common muscle of the ear. *Attollens auriculæ* of Albinus and Douglas; *Superior auris* of Winslow; and *Attollens auriculam* of Cowper. It arises thin, broad, and tendinous, from the tendon of the occipito-frontalis, from which it is almost inseparable, where it covers the aponeurosis of the temporal muscle: and is inserted into the upper part of the ear, opposite to the antihelex. Its use is to draw the ear upwards, and to make the parts into which it is inserted, tense.

Attollens occuli. One of the muscles which pulls up the eye.—See *Rutus superior occuli.*

Atto'nitus morbus. (From *attono*, to surprise; so called because the person falls down suddenly.) *Attonitus stupor.* The apoplexy and epilepsy.

ATTRACTION. (*Attractio;* from *attraho*, to attract.) Affinity. The terms attraction, or affinity, and repulsion, in the language of modern philosophers, are employed merely as the expression of the general facts, that the masses or particles of matter have a tendency to approach and unite to, or to recede from one another, under certain circumstances. The term attraction is used synonymously with affinity. See *Affinity.*

All bodies have a tendency or power to attract each other more or less, and it is this power which is called attraction.

Attraction is mutual: it extends to indefinite distances. All bodies whatever, as well as their component elementary particles, are endued with it. It is not annihilated, at how great a distance soever, we suppose them to be placed from each other; neither does it disappear though they be arranged ever so near each other.

The nature of this reciprocal attraction, or at least the cause which produces it, is altogether unknown to us. Whether it be inherent in all matter, or whether it be the consequence of some other agent, are questions beyond the reach of human understanding; but its existence is nevertheless certain.

"The instances of attraction which are exhibited by the phenomena around us, are exceedingly numerous, and continually present themselves to our observation. The effect of gravity, which causes the weight of bodies, is so universal, that we can scarcely form an idea how the universe could subsist without it. Other attractions, such as those of magnetism and electricity, are likewise observable; and every experiment in chemistry tends to show, that bodies are composed of various principles or substances, which adhere to each other with various degrees of force, and may be separated by known methods. It is a question among philosophers, whether all the attractions which obtain between bodies be referrible to one general cause modified by circumstances, or whether various original and distinct causes act upon the particles of bodies at one and the same time. The philosophers, at the beginning of the present century, were disposed to consider the several attractions as essentially different, because the laws of their action differ from each other; but the moderns appear disposed to generalize this subject, and to consider all the attractions which exist between bodies, or at least those which are permanent, as depending upon one and the same cause, whatever it may be, which regulates at once the motions of the immense bodies that circulate through the celestial spaces, and those minute particles that are transferred from one combination to another in the operations of chemistry. The earlier philosophers observed, for example, that the attraction of gravitation acts upon bodies with a force which is inversely as the squares of the distances; and from mathematical deduction they have inferred, that the law of attraction between the particles themselves follows the same ratio; but when their observations were applied to bodies very near each other, or in contact, an adhesion took place, which is found to be much greater than could be deduced from that law applied to the centres of gravity. Hence they concluded, that the cohesive attraction is governed by a much higher ratio, and probably the cubes of the distances. The moderns, on the contrary, have remarked, that these deductions are too general, because, for the most part, drawn from the consideration of spherical bodies, which admit of no contact but such as is indefinitely small, and exert the same powers on each other, whichever side may be obverted. They remark, likewise, that the consequence depending on the sum of the attractions in bodies not spherical, and at minute distances from each other, will not follow the inverted ratio of the square of the distance taken from any point assumed as the centre of gravity, admitting the particles to be governed by that law; but that it will greatly differ, according to the sides of the solid which are presented to each other, and their respective distances; insomuch that the attractions of certain particles indefinitely near each other will be indefinitely increased, though the ratio of the powers acting upon the remoter particles may continue nearly the same

That the parts of bodies do attract each other, is evident from that adhesion which produces solidity, and requires a certain force to overcome it. For the sake of perspicuity, the various effects of attraction have been considered as different kinds of affinity or powers. That power which physical writers call the attraction of cohesion, is generally called the *attraction of aggregation* by chemists. Aggregation is considered as the adhesion of parts of the same kind. Thus a number of pieces of brimstone, united by fusion, form an aggregate, the parts of which may be separated again by mechanical means These parts have been called integrant parts; that is to say, the minutest parts into which a body can be divided, either really or by the imagination, so as not to change its nature, are called integrant parts Thus, if sulphur and an alkali be combined together, and form liver of sulphur, we may conceive the mass to be divided and subdivided to an extreme degree, until at length the mass consists of merely a particle of brimstone and a particle of alkali. This then is an integrant part; and if it be divided further, the effect which chemists call decomposition will take place; and the particles, consisting no longer of liver of sulphur, but of sulphur alone, and of alkali alone, will be what chemists call component parts or principles.

The union of bodies in a gross way is called *mixture.* Thus sand and alkali may be mixed together. But when the very minute parts of a body unite with those of another so intimately as to form a body which has properties different from those of either of them, the union is called *combination* or *composition.* Thus, if sand and an alkali be exposed to a strong heat, the minute parts of the mixture combine and form glass.

If two solid bodies, disposed to combine together, be brought into contact with each other, the particles which touch will combine, and form a compound; and if the temperature at which this new compound assumes the fluid form be higher than the temperature of the experiment, the process will go no farther, because this new compound, being interposed between the two bodies, will prevent their farther access to each other; but if, on the contrary, the freezing point of the compound be lower than this temperature, liquefaction will ensue; and the fluid particles being at liberty to arrange themselves according to the law of their attractions, the process will go on, and the whole mass will gradually be converted into a new compound, in the fluid state. An instance of this may be exhibited by mixing common salt and perfectly dry pounded ice together. The crystals of the salt alone will not liquefy unless very much heated; the crystals of the water, that is to say, the ice, will not liquefy unless heated as high as thirty-two degrees of Fahrenheit; and we have, of course, supposed the temperature of the experiment to be lower than this, because our water is in the solid state. Now it is a well-known fact, that brine, or the saturated solution of sea-salt in water, cannot be frozen unless it be cooled thirty-eight degrees lower than the freezing point of pure water. It follows then, that if the temperature of the experiment be higher than this, the first combinations of salt and ice will produce a fluid brine, and the combination will proceed until the temperature of the mass has gradually sunk as low as the freezing point of brine; after which it would cease if it were not that surrounding bodies continually tend to raise the temperature. And accordingly it is found by experiment, that if the ice and the salt be previously cooled below the temperature of freezing brine, the combination and liquefaction will not take place.

The instances in which solid bodies thus combine together not being very numerous, and the fluidity which ensues immediately after the commencement of this kind of experiment, have induced several chemists to consider fluidity in one or both of the bodies applied to each other, to be a necessary circumstance, in order that they may produce chemical action upon each order. *Corpora non agunt nisi sint fluida.*

If one of two bodies applied to each other be fluid at the temperature of the experiment, its parts will successively unite with the parts of the solid, which will by that means be suspended in the fluid, and disappear. Such a fluid is called a *solvent* or *menstruum;* and the solid body is said to be dissolved.

Some substances unite together in all proportions. In this way the acids unite with water. But there are likewise many substances which cannot be dissolved in a fluid, at a settled temperature, in any quantity beyond a certain portion. Thus, water will dissolve only about one-third of its weight of common salt; and if more salt be added, it will remain solid. A fluid which holds in solution as much of any substance as it can dissolve, is said to be *saturated* with it. But saturation with one substance is so far from preventing a fluid from dissolving another body, that it very frequently happens, that the solvent power of the compound exceeds that of the original fluid itself. Chemists likewise use the word saturation in another sense; in which it denotes such a union of two bodies as produces a compound th: most remote in its properties from the properties of the component parts themselves. In combinations where one of the principles predominate, the one is said to be supersaturated, and the other principle is said to be subsaturated.

Heat in general increases the solvent power of fluids, probably by preventing part of the dissolved substance from congealing or assuming the solid form.

It often happens, that bodies which have no tendency to unite are made to combine together by means of a third, which is then called *the medium.* Thus water and fat oils are made to unite by the medium of an alkali, in the combination called soap. Some writers, who seem desirous of multiplying terms, call this tendency to unite *the affinity of intermedium.* This case has likewise been called *disposing affinity;* but Berthollet more properly styles it *reciprocal affinity.* He likewise distinguishes affinity into *elementary,* when it is between the elementary parts of bodies; and *resulting*, when it is a compound only, and would not take place with the elements of that compound.

It very frequently happens, on the contrary, that the tendency of two bodies to unite, or remain in combination together, is weakened or destroyed by the addition of a third. Thus alkohol unites with water in such a manner as to separate most salts from it. A striking instance of this is seen in a saturated or strong solution of nitre in water. If to this there be added an equal measure of alkohol, the greater part of the nitre instantly falls down. Thus magnesia is separated from a solution of Epsom salt, by the addition of an alkali, which combines with the sulphuric acid, and separates the earth. The principle which falls down is said to be *precipitated*, and in many instances is called a *precipitate.* Some modern chemists use the term precipitation in a more extended, and rather forced sense; for they apply it to all substances thus separated. In this enunciation, therefore, they would say, that potassa precipitates soda from a solution of common salt, though no visible separation or precipitation takes place; for the soda, when disengaged from its acid, is still suspended in the water by reason of its solubility.

From a great number of facts of this nature, it is clearly ascertained, not as a probable hypothesis, but as simple matter of fact, that some bodies have a stronger tendency to unite than others; and that the union of any substance with another will exclude, or separate, a third substance, which might have been previously united with one of them; excepting only in those cases wherein the new compound has a tendency to unite with that third substance, and form a triple compound. This preference of uniting, which a given substance is found to exhibit with regard to other bodies, is by an easy metaphor called elective attraction, and is subject to a variety of cases, according to the number and the powers of the principles which are respectively presented to each other. The cases which have been most frequently observed by chemists, are those called simple elective attractions, and double elective attractions.

When a simple substance is presented or applied to another substance compounded of two principles, and unites with one of these two principles so as to separate or exclude the other, this effect is said to be produced by *simple elective attraction.*

It may be doubted whether any of our operations have been carried to this degree of simplicity. All the chemical principles we are acquainted with are simple only with respect to our power of decomposing them; and the daily discoveries of our contemporaries tend to decompose those substances, which chemists a few years ago considered as simple. Without insisting, however, upon this difficulty, we may observe, that water is concerned in all the operations which are called humid, and beyond a doubt modifies all the effects of such bodies as are suspended in it; and the variations of temperature, whether arising from an actual igneous fluid, or from a mere modification of the parts of bodies, also tend greatly to disturb the effects of elective attraction. These causes render it difficult to point out an example of simple elective attraction, which may in strictness be reckoned as such.

Double elective attraction takes place when two bodies, each consisting of two principles, are presented to each other, and mutually exchange a principle of each; by which means two new bodies, or compounds, are produced of a different nature from the original compounds.

Under the same limitations as were pointed out in speaking of simple elective attraction, we may offer instances of double elective attraction. Let oxyde of mercury be dissolved to saturation in the nitric acid, the water will then contain nitrate of mercury. Again, let potassa be dissolved to saturation in the sulphuric acid, and the result will be a solution of sulphate of potassa. If mercury were added to the latter solution, it would indeed tend to unite with the acid, but, would produce no decomposition; because the elective attraction of the acid to the alkali is the strongest. So likewise, if the nitric acid alone be added to it, its tendency to unite with the alkali, strong as it is, will not effect any change, because the alkali is already in combination with a stronger acid. But if the nitrate of mercury be added to the solution of sulphate of potassa, a change of principles will take place; the sulphuric acid will quit the alkali, and unite with the mercury, while the nitric acid combines with the alkali; and these two new salts, namely, nitrate of potassa, and sulphate of mercury, may be obtained separately by crystallization. The most remarkable circumstance in this process, is that the joint effects of the attractions of the sulphuric acid to mercury, and the nitric acid to alkali, prove to be stronger than the sum of the attractions between the sulphuric acid and the alkali, and between the nitrous acid and the mercury; for if the sum of these two last had not been weaker, the original combinations would not have been broken.

Mr. Kirwan, who first, in the year 1782, considered this subject with that attention it deserves, called the affinities which tend to preserve the original combinations, the *quiescent affinities*. He distinguished the affinities or attractions which tend to produce a change of principles, by the name of the *divellent affinities*.

Some eminent chemists are disposed to consider as effects of double affinities, those changes of principles only which would not have taken place without the assistance of a fourth principle. Thus, the mutual decomposition of sulphate of soda and nitrate of potassa, in which the alkalies are changed, and sulphate of potassa and nitrate of soda are produced, is not considered by them as an instance of double decomposition; because the nitre would have been decomposed by simple elective attraction, upon the addition of the acid only.

There are various circumstances which modify the effects of elective attraction, and have from time to time misled chemists in their deductions. The chief of these is the temperature, which, acting differently upon the several parts of compounded bodies, seldom fails to alter, and frequently reverses the effects of the affinities. Thus, if alkohol be added to a solution of nitrate of potassa, it unites with the water, and precipitates the salt at a common temperature. But if the temperature be raised, the alkohol rises on account of its volatility, and the salt is again dissolved. Thus again, if sulphuric acid be added, in a common temperature, to a combination of phosphoric acid and lime, it will decompose the salt, and disengage the phosphoric acid; but if this same mixture of these principles be exposed to a considerable heat, the sulphuric acid will have its attraction to the lime so much diminished, that it will rise, and give place again to the phosphoric, which will combine with the lime. Again, mercury kept in a degree of heat very nearly equal to volatilizing it will absorb oxygen, and become converted into the red oxyde formerly called precipitate *per se*; but if the heat be augmented still more, the oxygen will assume the elastic state, and fly off, leaving the mercury in its original state. Numberless instances of the like nature continually present themselves to the observation of chemists, which are sufficient to establish the conclusion, that the elective attractions are not constant but at one and the same temperature.

Many philosophers are of opinion, that the variations produced by change of temperature arise from the elective attraction of the matter of heat itself. But there are no decisive experiments either in confirmation or refutation of this hypothesis.

If we except the operation of heat, which really produces a change in the elective attractions, we shall find, that most of the other difficulties attending this subject arise from the imperfect state of chemical science. If to a compound of two principles a third be added, the effect of this must necessarily be different according to its quality, and likewise according to the state of saturation of the two principles of the compounded body. If the third principle which is added be in excess, it may dissolve and suspend the compound which may be newly formed, and likewise that which might have been precipitated. The metallic solutions, decomposed by the addition of an alkali, afford no precipitate in various cases when the alkali is in excess; because this excess dissolves the precipitate, which would else have fallen down. If, on the other hand, one of the two principles of the compound body be in excess, the addition of a third substance may combine with that excess, and leave a neutral substance, exhibiting very different properties from the former. Thus, if cream of tartar, which is a salt of difficult solubility, consisting of potassa united to an excess of the acid of tartar, be dissolved in water, and chalk be added, the excess unites with part of the lime of the chalk, and forms a scarcely soluble salt; and the neutral compound, which remains after the privation of this excess of acid, is a very soluble salt, greatly differing in taste and properties from the cream of tartar. The metals and the acids likewise afford various phenomena, according to their degree of oxy dation. A determinate oxydation is in general necessary for the solution of metals in acids; and the acids themselves act very differently, accordingly as they are more or less acidified. Thus, the nitrous acid gives place to acids which are weaker than the nitric acid; the sulphurous acid gives place to acids greatly inferior in attractive power or affinity to the sulphuric acid. The deception arising from effects of this nature is in a great measure produced by the want of discrimination on the part of chemical philosophers; it being evident that the properties of any compound substance depend as much upon the proportion of its ingredients, as upon their respective nature.

The presence and quantity of water is probably of more consequence than is yet supposed. Thus, bismuth is dissolved in nitrous acid, but falls when the water is much in quantity.

The power of double elective attractions, too, is disturbed by this circumstance: If muriate of lime be added to a solution of carbonate of soda, they are both decomposed, and the results are muriate of soda and carbonate of lime. But if lime and muriate of soda be mixed with just water sufficient to make them into a paste, and this be exposed to the action of carbonic acid gas, a saline efflorescence, consisting of carbonate of soda, will be formed on the surface, and the bottom of the vessel will be occupied by muriate of lime in a state of deliquescence.

Berthollet made a great number of experiments, from which he deduced the following law:—that in elective attractions the power exerted is not in the ratio of the affinity simple, but in a ratio compounded of the force of affinity and the quantity of the agent; so that quantity may compensate for weaker affinity. Thus an acid which has a weaker affinity than another for a given base, if it be employed in a certain quantity, is capable of taking part of that base from the acid which has a stronger affinity for it; so that the base will be divided between them in the compound ratio of their affinity and quantity. This division of one substance between two others, for which it has different affinities, always takes place, according to him, when three such are present under circumstances in which they can mutually act on each other. And hence it is, that the force of affinity acts most powerfully when two substances first come into contact, and continues to decrease in power as either approaches the point of saturation. For the same reason it is so difficult to separate the last portions of any substance adhering to another. Hence, if the doctrine laid down by M. Berthollet be true, to its utmost extent, it must be impossible ever to free a compound completely from any one of its constituent parts by the agency of elective attraction; so that all our best established analyses are more or less inaccurate.

The solubility or insolubility of principles, at the temperature of any experiment, has likewise tended to mislead chemists, who have deduced consequences from the first effects of their experiments. It is evident, that many separations may ensue without precipitation; because this circumstance does not take place unless the separated principle be insoluble, or nearly so. The soda cannot be precipitated from a solution of sulphate of soda, by the addition of potassa, because of its great solubility; but, on the contrary, the new compound itself, or sulphate of potassa, which is much less soluble, may fall down, if there be not enough of water present to suspend it. No certain knowledge can therefore be derived from the appearance or the want of precipitation, unless the products be carefully examined. In some instances all the products remain suspended; and in others, they all fall down, as may be instanced in the decomposition of sulphate of iron by lime. Here the acid unites with the lime, and forms sulphate of lime, which is scarcely at all soluble; and the still less soluble oxyde of iron, which was disengaged, falls down along with it.

Many instances present themselves, in which decom

position does not take place, but a sort of equilibrium of affinity is perceived. Thus, soda, added to the supertartrate of potassa, forms a triple salt by combining with its excess of acid. So likewise ammonia combines with a portion of the acid of muriate of mercury, and forms the triple compound formerly distinguished by the barbarous name of "sal alembroth."

Attraction, double elective. See *Affinity, double.*

AUA'NTE. (From αυαινω, to dry.) A dry disease, proceeding from a fermentation in the stomach, described by Hippocrates de Morbis.

AUA'PSE. The same.

AU'CHEN. (From αυχεω, to be proud.) The neck, which in the posture of pride, is made stiff and erect.

AUDITORY. (*Auditorius; from audio*, to hear.) Belonging to the organ of hearing; as auditory nerve, passage, &c.

Auditory nerve. See *Portio mollis.*

Auditory passage. See *Ear*, and *Meatus auditorius internus.*

AUGITE. Pyroxene of Haüy. A green, brown, or black mineral, found crystallized, and in grains in volcanic rocks in basaltes. It consists of silica, lime, oxyde of iron, magnesia, alumina, and manganese.

[It occurs in crystals, amorphous, in rounded fragments, or in grains. The Augite has a foliated structure in two directions, parallel to the sides of the primitive form. It is harder than hornblende or olivine, scratches glass, and gives sparks with steel. Its specific gravity varies from 3.10 to 3.47.

It is fused with difficulty by the blow-pipe; but in small fragments melts into an enamel, which, in the coloured varieties, is black. Its greater hardness, the results of mechanical division, and its difficult fusibility, will in general be sufficient to distinguish it from hornblende, which it often resembles. It cannot easily be confounded with schorl. It has two varieties. 1. Common Augite. 2. Coccolite.—*Cl. Min.* A.]

AUGU'STUM. An epithet formerly given to several compound medicines.

AULI'SCOS. (From αυλος, a pipe.) A catheter, or clyster-pipe.

AU'LOS. (Αυλος, a pipe.) A catheter, canula, or clyster-pipe.

AU'RA. (*Aura, æ.* f.; from αω, to breathe.) Any subtile vapour or exhalation.

AURA EPILEPTICA. A sensation which is felt by epileptic patients, as if a blast of cold air ascended from the lower parts towards the heart and head.

AURA SEMINIS. The extremely subtile and vivifying portion of the semen virile, that ascends through the Fallopian tubes, to impregnate the ovum in the ovarium.

AURA VITALIS. So Van Helmont calls the vital heat.

AURA'NTIUM. (*Aurantium, i.* n.; so called, *ab aureo colore*, from its golden colour, or from *Arantium*, a town of Achaia.) The orange. See *Citrus aurantium.*

AURANTIUM CURASSAVENTE. The Curassoa, or Curassao apple, or orange. The fruit so called seems to be the immature oranges, that by some accident have been checked in their growth. They are a grateful aromatic bitter, of a flavour very different from that of the peel of the ripe fruit, and without any acid; what little tartness they have when fresh, is lost in drying. Infused in wine, or brandy, they afford a good bitter for the stomach. They are used to promote the discharge in issues, whence their name of *issue peas*, and to give the flavour of hops to beer.

AURANTII BACCÆ. See *Citrus aurantium.*

AURANTII CORTEX. See *Citrus aurantium.*

AURICHALCUM. Brass.

AURI'CULA. (*Auricula, æ.* f. dim. of *auris*, the ear.) 1. An auricle or little ear.

2. The external ear, upon which are several eminences and depressions; as the *helix, antihelix, tragus, antitragus, conchæ auriculæ, scapha*, and *lobulus*. See *Ear.*

3. Applied to some parts which resemble a little ear, as the auricles of the heart.

4. In botany, applied to parts of plants, which resemble an ear in figure, as *Auricula judæ*, and *Auricula muris, &c.*

AURICULA JUDÆ. See *Petiza auricula.*

AURICULA MURIS. See *Hieracium.*

AURICULÆ CORDIS The auricles of the heart. See *Heart.*

AURICULA'RIS. (*Auricularis*, from *auris*, the ear.) Pertaining to the ear.

AURICULARIS DIGITUS. The little finger; so called because people generally put it into the ear, when the hearing is obstructed.

AURICULATUS. Auricled. A leaf is said to be so, when furnished at its base with a pair of leaflets, properly distinct, but occasionally liable to be joined to it, as in *Citrus aurantium.*

AURI'GA. (*Auriga*, a wagoner.) A bandage for the sides is so called because it is made like the traces of a wagon-horse.—*Galen.*

AURI'GO. (*Ab aureo colore;* from its yellow colour.) The jaundice. See *Icterus*

AURIPI'GMENTUM. (From *aurum*, gold, and *pigmentum*, paint; so called from its colour and its use to painters.) Yellow orpiment. See *Arsenic.*

AU'RIS. (*Auris, is.* f.; from *aura*, air, as being the medium of hearing.) The ear, or organ of hearing See *Ear.*

AURISCA'LPIUM. (From *auris*, the ear, and *scalpo*, to scrape.) An instrument for cleansing the ear.

AURU'GO The jaundice. See *Aurigo.*

AU'RUM. 1. Gold.

2. This term was applied to many substances by alchemists and chemists, which resembled gold in colour or virtues.

AURUM FULMINANS. The precipitate formed by putting ammonia into a solution of gold.

AURUM GRAPHICUM. An ore of gold.

AURUM HORIZONTALE. Oil of cinnamon and sugar

AURUM LEPROSUM. Antimony.

AURUM MUSIVUM. Mosaic gold. "A combination of tin and sulphur, which is thus made; Melt twelve ounces of tin, and add to it three ounces of mercury; triturate this amalgam with seven ounces of sulphur, and three of muriate of ammonia. Put the powder into a mattress, bedded rather deep in sand, and keep it for several hours in a gentle heat; which is afterward to be raised, and continued for several hours longer. If the heat have been moderate, and not continued too long, the golden-coloured scaly porous mass, called *aurum musivum*, will be found at the bottom of the vessel; but if it have been too strong, the *aurum musivum* fuses to a black mass of a striated texture. This process is thus explained: as the heat increases, the tin, by stronger affinity, seizes and combines with the muriatic acid of the muriate of ammonia; while the alkali of that salt, combining with a portion of the sulphur, flies off in the form of a sulphuret. The combination of tin and muriatic acid sublimes; and is found adhering to the sides of the mattress. The mercury, which served to divide the tin, combines with part of the sulphur, and forms cinnabar, which also sublimes; and the remaining sulphur, with the remaining tin, forms the *aurum musivum* which occupies the lower part of the vessel. It must be admitted, however, that this explanation does not indicate the reasons why such an indirect and complicated process should be required to form a simple combination of tin and sulphur.

Aurum musivum has no taste, though some specimens exhibit a sulphureous smell. It is not soluble in water, acids, or alkaline solutions. But in the dry way it forms a yellow sulphuret, soluble in water. It deflagrates with nitre. Bergman mentions a native *aurum musivum* from Siberia, containing tin, sulphur, and a small proportion of copper.

This substance is used as a pigment for giving a golden colour to small statue or plaster figures. It is likewise said to be mixed with melted glass to imitate *lapis lazulii.*

AURUM POTABILE. Gold dissolved and mixed with oil of rosemary, to be drunk.

AUTHE'MERON. (From αυτος, the same, and ημερα, a day.) A medicine which gives relief, or is to be administered the same day.

AUTOCRATE'IA. The healing power of nature —*Hippocrates.*

[AUTOMALITE. This mineral substance is otherwise called *Gahnite.* It is always crystallized in small, but very regular octaedrons, which are sometimes double, like those of spinelle. Its colour is deep green, or greenish black, and its fragments are translucent. It scratches quartz, and has an uneven or conchoidal fracture. Its specific gravity varies from 4.26 to 4.69. It is not a conductor of electricity.

Before the blow-pipe it is infusible; but with borax, according to Eckeberg, it gives a green glass, while hot, which becomes colourless when cold. It contains Alumine 60., oxide of zinc 24.25, oxide of iron 9.25, silex, 4.75=98.25. According to Vauquelin, Alumine 42., oxide of zinc 28., oxide of iron 5., silex 4., sulphur 17., insoluble residue 4. It has been found at a mine of Fahlun, in Sweden, in a rock abounding in talc. —*Cl. Min.* A.]

AUTO'PSIA. (From αυτος, himself, and οπτομαι, to see.) Ocular evidence.

Auto'pyros. (From αυτος, itself, and πυρος, wheat.) Bread made with the meal of wheat, from which the bran has not been removed.—*Galen.*

AUXILIARY. Assisting. This term is applied to the means which co-operate in curing diseases, and to parts which assist others in performing certain functions. The pyramidales were called auxiliary muscles.

AVANTURINE. A variety of quartz rock containing mica spangles. It is found in Spain and Scotland

AVELLA'NA. (From *Abella*, or *Avella*, a town in Campania, where they grow.) The specific name of the hazel-nut. See *Corylus avellana.*

Avellana cathartica. A purgative seed or nut, from Barbadoes, the produce of the *Jatropha curcas.* See *Jatropha curcas.*

Avellana mexicana. Cocoa and chocolate nut.

Avellana purgatrix. Garden spurge.

AVE'NA. (*Avena, æ.* f.; from *aveo*, to covet; because cattle are so fond of it.) The oat. 1. The name of a genus of plants in the Linnæan system. Class, *Triandria;* Order, *Digynia.*

2. The pharmacopœial name of the oat.

Avena sativa. The systematic name for the *avena* of the pharmacopœias. It is the seed which is commonly used, and called the oat. There are two kinds of oats: the black and the white. They have similar virtues, but the black are chiefly sown for horses. They are less farinaceous, and less nourishing, than rice, or wheat; yet afford sufficient nourishment, of easy digestion, to such as feed constantly on them. In Scotland, and some of the northern counties of England, oats form the chief bread of the inhabitants. They are much used in Germany; but, in Norway, oat bread is a luxury among the common people. Gruels, made with the flour, or meal, called oatmeal, digest easily, have a soft mucilaginous quality, by which they obtund acrimony, and are used for common drink and food in fevers, inflammatory disorders, coughs, hoarseness, roughness, and exulceration of the fauces; and water gruels answer all the purposes of Hippocrates's ptisan. Externally, poultices, with oatmeal, vinegar, and a very little oil, are good for sprains and bruises. Stimulant poultices, with the grounds of strong beer, mixed up with oatmeal, are made for tumours, &c. of a gangrenous tendency.

Avenacu. A Molucca tree, of a caustic quality.

AVENS. (*Avens, entis;* from *aves*, to desire.) 1. The specific name of a species of dipsosis in Good's Nosology: immoderate thirst.

2. The name of a plant. See *Geum.*

AVENIUS. Veinless. Without a vein. A term applied by botanists to a leaf which is without what they call a vein; as in *Clusia alba.*

AVENZOAR. A native of Seville, in Spain, who flourished about the beginning of the twelfth century; he was made physician to the king, and is said, but on imperfect evidence, to have attained the uncommon age of 135. He prepared his own medicines, and practised surgery, as well as physic. His principal work was a compendium of the practice of medicine, called, "Al-Theiser," containing some diseases not elsewhere described, and numerous cases candidly related. He was called the Experimenter, from his careful investigation of the powers of medicines by actual trial.

AVERROES. An eminent philosopher and physician, born about the middle of the 12th century, at Corduba, in Spain. He studied medicine under Avenzoar, but does not appear to have been much engaged in the practice of it, his life exhibiting the most extraordinary vicissitudes of honours bestowed upon him as a magistrate, and persecutions, which he underwent for religion. He appears to have first observed, that the small-pox occurs but once in the same person. His principal medical work called the "Universal," is a compendium of physic, mostly collected from other authors. He died about the year 1206.

AVICENNA. A celebrated philosopher and physician, born in Chorasan, in the year 980. He studied at Bagdat, obtained a degree, and began to practise at 18: and he soon attained great wealth and honour in the court of the caliph. But during the latter part of his life, residing at Ispahan, after several years spent in travelling, he impaired his constitution by intemperance, and died of a dysentery in his 58th year. His chief work on medicine, called "Canon Medicinæ," though mostly borrowed from the Greek or other preceding writers, and in a very diffuse style, acquired great reputation, and was taught in the European colleges till near the middle of the 17th century.

AVICE'NNIA. (Named after the celebrated physician of that name.) The name of a genus of plants in the Linnæan system. Class, *Didynamia;* Order, *Angiospermia.*

Avicennia tomentosa. The systematic name for the *Avicennia—foliis cordato ovatis, subtus tomentosis,* of Linnæus, which affords the Malacca bean, or *Anacardium orientale* of the pharmacopœias. The fruit, or nut, so called, is of a shining black colour, heart-shaped, compressed, and about the size of the thumb-nail. It is now deservedly forgot in this country.

Avigato pear. See *Laurus persea.*

Awl-shaped. See *Leaf.*

AWN. See *Arista.*

AXE-STONE. A species of nephrite, and a subspecies of jade, from which it differs in not being of so light a green, and in having a somewhat slaty texture.

[The fracture of this mineral is more or less splintery and glimmering. The structure of large specimens is a little slaty. Its hardness is less than that of nephrite; it is more easily broken, and often falls into tabular fragments. It is usually translucent, sometimes at the edges only. Its colour varies from a dark or leek green, to grass and olive green, or even greenish gray It occurs amorphous, sometimes in rolled fragments.

It is less easily fusible than nephrite or Saussurite, and melts with efferverscence into a black enamel. It often appears to be nearly allied to serpentine This mineral has been found chiefly in South America, New Zealand, and the islands of the South sea. It receives a tolerable polish; and is employed by the natives of the aforesaid islands for making *hatchets,* and other instruments; and hence its name.—*Cleav Min.* A.]

AXI'LLA. (*Axilla, æ.* f. *Atzil*, Heb. Scaliger deduces it from *ago*, to act; in this manner, *ago, axo axa, axula, axilla.*) 1. In anatomy, the cavity under the upper part of the arm, called the arm-pit.

2. In botany, the angle formed by the branch and stem of a plant, or by the leaf with either.

AXILLARIS. (From *axilla*, the arm-pit.) Axillary. 1. Of, or belonging to the *axilla*, or arm-pit.

2. In botany, leaves, &c. are said to be axillary which proceed from the angles formed by the stem and branch.

AXILLARIS. See *Axillary.*

Axillaris gemma. Axillary gem. The gem which comes out of the axilla of a plant. It is this which bears the fruit.

AXILLARY. (*Axillaris;* from *axilla*, the arm-pit.) Of or belonging to the axilla, or arm-pit.

Axillary arteries. *Arteriæ axillares.* The axillary arteries are continuations of the subclavians, and give off, each of them, in the axilla, four mammary arteries, the subscapular, and the posterior and anterior circumflex arteries, which ramify about the joint.

Axillary nerves. *Nervis axillares.* Articular nerve. A branch of the brachial plexus, and sometimes of the radial nerve. It runs outwards and backwards, around the neck of the humerus, and is lost in the muscles of the scapula.

Axillary veins. *Venæ axillares.* The axillary veins receive the blood from the veins of the arm, and evacuate it into the subclavian vein.

AXINITE. *Thumerstone.* A massive or crystallized mineral, the crystals of which resemble an axe in the form and sharpness of their edges. It is found in beds at Thum, in Saxony, and in Cornwall.

[This mineral is sometimes in tabular masses, but most commonly in crystals, which are easily recognised. The general form of these crystals is a very oblique romb, or rather four-sided prism, so flattened, that some of its edges become thin and sharp, like the edge of an axe. The primitive form is a four-sided prism, whose bases are parallelograms with angles of 101° 30′ and 78° 30′. The integrant particles are oblique triangular prisms. M. Haüy has described five secondary forms.

Before the blow-pipe it easily melts with ebullition, into a dark gray enamel, which with borax becomes olive green. It contains, according to Vauquelin, silex 44, alumine 18, lime 19, iron 14, manganese 4,=99.

Axinite is a rare mineral. It is found in primitive rocks, more particularly in fissures or veins which traverse them. In Dauphiny, it is associated with quartz, feldspar, epidote, and asbestus. In the Pyrenees with quartz and limestone. In Norway, near Arendal, with feldspar and epidote; and near Konsberg it exists in limestone with mica, quartz, &c. It occurs in lamellar masses near *Thum* in Saxony, whence the name Thumerstone.—*Cl. Min.* A.]

A'XIS. (From *ago*, to act.) The second vertebra. See *Dentatus*.

AXU'NGIA. (*Axungia*, *æ*. f.; from *axis*, an axletree, and *unguo*, to anoint.) Hog's lard.

AXUNGIA CURATA. Purified hog's lard.

AXUNGIA DE MUMMIA. Marrow.

A'ZAC. (Arabian.) Gum ammoniac.

AZA'GOR. Verdigris.

AZALÆA. (From αζαλεος, dry, from its growing in a dry soil.) The name of a genus of plants in the Linnæan system. Class, *Pentandria*; Order, *Monogynia*.

AZALÆA PONTICA. The Pontic azalea.

AZAMAR. Native cinnabar. Vermilion.

AZED. A fine kind of camphire.

AZOTE. (From *a*, priv. and ζεω, to live; because it is unfit for respiration.) Azot. See *Nitrogen*.

Azotane. The chloride of azote.

Azote, chloride of. See *Nitrogen*.

Azote, deutoxyde of. See *Nitrogen*

Azote, gaseous oxyde of. See *Nitrogen*.

Azote, iodide of. See *Nitrogen*.

Azote, protoxyde of. See *Nitrogen*.

A'ZOTH. An imaginary universal remedy

A'ZUB. Alum.

Azurestone. See *Lapis lazuli*.

Azure spar, prismatic. See *Azurite*

AZURITE. Prismatic azure spar. Lazulite of Werner. A mineral of a fine blue colour, composed of alumina, magnesia, silica, oxyde of iron, and lime. It occurs in Vorau, in Stiria, and the bishopric of Salzburg.

AZU'RIUM. Quicksilver, sulphur, and sal-ammoniac.

A'ZYGES. (From *a*, priv. and ζυγος, a yoke.) The os sphenoides was so called, because it has no fellow.

A'ZYGOS. (From *a*, priv. and ζυγος, a yoke; because it has no fellow.) Several single muscles, veins, bones, &c. are so called.

AZYGOS PROCESSUS. A process of the os sphenoides.

AZYGOS UVULÆ. A muscle of the uvula. *Palato staphilinus* of Douglas. *Staphilinus*, or *Epistaphilinus* of Winslow. It arises at one extremity of the suture which joins the palate bones, runs down the whole length of the velum and uvula, resembling an earth-worm, and adhering to the tendons of the circumflexi. It is inserted into the tip of the uvula. Its use is to raise the uvula upwards and forwards, and to shorten it.

AZYGOS VENA. Azygos vein. *Vena sine pari*. This vein is situated in the right cavity of the thorax, upon the dorsal vertebræ. It receives the blood from the vertebral, intercostal, bronchial, pericardiac, and diaphragmatic veins, and evacuates it into the vena cava superior.

B.

BABUZICA'RIUS. (Βαβουζικαριος; from βαβαζω, to speak inarticulately.) The incubus, or nightmare: so called, because, in it, the person is apt to make an inarticulate or confused noise.

BA'CCA. (*Bacca*, *æ*. f., a berry.) A pulpy pericarpium, or seed-vessel, enclosing several naked seeds, connected by a slender membrane, and dispersed through the pulp. It is distinguished by its figure into,

1. *Bacca rotunda*, round; as in *Ribes rubrum*, the currant, and *Grossularia*, the gooseberry.
2. *Bacca oblonga*, oblong; as in *Barbaria vulgaris*, common barberry.
3. *Bacca dicocca*, double, as in *Jasminum*.
4. *Bacca recutita*, circumcised like the prominent glans penis, without the prepuce; as in *Taxus baccata*.

From the substances it is denominated,

1. *Bacca succosa*, juicy; as in *Ribes rubrum*.
2. *Bacca corticosa*, covered with a hard bark; as in *Garcinia mangostana*.
3. *Bacca exsicca*, dry; as in *Hedera helix*.

From the number of loculaments into,

1. *Bacca unilocularis*, with one; as in the *Actæa* and *Cactus*.
2. *Bacca bilocularis*, with two; as in *Lonicera*.
3. *Bacca trilocularis*, with three; as in *Asparagus* and *Ruscus*.
4. *Bacca quadrilocularis*, with four; as *Caris quadrifolia*.
5. *Bacca quinquelocularis*, with five; as in *Melastoma*.
6. *Bacca multilocularis*, with many; as in *Nymphæa*.

From the number of the seeds into,

1. *Bacca monosperma*, with one only; as in *Daphne*, *Viscum*, and *Viburnum*.
2. *Bacca disperma*, with two seeds; as *Barbarea vulgaris*, and *Coffea arabica*.
3. *Bacca trisperma*, with three; as in *Sambucus*, and *Juniperus*.
4. *Bacca quadrisperma*, with four; as in *Ligustrum*, and *Ilex*.
5. *Bacca polysperma*, with many seeds; as in *Arbutus unedo*, *Ribes*, and *Gardenia*.

The *Bacca* is also distinguished into *simple* and *compound*, when it is composed of several berries, which are called *acini*; as in *Rubus fruticosus*.

BACCA BERMUDENSIS. The Bermuda berry. See *Sapindus saponaria*.

BACCA JUNIPERI. The juniper berry. See *Juniperus communis*.

BACCA LAURI. The laurel berry. See *Laurus nobilis*.

BACCA MONSPELIENSIS. See *Inula dysenterica*.

BACCA NORLANDICA. The shrubby strawberry. See *Rubus arcticus*.

BACCA PISCATORIA. So named because fish are caught with them. See *Menispermum cocculus*.

BACCA'LIA. (From *baccharum copia*, because it abounds in berries.) The bay, or laurel-tree. See *Laurus nobilis*.

BA'CCHARIS. (From *bacchus*, wine; from its fragrance resembling that liquor.) See *Inula dysenterica*.

BACCIFERUS. (From *bacca*, a berry, and *fero*, to bear.) Berry bearing.

BACCIFERÆ PLANTÆ. Plants are so called which have a berry or pulpy pericarpium.

BA'CCHIA. (From *bacchus*, wine; because it generally proceeds from hard drinking and intemperance.) A name given by Linnæus to the pimpled face, which results from free living.

BACCILLUM. A little berry.

BACCIUS, ANDREW, a native of Ancona, practised medicine at Rome towards the end of the 16th century, and became physician to Pope Sixtus V. He appears to have had great industry and learning from his numerous publications; of which the chief, "De Thermis," gives an extensive examination of natural waters.

BA'CCULI. 1. Is used, by some writers, for a particular kind of lozenges, shaped into little short rolls.

2. Hildanus likewise uses it for an instrument in surgery.

Bacher's Pills. Pilulæ tonicæ Bacheri. A celebrated medicine in France, employed for the cure of dropsies. Their principal ingredient is the extract of melampodium, or black hellebore.

BA'COBA. The *Banana.*

BACTISHUA, GEORGE, was a celebrated physician of Chorasan, distinguished also for his literary attainments. He was successful in curing the reigning caliph of a complaint of the stomach, which brought him into great honour; he translated several of the ancient medical authors into the Arabian language; and many of his observations are recorded by Rhazes and other succeeding physicians. His son, *Gabriel*, was in equal estimation with the famous Haroun Al Raschid, whom he cured of apoplexy by blood-letting, in opposition to the opinion of the other physicians.

BADIA'GA. A kind of sponge usually sold in Russia, the powder of which is said to take away the livid marks of blows and bruises within a few hours. It is only described by Bauxbaum, and its nature is not properly understood.

BADIAN SEMEN. The seed of a tree which grows in China, and smells like aniseed. The Chinese, and Dutch, in imitation of them, sometimes use the badian to give their tea an aromatic taste.

BADI'ZA AQUA. See *Bath waters.*

BADRANUM SEMEN. Indian aniseed.

BADU'CCA. The Indian name for a species of capparis.

BA'DZCHER. An antidote.

BÆ'OS. Βαιος. In Hippocrates it means few; but in P. Ægineta, it is an epithet for a poultice.

BAGLIVI, GEORGE, born at Ragusa in 1668, after graduating at Padua, and improving himself greatly by travelling throughout Italy, was made professor of medicine and anatomy at Rome. In 1696, he published an excellent work on the practice of physic, condemning the exclusive attachment to theory, and earnestly recommending the Hippocratic method of observation; which, he maintained, assisted by the modern improvements in anatomy and physiology, would tend greatly to the advancement of medicine. He has left also several other tracts, though he died at the early age of thirty-eight.

BAGNIGGE WELLS. A saline mineral spring, near Clerkenwell, in London, resembling the Epsom water. In most constitutions, three half-pints is considered a full dose for purging.

BA'GNIO. (From *bagno*, Italian.) A bathing or sweating-house.

BA'HEI COYOLLI. Ray takes it to be the *Areca*, or *Faufel.*

BA'HEL SCHULLI. An Indian tree. See *Genista spinosa indica.*

BAHODAL. See *Adansonia.*

BAIKALITE. The asbestiform species of tremolite.

[It is a variety of tremolite which Kirwan named Baikalite, because it was first found near lake Baikal in Siberia, in foliated limestone.—In Chinese Tartary it occurs in dolomite.

It is found in groups of acicular prisms, sometimes very long, and sometimes radiating from a centre. Its colour is greenish, often with a shade of yellow; and its lustre sometimes silky. According to Kirwan, its spec. grav. is only 2.20, and it melts into a dark green glass. It contains silex 44, lime 20, magnesia 30, oxyde of iron 6.—See *Cl. Min.* A.]

BAILLIE, MATTHEW, born in Scotland, in the year 1760. His mother was sister of the two celebrated Hunters, Dr. William and Mr. John; his father, a clergyman. In the early part of his education he enjoyed great advantages. After studying at Glasgow, where his father was Professor of Divinity, he was sent to one of the exhibitions of that university at Baliol College, Oxford, where he took his degrees in physic, by which he became a Fellow of the College of Physicians in London, and was soon after elected Fellow of the Royal Society. At an early period he came to London and was an inmate with his uncle, Dr. William Hunter, at that time lecturing to a numerous class of pupils, and who had the superintendence of his education. After demonstrating in the dissecting room with the celebrated and learned Mr. Cruickshanks, he became, on the death of his uncle, joint lecturer with him, and continued to lecture until 1799

Dr. Baillie's practice as a physician was for several years extremely small, and he often complained of the little he had to do; indeed, at one time, he thought of leaving the metropolis. In the year 1787, he was elected physician to St. George's Hospital; and he now began to find his practice increase. About this period he married.

Dr. Denman, the celebrated accoucheur of the day, had two daughters; Mr. Croft, afterward Sir Richard, married one, Dr. Baillie, the other. The confidence which the two first obtained in the higher circles of society, was great and extensive; and they lost no opportunity of requiring the opinion and attendance of their relation. Dr. Baillie's pupils had now gone yearly to every part of England, and the Indies, and were not merely enforcing the principles and doctrines of their master, whose lectures they had heard delivered with such lucid order, and clearness of expression, as to convey information in the most simple and intelligible manner; but were sending their patients from the most distant parts to profit by his advice and experience. Two other circumstances soon occurred, which at once placed Dr. Baillie in a practice before unheard of. His uncle's, and his own great friend, Dr. Pitcairn, who was in great practice, was, from ill health, obliged to leave England for a more temperate climate, and he previously introduced him to all his patients; and Dr. Warren, who had enjoyed the greater part of the practice of the nobility, was suddenly cut off. There was no practitioner left whose opportunities had fitted him to take the lead, and thus a field was opened for aspiring genius, ability, skill, and perseverance, which Dr. Baillie soon occupied, and from which he reaped an abundant harvest for more than twenty years.

Before he discontinued his lectures in 1799, he published an octavo volume, on Morbid Anatomy, in which is compressed more accurate and more useful information than is to be found in the elaborate works of Bonetus, Morgagni, and Lieutaud. This was followed by a large work, consisting of a series of splendid engravings to illustrate Morbid Anatomy. He also gave a description of the gravid uterus, and many important contributions to the transactions and medical collections of the time.

Dr. Baillie presented his collection of specimens of morbid parts to the college of physicians, with a sum of money to be expended in keeping them in order.

The professional and moral character of this great physician cannot be too highly appreciated. To his brethren, among whom he might, from his extensive and peculiar practice, have exercised a high and reserved deportment, he was humble, attentive, communicative, and kind; and he never permitted the caprice of a patient or friends to interfere with the conduct of, or injure a practitioner, when unjustly censured.

In the exercise of his practice, he displayed a discriminating and profound knowledge; happy in the conception of the cause of symptoms, he distinguished diseases from those with which they might have been confounded, and pointed out their probable progress and termination; and in delivering his opinion, he expressed himself with clearness, decision, and candour

His moral character was adorned by the strictest virtues, and amplest charities. He died in the year 1823, in the sixty-third year of his age, from a gradual decay of the powers of nature, continuing to practise until about a year before his death, leaving a wife, a son, a daughter, and a sister, Miss Joanna Baillie, who has acquired a degree of eminence surpassed by none of her sex in any age. A few of his private professional friends have directed a simple tablet and bust from the chisel of Chantry, to be placed in Westminster Abbey, to perpetuate his high and honourable professional character, and his many private virtues.

BAILLOU, GUILLAUME DE, commonly called *Ballonius*, was born in 1538 at Paris, where he graduated, and attained considerable eminence. He was very active in the contest for precedence between the physicians and surgeons, which was at length decided in favour of the former. His writings are numerous, though not now much esteemed; but he appears to have been the first, who properly discriminated between gout and rheumatism.

Ba'la. The plaintain-tree.

BALÆ'NA. (Βαλαινα; from βαλλω, to cast, from its power in casting up water.) The name of a genus of animals. Class, *Mammalia;* Order, *Cete.*

[Balæna mysticetus. The systematic and Linnæan name for the common or right whale, which is pursued in the icy and Greenland seas, on the coast of Brazil, and in the Pacific Ocean, supplying, when taken, blubber and whalebone. The blubber is the fat cut from the body of the whale, and being afterward tried, produces common whale or lamp oil. The *whalebone* is a horny substance projecting from the jaws, and does not partake of the nature of bone. The ends are split into numerous fibres, and the animal uses them as a filtering machine. The right-whale lives upon the small worms and molluscous animals which abound in the ocean. When it feeds, it opens the mouth, and swims forward, and when it has collected a large quantity of these vermes, the mouth is closed, and the water is forced through the fibrous ends of the whalebone, while the small animals are retained within and swallowed.—See *Scoresby's North. Whale Fishery.* A.]

Balæna macrocephala. The systematic name of a species of whale.

[This is the *cacholet* or large-headed whale, the true spermaceti-whale, principally taken in the Pacific ocean. It is called *macrocephalus*, from μακρος, large, and κεφαλη, the head, because the head constitutes two-thirds of the animal. The blubber or fat is stripped off this as it is from the right-whale, and affords abundant oil. There is however a cavity in the skull of the marcrocephalus containing a large quantity of pure oil called head-matter, which affords the best of spermaceti. In the natural state it is so liquid that it can be dipped out with a bucket. A.]

Balais ruby. See *Spinelle.*

BALANCE. "The beginning and end of every exact chemical process consists in weighing. With imperfect instruments this operation will be tedious and inaccurate; but with a good balance, the result will be satisfactory; and much time, which is so precious in experimental researches, will be saved.

The balance is a lever, the axis of motion of which is formed with an edge like that of a knife; and the two dishes at its extremities are hung upon edges of the same kind. These edges are first made sharp, and then rounded with a fine hone, or a piece of buff leather. The excellence of the instrument depends, in a great measure, on the regular form of this rounded part. When the lever is considered as a mere line, the two outer edges are called points of suspension, and the inner the fulcrum. The points of suspension are supposed to be at equal distances from the fulcrum, and to be pressed with equal weights when loaded.

1. If the fulcrum be placed in the centre of gravity of the beam, and the three edges lie all in the same right line, the balance will have no tendency to one position more than another, but will rest in any position it may be placed in, whether the scales be on or off, empty or loaded.

2. If the centre of gravity of the beam, when level, be immediately above the fulcrum, it will overset by the smallest action; that is, the end which is lowest will descend: and it will do this with more swiftness, the higher the centre of gravity, and the less the points of suspension are loaded.

3. But if the centre of gravity of the beam be immediately below the fulcrum, the beam will not rest in any position but when level; and, if disturbed from this position, and then left at liberty, it will vibrate, and at last come to rest on the level. Its vibrations will be quicker, and its horizontal tendency stronger, the lower the centre of gravity, and the less the weights upon the points of suspension.

4. If the fulcrum be below the line joining the points of suspension, and these be loaded, the beam will overset, unless prevented by the weight of the beam tending to produce a horizontal position. In this last case, small weights will equilibrate; a certain exact weight will rest in any position of the beam; and all greater weights will cause the beam to overset. Many scales are often made this way, and will overset with any considerable load.

5. If the fulcrum be above the line joining the points of suspension, the beam will come to the horizontal position, unless prevented by its own weight. If the centre of gravity of the beam be nearly in the fulcrum, all the vibrations of the loaded beam will be made in times nearly equal, unless the weights be very small, when they will be slower. The vibrations of balances are quicker, and the horizontal tendency stronger, the higher the fulcrum.

6. If the arms of a balance be unequal, the weights in equipoise will be unequal in the same proportion. It is a severe check upon a workman to keep the arms equal, while he is making the other adjustments in a strong and inflexible beam.

7. The equality of the arms of a balance is of use, in scientific pursuits, chiefly in making weights by bisection. A balance with unequal arms will weigh as accurately as another of the same workmanship with equal arms, provided the standard weight itself be first counterpoised, then taken out of the scale, and the thing to be weighed be put into the scale, and adjusted against the counterpoise; or when proportional quantities only are considered, as in chemical and in other philosophical experiments, the bodies and products under examination may be weighed against the weights, taking care always to put the weights into the same scale. For then, though the bodies may not be really equal to the weights, yet their proportions among each other may be the same as if they had been accurately so.

8. But though the quality of the arms may be well dispensed with, yet it is indispensably necessary that their relative lengths, whatever they may be, should continue invariable. For this purpose, it is necessary, either that the three edges be all truly parallel, or that the points of suspension and support should be always in the same part of the edge. This last requisite is the most easily obtained.

The balances made in London are usually constructed in such a manner, that the bearing parts form notches in the other parts of the edges; so that the scales being set to vibrate, all the parts naturally fall into the same bearing. The balances made in the country have the fulcrum edge straight, and confined to one constant bearing by two side plates. But the points of suspension are referred to notches in the edges, like the London balances. The balances here mentioned, which come from the country, are enclosed in a small iron japanned box; and are to be met with at Birmingham and Sheffield ware-houses, though less frequently than some years ago; because a pocket contrivance for weighing guineas and half-guineas has got possession of the market. They are, in general, well made and adjusted, turn with the twentieth of a grain when empty, and will sensibly show the tenth of a grain, with an ounce in each scale. Their price is from five shillings to half a guinea; but those which are under seven shillings, have not their edges hardened, and consequently are not durable. This may be ascertained by the purchaser, by passing the point of a penknife across the small piece which goes through one of the end boxes: if it make any mark or impression, the part is soft.

9. If a beam be adjusted so as to have no tendency to any one position, and the scales be equally loaded, then, if a small weight be added in one of the scales, that balance will turn, and the points of suspension will move with an accelerated motion, similar to that of falling bodies, but as much slower, in proportion, very nearly, as the added weight is less than the whole weight borne by the fulcrum.

10. The stronger the tendency to a horizontal position in any balance, or the quicker its vibrations, the greater additional weight will be required to cause it to turn, or incline to any given angle. No balance, therefore, can turn so quick as the motion deduced. Such a balance as is there described, if it were to turn with the ten-thousandth part of the weight, would move at quickest ten thousand times slower than falling bodies; that is, the dish containing the weight, instead of falling through sixteen feet in a second of time, would fall through only two hundred parts of an inch, and it would require four seconds to move through one-third part of an inch; consequently all accurate weighing must be slow. If the indices of two balances be of equal lengths, that index which is connected with the shorter balance will move proportionally quicker than the other. Long beams are the most in request, because they are thought to have less friction: this is doubtful, but the quicker angular motion,

greater strength, and less weight of a short balance, are certainly advantages.

11. Very delicate balances are not only useful in nice experiments, but are likewise much more expeditious than others in common weighing. If a pair of scales with a certain load be barely sensible to one-tenth of a grain, it will require a considerable time to ascertain the weight to that degree of accuracy, because the turn must be observed several times over, and is very small. But if no greater accuracy were required, and scales were used which would turn with the hundredth of a grain, a tenth of a grain, more or less, would make so great a difference in the turn, that it would be seen immediately.

12. If a balance be found to turn with a certain addition, and is not moved by any smaller weight, a greater sensibility may be given to that balance, by producing a tremulous motion in its parts. Thus, if the edge of a blunt saw, a file, or other similar instrument, be drawn along any part of the case or support of a balance, it will produce a jarring, which will diminish the friction on the moving parts so much, that the turn will be evident with one-third or one-fourth of the addition that would else have been required. In this way, a beam which would barely turn by the addition of one-tenth of a grain, will turn with one-thirtieth or fortieth of a grain.

13. A balance, the horizontal tendency of which depends only on its own weight, will turn with the same addition, whatever may be the load; except so far as a greater load will produce a greater friction.

14. But a balance, the horizontal tendency of which depends only on the elevation of the fulcrum, will be less sensible the greater the load; and the addition requisite to produce an equal turn will be in proportion to the load itself.

15. In order to regulate the horizontal tendency in some beams, the fulcrum is placed below the points of suspension, and a sliding weight is put upon the cock or index, by means of which the centre of gravity may be raised or depressed. This is a useful contrivance.

16. Weights are made by a subdivision of a standard weight. If the weight be continually halved, it will produce the common pile, which is the smallest number for weighing between its extremes, without placing any weight in the scale with the body under examination. Granulated lead is a very convenient substance to be used in this operation of halving, which, however, is very tedious. The readiest way to subdivide small weights, consists in weighing a certain quantity of small wire, and afterward cutting it into such parts, by measure, as are desired; or the wire may be wrapped close round two pins, and then cut asunder with a knife. By this means it will be divided into a great number of equal lengths, or small rings. The wire ought to be so thin, as that one of these rings may barely produce a sensible effect on the beam. If any quantity (as, for example, a grain) of these rings be weighed, and the number then reckoned, the grain may be subdivided in any proportion, by dividing that number, and making the weights equal to as many of the rings as the quotient of the division denotes. Then, if 750 of the rings amounted to a grain, and it were required to divide the grain decimally, downwards, 9-10ths would be equal to 675 rings, 8-10ths would be equal to 600 rings, 7-10ths to 525 rings, &c. Small weights may be made of thin leaf brass. Jewellers' foil is a good material for weights below 1-10th of a grain, as low as to 1-100th of a grain; and all lower quantities may be either estimated by the position of the index, or shown by actually counting the rings of wire, the value of which has been determined.

17. In philosophical experiments, it will be found very convenient to admit no more than one dimension of weight. The grain is of that magnitude as to deserve the preference. With regard to the number of weights the chemists ought to be provided with, writers have differed according to their habits and views. Mathematicians have computed the least possible number, with which all weights within certain limits might be ascertained; but their determination is of little use. Because, with so small a number, it must often happen, that the scales will be heavily loaded with weights on each side, put in with a view only to determine the difference between them. It is not the least possible number of weights which it is necessary an operator should buy to effect his purpose, that we ought to inquire after, but the most convenient number for ascertaining his inquiries with accuracy and expedition. The error of adjustment is the least possible, when only one weight is in the scale; that is, a single weight of five grains is twice as likely to be true, as two weights, one of three, and the other of two grains, put into the dish to supply the place of the single five; because each of these last has its own probability of error in adjustment. But since it is as inconsistent with convenience to provide a single weight, as it would be to have a single character for every number; and as we have nine characters, which we use in rotation, to express higher values according to their position, it will be found very serviceable to make the set of weights correspond with our numerical system. This directs us to the set of weights as follows: 1000 grains, 900 g. 800 g. 700 g. 600 g. 500 g. 400 g. 300. 200 g. 100 g. 90 g. 80 g. 70 g. 60 g. 50 g. 40 g. 30 g. 20 g. 10 g. 9 g. 8 g. 7 g. 6 g. 5 g. 4 g. 3 g. 2 g. 1 g. 9-10 g. 8-10 g. 7-10 g. 6-10 g. 5-10 g. 4-10 g. 3-10 g. 2-10 g. 1-10 g. 9-100 g. 8-100 g. 7-100 g. 6-100 g. 5-100 g. 4-100 g. 3-100 g. 2-100 g. 1-100 g. With these the philosopher will always have the same number of weights in his scales as there are figures in the number expressing the weights in grains. Thus 742.5 grains will be weighed by the weights 700, 40, 2, and 5-10ths."—*Ure's Chemical Dictionary.*

BALANI'NUM OLEUM. Oil of the ben-nut.

BALANOCA'STANUM. (From βαλανος, a nut, and καςανον, a chesnut; so called from its tuberous root.) The earth-nut. See *Bunium bulbocastanum.*

BA'LANOS. (From βαλλω, to cast; because it sheds its fruit upon the ground.) *Balanus.* 1. An acorn.

2. The oak-tree. See *Quercus robur.*

3. Theophrastus uses it sometimes to express any glandiferous tree.

4. From the similitude of form, this word is used to express suppositories and pessaries, βαλανος signifying a nut.

5. A name of the glans penis.

Balas ruby. See *Spinelle.*

BALAU'STIUM. (From βαλιος, various, and αυω, to dry; so called from the variety of its colours, and its becoming soon dry; or from βλαςανω, to germinate.) *Balaustia.* A large rose-like flower, of a red colour, the produce of the plant from which we obtain the granate. See *Punica granatum.*

BALBU'TIES. (From βαβαζω, to stammer; or from *balbel*, Heb. to stammer.) A defect of speech; properly, that sort of stammering where the patient sometimes hesitates, and immediately after, speaks precipitately. It is the *Psellismus balbutiens* of Cullen.

Baldmoney. See *Æthusa meum.*

Baldwin's phosphorus. Ignited nitrate of lime.

BALISMUS. (Βαλλισμος; from βαλλιζω, *tripudio pedibus plando.*) The specific name of a disease in Good's genus *Synclonus* for shaking palsy. See *Chorea* and *Tremor.*

BALI'STA. (From βαλλω, to cast.) The astragalus, a bone of the foot, was formerly called os balistæ, because the ancients used to cast it from their slings.

BALLOO'N. (*Ballon*, or *balon*, French.) 1. A large glass receiver in the form of a hollow globe. For certain chemical operations *balloons* are made with two necks, placed opposite to each other; one to receive the neck of a retort, and the other to enter the neck of a second *balloon:* this apparatus is called *enfiladed balloons.* Their use is to increase the whole space of the receiver, because any number of these may be adjusted to each other. The only one of these vessels which is generally used, is a small oblong *balloon* with two necks, which is to be luted to the retort, and to the receiver, or great *balloon;* it serves to remove this receiver from the body of the furnace, and to hinder it from being too much heated.

2. A spherical bag filled with a gas of a small specific gravity, or with heated air, by the buoyancy of which it is raised into the atmosphere.

BALLO'TE. (From βαλλω, to send forth, and ους ωτος the ear; because it sends forth flowers like ears.) *Ballota.* The name of a genus of plants. Class, *Didynamia;* Order, *Gymnospermia.*

BALLOTE NIGRA. Stinking horehound. A nettle-like plant, used, when boiled, by the country people against scurvy and cutaneous eruptions.

BALM. See *Melissa*.

Balm of Gilead. See *Dracocephalum.*

Balm of Mecca. See *Amyris gileadensis.*

Balm, Turkey. See *Dracocephalum.*

BA'LNEUM. (*Balneum, ei.* n. βαλανειον, a bath.) A bath, or bathing-house. See *Bath.*

BALNEUM ANIMALE. The wrapping any part of an animal just killed, round the body, or a limb.

BALNEUM ARENÆ. A sand-bath for chemical purposes. See *Bath.*

BALNEUM CALIDUM. A hot-bath. See *Bath.*

BALNEUM FRIGIDUM. A cold-bath. See *Bath.*

BALNEUM MARIÆ. *Balneum maris.* A warm-water bath. See *Bath.*

BALNEUM MEDICATUM. A bath impregnated with drugs.

BALNEUM SICCUM. *Balneum cinereum.* A dry bath, either with ashes, sand, or iron filings.

BALNEUM SULPHUREUM. A sulphurous bath.

BALNEUM TEPIDUM. A tepid bath. See *Bath.*

BALNEUM VAPORIS. A vapour bath.

BA'LSAM. (*Balsamum;* from *baal samen,* Hebrew.) The term balsam was anciently applied to any strong-scented, natural vegetable resin of about the fluidity of treacle, inflammable, not miscible with water, without addition, and supposed to be possessed of many medical virtues. All the turpentines, the Peruvian balsam, copaiba balsam, &c. are examples of natural balsams. Besides, many medicines compounded of various resins, or oils, and brought to this consistence, obtained the name of balsam. Latterly, however, chemists have restricted this term to vegetable juices, either liquid, or which spontaneously become concrete, consisting of a substance of a resinous nature, combined with benzoic acid, or which are capable of affording benzoic acid, by being heated alone, or with water. They are insoluble in water, but readily dissolve in alkohol and æther. The liquid balsams are copaiva, opo-balsam, Peru, styrax, Tolu; the concrete are benzoin, dragon's blood, and storax.

Balsam apple, male. The fruit of the *elaterium.* See *Momordica elaterium.*

Balsam, artificial. Compound medicines are thus termed which are made of a balsamic consistence and fragrance. They are generally composed of expressed or ethereal oils, resins, and other solid bodies, which give them the consistence of butter. The basis, or body of them, is expressed oil of nutmeg, and frequently wax, butter, &c. They are usually tinged with cinnabar and saffron.

Balsam of Canada. See *Pinus Balsamea.*

Balsam, Canary. See *Dracocephalum.*

Balsam of Copaiba. See *Copaifera officinalis.*

Balsam, natural. A resin which has not yet assumed the concrete form, but still continues in a fluid state, is so called, as common turpentine, balsamum copaiva, peruvianum, tolutanum, &c.

Balsam, Peruvian. See *Myroxylon Peruiferum.*

Balsam of sulphur. See *Balsamum sulphuris.*

Balsam of Tolu. See *Toluifera balsamum.*

Balsam, Turkey. See *Dracocephalum.*

BALSAMA'TIO. (From *balsamum,* a balsam.) The embalming of dead bodies.

BALSA'MEA. (From *balsamum,* balsam.) The balm of Gilead fir; so called from its odour. See *Pinus balsamea.*

BALSAMELÆ'ON. (From *balsamum,* balsam, and ελαιον, oil.) Balm of Gilead, or true balsamum Judaicum.

BA'LSAMI OLEUM. Balm of Gilead.

BALSA'MIC. (*Balsamica,* sc. *medicamenta;* from βαλσαμον, balsam.) A term generally applied to substances of a smooth and oily consistence, which possess emollient, sweet, and generally aromatic qualities. Hoffman calls those medicines by this name, which are hot and acrid, and also the natural balsams, stimulating gums, &c. by which the vital heat is increased. Dr. Cullen speaks of them under the joint title of *balsamica et resinosa,* considering that turpentine is the basis of all balsams.

BALSAMI'FERA. (From *balsamum,* balsam, and *fero,* to bear.) Balsam berry.

BALSAMIFERA BRAZILIENSIS. The copaiba tree. See *Copaifera officinalis.*

BALSAMIFERA INDICANA. Peruvian balsam tree. See *Myroxylon peruiferum.*

BALSAMITA FŒMINEA. See *Achillea ageratum*

BALSAMITA LUTEA. See *Polygonum persicaria.*

BALSAMITA MAJOR. See *Tanacetum balsamita.*

BALSAMITA MAS. See *Tanacetum balsamita.*

BALSAMITA MINOR. Sweet maudlin.

BA'LSAMUM. (From *baal samen,* the Hebrew for the prince of oils.) A Balsam. See *Balsam.*

BALSAMUM ÆGYPTIACUM. See *Amyris gileadensis*

BALSAMUM ALPINUM. See *Amyris gileadensis.*

BALSAMUM AMERICANUM. See *Myroxylon peruiferum.*

BALSAMUM ANODYNUM. A preparation made from tacamahacca, distilled with turpentine and soap liniment; and tincture of opium, but there were a great number of balsams sold under this name formerly.

BALSAMUM ARCÆI. A preparation composed of gum-elemi and suet.

BALSAMUM ASIATICUM. See *Amyris gileadensis.*

BALSAMUM BRAZILIENSE. See *Pinus balsamea.*

BALSAMUM CANADENSE. See *Pinus balsamea.*

BALSAMUM CEPHALICUM. A distillation from oils, nutmegs, cloves, amber, &c.

BALSAMUM COMMENDATORIS. A composition of storax, benzoe, myrrh, aloes.

BALSAMUM COPAIBÆ. See *Copaifera officinalis.*

BALSAMUM EMBRYONUM. A preparation of aniseed, fallen into disuse.

BALSAMUM GENUINUM ANTIQUORUM. See *Amyris gileadensis.*

BALSAMUM GILEADENSE. See *Amyris gileadensis*

BALSAMUM GUAIACINUM. Balsam of Peru and spirits of wine.

BALSAMUM GUIDONIS. The same as balsamum anodynum.

BALSAMUM HUNGARICUM. A balsam prepared from a coniferous tree on the Carpathian mountains.

BALSAMUM JUDAICUM. See *Amyris gileadensis.*

BALSAMUM LUCATELLI. (*Lucatelli;* so called from its inventor Lucatellus.) A preparation made of oil, turpentine, wax, and red saunders; now disused; formerly exhibited in coughs of long standing.

BALSAMUM MAS. The herb costmary. See *Tanacetum balsamita.*

BALSAMUM E MECCA. See *Amyris gileadensis.*

BALSAMUM MEXICANUM. See *Myroxylon peruiferum.*

BALSAMUM NOVUM. A new balsam from a red fruit in the West Indies.

BALSAMUM ODORIFERUM. A preparation of oil, wax, and any essential oil.

BALSAMUM PERSICUM. A balsam composed of storax, benzoe, myrrh, and aloes.

BALSAMUM PERUVIANUM. See *Myroxylon peruiferum.*

BALSAMUM RACKASIRA. This balsam, which is inodorous when cold, but of a smell approaching to that of Tolu balsam when heated, is brought from India in gourd-shells. It is slightly bitter to the taste, and adheres to the teeth, on chewing. It is supposed to be one of the factitious balsams, and is scarcely ever prescribed in this country.

BALSAMUM SAMECH. A factitious balsam, composed of tartar, and spirits of wine.

BALSAMUM SAPONACEUM. A name given to the preparation very similar to the compound soap liniment.

BALSAMUM SATURNI. The remedy so named is prepared by dissolving the acetate of lead in oil of turpentine, by digesting the mixture till it acquires a red colour. This is found to be a good remedy for cleansing foul ulcers; but it is not acknowledged in our dispensatories.

BALSAMUM STYRACIS BENZOINI. See *Styrax benzoin*

BALSAMUM SUCCINI. Oil of amber.

BALSAMUM SULPHURIS. A solution of sulphur in oil

BALSAMUM SULPHURIS ANISATUM. Terebinthinated balsam of sulphur, and oil of aniseed.

BALSAMUM SULPHURIS BARBADENSE. Sulphur boiled with Barbadoes tar.

BALSAMUM SULPHURIS CRASSUM. Thick balsam of sulphur.

BALSAMUM SULPHURIS SIMPLEX. Sulphur boiled with oil.

BALSAMUM SULPHURIS TEREBINTHINATUM. This is made by digesting the sulphur with oil of turpentine, it is now confined to veterinary medicine.

BALSAMUM SYRIACUM. See *Amyris gileadensis.*

BALSAMUM TOLUTANUM. See *Toluifera balsamum*

Balsamum traumaticum. Vulnerary balsam. A form of medicine intended to supply the place of the tincture commonly called Friar's balsam, so famous for curing old ulcers. The London College have named it Tinctura Benzoini composita.

Balsamum universale. The unguentum saturninum of old pharmacopœias. See *Ceratum plumbi compositum.*

Balsamum verum. See *Amyris gileadensis.*

Balsamum viride. Linseed-oil, turpentine, and verdigris mixed together.

Balsamum vitæ hoffmanni. *Beaume de vie.* An artificial balsam, so named from its inventor, and composed of a great variety of the warmest and most grateful essential oils, such as nutmegs, cloves, lavender, &c., with balsam of Peru, dissolved in highly rectified spirit of wine; but it is now greatly abridged in the number of ingredients, and but little used.

Balzoi'num. The gum-benjamin.

BAMBA'LIO. (From βαμβαινω, to speak inarticulately.) A person who stammers, or lisps.

Bambo'o. (An Indian root.) See *Arundo bambos.*

Ba'mia moschata. See *Hibiscus.*

Bamier. The name of a plant common in Egypt, the husk of which they dress with meat, and, from its agreeable flavour, make great use of it in their ragouts.

Ban a'rbor. The coffee-tree.

Bana'na. An Indian word. See *Musa sapientum.*

Bananei'ra. See *Banana.*

Ba'ncia. The wild parsnip.

BANDAGE. *Deligatio. Fascia.* An apparatus consisting of one or several pieces of linen, or flannel, and intended for covering or surrounding parts of the body for surgical purposes. Bandages are either simple or compound. The chief of the simple are the circular, the spiral, the uniting, the retaining, the expellent, and the creeping. The compound bandages used in surgery, are the T bandage, the suspensory one, the capistrum, the eighteen-tail bandage, and others, to be met with in surgical treatises.

Bandu'ra. A plant which grows in Ceylon, the root of which is said to be astringent.

Bangu'e. *Bange.* A species of opiate in great use throughout the East, for its intoxicating qualities. It is the leaf of a kind of wild hemp, growing in the countries of the Levant, and made into powder, pills, or conserves.

Ba'nica. The wild parsnip.

Bani'las. See *Epidendrum vanilla.*

Bani'lia. See *Epidendrum vanilla.*

Bao'bab. See *Adansonia digitata.*

Ba'ptica coccus. Kermes berries.

BAPTISTE'RIUM. (From βαπ7ω, to immerge.) A bath, or repository of water, to wash the body.

Bapti'strum. (From βαπ7ω, to dye.) A species of wild mustard, so called from its reddish colour.

BA'RBA. (From *barbarus*, because wild nations are usually unshaven.) 1. The beard of man.

2. In botany a species of pubescence, or down, with which the surface of some plants are covered sometimes in patches; as in the leaves of the *Mesembryanthemum barbatum.*

3. Some vegetables have the specific name of *barba*, the ramifications of which are bushy, like a beard, as *Barba, jovis*, &c.

Barba aronis. See *Arum maculatum.*

Barba capræ. See *Spirea ulmaria.*

Barba hirci. See *Tragopogon.*

Barba jovis. Jupiter's beard. This name is given to several plants, as the silver bush; the *Sempervivum majus;* and of a species of anthyllis.

BARBADOES. The name of an island in the West, from which we obtain a mineral tar, and several medicinal plants.

Barbadoes cherry. See *Malphigia glabra.*

Barbadoes nut. See *Jatropha curcas.*

Barbadoes tar. See *Petroleum barbadense*, the use of which in medicine is limited to its external application, at times, in paralytic cases.

Barba'rea. (From St. Barbary, who is said to have found its virtues.) See *Erysimum barbarea.*

Barbaro'ssæ pilula. Barbarossa's pill. An ancient composition of quicksilver, rhubarb, diagridium, musk, amber, &c. It was the first internal mercurial medicine which obtained any real credit.

Ba'rbarum. The name of a plaster in Scribonius Largus.

Barbatina. A Persian vermifuge seed.

BARBA'TUS. (From *barba*, a beard.) Bearded; applied to a leaf which has a hairy or beard-like pubescence; as *Mesembryanthemum barbatum*, and *Spananthe paniculata.*

BA'RBEL *Barbo.* An oblong fish, resembling the pike, the eating of the roe of which often brings on the cholera.

BARBERRY. See *Berberis.*

BARBEYRAC, Charles. A French physician of the 17th century, who graduated and settled at Montpelier, where he acquired great celebrity. He died in 1699, at the age of about 70, having published little, except a good account of the diseases of the chest and stomach in females. Mr. Locke, who became intimate with him abroad, considered him very similar in his manners and opinions to Sydenham. His practice is said to have been distinguished for simplicity and energy.

Barbo'ta. The barbut. A small river-fish. It is remarkable for the size of its liver, which is esteemed the most delicate part of it.

[**BARD, Dr. John.** Dr. Bard was of French descent. His ancestors preferring their faith to their country, became exiles under the provisions of the revocation of the edict of Nantes. Dr. Bard first settled in his profession in Philadelphia, but after practising in that city about five or six years, he was induced to remove to New-York in the year 1746. By the urbanity of his manners, his professional talents, and the charms of his conversation, which was enlivened by an uncommon flow of cheerfulness, enriched by sound sense, and adorned by a large fund of anecdote, he so effectually recommended himself to the notice and friendship of the most respectable families, that he was almost immediately introduced into a valuable scene of business, and very soon arrived at the first rank of professional eminence, which he retained through a long life of more than fourscore years. He died in March, 1799, leaving a son who afterward eclipsed his father in his professional career.—See *Thach. Med. Biog.* A.]

[**BARD, Samuel,** M.D. LL.D. was the son of Dr. John Bard, and was born in Philadelphia, April 1, 1742. He acquired his classical education at Kings, now Columbia College, in the city of New-York. He spent five years abroad, and acquired his medical education principally in Edinburgh, where he received his degree of Doctor in Medicine in May, 1765. He commenced practice in New-York, but the events of the revolution prevented his success until the close of the war in 1783, after which he rose in professional eminence until he retired from practice in 1798. After his return from Europe, he was instrumental in establishing the medical faculty which was annexed to Columbia College, his alma mater, and he was appointed the first professor of the practice of physic. The establishment of the New-York hospital was effected principally by his exertions, and he was for many years one of the physicians to the institution. He was author of several medical essays, but the principal work of his is a system of midwifery, published after he retired from practice. Princeton College in New Jersey conferred upon him the degree of (LL.D.) Doctor of Laws, on account of the high reputation of his professional skill, learning, and abilities.—See *Thach. Med. Biog.* A.]

BARDA'NA. (From *bardus*, foolish; because silly people are apt to throw them on the garments of passengers, having the property of sticking to whatever they touch.) Burdock. See *Arctium lappa.*

BARE'GE. The small village of Barege, celebrated for its thermal waters, is situated on the French side of the Pyrenees, about half way between the Mediterranean and the Bay of Biscay. The hot springs are four in number. They have all the same component parts, but differ somewhat in their temperature, and in the quantity of sulphur, the hottest being most strongly penetrated with this active ingredient. The coolest of these waters raises Fahrenheit's thermometer to 73 deg.; the hottest to 120 deg. Barege waters are remarkable for a very smooth, soapy feel; they render the skin very supple and pliable, and dissolve perfectly well soap and animal lymph; and are resorted to as a bath in resolving tumours of various kinds, rigidities, and contractions of the tendons, stiffness of the joints, left by rheumatic and gouty com-plants, and are highly serviceable in cutaneous eruptions. Internally taken, this water gives considerable relief in disorders of the stomach, especially attended with acidity and heart-burn, in obstinate colics, jaundice, and in gravel, and other affections of the urinary organs.

Bari'glia. See *Barilla.*

BARI'LLA. *Barillor; Bariglia* The term given in commerce to the impure soda imported from Spain and the Levant. It is made by burning to ashes different plants that grow on the sea-shore, chiefly of the genus *salsola*, and is brought to us in hard porous masses, of a speckled brown colour. Kelp, which is made in this country by burning sea-weeds, and is called *British barilla*, is much more impure.

[Barilla is much used in the arts on account of the soda it contains.

"Carbonate of soda is chiefly obtained by the combustion of marine plants, the ashes of which afford, by lixiviation, the impure alkali called *soda*. Two kinds of rough soda occur in the market; *barilla* and *kelp*; besides which some *native carbonate of soda* is also imported. Barilla is the semifused ashes of the *salsola soda*, which is largely cultivated upon the Mediterranean shores of Spain, in the vicinity of Alicant. Kelp consists of the ashes of sea-weeds which are collected upon the sea coast and burned in kilns, or merely in excavations made in the ground and surrounded by stones. It seldom contains more than five per cent. of carbonated alkali, and about 24 tons of sea-weed are required to produce one ton of kelp. The best produce is from the hardest *fuci*, such as the *serratus, digitatus, nodosus, and vesiculosus.* The rough alkali is contaminated by common salt, and impurities, from which it may be separated by solution in a small portion of water, filtrating the solution, and evaporating it at a low heat; the common salt may be skimmed off as its crystals form upon the surface."—See *Webster's Man. of Chem.* A.]

BARIUM. (From *barytes*, from which it is obtained.) The metallic basis of the earth barytes, so named by Sir Humphrey Davy, who discovered it.

Take pure barytes, make it into a paste with water, and put this on a plate of platinum. Make a cavity in the middle of the barytes, into which a globule of mercury is to be placed. Touch the globule with the negative wire, and the platinum with the positive wire, of a voltaic battery of about 100 pairs of plates in good action. In a short time an amalgam will be formed, consisting of mercury and barium. This amalgam must be introduced into a little bent tube, made of glass free from lead, sealed at one end, which being filled with the vapour of naphtha, is then to be hermetically sealed at the other end. Heat must be applied to the recurved end of the tube, where the amalgam lies. The mercury will distil over, while the barium will remain.

This metal is of a dark gray colour, with a lustre inferior to that of cast iron. It is fusible at a red heat. Its density is superior to that of sulphuric acid; for though surrounded with globules of gas, it sinks immediately in that liquid. When exposed to air, it instantly becomes covered with a crust of barytes; and when gently heated in air, burns with a deep red light. It effervesces violently in water, converting this liquid into a solution of barytes."

BARK. A term very frequently employed to signify, by way of eminence, Peruvian bark. See *Cinchona.*

Bark, Carribæan. See *Cinchona Carribæa.*

Bark, Jamaica. See *Cinchona Carribæa.*

Bark, Peruvian. See *Cinchona.*

Bark, red. See *Cinchona oblongifolia.*

Bark, yellow. See *Cinchona cordifolia.*

BARLEY. See *Hordeum.*

Barley, caustic. See *Cevadilla.*

Barley, pearl. See *Hordeum.*

BARM. See *Fermentum cerevisiæ.*

BARNET. A town near London, where there is a mineral water; of a purging kind, of a similar quality to that of Epsom, and about half its strength.

[BAROLITE. The name given by Kirwan to the carbonate of barytes. A.]

BARO'METER. (From Βαρος, weight, and μετρον, measure.) An instrument to determine the weight of the air; it is commonly called a weather-glass.

Barolyte. A carbonate of barytes

Baro'nes. Small worms; called also Nepones.

BA'ROS. (Βαρος.) Gravity. 1. Hippocrates uses this word to express by it, an uneasy weight in any part.

2. It is also the Indian name for a species of camphire, which is distilled from the roots of the true cinnamon-tree.

[BAROSELENITE. Kirwan's name for the sulphate of barytes. A.]

Barras. Galipot. The resinous incrustation on the wounds made in fir-trees.

Barren Flower. See *Flos.*

BA'RRENNESS. See *Sterility.*

BA'RTHOLINE, Thomas, was born at Copenhagen in 1616. After studying in various parts of Europe, particularly Padua, and graduating at Basil, he became professor of anatomy in his native city; in which office he greatly distinguished himself, as well as in many other branches of learning. He was the first who described the lymphatics with accuracy; though some of these vessels, as well as the lacteals and thoracic duct, had been before discovered by other anatomists. Besides many learned works which he published, several others were unfortunately destroyed by fire in 1670; and he particularly regretted a dissertation on the ancient practice of midwifery, of which an outline was afterward published by his son *Caspar.* Of those which remain, the most esteemed are, his epistolary correspondence with the most celebrated of his cotemporaries: his collection of cases where fœtuses have been discharged by preternatural outlets; and the "Medical and Philosophical Transactions of Copenhagen," enriched by the communications of many correspondents. This last work was in four volumes, published within the ten years preceding his death, which happened 1680; and a fifth was afterward added by his son.

Bartholinia'næ glandulæ. See *Sublingual glands.*

[BARTLETT, Josiah, M. D. Dr. Bartlett was born in Amesbury in Massachusetts in 1729, and after acquiring his profession commenced practice in the town of Kingston in New-Hampshire, where he had acquired considerable reputation before the commencement of the American revolution, in which he took an active and decided part in favour of his country. "From his integrity and decision of character, Dr. Bartlett was soon designated as a magistrate, and sustained various offices from the lowest to the highest. In 1775 he was chosen a delegate to the continental congress. He attended in that honourable assembly, and when the vote for American Independence was taken, Dr. Bartlett's name was first called, as representing the most easterly province, and he boldly answered in the affirmative." After the revolution he was elected governor of the state of New-Hampshire under the new form of government.

"His mind was quick and penetrating, his memory tenacious, his judgment sound and prospective; his natural temper was open, humane, and compassionate. In all his dealings he was scrupulously just, and faithful in the performance of all his engagements. These shining talents accompanied with distinguished probity, early in life recommended him to the esteem and confidence of his fellow-citizens. But few persons, by their own merit, without the influence of family or party connexions, have risen from one degree of honour to another as he did; and fewer still have been the instances in which a succession of honourable and important offices, have been held by any man with less envy, or executed with more general approbation."—See *Thach. Med. Biog.* A.]

[BARTON, Benjamin Smith, M. D. Dr. Barton was born at Lancaster in Pennsylvania in 1766. In 1786 he went to Great Britain, and prosecuted his medical studies at Edinburgh and London. He afterward visited Gottingen, and there obtained the degree of doctor in medicine. On returning to Philadelphia, in 1789, he established himself as a physician in that city, and his superior talents and education soon procured him competent employment. He was that year appointed Professor of Natural History and Botany in the College of Philadelphia, and continued in the office on the incorporation of the college with the university, in 1791. He was appointed Professor of Materia Medica on the resignation of Dr. Griffiths, and on the death of Dr. Rush, succeeded him in the department of the Theory and Practice of Medicine. He died in December, 1815.

He published, "Elements of Zoology and Botany," "Elements of Botany, or Outlines of the Natural History of Vegetables," "Collections for an Essay towards a Materia Medica of the United States;" besides numerous essays and communications contributed to the "Medical and Physical Journal."—See *Thacker's Med. Biog.* A.]

BARYCOI'A. (From βαρυς, heavy, and ακουω, to bear.) Deafness, or difficulty of hearing.

BARYOCO'CCALON. (From βαρυς, heavy, and κοκκαλος, a nut; because it gives a deep sound.) A name for the stramonium.

BARYPHO'NIA. (From βαρυς, dull, and φωνη, the voice.) A difficulty of speaking.

BARYTE. See *Heavy spar.*

BARY'TES. (From βαρυς, heavy; so called because it is very ponderous.) *Cauk; Calk; Terra ponderosa; Baryta.* Ponderous earth; Heavy earth. United with the sulphuric acid, it forms the mineral called *sulphate of barytes*, or *baroselenite.* When united to carbonic acid, it is called *aërated barytes*, or *carbonate of barytes.* See *Heavy spar.*

Barytes, is a compound of barium and oxygen. Oxygen combines with two portions of barium, forming, 1. *Barytes.* 2. *Deutoxyde of barium.*

1. *Barytes*, or *protoxyde of barium*, "is best obtained by igniting, in a covered crucible, the pure crystallized nitrate of barytes. It is procured in the state of hydrate, by adding caustic potassa or soda to a solution of the muriate of nitrate. And barytes, slightly coloured with charcoal, may be obtained by strongly igniting the carbonate and charcoal mixed together in fine powder. Barytes obtained from the ignited nitrate is of a whitish-gray colour; more caustic than strontites, or perhaps even lime. It renders the syrup of violets green, and the infusion of tumeric red. Its specific gravity by Fourcroy is 4. When water in small quantity is poured on the dry earth, it slakes like quicklime, but perhaps with evolution of more heat. When swallowed it acts as a violent poison. It is destitute of smell.

When pure barytes is exposed, in a porcelain tube, at a heat verging on ignition, to a stream of dry oxygen gas, it absorbs the gas rapidly, and passes to the state of deutoxyde of barium. But when it is calcined in contact with atmospheric air, we obtain at first this deutoxyde and carbonate of barytes; the former of which passes very slowly into the latter, by absorption of carbonic acid from the atmosphere.

2. The *deutoxyde of barium* is of a greenish-gray colour, it is caustic, renders the syrup of violets green, and is not decomposable by heat or light. The voltaic pile reduces it. Exposed at a moderate heat to carbonic acid, it absorbs it, emitting oxygen, and becoming carbonate of barytes. The deutoxyde is probably decomposed by sulphuretted hydrogen at ordinary temperatures. Aided by heat, almost all combustible bodies, as well as many metals, decompose it. The action of hydrogen is accompanied with remarkable phenomena.

Water at 50° F. dissolves one-twentieth of its weight of barytes, and at 212° about one half of its weight. It is colourless, acrid, and caustic. It acts powerfully on the vegetable purples and yellows. Exposed to the air, it attracts carbonic acid, and the dissolved barytes is converted into carbonate, which falls down in insoluble crusts.

Sulphur combines with barytes, when they are mixed together, and heated in a crucible. The same compound is more economically obtained by igniting a mixture of sulphate of barytes and charcoal in fine powder. This sulphuret is of a reddish yellow colour, and when dry without smell. When this substance is put into hot water, a powerful action is manifested. The water is decomposed, and two new products are formed, namely, hydrosulphuret, and hydroguretted sulphuret of barytes. The first crystallizes as the liquid cools, the second remains dissolved. The *hydrosulphuret* is a compound of 9.75 of barytes with 2.125 sulphuretted hydrogen. Its crystals should be quickly separated by filtration, and dried by pressure between the folds of porous paper. They are white scales, have a silky lustre, are soluble in water, and yield a solution having a greenish tinge. Its taste is acrid, sulphureous, and when mixed with the hydroguretted sulphuret, eminently corrosive. It rapidly attracts oxygen from the atmosphere, and is converted into the sulphate of barytes. The *hydroguretted sulphuret* is a compound of 9.75 barytes with 4.125 bisulphuretted hydrogen: but contaminated with sulphite and hypo sulphite in unknown proportions. The dry sulphuret consists probably of 2 sulphur + 9.75 barytes. The readiest way of obtaining barytes water is to boil the solution of the sulphuret with deutoxyde of copper, which seizes the sulphur, while the hydrogen flies off, and the barytes remains dissolved.

Phosphuret of barytes may be easily formed by exposing the constituents together to heat in a glass tube. Their reciprocal action is so intense as to cause ignition. Like phosphuret of lime, it decomposes water, and causes the disengagement of phosphuretted hydrogen gas, which spontaneously inflames with contact of air. When sulphur is made to act on the deutoxyde of barytes, sulphuric acid is formed, which unites to a portion of the earth into a sulphate.

The salts of barytes are white, and more or less transparent. All the soluble sulphates cause in the soluble salts of barytes a precipitate insoluble in nitric acid. They are all poisonous except the sulphate; and hence the proper counter-poison is dilute sulphuric acid for the carbonate, and sulphate of soda for the soluble salts of barytes."

Pure barytes has a much stronger affinity than any other body for sulphuric acid; it turns blue tincture of cabbage green. It is entirely infusible by heat alone, but melts when mixed with various earths. Its specific gravity is 4.000. It changes quickly in the air, swells, becomes soft, and falls into a white powder, with the acquisition of about one-fifth of its weight. This slaking is much more active and speedy than that of lime. It combines with phosphorus, which compound decomposes water rapidly. It unites to sulphur by the dry and humid way. It has a powerful attraction for water, which it absorbs with a hissing noise, and consolidates it strongly. It is soluble in twenty times its weight of cold, and twice its weight of boiling water. Its crystals are long four-sided prisms of a satin-like appearance. It is a deadly poison to animals.

Other Methods of obtaining Barytes.—1. Take native carbonate of barytes; reduce it to a fine powder, and dissolve it in a sufficient quantity of diluted nitric acid; evaporate this solution till a pellicle appears, and then suffer it to crystallize in a shallow basin. The salt obtained is nitrate of barytes; expose this nitrate of barytes to the action of heat in a china-cup, or silver crucible, and keep it in a dull red heat for at least one hour; then suffer the vessel to cool, and transfer the greenish solid contents, which are pure barytes, into a well-stopped bottle. When dissolved in a small quantity of distilled water, and evaporated, it may be obtained in a beautiful crystalline form.

In this process the nitric acid, added to the native carbonate of barytes, unites to the barytes, and expels the carbonic acid, and forms nitrate of barytes; on exposing this nitrate to heat, it parts with its nitric acid, which becomes decomposed into its constituents, leaving the barytes behind.

2. Pure barytes may likewise be obtained from its sulphate. For this purpose, boil powdered sulphate of barytes in a solution of twice or three times its weight of carbonate of potassa, in a Florence flask, for about two hours; filter the solution, and expose what remains on the filter to the action of a violent heat.

In this case, the sulphuric acid of the barytes unites to the potassa, and the carbonic acid of the latter joins to the barytes; hence sulphate of potassa and carbonate of barytes are obtained. The former is in solution, and passes through the filter; the latter is insoluble, and remains behind. From this artificial carbonate of barytes, the carbonic acid is driven off by heat.

BARYTÆ MURIAS. *Terra ponderosa salita.* The muriate of barytes is a very acrid and poisonous preparation. In small doses it proves sudorific, diuretic, deobstruent, and alterative; in an over-dose, emetic, and violently purgative. The late Dr. Crawford found it very serviceable in all diseases connected with scrofula; and the Germans have employed it with great success in some diseases of the skin and viscera, and obstinate ulcers. The dose of the saturated solution in distilled water, is from five to fifteen drops for children, and from fifteen to twenty for adults.

BASAAL. (Indian.) The name of an Indian tree. A decoction of its leaves, with ginger, in water, is used as a gargle in disorders of the fauces. The kernels of the fruit kill worms.—*Ray's Hist.*

BASA'LTES. (In the Æthiopic tongue, this word means *iron*, which is the colour of the stone.) A heavy and hard kind of stone, found standing up in the form of regular angular columns, composed of a number of joints, one placed upon and nicely fitted to another as if formed by the hands of a skilful architect. It is found in beds and veins in granite and mica slate, the old red sandstone, limestone, and coal formations. It is distributed over the whole world; but nowhere is it met with in greater variety than in Scotland. The German basalt is supposed to be a watery deposite; and that of France to be of volcanic origin.

The most remarkable is the columnar basaltes, which forms immense masses, composed of columns thirty, forty, or more feet in height, and of enormous thickness. Nay, those at Fairhead are two hundred and fifty feet high. These constitute some of the most astonishing scenes in nature, for the immensity and regularity of their parts. The coast of Antrim in Ireland, for the space of three miles in length, exhibits a very magnificent variety of columnar cliffs: and the Giant's Causeway consists of a point of that coast formed of similar columns, and projecting into the sea upon a descent for several hundred feet. These columns are, for the most part, hexagonal, and fit very accurately together; but most frequently not adherent to each other, though water cannot penetrate between them. And the basaltic appearances on the Hebrides Islands on the coast of Scotland, as described by Sir Joseph Banks, who visited them in 1772, are upon a scale very striking for their vastness and variety.

[Basaltes belongs to a class of rocks now called *superincumbent.* They are always found in a vertical position, resting upon other strata of rocks which are horizontal. Some of the most remarkable of these are the *Pallisado rocks*, extending forty miles or more along the Hudson river, on its west bank, partly in New-Jersey and partly in the state of New-York. There are other ridges of the same formation in other parts of New-Jersey, all resting upon sandstone. On the south shore of Lake Superior, the basaltic rocks, as they have been described by travellers, particularly by Mr. Schoolcraft, have a grand and imposing appearance. There is a ridge of this kind of rock extending a number of miles north from New-Haven, in the state of Connecticut. A singular formation of basaltic rocks is found in North Carolina, constituting a wall many miles in extent, which has given rise to much controversy; but Dr. Woodhouse, of Philadelphia, settled the question, as to the true nature of this formation.

"Basalt (says professor Eaton) is a hornblende rock, not primitive, probably of volcanic origin. Subdivisions—*Amygdaloid*, when amorphous, of a compact texture, but containing cellules, empty or filled. *Greenstone trap*, when of a columnar structure, or in angular blocks, often coarse-grained. Variety—*Toadstone*, when the amygdaloid has a warty appearance, and resembles slag." A.]

Basaltic hornblende. See *Hornblende.*

BASANITE. See *Flinty slate.*

BASANI'TES. (From βασανιζω, to find out.) A stone said, by Pliny, to contain a bloody juice, and useful in diseases of the liver: also a stone upon which, by some, the purity of gold was formerly said to be tried, and of which medical mortars were made.

BASE. See *Basis.*

Base, acidifiable. See *Acid.*

Base, acidifying. See *Acid.*

BASIA'TIO. (From *basio*, to kiss.) Venereal connexion between the sexes.

BASIA'TOR. See *Orbicularis oris*

BASIL. See *Ocimum basilicum.*

BASILA'RIS. See *Basilary.*

BASILARIS ARTERIA. Basilary artery. An artery of the brain; so called, because it lies upon the basilary process of the occipital bone. It is formed by the junction of the two vertebral arteries within the skull, and runs forwards to the sella turcica along the pons varolii, which it supplies, as well as the adjacent parts, with blood

BASILARIS PORCESSUS. See *Occipital bone.*

BASILARIS APOPHYSIS. See *Occipital bone.*

BASILA'RY. (*Basilaris*; from βασιλευς, a king.) Several parts of the body, bones, arteries, veins, processes, &c. were so named by the ancients, from their situation being connected with or leading to the liver or brain, which they considered as the seat of the soul or royalty.

BASI'LICA MEDIANA. See *Basilica vena.*

BASILICA NUX. The walnut.

BASILICA VENA. The large vein that runs in the internal part of the arm, and evacuates its blood into the axillary vein. The branch which crosses, at the head of the arm, to join this vein, is called the *basilic median.* They may either of them be opened in the operation of bloodletting.

Basilicon. See *Basilicum unguentum.*

BASI'LICUM. (From βασιλικος, royal; so called from its great virtues.) See *Ocimum basilicum.*

BASILICUM UNGUENTUM. *Unguentum basilicum flavum.* An ointment popularly so called from its having the ocimum basilicum in its composition. It came afterward to be composed of wax, resin, &c. and is now called *ceratum resinæ.*

BASILICUS. (From βασιλευς, a king. See *Basilary.*) Basilic.

BASILICUS PULVIS. The royal powder. A preparation formerly composed of calomel, rhubarb, and jalap. Many compositions were, by the ancients, so called from their supposed pre-eminence.

BASILI'DION. An itchy ointment was formerly so called by Galen.

BA'SILIS. A name formerly given to collyriums of supposed virtues, by Galen.

BASILI'SCUS. (From βασιλευς, a king.) 1. The basilisk, or cockatrice, a poisonous serpent; so called from a white spot upon its head, which resembles a crown.

2. The philosopher's stone.

3. Corrosive sublimate.

BASIO. Some muscles so have the first part of their names, because they originate from the basilary process of the occipital bone.

BASIO-CERATO-CHONDRO-GLOSSUS. See *Hyoglossus.*

BASIO-GLOSSUM. See *Hyoglossus.*

BASIO-PHARYNGÆUS. See *Constrictor pharyngis medius.*

BA'SIS. (From βαινω, to go: the support of any thing, upon which it stands or goes.) Base. 1. This word is frequently applied anatomically to the body of any part, or to that part from which the other parts appear, as it were, to proceed, or by which they are supported.

2. In pharmacy it signifies the principal ingredient.

3. In chemistry, usually applied to alkalies, earths, and metallic oxydes, in their relations to the acids and salts. It is sometimes also applied to the particular constituents of an acid or oxyde, on the supposition that the substance combined with the oxygen, &c. is the basis of the compound to which it owes its particular qualities. This notion seems unphilosophical, as these qualities depend as much on the state of combination as on the nature of the constituent.

BASI COLICA. The name of a medicine in Scribonius Largus, compounded of aromatics and honey.

BASSORINE. This substance is extracted from the gum resins which contain it, by treating them successively with water, alkohol, and æther. Bassorine being insoluble in these liquids, remains mixed merely with the woody particles, from which it is easy to separate it, by repeated washings and decantations: because one of its characteristic properties is to swell extremely in the water and to become very buoyant. This substance swells up in cold as well as in boiling water, without any of its parts dissolving. It is soluble however almost completely by the aid of heat, in water sharpened with nitric or muriatic acid. If after concentrating with a gentle heat the nitric solution, we add highly rectified alkohol, there results a white precipitate, flocculent and bulky, which, washed with much alkohol and dried, does not form, at the utmost, the tenth of the quantity of bassorine employed, and which presents all the properties of gum arabic. *Vauquelin, Bulletin de Pharmacie*, iii. 56.

BASTARD. A term often employed in medicine, and botany, to designate a disease or plant which has the appearance of, but is not in reality what it seem bles: The name of that which it similates is generally attached to it, as bastard peripneumony, bastard pellitory, &c.

Bastard pellitory. See *Achillæa ptarmica.*

Bastard pleurisy. See *Peripneumonia notha.*

BATA'TAS. (So the natives of Peru call the root of a convolvulus falso. The potato, which is a native of that country. See *Solanum tuberosum*, and *Convolvulus batatas.*

[The *Solanum tuberosum* is the common potato, from which all the edible varieties are derived The *Convolvulus batatas* is the Carolina or sweet potato of the United States. A.]

BATATAS PEREGRINA. The purging potato.

BATH. Βαλανειον *Balneum.* A bath.

1. A convenient receptacle of water, for persons to wash or plunge in, either for health or pleasure. These are distinguished into hot and cold; and are either natural or artificial. The natural hot baths are formed of the water of hot springs, of which there are many in different parts of the world; especially in those countries where there are, or have evidently been, volcanoes. The artificial hot baths consist either of water, or of some other fluid, made hot by art. The cold bath consists of water, either fresh or salt, in its natural degree of heat; or it may be made colder by art, as by a mixture of nitre, sal-ammoniac, &c. The chief hot baths in our country are those of Bath and Bristol, and those of Buxton and Matlock; which latter, however, are rather warm, or tepid, than hot. The use of baths is found to be beneficial in diseases of the head, as palsies, &c.; in cuticular diseases, as leprosies, &c.; obstructions and constipations of the bowels, the scurvy, and stone; and in many diseases of women and children. The cold bath, though popularly esteemed one of the most innocent remedies yet discovered, is not, however, to be adopted indiscriminately. On the contrary, it is liable to do considerable mischief in some cases of diseased viscera, and is not, in any case, proper to be used during the existence of costiveness. As a preventive remedy for the young, and as a general bracer for persons of a relaxed fibre, especially of the female sex, it often proves highly advantageous; and, in general, the popular idea is a correct one, that the *glow* which succeeds the use of cold or temperate bath, is a test of their utility; while, on the other hand, their producing *chilliness*, headache, &c. is a proof of their being pernicious.

1. *The Cold Bath.* The diseases and morbid symptoms, for which the cold bath, under one form or another, may be applied with advantage, are very numerous; and some of them deserve particular attention. One of the most important of its uses is in *ardent fever;* and, under proper management, it forms a highly valuable remedy in this dangerous disorder. It is highly important, however, to attend to the precautions which the use of this vigorous remedial process requires. "Affusion with cold water," Dr. Currie observes, "may be used whenever the heat of the body is steadily above the natural standard, when there is no sense of chilliness, and especially when there is no general nor profuse perspiration. If used during the cold stage of a fever, even though the heat be higher than natural, it brings on interruption of respiration, a fluttering, weak, and extremely quick pulse, and certainly might be carried so far as to extinguish animation entirely." The most salutary consequence which follows the proper use of this powerful remedy, is the production of free and general perspiration. It is this circumstance that appears to give so much advantage to a general affusion of cold water in fevers, in preference to any partial application. The cold bath is better known, especially in this country, as a general tonic remedy in various chronic diseases. The general circumstances of disorder for which cold bathing appears to be of service, according to Dr. Saunders, are a langour and weakness of circulation, accompanied with profuse sweating and fatigue, on very moderate exertion; tremors in the limbs, and many of those symptoms usually called nervous; where the moving powers are weak, and the mind listless and indolent; but, at the same time, where no permanent morbid obstruction, or visceral disease, is present. Such a state of body is often the consequence of a long and debilitating sickness, or of a sedentary life, without using the exercise requisite to keep up the activity of the bodily powers. In all these cases, the great object to be fulfilled, is to produce a considerable reaction, from the shock of cold water, at the expense of as little heat as possible; and when cold bathing does harm, it is precisely where the powers of the body are too languid to bring on reaction, and the chilling effects remain unopposed. When the patient feels the shock of immersion very severely, and, from experience of its pain, has acquired an insuperable dread of this application; when he has felt little or no friendly glow to succeed the first shock, but on coming out of the bath remains cold, shivering, sick at the stomach, oppressed with headache, languid, drowsy, and listless, and averse to food and exercise during the whole of the day, we may be sure that the bath has been too cold, the shock too severe, and no reaction produced as all adequate to the impression on the surface of the body.

There is a kind of slow, irregular fever, or rather febricula, in which Dr. Saunders has often found the cold bath of singular service. This disorder principally affects persons naturally of a sound constitution, but who lead a sedentary life, and at the same time are employed in some occupation which strongly engages their attention, requires much exertion of thought, and excites a degree of anxiety. Such persons have constantly a pulse rather quicker than natural, hot hands, restless nights, and an impaired appetite, but without any considerable derangement in the digestive organs. This disorder will continue for a long time in an irregular way, never entirely preventing their ordinary occupation, but rendering it more than usually anxious and fatiguing, and often preparing the way for confirmed hypochondriasis. Persons in this situation are remarkably relieved by the cold bath and, for the most part, bear it well; and its use should also, if possible, be aided by that relaxation from business, and that diversion of the mind from its ordinary train of thinking, which are obtained by attending a watering place. The Doctor also found cold bathing hurtful in chlorosis, and observes, that it is seldom advisable in those cases of disease in the stomach which are brought on by high living, and constitute what may be termed the true dyspepsia.

The topical application of cold water, or of a cold saturnine lotion, in cases of local inflammation, has become an established practice; the efficacy of which is daily experienced. Burns of every description will bear a most liberal use of cold water, or even of ice: and this may be applied to a very extensive inflamed surface, without even producing the ordinary effects of general chilling, which would be brought on from the same application to a sound and healthy skin. Another very distressing symptom, remarkably relieved by cold water, topically applied, is that intolerable itching in the vagina, which women sometimes experience, entirely unconnected with any general cause, and which appears to be a kind of herpes confined to that part. Cold water has also been used topically in the various cases of strains, bruises, and similar injuries, in tentinous and ligamentous parts, with success, also in rigidity of muscles, that have been long kept at rest, in order to favour the union of bone, where there appears to have been no organic injury, but only a deficiency of nervous energy, and in mobility of parts, or at most, only slight adhesions, which would give way to regular exercise of the weakened limb. Another very striking instance of the powerful effects of topical cold, in stimulating a part to action, is shown in the use of cold, or even iced water, to the vagina of parturient women, during the dangerous hæmorrhages that take place from the uterus, on the partial separation of the placenta.

2. *The Shower Bath.* A species of cold bath. A modern invention, in which the water falls through numerous apertures on the body. A proper apparatus for this purpose is to be obtained at the shops. The use of the shower bath applies, in every case, to the same purposes as the cold bath, and is often attended with particular advantages. 1. From the sudden contact of the water, which, in the common cold bath, is only momentary, but which, in the shower bath, may be prolonged, repeated, and modified, at pleasure; and, secondly, from the head and breast, which are exposed to some inconvenience and danger in the common bath, being here effectually secured, by receiving the first shock of the water.

3 *The Tepid Bath* The range of temperature

from the lowest degree of the hot bath to the highest of the cold bath, forms what may be termed the tepid. In general, the heat of water which we should term tepid, is about 90 deg. In a medicinal point of view, it produces the greatest effect in ardent fever, where the temperature is little above that of health, but the powers of the body weak, not able to bear the vigorous application of cold immersion. In cutaneous diseases, a tepid bath is often quite sufficient to produce a salutary relaxation, and perspirability of the skin.

4. *The Hot Bath.* From 93 to 96 deg. of Fahrenheit, the hot bath has a peculiar tendency to bring on a state of repose, to alleviate any local irritation, and thereby induce sleep. It is, upon the whole, a safer remedy than the cold bath, and more peculiarly applicable to very weak and irritable constitutions, whom the shock produced by cold immersion would overpower, and who have not sufficient vigour of circulation for an adequate reaction. In cases of topical inflammation, connected with a phlogistic state of body, preceded by rigour and general fever, and where the local formation of matter is the solution of the general inflammatory symptoms, experience directs us to the use of the warm relaxing applications, rather than those which, by exciting a general reaction, would increase the local complaint. This object is particularly to be consulted when the part affected is one that is essential to life. Hence it is that in fever, where there is a great determination to the lungs, and the respiration appears to be locally affected, independently of the oppression produced by mere febrile increase of circulation, practitioners have avoided the external use of cold, in order to promote the solution of the fever; and have trusted to the general antiphlogistic treatment, along with the topically relaxing application of warm vapour, inhaled by the lungs. Warm bathing appears to be peculiarly well calculated to relieve those complaints that seem to depend on an irregular or diminished action of any part of the alimentary canal; and the state of the skin, produced by immersion in warm water, seems highly favourable to the healthy action of the stomach and bowels. Another very important use of the warm bath, is in herpetic eruptions, by relaxing the skin, and rendering it more pervious, and preparing it admirably for receiving the stimulant applications of tar ointment, mercurials, and the like, that are intended to restore it to a healthy state. The constitutions of children seem more extensively relieved by the warm bath than those of adults; and this remedy seems more generally applicable to acute fevers in them than in persons of a more advanced age. Where the warm bath produces its salutary operation, it is almost always followed by an easy and profound sleep. Dr. Saunders strongly recommends the use of the tepid bath, or even one of a higher temperature, in the true menorrhagia of females. In paralytic affections of particular parts, the powerful stimulus of heated water is generally allowed; and in these cases, the effect may be assisted by any thing which will increase the stimulating properties of the water; as, for instance, by the addition of salt. In these cases, much benefit may be expected from the use of warm sea-baths. The application of the warm bath topically, as in pediluvia, or fomentations to the feet, often produces the most powerful effects in quieting irritations in fever, and bringing on a sound and refreshing repose. The cases in which the warm bath is likely to be attended with danger, are particularly those where there exists a strong tendency to a determination of blood to the head; and apoplexy has sometimes been thus brought on. The lowest temperature will be required for cutaneous complaints, and to bring on relaxation in the skin, during febrile irritation; the warmer will be necessary in paralysis: more heat should be employed on a deep-seated part than one that is superficial.

5. *The Vapour Bath.* The vapour bath, called also *Balneum laconicum*, though not much employed in England, forms a valuable remedy in a variety of cases. In most of the hot natural waters on the Continent, the vapour bath forms a regular part of the bathing apparatus, and is there highly valued. In no country, however, is this application carried to so great an extent as in Russia, where it forms the principal and almost daily luxury of all the people, in every rank; and it is employed as a sovereign remedy for a great variety of disorders. The Hon. Mr. Basil Cochrane has lately published a Treatise on the Vapour Bath, from which, it appears, he has brought the apparatus to such perfection, that he can apply it to all degrees of temperature, partially or generally, by shower, or by steam, with a great force or a small one; according to the particular circumstances under which patients are so variously placed, who require such assistance. See *Cochrane on Vapour Baths.* Connected with this article, is the *air-pump vapour bath*, a species of vapour bath, or machine, to which the inventor has given this name. This apparatus has been found efficacious in removing paroxysms of the gout and preventing their recurrence; in acute and chronic rheumatism, palsy, cutaneous diseases, ulcers, &c. It has also been proposed in chilblains, leprosy, yaws, tetanus, amenorrhea, and dropsy.

[The vapour bath has been introduced and successfully applied in many cutaneous and other diseases, in the city of New-York. This bath may be either aqueous or spirituous. Its immediate effect is to produce relaxation of the skin and copious perspiration. It may be made a medicated bath by passing the steam or vapour through a quantity of herbs, before it is applied to the body of the person requiring it. A.]

II. Those applications are called *dry baths*, which are made of ashes, salt, sand, &c. The ancients had many ways of exciting a sweat, by means of a dry heat, as by the use of hot sand, stove rooms, or artificial bagnios; and even from certain natural hot steams of the earth, received under a proper arch, or hot-house, as we learn from Celsus. They had also another kind of bath by insolation, where the body was exposed to the sun for some time, in order to draw forth the superfluous moisture from the inward parts; and to this day it is a practice, in some nations, to cover the body over with horse-dung, especially in painful chronic diseases. In New-England, they make a kind of stove of turf, wherein the sick are shut up to bathe, or sweat. It was probably from a knowledge of this practice, and of the exploded doctrines of Celsus, that the noted empiric Dr. Graham drew his notions of the salutary effects of what he called *earth bathing;* a practice which, in the way he used it, consigned some of his patients to a perpetual mansion under the ground. The like name of *dry* bath, is sometimes also given to another kind of bath, made of kindled coals, or burning spirit of wine. The patient being placed in a convenient close chair, for the reception of the fume, which rises and provokes sweat in a plentiful manner; care being taken to keep the head out, and to secure respiration. This bath has been said to be very effectual in removing old obstinate pains in the limbs.

III. *Medicated baths* are such as are saturated with various mineral, vegetable, or sometimes animal substances. Thus we have sulphur and iron baths, aromatic and milk baths. There can be no doubt that such ingredients, if duly mixed, and a proper temperature given to the water, may, in certain complaints, be productive of effects highly beneficial. Water, impregnated with sulphate of iron, will abound with the bracing particles of that metal, and may be useful for strengthening the part to which it is applied, re-invigorating debilitated limbs, stopping various kinds of bleeding, restoring the menstrual and hæmorrhoidal discharges when obstructed, and, in short, as a substitute for the natural iron bath. There are various other medicated baths, such as those prepared with alum, and quick-lime, sal-ammoniac, &c. by boiling them together, or separately, in pure rain water. These have long been reputed as eminently serviceable in paralytic, and all other diseases arising from nervous and muscular debility.

IV. A term in chemistry, when the vessels in which bodies are exposed to the action of heat, are not placed in immediate contact with the fire, but receive the required degree of heat by another intermediate body, such apparatus is termed a bath. These have been variously named, as dry, vapour, &c. Modern chemists distinguish three kinds:

1. *Balneum arenæ*, or the sand bath. This consists merely of an open iron, or baked clay sand-pot, whose bottom is mostly convex, and exposed to the furnace. Finely sifted sea-sand is put into this, and the vessel containing the substance to be heated, &c. in the sand bath, immersed in the middle.

2. *Balneum mariæ*, or the water bath. This is very

simple, and requires no particular apparatus. The object is to place the vessel containing the substance to be heated, in another, containing water; which last must be of such a nature as to be fitted for the application of fire, as a common still, or kettle.

3. *The vapour bath.* When any substance is heated by the steam, or vapour, of boiling water, chemists say it is done by means of a vapour bath.

BATH WATERS. *Bathoniæ aquæ; Solis aquæ; Badiguæ aquæ.* Bath is the name of a city in Gloucestershire, that has been celebrated, for a long series of years, for its numerous hot springs, which are of a higher temperature than any in this kingdom, (from 112° to 116°,) and, indeed, are the only natural waters which we possess that are at all hot to the touch; all the other thermal waters being of a heat below the animal temperature, and only deserving that appellation from being invariably warmer than the general average of the heat of common springs. By the erection of elegant baths, these waters are particularly adapted to the benefit of invalids, who find here a variety of establishments, contributing equally to health, convenience, and amusement. There are three principal springs in the city of Bath, namely, those called the *King's Bath*, the *Cross Bath*, and the *Hot Bath;* all within a short distance of each other, and emptying themselves into the river Avon, after having passed through the several baths. Their supply is so copious, that all the large reservoirs used for bathing are filled every evening with fresh water from their respective fountains. In their sensible and medicinal properties, there is but a slight difference. According to Dr. Falconer, the former are—1. That the water, when newly drawn, appears clear and colourless, remains perfectly inactive, without bubbles, or any sign of briskness, or effervescence. 2. After being exposed to the open air for some hours, it becomes rather turbid, by the separation of a pale yellow, ochery precipitate, which gradually subsides. 3. No odour is perceptible from a glass of the fresh water, but a slight pungency to the taste from a large mass of it, when fresh drawn: which, however, is neither fœtid nor sulphureous. 4. When hot from the pump, it affects the mouth with a strong chalybeate impression, without being of a saline or pungent taste. And, fifthly, on growing cold, the chalybeate taste is entirely lost, leaving only a very slight sensation on the tongue, by which it can scarcely be distinguished from common hard spring-water. The temperature of the King's Bath water, which is usually preferred for drinking, is, when fresh drawn in the glass, above 116°; that of the Cross Bath, 112°. But, after flowing into the spacious bathing vessels, it is generally from 100° to 106° in the hotter baths, and from 92° to 94° in the Cross Bath; a temperature which remains nearly stationary, and is greater than that of any other natural spring in Britain. A small quantity of gas is also disengaged from these waters, which Dr. Priestley first discovered to contain no more than one-twentieth part of its bulk of fixed air, or carbonic acid. The chemical properties of the Bath waters, according to the most accurate analyzers, Doctors Lucas, Falconer, and Gibbs, contain so small a proportion of iron, as to amount only to one-twentieth or one-thirty-eighth of a grain in the pint; and, according to Dr. Gibbs, fifteen grains and a quarter of siliceous earth in the gallon. Dr. Saunders estimates a gallon of the King's Bath water to contain about eight cubic inches of carbonic acid, and a similar quantity of air, nearly azotic, about eighty grains of solid ingredients, one-half of which probably consists of sulphate and muriate of soda, fifteen grains and a half of siliceous earth, and the remainder is selenite, carbonate of lime, and so small a portion of oxyde of iron as to be scarcely calculable. Hence he concludes, that the King's Bath water is the strongest chalybeate; next in order, the Hot Bath water; and, lastly, that of the Cross Bath, which contains the smallest proportions of chalybeate, gaseous and saline, but considerably more of the earthy particles; while its water, in the pump, is also two degrees lower than that of the others. It is likewise now ascertained, that these springs do not exhibit the slightest traces of sulphur, though it was formerly believed, and erroneously supported, on the authority of Dr. Charleton, that the subtile aromatic vapour in the Bath waters, was a sulphureous principle entirely similar to common brimstone.

With regard to the effect of the Bath waters on the human system, independent of their specific properties, as a medicinal remedy not to be imitated completely by any chemical process, Dr. Saunders attributes much of their salubrious influence to the natural degree of warmth peculiar to these springs, which, for ages, have preserved an admirable degree of uniformity of temperature. He thinks too, that one of their most important uses is that of an external application, yet supposes that, in this respect, they differ little from common water, when heated to the same temperature, and applied under similar circumstances.

According to Dr. Falconer, the Bath water, when drunk fresh from the spring, generally raises, or rather accelerates the pulse, increases the heat, and promotes the different secretions. These symptoms in most cases, become perceptible soon after drinking it, and will sometimes continue for a considerable time. It is, however, remarkable, that they are only produced in invalids. Hence we may conclude, that these waters not only possess heating properties, but their internal use is likewise attended with a peculiar stimulus, acting more immediately on the nerves.

One of the most salutary effects of the Bath water, consists in its action on the urinary organs, even when taken in moderate doses. Its operation on the bowels varies in different individuals, like that of all other waters, which do not contain any cathartic salt; but, in general, it is productive of costiveness: an effect resulting from the want of an active stimulus to the intestines, and probably also from the determination this water occasions to the skin, more than from any astringency which it may possess; for, if perspiration be suddenly checked during the use of it, a diarrhœa is sometimes the consequence. Hence it appears that its stimulant powers are primarily, and more particularly exerted in the stomach, where it produces a variety of symptoms, sometimes slight and transient, but, occasionally, so considerable and permanent, as to require it to be discontinued. In those individuals with whom it is likely to agree, and prove beneficial, the Bath waters excite, at first, an agreeable glowing sensation in the stomach, which is speedily followed by an increase both of appetite and spirits, as well as a quick secretion of urine. In others, when the use of them is attended with headache, thirst, and constant dryness of the tongue, heaviness, loathing of the stomach, and sickness; or if they are not evacuated, either by urine or an increased perspiration, it may be justly inferred that their further continuance is improper.

The diseases for which these celebrated waters are resorted to, are very numerous, and are some of the most important and difficult to cure of all that come under medical treatment. In most of them, the bath is used along with the waters, as an internal medicine. The general indications, of the propriety of using this medicinal water, are in those cases where a gentle, gradual, and permanent stimulus, is required. Bath water may certainly be considered as a chalybeate, in which the iron is very small in quantity, but in a highly active form; and the degree of temperature is in itself a stimulus, often of considerable powers. These circumstances again point out the necessity of certain cautions, which, from a view of the mere quantity of foreign contents, might be thought superfluous. Although, in estimating the powers of this medicine, allowance must be made for local prejudice in its favour, there can be no doubt but that its employment is hazardous, and might often do considerable mischief, in various cases of active inflammation, especially in irritable habits, where there exists a strong tendency to hectic fever; and even in the less inflammatory state of diseased and suppurating viscera; and, in general, wherever a quick pulse and dry tongue indicate a degree of general fever. The cases, therefore, to which this water are peculiarly suited, are mostly of the chronic kind; and by a steady perseverance in this remedy, very obstinate disorders have given way The following, Dr. Saunders, in his Treatise on Mineral Waters, considers as the principal, viz. 1. Chlorosis a disease which, at all times, is much relieved by steel, and will bear it, even where there is a considerable degree of feverish irritation, receives particular benefit from the bath water; and its use, as a warm bath, excellently contributes to remove that languor of circulation, and obstruction of the natural evacuations, which constitute the leading features of this common and troublesome disorder. 2. The complicated diseases, which are often brought on by a long residence in hot climates, affecting the secretion of bile, the functions of the stomach, and alimentary canal, and which generally produce organic derangement in some part of the hepatic system, often receive much benefit from the bath water, if used at a time when suppurative inflammation is not actually present. 3. Another and less active disease of the biliary organs, the jaundice, which arises from a simple obstruction of the gall-ducts, is still oftener removed by both the internal and external use of these waters. 4. In rheumatic complaints, the power of this water, as Dr. Charleton well observes, is chiefly confined to that species of rheumatism which is unattended with inflammation, or in which the patient's pains are not increased by the warmth of his bed A great number of the patients that resort to Bath, especially those that are admitted into the hospital, are affected with rheumatism in all its stages; and it appears, from the most respectable testimony, that a large proportion of them receive a permanent cure. (See *Falconer on Bath Water in Rheumatic Cases.*) 5. In gout, the greatest benefit is derived from this water, in those cases where it produces anomalous affections of the head, stomach, and bowels; and it is here a principal advantage to be able to bring, by warmth, that active local inflammation in any limb, which relieves all the other troublesome and dangerous symptoms. Hence it is that Bath water is commonly said to produce the gout; by which is only meant that, where persons have a gouty ffection, shifting from place to place, and thereby much disordering the system, the internal and external use of the bath water will soon bring on a general increase of action, indicated by a flushing in the face, fulness in the circulating vessels, and relief of the dyspeptic symptoms; and the whole disorder will terminate in a regular fit of the gout in the extremities, which is the crisis always to be wished for. 6. The colica pictonum, and the paralysis or loss of nervous power in particular limbs, which is one of its most serious consequences, is found to be peculiarly relieved by the use of the Bath waters, more especially when applied externally, either generally, or upon the part affected.

The quantity of water taken daily, during a full course, and by adults, is recommended by Dr. Falconer, not to exceed a pint and a half, or two pints; and in chlorosis, with irritable habits, not more than one pint is employed; and when the bath is made use of, it is generally two or three times a week, in the morning. The Bath waters require a considerable time to be persevered in, before a full and fair trial can be made. Chronic rheumatism, habitual gout, dyspepsia, from a long course of high and intemperate living, and the like, are disorders not to be removed by a short course of any mineral water, and many of those who have once received benefit at the fountains, find it necessary to make an annual visit to them, to repair the waste in health during the preceding year.

BATH, CAUTERES. A sulphureous bath near Barege, which raises the mercury in Fahrenheit's thermometer to 131°.

BATH, ST. SAVIOUR'S. A sulphureous and alkaline bath, in the valley adjoining Barege, the latter of which raises Fahrenheit's thermometer as high as 131°. It is much resorted to from the South of France, and used chiefly externally, as a simple thermal water.

Bath, cold. See *Bath.*

Bath, hot. See *Bath.*

Bath, tepid. See *Bath.*

Bath, vapour. See *Bath.*

BA'THMIS. (From βαινω, to enter.) *Bathmus.* The seat, or base; the cavity of a bone, with the protuberance of another, particularly those at the articulation of the humerus and ulna, according to Hippocrates and Galen.

BATHO'NIÆ AQUÆ. See *Bath waters.*

BA'THRON. (From βαινω, to enter.) *Bathrum.* The same as bathmis; also an instrument used in the extension of fractured limbs, called *scamnum.—Hippocrates.* It is described by Oribasius and Scultetus.

BA'TIA. A retort. Obsolete.

BATI'NON-MORON. (From βατος, a bramble, and μορον, a raspberry.) The raspberry.

BATRA'CHIUM. (From βατραχος, a frog; so called from its likeness to a frog.) The herb crow's foot, or ranunculus.

BA'TRACHUS. (From βατραχος, a frog; so called because they who are infected with it croak like a frog.) An inflammatory tumour under the tongue See *Ranula.*

[BATRACHIAN. Batrachian animals. A term used in natural history, intended to include all animals of the frog, toad, or lizard kind. A.]

BATTARI'SMUS. (From Βαττος, a Cyrenæan prince who stammered.) Stammering; a defect in pronunciation. See *Psellismus.*

BATTA'TA VIRGINIANA. See *Batatas,* and *Convolvulus batatas.*

BATTA'TA PEREGRINA. The cathartic potato; perhaps a species of *ipomæa.* If about two ounces of them are eaten at bed-time, they greatly move the belly the next morning.

BATTIE, WILLIAM, was born in Devonshire, in 1704. He graduated at Cambridge, and after practising some years successfully at Uxbridge, settled in London, and became a fellow of the College of Physicians, as well as of the Royal Society. The insufficiency of Bethlehem hospital to receive all the indigent objects labouring under insanity in this metropolis, naturally led to the establishment of another similar institution; and Dr. Battie having been very active in promoting the subscription for that purpose, he was appointed physician to the new institution, which was called St. Luke's Hospital, then situated on the north side of Moorfields. In 1757 he published a treatise on madness; and a few years after, having exposed before the House of Commons the abuses often com mitted in private mad-houses, they became the subject of legislative interference, and were at length placed under the control of the College of Physicians, and the magistrates in the country. He died at the age of 72.

BAUHIN, JOHN, was born at Lyons, in 1541. Being greatly attached to botany, he accompanied the celebrated Gesner in his travels through several countries of Europe, and collected abundant materials for his principal work, the "Historia Plantarum," which contributed greatly to the improvement of his favourite science. He was, at the age of 32, appointed physician to the duke of Wirtemberg, and died in 1613. A Treatise on Mineral Waters, and some other publications by him also remain.

BAUHIN, GASPARD, was brother to the preceding, but younger by 20 years. He graduated at Basle, after studying at several universities, and was chosen Greek professor at the early age of 22; afterward professor of anatomy and botany; then of medicine, with other distinguished honours, which he retained till his death in 1624. Besides the plants collected by himself, he received material assistance from his pupils and friends, and was enabled to add considerably to the knowledge of botany; on which subject, as well as anatomy, he has left numerous publications. Among other anatomical improvements, he claims the discovery of the valve of the colon. His "Pinax" contains the names of six thousand plants mentioned by the ancients, tolerably well arranged; and being continually referred to by Linnæus, must long retain its value.

BAULMONEY. See *Æthusa meum.*

BAUME, ANTHONY, an apothecary, born at Senlis, in 1728. He distinguished himself at an early age by his skill in chemistry and pharmacy: and was afterward admitted a member of the Royal Academy of Sciences of Paris. He also gave lectures on chemistry for several years with great credit. Among other works, he published "Elements of Pharmacy," and a "Manual of Chemistry," which met with considerable approbation; also a detailed account of the different kinds of soil, and the method of improving them for the purposes of agriculture.

BAXA'NA. (Indian.) *Rabuxit.* A poisonous tree growing near Ormuz.

BAY. A name of several articles; as bay-cherry bay-leaf, bay-salt, &c.

Bay-cherry. See *Prunus Lauro-cerasus.*

Bay-leaves. See *Laurus.*

Bay-leaved Passion-flower. See *Passiflora lauri folia.*

Bay-salt. A very pure salt, prepared from sea-water by spontaneous evaporation.

[BAYLEY, DR. RICHARD, a celebrated surgeon and

practitioner in the city of New-York. Dr. Bayley was born at Fairfield, Connecticut, in the year 1745. His father was of English, and his mother of French, descent. After returning from London, where he studied anatomy under Dr. John Hunter, he commenced practice in connexion with Dr. Charleton of New-York, with whom he had previously studied. At that time the croup (cynanche trachealis) was confounded with the angina maligna, or putrid sore throat, and both treated with stimulants. Dr. Bayley was the first to point out the difference, and demonstrate that the croup was an inflammatory disease, and required a different treatment.

"In the year 1782, he successfully removed the arm from its glenoid cavity by the operation at the shoulder joint; an operation at which Dr. Wright Post, then a student, assisted; and which, as far as it has been in our power to examine, is the first instance of its being practised in the United States." His surgical skill was often displayed in operations upon the eye. With Dr. Bard and others, he was one of the earliest promoters of the New York City Dispensary. In 1797, he published his work on yellow fever, in which he advocates the opinion of its local origin and noncontagiousness. He afterward, while health officer of the port of New-York, published a series of letters on the same subject, addressed to the New-York common council, or corporation of the city. He died in August, 1801, "leaving behind him a high character as a clinically instructed physician, an excellent and bold operator, a prompt practitioner, of rapid diagnosis, and unhesitating decision."—See *Thach. Med. Biog.* A.]

BDE'LLA. (From βδαλλω, to suck.) *Bdellerum.* A horse-leech.

BDE'LLIUM. (From *bedallah*, Arab.) *Adrabolon; Madeleon; Bolchon; Balchus.* Called by the Arabians, *Mokel.* A gum resin, like very impure myrrh. The best bdellium is of a yellowish-brown, or dark-brown colour, according to its age; unctuous to the touch, brittle, but soon softening, and growing tough between the fingers; in some degree transparent, not unlike myrrh; of a bitterish taste, and a moderately strong smell. It does not easily take flame, and, when set on fire, soon goes out. In burning, it sputters a little, owing to its aqueous humidity. Its sp. grav. is 1.371. Alkohol dissolves about three-fifths of bdellium, leaving a mixture of gum and cerasin. Its constituents, according to Pelletier, are 59 resin, 9.2 gum, 30.6 cerasin, 1.2 volatile oil and loss. It is one of the weakest of the deobstruent gums. It was sometimes used as a pectoral and an emmenagogue. Applied externally, it is stimulant, and promotes suppuration. It is never met with in the shops of this country.

BEAK. See *Rostrum.*

BEAN. See *Vicia faba.*

Bean, French. See *Phaseolus vulgaris.*

Bean, Kidney. See *Phaseolus vulgaris.*

Bean, Malacca. See *Avicennia tomentosa.*

Bean of Carthagena. See *Bejuio.*

Bean, St. Ignatius. See *Ignatia amara.*

BEAR. *Ursa.* The name of a well-known animal. Several things are designated after it, or a part of it.

Bear's berry. See *Arbutus uva ursi.*

Bear's bilberry. See *Arbutus uva ursi.*

Bear's breech. See *Acanthus.*

Bear's foot. See *Helleborus fœtidus.*

Bear's whortleberry. See *Arbutus uva ursi.*

Bear's whorts. See *Arbutus uva ursi.*

BEARD. 1. The hair growing on the chin and adjacent parts of the face, in adults of the male sex.

2. In botany. See *Barba; Arista.*

BE'CCA. A fine kind of resin from the turpentine and mastich trees of Greece and Syria, formerly held in great repute.

BECCABU'NGA. (From *bach bungen*, water-herb. German, because it grows in rivulets.) See *Veronica beccabunga.*

BE'CHA. See *Bechica.*

BE'CHICA. (*Bechicus;* from βηξ, a cough.) *Bechita.* Medicines to relieve a cough. An obsolete term. The *trochisci bechici albi* consist of starch and liquorice, with a small proportion of Florentine orris root made into lozenges, with mucilage of gum tragacanth. They are a soft pleasant demulcent. The *trochisci bechici nigri* consist chiefly of the juice of liquorice, with sugar and gum tragacanth.

BE'CHION. (From βηξ, a cough; so called from its supposed virtues in relieving coughs.) See *Tusilago farfara.*

BECUI'BA NUX. A large nut growing in Brazil, from which a balsam is drawn that is held in estimation in rheumatisms.

BEDE'GUAR. (Arabian.) *Bedeguar.* The *Carduus lacteus syriacus* is so called, and also the *Rosa canina.*

BEDENGIAN. The name of the love-apples in Avicenna.

BEDSTRAW. See *Galium aparine.*

BEE. See *Apis mellifica.*

BEECH. See *Fagus.*

BEER. The wine of grain made from malt and hops in the following manner. The grain is steeped for two or three days in water, until it swells, becomes somewhat tender, and tinges the water of a bright reddish brown colour. The water being then drained away, the barley is spread about two feet thick upon a floor, where it heats spontaneously, and begins to grow, by first shooting out the radical. In this state the germination is stopped by spreading it thinner, and turning it over for two days; after which it is again made into a heap, and suffered to become sensibly hot, which usually happens in little more than a day. Lastly, it is conveyed to the kiln, where, by a gradual and low heat, it is rendered dry and crisp. This is malt; and its qualities differ according as it is more or less soaked, drained, germinated, dried, and baked. In this, as in other manufactories, the intelligent operators often make a mystery of their processes from views of profit; and others pretend to peculiar secrets who really possess none.

Indian corn, and probably all large grain, requires to be suffered to grow into the blade, as well as root, before it is fit to be made into malt. For this purpose it is buried about two or three inches deep in the ground, and covered with loose earth; and in ten or twelve days it springs up. In this state it is taken up and washed, or fanned, to clear it from its dirt; and then dried in the kiln for use.

Barley, by being converted into malt, becomes one-fifth lighter, or 20 per cent.; 12 of which are owing to kiln-drying, 1.5 are carried off by the steep-water, 3 dissipated on the floor, 3 loss in cleaning the roots, and 0.5 waste or loss.

The degree of heat to which the malt is exposed in this process, gradually changes its colour from very pale to actual blackness, as it simply dries it, or converts it to charcoal.

The colour of the malt not only affects the colour of the liquor brewed from it; but, in consequence of the chemical operation, of the heat applied, on the principles that are developed in the grain during the process of malting, materially alters the quality of the beer, especially with regard to the properties of becoming fit for drinking and growing fine.

Beer is made from malt previously ground, or cut to pieces by a mill. This is placed in a tun, or tub with a false bottom; hot water is poured upon it, and the whole stirred about with a proper instrument. The temperature of the water in this operation, called mashing, must not be equal to boiling; for, in that case, the malt would be converted into a paste, from which the impregnated water could not be separated. This is called setting. After the infusion has remained for some time upon the malt, it is drawn off, and is then distinguished by the name of Sweet Wort. By one or more subsequent infusions of water, a quantity of weaker wort is made, which is either added to the foregoing, or kept apart, according to the intention of the operator. The wort is then boiled with hops, which gives it an aromatic bitter taste, and is supposed to render it less liable to be spoiled in keeping; after which it is cooled in shallow vessels, and suffered to ferment, with the addition of a proper quantity of yest. The fermented liquor is beer; and differs greatly in its quality, according to the nature of the grain, the malting, the mashing, the quantity and kind of the hops and the yest, the purity or admixtures of the water made use of, the temperature and vicissitudes of the weather, &c.

Beside the various qualities of malt liquors of a similar kind, there are certain leading features by which they are distinguished, and classed under different names, and to produce which, different modes of management must be pursued. The principal distinctions are into beer, properly so called; ale; table, or small beer; and porter, which is commonly termed beer in London. Beer is a strong, fine, and thin liquor; the greater part of the mucilage having been separated by boiling the wort longer than for ale, and carrying the fermentation farther, so as to convert the saccharine matter into alkohol. Ale is of a more syrupy consistence, and sweeter taste; more of the mucilage being retained in it, and the fermentation not having been carried so far as to decompose all the sugar. Small beer, as its name implies, is a weaker liquor; and is made, either by adding a large portion of water to the malt, or by mashing with a fresh quantity of water what is left after the beer or ale wort is drawn off. Porter was probably made originally from very high dried malt; but it is said, that its peculiar flavour cannot be imparted by malt and hops alone.

Mr. Brande obtained the following quantities of alkohol from 100 parts of different species of beers. Burton ale, 8.88; Edinburgh ale, 6.2; Dorchester ale, 5.56; the average being = 6.87. Brown stout, 6.8; London porter (average) 4.2; London small beer (average) 1.28.

As long ago as the reign of Queen Anne, brewers were forbid to mix sugar, honey, Guinea pepper, essentia bina, cocculus indicus, or any other unwholesome ingredient, in beer, under a certain penalty; from which we may infer, that such at least was the practice of some; and writers, who profess to discuss the secrets of the trade, mention most of these, and some other articles, as essentially necessary. The essentia bina is sugar boiled down to a dark colour, and empyreumatic flavour. Broom tops, wormwood, and other bitter plants, were formerly used to render beer fit for keeping, before hops were introduced into this country; but are now prohibited to be used in beer made for sale.

By the present law of this country, nothing is allowed to enter into the composition of beer, except malt and hops. Quassia and wormwood are often fraudulently introduced; both of which are easily discoverable by their nauseous bitter taste. They form a beer which does not preserve so well as hop beer. Sulphate of iron, alum, and salt, are often added by the publicans, under the name of *beer heading*, to impart a frothing property to beer, when it is poured out of one vessel into another. Molasses and extract of gentian root are added with the same view. Capsicum, grains of paradise, ginger root, coriander seed, and orange peel, are also employed to give pungency and flavour to weak or bad beer. The following is a list of some of the unlawful substances seized at different breweries, and brewers' druggists' laboratories, in London, as copied from the minutes of the committee of the house of commons. Cocculus indicus multum, (an extract of the cocculus) colouring, honey, hartshorn shavings, Spanish juice, orange powder, ginger, grains of paradise, quassia, liquorice, caraway seeds, copperas, capsicum, mixed drugs. Sulphuric acid is very frequently added to *bring beer forward*, or make it hard, giving new beer instantly the taste of what is 18 months old. According to Mr. Accum, the present *entire* beer of the London brewer is composed of all the waste and spoiled beer of the publicans, the bottoms of butts, the leavings of the pots, the drippings of the machines for drawing the beer, the remnants of beer that lay in the leaden pipes of the brewery, with a portion of brown stout, bottling beer, and mild beer. He says that opium, tobacco, nux vomica, and extract of poppies, have been likewise used to adulterate beer. By evaporating a portion of beer to dryness, and igniting the residuum with chlorate of potassa, the iron of the copperas will be procured in an insoluble oxyde. Muriate of barytes will throw down an abundant precipitate from beer contaminated with sulphuric acid or copperas; which precipitate may be collected, dried, and ignited. It will be insoluble in nitric acid.

Beer appears to have been of ancient use, as Tacitus mentions it among the Germans, and has been usually supposed to have been peculiar to the northern nations; but the ancient Egyptians, whose country was not adapted to the culture of the grape, had also contrived this substitute for wine; and Mr. Park has found the art of making malt, and brewing from it very good beer, among the negroes in the interior parts of Africa. See *Wheat*.

Bees' wax. See *Cera.*

BEET. See *Beta.*

Beet, red. See *Beta.*

Beet, white. A variety of red beet. The juice and powder of the root are said to be good to excite sneezing, and will bring away a considerable quantity of mucus.

BE'GMA. (From βησσω, to cough.) A cough; also expectorated mucus, according to Hippocrates.

BE'HEN. The Arabian for finger.

BEHEN ALBUM. (From *behen*, a finger, Arabian See *Centaurea behen.*

BEHEN OFFICINARUM. See *Cucubalus behen.*

BEHEN RUBRUM. See *Statice Limonium.*

BEIDE'LSAR. *Beidellopar.* A species of Asclepias, used in Africa as a remedy for fevers and the bites of serpents. The caustic juice which issues from the roots when wounded, is used by the negroes to destroy venereal and similar swellings.

BEJU'IO. *Habilla de Carthagenâ.* Bean of Carthagena. A kind of bean in South America, famed for being an effectual antidote against the poison of all serpents, if a small quantity is eaten immediately. This bean is the peculiar product of the jurisdiction of Carthagena.

BELA-AYE. (An Indian word.) See *Nerium antidysentericum.*

BELEMNOI'DES. (From βελεμνον, a dart, and ειδος, form; so named from their dart-like shape. *Belonoides; Beloides.* The styloid process of the temporal bone, and the lower end of the ulna, were formerly so called.

BELE'SON. (An Indian word.) *Belilia.* See *Mussenda frondosa.*

BELL METAL. A mixture of tin and copper.

BELLADO'NNA. (From *bella donna*, Italian, a handsome lady; so called because the ladies of Italy use it, to take away the too florid colour of their faces See *Atropa belladonna.*

BE'LLEGU. See *Myrobalanus bellirica.*

BELLERE'GI. See *Myrobalanus bellirica.*

BELLE'RICÆ. See *Myrobalanus bellirica.*

BELLIDIOI'DES. (From *bellis*, a daisy, and ειδος, form.) See *Chrysanthemum.*

BELLI'NI, LAURENCE, an ingenious physician, born at Florence in 1643. He was greatly attached to the mathematics, of which he was made professor at Pisa, when only twenty years of age. He was soon after appointed professor of anatomy, which office he filled with credit for nearly thirty years. He was one of the chief supporters of the mathematical theory of medicine, which attempted to explain the functions of the body, the causes of diseases, and the operations of medicines on mechanical principles: and having imprudently regulated his practice accordingly, he was generally unsuccessful, and lost the confidence of the public, as well as of Cosmo III. of Florence, who had appointed him his physician. In his anatomical researches he was more successful, having first accurately described the nervous papillæ of the tongue, and discovered them to be the organ of taste; and also having made better known the structure of the kidney. He was author of several other publications, and died in 1704

BE'LLIS. (*A' bello colore*, from its fair colour.) The name of a genus of plants in the Linnæan system. Class, *Syngenesia;* Order, *Polygamia superflua.* The daisy.

BELLIS MAJOR. See *Chrysanthemum.*

BELLIS MINOR. See *Bellis perennis.*

BELLIS PERENNIS. The systematic name of the common daisy. *Bellis; Bellis minor; Bellis perennis—scapo nudo*, of Linnæus, or bruisewort, was formerly directed in the pharmacopœias by this name. Although the leaves and flowers are rather acrid, and are said to cure several species of wounds, they are never employed by modern surgeons.

BELLO'CULUS. (From *bellus*, fair, and *oculus*, the eye.) A precious stone, resembling the eye, and formerly supposed to be useful in its disorders.

BE'LLON. The Colica pictonum.

BELLONA'RIA. (From *Bellona*, the goddess of war.) An herb which, if eaten, makes people mad, and act outrageously, like the votaries of Bellona.

BELLOSTE, AUGUSTIN, a surgeon, born at Paris in 1654. After practising several years there, and as an army surgeon, he was invited to attend the mother of the Queen of Sardinia, and continued at Turin till his death in 1730. He was inventor of a mercurial pill, called by his name, by which he is said to have acquired a great fortune. The work by which he is principally known, is called the "Hospital Surgeon," which passed through numerous editions, and was translated into most of the European languages.—Among other useful observations, he recommended piercing carious bones, to promote exfoliation, which indeed Celsus had advised before; and he blamed the custom of frequently changing the dressings of wounds, as retarding the cure.

BELMU'SCHUS. A name of the Abelmoschus. See *Hibischus abelmoschus.*

BE'LNILEG. See *Myrobalanus Bellirica.*

BELO'ERE. (Indian.) An evergreen plant of America, the seeds of which purge moderately, but the leaves roughly.

BELONOI'DES. See *Belemnoides.*

BELU'LCUM. (From βελος, a dart, and ελκω, to draw out.) A surgeon's instrument for extracting thorns, or darts.

BELZO'E. See *Styrax benzoin.*

BELZOI'NUM. See *Styrax Benzoin.*

BEM-TA'MARA. The faba Ægyptiaca.

BEN. An Arabian word formerly very much used. See *Guilandina moringa.*

BEN MAGNUM. Monardus calls a species of esula, or garden spurge, by this name, which purges and vomits violently.

BEN TAMARA. The Egyptian bean.

BE'NEDICT. *Benedictus.* A specific name prefixed to many compositions and herbs on account of their supposed good qualities; as *Benedicta herba, Benedicta aqua,* &c.

BENEDICTA AQUA. Many compound waters have been so called, especially lime-water, and a water distilled from *Serpyllum.* In Schroeder, it is the name for an emetic.

BENEDICTA HERBA. See *Geum urbanum.*

BENEDICTA LAXATIVA. A compound of turbeth, scammony, and spurges, with some warm aromatics.

BENEDICTUM LAXATIVUM. Rhubarb, and sometimes the lenitive electuary.

BENEDICTUM LIGNUM. Guaiacum.

BENEDICTUM VINUM. Antimonial wine.

BENEDI'CTUS. (From *benedico,* to bless.) See *Benedict.*

BENEDICTUS CARDUUS. See *Centaurea benedicta.*

BENEDICTUS LAPIS. A name for the philosopher's stone.

BENEOLE'NTIA. (From *bene,* well, and *oleo,* to smell.) Sweet-scented medicines.

BENG. A name given by the Mahomedans to the leaves of hemp, formed into pills, or conserve. They possess exhilarating and intoxicating powers.

Bengal quince. See *Erateva marmelos.*

BENGA'LÆ RADIX. (From *Bengal,* its native place.) See *Cassumuniar.*

BENGA'LÆ INDORUM. (From *Bengal,* its native place.) See *Cassumuniar.*

BE'NGI EIRI. A species of evergreen. Indian *ricinus,* which grows in Malabar.

BENIT. See *Geum urbanum.*

BENI'VI ARBOR. See *Styrax benzoin.*

BENJAMIN. See *Styrax benzoin.*

Benjamin flowers. See *Benzoic acid.*

[BENNE SEED. Among the negroes, in Georgia, a plant is cultivated which appears to be a species of *sesamum.* They call it benne, which is probably its African name. The seeds are of a brownish-white, and about the size of flaxseed, abounding in oil.

Several barrels of *benne seeds* were shipped by John Milledge, from Savannah to New-York, in 1807, consigned to Col. Few. By direction of this latter gentleman, they were pressed, and have been found to yield plenty of oil; three gallons, at least, to a bushel. The benne plant is an annual, and may hereafter become of some importance to this country. One difficulty in its cultivation, since ascertained, arises from the facility with which the plant sheds its seeds before the whole are mature.—See *Med. Repos.* vol. ii. A.]

[BENNE OIL. This vegetable oil is clear, mild, and well-flavoured, and excellent for salads. Its qualities are so good and wholesome that it may be employed in lieu of the oil of olives, both in medicine and diet. Instead of importing this article from the south of Europe, the Americans may prepare the oil of sesamum from their own fields. The grains are of a tender structure, and may be crushed under the screw without previous grinding. In addition to all which circumstances it may be added, that the oil separates freely by cold expression; and it may hence be hoped that our tables will, in process of time, be furnished with plentiful supplies of this sweet and nutritious substance.—See *Med. Repos.* vol. ii, p. 88.

The *sesamum orientale* is cultivated in Asia, Africa, and the West Indies, principally on account of its oil. Its seeds were used by the ancient Egyptians for food, and are still employed by the negroes and Asiatics for this purpose. The plant is now cultivated in the southern parts of the United States. The seeds afford a copious quantity of oil, amounting, according to some authors, to nearly one half of their weight. This oil is bland, sweet, and is said to keep some years without turning rancid. It is applicable to the same purposes as olive oil, and in sufficient doses proves purgative on the same principle as other animal and vegetable fixed oils."—See *Big. Mat. Med.* A.]

BENZO'AS. A benzoate. A salt formed by the union of benzoic acid with salifiable bases; as benzoate of alumine, &c.

BENZO'E. See *Styrax benzoin.*

BENZOE AMYGDALOIDES. See *Styrax benzoin.*

BENZOES FLORES. See *Benzoic acid.*

BENZOIC ACID. See *Acidum benzoicum.* "This acid was first described in 1608, by Blaise de Vigenere, in his Treatise on Fire and Salt, and has been generally known since by the name of flowers of benjamin or benzoin, because it was obtained by sublimation from the resin of this name. As it is still most commonly procured from this substance, it has preserved the epithet of benzoic, though known to be a peculiar acid, obtainable not from benzoin alone, but from different vegetable balsams, venello, cinnamon, ambergris, the urine of children, frequently that of adults, and always, according to Fourcroy and Vauquelin though Giese denies this, from that of quadrupeds living on grass and hay, particularly the camel, the horse, and the cow. There is reason to conjecture that many vegetables, and among them some of the grasses, contain it, and that it passes from them into the urine. Fourcroy and Vauquelin found it combined with potassa and lime in the liquor of dunghills, as well as in the urine of the quadrupeds above-mentioned; and they strongly suspect it to exist in the *Anthoxanthum odoratum,* or sweet-scented vernal-grass, from which hay principally derives its fragrant smell. Giese, however, could find none either in this grass or in oats.

The usual method of obtaining it affords a very elegant and pleasing example of the chemical process of sublimation. For this purpose a thin stratum of powdered benzoin is spread over the bottom of a glazed earthen pot, to which a tall conical paper covering is fitted: gentle heat is then to be applied to the bottom of the pot, which fuses the benzoin, and fills the apartment with a fragrant smell, arising from a portion of essential oil and acid of benzoin, which are dissipated into the air, at the same time the acid itself rises very suddenly in the paper head, which may be occasionally inspected at the top, though with some little care, because the fumes will excite coughing. This saline sublimate is condensed in the form of long needles, or straight filaments of a white colour, crossing each other in all directions. When the acid ceases to rise, the cover may be changed, a new one applied, and the heat raised: more flowers of a yellowish colour will then rise, which will require a second sublimation to deprive them of the empyreumatic oil they contain.

The sublimation of the acid of benzoin may be conveniently performed by substituting an inverted earthen pan instead of the paper cone. In this case the two pans should be made to fit, by grinding on a stone with sand, and they must be luted together with paper dipped in paste. This method seems preferable to the other, where the presence of the operator is required elsewhere; but the paper head can be more easily inspected and changed. The heat applied must be gentle, and the vessels ought not to be separated till they have become cool.

The quantity of acid obtained in these methods differs according to the management, and probably also from difference of purity, and in other respects, of the resin itself. It usually amounts to no more than about one-eighth part of the whole weight. Indeed Scheele says, not more than a tenth or twelfth. The whole acid of benzoin is obtained with greater certainty in the humid process of Scheele: this consists in boiling the powdered balsam with lime water, and afterward separating the lime by the addition of muriatic acid. Twelve ounces of water are to be poured upon four ounces of slaked lime; and, after the ebullition is over, eight pounds, or ninety-six ounces, more of water are to be added; a pound of finely-powdered benzoin being then put into a tin vessel, six ounces of the lime water are to be added, and mixed well with the powder; and afterward the rest of the lime water in the same gradual manner, because the benzoin would coagulate into a mass, if the whole were added at once. This mixture must be gently boiled for half an hour with constant agitation, and afterward suffered to cool and subside during an hour. The supernatant liquor must be decanted, and the residuum boiled with eight pounds more of lime water; after which the same process is to be once more repeated: the remaining powder must be edulcorated on the filter by affusions of hot water. Lastly, all the decoctions, being mixed together, must be evaporated to two pounds, and strained into a glass vessel. This fluid consists of the acid of benzoin combined with lime. After it is become cold, a quantity of muriatic acid must be added, with constant stirring, until the fluid tastes a little sourish. Duirng this time the last-mentioned acid unites with the lime, and forms a soluble salt, which remains suspended, while the less soluble acid of benzoin being disengaged, falls to the bottom in powder. By repeated affusions of cold water upon the filter, it may be deprived of the muriate of lime and muriatic acid with which it may happen to be mixed. If it be required to have a shining appearance, it may be dissolved in a small quantity of boiling water, from which it will separate in silky filaments by cooling. By this process the benzoic acid may be procured from other substances, in which it exists.

Mr. Hatchell has shown, that, by digesting benzoin in hot sulphuric acid, very beautiful crystals are sublimed. This is perhaps the best process for extracting the acid. If we concentrate the urine of horses or cows, and pour muriatic acid into it, a copious precipitate of benzoic acid takes place. This is the cheapest source of it."—*Ure's Chem. Dict.*

As an economical mode of obtaining this acid, Fourcroy recommends the extraction of it from the water that drains from dunghills, cowhouses, and stables, by means of the muriatic acid, which decomposes the benzoate of lime contained in them, and separates the benzoic acid, as in Scheele's process. He confesses the smell of the acid thus obtained differs a little from that of the acid extracted from benzoin; but this, he says, may be remedied, by dissolving the acid in boiling water, filtering the solution, letting it cool, and thus suffering the acid to crystallize, and repeating this operation a second time.

The acid of benzoin is so inflammable, that it burns with a clear yellow flame without the assistance of a wick. The sublimed flowers in their purest state, as white as ordinary writing paper, were fused into a clear transparent yellowish fluid, at the two hundred-and-thirtieth degree of Fahrenheit's thermometer, and at the same time began to rise in sublimation. It is probable that a heat somewhat greater than this may be required to separate it from the resin. It is strongly disposed to take the crystalline form in cooling. The concentrated sulphuric and nitric acids dissolve this concrete acid, and it is again separated without alteration, by adding water. Other acids dissolve it by the assistance of heat, from which it separates by cooling, unchanged. It is plentifully soluble in ardent spirit, from which it may likewise be separated by diluting the spirit with water. It readily dissolves in oils, and in melted tallow. If it be added in a small proportion to this last fluid, part of the tallow congeals before the rest, in the form of white opaque clouds. If the quantity of acid be more considerable, it separates in part by cooling, in the form of needles or feathers. It did not communicate any considerable degree of hardness to the tallow, which was the object of this experiment. When the tallow was heated nearly to ebullition, it emitted fumes which affected the respiration, like those of the acid of benzoin, but did not possess the peculiar and agreeable smell of that substance, being probably the sebacic acid. A stratum of this tallow, about one-twentieth of an inch thick, was fused upon a plate of brass, together with other fat substances, with a view to determine its relative disposition to acquire and retain the solid state. After it had cooled, it was left upon the plate, and, in the course of some weeks, it gradually became tinged throughout of a bluish-green colour. If this circumstance be not supposed to have arisen from a solution of the copper during the fusion, it seems a remarkable instance of the mutual action of two bodies in the solid state, contrary to that axiom of chemistry which affirms, that bodies do not act on each other, unless one or more of them be in the fluid state. Tallow itself, however, has the same effect.

Pure benzoic acid is in the form of a light powder, evidently crystallized in fine needles, the figure of which is difficult to be determined from their smallness. It has a white and shining appearance; but when contaminated by a portion of volatile oil, is yellow or brownish. It is not brittle, as might be expected from its appearance, but has rather a kind of ductility and elasticity, and, on rubbing in a mortar, becomes a sort of paste. Its taste is acrid, hot, acidulous, and bitter. It reddens the infusion of litmus, but not syrup of violets. It has a peculiar aromatic smell, but not strong unless heated. This, however, appears not to belong to the acid; for Mr. Giese informs us, that on dissolving the benzoic acid in as little alkohol as possible, filtering the solution, and precipitating by water, the acid will be obtained pure, and void of smell, the odorous oil remaining dissolved in the spirit. Its specific gravity is 0.667. It is not perceptibly altered by the air, and has been kept in an open vessel twenty years without losing any of its weight. None of the combustible substances have any effect on it; but it may be refined by mixing it with charcoal powder and subliming, being thus rendered much whiter and better crystallized. It is not very soluble in water. Wenzel and Lichtenstein say four hundred parts of cold water dissolve but one, though the same quantity of boiling water dissolves twenty parts, nineteen of which separate on cooling.

The benzoic acid unites without much difficulty with the earthy and alkaline bases. These compounds are called *benzoates.*

The *benzoate of barytes* is soluble, crystallizes tolerably well, is not affected by exposure to the air, but is decomposable by fire, and by the stronger acids. That of *lime* is very soluble in water, though much less in cold than in hot, and crystallizes on cooling. It is in like manner decomposable by the acids and by barytes. The *benzoate of magnesia* is soluble, crystallizable, a little deliquescent, and more decomposable than the former. That of *alumina* is very soluble, crystallizes in dendrites, is deliquescent, has an acerb and bitter taste, and is decomposable by fire, and even by most of the vegetable acids. The *benzoate of potassa* crystallizes on cooling in little compacted needles. All the acids decompose it, and the solution of barytes and lime form with it a precipitate. The *benzoate of soda* is very crystallizable, very soluble, and not deliquescent like that of potassa, but it is decomposable by the same means. It is sometimes found native in the urine of graminivorous quadrupeds, but by no means so abundantly as that of lime. The *benzoate of ammonia* is volatile, and decomposable by all the acids and all the bases. The solutions of all the benzoates, when drying on the sides of a vessel wetted with them, form dendritical crystallizations.

Trommsdorf found in his experiments, that benzoic acid united readily with *metallic oxydes.*

The benzoates are all decomposable by heat, which, when it is slowly applied, first separates a portion of the acid in a vapour, that condenses in crystals. The soluble benzoates are decomposed by the powerful acids, which separate their acid in a crystalline form.

The benzoic acid is occasionally used in medicine, but not so much as formerly; and enters into the composition of the camphorated tincture of opium of the London college, heretofore called paregoric elixir.

BENZOI'FERA. See *Styrax benzoin.*

BENZOI'NUM. (From the Arabic term *benzoah.*) See *Styrax benzoin.*

BENZOINI MAGISTERIUM. Magistery, or precipitate of gum-benjamin.

Benzoini oleum. Oil of benjamin.

BERBERIA. (Origin uncertain.) *Berberi.* The name of a species of disease in the genus *Synclonus* of Good's Nosology See *Beriberia.*

BE'RBERIS. (*Berberi*, wild Arab. used by Averrhoes, and officinal writers.)

1. The name of a genus of plants in the Linnæan system. Class, *Hexandria;* Order, *Monogynia.* The barbery, or pepperidge bush.

2. The pharmacopœial name for the barberry. See *Berberis vulgaris.*

Berberis gelatina. Barberry jelly. Barberries boiled in sugar.

Berberis vulgaris. The systematic name for the barberry of the pharmacopœias. *Oxycantha Galeni; Spina acida; Crespinus.* This tree, *Berberis; pedunculis racemosis, spinus triplicibus*, of Linnæus, is a native of England. The fruit, or berries, which are gratefully acid, and moderately astringent, are said to be of great use in biliary fluxes, and in all cases where heat, acrimony, and putridity of the humours prevail. The filaments of this shrub possess a remarkable degree of irritability; for on being touched near the base with the point of a pin, a sudden contraction is produced, which may be repeated several times.

BERENGA'RIUS, James, born about the end of the 15th century at Carpi, in Modena, whence he is often called *Carpus.* He was one of the restorers of anatomy, of which he was professor, first at Padua, afterward at Bologna, which he was in a few years obliged to quit, being accused of having opened the bodies of two Spaniards alive. By his numerous dissections, he corrected many previous errors concerning the structure of the human body, and paved the way for his successor Vesalius. He was among the first to use mercurial frictions in syphilis, whereby he acquired a large fortune, which he left to the Duke of Ferrara, into whose territory he retired, at his death in 1527. His principal works are an enlarged Commentary on Mundinus, and a Treatise on Fracture of the Cranium.

Bereni secum. See *Artemisia vulgaris.*

Bereni'ce. (The city from whence it was formerly brought.) Amber.

Bereni'cium. (From φερω, to bring, and νικη victory.) A term applied by the old Greek writers to nitre, from its supposed power in healing wounds.

BERGAMO'TE. A species of citron. See *Citrus medica.*

BERGMANITE. A massive mineral of a greenish, grayish-white, or reddish colour, which fuses into a transparent glass, or a semitransparent enamel. It is found in Fredrickswam, in Norway, in quartz and in felspar.

[This mineral has not yet been satisfactorily analyzed. Its masses are composed of fibres, or little needles, confusedly grouped, and often so closely applied to each other, that the texture becomes nearly compact. Some of the needles have a foliated shining fracture. Its colour is a deep gray. Its sharp fragments scratch glass, and even quartz in a slight degree. Its spec. grav. is 2.30. When moistened by the breath, it yields an argillaceous odour. A fragment exposed to the flame of a candle, or placed on a hot coal, becomes white and friable. It melts by the blow-pipe into a white translucent glass.—See *Cleav. Min.* A.]

BERIBE'RI. (An Hindostan word signifying a sheep.) *Beriberia.* A species of palsy, common in some parts of the East Indies, according to Bontius. In this disease, the patients lift up their legs very much in the same manner as is usual with sheep. Bontius adds, that this palsy is a kind of trembling, in which there is deprivation of the motion and sensation of the hands and feet, and sometimes of the body.

BERKENHOUT, John, born at Leeds, about the year 1730. His medical studies were commenced late in life, having graduated at Leyden only in 1765; nor did he long continue the practice of medicine. His "Pharmacopœia Medica," however, was very much approved, and has since passed through many editions; his other medical publications are of little importance. He died in 1791.

Bermudas berry. See *Sapindus saponaria.*

BERRY. See *Bacca.*

Bers. Formerly the name of an exhilarating electuary.

Be'rula. An old name for brooklime.

Be'rula gallica. Upright water parsnip.

BERYL. Aqua marine. A precious mineral, harder than the emerald, of a green, or greenish-yellow colour, found in Siberia, France, Saxony, Brasil, Scotland, and Ireland.

Bessa'nen. (An Arabian word.) A redness of the external parts, resembling that which precedes the leprosy; it occupies the face and extremities.—*Avicenna.*

Be'sto. A name in Oribasius for a species of saxifrage.

BE'TA (So called from the river *Bœtis*, in Spain, where it grows naturally; or, according to Blanchard, from the Greek letter βητα, which it is said to resemble when turgid with seed.) The beet.

1. The name of a genus of plants in the Linnæan system. Class, *Pentandria;* Order, *Digynia.* The beet.

2. The pharmacopœial name of the common beet. See *Beta vulgaris.*

Beta hybrida. The plant which affords the root of scarcity. *Mangel wurzel* of the Germans; a large root. It contains much of the saccharine principle, and is very nourishing. Applied externally it is useful in cleaning foul ulcers; and is a better application than the carrot.

Beta vulgaris. The systematic name for the beet of the pharmacopœias. *Beta:—floribus congestis* of Linnæus. The root of this plant is frequently eaten by the French; it may be considered as nutritious and antiscorbutic, and forms a very elegant pickle with vinegar. The root and leaves, although formerly employed as laxatives and emollients, are now forgotten. A considerable quantity of sugar may be obtained from the root of the beet. It is likewise said, that if beet roots be dried in the same manner as malt, after the greater part of their juice is pressed out very good beer may be made from them. It is occasionally used to improve the colour of claret.

Betele. *Bethle; Betle; Betelle.* An oriental plant, like the tail of a lizard. It is chewed by the Indians, and makes the teeth black; is cordial and exhilarating, and in very general use throughout the east. It is supposed to be the long pepper.

BETO'NICA. (Corrupted from *Vettonica*, which is derived from the *Vectones*, an ancient people of Spain.) Betony.

1. The name of a genus of plants in the Linnæan system. Class, *Didynamia;* Order, *Gymnospermia.*

2. The pharmacopœial name of the wood betony See *Betonica officinalis.*

Betonica aquatica. See *Scrophularia aquatica.*

Betonica officinalis. The systematic name of the betony of the pharmacopœias. *Betonica purpurea; Betonica vulgaris; Cestrum; Vetonica cordi; Betonica—spica interrupta, corollarum labii lacinia intermedia emarginata* of Linnæus. The leaves and tops of this plant have an agreeable, but weak smell; and to the taste they discover a slight warmth, accompanied with some degree of adstringency and bitterness. The powder of the leaves of betony, snuffed up the nose, provokes sneezing; and hence it is sometimes made an ingredient in sternutatory powders. Its leaves are sometimes smoked like tobacco. The roots differ greatly, in their quality, from the other parts; their taste is very bitter and nauseous; taken in a small dose, they vomit and purge violently, and are supposed to have somewhat in common with the roots of hellebore. Like many other plants, formerly in high medical estimation, betony is now almost entirely neglected. Antonius Musa, physician to the emperor Augustus, filled a whole volume with enumerating its virtues, stating it as a remedy for no less than forty-seven disorders; and hence in Italy the proverbial compliment, *You have more virtues than betony.*

Betonica pauli. A species of veronica.

Betonica vulgaris. See *Betonica officinalis*

BETONY. See *Betonica.*

Betony, water. See *Scrophularia aquatica*

BETULA. 1. The name of a genus of plants in the Linnæan system. Class, *Monœcia;* Order, *Tetrandria.* Alder and birch.

2. The pharmacopœial name of the white birch. See *Betula alba.*

Betula alba. The systematic name of the *betula* of the pharmacopœias. *Betula:—foliis ovatis, acuminatis, serratis*, of Linnæus. The juice, leaves, and bark have been employed medicinally. If the tree be bored early in the spring, there issues, by degrees, a large quantity of limpid, watery, sweetish juice; it is said that one tree will afford from one to two gallons a day. This juice is esteemed as an antiscorbutic, deobstruent, and diuretic. When well fermented, and having a proper addition of raisins in its composition, it is frequently a rich and strong liquor; it keeps better than many of the other made-wines, often for a number of years, and was formerly supposed to possess many medical virtues; but these experience does not seem to sanction; and the virtues of the alder, like those of many other simples formerly prized, have sunk into oblivion. The leaves and bark were used externally as resolvents, detergents, and antiseptics.

Betula alnus. The systematic name for the *alnus* of the pharmacopœias. The common alder.

BEX. (From βησσω, to cough.) A cough. Dr. Good, in his Nosology, has applied this term to a genus of diseases, which embraces three species, *bex humida, sicca, convulsiva.*

Bexagui'llo. A name given to the white ipecacuanha, which the Spaniards bring from Peru, as the Portuguese do the brown from Brazil.

Bexu'go. The root of the *Æmatitis peruviana* of Caspar Bauhin; one drachm of which is sufficient for a purge.

Be'zahan. The fossile bezoar.

Beze'tta cœrulea. See *Croton tinctorium*

BE'ZOAR. (From *pa-zahar*, Persian, a destroyer of poison.) *Lapis bezoardicus.* Bezoard. A preternatural or morbid concretion formed in the bodies of land-animals. Several of these kinds of substances were formerly celebrated for their medicinal virtues, and distinguished by the names of the countries from whence they came, or the animal in which they were found. There are eight kinds, according to Fourcroy, Vauquelin, and Berthollet.

1. Superphosphate of lime, which forms concretions in the intestines of many *mammalia.*

2. Phosphate of magnesia, semitransparent and yellowish, and of sp. grav. 2.160.

3. Phosphate of ammonia and magnesia. A concretion of a gray or brown colour, composed of radiations from a centre. It is found in the intestines of herbivorous animals, the elephant, horse, &c.

4. Biliary, colour reddish-brown, found frequently in the intestines and gall-bladder of oxen, and used by painters for an orange-yellow pigment. It is inspissated bile.

5. Resinous. The oriental bezoars, procured from unknown animals, belong to this class of concretions. They consist of concentric layers, are fusible, combustible, smooth, soft, and finely polished. They are composed of bile and resin.

6. Fungous, consisting of pieces of the *Boletus igniarius*, swallowed by the animal.

7. Hairy.

8. Ligniform. Three bezoars sent to Bonaparte by the king of Persia, were found by Berthollet to be nothing but woody fibre agglomerated.

Bezoars were formerly considered as very powerful alexipharmics, so much so, indeed, that other medicines, possessed, or supposed to be possessed, of alexipharmic powers, were called *bezoardics;* and so efficacious were they once thought, that they were bought for ten times their weight in gold. These virtues, however, are in the present day justly denied them, as they produce no other effects than those common to the saline particles which they contain, and which may be given to greater advantage from other sources. A composition of bezoar with absorbent powders, has been much in repute, as a popular remedy for disorders in children, by the name of Gascoigne's powder, and Gascoigne's ball; but the real bezoar was rarely, if ever, used for these, its price offering such a temptation to counterfeit it. Some have employed for this purpose, a resinous composition, capable of melting in the fire, and soluble in alkohol; but Newmann supposed that those nearest resembling it, were made of gypsum, chalk, or some other earth, to which the proper colour was imparted by some vegetable juice. We understand, however, that tobacco-pipe clay, tinged with ox-gall, is commonly employed, at least for the Gascoigne's powder; this giving a yellow tint to paper, rubbed with chalk, and a green to paper rubbed over with quick-lime; which are considered as proofs of genuine bezoar, and which a vegetable juice would not effect.

Bezoar bovinum. Bezoar of the ox.

Bezoar germanicum. The bezoar from the alpine goat.

Bezoar hystricis. *Lapis porcinus; Lapis malacensis; Petro del porco.* The bezoar of the Indian porcupine; said to be found in the gall-bladder of an Indian porcupine, particularly in the province of Malacca. This concrete differs from others: it has an intensely bitter taste; and on being steeped in water, for a very little time, impregnates the fluid with its bitterness, and with aperient, stomachic, and, as it is supposed, with alexipharmic virtues. How far it differs in virtue from the similar concretions found in the gall-bladder of the ox, and other animals, does not appear.

Bezoar microcosmicum. The calculus found in the human bladder.

Bezoar occidentale. Occidental bezoar. This concretion is said to be found in the stomach of an animal of the stag or goat kind, a native of Peru, &c. It is of a larger size than the oriental bezoar, and sometimes as large as a hen's egg; its surface is rough, and the colour green, grayish, or brown.

Bezoar orientale. *Lapis bezoar orientalis.* Oriental bezoar stone. This concretion is said to be found in the pylorus, or fourth stomach of an animal of the goat kind, which inhabits the mountains of Persia. It is generally about the size of a kidney bean, of a roundish or oblong figure, smooth, and of a shining olive or dark greenish colour.

Bezoar porcinum. See *Bezoar hystricis.*

Bezoar simiæ. The bezoar from the monkey.

Bezoardica radix. See *Dorstenia.*

Bezoardicum joviale. *Bezoar* with tin. It differed very little from the *Antihecticum Poterii.*

Bezoardicum lunale. A preparation of antimony and silver.

Bezoardicum martiale. A preparation of iron and antimony.

Bezoardicum minerale. A preparation of antimony, made by adding nitrous acid to butter of antimony.

Bezoardicum saturni. A preparation of antimony and lead.

Bezo'ardicus lapis. See *Bezoar.*

Bezoardicus pulvis. The powder of the oriental bezoar.

Bezoarticum minerale. A calx of antimony.

BI. (From *bis*, twice.) In composition signifies twice or double, and is frequently attached to other words in anatomy, chemistry, and botany; as *biceps*, having two heads; *bicuspides*, two points, or fangs; *bilocular*, with two cells; *bivalve*, with two valves, &c.

Biæon. Wine made from sun-raisins, fermented in sea water.

Bibine'lla. See *Pimpinella.*

BIBITO'RIUS. (*Bibitorius*, from *bibo*, to drink, because by drawing the eye inwards towards the nose, it causes those who drink to look into the cup.) See *Rectus internus oculi.*

BIBULUS. Bibulous; attracting moisture; *charta bibula*, blotting paper.

BICAPSULARIS. Having two capsules. *Pericarpium bicapsulare.* See *Capsula.*

BI'CEPS. (From *bis*, twice, and *caput*, a head.) Two heads. Applied to muscles from their having two distinct origins or heads.

Biceps brachii. See *Biceps flexor cubiti.*

Biceps cruris. See *Biceps flexor cruris.*

Biceps cubiti. See *Biceps flexor cubiti.*

Biceps externus. See *Triceps extensor cubiti.*

Biceps flexor cruris. *Biceps cruris* of Albinus. *Biceps* of Winslow, Douglas, and Cowper; and *Ischio-femoroperonien* of Dumas. A muscle of the leg, situated on the hind part of the thigh. It arises by two distinct heads; the first, called *longus*, arises in common with the semitendinosus, from the upper and posterior part of the tuberosity of the os ischium. The second, called *brevis*, arises from the linea aspera, a little below the termination of the glutæus maximus, by a fleshy acute beginning, which soon grows broader, as it descends to join with the first head, a little above the external condyle of the os femoris. It is inserted by a strong tendon, into the upper part of the head of the fibula. Its use is to bend the leg. This muscle forms what is called the outer hamstring; and, between it and the inner, the nervous popliteus, arteria and vena poplitea, are situated.

BICEPS FLEXOR CUBITI. *Biceps brachii* of Albinus. *Coraco-radialis, seu biceps* of Winslow. *Biceps internus* of Douglas. *Biceps internus humeri* of Cowper. *Scapulo coracoradial* of Dumas. A muscle of the forearm, situated on the forepart of the *os humeri*. It arises by two heads. The first and outermost, called *longus*, begins tendinous from the upper edge of the glenoid cavity of the scapula, passes over the head of the os humeri within the joint, and in its descent without the joint, is enclosed in a groove near the head of the os humeri, by a membraneous ligament that proceeds from the capsular ligament and adjacent tendons. The second, or innermost head, called *brevis*, arises, tendinous and fleshy, from the coracoid process of the scapula, in common with the coracobrachialis muscle. A little below the middle of the forepart of the os humeri, these heads unite. It is inserted by a strong roundish tendon into the tubercle on the upper end of the radius internally. Its use is to turn the hand supine, and to bend the forearm. At the bending of the elbow, where it begins to grow tendinous, it sends off an aponeurosis, which covers all the muscles on the inside of the forearm, and joins with another tendinous membrane, which is sent off from the triceps extensor cubiti, and covers all the muscles on the outside of the forearm, and a number of the fibres, from opposite sides, decussate each other. It serves to strengthen the muscles, by keeping them from swelling too much outwardly when in action, and a number of their fleshy fibres take their origin from it.

BICEPS INTERNUS. See *Biceps flexor cubiti.*

BICHI'CHIÆ. An epithet of certain pectorals, or rather troches, described by Rhazes, which were made of liquorice, &c.

BI'CHOS. A Portuguese name for the worms that get under the toe of the people in the Indies, which are destroyed by the oil of cashew nut.

BICI. The Indian name of an intoxicating liquor, made from Turkey wheat in South America. See *wheat, Turkey.*

BI'CORNIS. (From *bis*, twice, and *cornu*, a horn.) 1. An epithet sometimes applied to the os hyoides, which has two processes, or horns.

2. In former times, to muscles that had two terminations.

3. A name given to those plants, the antheræ of which have the appearance of two horns.

BICORNES PLANTÆ. The name of an order of plants in the natural method of Linnæus and Gerard.

BICUSPIDATUS. Having two points. See *Bicuspis.*

BICU'SPIS. (From *bis*, twice, and *cuspis*, a spear.) 1. The name of those teeth which have double points, or fangs. See *Teeth.*

2. Applied to leaves which terminate by two points; *folia bicuspida*, or *bicuspidata.*

BI'DENS. (From *bis*, twice, and *dens*, a tooth; so called from its being deeply serrated, or indented.) The name of a genus of plants in the Linnæan system. Class, *Syngenesia;* Order, *Polygamia æqualis.*

BIDENS TRIPARTITA. The systematic name of the hemp agrimony, formerly used as a bitter and aperient, but not in the practice of the present day.

BIDLOO, GODFREY, a celebrated anatomist, born at Amsterdam, in 1649. After practising several years as a surgeon, he was appointed physician to William III., and in 1694, made professor of anatomy and surgery at Leyden. He published 105 very splendid, though rather inaccurate anatomical tables, with explanations; and several minor works. His nephew, *Nicholas*, was physician to the Czar Peter I.

BIENNIS. Biennial. A biennial plant is one, as the term imports, of two year's duration. Of this tribe there are numerous plants, which being raised one year from the seed, generally attain perfection the same year, or within about twelve months, shooting up stalks, producing flowers, and perfecting seeds in the following spring or summer, and soon after commonly perish.

BIFARIAM. In two parts.

BIFER. (From *bis*, twice, and *fero*, to bear.) A plant is so called, which bears twice in the year, in spring and autumn, as is common between the tropics.

BIFIDUS. Forked. Divided into two; as a bifid seed-vessel in *Adoxa moschatellina, petala bifida* in the *Silene nocturna* and *Alyssum incanum.*

BIFLORUS. Bearing two flowers; as *pedunculus biflorus.*

BIFORIUM. Applied to a leaf which points two ways.

BIFORUS. (From *bis*, twice, and *forus*, a door.) Two-doored, or bivalved. A class of plants is so denominated in some natural arrangements, constituted by those which have a pericarp, or seed-vessel, furnished with two valves.

BIFURCATE. (*Bifurcus;* from *bis*, twice, and *furca*, a fork.) A vessel, or nerve, stem, root, &c. is said to bifurcate when it divides into two branches; thus the bifurcation of the aorta, &c.

BIFURCATIO. Bifurcation.

BIFURCATUS. (From *bis*, twice, and *furca*, a fork.) Forked. See *Bifurcate* and *Dichotomus.*

BIGA'STER. (*Bigaster:* from *bis*, twice, and γαστηρ, a belly.) A name given to muscles which have two bellies.

BIGEMINATUS. (From *bis*, and *gemini*, twins.) Twice paired. *Biconjugatus.* A leaf is so called when near the apex of the common petiole there is a single pair of secondary petioles, each of which support a pair of opposite leaflets; as in *Mimosa unguis cati.*

BIH'ERNIUS. (From *bis*, double, and *hernia*, a disease so called.) Having a double hernia or one on each side.

Bihydroguret of carbon. See *Carburetted hydrogen.*

BIJUGUS. A winged leaf is termed *folium bijugum*, which bears two pairs of leaflets.

BILABIATUS. Two-lipped. Often used in botany; as *pericarpium bilabiatum; corolla bilabeata*, &c.

BILACINIATUS. Applied to a leaf *Folium bilaciniatum;* when cut into two segments.

BILA'DEN. A name of iron.

BILAMELLATUS. Composed of two lamina.

Bilberry bean. See *Arbutus uva ursi.*

BILDSTEIN. See *Figurestone.*

BILE. (*Bilis.* Nævius derives it from *bis*, twice and *lis*, contention; as being supposed to be the cause of anger and dispute.) The gall. A bitter fluid, secreted in the glandular substance of the liver; in part flowing into the intestines, and in part regurgitating into the gall-bladder. The secretory organs of this fluid are the penicilli of the liver, which terminate in very minute canals, called biliary ducts. The biliary ducts pour their bile into the *ductus hepaticus*, which conveys it into the *ductus communis choledochus*, from whence it is in part carried into the duodenum. The other part of the bile regurgitates through the cystic duct into the gall-bladder: for hepatic bile, except during digestion, cannot flow into the duodenum, which contracts when empty; hence it necessarily regurgitates into the gall-bladder. The branches of the *vena portæ* contribute most to the secretion of bile; its peculiar blood, returning from the abdominal viscera, is supposed to be, in some respects, different from other venal blood, and to answer exactly to the nature of bile. It is not yet ascertained clearly whether the florid blood in the hepatic artery, merely nourishes the liver, or whether, at the same time, it contributes a certain principle, necessary for the formation of bile. It has been supposed, by physiologists, that cystic bile was secreted by the arterial vessels of the gall-bladder; but the fallacy of this opinion is proved by making a ligature on the cystic duct of a living animal. From what has been said, it appears that there are, as it were, two kinds of bile in the human body:—

1. *Hepatic bile*, which flows from the liver into the duodenum: this is thin, of a faint yellow colour, inodorous, and very slightly bitter, otherwise the liver of animals would not be eatable.

2. *Cystic bile*, which regurgitates from the hepatic duct into the gall-bladder, and there, from stagnating, becomes thicker, the aqueous part being absorbed by lymphatic vessels, and more acrid from concentration. Healthy bile is of a yellow, green colour; of a plastic consistence, like thin oil, and when very much agitated, it froths like soap and water: its smell is fatuous, somewhat like musk, especially the putrefying or evaporating bile of animals: its taste is bitter.

The primary uses of this fluid, so important to the animal economy, are:

1. *To separate the chyle from the chyme:* thus chyle is never observed in the duodenum before the chyme has been mixed with the bile: and thus it is that oil is extricated from linen by the bile of animals.

2. By its *acridity* it excites the peristaltic motion of the intestines; hence the bowels are so inactive in people with jaundice.

3. It imparts a *yellow colour* to the excrements: thus we observe the white colour of the fæces in jaundice, in which disease the flow of bile into the duodenum is entirely prevented.

4. It prevents the *abundance of mucus and acidity* in the primæ viæ; hence acid, pituitous, and verminous saburra are common from deficient or inert bile.

The chemical analysis of bile has been principally illustrated by Mons. Thenard. "Ox bile is usually of a greenish-yellow colour, rarely of a deep green. By its colour it changes the blue of turnsole and violet to a reddish-yellow. At once very bitter, and slightly sweet, its taste is scarcely supportable. Its smell, though feeble, is easy to recognise, and approaches somewhat to the nauseous odour of certain fatty matters, when they are heated. Its specific gravity varies very little. It is about 1.026 at 43° F. It is sometimes limpid, and at others disturbed with a yellow matter, from which it may be easily separated by water: its consistence varies from that of a thin mucilage, to viscidity." Cadet regarded it as a kind of soap. This opinion was first refuted by Thenard. According to this able chemist, 800 parts of ox bile are composed of 700 water, 15 resinous matters, 69 picromel, about 4 of a yellow matter, 4 of soda, 2 phosphate of soda, 3.5 muriates of soda and potassa, 0.8 sulphate of soda, 1.2 phosphate of lime, and a trace of oxide of iron. When distilled to dryness, it leaves from 1-8th to 1-9th of solid matter, which, urged with a higher heat, is resolved into the usual igneous products of animal analysis; only with more oil and less carbonate of ammonia.

Exposed for some time in an open vessel, the bile gradually corrupts, and lets fall a small quantity of a yellowish matter; then its mucilage decomposes. Thus the putrefactive process is very inactive, and the odour it exhales is not insupportable, but in some cases has been thought to resemble that of musk. Water and alkohol combine in all proportions with bile. When a very little acid is poured into bile, it becomes slightly turbid, and reddens litmus; when more is added, the precipitate augments, particularly if sulphuric acid be employed. It is formed of a yellow animal matter, with very little resin. Potassa and soda increase the thinness and transparency of bile. Acetate of lead precipitates the yellow matter, and the sulphuric and phosphoric acids of the bile. The solution of the subacetate precipitates not only these bodies, but also the picromel and the muriatic acid, all combined with the oxide of lead. The acetic acid remains in the liquid united to the soda. The greater number of fatty substances are capable of being dissolved by bile. This property, which made it be considered a soap, is owing to the soda, and to the triple compound of soda, resin, and picromel. Scourers sometimes prefer it to soap, for cleansing woollen. The bile of the calf, the dog, and the sheep, are similar to that of the ox. The bile of the sow contains no picromel. It is merely a soda-resinous soap. Human bile is peculiar. It varies in colour, sometimes being green, generally yellowish-brown, occasionally almost colourless. Its taste is not very bitter. In the gall-bladder it is seldom limpid, containing often, like that of the ox, a certain quantity of yellow matter in suspension. At times this is in such quantity, as to render the bile somewhat grumous. Filtered and boiled, it becomes very turbid, and diffuses the odour of white of egg. When evaporated to dryness, there results a brown extract, equal in weight to 1-11th of the bile. By calcination we obtain the same salts as from ox bile.

All the acids decompose human bile, and occasion an abundant precipitate of albumen and resin, which are easily separable by alkohol. One part of nitric acid, sp. grav. 1.210, saturates 100 of bile. On pouring into it a solution of sugar of lead, it is changed into a liquid of a light-yellow colour, in which no picromel can be found, and which contains only acetate of soda and some traces of animal matter. Human bile appears hence to be formed, by Thenard, in 1100 parts; of 1000 water; from 2 to 10 yellow insoluble matter; 42 albumen; 41 resin; 5.6 soda; and 45 phosphates of soda of lime, sulphate of soda, muriate of soda, and oxide of iron. But by Berzelius, its constituents are in 1000 parts: 908.4 water; 80 picromel; 3 albumen; 4.1 soda; 0.1 phosphate of lime; 3.4 common salt; and 1 phosphate of soda, with some phosphate of lime.

BILGUER, JOHN ULRICK, was born at Coire, in Swisserland. He practised surgery at Berlin with such reputation, that he was appointed, by the great Frederick, Surgeon-General to the Prussian army. It was then the general practice to amputate in bad compound fractures; and being struck with the small proportion of those who recovered after the operation, he was led to try more lenient methods; from which meeting with much better success, he published as a thesis, on graduating at Halle, in 1761, a pretty general condemnation of amputation. This work attracted much notice throughout Europe, and materially checked the unnecessary use of the knife. In his "Instructions for Hospital Surgeons," which appeared soon after, he insisted farther on the same subject; and where amputation was unavoidable, he advised leaving a portion of the integuments, which is now generally adopted.

BI'LIARY. (*Biliaris;* from *bilis*, the bile.) Of or belonging to the bile.

BILIARY DUCT. *Ductus biliosus.* The very vascular *glandules*, which compose almost the whole substance of the liver, terminate in very small canals, called *biliary ducts*, which at length form one trunk, the *ductus hepaticus.* Their use is to convey the bile, secreted by the liver, into the hepatic duct; this uniting with a duct from the gall-bladder, forms one common canal, called the *ductus communis choledochus*, which conveys the bile into the intestinal canal.

BILI'MBI. (Indian.) See *Malus Indica.*

BI'LIOUS. (*Biliosus*, from *bilis*, bile.) A term very generally made use of, to express diseases which arise from too copious a secretion of bile: thus bilious colic, bilious diarrhœa, bilious fever, &c.

BI'LIS. See *Bile.*

BILIS ATRA. Black bile. The supposed cause among the ancients of melancholy.

BILIS CYSTICA. *Bilis fellea.* Cystic bile. The bile when in the gall-bladder is so called to distinguish it from that which is found in the liver. See *Bile.*

BILIS HEPATICA. Hepatic bile. Bile that has not entered the gall-bladder. See *Bile.*

BI'LOBUS. (From *bis*, double, and *lobus*, the end of the ear.) Having two lobes, resembling the tips of ears; applied to a leaf, *folium bilobum*, when it is deeply divided into rounded segments, as the petals of the *Geranium pyrenaicum* and *striatum* which are bilobed.

BILOCULARIS (From *bis*, twice, and *loculus*, a little cell.) Two-celled; applied to a capsule which has two cells.

BILOCULARES. Is the name of a natural order of plants.

BIME'STRIS. (From *bis*, twice, and *mensis*, month.) Two months old.

BINATUS. *Binus.* Binate. A term applied to compound leaves, when consisting of a pair of leaflets only, on one footstalk as in the great everlasting pea and other species of *lathyrus.*

BINDWEED. See *Convolvulus sepium.*

BINERVIUS. Two-nerved. Having two ribs or nerves very apparent. Hence, *folium binerium.*

BINGA'LLE. See *Casumuniar.*

BINO'CULUS. (From *binus*, double, and *oculus*, the eye.) A bandage for securing the dressings on both eyes.

BI'NSICA. A disordered mind.—*Helmont.*

BINSICA MORS. The binsical, or that death which follows a disordered mind.

BINUS. (From *bis*, twice.) Two by two; by couplets; applied to leaves when there are only two upon a plant, *folia bina;* as in *Convallaria majalis*, &c.

BIOLY'CHNIUM. (From βιος, life, and λυχνιον, a lamp.) Vital heat: also the name of an officinal nostrum.

BI'OTE. (From βιος, life.) Life. Also light food.

BIOTHA'NATI. (From βια, violence, or βιος, life, and θανατος, death.) Those who die a violent death, or suddenly, as if there were no space between life and death.

BIPARTITUS. Bipartite. Deeply divided almost

to the basis; as *calyx bipartitus; folium bipartitum; perianthium bipartitum;* and *petala bipartita.*

BIPEMU'LLA. See *Pimpinella.*

BIPENE'LLA. See *Pimpinella.*

BIPINATIFIDUS. Doubly pinnatifid; as in the long rough-headed poppy, *Papaver arzemone.* See *Pinnatifidus.*

BIPINNATIFIDUS. Doubly pinnatifid; applied to a leaf. See *Leaf.*

BIPINNATUS. Doubly pinnate. A compound leaf is so termed when the secondary petioles are arranged in pairs on the common petiole, and each secondary petiole is pinnate.

BI'RA. Malt liquor or beer.

BIRA'O. Stone Parsley.

BIRCH. See *Betula.*

BIRDLIME. The best birdlime is made of the middle bark of the holly, boiled seven or eight hours in water, till it is soft and tender; then laid in heaps in pits in the ground and covered with stones, the water being previously drained from it; and in this state left for two or three weeks to ferment, till it is reduced to a kind of mucilage. This being taken from the pit is pounded in a mortar to a paste, washed in river water, and kneaded, till it is freed from extraneous matters. In this state it is left four or five days in earthen vessels, to ferment and purify itself, when it is fit for use.

It may likewise be obtained from the misletoe, the *Viburnum lantana*, young shoots of elder, and other vegetable substances.

It is sometimes adulterated with turpentine, oil, vinegar, and other matters.

Good birdlime is of a greenish colour, and sour flavour; gluey, stringy, and tenacious; and in smell resembling linseed oil. By exposure to the air it becomes dry and brittle, so that it may be powdered; but its viscidity is restored by wetting it. It reddens tincture of litmus. Exposed to a gentle heat it liquefies slightly, swells in bubbles, becomes grumous, emits a smell resembling that of animal oils, grows brown, but recovers its properties on cooling, if not heated too much. With a greater heat it burns, giving out a brisk flame and much smoke. The residuum contains sulphate and muriate of potassa, carbonate of lime and alumina, with a small portion of iron.

BIRDSTONGUE. A name given to the seeds of the *Flaxinus excelsior* of Linnæus.

BI'RSEN. (Hebrew for an aperture.) A deep ulcer, or imposthume in the breast.

BIRTHWORT. See *Aristolochia.*

Birthwort, climbing. See *Aristolochia clematitis.*

Birthwort, long-rooted. See *Aristolochia longa.*

Birthwort, snake-killing. See *Aristolochia anguicida.*

Birthwort, three-lobed See *Arislolochia trilobata.*

BISCO'CTUS. (From *bis*, twice, and *coquo*, to boil.) Twice dressed. It is chiefly applied to bread much baked, as biscuit.

BISCUTE'LLA. Mustard.

BISE'RMAS. A name formerly given to clary, or garden clary.

BISHOP'S WEED. See *Ammi.*

BISILI'NGUA. (From *bis*, twice, and *lingua*, a tongue; so called from its appearance of being double-tongued; that is, of having upon each leaf a less leaf.) The Alexandrian laurel.

BISMA'LVA. From *vismalva*, *quasi viscum malva*, from its superior viscidity. The water, or marsh-mallow.

BI'SMUTH. (*Bismuthum*, from *Bismut*, Germ.) A metal which is found in the earth in very few different states, more generally native or in the metallic state. *Native bismuth* is met with in solid masses, and also in small particles dispersed in and frequently deposited on different stones, at Schreeberg, in Saxony, Sweden, &c. Sometimes it is crystallized in four-sided tables, or indistinct cubes. It exists combined with oxygen in the *oxide of bismuth* (*bismuth hochre*,) found in small particles, dispersed, of a bluish or yellowish-gray colour, needle-shaped and capillary; sometimes laminated, forming small cells. It is also, though more seldom, united to sulphur and iron in the form of a sulphuret in the *martial sulphuretted bismuth ore.* This ore has a yellowish-gray appearance, resembling somewhat the martial pyrites. And it is sometimes combined with arsenic.

Bismuth is a metal of a yellowish or reddish-white colour, little subject to change in the air. It is somewhat harder than lead, and is scarcely, if at all malleable; being easily broken, and even reduced to powder, by the hammer. The internal face, or place of fracture, exhibits large shining plates, disposed in a variety of positions; thin pieces are considerably sonorous. At a temperature of 480° Fahrenheit, it melts, and its surface becomes covered with a greenish-gray or brown oxide. A stronger heat ignites it, and causes it to burn with a small blue flame; at the same time that a yellowish oxide, known by the name of flowers of bismuth, is driven up. The oxide appears to rise in consequence of the combustion; for it is very fixed, and runs into a greenish glass when exposed to heat alone.

Bismuth urged by a strong heat in a close vessel, sublimes entire, and crystallizes very distinctly when gradually cooled.

The sulphuric acid has a slight action upon bismuth, when it is concentrated and boiling. Sulphurous acid gas is exhaled, and part of the bismuth is converted into a white oxide. A small portion combines with the sulphuric acid, and affords a deliquescent salt in the form of small needles.

The nitric acid dissolves bismuth with the greatest rapidity and violence; at the same time that much heat is extricated, and a large quantity of nitric oxide escapes. The solution, when saturated, affords crystals as it cools; the salt detonates weakly, and leaves a yellow oxide behind, which effloresces in the air Upon dissolving this salt in water, it renders that fluid of a milky white, and lets fall an oxide of the same colour.

The nitric solution of bismuth exhibits the same property when diluted with water, most of the metal falling down in the form of a white oxide, called magistery of bismuth. This precipitation of the nitric solution, by the addition of water, is the criterion by which bismuth is distinguished from most other metals. The magistery or oxide is a very white and subtile powder; when prepared by the addition of a large quantity of water, it is used as a paint for the complexion, and is thought gradually to impair the skin. The liberal use of any paint for the skin seems indeed likely to do this; but there is reason to suspect, from the resemblance between the general properties of lead and bismuth, that the oxide of this metal may be attended with effects similar to those which the oxides of lead are known to produce. If a small portion of muriatic acid be mixed with the nitric, and the precipitated oxide be washed with but a small quantity of cold water, it will appear in minute scales of a pearly lustre, consisting the *pearl powder* of perfumers. These paints are liable to be turned black by sulphuretted hydrogen gas.

The muriatic acid does not readily act upon bismuth.

When bismuth is exposed to chlorine gas it takes fire, and is converted into a chloride, which, formerly prepared by heating the metal with corrosive sublimate, was called butter of bismuth. The chloride is of a grayish-white colour, a granular texture, and is opaque. It is fixed at a red heat. When iodine and bismuth are heated together, they readily form an iodide of an orange yellow colour, insoluble in water, but easily dissolved in potassa ley.

Alkalis likewise precipitate its oxide; but not of so beautiful a white colour as that afforded by the affusion of pure water.

The gallic acid precipitates bismuth of a greenish yellow, as ferroprussiate of potassa does of a yellowish colour.

There appears to be two sulphurets, the first a compound of 100 bismuth to 22.34 sulphur; the second of 100 to 46.5: the second is a bisulphuret.

The metal unites with most metallic substances, and renders them in general more fusible. When calcined with the imperfect metals, its glass dissolves them, and produces the same effect as lead in cupillation; in which process it is even said to be preferable to lead.

Bismuth is used in the composition of pewter, in the fabrication of printers' types, and in various other metallic mixtures. With an equal weight of lead, it forms a brilliant white alloy, much harder than lead, and more malleable than bismuth, though not ductile and if the proportion of lead be increased, it is rendered still more malleable. Eight parts of bismuth five of lead, and three of tin, constitute the fusible metal, sometimes called Newton's, from its discoverer, which melts at the heat of boiling water, and may be fused over a candle in a piece of stiff paper without burning the paper. One part of bismuth, with five of lead, and three of tin, forms plumbers' solder. It forms the basis of a sympathetic ink. The oxide of bismuth precipitated by potassa from nitric acid, has been recommended in spasmodic disorders of the stomach, and given in doses of four grains, four times a day. A writer in the Jena Journal says he has known the dose carried gradually to one scruple without injury.

Bismuth is easily separable, in the dry way, from its ores, on account of its great fusibility. It is usual, in the processes at large, to throw the bismuth ore into a fire of wood; beneath which a hole is made in the ground to receive the metal, and defend it from oxidation. The same process may be imitated in the small way, in the examination of the ores of this metal; nothing more being necessary, than to expose it to a moderate heat in a crucible, with a quantity of reducing flux; taking care, at the same time, to perform the operation as speedily as possible, that the bismuth may be neither oxidized nor volatilized.

["In the United States, native bismuth has been found in Connecticut. The official preparation of this metal is the *subnitrate*. As a small portion of nitric acid remains combined with the oxide of bismuth in its preparation, it is properly called a subnitrate. The precipitation which takes place from the nitric solution, by adding mere water, is a criterion by which bismuth is distinguished from most other metals. Subnitrate of bismuth is a fine, soft powder, of a pearly white colour, and nearly destitute of taste and smell. It changes to a dark colour on the contact of sulphuretted or carburetted hydrogen.

Under the name of *magistery* of bismuth, this substance was formerly regarded as noxious to the human system. But during the last forty years it has been brought into the practice of medicine, and found to be a salutary tonic to the stomach and organs of digestion. Its use commenced in Geneva, and it has since had the testimony of some of the most distinguished physicians in France and England in its favour. It has also in this country generally satisfied the expectations formed of it. In dyspeptic complaints, especially in patients of a nervous temperament, it is found a very useful palliative, and sometimes does much toward promoting a cure. It is an important medicine in the case of persons habitually subject to cramp of the stomach, and does more to fortify that organ against the returns of the disease than perhaps any of the tonics in common use. In habitual vomiting or nausea, both from a primary affection of the stomach, and from sympathy with other parts, it frequently gives great relief. Its tonic effect appears not to be confined to the stomach, since it is found to do good in different spasmodic affections, such as palpitations and chorea. Recently, it has been announced to cure intermittents.

A drachm of the bismuth, with an equal quantity of liquorice powder, divided into twelve papers, three of which are to be taken during the day, will commonly be sufficient to display the activity of the medicine. Large quantities taken at once are unsafe."—*Big. Mat. Med.* A.]

BISMU'THUM. (From *bismut*, German.) See *bismuth*.

BISSET, CHARLES, was born about the year 1716. After studying at Edinburgh, and practising some years as an hospital-surgeon in Jamaica, he entered the army; but soon after settled in Yorkshire, and in 1755, published a Treatise on the Scurvy. But his most celebrated work is an "Essay on the Medical Constitution of Great Britain," in 1762. He obtained three years after a diploma from St. Andrew's, and reached his 75th year.

BISTORT. See *Bistorta*.

BISTO'RTA. (From *bis*, twice, and *torqueo*, to bend; so called from the contortions of its roots.) Bistort. See *Polygonum bistorta*.

BISTOURY. (*Bistoire*, French.) Any small knife for surgical purposes.

BISTRE. A brown pigment, consisting of the finer parts of wood soot, separated from the grosser by washing. The soot of the beech is said to make the best.

BISULPHATE. A sulphate with an additional quantity of sulphuric acid.

BIT NOBEN. Salt of bitumen. A white saline substance has lately been imported from India by this name, which is not a natural production, but a Hindoo preparation of great antiquity. It is called in the country, *bit noben*, *padanoon*, and *soucherloon*, and popularly *khala mimuc*, or black salt. Mr. Henderson, of Bengal, conjectures it to be the *sal asphaltites* and *sal sodomenus* of Pliny and Galen. This salt is far more extensively used in Hindostan than any other medicine whatever. The Hindoos use it to improve their appetite and digestion. They consider it as a specific for obstructions of the liver and spleen; and it is in high estimation with them in paralytic disorders, particularly those that affect the organs of speech, cutaneous affections, worms, old rheumatisms, and indeed all chronic disorders of man and beast.

BITERNATUS. Twice-ternate. Applied to compound leaves, when the common footstalk supports three secondary petioles on its apex, and each of these support three leaflets; as in *Ægopodium*.

BITHI'NICI EMPLASTRUM. A plaster for the spleen.

BI'THINOS. A Galenical plaster.

BITTER. *Amarus*.

BITTER APPLE. See *Cucumis Colocynthis*.

BITTERN. The mother water which remains after the crystallization of common salt in sea-water, or the water of salt springs. It abounds with sulphate and muriate of magnesia, to which its bitterness is owing.

BITTERSPAR. Rhombspar. A mineral of a grayish or yellowish colour, and somewhat pearly lustre, usually found embedded in serpentine, chlorite, or steatite, and found in the Tyrol, Salsburg, Dauphiny, Scotland, and the Isle of Man.

BITU'MEN. (Πιʇυμα, πιʇυς, pine; because it flows from the pine-tree; or, *quòd vi tumeat è terra*, from its bursting forth from the earth.) This term includes a considerable range of inflammable mineral substances, burning with flame in the open air. They are of different consistency, from a thin fluid to a solid; but the solids are for the most part liquefiable at a moderate heat. The fluid are,

1. Naphtha; a fine, white, thin, fragrant, colourless, oil, which issues out of white, yellow, or black clays in Persia and Media. This is highly inflammable, and is decomposed by distillation. It dissolves resins, and the essential oils of thyme and lavender; but is not itself soluble either in alkohol or æther. It is the lightest of all the dense fluids, its specific gravity being 0.708. See *Naphtha*.

2. Petroleum, which is a yellow, reddish, brown, greenish, or blackish oil, found dropping from rocks, or issuing from the earth, in the dutchy of Modena, and in various other parts of Europe and Asia. This likewise is insoluble in alkohol, and seems to consist of naphtha, thickened by exposure to the atmosphere. It contains a portion of the succinic acid. See *Petroleum*.

3. Barbadoes tar, which is a viscid, brown, or black inflammable substance, insoluble in alkohol, and containing the succinic acid. This appears to be the mineral oil in its third state of alteration.

The solid are, 1. Asphaltum, mineral pitch, of which there are three varieties: the cohesive; the semi-compact, maltha; the compact, or asphaltum. These are smooth, more or less hard or brittle, inflammable substances, which melt easily, and burn without leaving any or but little ashes, if they be pure. They are slightly and partially acted on by alkohol and æther. See *Asphaltum*.

2. Mineral tallow, which is a white substance of the consistence of tallow, and as greasy, although more brittle. It was found in the sea on the coasts of Finland, in the year 1736; and is also met with in some rocky parts of Persia. It is near one-fifth lighter than tallow; burns with a blue flame, and a smell of grease, leaving a black viscid matter behind, which is more difficultly consumed.

3. Elastic bitumen, or mineral caoutchouc, of which there are two varieties. Besides these, there are other bituminous substances, as jet and amber, which approach the harder bitumens in their nature; and all the varieties of pit coal, and the bituminous schistus, or shale, which contain more or less of bitumen in their composition.

Bitumen barbadense. See *Petroleum barbadense.*

Bitumen judaicum. *Asphaltus.* Jews' pitch. A solid, light, bituminous substance; of a dusky colour on the outside, and a deep shining black within; of very little taste, and scarcely any smell, unless heated; when it emits a strong pitchy one. It is said to be found plentifully in the earth in several parts of Egypt, and floating on the surface of the Dead sea. It is now wholly expunged from the catalogue of officinals of this country; but was formerly esteemed as a discutient, sudorific, and emmenagogue.

Bitumen liquidum. See *Petroleum.*

BITUMINOUS. Of the nature of bitumen.

[**Bituminous coal.** In the United States, coal has been explored in several districts, and undoubtedly exists in great abundance. In Virginia, near Richmond, is a deposite of coal about 20 miles in length, and ten miles in breadth; it is accompanied by a whitish sandstone and shale, with vegetable impressions, as is usual in the independent coal formation, which here lies over, and is surrounded by, primitive rocks. In Pennsylvania, coal is found on the west branch of the Susquehannah; in various places west of that branch; also on the Juniata, and on the waters of the Alleghany and Monongahela. Indeed, according to Mr. Maclure, the independent coal formation extends from the head waters of the Ohio, with some interruptions, to the waters of the Tombigbee river, in Alabama.—See *Cl. Min.* A.]

Bituminous limestone. Found near Bristol, and in Galway, in Ireland. The Dalmatian is so charged with bitumen, that it may be cut like soap, and is used for building houses. When the walls are reared, fire is applied to them, and they burn white.

BIVALVIS. Two-valved. Applied to the valves of the absorbents in anatomy, and in botany to capsules.—*Capsula bivalvis.*

BIVASCULARIS. (From *bis*, twice, and *vasculum*, a little vessel.) Having two cells.

BIVE'NTER. (From *bis*, twice, and *venter*, a belly.) A muscle is so termed, which has two bellies.

Biventer cervicis. A muscle of the lower jaw.

Biventer maxillæ inferioris. See *Digastricus.*

BI'XA. The name of a genus of plants. Class, *Polyandria.* Order, *Monogynia.*

Bixa orellana. The systematic name for the plant affording the *terra orellana* or *annotto* of the shops and pharmacopœias. The substance so called is a ceraceous mass obtained from the pellicles of the seeds. In Jamaica and other warm climates, it is considered as a useful remedy in dysentery, possessing adstringent and stomachic qualities; but here it is only used to colour cheese, and some other articles.

Bla'cciæ. The measles.—*Rhazes.*

BLA'CKBERRY. The fruit of the common brambles.—See *Rubus fruticosus.*

[In the United States, there are two species of the blackberry, the fruit of which is eaten, and the roots used as astringents. They are the *Rubus trivialis*, or Dewberry, or running blackberry, and the *Rubus villosus*, or standing blackberry.

"The bark of the root of the *dewberry*, or *low blackberry*, a common native briar, is highly astringent, possessing both tannin and gallic acid in large quantity. It is a popular remedy in cholera infantum, to which disease it appears well suited after liberal evacuations have been made. In the secondary stages of dysentery, and in diarrhœa, after the removal of offending causes from the alimentary canal, it has been resorted to with success in controlling the discharges, and giving tone to the bowels. It is usually exhibited in strong decoction.

The *Rubus villosus* is commonly distinguished from the preceding by the name of *high*, or *tall blackberry.* The properties of the two are the same."—See *Big. Mat. Med.*

A jelly made of the fruit is an excellent domestic remedy for young children in cholera infantum, after proper evacuations. A.]

BLACK CHALK. A mineral of a bluish black colour, and slaty texture, which soils the fingers. It is found in primitive mountains, and occurs in Caernarvonshire, and the island of Isla.

[**Black drop.** "The formula for this preparation in the Pharmacopœia, is essentially the same with the one made public by Dr. Armstrong, and which, under the name of *Black Drop*, has been known and prized in England for a century and upwards. As the recipe wants the usual precision of pharmaceutical formulæ, it may be proper to secure a tolerable uniformity of strength, by boiling the first ingredients no longer than is necessary to blend them together, and by afterward exposing them in a warm place, until about one-fourth of their original volume is evaporated. The compound directed in the Pharmacopœia should afford about two pints of strained liquor. As the filtration of so viscid a liquor is difficult, it may be strained without pressure through a double linen bag.

The black drop is a fermented aromatic vinegar of opium. Its taste, when properly prepared, is bitter and acid, the saccharine principle being changed by the fermentation. Its consistence is moderately viscid.

Acetous solutions of opium have been in use since the days of Van Helmont, and even earlier. Our medical chemists of the present day consider that the peculiarities which attend the operation of these preparations depend upon the formation of an acetate of morphia. The black drop has sustained its popularity for a great length of time on account of its favourable operation. According to Dr. Armstrong, it often stays in the stomach when other preparations will not, and it also affects the head less than laudanum. Dr. Paris and other medical writers give their testimony to its usefulness.

About ten or twelve minims form a dose. Notwithstanding the advantages ascribed to this preparation, it is not always uniform in its strength, or in the amount of sediment it deposites. It is probable that a better vinegar of opium might be prepared."—*Big. Mat. Med.* A.]

BLACK JACK. Blende, or mock lead: an ore of zinc.

BLACK LEAD. See *Plumbago.*

BLACKMORE, Sir Richard, was born in Wiltshire about the year 1650. After studying at Oxford, he took his degree in medicine at Padua, then settled in London, and met with considerable success, insomuch that he was appointed physician to William III. and retained the same office under Queen Anne. He then published several long and dull epic poems, which appear to have materially lessened his reputation; so that his opposition to the inoculation for small-pox had very little weight. He wrote also several medical tracts, which are little known at present.

BLACK WADD. One of the ores of manganese.

[**Black vomit.** This is one of the fatal symptoms of yellow fever, it being a very rare case for a patient to recover after its occurrence.

"A memoir on the analysis of black vomit, by Dr. Cathral, was read before the American Philosophical Society at Philadelphia, on the 20th June, 1800. The experienced and intrepid author has given a description of the black vomit, has analyzed the fluids ejected a few hours before the commencement of black vomiting itself, to which he has added experiments to ascertain the effects of black vomit on the living system of man and other animals, and a synopsis of the opinions of authors concerning its formation and qualities. The experiments show that this singular morbid excretion contains an *acid*, which is neither *carbonic*, *phosphoric*, nor *sulphuric*; and, what our readers will hardly expect, that the black vomit may be *smelled*, *tasted*, and *swallowed*, without inducing yellow fever, or even any sickness at all—so little infection or contagion does it seem to contain. He concludes it to be an altered secretion from the liver."—*New-York Med. Repos* vol. iv. p. 75.

"Dr. May, of Philadelphia, dropped the matter of black vomit into his eyes, and never experienced inconvenience or sickness."—*Med. Rep.* vol. v. p. 131.

"Dr. Ffirth of Salem, in New-Jersey, has published a Dissertation on Malignant Fever, with an attempt to prove that it is *not contagious.* In this he relates a number of experiments which he has made upon the matter of black vomit, as discharged by persons labouring under that disease. He inoculated himself in the left fore-arm with black vomit just discharged from a moribund patient; a slight inflammation ensued, which subsided in three days, and the wound readily healed, and without the formation of pus. To avoid cavil and deception, he repeated these experiments above twenty times on various parts of his body, with the black matter collected in Philadelphia during the seasons of 1802 and 1803. He put it into his eye, without experiencing more inconvenience than cold water produces. He exposed himself to the exhalations of it while acted upon by heat in an iron skillet, and experienced no unpleasant sensation. He swallowed the thick extractive matter which remained after evaporation, in the form of pills, without incommoding his stomach. He even went so far as to mix half an ounce of fresh black vomit with an ounce and a half of water and to drink it. It produced no more effect upon his stomach than so much water. He increased the dose to two ounces, and finally swallowed the black vomit in like quantity without any dilution at all, and without sustaining the least injury. He inoculated himself with saliva and serum, with as little inconvenience!!"—*Med. Rep.* vol. viii. p. 70. A.]

BLADDER. See *Urinary bladder*, and *Gall-bladder*.

Bladder, inflamed. See *Cystitis*.

BLADE-BONE. See *Scapula*.

BLÆ'SITAS. (From *blæsus*.) A defect in speech, called stammering.

Blæ'sus. (From βλαπ7ω, to injure.) A stammerer.

Bla'nca. (*Blanc*, French.) A purging mixture; so called because it was supposed to evacuate the white phlegmatic humours. Also white lead.

BLANCARD, Stephen, was born at Leyden, and graduated at Franeker, in 1678. He settled at Amsterdam, and published many anatomical and medical works; especially one on morbid anatomy, containing 200 cases, and a "Lexicon Medicum," which passed through numerous editions.

Bla'sa. (Indian.) A tree, the fruit of which the Indians powder, and use to destroy worms.

BLASIUS, Gerard, son of a physician at Amsterdam, from whom he derived a great predilection for comparative anatomy. After graduating at Leyden about the year 1646, he returned to his native city, and acquired so much reputation, that he was made professor of medicine in 1660, and soon after physician to the hospital. Besides publishing new editions of several useful works, with notes comprehending subsequent improvements, he was author of various original ones, especially relating to comparative and morbid anatomy. He claimed the discovery of the ductus salivaris, asserting he had pointed it out to Steno; to whom it has been commonly ascribed.

Blaste'ma. (From βλαςανω, to germinate.) A bud or shoot. Hippocrates uses it to signify a cutaneous pimple like a bud.

Bla'stum mosylitum. Cassia bark kept with the wood.

Bla'tta. (From βλαττω, to hurt.) A sort of beetle, or bookworm; so called from its injuring books or clothes; the kermes insect.

[Blatta is the generic name given by Linnæus to the cock-roach, which infests houses, and preys upon provisions, and not upon clothes. A.]

Blatta'ria lutea. (From *blatta*; so called, because, according to Pliny, it engenders the blatta.) The *Verbascum blattaria*, or herb yellow moth-mullein.

BLEACHING. The chemical art by which the various articles used for clothing are deprived of their natural dark colour, and rendered white.

Bleaching powder. The chloride of lime.

Ble'chon. (From βληχαομαι, to bleat; so called according to Pliny, because if sheep taste it they bleat.) The herb, wild penny-royal. See *Mentha pulegium*.

BLEEDING. See *Blood-letting* and *Hæmorrhage*.

BLE'MA. (From βαλλω, to inflict.) A wound.

BLE'NDE. A species of zinc ore, formed of zinc in combination with sulphur, forming a sulphuret of zinc.

BLE'NNA. Βλεννα. *Blena*. Mucus, a thick excrementitious humour.

BLENNORRHA'GIA. (From βλεννα, mucus, and ῥεω, to flow.) The discharge of mucus from the urethra.

BLENNORRHŒ'A. (From βλεννα, mucus, and ῥεω, to flow.) 1. A gleet; *Gonorrhœa mucosa*. A discharge of mucus from the urethra, arising from weakness.

2 The name of a genus of diseases in Good's Nosology, embracing three species, *Blennorrhœa simplex, luodes*, and *chronica*.

BLE'PHARA. (*Quasi* βλεπους φαρος, as being the cover and defence of the sight.) The eyelids.

Blepha'rides. (From βλεφαρον.) The hair upon the eyelids; also the part of the eyelids where the hair grows.

BLEPHAROPHTHA'LMIA. (From βλεφαρον, the eyelid, and οφθαλμια, a disease of the eye.) An inflammation of the eyelid.

BLEPHAROPTO'SIS. (From βλεφαρον, the eyelid, and πτωσις, from πιπ7ω, to fall.) A prolapse, or falling down of the upper eyelid, so as to cover the cornea. See *Ptosis*.

BLEPHARO'TIS. (From βλεφαρον, the eyelid.) An inflammation of the eyelids.

Blepharo'xysis. (From βλεφαρον, the eyelid, and ξεω, to scrape off.) 1. The cleansing of the eyelids.

2. Inflammation of the eyelids.

Blepharoxy'ston. (From βλεφαρον, the eyelid, and ξεω, to scrape off.) A brush for the eyes. An instrument for cleansing or scraping off foul substances from the eyelids.

BLESSED. *Benedictus*. Applied to remedies and plants from their supposed virtues. See *Benedictus*.

Blessed Thistle. See *Centaurea benedicta*.

Blestri'smus. (From βαλλω, to throw about.) Phrenitic restlessness.

Ble'ta. A word used by Paracelsus to signify white, and applied to urine when it is milky, and proceeds from a disease of the kidneys.

Ble'ti. (*Bletus*, from βαλλω, to strike.) Those seized with dyspnœa or suffocation.

BLISTER. *Vesicatorium; Epispasticum*. 1. The name of a topical application, *Emplastrum vesicatorium*, which when put on the skin raises the cuticle in the form of a vesicle, filled with a serous fluid. Various substances produce this effect on the skin; but the powder of the *cantharis*, or blistering fly, is what operates with most certainty and expedition, and is now invariably made use of for the purpose.

It is a principle sufficiently established with regard to the living system, that where a morbid action exists, it may often be removed by inducing an action of a different kind in the same or neighbouring part. On this principle is explained the utility of blisters in local inflammation and spasmodic action, and it regulates their application in pneumonia, gastritis, hepatitis, phrenitis, angina, rheumatism, colic, and spasmodic affections of the stomach; diseases in which they are employed with the most marked advantage. A similar principle exists with respect to pain; exciting one pain often relieves another. Hence blisters often give relief in toothache, and some other painful affections Lastly, blisters, by their operation, communicate a stimulus to the whole system, and raise the vigour of the circulation. Hence, in part, their utility in fevers of the typhoid kind, though in such cases they are used with still more advantage to obviate or remove local inflammation.

When it is not wished to maintain a discharge from the blistered part, it is sufficient to make a puncture in the cuticle to let out the fluid; but when the case requires keeping up a secretion of pus, the surgeon must remove the whole of the detached cuticle with a pair of scissors, and dress the excoriated surface in a particular manner. Practitioners used formerly to mix powder of cantharides with an ointment, and dress the part with this composition. But such a dressing not unfrequently occasioned very painful affections of the bladder, a scalding sensation in making of water, and very afflicting stranguries. The treatment of such complaints consists in removing every particle of the fly from the blistered part, making the patient drink abundantly of mucilaginous drinks, giving emulsions and some doses of camphor.

These objections to the employment of salves containing the lytta, for dressing blistered surfaces, led to the use of mezereon, euphorbium, and other irritating substances, which, when incorporated with ointment, form very proper compositions for keeping blisters open, which they do without the inconvenience of irritating the bladder, like the blistering fly. The favourite application, however, for keeping open blisters, is the savine cerate, which was brought into notice by Mr. Crowther in his book on white swellings. (See *Ceratum Sabinæ*.) On the use of the savine cerate, immediately after the cuticle raised by the blister is removed, says Mr. Crowther, it should be observed that experience has proved the advantage of using the application lowered by a half or two-thirds of the unguentum ceræ. An attention to this direction will produce less irritation and more discharge, than if the savine cerate were used in its full strength. Mr. Crowther says also, that he has found fomenting the part with flannel, wrung out of warm water, a more easy and preferable way of keeping the blistered surface clean, and fit for the impression of the ointment, than scraping the part, as has been directed by others. An occasional dressing of unguentum resinæ flavæ, he has found a very useful application for rendering the sore free from an appearance of slough, or rather dense lymph, which has sometimes been so firm in its texture as to be separated by the probe, with as much readiness as the cuticle is detached after blistering. As the discharge diminishes, the strength of the savine dressing should be proportionably increased. The ceratum sabinæ must be used in a stronger, or weaker degree, in proportion to the excitement produced on the patient's skin.

2. The name of a vesicle on the skin, whether formed by a blistering application, or arising from any other cause.

BLISTER-FLY. See *Cantharis*.

BLI'TUM FŒTIDUM. See *Chenopodium vulvaria*.

BLONDEL, JAMES AUGUSTUS, was born in England of a French family, and admitted licentiate of the College of Physicians about 1720. He chiefly distinguished himself by controverting, in a very able manner, the opinion then generally received, that marks could be imprinted on the fœtus by the imagination of the mother, and he has the merit of contributing very largely to the removal of this prejudice, which had prevailed for ages, and often produced much mischief.

BLOOD. *Sanguis.* A red homogeneous fluid, of a saltish taste, and somewhat urinous smell, and glutinous consistence, which circulates in the cavities of the heart, arteries, and veins. The quantity is estimated to be about twenty-eight pounds in an adult; of this, four parts are contained in the veins, and a fifth in the arteries. The colour of the blood is red: in the arteries it is of a florid hue, in the veins darker; except only the pulmonary vessels in which the colour is reversed. The blood is the most important fluid of our body. Some physicians and anatomists have considered it as alive, and have formed many ingeni us hypotheses in support of its vitality. The temperature of this fluid is of considerable importance, and appears to depend upon the circulation and respiration. The blood of man, quadrupeds, and birds is hotter than the medium they inhabit; hence they are termed animals of *warm blood;* while in fishes and reptiles, animals with *cold blood*, it is nearly of the temperature of the medium they inhabit. The blood possesses remarkable physical properties. Its colour is of a dark red, it is less deep in certain cases, and perhaps even scarlet. Its odour is insipid, and *sui generis;* its taste is also peculiar; however, it is known to contain salts, and principally the muriate of soda. Its specific gravity is a little more than that of water. Haller found its *medium* as 1.0527 : 1.0000. Its capacity for caloric may be expressed by 934, that of arterial blood being 921. Its mean temperature is 31 degrees of Reaumur, = 102 F.

Venous blood, being extracted from its proper vessels, and left to itself, in a short time forms a soft mass; this mass *separates spontaneously* into two parts, the one liquid, yellowish, transparent, called *serum*: the other soft, almost solid, of a deep brown red, entirely opaque: this is the *cruor*, or *clot*. This occupies the bottom of the vessel; the serum is placed above. Sometimes a thin layer forms at the top of the serum, which is soft and reddish, and to which has been very improperly given the name of *rind*, *buff*, or *crust* of the blood.

This *spontaneous separation* of the elements of the blood does not take place quickly, except when it is in repose. If it is agitated it remains liquid, and preserves its homogeneity much longer.

If the venous blood is placed in contact with the atmosphere, or with oxygen gas, it takes a vermilion red colour; with ammonia it becomes cherry red; with azote a deeper brown red, &c. In changing colour it absorbs a considerable quantity of these different gases; it exhales a considerable quantity of carbonic acid, when kept some time under a bell upon mercury.

The serum sometimes presents a whitish tint, as if milky, which has made it be supposed that it contained chyle: it appears to be a fatty matter which gives it this appearance.

The cruor, or clot of the blood is essentially formed of fibrin, and colouring matter.

The fibrin, separated from the colouring matter, is whitish, insipid, and inodorous; heavier than water, without action upon vegetable colours, elastic when humid, it becomes brittle by being dried.

In distillation it gives out a great deal of carbonate of ammonia, and a vast quantity of carbon, the ashes of which contain much phosphate of lime, a little phosphate of magnesia, carbonate of lime, and carbonate of soda. A hundred parts of fibrin are composed of,

Carbon	53.360
Oxygen	19.685
Hydrogen	7.021
Azote	19.934
Total	100.000

The colouring matter is soluble in water and in the serum of the blood. Examined with the microscope in solution with these liquids, it appears like most fluids of the animal economy, formed of small globules; dried and calcined in contact with the air, it melts and swells up, burns with flame, and yields a coal that is difficultly reduced to ashes.

It is of importance to remark, that in none of the parts of the blood are any gelatine or phosphate of iron found, as was at first supposed.

The respective relations in quantity of the serum to the coagulum, and those of the colouring matter to the fibrin, have not yet been carefully examined. It is to be presumed, as we shall see afterward, that they are variable according to an infinity of circumstances.

The coagulation of the blood has been, by turns, attributed to refrigeration, to the contact of the air, to the state of repose, &c.; but J. Hunter and Hewson have demonstrated by experiments, that this phenomenon cannot be attributed to any of these causes. Hewson took fresh blood, and froze it, by exposing it to a low temperature. He afterward thawed it: the blood appeared fluid at first, and shortly afterward it coagulated as usual. An experiment of the same kind was made by J. Hunter, with a similar result. Thus, blood does not coagulate because it is cooled. It even appears that a temperature a little elevated is favourable to its coagulation. We also know by experience that the blood thickens when it is deprived of the contact of the air, and agitated; its coagulation is, however, generally favoured by repose and the contact of the air.

The elements of venous blood, such as we have noticed, are known by its analysis; but as all the matters absorbed from the intestinal canal, the serous membranes, the cellular tissue, &c., are immediately mixed with the venous blood, the composition of this liquid must vary in proportion to the matter absorbed There will be found in it, in different circumstances, alkohol, æther, camphor, and salts, which it does not usually contain, &c., when these substances have been submitted to absorption in any part of the body

When, by the aid of a strong lens, or a microscope, we observe the transparent parts of cold-blooded animals, we see in the blood-vessels an immense multitude of small, rounded molecules, which swim in the serum, and roll upon each other, while they flow through the arteries and the veins

Similar observations have never been made upon the hot-blooded animals; the membranes and sides of the vessels being opaque. But as, in separating a drop of blood in water, rounded particles are often seen with the microscope, the existence of globules has been admitted for the blood of animals, and consequently for that of man.

Authors have related marvellous things of these globules. According to *Leuwenhoeck*, a thousand millions of those globules are not larger than a grain of sand. Haller, in speaking of cold-blooded animals, for he never could see those of hot-blooded animals, says, that they are to an inch as one inch is to five thousand. Some will have them of the same form and diameter in all animals: others, on the contrary, assert, that they have a particular form and size for each animal; some declare that they are spherical and solid, others that they are flattened, and pierced with a small hole in the centre; lastly, many believe that a globule is a species of small bladder, which contains a certain number of smaller globules.

Probably many errors of imagination and optical illusions, have slid into these different opinions. Dr. Magendie made a great number of microscopic experiments, in order to satisfy himself in this respect.

He has never seen, in the blood of man diluted in water, any thing but particles of colouring matter, generally rounded, of different sizes, which, according as they are placed exactly or not in the focus of the microscope, appear sometimes spherical, sometimes flat, and, at other times, of the figure of a disc, pierced in the centre. All these appearances, he says, can be produced at pleasure, by varying the position of the particles relatively to the instrument, and he believes that bubbles of air have often been described and drawn for globules of blood; at least, nothing has more resemblance to certain figures of Hewson, than very small bubbles of air that are produced by slightly agitating the liquid submitted to the microscope.

The latest and most accurate chemical analysis of blood is as follows:

The specific gravity of the serum is about 1.029, while that of blood itself is 1.058. It changes syrup of violets to a green, from its containing free soda. At 156° serum coagulates, and resembles boiled white of egg. When this coagulated albumen is squeezed, a muddy fluid exudes, which has been called the serosity. According to Berzelius, 1000 parts of the serum of bullock's blood consist of 905 water, 79.99 albumen, 6.175 lactate of soda and extractive matter, 2.565 muriates of soda and potassa, 1.52 soda and animal matter, and 4.75 loss. 1000 parts of serum of human blood consist, by the same chemist, of 905 water, 80 albumen, 6 muriates of potassa and soda, 4 lactate of soda with animal matter, and 4.1 of soda, and phosphate of soda with animal matter. There is no gelatin in serum.

The cruor has a specific gravity of about 1.245. By making a stream of water flow upon it till the water runs off colourless, it is separated into insoluble fibrin, and the soluble colouring matter. A little albumen has also been found in cruor. The proportions of the former two are, 64 colouring matter, and 36 fibrin in 100. To obtain the colouring matter pure, we mix the cruor with 4 parts of oil of vitriol previously diluted with 8 parts of water, and expose the mixture to a heat of about 160° for 5 or 6 hours. Filter the liquid while hot, and wash the residue with a few ounces of hot water. Evaporate the liquid to one-half, and add ammonia, till the acid be almost, but not entirely saturated. The colouring matter falls. Decant the supernatant liquid, filter and wash the residuum from the whole of the sulphate of ammonia. When it is well drained, remove it with a platina blade, and dry it in a capsule.

When solid, it appears of a black colour, but becomes wine-red by diffusion through water, in which, however, it is not soluble. It has neither taste nor smell. Alkohol and æther convert it into an unpleasant smelling kind of adipocire. It is soluble both in alkalies and acids. It approaches to fibrin in its constitution, and contains iron in a peculiar state, $\frac{1}{3}$ of a per cent. of the oxide of which may be extracted from it by calcination. The incinerated colouring matter weighs 1-80th of the whole; and these ashes consist of 50 oxide of iron, 7.5 subphosphate of iron, 6 phosphate of lime, with traces of magnesia, 20 pure lime, 16.5 carbonic acid and loss; or the two latter ingredients may be reckoned 32 carbonate of lime. Berzelius imagines that none of these bodies existed in the colouring matter, but only their bases, iron, phosphorus, calcium, carbon, &c.; and that they were formed during the incineration. From the albumen of blood, the same proportion of ashes may be obtained, but no iron.

The importance of the blood is very considerable; it distends the cavities of the heart and blood-vessels, and prevents them from collapsing; it stimulates to contraction the cavities of the heart and vessels, by which means the circulation of the blood is performed; it generates within itself animal heat, which it propagates throughout the body; it nourishes the whole body; and, lastly, it is that source from which every secretion of the body is separated.

[In the winter of 1824-5, Dr. Mitchill then Professor of Materia Medica in the College of Physicians and Surgeons of New-York, read the following letter to his class, while speaking on the operation of remedies, and their effects upon the blood.

Dr. Akerly to Dr. Samuel L. Mitchill, Professor, &c.

Dear Sir.—While speaking on the operation of remedies, it reminds me of an occurrence which took place in 1819, connected with this subject. A man called on me in the summer of that year, stating that he had fallen in the street in a fit, from which having recovered he requested to be bled to relieve his head, as from the distress there he was apprehensive of another. Mr. Knapp having just commenced the study of medicine with me, I desired him to take a stick and stir the blood to collect the fibrin, and to show him that the blood would not coagulate after being deprived of it. His attention as soon as he began to stir the blood was attracted by the strong smell of spirituous liquor arising from it. We both satisfied ourselves that the alkoholic odour actually arose from the blood, and that it was more perceptible when agitated, than when undisturbed. I immediately went out and made inquiries at a neighbouring store of the character and habits of the man, and ascertained that he was a great lover of ardent spirits, and daily drank a quart or more by small glasses. This appeared to me a case in which the fluid taken into the stomach reached the blood vessels without change, and as it may throw some light on the operation of remedies upon the human constitution, I communicate the fact for your consideration. A.]

Blood, dragon's. See *Calamus rotang.*

Blood, spitting of. See *Hæmoptysis.*

Blood, vomiting of. See *Hæmatemesis.*

BLOOD-LETTING. Under this term is comprehended every artificial discharge of blood made with a view to cure or prevent a disease. Blood-letting is divided into *general* and *topical.* As examples of the former, *venæsection* and *arteriotomy* may be mentioned; and of the latter, the *application* of *leeches, cupping-glasses,* and *scarification.*

[BLOOD-ROOT. "This is an indigenous article, derived from the *Sanguinaria Canadensis,* one of our earliest flowering plants, common in woods in various parts of the United States.

The root is brownish externally; but, when broken, emits a bright vermilion or orange-coloured juice. This root has a bitter taste, leaving a sense of acrimony in the throat when swallowed. Besides fibrous matter, it contains resin, fæcula, bitter extractive, and an acrid principle.

The medicinal properties of blood-root are those of an acrid narcotic. When taken in a large dose, it irritates the fauces, leaving a disagreeable sensation in the throat for some time after it is swallowed. It occasions heartburn, nausea, fainting, and frequently vertigo, and diminished vision. It also vomits; but in this operation it is less certain than many other emetics in common use. When given in smaller doses, such as produce nausea without vomiting, and repeated at frequent intervals, it lessens the frequency of the pulse in a manner somewhat analagous to the operation of digitalis. This, however, is a secondary effect, since, in its primary operation, it seems to accelerate the circulation. In still smaller doses, such as do not disturb the stomach, it has required some reputation as a tonic. It has been given in phthisis, both as a preventive in the early symptoms and as a palliative in the confirmed disease; also in catarrh, typhoid pneumonia, dyspepsia and various other complaints; in which, however, its use should not exclude the employment of more active means. It should be dried a short time before it is to be used, as the virtues are much impaired by age.

From ten to twenty grains ordinarily produce vomiting. Many country physicians prefer an infusion made with a drachm of the powder to a gill of water, of which a table-spoonful may be repeated till the effect of the medicine is obtained. As a tonic, the *tincture* is more frequently used."—See *Big. Mat Med.* A.]

Blood-stone. See *Hæmatites,* and *Calcedony.*

Bloody flux. See *Dysenteria.*

BLOWPIPE. A very simple and useful instrument. That used by the anatomist is made of silver or brass, of the size of a common probe, or larger, to inflate vessels and other parts.

The chemical blowpipe is made of brass, is of about one-eighth of an inch diameter at one end, and the other tapering to a much less size, with a very small perforation for the wind to escape. The smaller end is beveled on one side.

[BLUE IRON EARTH. This is the earthy phosphate of iron of some mineralogists. "The original colour of this variety is generally grayish, yellowish, or greenish white, or with a very slight tinge of blue; but by exposure to the air it absorbs oxygen, becomes indigo blue of different shades, sometimes pale. It is sometimes in small masses, considerably compact and solid, but more frequently it is friable, or even loose, and soils the fingers. It is often a mere coat.

Before the blowpipe it becomes reddish-brown, and then melts into a magnetic, blackish globule. In oil it usually acquires a shade of brown. A specimen yielded klaproth iron slightly oxidated 47.5, phosphoric acid 32.0, water 20.0; =99.5. But the proportion of acid appears to be extremely variable in different specimens. This mineral is sometimes employed with advantage as a pigment. It has been found in Maine and Massachusetts, but principally in New-Jersey. It generally accompanies bog ore, or certain argillaceous deposites. It is sometimes in masses weighing 30lbs. or more, with a texture more or less compact and solid. When first obtained it is yellowish white; but by exposure to the air, it assumes a fine blue colour. In some instances it appears to contain very little phosphoric acid.—See *Cl. Min.* A.]

BLUE, PRUSSIAN. A combination of oxide of iron with the ferro-prussic acid.

BLUE, SAXON. Made by digesting sulphuric acid and water, on powdered indigo.

BO'A. (From βους, an ox.) 1. A pustulous eruption like the small-pox, so called because it was cured, according to Pliny, by anointing it with hot ox-dung.

2. The name of a genus of serpents.

BOCHE'TUM. *Decoctum secundarium.* A decoction of the woods prepared by a second boiling with fresh water.

BO'CHIA. A subliming vessel.

BO'CHIUM. A swelling of the bronchial glands.

BODY. Whatever is capable of acting on our senses may be so denominated.

Bodies in *Natural Philosophy* are divided into *Ponderable* and *Imponderable.*

The first are those which may act upon several of our senses, and of which the existence is sufficiently established; of this kind are solids, fluids, and gases. The second are those which, in general, only act on one of our senses, the existence of which is by no means demonstrated, and which, perhaps, are only forces, or a modification of other bodies; such are caloric, light, the electric and magnetic fluids.

Ponderable bodies are endowed with common or general properties, and likewise with particular or secondary properties.

The general properties of bodies are,—extent, divisibility, impenetrability, mobility. A ponderable body, of whatever kind, always presents these four properties combined. Secondary properties are variously distributed among different bodies; as hardness, porosity, elasticity, fluidity, &c. They constitute, by their combination with the general properties, the condition or state of bodies. It is by gaining or losing some of these secondary properties that bodies change their state: for instance, water may appear under the form of ice, of a fluid, or of vapour, although it is always the same body. To present itself successively under these three forms, nothing more is necessary than the addition or abstraction of some of its secondary qualities.

Bodies are *simple*, or *compound.*

Simple bodies are rarely met with in nature; they are almost always the product of art, and we even name them simple, only because art has not arrived at their decomposition. At present, the bodies regarded as simple are the following:—Oxygen, chlorine, iodine, fluorine, sulphur, hydrogen, boracium, carbon, phosphorus, azote, silicium, zirconium, aluminum, yttrium, glucinum, magnesium, calcium, strontium, barium, sodium, potassium, manganese, zinc, iron, tin, arsenic, molybdenum, chromium, tungsten, columbium, antimony, uranium, cerium, cobalt, titanium, bismuth, copper, tellurium, nickel, lead, mercury, osmium, silver, rhodium, palladium, gold, platinum, iridium, selenium, lithium, thorenum, wood, anium, cadmium.

Compound bodies occur every where; they form the mass of the globe, and that of all the beings which are seen on its surface. Certain bodies have a constant composition; that is to say, a composition that never is changed, at least from accidental circumstances: there are, on the contrary, bodies, the composition of which is changed at every instant.

This diversity of bodies is extremely important; it divides them naturally into two classes; bodies, the composition of which is constant, are named brute, or gross, inert, inorganic; but those, the elements of which continually vary, are called living, organized bodies.

Brute and organized bodies differ from each other in respect, 1st, of form; 2d, of composition; 3d, of the laws which regulate their changes of state. The following table presents the differences which are best marked.

TABLE I.

DIFFERENCES BETWEEN INORGANIC AND LIVING BODIES.

1. *Form.*

	Inorganic Bodies.		Living Bodies.
1. *Form.*	Angular form. Indeterminate Volume.		Rounded form. Determinate Volume.
2. *Composition*	Sometimes simple. Seldom of more than 3 elements. Constant. Each part capable of existing, independent of the others. Capable of being decomposed and recomposed.		Never simple. At least 4 elements, often 8 or 10. Variable. Each part more or less depending on the whole. Capable of decomposition, but totally incapable of recomposition.
3. *Regulating Laws*	Entirely subject to attraction, and chemical affinity		In part subject to attraction and chemical affinity. In part subject to a power unknown

Living bodies are divided into two classes, one of which comprehends *Vegetables*, the other *Animals.*

TABLE II.

DIFFERENCES BETWEEN VEGETABLES AND ANIMALS.

Vegetables,	*Animals,*
Are fixed to the ground.	Move on the surface of the ground.
Have carbon for the principal base of their composition.	Have azot for the base of their composition.
Composed of four or five elements.	Often composed of eight or ten elements.
Find and assume in their vicinity their nourishment in a state of preparation.	Must act on their aliments, in order to render them fit for nourishment.
Are nourished by tubes opening externally.	Are nourished by an internal canal

In Anatomy. The human body is divided by anatomists into the trunk and extremities: *i. e.* the head, and inferior and superior extremities, each of which have certain regions before any part is removed, by which the physician is enabled to direct the application of blisters and the like, and the situation of diseases is better described.

The head is distinguished into the hairy part and the face. The former has five regions, viz. the crown of the head or *vertex*, the fore-part of the head or *sinciput*, the hind-part or *occiput*, and the sides, *partes laterales capitis*. In the latter are distinguished, the region of the forehead, *frons;* temples, or *tempora;* the nose, or *nasus;* the eyes, or *oculi;* the mouth, or *os;* the cheeks, *buccæ;* the chin, or *mentum;* and the ears, or *aures*.

The trunk is distinguished into three principal parts, the neck, thorax, and abdomen. The neck is divided into the anterior region or *pars antica*, in which, in men, is an eminence called *pomum Adami;* the posterior region is called *nucha colli;* and the lateral regions, *partes laterales colli*.

The thorax is distinguished into the anterior region, in which are the *sternum* and *mammæ*, and at the inferior part of which is a pit or hollow called *scrobiculus cordis;* a posterior region, called *dorsum;* and the sides, or *latera thoracis*.

The abdomen is distinguished into an anterior region, properly the *abdomen;* a posterior region, called the loins, or *lumbi;* and lateral regions or flanks, called *latera abdominis*. The anterior region of the abdomen being very extensive, is subdivided into the *epigastric*, *hypochondriac*, *umbilical*, and *hypogastric* regions, which are described under their respective names. Immediately below the abdomen is the *mons veneris*, and at its sides the groins or *inguina*. The space between the organs of generation and the *anus*, or fundament, is called the *perinæum*.

The superior extremity is distinguished into the shoulder, *summitas humeri*, under which is the arm-pit, called *axilla* or *fovea axillaris;* the *brachium*, or arm; the *antibrachium*, or fore-arm, in which anteriorly is the bend of the arm, where the veins are generally opened, called *flexura antibrachii;* and posteriorly the elbow, called *angulus cubiti;* and the hand, in which are the *carpus* or wrist, the back or *dorsum manûs*, and the palm or *vola*.

The inferior extremity is divided into, 1. the region of the femur, in which is distinguished the *coxa* or *regio-ischiadica*, forming the outer and superior part; 2. the leg, in which are the knee or *genu*, the bend or *cavum poplitis*, and the calf or *sura* · 3. the foot, in which are the outer and inner ankle, or *malleolus externus* and *internus*, the back or *dorsum*, and the sole or *planta*.

BODY, COMBUSTIBLE. This term is given by chemists to all substances which, on account of their affinity for oxygen, are capable of burning.

BODY, GASEOUS. See *Gas*.

BODY, INFLAMMABLE. Chemists give this name to such bodies as burn with facility, and flame in an increased temperature, although, strictly speaking, all combustible bodies are inflammable bodies; such are the diamond, sulphur, bitumens, &c.

BODY, PHOSPHORESCENT. Bodies which produce light, though their temperature be not increased.

BO'E. (From βοαω, to exclaim.) Clamour, or moaning made by a sick person.

BOERHAAVE, HERMAN, was born at Voorhout, in Holland, December 31, 1668. His father, the pastor of the village, having nine children, educated them himself, and intending Herman for the church, was careful to ground him well in the learned languages; in which he made such rapid progress, that he was sent at 14 to Leyden. His father dying soon after in slender circumstances, he was fortunately supported by the burgomaster, Daniel Van Alphin; which Boerhaave ever remembered with gratitude. Among other studies, he was very partial to the mathematics, and improved so much, as to be able to give private instructions in them, whereby he partly maintained himself. In 1690, he took his degree in philosophy, and in an inaugural thesis refuted the errors of the materialists. But he soon after turned his mind to the study of medicine, and attended dissections under Nuck; he greatly preferred Hippocrates among the ancient, and Sydenham among the modern physicians. He was made doctor of medicine at Harderwyck, in 1693; and in his dissertation on that occasion, insisted on the utility of observing the excretions in disease, especially the urine. He was then engaged in forming a new theory of medicine, by a judicious selection from all that had been before advanced; which was so well arranged, and so ably supported by him, that it became generally adopted, and prevailed throughout Europe for more than half a century. He also gave lectures on chemistry, with considerable reputation, about the same period. The university of Leyden therefore appointed him, in 1701, professor of the theory of medicine; when he read an oration recommending the study of Hippocrates; and, as he declined some very advantageous offers from other parts, they afterward augmented his salary. About this time, he published another Latin oration, "On the Use of mechanical Reasoning in Medicine," which contributed to extend his fame. In 1709, he was appointed professor of botany, to which study he was ever after eminently attached. On that occasion, he produced another oration, maintaining that medicine would be best improved by observation, and by simplicity in prescriptions. His "Aphorisms," had appeared the year before, giving a brief account of the history and cure of diseases, a work universally admired; to which his pupil Van Swieten afterward attached a very ample commentary. About the same time he published his "Institutes," treating of physiology. These two works, with successive improvements, passed through numerous editions, and were translated into every European, nay, even into the Arabic language. In the year after, he printed a catalogue of the plants in the university garden. In 1714, he was made rector of the university, and at the end of the year for which he held the office, delivered a discourse "On attaining Certainty in Physics." About this period he was made professor of the practice of medicine, and in 1718, of chemistry also. His lectures on these subjects, and on botany, were delivered with such clearness and precision, that students thronged from every part to hear him; insomuch that Leyden could scarcely afford accommodations for them. He was also often consulted in difficult cases by physicians even in distant parts of the world. When appointed to the chemical chair, he had published a short work on that subject, but some of his pupils having printed his lectures without authority, and very incorrectly, he was led to prepare them for the press in 1732. In his conversation, Boerhaave was generally familiar, in his demeanour grave, but disposed to occasional pleasantry: he was distinguished for piety, and on his moral character, his disciple Haller has passed a very high eulogium. Having acquired considerable wealth by his exertions, and being plain in his dress, as well as abstemious in his diet, he was by some accused of parsimony: but he spared no reasonable expense in procuring rare books, and foreign plants. Being of a vigorous constitution, and accustomed to much exercise abroad, he met with little interruption from illness; but in 1729, having become corpulent, and incapable of riding, his health began to suffer, and he was induced to resign his botanical and chemical appointments. In an oration then delivered, he recounted the chief events of his life, expressing himself grateful for the patronage which he had received from individuals; as well as to his own profession, for the little opposition shown to his opinions. It perhaps never happened, that so great a revolution in science was so readily brought about. The great reputation acquired by his extensive abilities, and the moderation of his character, particularly averse from contention, no doubt contributed materially to this result. In the year following, he was again made rector of the university of Leyden; and also elected a fellow of the Royal Society in London, having been previously admitted to the Royal Academy of Sciences in Paris. The remainder of his life was chiefly occupied in revising his own numerous productions, in publishing more correct editions of several esteemed authors, and in domestic recreations at his seat near Leyden, with his wife and daughter. Toward the end of 1737, he was attacked with symptoms of disease in the chest, which terminated his existence in the September following. His fellow-citizens erected an elegant monument to his memory.

BOETHE'MA. (From βοηθεω, to assist.) A remedy

Boethema'tica. (From $\beta o\eta\theta\epsilon\omega$, to assist.) Favourable symptoms.

BOG-BEAN. See *Menyanthes trifoliata.*

Bo'gia gummi. Gamboge.

BOHEA. See *Thea.*

BOHN, John, was born at Leipsic, in 1640; and after studying in many parts of Europe, graduated there, and was made successively professor of anatomy, and of therapeutics, public physician to the city, &c. Among numerous publications, he chiefly distinguished himself by his "Circulus anatomico physiologicus," and a treatise "De officio medici clinico et forensi," which latter particularly has great merit. He also well explained the judgment to be formed concerning wounds; and recommended purging with calomel in the beginning of small-pox. He died in 1718.

Bois de coissi. See *Quassia.*

Bolar earths. See *Bole.*

BOLE, ($\beta\omega\lambda o\varsigma$, a mass,) in chemistry, is a massive mineral, having a perfectly conchoidal fracture, a glimmering internal lustre, and a shining streak. Its colours are yellow-red, and brownish black, when it is called mountain soap. It is translucent or opaque. Soft, so as to be easily cut, and to yield to the nail. It adheres to the tongue, has a greasy feel, and falls to pieces in water. Sp. grav. 1.4 to 2. It may be polished. If it be immersed in water after it is dried, it falls asunder with a crackling noise. It occurs in wacke and basalt, in Silesia, Hessia, and Sienna in Italy, and also in the cliffs of the Giant's Causeway, Ireland. The black variety is found in the trap rocks of the isle of Sky. Several compounds were formerly used in medicine, particularly the Armenian and French; and in old pharmacopœias mention is made of red boles from Armenia, Lemnos, Strigonium, Portugal, Tuscany, and Livonia; yellow boles from Armenia, Tockay, Silesia, Bohemia, and Blois; white boles from Armenia, Lemnos, Nocera, Eretria, Lamos, Chio, Malta, Tuscany, and Goltberg. Several of these earths have been commonly made into little cakes or flat masses, and stamped with certain impressions; from which circumstance they received the name of *terræ sagillatæ*, or sealed earths.

Bole, Armenian. *Bolus Armeniæ.* Bole armenic. A pale but bright red-coloured earth, which is occasionally mixed with honey, and applied to children's mouths when afflicted with aphthæ. It forms, like all argillaceous earths, a good tooth-powder, when mixed with some aromatic.

BOLETIC ACID. *Acidum boleticum.* An acid extracted from the expressed juice of the *Boletus pseudo-igniarius*, by M. Braconnot. The juice concentrated to a syrup by a very gentle heat, was acted on by strong alkohol. What remained was dissolved in water. When nitrate of lead was dropped into this solution, a white precipitate fell, which, after being well washed with water, was decomposed by a current of sulphuretted hydrogen gas. Two different acids were found in the liquid after filtration and evaporation. One in permanent crystals was boletic acid; the other was a small proportion of phosphoric acid. The former was purified by a solution in alkohol, and subsequent evaporation.

It consists of irregular four-sided prisms, of a white colour, and permanent in the air. Its taste resembles cream of tartar; at the temperature of 68° it dissolves in 180 times its weight of water, and in 45 of alkohol. Vegetable blues are reddened by it. Red oxide of iron, and the oxides of silver and mercury, are precipitated by it from their solutions in nitric acid; but lime and barytes waters are not affected. It sublimes when heated, in white vapours, and is condensed in a white powder.—*Ann. de Chimie*, lxxx.

BOLE'TUS. (From $\beta\omega\lambda o\varsigma$, a mass, or $\beta\omega\lambda\iota\tau\eta\varsigma$, from its globular form.) The name of a genus of plants in the Linnean system. Class, *Cryptogamia;* Order, *Fungi.* Boletus; Spunk.

Boletus cervi. The mushroom.

Boletus igniarius. The systematic name for the *agaricus* of the pharmacopœias. *Agaricus chirurgorum; Agaricus quercûs; Fungus igniarius.* Agaric of the oak; Touchwood boletus; Female agaric. This fungus *Boletus:—acaulis pulvinatus levis, poris tenuissimis* of Linnæus, has been much used by surgeons as an external styptic. Though still employed on the continent, the surgeons in this country have not much confidence in it.

Boletus laricis. The systematic name for the officinal *agaricus albus*, which is met with on old larch trees, in different parts of Europe. Several preparations, as troches, an extract, and pills, are ordered to be made with it in foreign pharmacopœias, which are administered against phthisical complaints.

Boletus pini laricis. A species of agaric which grows on the larch.

Boletus suaveolens. The systematic name for the *fungus salicis* of the pharmacopœias. This species of fungus, *Boletus—acaulis superne lævis, salicibus*, of Linnæus, and the *Boletus albus* of Hudson, when fresh, has a suburinous smell, and at first an acid taste, followed by a bitter. It is seldom used at present, but was formerly given in phthisical complaints.

Boli'smus. A voracious appetite, according to Avicenna; but most probably meant for bulimus.

BOLOGNIAN STONE. A mixture of mucilage and powdered sulphate of barytes.

[Bolognian phosphorus. When native sulphate of baryta is heated it decrepitates, and at a high temperature, fuses into an opaque white enamel: it was employed in the manafacture of *Jasper ware* by the late Mr. Wedgewood. When heated to redness, it acquires the property of phosphorescence. This was first ascertained by Vincenzo Cascarioli, of Bologna, whence the term Bologna phosphorus is applied to it. This kind of phosphorus, after being exposed for a few minutes to the sun's rays, shines in the dark sufficiently to render visible the dial of a watch. This prosperty is lost by repeated uses, in consequence of the oxygenation of the sulphur: but it may be restored by a second calcination.—See *Webster's Man. of Chem.* A.]

BO'LUS. ($B\omega\lambda o\varsigma$, a bole, or bolus.) Any medicine, rolled round, that is larger than an ordinary sized pea, and yet not too large to be swallowed.

Bolus armena. See *Bole, Armenian.*

Bolus armena alba. The white Armenian bole.

Bolus armoniac. See *Bole, Armenian.*

Bolus blessensis. Bole of Blois. See *Bole.*

Bolus gallica. French bole. A pale red-coloured bolar earth, variegated with irregular specks and veins of white and yellow. It is occasionally administered as an absorbent and antacid.

BOMBAX. See *Gossypium.*

BOMBIATE. *Bombias.* A salt formed by the union of the bombic acid with salifiable bases; thus, *bombiate of alumine*, &c.

BO'MBIC ACID. *Acidum bombicum.* Acid of the silkworm. Silkworms contain, especially when in the state of chrysalis, an acid liquor in a reservoir placed near the anus. It is obtained by expressing their juice in a cloth, and precipitating the mucilage by spirit of wine, and likewise by infusing the chrysalides in that liquor. This acid is very penetrating, of a yellow amber colour, but its nature and combinations are not yet well known.

BO'MBUS. $Bo\mu\beta o\varsigma$. 1. A resounding noise, or ringing of the ears.

2. A sonorous expulsion of flatus from the intestines.

3. Dr. Good gives this name to that variety of imaginary sound, *parapsis illusoria*, which is characterized by a dull, heavy, intermitting sound.

Bon arbor. A name given to the coffee-tree.

Bo'na. *Boona.* The phaseolus, or kidney-beans.

[BOND, Thomas, M.D. This celebrated physician and surgeon was a native of Maryland, and studied his profession there under Dr. Hamilton, a very learned practitioner. Afterward he travelled in Europe and spent a considerable time in Paris, where he attended the practice of the Hôtel Dieu. He began the practice of medicine in Philadelphia about the year 1734, and soon attracted the public attention. He was the founder of the College and Academy, and one of the most active managers of the Pennsylvania Hospital, at its commencement. He was a contributor to some of the Medical Journals of Great Britain before the establishment of one in this country. In 1782 he delivered the annual address before the American Philosophical Society. The subject was, "The rank and dignity of man in the scale of being, and the conveniences and advantages he derives from the Arts and Sciences, and the prognostic of the unceasing grandeur and glory of America, founded on the nature of its climate." He was for half a century in the first practice in Philadelphia, and remarkable for attention to the cases under his care, and his sound judgment. He died in the year 1784, aged 72.—See *Thach. Med. Biog.* A.]

Bo'nduch indorum. See *Guilandina*.

BONE. *Os.* Bones are hard, dry, and insensible parts of the body, of a whitish colour, and composed of a spongy, compact, or recticular substance. They vary much in their appearances, some being long and hollow, others flat and compact, &c. The greater number of bones have several processes and cavities, which are distinguished from their figure, situation, use, &c. Thus, processes extended from the end of a bone, if smooth and round, are called *heads;* and *condyles*, when flattened either above or laterally. That part which is beneath the head, and which exceeds the rest of the bone in smallness and levity, is called the neck. Rough, unequal processes are called *tuberosities*, or tubercles: but the longer and more acute, *spinous*, or *styloid* processes, from their resemblance to a thorn. Thin broad processes, with sharp extremities, are known by the name of *cristæ*, or *sharp edges.* Other processes are distinguished by their form, and called *alar*, or *ptergoid; mamillary*, or *mastoid; dentiform*, or *odontoid*, &c. Others, from their situation, are called *superior*, *inferior*, *exterior*, and *interior.* Some have their name from their direction; as *oblique*, *straight*, *transverse*, &c.; and some from their use, as *trochanters*, *rotators*, &c. *Furrows*, *depressions*, and *cavities*, are destined either for the reception of contiguous bones, to form an articulation with them, when they are called *articular cavities*, which are sometimes deeper, sometimes shallower; or they receive hard parts, but do not constitute a joint with them. Cavities serve also for the transmission and attachment of soft parts. Various names are given to them, according to the magnitude and figure of bones. If they be broad and large at the beginning, and not deep, but contracted at their ends, they are called *foveæ*, or *pits.* Furrows are open canals, extending longitudinally in the surface of bones. A hollow, circular tube, for the most part of the same diameter from beginning to end, and more or less crooked or straight, long or short, is named a *canal.* *Foramina* are the apertures of canals, or they are formed of the excavated margins of two bones, placed against each other. If such be the form of the margin of a bone, as if a portion were taken out of it, it is called a *notch.*

With respect to the formation of bone, there have been various opinions. Physiologists of the present day assert, that it is from a specific action of small arteries, by which ossific matter is separated from the blood, and deposited where it is required. The first thing observable in the embryo, where bone is to be formed, is a transparent *jelly*, which becomes gradually firmer, and is formed into *cartilage.* The cartilage gradually increases to a certain size, and when the process of ossification commences, vanishes as it advances. Cartilages, previous to the ossific action, are solid, and without any cavity; but when the ossific action of the arteries is about to commence, the absorbents become very active, and form a *small cavity* in which the bony matter is deposited; bone continues to be separated, and the absorbents model the mass into its required shape. The process of ossification is extremely rapid in utero: it advances slowly after birth, and is not completed in the human body till about the twentieth year. Ossification in the flat bones, as those of the skull, always begin from *central points*, and the radiated fibres meet the radii of other ossifying points, or the edges of the adjoining bone. In long bones, as those of the arm and leg, the clavical, metacarpal, and metatarsal bones, a *central ring* is formed in the body of the bone, the head and extremities being cartilage, in the centre of which ossification afterward begins. The central ring of the body shoots its bony fibres towards the head and extremities, which extend towards the body of the bone. The head and extremities at length come so close to the body as to be merely separated by a cartilage, which becomes gradually thinner until the twentieth year. Thick and round bones, as those of the tarsus, carpus, sternum, and patella, are, at first, all cartilage: ossification begins in the *centre* of each. When the bones are deprived of their soft parts, and are hung together in their natural situation, by means of wire, the whole is termed an *artificial* skeleton; but when they are kept together by means of their ligaments, it is called a *natural* skeleton.—The uses of the bones are various, and are to be found in the account of each bone; it is, therefore, only necessary to observe, in this place, that they give shape to the body, contain and defend the vital viscera, and afford an attachment to all the muscles.

A Table of the Bones.

				No
Bones of the Head.	Bones of the *cranium* or *skull*		Frontal	1
			Parietal	2
			Occipital	1
			Temporal	2
			Ethmoid	1
			Sphenoid	1
	Bones of the *face*		Superior maxil	2
			Jugal	2
			Nasal	2
			Lachrymal	2
			Palatine	2
			Inferior spongy	2
			Vomer	1
			Inferior maxil	1
	Dentes or *teeth*		Incisores	8
			Cuspidati	4
			Molares	20
	Bone of the *tongue*		Hyoides os	1
	Bones of the *ear*, within the temporal bones		Malleus	2
			Incus	2
			Stapes	2
			Orbiculare os	2
Bones of the Trunk.	The *spine.*	Vertebræ	Cervical	7
			Dorsal	12
			Lumbar	5
		Sacrum		1
		Coccygis os		1
	The *thorax*		Sternum	1
			Ribs	24
	The *pelvis*		Innominata ossa	2
Bones of the Upper Extrem.	The *shoulder*		Clavicle	2
			Scapula	2
	The *arm*		Humeri os	2
	The *fore-arm*		Ulna	2
			Radius	2
	The *hand.*	*Carpus* or *wrist*	Naviculare os	2
			Lunare os	2
			Cuneiforme os	2
			Orbiculare os	2
			Trapezium os	2
			Trapezoides os	2
			Magnum os	2
			Unciforme os	2
		Metacarpus		10
		Phalanges		28
Bones of the Low. Extr.	The *thigh*		Femur	2
	The *leg*		Patella	2
			Tibia	2
			Fibula	2
	The *foot.*	*Tarsus* or *instep*	Calcaneus	2
			Astragalus	2
			Cuboides os	2
			Naviculare os	2
			Cuneiformia ossa	6
		Metatarsus		10
		Phalanges		28
Sesamoid bones of the thumb and great toe, occasionally found				8
			Total	248

Calcined human bones, according to Berzelius, are composed, in 100 parts, of 81.9 phosphate of lime, 3 fluate of lime, 10 lime, 1.1 phosphate of magnesia, 2 soda, and 2 carbonic acid. 100 parts of bones by calcination are reduced to 63. Fourcroy and Vauquelin found the following to be the composition of 100 parts of ox bones: 51 solid gelatin, 37.7 phosphate of lime, 10 carbonate of lime, and 1.3 phosphate of magnesia; but Berzelius gives the following as their constituents: 33.3 cartilage, 55.35 phosphate of lime, 3 fluate of lime, 3.85 carbonate of lime, 2.05 phosphate of magnesia, and 2.45 soda, with a little common salt.

About 1-30th of phosphate of magnesia was obtained from the calcined bones of fowls, by Fourcroy and

Vauquelin. When the enamel of teeth, rasped down, is dissolved in muriatic acid, it leaves no albumen, like the other bones. Fourcroy and Vauquelin state its components to be, 27.1 gelatin and water, 72.9 phosphate of lime. Messrs. Hatchett and Fepys rate its composition at 78 phosphate of lime, 6 carbonate of lime, and 16 water and loss. Berzelius, on the other hand, found only 2 per cent. of combustible matter in teeth. The teeth of adults, by Mr. Pepys, consist of 64 phosphate of lime, 6 carbonate of lime, 20 cartilage, and 10 water or loss. The fossil bones of Gibraltar are composed of phosphate of lime and carbonate, like burnt bones. Much difference of opinion exists with regard to the existence of fluoric acid in the teeth of animals; some of the most eminent chemists taking opposite sides of the question. It appears that bones buried for many centuries still retain their albumen, with very little diminution of its quantity.

Fourcroy and Vauquelin discovered phosphate of magnesia in all the bones they examined, except human bones. The bones of the horse and sheep afford about 1-36th of phosphate of magnesia; those of fish nearly the same quantity as those of the ox. They account for this by observing, that phosphate of magnesia is found in the urine of man, but not in that of animals, though both equally take in a portion of magnesia with their food.

The experiments of Mr. Hatchett show, that the membranous or cartilaginous substance, which retains the earthy salts within its interstices, and appears to determine the shape of the bone, is albumen. Mr. Hatchett observes, that the enamel of tooth is analogous to the porcellaneous shells, while mother of pearl approaches in its nature to true bone.

A curious phenomenon with respect to bones is the circumstance of their acquiring a red tinge, when madder is given to animals with their food. The bones of young pigeons will thus be tinged of a rose colour in twenty-four hours, and of a deep scarlet in three days; but the bones of adult animals will be a fortnight in acquiring a rose colour. The bones most remote from the heart are the longest in acquiring this tinge. Mr. Gibson informs us, that extract of logwood too, in considerable quantity, will tinge the bones of young pigeons purple. On desisting from the use of this food, however, the colouring matter is again taken up into the circulation, and carried off, the bones regaining their natural hue in a short time. It was said by Du Hamel, that the bones would become coloured and colourless in concentric layers, if an animal were fed alternately one week with madder, and one week without; and hence he inferred, that the bones were formed in the same manner as the woody parts of trees. But he was mistaken in the fact; and indeed had it been true, with the inference he naturally draws from it, the bones of animals must have been out of all proportion larger than they are at present.

Bones are of extensive use in the arts. In their natural state, or dyed of various colours, they are made into handles of knives and forks, and numerous articles of turnery. We have already noticed the manufacture of volatile alkali from bones, the coal of which forms bone-black; or, if they be afterward calcined to whiteness in the open air, they constitute the bone ashes of which cupels are made, and which, finely levigated, are used for cleaning articles of paste, and some other trinkets, by the name of burnt hartshorn. The shavings of hartshorn, which is a species of bone, afford an elegant jelly; and the shavings of other bones, of which those of the calf are the best, are often employed in their stead.

On this principle, Mr. Proust has recommended an economical use of bones, particularly with a view to improve the subsistence of the soldier. He first chops them into small pieces, throws them into a kettle of boiling water, and lets them boil about a quarter of an hour. When this has stood till it is cold, a quantity of fat, excellent for culinary purposes when fresh, and at any time fit for making candles, may be taken off the liquor. This, in some instances, amounted to an eighth, and in others even to a fourth, of the weight of the bones. After this the bones may be ground, and boiled in eight or ten times their weight of water, of which that already used may form a part, till about half is wasted, when a very nutritious jelly will be obtained. The boiler should not be of copper, as this metal is easily dissolved by the jelly; and the cover should fit very tight, so that the heat may be greater than that of boiling water, but not equal to that of Papin's digester, which would give it an empyreuma The bones of meat that have been boiled are nearly as productive as fresh bones; but Dr. Young found those of meat that had been roasted afforded no jelly, at least by simmering, or gentle boiling.

Bones, growth of. See *Osteogeny*.

BONEBINDER. See *Osteocolla*.

[BONESET. Thoroughwort. Eupatorium perfoliatum. This is an indigenous vegetable, growing in wet meadows throughout the United States. The whole plant is medicinal, but the leaves and flowers are most active. See Eupatorium perfoliatum. A.]

BONET, THEOPHILUS, was born at Geneva in 1620, and graduated at Bologna. He had considerable practice, and was extremely zealous in the pursuit of morbid anatomy, as well as in extracting valuable observations from authors. His hearing becoming impaired, he devoted the latter part of his life to the arrangement of the materials which he had prepared. His principal work, entitled "Sepulchretum," published 1679, was highly approved: and laid the foundation of Morgagni's excellent treatise, "De Sedibus et Causis Morborum." Another publication of his, "Mercurius compilatitius," is an index of medical literature to the time of its appearance, 1682. His death occurred seven years after.

BONONIE'NSIS LAPIS. The Bononian stone. Called also *phosphorus bononiensis*, *phosphorus kircheri*, the light carrier, or Bononian phosphorus. As a medicine, the stone is caustic and emetic.

BONTIUS, JAMES, was born at Leyden, where he studied medicine, and then went to practice in India. After his return, he wrote several valuable works on the diseases and practice of that country, as well as on its natural productions, animal and vegetable. The most esteemed is entitled "De Medicina Indorum," and appeared in 1642.

BO'NUS. Good. A term applied to plants, and remedies from their supposed efficacy.

BONUS HENRICUS. (*Henricus;* so called, because its virtues were detected by some one whose name was Henry.) See *Chenopodium bonus Henricus.*

BONY. *Osseus.* Of, or belonging to, or resembling bone.

BORACIC ACID. *Acidum boracicum.* Sedative salt of Homberg. Acid of Borax. Boracine acid. "The salt composed of this acid and soda had long been used both in medicine and the arts under the name of borax, when Homberg first obtained the acid separate in 1702, by distilling a mixture of borax and sulphate of iron. He supposed, however, that it was a product of the latter; and gave it the name of *volatile narcotic salt of vitriol*, or *sedative salt.* Lemery the younger, soon after discovered that it could be obtained from borax equally by means of the nitric or muriatic acid; Geoffroy detected soda in borax: and at length Baron proved, by a number of experiments, that borax is a compound of soda and a peculiar acid. Cadet has disputed this; but he has merely shown, that the borax of the shops is frequently contaminated with copper; and Struve and Exchaquet have endeavoured to prove that the boracic and phosphoric acids are the same; yet their experiments only show, that they resemble each other in certain respects, not in all.

To procure the acid, dissolve borax in hot water, and filter the solution, then add sulphuric acid by little and little, till the liquid has a sensibly acid taste. Lay it aside to cool, and a great number of small shining laminated crystals will form. These are the boracic acid. They are to be washed with cold water, and drained upon brown paper.

Boracic acid thus procured is in the form of thin irregular hexagonal scales, of a silvery whiteness, having some resemblance to spermaceti, and the same kind of greasy feel. It has a sourish taste at first, then makes a bitterish cooling impression, and at last leaves an agreeable sweetness. Pressed between the teeth, it is not brittle but ductile. It has no smell; but, when sulphuric acid is poured on it, a transient odour of musk is produced. Its specific gravity in the form of scales is 1.479; after it has been fused, 1.803. It is not altered by light. Exposed to the fire it swells up, from losing its water of crystallization, and in this state is called calcined boracic acid. It melts a little before it is red-hot, without perceptibly losing any water, but it does not flow freely till it is red, and then less than the borate of soda. After this fusion it is a hard transparent glass, becoming a little opaque on exposure to the air, without abstracting moisture from it, and unaltered in its properties, for on being dissolved in boiling water it crystallizes as before. This glass is used in the composition of false gems.

Boiling water scarcely dissolves one-fiftieth part, and cold water much less. When this solution is distilled in close vessels, part of the acid rises with the water, and crystallizes in the receiver. It is more soluble in alkohol, and alkohol containing it burns with a green flame, as does paper dipped in a solution of boracic acid.

Neither oxygen gas, nor the simple combustibles, nor the common metals, produce any change upon boracic acid, as far as is at present known. If mixed with finely powdered charcoal, it is nevertheless capable of vitrification; and with soot it melts into a black bitumen-like mass, which however is soluble in water, and cannot easily be burned to ashes, but sublimes in part. With the assistance of a distilling heat it dissolves in oils, especially mineral oils; and with these it yields fluid and solid products, which impart a green colour to spirit of wine. When rubbed with phosphorus it does not prevent its inflammation, but an earthy yellow matter is left behind. It is hardly capable of oxiding or dissolving any of the metals except iron and zinc, and perhaps copper; but it combines with most of the metallic oxides, as it does with the alkalies, and probably with all the earths, though the greater part of its combinations have hitherto been little examined. It is of great use in analyzing stones that contain a fixed alkali.

Crystallized boracic acid is a compound of 57 parts of acid and 43 of water. The honour of discovering the *radical* of *boracic acid*, is divided between Sir H. Davy and Gay Lussac and Thenard. The first, on applying his powerful voltaic battery to it, obtained a chocolate-coloured body in small quantity; but the two latter chemists, by acting on it with potassium in equal quantities, at a low red-heat, formed *boron* and sub-borate of potass. For a small experiment, a glass tube will serve, but on a greater scale a copper tube is to be preferred. The potassium and boracic acid, perfectly dry, should be intimately mixed before exposing them to heat. On withdrawing the tube from the fire, allowing it to cool, and removing the cork which loosely closed its mouth, we then pour successive portions of water into it, till we detach or dissolve the whole matter. The water ought to be heated each time. The whole collected liquids are allowed to settle; when, after washing the precipitate till the liquid ceases to affect syrup of violets, we dry the boron in a capsule, and then put it into a phial out of contact of air. *Boron* is solid, tasteless, inodorous, and of a greenish-brown colour. Its specific gravity is somewhat greater than water. The prime equivalent of boracic acid has been inferred from the borate of ammonia, to be about 2.7 or 2.8; oxygen being 1.0; and it probably consists of 2.0 of oxygen + 0.8 of boron. But by Gay Lussac and Thenard, the proportions would be 2 of boron to 1 of oxygen.

The boracic acid has a more powerful attraction for lime than for any other of the bases, though it does not readily form *borate of lime* by adding a solution of it to lime water, or decomposing by lime water the soluble alkaline borates. In either case an insipid white powder, nearly insoluble, which is the borate of lime, is, however, precipitated. The borate of barytes is likewise an insoluble, tasteless, white powder.

Bergman has observed, that magnesia, thrown by little and little into a solution of boracic acid, dissolved slowly, and the liquor on evaporation afforded granulated crystals, without any regular form: that these crystals were fusible in the fire without being decomposed; but that alkohol was sufficient to separate the boracic acid from the magnesia. If, however, some of the soluble magnesian salts be decomposed by alkaline borates in a state of solution, an insipid and insoluble borate of magnesia is thrown down. It is probable, therefore, that Bergman's salt was a borate of magnesia dissolved in an excess of boracic acid; which acid being taken up by the alkohol, the true borate of magnesia was precipitated in a white powder, and mistaken by him for magnesia.

One of the best known combinations of this acid is the native *magnesio-calcareous borate* of Kalkberg, near Lunenburg; the *wurfelstein* of the Germans, *cubic quartz* of various mineralogists, and boracite of Kirwan.

The *borate of potassa* is but little known, though it is said to be capable of supplying the place of that of soda in the arts; but more direct experiments are required to establish this effect. Like that, it is capable of existing in two states, neutral and with excess of base, but it is not so crystallizable, and assumes the form of parallelobipeds.

With *soda* the boracic acid forms two different salts. One, in which the alkali is more than triple the quantity necessary to saturate the acid, is of considerable use in the arts, and has long been known by the name of borax; under which its history and an account of its properties will be given. The *other* is a neutral salt, not changing the syrup of violets green like the borate with excess of base; differing from it in taste and solubility; crystallizing neither so readily, nor in the same manner; not efflorescent like it; but, like it, fusible into a glass, and capable of being employed for the same purposes. This salt may be formed by saturating the superabundant soda in borax with some other acid, and then separating the two salts; but it is obviously more eligible to saturate the excess of soda with an additional portion of the boracic acid itself.

Borate of ammonia forms in small rhomboidal crystals, easily decomposed by fire; or in scales, of a pungent urinous taste, which lose the crystalline form, and grow brown on exposure to the air.

It is very difficult to combine the boracic acid with *alumina*, at least in the direct way.

The boracic acid unites with *silex* by fusion, and forms with it a solid and permanent vitreous compound. This *borate of silex*, however, is neither sapid, nor soluble, nor perceptibly alterable in the air; and cannot be formed without the assistance of a violent heat. In the same manner, triple compounds may be formed with silex and borates already saturated with other bases.

The boracic acid has been found in a disengaged state in several lakes of hot mineral waters near Monte Rotondo, Berchiaio, and Castellonuovo, in Tuscany, in the proportion of nearly nine grains in a hundred of water, by Hoeffer. Mascagni also found it adhering to schistus, on the borders of lakes, of an obscure white, yellow, or greenish colour, and crystallized in the form of needles. He has likewise found it in combination with ammonia.

BORACITE. Borate of magnesia. A crystallized mineral found in gypsum in the Kalberg, in Brunswick, and at Segeberg, in Holland. It is translucent, and of a shining greasy lustre, yellowish, grayish, or of a greenish-white colour. Vauquelin's Analysis gives 33.4 boracic acid, and 16.6 magnesia.

BO'RAGE. See *Borago.*

BORA'GO. (Formerly written *Corago;* from *cor*, the heart, and *ago*, to affect; because it was supposed to comfort the heart and spirits.) Borage. 1. The name of a genus of plants in the Linnæan system. Class, *Pentandria;* Order, *Monogynia.*

2. The pharmacopœial name of the officinal borage. See *Borago officinalis.*

BORAGO OFFICINALIS. The systematic name for the borage of the shops. *Corrago; Buglossum verum; Buglossum latifolium; Borago hortensis.* The leaves and flowers of this plant, *Borago—foliis omnibus alternis, calycibus patentibus* of Linnæus, are esteemed in some countries as refrigerant and cordial. A syrup is prepared from the leaves in France, and used in pleurisies and inflammatory fevers. Their principal use in this island is in that grateful summer beverage, known by the name of cool tankard.

BO'RAS. See *Borate.*

BORAS SODÆ. Borate of soda. See *Borax.*

BO'RATE. *Boras.* A salt formed of boracic acid with an earthy, alkaline, or metallic base; as borate of soda, &c.

BO'RAX. (*Borak*, Arabian.) *Boras sodæ; Subboras sodæ.* The obsolete synonyms are, *Chrysocolla; Capistrum auri; Ancinar; Borax-trion; Acestis anucar; Antincar; Tincal; Amphitane; Baurach; Nitrum factitium; Santerna,* and *Nitrum nativum.* "It does not appear that borax was known to the ancients; their chrysocolla being a very different substance, composed of the rust of copper, triturated with urine. The word borax occurs for the first time in the works of Geber.

Borax is found in the East, and likewise in South America.

The purification of borax by the Venetians and the Hollanders, was, for a long time, kept secret. Chaptal finds, after trying all the processes in the large way, that the simplest method consists in boiling the borax strongly, and for a long time, with water. This solution being filtered, affords by evaporation crystals, which are somewhat foul, but may be purified by repeating the operation.

Purified borax is white, transparent, rather greasy in its fracture, affecting the form of six-sided prisms, terminating in three-sided or six-sided pyramids. Its taste is styptic; it converts syrup of violets to a green; and when exposed to heat, it swells up, boils, loses its water of crystallization, and becomes converted into a porous, white, opaque mass, commonly called Calcined Borax. A stronger heat brings it into a state of quiet fusion; but the glassy substance thus afforded, which is transparent, and of a greenish yellow colour, is soluble in water, and effloresces in the air. It requires about eighteen times its weight of water to dissolve it at the temperature of sixty degrees of Fahrenheit; but water at the boiling heat dissolves three times this quantity. Its component parts, according to Kirwan, are, boracic acid 34, soda 17, water 47.

Borax is rarely used internally in modern practice; and, according to Murray, it does not appear to possess any activity, although it is supposed by some to be, in doses of half a drachm or two scruples, diuretic and emmenagogue. It is occasionally given in cardialgia as an antacid. Its solution is in common use as a cooling gargle, and to detach mucus, &c. from the mouth in putrid fever; and mixed with an equal quantity of sugar, it is used in the form of powder to remove the aphthous crust from the tongue in children. The salts formed by the union of the acid of borax with different bases are called borates.

BORBORY'GMUS. (From βορβορυζω, to make a noise.) The rumbling noise occasioned by flatus in the intestines. It frequently precedes hysterical affections. Dr. Good gives this name to that variety of his *Limotis flatus*, which is known by frequent rumbling of the bowels.

BORDEU, Theophilus de, a French physician, born in 1722. He graduated at Montpelier, and was soon after appointed inspector of the mineral waters at Bareges, and professor of anatomy. Subsequently, he went to Paris, and was admitted to the faculty there in 1754. He died of apoplexy in his 55th year. His most esteemed work is on the cellular membrane; his distinctions of the pulse appear too nice for practical utility.

BORELLI, John Alphonsus, was born at Castelnuovo, in 1608. He first taught the mathematics in Sicily, then as professor at Pisa; and being soon after admitted to the celebrated academy del Cimento, he formed the design of explaining the functions of animal bodies, on mathematical principles. For this purpose he applied himself diligently to dissection. His grand work, "De Motu Animalium," was published after his death, which happened in 1679, at the expense of Christina, queen of Sweden. The imposing appearance of his opinions gained them many converts at first, but they have been found very defective on maturer examination. He was author of many other publications on different subjects.

BORON. The combustible basis of boracic acid. See *Boracic acid.*

Boro'zail. An Ethiopian word for an epidemic disease, in appearance similar to the lues venerea.

Borra'go. See *Borago.*

Bo'rri. (Indian.) *Borri-borri. Boberri.* The Indian name for turmeric; also an ointment used there, in which the roots of turmeric are a chief ingredient.

Bota'le foramen. A name formerly applied to the foramen ovale of the heart.

BOTALLUS, Leonard, an eminent physician of Piedmont, flourished about the middle of the 16th century. He graduated at Padua; and attained considerable reputation, as well in surgery as in medicine; having the honour of attending two of the French kings, and the Prince of Orange; the latter of whom he cured of a wound, in which the carotid artery had been injured. He published a treatise on gun-shot wounds, which long remained in high estimation. But that which chiefly gained him celebrity, was a work on bleeding, general and local, which he recommended to be freely practised in a great variety of diseases, both acute and chronic. His opinions were adopted by many, and carried to an extravagant length, particularly in France; but more enlarged experience has tended greatly to lessen their prevalence.

Bota'nicon. (From βοτανη, an herb.) A plaster made of herbs, and described by Paulus Ægineta.

BOTANIST. *Botanicus.* One who understands the nature, history, and distinction of vegetables, on settled and certain principles, and can call every plant by a distinct, proper, and intelligible name.

BO'TANY. (*Botanica.* Βοτανικη; from βοτανη, an herb or grass, which is derived from βοω, or βοσκω, to feed, because grass is the chief food of the animals which are most useful to man.) That branch of natural history which relates to the vegetable kingdom, the second of the three grand assemblages into which all terrestrial objects are divided. It is a science not confined to the description and classification of plants, as has often been represented, but it comprehends many other important particulars. Its various objects may be conveniently arranged under the following general heads:—

1. The *terminology*, or description and nomenclature of the several parts of a plant, which are externally visible.

If all natural objects were simple in their form, it would not be easy to distinguish one from another, nor would it be possible to describe them so as to give a clear and precise idea of them. Hence a boundless variety, connected with general resemblances, is wisely and benevolently made their universal character. Every plant is composed of several parts, which differ from each other in their outward appearance, and which cannot fail to strike the most careless spectator. Many of them also are themselves compound, and are obviously capable of being divided into subordinate parts.

2. The *classification* or arrangement. A knowledge of the different parts of a plant must necessarily be gained before it is described. But amidst the numerous vegetable productions of even a single country, this of itself would avail but little. To give a peculiar name to every individual would be a labour which no invention or diligence can perform; and, if performed, would produce a burden which no memory can sustain. It is necessary, therefore, to pursue resemblances and differences through a number of gradations, and to found on them primary and subordinate divisions, either ascending from particulars to generals, or descending from generals to particulars. The former is the method in which science of every kind is slowly formed and extended; the latter that in which it is most easily taught. The number of stages through which these subdivisions should be carried is either not pointed out by nature, or enough of nature is not known to fix them with precision. They differ, therefore, in different systems; and, unfortunately, corresponding ones have not always been called by the same names.

3. The *synonymes* of plants, or the names by which they are distinguished in the writings of professed botanists and others, from the earliest times to the present.

4. The *sensible qualities* of plants, or the different manner in which they severally affect the organs of sight, smell, taste, and touch.

5. The *anatomy of plants*, or description of the different visible parts of which their substance is composed.

6. The *physiology of plants*. A plant, like an animal, is a very compound, organized, living being, in which various operations, both chemical and mechanical, are continually carrying on, from its first production to its final dissolution. It springs from a seed fertilized by the pollen of its parent plant. It takes in foreign substances by its inhaling and absorbent vessels. It elaborates and assimilates to its own substance those parts of them that are nutritious, and throws off the rest. It secretes a variety of fluids by the means of glands, and other unknown organs. It gives that motion to its sap on which a continuance of its life depends.

7. The *purposes* to which different plants are *applied*, either as articles of food, ingredients in the composition of medicine, or materials and instruments in the useful and elegant arts; the soil and situation in which they are generally found, and which are most favourable to their growth, the time of year in which they open their flowers, and ripen their fruit, with many other incidental particulars, are properly within the province of the botanist. But as a botanist he is concerned with nothing more than the simple facts. The first methods of cultivating such as are raised in considerable quantities for the special use or amusement of man; the theory of their nutritious or medicinal properties; and the manner in which they are to be prepared, so as to effect the intended purposes; are the province either of the gardener, farmer, physician, chemist, or the artist.

8. The *history* of botany.

BOTANY BAY. An English settlement in New Holland, so called because it afforded the botanist numerous plants. A yellow resin goes by the name of Botany Bay gum, which exudes spontaneously from the trunk of the tree called *Acarois resinifera*, and also from the wounded bark. All the information that has been hitherto collected respecting the history of the yellow gum is the following:—The plant that produces it is low and small, with long grassy leaves; but the fructification of it shoots out in a singular manner from the centre of the leaves, on a single straight stem, to the height of twelve or fourteen feet. Of this stem, which is strong and light, like some of the reed class, the natives usually make their spears. The resin is generally dug up out of the soil under the tree, not collected from it, and may, perhaps, be that which Tasman calls "gum lac of the ground." Mr. Boles, surgeon of the Lady Penrhyn, gives a somewhat different account; and as this gentleman appears to have paid considerable attention to the subject, his account may certainly be relied upon. After describing the tree in precisely the same manner as above, he observes, that at the top of the trunk of the tree, long grassy leaves grow in great abundance. The gum is found under these leaves in considerable quantities: it commonly exudes in round tears, or drops, from the size of a large pea to that of a marble, and sometimes much larger. These are, by the heat of the sun, frequently so much softened, that they fall on the ground, and in this soft state adhere to whatever they fall upon: hence the gum is frequently found mixed with dirt, wood, the bark of the tree, and various other substances; so that one lump has been seen composed of many small pure pieces of various sizes, united together, which weighed nearly half a hundred-weight. It is produced in such abundance, that one man may collect thirty or forty pounds in the space of a few hours. The convicts have another method of collecting it; they dig round the tree, and break off pieces of the roots, which always have some, and frequently considerable quantities of the gum in them. This gum appears nearly, but not entirely, the same as that which exudes from the trunk of the tree; the former is often mixed with a strong-smelling resinous substance of a black nature, and is so interwoven in the wood itself, that it is with difficulty separated. The latter appears a pure, unmixed, resinous substance.

Several experiments have been made, principally with the view of determining what menstruum would dissolve the gum the most readily, and in the greatest quantity, from which it appears alkohol and æther dissolve the most.

The diseases in which this resin is administered are those of the primæ viæ, and principally such as arise from spasm, a debility, a loss of tone, or a diminished action in the muscular fibres of the stomach and bowels, such as loss of appetite, sickness, vomiting, flatulency, heart-burn, pains in the stomach, &c. when they were really idiopathic complaints, and not dependent upon any disease in the stomach, or affections of other parts of the body communicated to the stomach. In debilities and relaxations of the bowels, and the symptoms from thence arising, such as purging and flatulency, it has been found of good effect. In certain cases of diarrhœa, however, (and it seemed those in which an unusual degree of irritability prevailed) it did not answer so well, unless given in small doses, and combined with opiates, when the patient seemed to gain greater advantage than when opiates only were had recourse to. In cases of amenorrhœa. depending on (what most of those cases do depend upon) a sluggishness, a debility, and flaccidity of the system, this medicine, when assisted by proper exercise and diet, has, by removing the symptoms of dyspepsia, and by restoring the tone and action of the muscular fibres, been found very serviceable. This medicine does not, in the dose of about half a drachm, appear to possess any remarkably sensible operation It neither vomits, purges, nor binds the belly, nor does it materially increase the secretion of urine or perspiration. It has, indeed, sometimes been said to purge and at others to occasion sweating; but they are not constant effects, and, when they do occur, it generally depends on some accidental circumstance. It should seem to possess, in a very extensive degree, the property of allaying morbid irritability, and of restoring tone, strength, and action, to the debilitated and relaxed fibre. When the gum itself is given, it should always be the pure unmixed part, if given in the form of a draught, it should be mixed in water with mucilage of gum-arabic; if made into pills, a small portion of Castile soap may be employed; it was found the lixiv. sapon. dissolved it entirely. It is commonly, however, made into a tincture by mixing equal parts of the gum and rectified spirit; one drachm of this tincture, (containing half a drachm of the pure gum) made into a draught with water and syrup, by the assistance of fifteen grains of gum-arabic in mucilage forms an elegant medicine, and at the same time very palatable. It soon solidifies by the sun, into pieces of a yellow colour of various sizes. It pulverizes easily without caking; nor does it adhere to the teeth when chewed. It has a slightly sweet astringent taste. It melts at a moderate heat. When kindled, it emits a white fragrant smoke. It is insoluble in water, but imparts to it the flavour of storax. Out of nine parts, six are soluble in water, and astringent to the taste, and two parts are woody fibre.

Bo'thrion. (From βοθριον, a little pit.) *Botrium* 1. The socket for the tooth.

2. An ulceration of the cornea.

Botri'tis. (From βοτρυς, a bunch of grapes.) *Botryites.* A sort of burnt cadmia, collected in the top of the furnace, and resembling a bunch of grapes.

BOTRYOLITE. A brittle and moderately hard mineral, which occurs in mamillary concretions of a pearly or grayish-white colour, composed of silica, boracic acid, lime, oxide of iron and water. It comes from Norway.

BO'TRYS. (Βοτρυς, a cluster of grapes: so called because its seeds hang down like a bunch of grapes. The oak of Jerusalem.

Botrys mexicana. See *Chenopodium ambrosioides.*

Botrys vulgaris. See *Chenopodium botrys.*

Bouba'lios. See *Momordica Elaterium*, and *Pudendum muliebre.*

Bou'bon. See *Bubo.*

BOUGI'E. (French for wax candle.) *Candela cerea; Candela medicata; Catheteres* of Swediaur *Cerei medicati* of Le Dran; *Cereolus Chirurgorum* A term applied by surgeons to a long, slender instrument, that is introduced through the urethra into the bladder. Bougies made of the elastic gum are preferable to those made of wax. The caustic bougie differs from the ordinary one in having a thin roll of caustic in its middle, which destroys the stricture, or any part it comes in contact with. Those made of catgut are very seldom used, but are deserving of the attention of the surgeon. Bougies are chiefly used to overcome strictures in the urethra, and the introduction of them requires a good deal of address and caution. They should not be kept in the urethra so long at one time as to excite much pain or irritation. Before their use is discontinued, they should, if practicable, be carried the length of the bladder, in order to ascertain the extent of the strictures, taking care that this be performed not at once, but in a gradual manner, and after repeated trials, for much injury might arise from any hasty or violent efforts to remove the resistance that may present itself. There are bougies also for the œsophagus and rectum.

BOU'LIMUS. (From βου, greatly, and λιμος, hunger; or from βουλομαι, to desire.) A canine or voracious appetite.

BOURNONITE. An antimonial sulphuret of lead.

Bovey coal. Of a brownish-black colour and lamellar texture, formed of wood, penetrated with petroleum or bitumen, and found in England, France, Italy, &c.

BOVI'LLÆ. (From *bos*, an ox, because cattle were supposed subject to it.) The measles.

BOVI'NA FAMES. The same as bulimia.

BOVI'STA. See *Lycoperdon.*

[BOWEN, PARDON, M.D. This accomplished physician and excellent man was born in Providence, Rhode Island, 22d of March, in the year 1757.

The incidents of Dr. Bowen's early life, we have been unable to collect with sufficient accuracy to warrant us in committing them to the pages of an authentic memoir.

During the prevalence of the yellow fever in Providence, when dejection and dismay sat upon many a brow, and the sense of personal danger threatened to absorb the sympathies of our common nature, and death mocked at the expedients of human science to avert his blow, Dr. Bowen shrunk not from the perils in his way. More than once was his life endangered by an attack of that fearful malady, but God preserved him from thus becoming a victim to his noble intrepidity in the service of humanity.

Dr. Bowen confined his attention to no particular department of his profession, but aimed at excellence in all. For his skill in operative surgery he was highly respected, and during many years most of the surgical operations, in and around Providence, were performed by him. In medical surgery he was thought extremely judicious; and his uncommon science, experience, and success in obstetrics, left him without a superior in that difficult branch of his profession.

Dr. Bowen contributed occasionally to the medical journals of the day; and in the fourth volume of Hosack and Francis's Medical and Philosophical Register may be found an elaborate account from his pen of the yellow fever, as it prevailed in Providence in the year 1805. He died in October 1826, aged 69 years. His life, in all its stages, was a beautiful exhibition of the virtues, and at its close, an example of Christian holiness.—See *Thach. Med. Biog.* A.]

BOX-TREE. See *Buxus.*

BOYLE'S FUMING LIQUOR. The hydroguretted sulphuret of ammonia.

[BOYLSTON, DR. ZABDIEL, was born in Massachusetts in 1680, and was the eldest son of an English physician of the same name, one of the early settlers of that province under the British government. Dr. Boylston is represented as a skilful physician, bold, persevering, courageous and benevolent. "In the year 1721 the small-pox appeared in Boston, and pursued its usual desolating career, carrying with it the utmost terror and confusion. On this alarming occasion Dr. Cotton Mather, the learned and distinguished divine, communicated to Dr. Boylston a publication in the Transactions of the Royal Society, announcing the discovery of a new method of mitigating the virulence of this fatal disease. Dr. Boylston was forcibly impressed with the benefit of the discovery, and accordingly after deliberating on the most safe and expeditious mode of thus artificially introducing the disease into the system, he communicated to the medical gentlemen in Boston the plan he proposed to adopt, and the source whence he derived the first hints of the operation, desiring their concurrence in the undertaking." In this measure he was opposed by the physicians and clergy, some of whom denounced him from the pulpit; and the inhabitants became enraged, and were excited to commit atrocious acts of outrage on the person of Dr. Boylston, extending their rancour even to his family.

"Undismayed, however, by all this violence, and unsupported by the friendship of any but Dr. Mather, he commenced, on the 27th June 1721, while the small-pox was in its most destructive progress through the town, this untried experiment of inoculation on his own son, a child of thirteen years of age, and two blacks in his family, one of thirty-six, and the other of two years of age, and on all with complete success. This rekindled the fury of the populace, and induced the authorities of the town to summon him before them to answer for his practice. He underwent repeated examinations; and although he invited all the practitioners in Boston to visit his patients and judge for themselves, he received only insults and threats in reply The facts we have thought worthy of notice, as remarkable in themselves, and as in some degree characteristic of the excitable spirit of the times. In thus encountering obloquy and reproach, however, Dr. Boylston but experienced the fortune of most of those who have attempted to innovate on long established usages, or to take the lead in the career of public improvement. The small-pox ceased its ravages in May 1722; and during its prevalence Dr. Boylston continued the practice of inoculation to all who could be induced to submit to it. He inoculated with his own hand two hundred and forty-seven of both sexes from nine months to sixty-seven years of age in Boston and in the neighbouring towns; thirty-nine were inoculated by other physicians, after the tumult had in some measure subsided, making in the whole two hundred and eighty-six, of whom only six died; and of these, three were supposed to have taken the disease the natural way, some days previous to their being inoculated; three of those who died were his oldest patients. It appears, by the account published by the select men, that during the same period five thousand seven hundred and fifty-nine had taken the natural small-pox; eight hundred and forty-four of whom fell victims to the disease, being more than one in six. In the vicinity of Boston it had been still more malignant and fatal. The utility of the practice was now established without dispute; and its success encouraged its more general practice in England, in which country it had been tried upon but few persons, most of whom were condemned convicts and charity children. The daughter of Lady Mary W. Montague was inoculated in London, in April 1721, being the first instance in Europe, and the convicts were made the subjects of the experiment in August of the same year. Dr. Boylston therefore is justly entitled to the honour of being the first inoculator in America; and this, even before the single instance of the experiment in Europe had come to his knowledge.

Dr. Boylston, during his unjust persecution, held a correspondence with Sir Hans Sloane, of London, the court physician; who, being apprised of his very eminent services in first introducing inoculation into America, honoured him with an invitation to visit London. He accordingly embarked for that city, and on his arrival was greeted with the most cordial affection and respect. He was elected a member of the Royal Society, the first American, we believe, ever admitted to that honour. He was moreover honoured by being introduced to the royal family, and received the most flattering attentions and friendship of some of the most distinguished characters of the nation. After his return to his native country, Dr. Boylston continued at the head of his profession, and engaged in literary pursuits, making many ingenious and useful communications to the Royal Society, and corresponding with his numerous friends, among whom he used to mention with great respect and affection the Rev. Dr. Watts, who appears by his letters to have been a warm advocate for inoculation.

Dr. Boylston possessed a strong and reflecting mind and acute discernment. His character through life was one of unimpeached integrity. He was charitable in his opinions of others, patient under the severest persecution, and forgiving of his bitterest enemies. These qualities, added to the natural ease and suavity of his manners, which had been improved by intercourse with the world, caused his society to be much sought, and to his family and his friends rendered him a most interesting and instructive companion. His health was often interrupted by severe attacks of asthma, to which he was subject for the last forty years of his life. He met death with calmness and perfect resignation in the eighty-seventh year of his age, saying to his friends, 'my work in this world is done, and my hopes of futurity are brightening.' He was buried in the family tomb at Brooklyn, on which is inscribed the following appropriate and just language: 'Sacred to the memory of Dr. Zabdiel Boylston, Esq., physician and F.R.S., who first introduced the practice of inoculation into America. Through a life of extensive benevolence, he was always faithful to his word, just in his dealings, affable in his manners; and after a long sickness, in which he was exemplary for his patience and resignation to his Maker, he quitted this mortal life in a just expectation of a happy immortality, March 1st, 1766' His wife died a few years before him."—See *Thach. Med. Biog.* A.]

BRACHE'RIUM. (From *brachiale*, a bracelet.) A truss or bandage for hernia; a term used by the barbarous Latin writers.

BRACHIÆ'US. Brachial; belonging to the arm.

BRACHIÆUS EXTERNUS. See *Triceps extensor cubiti.*

BRACHIÆUS INTERNUS. See *Brachialus internus.*

BRACHIÆUS MUSCULUS. See *Brachialis internus.*

BRACHIAL. *Brachialis.* Of or belonging to the arm.

BRACHIAL ARTERY. *Arteria brachialis.* The brachial artery is the continuation of the axillary artery. which, as it passes behind the tendon of the pectoralis major, receives the name of *brachial.* It runs down on the inside of the arm, over the musculus coracobrachialis, and anconæus internus, and along the inner edge of the biceps, behind the vena basilica, giving out small branches as it goes along. Below the bend of the arm it divides into the cubitalis and radialis. Sometimes, though rarely, the *brachial artery* is divided from its origin into two large branches, which run down on the arm, and afterward on the fore-arm, where they are called *cubitalis* and *radialis.*

BRACHIA'LE. The word means a bracelet; but the ancient anatomical writers apply this term to the carpus, the part on which the bracelet was worn.

BRACHIA'LIS. See *Brachial.*

BRACHIALIS EXTERNUS. See *Triceps extensor cubiti.*

BRACHIALIS INTERNUS. *Brachiæus* of Winslow. *Brachiæus internus* of Cowper; and *Humero-cubital* of Dumas. A muscle of the fore-arm, situated on the fore-part of the os humeri. It arises fleshy from the middle of the os humeri, at each side of the insertion of the deltoid muscle, covering all the inferior and fore-part of this bone, runs over the joint, and adheres firmly to the ligament; is inserted, by a strong short tendon, into the coronoid process of the ulna. Its use is to bend the fore-arm, and to prevent the capsular ligament of the joint from being pinched.

BRACHIATUS. Brachiate. Applied to branches, panicles, &c. spread in four directions, crossing each other alternately in pairs; a common mode of growth in the branches of shrubs that have opposite leaves, as the lilac, syringa, &c.

BRA'CHII OS. See *Humeri os.*

BRACHIO-CUBITAL LIGAMENT. *Ligamentum brachio-cubitale.* The expansion of the lateral ligament, which is fixed in the inner condyle of the os humeri, runs over the capsular, to which it closely adheres, and is inserted like radii on the side of the great sigmoid cavity of the ulna; it is covered on the inside by several tendons, which adhere closely to it, and seem to strengthen it very considerably.

BRACHIO-RADIAL LIGAMENT. *Ligamentum brachio-radiale.* The expansion of the lateral ligament, which runs over the external condyle of the os humeri, is inserted round the coronary ligament from thence all the way down to the neck of the radius, and also in the neighbouring parts of the ulna. Through all this passage it covers the capsular ligament, and is covered by several tendons adhering closely to both.

BRA'CHIUM. (Βραχιον, the arm.) The arm, from the shoulder to the wrist.

BRACHIUM MOVENS QUARTUS. See *Latissimus dorsi.*

BRACHU'NA. According to Avicenna, a species of furor uterinus.

BRACHYCHRO'NIUS. (From βραχυς, short, and χρονος, time.) A disease which continues but a short time.

BRACHYPNŒ'A. (From βραχυς, short, and πνεω, to breathe.) Shortness and difficulty of breathing.

BRA'CHYS. (From βραχυς, short.) A muscle of the scapula.

BRACTEA. (*Bractea*, a thin leaf or plate of metal.) A floral leaf. One of the seven fulcra or props of plants, according to Linnæus. A bractea is a little leaf-like appendage to some flowers, lying under or interspersed in the flower, but generally different in colour from the true leaves of the plant.

1. It is *green* in some; as in *Ocymum basilicum majus.*
2. *Coloured* in others; as in *Salvia horminum*, &c.
3. In some it is *caducous*, falling off before the flowers.
4. In others in remains; as in *Tibia europæa.*

Coma bracteata is, when the flower-stem is terminated with a number of very large bracteæ, resembling a bush of hair.

BRACTEATÆ. (From *bractea*, here meaning a corolla.) The name of a class of Boerhaave's method of plants, consisting of herbaceous vegetables, which have petals, and the seeds of which are furnished with a single lobe or cotyledon.

BRACTEATUS (From *bractea*, a floral leaf.) Having a floral leaf; as *pedunculus bracteatus.*

BRACTEIFORMIS Resembling a bractea or floral leaf.

BRADYPE'PSIA. (From βραδυς, slow, and πεπτω, to concoct.) Weak digestion.

BRA'GGAT. A name formerly applied to a ptisan of honey and water.

BRAIN. See *Cerebrum*

Brain, little. See *Cerebellum.*

BRAN. *Furfur.* The husks or shells of wheat, which remain in the bolting machine. It contains a portion of the farinaceous matter, and is said to have a laxative quality. Decoctions of bran, sweetened with sugar, are used by the common people, and sometimes with success, against coughs, hoarseness, &c.

BRA'NCA. (*Branca*, the Spanish for a foot, or branch.) A term applied to some herbs, which are supposed to resemble a particular foot; as *branca leonis*, lion's foot; *branca ursina*, bear's foot.

BRANCA LEONINA. See *Alchemilla.*

BRANCA LEONIS. See *Alchemilla.*

BRANCA URSINA. See *Acanthus* and *Heracleum*

BRA'NCHÆ. (From βρεχω, to make moist.) *Branchi.* Swelled tonsils, or glandulous tumours, of the fauces, which secrete saliva.

BRA'NCHUS. (From βρεχω, to moisten.) A defluxion of humours from the fauces.

BRANDY. *Spiritus Gallicus.* A colourless, slightly opaque, and milky fluid, of a hot and penetrating taste, and a strong and agreeable smell, obtained by distilling from wine. It consists of water, ardent spirit, and a small portion of oil, which renders it milky at first, and, after a certain time, colours it yellow. It is the fluid from which rectified or ardent spirit is obtained. Its peculiar flavour depends on the nature of the volatile principles, or essential oil, which come over along with it in the distillation, and likewise, in some measure, upon the management of the fire, the wood of the cask in which it is kept, &c. It is said, that our rectifiers imitate the flavour of brandy, by adding a small proportion of nitrous æther to the spirit of malt, or molasses. The utility of brandy is very considerable, but, from its pleasant taste and exhilarating property, it is two often taken to excess. It gives energy to the animal functions; it is a powerful tonic, cordial, and antispasmodic; and its utility with camphire, in gangrenous affections, is very great.

BRANKS. The name in Scotland for the mumps See *Cynanche parotidæa.*

BRANKURSINE. See *Acanthus.*

BRASI'LIA. Brazil wood.

BRASILIENSE LIGNUM. See *Hæmatoxylum campechianum.*

BRASILIENSIS RADIX. The ipecacuanha root is sometimes so called.

BRA'SIUM. (From βρασσω, to boil.) Malt, or germinated barley.

BRA'SMA. (From βρασσω, to boil.) The unripe black pepper. Fermentation.

BRA'SMOS. The same.

BRASS. *Æs.* A combination of copper and zinc.

BRASSADE'LLA. *Brassatella.* The *Ophioglossum*, or herb, adder's tongue.

BRA'SSICA. (Varro says, *quasi præsica;* from *præseco*, to cut off; because it is cut from the stalk for use; or from πρασια, a bed in a garden where they are cultivated, or from βρασσω, to devour, because it is eagerly eaten by cattle.) The name of a genus of plants in the Linnæan system. Class, *Tetradynamia;* Order, *Siliquosa.* Crambe. Cabbage. Colewort.

BRASSICA ALBA. The white cabbage.

BRASSICA APIANA. Jagged or crimpled colewort.

BRASSICA CANINA. *Mercurialis sylvestris.* See *Mercurialis annua.*

BRASSICA CAPITATA. Cabbage. There are several varieties of cabbage, all of which are generally hard of digestion, producing flatulencies, and afford very little nourishment. These inconveniences are not expe nenced by those whose stomachs are strong and accustomed to them. Few vegetables run into a state of putrefaction so quickly as cabbages; they ought, therefore, always to be used immediately after cutting. In Holland and Germany there is a method of preserving them, by cutting them into pieces, and sprinkling salt and some aromatic herbs among them; this mass is put into a tub, where it is pressed close, and left to ferment, when it is called *sour crout*, or *sauer kraut*. These, and all pickles of cabbage, are considered as wholesome and antiscorbutic, from the vinegar and spices they contain.

Brassica congylodes. Turnip cabbage.

Brassica cumana. Red colewort.

Brassica eruca. *Brassica erucastrum. Eruca sylvestris.* The systematic name for the plant which affords the semen erucæ. Garden rocket. Roman rocket. Rocket gentle. *Brassica—foliis lyartis, caule hirsuto siliquis glabris*, of Linnæus. The seeds of this plant, and of the wild rocket, have an acrid taste, and are eaten by the Italians in their pickles, &c. They are said to be good aperients and antiscorbutics, but are esteemed by the above-mentioned people for their supposed aphrodisiac qualities.

Brassica erucastrum. See *Brassica eruca.*

Brassica florida. The cauliflower.

Brassica gonylicodes. The turnip cabbage.

Brassica lacuturria. *Brassica lacuturris.* The Savoy plant.

Brassica marina. See *Convolvulus soldanella.*

Brassica napus. The systematic name for the plant from which the *semen napi* is obtained. *Napus sylvestris. Bunias.* Wild navew, or rape. The seeds yield, upon expression, a large quantity of oil called rape oil, which is sometimes ordered in stimulating liniments.

Brassica oleracea. The systematic name for the *brassica capitata* of the shops. See *Brassica capitata.*

Brassica rapa. The systematic name for the plant whose root is called turnip. *Rapum. Rapus. Napus. Napus dulcis.* The turnip. Turnips are accounted a salubrious food, demulcent, detergent, somewhat laxative and diuretic, but liable, in weak stomachs, to produce flatulencies, and prove difficult of digestion. The liquor pressed out of them, after boiling, is sometimes taken medicinally in coughs and disorders of the breast. The seeds are occasionally taken as diuretics; they have no smell, but a mild acrid taste.

Brassica rubra. Red cabbage. A very excellent test both for acids and alkalies in which it is superior to litmus, being naturally blue, turning green with alkalies, and red with acids.

Brassica sabauda. The Savoy plant.

Brassica sativa. The common garden cabbage.

Brasside'llica ars. A way of curing wounds, mentioned by Paracelsus, by applying the herb *Brassidella* to them.

Bra'thu Βραθυ. An old name for savine.

BRAZIL WOOD. See *Cæsalpina crista.*

["Brazil wood is the produce of the *Cæsalpina crista*, growing in Brazil, in the Isle of France, Japan, and other countries. The wood is hard and heavy; and though pale when recent, it acquires a deep red colour by exposure. Digested in water, it affords a fine red infusion, of a sweetish flavour; the residue, which appears nearly black, imparts much of its colour to alkaline liquors. With alkohol it gives a deep red tincture: alkalies and soap convert its red colour to a fine purple; hence, paper tinged with Brazil wood is sometimes used as a test for alkalies; acids render it yellow: alum produces a fine crimson lake, with infusion of Brazil wood: muriate of tin forms with it a crimson precipitate, bordering on purple: the salts of iron give a dingy purple colour. Sulphuretted hydrogen destroys the colour of infusion of Brazil wood, but it reappears on expelling the gas."—See *Webster's Man. of Chem.* A.]

BREAD. *Panis.* "Farinaceous vegetables are converted into meal by trituration, or grinding in a mill; and when the husk or bran has been separated by sifting or bolting, the powder is called flour. This is composed of a small quantity of mucilaginous saccharine matter, soluble in cold water; much starch, which is scarcely soluble in cold water, but combines with that fluid by heat; and an adhesive gray substance insoluble in water, alkohol, oil, or æther, and resembling an animal substance in many of its properties.

When flour is kneaded together with water, it forms a tough paste, containing these principles very little altered, and not easily digested by the stomach. The action of heat produces a considerable change in the gluten, and probably in the starch, rendering the compound more easy to masticate, as well as to digest. Hence the first approaches towards the making of bread consisted in parching the corn, either for immediate use as food, or previous to its trituration into meal; or else in baking the flour into unleavened bread, or boiling it into masses more or less consistent; of all which we have sufficient indications in the histories of the earlier nations, as well as in the various practices of the moderns. It appears likewise from the Scriptures, that the practice of making leavened bread is of very considerable antiquity; but the additions of yest, or the vinous ferment, now so generally used, seems to be of modern date.

Unleavened bread in the form of small cakes, or biscuit, is made for the use of shipping in large quantities; but most of the bread used on shore is made to undergo, previous to baking, a kind of fermentation, which appears to be of the same nature as the fermentation of saccharine substances; but is checked and modified by so many circumstances, as to render it not a little difficult to speak with certainty and precision respecting it.

When dough or paste is left to undergo a spontaneous decomposition in an open vessel, the various parts of the mass are differently affected, according to the humidity, the thickness or thinness of the part, the vicinity or remoteness of fire, and other circumstances less easily investigated. The saccharine part is disposed to become converted into alkohol, the mucilage has a tendency to become sour and mouldy, while the gluten in all probability verges towards the putrid state. An entire change in the chemical attractions of the several component parts must then take place in a progressive manner, not altogether the same in the internal and more humid parts as in the external parts, which not only become dry by simple evaporation, but are acted upon by the surrounding air. The outside may therefore become mouldy or putrid, while the inner part may be only advanced to an acid state. Occasional admixture of the mass would of course not only produce some change in the rapidity of this alteration, but likewise render it more uniform throughout the whole. The effect of this commencing fermentation is found to be, that the mass is rendered more digestible and light; by which last expression it is understood, that it is rendered much more porous by the disengagement of elastic fluid, that separates its parts from each other, and greatly increases its bulk. The operation of baking puts a stop to this process, by evaporating great part of the moisture which is requisite to favour the chemical attraction, and probably also by still farther changing the nature of the component parts. It is then bread.

Bread made according to the preceding method will not possess the uniformity which is requisite, because some parts may be mouldy, while others are not yet sufficiently changed from the state of dough. The same means are used in this case as have been found effectual in promoting the uniform fermentation of large masses. This consists in the use of a leaven or ferment, which is a small portion of some matter of the same kind, but in a more advanced stage of the fermentation. After the leaven has been well incorporated by kneading into fresh dough, it not only brings on the fermentation with greater speed, but causes it to take place in the whole of the mass at the same time; and as soon as the dough has by this means acquired a due increase of bulk from the carbonic acid, which endeavours to escape, it is judged to be sufficiently fermented, and ready for the oven.

The fermentation by means of leaven or sour dough is thought to be of the acetous kind, because it is generally so managed, that the bread has a sour flavour and taste. But it has been ascertained that this acidity proceeds from true vinegar. Bread raised by leaven is usually made of a mixture of wheat and rye, not very accurately cleared of the bran. It is distinguished by the name of rye-bread; and the mixture of these two kinds of grain is called bread-corn, or meslin, in many parts of the kingdom, where it is raised on one the same piece of ground, and passes through all the processes of reaping, threshing, grinding, &c. in this mixed state.

Yest or barm is used as the ferment for the finer kinds of bread. This is the mucilaginous froth which rises to the surface of beer in its first stage of fermentation. When it is mixed with dough, it produces a much more speedy and effectual fermentation than that obtained by leaven, and the bread is accordingly much lighter, and scarcely ever sour. The fermentation by yest seems to be almost certainly of the vinous or spirituous kind.

Bread is much more uniformly miscible with water than dough; and on this circumstance its good qualities most probably do in a great measure depend.

A very great number of processes are used by cooks, confectioners, and others, to make cakes, puddings, and other kinds of bread, in which different qualities are required. Some cakes are rendered brittle, or as it is called *short*, by an admixture of sugar or of starch. Another kind of brittleness is given by the addition of butter or fat. White of egg, gum-water, isinglass, and other adhesive substances, are used, when it is intended that the effect of fermentation shall expand the dough into an exceedingly porous mass. Dr. Percival has recommended the addition of salep, or the nutritious powder of the orchis root. He says, that an ounce of salep, dissolved in a quart of water, and mixed with two pounds of flour, two ounces of yest, and eighty grains of salt, produced a remarkably good loaf, weighing three pounds two ounces; while a loaf made of an equal quantity of the other ingredients, without the salep, weighed but two pounds and twelve ounces. If the salep be in too large quantity, however, its peculiar taste will be distinguishable in the bread. The farina of potatoes, likewise, mixed with wheaten flour, makes very good bread. The reflecting chemist will receive considerable information on this subject from an attentive inspection of the receipts to be met with in treatises of cooking and confectionary.

Mr. Accum, in his late Treatise on Culinary Poisons, states, that the inferior kind of flour which the London bakers generally use for making loaves, requires the addition of alum to give them the white appearance of bread made from fine flour. 'The baker's flour is very often made of the worst kinds of damaged foreign wheat, and other cereal grains mixed with them in grinding the wheat into flour. In this capital, no fewer than six distinct kinds of wheaten flour are brought into the market. They are called fine flour, seconds, middlings, fine middlings, coarse middlings, and twenty-penny flour. Common garden beans and pease are also frequently ground up among the London bread flour.

'The smallest quantity of alum that can be employed with effect to produce a white, light, and porous bread from an inferior kind of flour, I have my own baker's authority to state, is from three to four ounces to a sack of flour weighing 240 pounds.'

'The following account of making a sack of five bushels of flour into bread, is taken from Dr. P. Markham's Considerations on the Ingredients used in the Adulteration of Flour and Bread, p. 21.

Five bushels flour,
Eight ounces of alum,
Four lbs. salt,
Half a gallon of yest, mixed with about
Three gallons of water.

'Another substance employed by fraudulent bakers is subcarbonate of ammonia. With this salt they realize the important consideration of producing light and porous bread from spoiled, or what is technically called *sour flour*. This salt, which becomes wholly converted into a gaseous substance during the operation of baking, causes the dough to swell up into air-bubbles, which carry before them the stiff dough, and thus it renders the dough porous; the salt itself is at the same time totally volatilized during the operation of baking.'—'Potatoes are likewise largely, and, perhaps, constantly used by fraudulent bakers, as a cheap ingredient to enhance their profit.'—'There are instances of convictions on record, of bakers having used gypsum, chalk, and pipe-clay, in the manufacture of bread.'

Mr. E. Davy, Prof. of Chemistry at the Cork Institution, has made experiments, showing that from twenty to forty grains of common carbonate of magnesia, well mixed with a pound of the worst *new seconds* flour, materially improved the quality of the bread baked with it.

The habitual and daily introduction of a portion of alum into the human stomach, however small, must be prejudicial to the exercise of its functions, and particularly in persons of a bilious and costive habit. And, besides, as the best sweet flour never stands in need of alum, the presence of this salt indicates an inferior and highly acescent food; which cannot fail to aggravate dyspepsia, and which may generate a calculous diathesis in the urinary organs. Every precaution of science and law ought, therefore, to be employed to detect and stop such deleterious adulterations. Bread may be analyzed for alum by crumbling it down when somewhat stale in distilled water, squeezing the pasty mass through a piece of cloth, and then passing the liquid through a paper filter. A limpid infusion will thus be obtained. It is difficult to procure it clear if we use new bread or hot water. A dilute solution of muriate of barytes dropped into the filtered infusion, will indicate by a white cloud, more or less heavy, the presence and quantity of alum. I find that genuine bread gives no precipitate by this treatment. The earthy adulterations are easily discovered by incinerating the bread at a red heat in a shallow earthen vessel, and treating the residuary ashes with a little nitrate of ammonia. The earths themselves will then remain, characterized by their whiteness and insolubility.

The latest chemical treatise on the art of making bread, except the account given by Mr. Accum in his work on the *Adulterations of Food*, is the article Baking, in the Supplement to the Encyclopædia Britannica.

Under *Process of Baking*, we have the following statement: 'An ounce of alum is then dissolved over the fire in a tin pot, and the solution poured into a large tub, called by the bakers the *seasoning-tub*. Four pounds and a half of salt are likewise put into the tub, and a pailful of hot water.' Note on this passage.—'In London, where the goodness of bread is estimated entirely by its whiteness, it is usual with those bakers who employ flour of an inferior quality, to add *as much* alum as common salt to the dough. Or, in other words, the quantity of salt added is diminished one-half, and the deficiency supplied by an equal weight of alum. This improves the look of the bread very much, rendering it much whiter and firmer.' "—*Ure's Chem. Dict.*

BREAD-FRUIT. The tree which affords this, grows in all the Ladrone islands in the South sea, in Otaheite, and now in the West Indies. The bread-fruit grows upon a tree the size of a middling oak. The fruit is about the size of a child's head, and the surface is reticulated, not much unlike the surface of a truffle. It is covered with a thin skin, and has a core about the size of a small knife. The eatable part is between the skin and the core: it is as white as snow, and somewhat of the consistence of new bread. It must be toasted before it is eaten, being first divided into three or four parts. Its taste is insipid, with a slight sweetness, nearly like that of wheaten bread and artichoke together. This fruit is the constant food of the inhabitants all the year, it being in season eight months.

Bread-nut. See *Brosimum alicastrum.*

BREAST. *Mamma.* The two globular projections, composed of common integuments, adipose substance, and lacteal glands and vessels, and adhering to the anterior and lateral regions of the thorax of females. On the middle of each breast is a projecting portion, termed the *papilla*, or *nipple*, in which the excretory ducts of the glands terminate, and around which is a coloured orb, or disc, called the *areola*. The use of the breasts is to suckle new-born infants.

BREAST-BONE. See *Sternum.*

BRECCIA. An Italian term, frequently used by our mineralogical writers to denote such compound stones as are composed of agglutinated fragments of considerable size. When the agglutinated parts are rounded, the stone is called pudding-stone. Breccias are denominated according to the nature of their component parts. Thus we have calcareous breccias, or marbles; and siliceous breccias, which are still more minutely classed, according to their varieties.

BRE'GMA. (From βρεχω, to moisten; formerly so

called, because, in infants, and sometimes even in adults, they are tender and moist.) An old name for the parietal bones.

BRE'VIS. Short. Applied to distinguish parts differing only in length, and to some parts, the termination of which is not far from their origin; as *brevia vasa*, the branches of the splenic vein.

BREY'NIA. (An American plant named in honour of Dr. Brennius.) A species of capparis.

BRIAR. See *Rosa*.

BRI'CUMUM. A name which the Gauls gave to the herb artemisia.

BRIMSTONE. See *Sulphur*.

BRISTLE. See *Seta*.

BRISTOL HOT-WELL. *Bristoliensis aqua*. A pure, thermal or warm, slightly acidulated, mineral spring, situated about a mile below Bristol. The fresh water is inodorous, perfectly limpid and sparkling, and sends forth numerous air-bubbles when poured into a glass. It is very agreeable to the palate, but without having any very decided taste, at least none that can be distinguished by a common observer. Its specific gravity is only 1.00077, which approaches so near to that of distilled water, that this circumstance alone would show that it contained but a very small admixture of foreign ingredients. The temperature of these waters, taking the average of the most accurate observations, may be reckoned at 74 deg.; and this does not very sensibly vary during winter or summer. Bristol water contains both solid and gaseous matter, and the distinction between the two requires to be attended to, as it is owing to the very small quantity of solid matter that it deserves the character of a very fine natural spring; and to an excess in gaseous contents that it seems to be principally indebted for its medical properties, whatever they may be, independent of those of mere water, with an increase of temperature. From the different investigations of chemists, it appears that the principal component parts of the Hot-Well water are, a large proportion of carbonic acid gas, or fixed air, and a certain portion of magnesia and lime, in various combinations, with the muriatic, vitriolic, and carbonic acids. The general inference is, that it is considerably pure for a natural fountain, as it contains no other solid matter than is found in almost all common spring water, and in less quantity.

On account of these ingredients, especially the carbonic acid gas, the Hot-Well water is efficacious in promoting salutary discharges, in green-sickness, as well as in the blind hæmorrhoids. It may be taken with advantage in obstructions, and weakness of the bowels, arising from habitual costiveness; and, from the purity of its aqueous part, it has justly been considered as a specific in diabetes, rendering the urinary organs more fitted to receive benefit from those medicines which are generally prescribed, and sometimes successful.

But the high reputation which this spring has acquired, is chiefly in the cure of pulmonary consumption. From the number of unsuccessful cases among those who frequent this place, many have denied any peculiar efficacy in this spring, superior to that of common water. It is not easy to determine how much may be owing to the favourable situation and mild, temperate climate which Bristol enjoys; but it cannot be doubted that the Hot-Well water, though by no means a cure for consumption, alleviates some of the most harassing symptoms of this formidable disease. It is particularly efficacious in moderating the thirst, the dry, burning heat of the hands and feet, the partial night sweats, and the symptoms that are peculiarly hectical; and thus, in the earlier stages of phthisis, it may materially contribute to a complete re-establishment of health; and even in the latter periods, mitigate the disease when the cure is doubtful, if not hopeless.

The sensible effects of this water, when drunk warm and fresh from the spring, are a gentle glow of the stomach, succeeded sometimes by a slight and transient degree of headach and giddiness. By a continued use, in most cases it is diuretic, keeps the skin moist and perspirable, and improves the appetite and health. Its effects on the bowels are variable. On the whole, a tendency to costiveness seems to be the more general consequence of a long course of this medicinal spring, and therefore the use of a mild aperient is requisite. These effects, however, are applicable only to invalids; for healthy persons who taste the water at the fountain, seldom discover any thing in it but a degree of warmth, which distinguishes it from the common element.

The season for the Hot-Well is generally from the middle of May to October: but as the medicinal properties of the water continue the same throughout the year, the summer months are preferred merely on account of the concomitant benefits of air and exercise.

It should be mentioned, that another spring, nearly resembling the Hot-Well, has been discovered at Clifton, which is situated on the summit of the same hill, from the bottom of which the Hot-Well issues. The water of Sion-Spring, as it is called, is one or two degrees colder than the Hot-Well; but in other respects it sufficiently resembles it to be employed for all similar purposes.

BRITANNICA HERBA. See *Rumex hydrolapathum*, and *Arctium lappa*.

BRITA'NNICUS. British. Applied to plants which grow in this country, and to some remedies.

BRITISH GUM. When starch is exposed to a temperature between 600° and 700° it swells, and exhales a peculiar smell; it becomes of a brown colour, and in that state is employed by calico-printers. It is soluble in cold water, and does not form a blue compound with iodine. Vauquelin found it to differ from gum in affording oxalic instead of mucous acid, when treated with nitric acid.—*Brande's Manuel*, iii. 34.

British Oil. A variety of the black species of petroleum, to which this name has been given as an empirical remedy.

BROCATELLO. A calcareous stone or marble, composed of fragments of four colours, white, gray, yellow, and red.

BRO'CCOLI. *Brassica Italica.* As an article of diet, this may be considered as more delicious than cauliflower and cabbage. Sound stomachs digest brocoli without any inconvenience; but in dyspeptic stomachs, even when combined with pepper, &c. it always produces flatulency, and nauseous eructations.

BROCHOS. (Βροχος, a snare.) A bandage.

BRO'CHTHUS. (From βρεχω, to pour.) The throat; also a small kind of drinking-vessel.

BRO'CHUS. Βροκος. One with a prominent upper-lip, or one with a full mouth and prominent teeth.

BROCKLESBY, RICHARD, was born in Somersetshire, though of an Irish family, in 1722. After studying at Edinburgh, he graduated at Leyden; then settled in London, but did not advance very rapidly in practice. About 1757, he was appointed physician to the army in Germany, and on his return after six years, published the result of his experience, in a work entitled "Economical and Medical Observations." His success now became more decided, and being prudent in his affairs, and without a family, he realized a considerable fortune. He proved himself however sufficiently liberal by presenting 1000*l.* to Mr. Edmund Burke, who had been his school-fellow; and by offering an annuity of 100*l.* to Dr. Johnson, to enable him to travel, which was not however accepted. He was author of several other works, and died in 1797.

BRO'DIUM. A term in pharmacy, signifying the same with *jusculum*, broth, or the liquor in which any thing is boiled. Thus, we sometimes read of *brodium salis*, or a decoction of salt.

BRO'MA. (From βρωσκω, to eat.) Food of any kind that is masticated, and not drank.

BROMA-THEON. (From βρωσκω, to eat.) Mushrooms.

BROMATO'LOGY. (*Bromatologia;* from βρωμα, food, and λογος, a discourse.) A discourse or treatise on food.

BROME'LIA. (So named in honour of Olaus Bromel, a Swede, author of *Lupologia*, &c. in 1687.) The name of a genus of plants. Class, *Hexandria*. Order, *Monogynia*.

BROMELIA ANANAS. The systematic name of the plant which affords the pine-apple, *Bromelia:—foliis ciliato spinosis, mucronatis, spica comosa* of Linnæus. It is used principally as a delicacy for the table, and is also given with advantage as a refrigerant in fevers.

BROMELIA KARATAS. The systematic name of the plant from which we obtain the fruit called penguin, which is given in the Spanish West Indies to cool and quench thirst in fevers, dysenteries, &c. It grows in a cluster, there being several of the size of one's finger together. Each portion is clothed with husk containing a white pulpy substance, which is the eatable part; and if it be not perfectly ripe, its flavour resembles that of the pine-apple. The juice of the ripe fruit is very austere, and is made use of to acidulate punch. The inhabitants of the West Indies make a wine of the penguin, which is very intoxicating, and has a good flavour.

BROMFIELD, William, was born in London, 1712; and attained considerable reputation as a surgeon. At the age of twenty-nine he began to give anatomical lectures, which were very well attended. About three years after, in conjunction with the Rev. Mr. Madan, he formed the plan of the Lock Hospital; and so ably enforced the advantages of such an institution, that a sufficient fund was raised for erecting the present building; and it has been since maintained by voluntary contributions. He was appointed surgeon, and held that office for many years: he was also surgeon to St. George's Hospital, and to Her Majesty's household. He wrote many works; the most considerable was entitled "Chirurgical Cases and Observations," in 1773, but reckoned not to answer the expectations entertained of him. He attained his eightieth year.

[BROMINE. In 1826, M. Balard of Montpelier discovered in sea-water a new substance, to which he gave the name *muride;* but it has since been changed to bromine, a word derived from the Greek βεωμος (graveolentia) signifying a strong or rank odour.

Bromine exists in sea-water in the form of hydrobromic acid. It is present, however, in very small quantity; and even the uncrystallizable residue called *bittern*, left after the muriate of soda has been separated from sea-water by evaporation, contains but little of it. On adding chlorine to this liquid, an orange yellow tint appears; and on heating the solution to the boiling point, the red vapours of bromine are expelled, which may be condensed by a freezing mixture. A better process is to transmit a current of chlorine gas through the bittern, and then to agitate a portion of æther with the liquid. The æther dissolves the whole of the bromine, from which it receives a beautiful hyacinth red tint, and on standing, rises to the surface. When the ethereal solution is agitated with caustic potassa, its colour entirely disappears, and on evaporation, cubic crystals of the hydro-bromate of potassa are deposited. On mixing these crystals, reduced to powder, with pure peroxide of manganese, and adding sulphuric acid diluted with its volume of water, the bromine is disengaged in a gaseous state. A small receiver, nearly filled with water, is attached to the retort, the beak of which and the receiver are kept cool by a frigorific mixture. The bromine condenses in the beak, runs into the receiver, and falls to the bottom on account of its great specific gravity. It is slightly soluble, but the water in its immediate vicinity soon becomes saturated. The water is decanted, and the remainder distilled with chloride of calcium, by which the bromine is obtained in a liquid state.

M. Balard has also detected bromine in marine plants which grow on the shores of the Mediterranean, and has procured it from the ashes of the sea-weeds that furnish iodine. He has likewise found it in the ashes of some animals, especially in those of the janthina violacea, one of the testaceous mollusca.

Bromine at common temperature is a liquid, the colour of which is blackish red, when viewed in mass and by reflected light, but appears hyacinth red when a thin stratum is interposed between the light and the observer. Its odour, which somewhat resembles that of chlorine, is very disagreeable; and its taste powerful. It acts with energy on organic matters, such as wood or cork, and corrodes the animal texture; but if applied to the skin for a short time only, it communicates a yellow stain less intense than that from iodine, and which soon disappears. It is highly destructive to animals: one drop of it placed on the beak of a bird proves fatal.—*Webster's Man. of Chem.* A.]

[Bromic acid. Bromine unites with oxygen and forms *Bromic acid*, which may be obtained in a separate state by decomposing a dilute solution of the bromate of baryta with sulphuric acid. From the analysis of the bromate of potassa, it appears to consist of 1 atom of bromine +5 atoms oxygen.

The bromates are analogous to the chlorates and iodates. Thus the bromate of potassa is converted by heat into the bromuret of potassium, with disengagement of pure oxygen, deflagrates when thrown on burning coals, and forms with sulphur a mixture which detonates by percussion. The acid of the bromates is decomposed by hydro-bromic and muriatic acids.—*Webst. Man. of Chem.* A.]

Bro'mion. (From βρωμος, the oat.) The name of a plaster, made with oaten flour, mentioned by Paulus Ægineta.

BRO'MUS. (From βρωμα, food.) The name of a genus of plants in the Linnæan system. Class, *Triandria;* Order, *Digynia.* Brome-grass.

Bromus sterilis. (From βρωσκω, to eat.) The wild oat.

BRO'NCHIA. (*Bronchia, orum.* neut. plur.; from βρογχος, the throat.) See *Trachea.*

BRONCHIAL. (*Bronchialis;* from *bronchia.*) Appertaining to the windpipe, or bronchia; as bronchial gland, artery, &c.

BRONCHIA'LIS. See *Bronchial.*

Bronchiales arteriæ. Bronchial arteries.—Branches of the aorta given off in the chest.

Bronchiales glandulæ. Bronchial glands.—Large blackish glands, situated about the bronchia and trachea.

BRONCHOCE'LE. (From βρογχος, the windpipe, and κηλη, a tumour.) *Botium; Hernia gutturis; Guttur tumidum; Trachelophyma; Gossum; Exechebronchos; Gongrona; Hernia bronchialis; Tracheocele.* Derbyshire neck. This disease is marked by a tumour on the fore-part of the neck, and seated between the trachea and skin. In general, it has been supposed principally to occupy the thyroid gland. We are given to understand that it is a very common disorder in Derbyshire; but its occurrence is by no means frequent in other parts of Great Britain, or in Ireland. Among the inhabitants of the Alps, and other mountainous countries bordering thereon, it is a disease very often met with, and is there known by the name of goitre. The cause which gives rise to it, is by no means certain, and the observations of different writers are of very little practical utility. Dr. Saunders controverts the general idea of the bronchocele being produced by the use of snow water. The swelling is at first without pain, or any evident fluctuation; when the disease is of long standing, and the swelling considerable, we find it in general a very difficult matter to effect a cure by medicine, or any external application; and it might be unsafe to attempt its removal with a knife, on account of the enlarged state of its arteries, and its vicinity to the carotids; but in an early stage of the disease, by the aid of medicine, a cure may be effected.

Although some relief has been obtained at times, and the disease probably somewhat retarded by external applications, such as blisters, discutient embrocations, and saponaceous and mercurial plasters, still a complete cure has seldom been effected without an internal use of medicine; and that which has always proved the most efficacious, is burnt sponge. The form under which this is most usually exhibited, is that of a lozenge. ℞. spongiæ ustæ ℥ss. mucilag. Arab gum. q. s. fiat trochiscus. When the tumour appears about the age of puberty, and before its structure has been too morbidly deranged, a pill consisting of a grain or two of calomel, must be given for three successive nights; and, on the fourth morning, a saline purge. Every night afterward, for three weeks, one of the troches should, when the patient is in bed, be put under the tongue, suffered to dissolve gradually, and the solution swallowed. The disgust at first arising from this remedy soon wears off. The pills and the purge are to be repeated at the end of three weeks, and the troches had recourse to as before; and this plan is to be pursued till the tumour is entirely dispersed. Some recommend the burnt sponge to be administered in larger doses. Sulphuretted potassa dissolved in water, in the proportion of 30 grains to a quart daily, is a remedy which has been employed by Dr Richter with success, in some cases, where calcined sponge failed. The sodæ subcarbonas being the basis of burnt sponge, is now frequently employed instead of it, and, indeed, it is a more active medicine.

[Bronchocele is said to have been cured by iodine; for which see that article. A.]

BRO'NCHOS. (Βρογχος, the windpipe.) A catarrh; a suppression of the voice from a catarrh.

BRONCHO'TOMY. (*Bronchotomia;* from βρογχος, the windpipe, and τεμνω, to cut.) Tracheotomy; Laryngotomy. This is an operation in which an opening is made into the larynx, or trachea, either for the purpose of making a passage for the air into and out of the lungs, when any disease prevents the patient from breathing through the mouth and nostrils, or of extracting foreign bodies, which have accidentally fallen into the trachea; or, lastly, in order to be able to inflate the lungs, in cases of sudden suffocation, drowning, &c. Its practicableness, and little danger, are founded on the facility with which certain wounds of the windpipe, even of the most complicated kind, have been healed, without leaving any ill effects whatever, and on the nature of the parts cut, which are not furnished with any vessel of consequence.

BRO'NCHUS. (From βρεχω, to pour.) The ancients believed that the solids were conveyed into the stomach by the œsophagus, and the fluids by the bronchia; whence its name. 1. The windpipe.

2. A defluxion from the fauces. See *Catarrhus.*

BRONZE. A mixed metal consisting chiefly of copper, with a small portion of tin, and sometimes other metals.

BRONZITE. A massive metal-like mineral, frequently resembling bronze, found in large masses in beds of serpentine in Upper Stiria, and in Perthshire.

BROOKLIME. See *Veronica beccabunga.*

[BROOKS, JOHN, M.D. LL.D. The honourable John Brooks was born in Medford, Massachusetts, in the year 1752. His father, Captain Caleb Brooks, was a respectable independent farmer, and the son spent his earliest years in the usual occupations of a farm. He received no education preparatory to his professional studies, but that of the town school; at which, however, he was able to acquire sufficient of the learned languages to qualify him for the profession of medicine. At the age of fourteen, he was placed under the tuition of Dr. Simon Tufts, of Medford, by a written indenture as an apprentice for seven years; this being the usual custom of that day.

Having finished his studies, he chose the neighbouring town of Reading as his residence, and commenced his practice there. But by this time, the storm of the revolutionary war was gathering; and, as its distant thunders rolled towards our shores, the hearts of the gallant youth of our country responded to the sound, and preparations for the field superceded the minor concerns of life.

Dr. Brooks accordingly entered into the military service of his country. As a Captain, he first exhibited his bravery in his attack upon the British at Lexington, in the neighbourhood of Boston. He shortly after received the commission of Major in the *Continental army*, as it was then called. In 1777, he was promoted to the rank of Colonel, and was a very efficient officer in the battles of Saratoga, which resulted in the capture of Burgoyne. In the battle of Monmouth, in New-Jersey, he was acting Adjutant-General, and on this, as on all occasions, conducted with great coolness and bravery, through the whole of the revolutionary war.

After the war, he recommenced the practice of physic, and continued for many years in high estimation as a practitioner. It is said of him, that, "As a physician, he ranked in the first class of practitioners. He possessed in an eminent degree those qualities which were calculated to render him the most useful in his professional labours, and the delight of those to whom he administered relief. His manners were dignified, courteous, and benign. He was kind, patient, and attentive. His kind offices were peculiarly acceptable from the felicitous manner in which he performed them. His mind was well furnished with scientific and practical knowledge. He was accurate in his investigations, and clear in his discernment. He therefore rarely failed in forming a true diagnosis. If he were not so bold and daring as some, in the administration of remedies, it was because his judgment and good sense led him to prefer erring on the side of prudence, rather than on that of rashness. He watched the operations of nature, and never interfered unless it was obvious he could aid and support her. He was truly the 'Hierophant of Nature,' studying her mysteries, and obeying her oracles."

Dr. Brooks became so great a favourite of his countrymen, that he was finally elected Governor of the state of Massachusetts. Dr. Thacher says of him:—

"Having faithfully and ably discharged the duties of chief magistrate for seven successive years, he expressed his determination to retire from the cares and anxieties of public life. How great were the public regrets, and how gladly would a large majority of his fellow-citizens have retained his valuable services; but they forbore urging him to any farther sacrifices for the good of his country. He retired to private life with dignity, and with the love and blessings of a grateful people." He died in March, 1825, in the 73d year of his age.—See *Thach. Med. Biog.* A.]

BROOM. See *Spartium scoparium.*

BROSIMUM. (From βρωσιμος, eatable.) The name of a genus of plants in the Linnæan system. Class, *Diœcia;* Order, *Monandria.*

BROSIMUM ALICASTRUM. The specific name of the tree, which affords the bread-nut.

BROWN, JOHN, born in the county of Berwick, in 1735. He made very rapid progress in his youth in the learned languages, and at the age of twenty went to Edinburgh to study theology; but before he could be ordained, became attached to free living and free thinking. About 1759, having translated the inaugural thesis of a medical candidate into Latin, and the performance being highly applauded, he was led to the study of medicine. The professors at Edinburgh allowed him to attend their lectures gratuitously; and he maintained himself by instructing the students in Latin, and composing or translating their dissertations. Dr. Cullen particularly encouraged him, notwithstanding his irregularities, employing him as tutor to his sons, and allowing him to repeat and enlarge upon his lectures in the evening, to those pupils who chose to attend. In 1765 he married, and his house was soon filled with boarders; but his imprudence brought on bankruptcy within four years after. About this period he was an unsuccessful candidate for one of the medical chairs; and attributing his failure to Dr. Cullen, became his declared enemy. This probably determined him to form his new system of medicine, afterward published under the title of "Elementa Medicinæ:" in which certainly much genius is displayed, but little acquaintance with practice, or with what had been written before on the subject. His chief object seems to have been to reduce the medical art to the utmost simplicity; whence he arranged all diseases under the two divisions of sthenic and asthenic, and maintained that all agents operate on the body as stimuli; so that we had only to increase or diminish the force of these according to circumstances. At the head of his stimulant remedies, he places wine, brandy, and opium, in the recommendation of which he is very liberal; and especially betrays his partiality to them by asserting, contrary to universal experience, that he found them in his own person the best preservatives against the gout. He is said to have prepared himself for his lectures by a large dose of laudanum in whiskey; and thus roused himself to a degree of enthusiasm bordering on frenzy. After completing his work, he procured a degree from St. Andrew's, and commenced public teacher. The novelty and imposing simplicity of his doctrines procured him at first a pretty numerous class: but being irregular in his attendance, and his habits of intemperance increasing, they fell off by degrees: and he was at length so embarrassed, as to be obliged to quit Edinburgh in 1786. He then settled in London, but met with little success, and in about two years after died. His opinions at first found many supporters, as well in this as in other countries; but they appear now nearly fallen into deserved oblivion.

BROWN SPAR. Pearl spar. Sideroculcite. A white, red, or brown, or black spar; harder than the calcareous, but yields to the knife.

BROWNE, SIR THOMAS, was born in Cheapside, 1605. After studying and practising for a short time at Oxford, he spent about three years in travelling, graduating at length at Leyden. He then came to London, and published his "Religio Medici;" which excited great attention as a work of genius, though blemished by a few of the popular superstitions then prevailing. He soon after settled at Norwich, and got into very good practice; and was admitted an honorary member of the London College of physicians. In 1646 appeared his most popular work "On Vulgar Errors," which added greatly to his fame; though he injudiciously ranked the Copernican system among them; he was knighted by Charles II.; and died at the termination of his 77th year. His son Edward was also a physician, and attained considerable eminence, having had the honour of attending Charles II. and William III., and being for three years president of the college.

[BRUCE, Archibald, M.D. A native of New-York, born in 1777, during the revolutionary war. He studied physic under Dr. Hosack, visited Europe, and graduated at Edinburgh in the year 1800. During a tour of two years in France, Switzerland, and Italy, Dr. Bruce collected a mineralogical cabinet of great value and extent. Upon his return to England, he married in London, and came out to New-York in the summer of 1803, to enter upon the duties of a practitioner of medicine. In 1807, he was appointed professor of Materia Medica and Mineralogy, in the *College of Physicians and Surgeons* of New-York. In 1810, he commenced the editorship of a Journal of American Mineralogy, after the manner of the well known work issued by the School of Mines, at Paris. It met with becoming success, and had many valuable contributors to its pages; but owing to various causes, was never carried beyond the completion of the first volume. The Mineralogical Journal contributed materially to extend the fame of Dr. Bruce, as well as his discovery of the hydrate of magnesia, at Hoboken. He died in February, 1818, in the 41st year of his age. —See *Thach. Med. Biog.* A.]

BRUCEA. (So named by Sir Joseph Banks, in honour of Mr. Bruce, the traveller in Abyssinia, who first brought the seeds thence into England.) The name of a genus of plants in the Linnæan system. Class, *Diœcia:* Order, *Tetrandria.*

Brucea antidysenterica. The systematic name of the plant from which it was erroneously supposed we obtained the Angustura bark. See *Cusparia.*

Brucea ferruginea. This plant was also supposed to afford the Angustura bark.

BRUCIA. Brucine. A new vegetable alkali, lately extracted from the bark of the false Angustura, or *Brucia antidysenterica*, by Pelletier and Caventou. After being treated with sulphuric æther, to get rid of a fatty matter, it was subjected to the action of alkohol. The dry residuum, from the evaporated alkoholic solution, was treated with Goulard's extract, or solution of acetate of lead, to throw down the colouring matter, and the excess of lead was separated by a current of sulphuretted hydrogen. The nearly colourless alkaline liquid was saturated with oxalic acid, and evaporated to dryness. The saline mass being freed from its remaining colouring particles by absolute alkohol, was then decomposed by lime or magnesia, when the *brucia* was disengaged. It was dissolved in boiling alkohol, and obtained in crystals, by the slow evaporation of the liquid. These crystals, when obtained by very slow evaporation, are oblique prisms, the bases of which are parallelograms. When deposited from a saturated solution in boiling water, by cooling, it is in bulky plates, somewhat similar to boracic acid in appearance. It is soluble in 500 times its weight of boiling water, and in 850 of cold. Its solubility is much increased by the colouring matter of the bark.

Its taste is exceedingly bitter, acrid, and durable in the mouth. When administered in doses of a few grains, it is poisonous, acting on animals like strychnia, but much less violently. It is not affected by the air. The dry crystals fuse at a temperature a little above that of boiling water, and assume the appearance of wax. At a strong heat it is resolved into carbon, hydrogen, and oxygen; without any trace of azote. It combines with the acids, and forms both neutral and super-salts.

Brucine. See *Brucia.*

BRUISEWORT. See *Saponaria.*

BRUMALIS. (From *Bruma*, winter.) *Hyemalis.* Belonging to winter.

Brumalles plantæ. Plants which flower in our winter, common about the cape.

Brune'lla. See *Prunella.*

BRUNNER, John Conrad, was born in Switzerland in 1653. He obtained his degree in medicine at Strasburg when only nineteen. He afterward spent several years in improving himself at different universities, particularly at Paris; where he made many experiments on the pancreas, and found that it might be removed from a dog with impunity. On his return he was made professor of medicine at Heidelburg; and gained great reputation, so as to be consulted by most of the princes of Germany. He discovered the mucous glands in the duodenum; and was author of several inconsiderable works. He died in 1727.

Brunner's glands. *Brunneri glandulæ.* Peyer's glands. The muciparous glands, situated between the villous and cellular coat of the intestinal canal; so named after Brunner, who discovered them.

BRUNSWICK GREEN. An ammoniaco-muriate of copper.

BRUNTKUP FERZ. Purple copper ore.

Bru'nus. An erysipelatous eruption.

Bru'scus. See *Ruscus.*

Brut'a. An Arabian word which means instinct, and is also applied to Savine.

Bru'tia. An epithet for the most resinous kind of pitch, and therefore used to make the *Oleum Picinum.* The *Pix Brucia* was so called from Brutia, a country in the extreme parts of Italy, where it was produced.

Bruti'no. Turpentine.

Bru'tobon. The name of an ointment used by the Greeks.

Brutua. See *Cissampelos Pareira.*

Bruxane'li. (Indian.) A tall tree in Malabar, the bark of which is diuretic.

Bry'gmus. (From βρυχω, to make a noise.) A peculiar kind of noise, such as is made by gnashing or grating the teeth; or, according to some, a certain kind of convulsion affecting the lower jaw, and striking the teeth together, most frequently observed in such children as have worms.

BRYO'NIA. (From βρυω, to abound, from its abundance.) Bryony. 1. The name of a genus of plants in the Linnæan system. Class, *Diœcia;* Order, *Syngenesia.*

2. The pharmacopœial name of the white bryony. See *Bryonia alba.*

Bryonia alba. The systematic name of the white bryony plant. *Vitis alba sylvestris; Agrostis; Ampelo sagria; Archeostris; Echetrosis* of Hippocrates. *Bryonia aspera; Cedrostis; Chelidonium; Labrusca; Melothrum; Ophrostaphylon; Psilothrum. Bryonia —foliis palmatis utrinque calloso-scabris* of Linnæus. This plant is very common in woods and hedges. The root has a very nauseous biting taste, and disagreeable smell. Bergius states the virtues of this root to be purgative, hydragogue, emmenagogue, and diuretic; the fresh root emetic. This powerful and irritating cathartic, though now seldom prescribed by physicians, is said to be of great efficacy in evacuating serous humours, and has been chiefly employed in hydropical cases. Instances of its good effects in other chronic diseases are also mentioned; as asthma, mania, and epilepsy. In small doses, it is reported to operate as a diuretic, and to be resolvent and deobstruent. In powder, from ℈j. to a drachm, it proves strongly purgative, and the juice, which issues spontaneously, in doses of a spoonful or more, has similar effects, but is more gentle in its operation. An extract prepared by water, acts more mildly, and with greater safety, than the root in substance, given from half a drachm to a drachm. It is said to prove a gentle purgative, and likewise to operate powerfully by urine. Of the expressed juice, a spoonful acts violently both upwards and downwards; but cream of tartar is said to take off its virulence. Externally, the fresh root has been employed in cataplasms, as are solvent and discutient: also in ischiadic and other rheumatic affections.

Bryonia mechoachana nigricans. A name given to the jalap root.

Bryonia nigra. See *Tamus communis*

Bryonia peruviana. Jalap.

BRY'ONY. See *Bryonia nigra.*

Bryony, black. See *Tamus.*

Bryony, white. See *Bryonia alba.*

Bry'thion. Βρυθιον. A malagma; so called and described by Paulus Ægineta.

Bry'ton. (From βρυω, to pour out.) A kind of ale, or wine, made of barley.

Bubasteco'rdium. (From *bubastus* and *cor*, the heart.) A name formerly given to artemisia, or mug wort.

BU'BO. (From βουβων, the groin; because they most frequently happen in that part.) Modern surgeons mean, by this term, a swelling of the lymphatic glands, particularly of those of the groin and axilla. The disease may arise from the mere irritation of some local disorder, when it is called *sympathetic bubo;* from the absorption of some irritating matter, such as the venereal poison; or from constitutional causes, as in the pestilential bubo, and scrophulous swellings, of the inguinal and axillary gland.

BU'BON. (From βουβων, the groin, or a tumour to which that part is liable, and which it was supposed to cure.) The name of a genus of plants in the Linnæan system. Class, *Pentandria;* Order, *Digynia.*

BUBON GALBANUM. The systematic name of the plant which affords the officinal galbanum. *Albetad; Chalbane; Gesor.* The plant is also named *Ferula Africana; Oreoselinum Africanum; Anisum fruticosum galbaniferum; Anisum Africanum fruticescens; Ayborzat.* The lovage-leaved bubon. *Bubon;—foliis rhombeis dentatis striatis glabris, umbellis paucis,* of Linnæus. Galbanum is the gummi-resinous juice, obtained partly by its spontaneous exudation from the joints of the stem, but more generally, and in greater abundance, by making an incision in the stalk, a few inches above the root, from which it immediately issues, and soon becomes sufficiently concrete to be gathered. It is imported into England from Turkey, and the East Indies, in large, softish, ductile, pale-coloured masses, which, by age, acquire a brownish-yellow appearance; these are intermixed with distinct whitish tears, that are the most pure part of the mass. Galbanum has a strong unpleasant smell, and a warm, bitterish, acrid taste. Like the other gummy resins, it unites with water, by trituration into a milky liquor, but does not perfectly dissolve, as some have reported, in water, vinegar, or wine. Rectified spirit takes up much more than either of these menstrua, but not the whole; the tincture is of a bright golden colour. A mixture of two parts of rectified spirit, and one of water, dissolves all but the impurities, which are commonly in considerable quantity. In distillation with water, the oil separates and rises to the surface, in colour yellowish, in quantity one-twentieth of the weight of the galbanum. Galbanum, medicinally considered, may be said to hold a middle rank between assafœtida and ammoniacum; but its fœtidness is very inconsiderable, especially when compared with the former: it is therefore accounted less antispasmodic, nor are its expectorant qualities equal to those of the latter: it however is esteemed more efficacious than either in hysterical disorders. Externally, it is often applied, by surgeons, to expedite the suppuration of inflammatory and indolent tumours, and, by physicians, as a warm stimulating plaster. It is an ingredient in the *pilulæ galbani compositæ,* the *emplastrum galbani compositum* of the London Pharmacopœia, and in the *emplastrum gummosum* of the Edinburgh.

BUBON MACEDONICUM. The systematic name of the plant which affords the *semen petroselini Macedonici* of the shops. *Apium petræum; Petrapium.* Macedonian parsley. This plant is similar in quality to the common parsley, but weaker and less grateful. The seeds enter the celebrated compounds mithridate and theriaca.

BUBO'NIUM. (From βουβων, the groin.) A name of the golden starwort; so called because it was supposed to be efficacious in diseases of the groin.

BUBONOCE'LE. (From βουβων, the groin, and κηλη, a tumour.) *Hernia inguinalis.* Inguinal hernia, or rupture of the groin. A species of hernia, in which the bowels protrude, at the abdominal ring. See *Hernia inguinalis.*

BU'CCA. (Hebrew.) The cheek. The hollow inner part of the cheek, that is inflated by the act of blowing.

BUCCACRA'TON. (From *bucca,* or *buccella,* and κραω, to mix.) A morsel of bread sopped in wine, which served in old times for a breakfast.

BU'CCAL. (From *bucca,* the cheek.) Belonging to the cheek.

BUCCINALES GLANDULÆ. The small glands of the mouth, under the cheek which assist in secreting saliva into that cavity.

BU'CCEA. (From *bucca,* the cheek; as much as can be contained at one time within the cheeks.) 1. A mouthful; a morsel.

2. A polypus of the nose.

BUCCELA'TON. (From *buccella,* a morsel.) A purging medicine, made up in the form of a loaf; consisting of scammony, &c. put into fermented flour, and then baked in an oven.

BUCCE'LLA. Paracelsus calls the polypus in the nose by this name, because he supposes it to be a portion of flesh parting from the bucca, and insinuating itself into the nose.

BUCCELLA'TIO. (From *bucellatus,* cut into small pieces.) *Baccellatio.* A method of stopping an hæmorrhage, by applying small pieces of lint to the vein, or artery.

BUCCINA'TOR. (From βουκανον, a trumpet; so named from its use in forcing the breath to sound the trumpet.) *Retractor anguli oris* of Albinus, and *alveolo-maxillaire* of Dumas. The trumpeter's muscle. The buccinator was long thought to be a muscle of the lower jaw, arising from the upper alveoli, and inserted into the lower alveoli, to pull the jaw upwards; but its origin and insertion, and the direction of its fibres, are quite the reverse of this. For this large flat muscle, which forms in a manner the walls of the cheek, arises chiefly from the coronoid process of the lower jaw-bone, and partly also from the end of the alveoli, or socket process of the upper-jaw, close by the pterygoid process of the sphenoid bone: it goes forward, with direct fibres, to be implanted into the corner of the mouth; it is thin and flat, covers in the mouth, and forms the walls of the cheek, and is perforated in the middle of the cheek by the duct of the parotid gland. These are its principal uses:—it flattens the cheek, and so assists in swallowing liquids; it turns, or helps to turn, the morsel in the mouth while chewing, and prevents it from getting without the line of the teeth; in blowing wind instruments, it both receives and expels the wind; it dilates like a bag, so as to receive the wind in the checks; and it contracts upon the wind, so as to expel the wind, and to swell the note. In blowing the strong wind-instruments, we cannot blow from the lungs, for it distresses the breathing, we reserve the air in the mouth, which we keep continually full; and from this circumstance, as mentioned above, it is named buccinator, from blowing the trumpet.

BU'CCULA. (Diminutive of *bucca,* the cheek.) The fleshy part under the chin.

Bucephalon, red-fruited. See *Trophis Americana.*

BU'CERAS. (From βους, an ox, and κερας, a horn; so called from the horn-like appearance of its seed.)

Buceros. See *Trigonella Fœnumgræcum.*

BUCHAN, WILLIAM, was born at Ancram, in 1729. After studying at Edinburgh, he settled in Sheffield, and was soon appointed physician to the Foundling Hospital at Ackworth: but that establishment being afterward given up, he went to practise at Edinburgh, where he remained several years. During that period he composed his celebrated work, called "Domestic Medicine," on the plan of Tissot's "Avis aux Peuples;" which has been very extensively circulated, translated into other languages, and obtained the author a gold medal, with a commendatory letter, from the Empress of Russia. It has been objected, that such publications tend to degrade and injure the medical profession; but it does not appear, that those who are properly qualified can suffer permanently thereby. There seems more foundation for the opinion, that imaginary diseases will be multiplied, and patients sometimes fall victims to their complaints, being treated by those who do not properly understand them. Dr. Buchan afterward practised in London, and published some other works; and died in 1805.

BUCK-BEAN. See *Menyanthes trifoliata.*

BUCK-THORN. See *Rhamnus catharticus.*

BUCK-WHEAT. See *Polygonum fagopyrum.*

Buck-wheat, eastern. See *Polygonum divaricatum.*

BUCNEMIA. (*Bucnemia;* from βου, a Greek augment, and κνημη, the leg.) A name in Good's Nosology for a genus of disease characterized by a tense, diffuse, inflammatory swelling of the lower extremity; usually commencing at the inguinal glands, and extending in the course of the lymphatics, it embraces two species; 1. *Bucnemia sparganosis,* the puerperal tumid leg.

2. *Bucnemia tropica,* the tumid leg of hot climates.

BUCRA'NION. (From βους, an ox, and κρανιον, the head; so called from its supposed resemblance to a calf's snout.) The Snap-dragon plant. See *Antirrhinum.*

BU'CTON. The hymen, according to Piræus.

BUGA'NTIA. Chilblains.

BUGLE. See *Prunella.*

[BUGLE WEED. This plant is the *Lycopus Vir-*

mica. It has of late been popular as a remedy in bleeding from the lungs, taken freely in the form of decoction. It is not, however, introduced as a medicinal plant into the American Pharmacopœia, nor in Bigelow's Materia Medica. Physicians in general place little confidence in its efficacy. A.]

BUGLOSS. See *Anchusa officinalis.*

Buglo'ssa. See *Anchusa officinalis.*

BUGLO'SSUM. (*Buglossum, i.* n.; from βους, an ox, and γλωσσα, a tongue: so called from the shape and roughness of its leaf.) See *Anchusa officinalis.*

Buglossum angustifolium. See *Anchusa officinalis.*

Buglossum majus. See *Anchusa officinalis.*

Buglossum sativum. See *Anchusa officinalis.*

Buglossum sylvestre. The stone bugloss.

Bu gula. (A diminutive of *buglossa.*) See *Ajuga pyramidalis.*

[BUHRSTONE. Millstone. "The exterior aspect of this mineral is somewhat peculiar. It occurs in amorphous masses, partly compact, but always containing a greater or less number of irregular cavities. Sometimes the mass is comparatively compact, and the cavities small and less frequent, but they always exist even in specimens of a moderate size. These cavities are sometimes crossed by siliceous threads or membranes, much resembling the interior structure of certain bones; and are sometimes lined by siliceous incrustations, or crystals of quartz.

Its fracture is nearly even, sometimes dull, and sometimes smooth, like that of flint. Its colour is gray or whitish, sometimes with a tinge of blue, and sometimes yellowish or reddish. Near Paris, the Buhrstone occurs in beds, unusually horizontal, and seldom more than 9 or 10 feet thick. It contains no organic remains. Its cavities are often crossed by threads, and filled with argillaceous marl or sand; but are very seldom lined by crystals of quartz.

In Georgia, (United States,) the Buhrstone is found near the boundary of South Carolina, about 40 miles from the sea. It is said to cover shell limestone. Some of its cavities are those of shells in a siliceous state, and lined by siliceous incrustations, or crystals of quartz. Others are traversed by minute threads, or contain a friable substance somewhat argillaceous. Its hardness and cavities, when not too numerous, render it peculiarly useful for making millstones. Hence also it is sometimes known by the name of Millstone."—See *Cleav. Min.* A.]

BULBIFERUS. (From *bulbus*, and *fero*, to bear.) Bulb-bearing. Having one or more bulbs; applied to stems. *Caulis bulbiferus.*

BULBOCA'STANUM. (From βολβος, a bulb, and καςανον, a chesnut: so called from its bulbous appearance.) See *Bunium bulbocastanam.*

BULBOCAVERNO'SUS. (So called from its origin and insertion.) See *Accelerator urinæ.*

Bu'lbonach. See *Lunaria rediviva.*

BULBOSUS. (From *bulba*, a bulb.) Bulbous: applied in anatomy to soft parts which are naturally enlarged, as the bulbous part of the urethra. In botany, to roots which have a bulb; as tulip, onion, lily, &c.

Bulbosæ. (From *bulbus.*) The name of a class of *Cæsalpinus's* systematic method, consisting of herbaceous vegetables, which have a bulbous root, and a pericarpium, divided into three cells; also, the name of one of the natural orders of plants.

BULBULUS. A litte bulb.

BUL'BUS. (Βολβος, a bulb, or somewhat rounded root.) A globular, or pyriform coated body, solid, or formed of fleshy scales or layers, constituting the lower part of some plants, and giving off radicals from the circumference of the flattened basis. A bulb differs from a *tuber*, which is a farinaceous root, and sends off radicles in every direction.

Bulbs are divided into,

1. The *solid*, which consists of a solid fleshy nutritious substance; as in *Crocus sativus, Colchicum autumnale, Tulipa gesneriana.*

2. The *scaly*, which consists of fleshy concentrical scales attached to a radical plate; as in *Allium cepa.*

3. The *squamose*, consisting of concave, overlapping scales; as in *Lilium candidum*, and *Lilium bulbiferum.*

4. The *compounded*, consisting of several lesser bulbs, lying close to each other: as in *Allium sativum.*

The bulbs of the orchis tribe differ from the common bulbs in not sending off radicles from the lower part, but from between the stem and basis. These are distinguished into,

5. The *testiculate*, having two bulbs of a round-oblong form; as in *Orchis morio*, and *Orchis mascula.*

6. *Palmate*, a compressed bulb, hand-like, divided below into finger-like lobes; as in *Orchis maculata.*

Bulbus esculentus. Such bulbous roots as are commonly eaten are so called.

Bulbus vomitorius. See *Hyacinthus muscari.*

BULGE-WATER-TREE. The *Geoffroya jamaicensis.*

BULI'MIA. (From βου, a particle of excess, and λιμος, hunger.) *Bulimiasis; Boulimos; Bulimus; Bolismos* of Avicenna. *Fames canina; Appetitus caninus; Phagedæna; Adephagia; Bupeina; Cynorexia.* Insatiable hunger, or canine appetite.

Dr. Cullen places this genus of disease in the class *Locales*, and order *Dysorexiæ;* and distinguishes three species. 1. *Bulimia helluonum;* in which there is no other disorder of the stomach, than an excessive craving of food. 2. *Bulimia syncopalis;* in which there is a frequent desire of food, and the sense of hunger is preceded by swooning. 3. *Bulimia emetica*, also *cynorexia;* in which an extraordinary appetite for food is followed by vomiting. The real causes of this disease are, perhaps, not properly understood. In some cases, it has been supposed to proceed from an acid in the stomach, and in others, from a superabundance of acid in the gastric juice, and from indigested sordes, or worms. Some consider it as depending more frequently on monstrosity than disease. An extraordinary and well attested case of this disease, is related in the third volume of the Medical and Physical Journal, of a French prisoner, who, in one day, consumed of raw cow's udder 4 lbs., raw beef 10 lbs., candles 2 lbs.; total, 16 lbs.; besides 5 bottles of porter.

Bulimia adephagia. A voracious appetite.

Bulimia canina. A voracious appetite, with subsequent vomiting.

Bulimia cardialgica. A voracious appetite, with heartburn.

Bulimia convulsorum. A voracious appetite, which attends some convulsive diseases.

Bulimia emetica. A voracious appetite, with vomiting.

Bulimia esurigio. Gluttony.

Bulimia helluonum. Gluttony.

Bulimia syncopalis. A voracious appetite, with fainting from hunger.

Bulimia verminosa. A voracious appetite from worms.

BULIMI'ASIS. See *Bulimia.*

BU'LIMUS. See *Bulimia.*

BULI'THUM. (From βους, an ox, and λιθος, a stone.) A bezoar, or stone found in the kidneys, or gall, or urinary bladder, of an ox, or cow.

BU'LLA. A bubble. A clear vesicle, which arises from burns, or scalds; or other causes.

[This word is also applied by Linnæus to a genus of univalve shells. A.]

BU'LLACE. The English name of the fruit of the *Prunus insitia* of Linnæus, which grows wild in our hedges. There are two varieties of bullace, the red and the white, which are used with the same intention as the common damsons.

BULLATUS. (From *bulla*, a bubble, or blister.) Blistery. Applied to a leaf which has its veins so tight, that the intermediate space appears blistered. This appearance is frequent in the garden cabbage.

Bullo'sa febris. An epithet applied to the vesicular fever, because the skin is covered with little vesicles, or blisters. See *Pemphigus.*

Buni'tes vinum. (From *bunium*, wild parsley.) Wine made of bunium and must.

BU'NIUM. (From βουνος, a little hill; so called from the tuberosity of its root.) 1. The name of a genus of plants in the Linnæan system. Class, *Pentandria;* Order, *Digynia.*

2. The name of the wild parsley.

Bunium bulbocastanum. The systematic name of a plant, the root of which is called the pig-nut. *Agriocastanum; Nucula terrestris; Bulbocastaneum; Bulbocastanum majus et minus.* Earth-nut; Hawknut; Kipper-nut; and Pig-nut. The root is as large as a nutmeg; hard, tuberous, and whitish; which is eaten raw, or roasted. It is sweetish to the taste, nourishing, and supposed to be of use against strangury and bloody urine. The roots, which are frequently ploughed up by the peasants of Burgundy, and called by them *arnotta;* and those found in Scotland, and called *arnots*, are most probably the roots of this species of bunium. They are roasted, and thus acquire the flavour of chesnuts.

Bu'nius. A species of turnip.

BU'PEINA. (From βου, a particle of magnitude, and πεινα, hunger.) A voracious appetite.

BU'PHAGOS. (From βου, a particle of excess, and φαγω, to eat.) The name of an antidote which created a voracious appetite in Marcellus Empericus.

BUPHTHA'LMUM. (From βους, an ox, an οφθαλμος, an eye; so called from its flowers, which are supposed to resemble an eye.) The herb, ox-eye daisy See *Chrysanthemum leucanthemum.*

Buphthalmum creticum. Pellitory of Spain. See *Anthemis pyrethrum.*

Buphthalmum germanicum. The common ox-eye daisy.

Buphthalmum majus. Great, or ox-eye daisy. See *Chrysanthemum leucanthemum.*

BUPHTHALMUS. (From βους, an ox, and οφθαλμος, an eye; so named from its large appearance like an ox's eye.)

1. Houseleek.
2. Diseased enlargement of the eye.

BUBLEU'RUM. (From βου, large, and πλευρον, a rib; so named from its having large rib-like filaments upon its leaves.) 1. The name of a genus of plants in the Linnæan system. Class, *Syngenesia;* Order, *Polygamia superflua.*

2. The pharmacopœial name of the herb hare's ear. See *Bupleurum rotundifolium.*

Bupleurum rotundifolium. The systematic name of the plant called *perfoliata*, in some pharmacopœias. *Bupleuron; Bupleuroides.* Round-leaved hare's ear, or thorow wax. This plant was formerly celebrated for curing ruptures, mixed into a poultice with wine and oatmeal.

BU'RDOCK. See *Arctium lappa.*

BU'RGUNDY PITCH. See *Pinus abies.*

Bu'ris. According to Avicenna, a scirrhous hernia, or hard abscess.

BURN. *Ambustio.* A burn, or scald, is a lesion of the animal body, occasioned by the application of heat, but the latter term is applicable only where this is conveyed through the medium of some fluid. The consequences are more or less serious according to the extent of the injury, or the particular part affected: sometimes even proving fatal, particularly in irritable constitutions. The life of the part may be at once destroyed by these accidents, or mortification speedily follow the violent inflammation excited; but when slighter, it usually produces an effusion of serum under the cuticle, like a blister. When the injury is extensive, considerable fever is apt to supervene, sometimes a comatose state; and a remarkable difficulty of breathing often precedes death. In the treatment of these accidents, two very different methods have been pursued. The more ancient plan consists in antiphlogistic means, giving cooling purgatives, &c. and even taking blood, where the irritation is great; employing at the same time cold applications, and where the skin is destroyed, emollient dressings; opium was also recommended to relieve the pain, notwithstanding stupor might attend.

Mr. Cleghorn, a brewer at Edinburgh, was very successful in these cases by a treatment materially different; first bathing the part with vinegar, usually a little warmed, till the pain abated; then, if there were any destruction of the parts, applying poultices, and finely powdered chalk immediately on the sore, to absorb the discharge: in the meantime allowing the patient to live pretty well, and abstaining from active purgatives, &c. More recently, a surgeon at Newcastle, of the name of Kentish, has deviated still more from the ancient practice; applying first oil of turpentine, alcohol, &c. heated as much as the sound parts could bear, and gradually lessening the stimulus; in the mean time supporting the patient by a cordial diet, æther, &c. and giving opium largely to lessen the irritation. Now, the cases chiefly under his care were of persons scorched very extensively by the explosion of carburetted hydrogen in mines; and probably where the injury is over a large part of the surface, or where the constitution is weakly, it may be hazardous to pursue the antiphlogistic plan, or to use cold applications, which, while intended to keep down action, are wearing out the power of the part. If any extraneous substance be forced into the burnt part, it should be of course removed: and sometimes where a limb is irrecoverably injured, amputation may be necessary.

Bu'rnea. Pitch.

Burnet saxifrage. See *Pimpinella.*

Burning. *Brenning.* An ancient medical term, denoting an infectious disease, got in the stews by conversing with lewd women, and supposed to be the same with what we now call the venereal disease.

Burnt hartshorn. See *Cornu ustum.*

Burnt sponge. See *Spongia usta.*

Bu'rrhi spiritus matricalis. Burrhus's spirit, for disorders of the womb. A compound of myrrh, olibanum, amber, and spirit of wine.

BU'RSA. From βυρσα, a bag.) A bag. 1. The scrotum.

2. An herb called *Thlaspi bursæ pastoris*, from the resemblance of its seminal follicles to a triangular purse.

Bursa mucosa. A mucous bag, composed of proper membranes, containing a kind of mucous fat, formed by the exhaling arteries of the internal coat. The bursæ mucosæ are of different sizes and firmness, and are connected by the cellular membrane with articular cavities, tendons, ligaments, or the periosteum. Their use is to secrete and contain a substance to lubricate tendons, muscles, and bones, in order to render their motions easy.

A Table of all the Bursæ Mucosæ.

In the Head.

1. *A bursa of the superior oblique muscle* of the eye, situated behind its trochlea in the orbit.
2. *The bursa of the digastricus*, situated in the internal surface of its tendon.
3. *A bursa of the circumflexus*, or tensor palati, situated between the hook-like process of the sphenoid bone and the tendon of that muscle.
4. *A bursa of the sterno-hyoideus muscle*, situated between the os hyoides and larynx.

About the Shoulder-joint.

1. *The external acromial*, situated under the acromion, between the coracoid process, deltoid muscle, and capsular ligament.
2. *The internal acromial*, situated above the tendon of the infra-spinatus and teres major: it often communicates with the former.
3. *The coracoid bursa*, situated near the root of the coracoid process; it is sometimes double and sometimes triple.
4. *The clavicula bursa*, found where the clavicle touches the coracoid process.
5. *The subclavian bursa*, between the tendon of the subclavius muscle and the first rib.
6. *The coraco-brachial*, placed between the common origin of this muscle and the biceps, and the capsular ligament.
7. *The bursa of the pectoralis major*, situated under the head of the humerus, between the internal surface of the tendon of that muscle, and another bursa placed on the long head of the biceps.
8. *An external bursa of the teres major*, under the head of the os humeri, between it and the tendon of the teres major.
9. *An internal bursa of the teres major*, found within the muscle where the fibres of its tendons diverge.
10. *A bursa of the latissimus dorsi*, between the tendon of this muscle and the os humeri.
11. *The humero-bicipital bursa*, in the vagina of the tendon of the biceps.

There are other bursæ mucosæ about the humerus, but their situation is uncertain.

Near the Elbow-joint

1. *The radio-bicipital* is situated between the tendon of the biceps, brachialis, and anterior tubercle of the radius.
2. *The cubito-radial* between the tendon of the biceps, supinator brevis, and the ligament common to the radius and ulna.
3. *The anconeal bursa*, between the olecranon and tendon of the anconous muscle.

4. *The capitulo-radial bursa*, between the tendon common to the extensor carpi radialis brevis, and extensor communis digitorum, and round head of the radius. There are occasionally other bursæ; but as their situation varies, they are omitted.

About the inferior part of the Fore-arm and Hand.

On the inside of the Wrist and Hand.

1. A very *large bursa*, for the tendon of the flexor pollicis longus.
2. *Four short bursæ* on the forepart of the tendons of the flexor sublimis.
3. *A large bursa* behind the tendon of the flexor pollicis longus, between it and the forepart of the radius, capsular ligament of the wrist and os trapezium.
4. *A large bursa* behind the tendons of the flexor digitorum profundus, and on the forepart of the end of the radius, and forepart of the capsular ligament of the wrist. In some subjects it communicates with the former.
5. *An oblong bursa* between the tendon of the flexor carpi radialis and os trapezium.
6. *A very small bursa* between the tendon of the flexor carpi ulnaris and os pisiforme.

On the back part of the Wrist and Hand.

7. *A bursa* between the tendon of the abductor pollicis longus and the radius.
8. *A large bursa* between the two extensores carpi radiales.
9. *Another* below it, common to the extensores carpi radiales.
10. *A bursa*, at the insertion of the tendon of the extensor carpi radialis.
11. *An oblong bursa*, for the tendon of the extensor pollicis longus, and which communicates with 9.
12. *A bursa*, for the tendon of the extensor pollicis longus, between it and the metacarpal bone of the thumb.
13. *A bursa* between the tendons of the extensor of the fore, middle, and ring fingers.
14. *A bursa* for the extensors of the little finger.
15. *A bursa* between the tendon of the extensor carpi ulnaris and ligament of the wrist.

There are also bursæ mucosæ between the musculi lumbricales and interossei.

Near the Hip-joint.

On the forepart of the joint.

1. *The ileo-puberal*, situated between the iliacus internus, psoas magnus, and the capsular ligament of the head of the femur.
2. *The pectineal*, between the tendon of the pectineus and the thigh-bone.
3. *A small bursa* of the gluteus mediu muscle, situated between it and the great trochanter, before the insertion of the pyriformis.
4. *A bursa* of the gluteus minimus muscle between its tendon and the great trochanter.
5. *The gluteo-fascial*, between the gluteu maximus and vastus externus.

On the posterior part of the Hip-joint.

6. *The tubero-ischiatic bursa*, situated between the obturator internus muscle, the posterior spine of the ischium, and its tuberosity.
7. *The obturatory bursa*, which is oblong and found between the obturator internu and gemini muscles, and the capsular ligament.
8. *A bursa of the semi-membranosu* under its origin and the long head of the biceps femoris.
9. *The gleuteo trochanteral bursa*, situated between the tendon of the psoas muscle and the root of the great trochanter.
10. *Two gluteo-femoral bursæ*, situated between the tendon of the gluteus maximus and os femoris.
11. *A bursa of the quadratus femoris*, situated between it and the little trochanter.
12. *The iliac bursa*, situated between the tendon of the iliacus internus and the little trochanter.

Near the Knee-joint.

1. *The suprá-genual*, which adheres to the tendons of the vastus and cruralis and the forepart of the thigh-bone.
2. *The infra-genual bursa*, situated under the ligament of the patella, and often communicating with the above.
3. *The anterior genual*, placed between the tendon of the sartorius, gracilis, and semitendinosus, and the internal and lateral ligament of the knee.
4. *The posterior genual*, which is sometimes double and is situated between the tendons of the semi-membranosus, the internal head of the gastrocnemius, the capsular ligament, and internal condyle.
5. *The popliteal*, conspicuous between the tendon of that muscle, the external condyle of the femur, the semilunar cartilage, and external condyle of the tibia.
6. *The bursa of the biceps cruris*, between the external part of the tendon, the biceps cruris, and the external lateral ligament of the knee.

In the Foot.

On the back, side, and hind part of the Foot

1. *A bursa of the tibialis anticus*, between its tendon, the lower part of the tibia, and capsular ligament of the ankle.
2. *A bursa* between the tendon of the extensor pollicis pedis longus, the tibia, and capsular ligament of the ankle.
3. *A bursa of the extensor digitorum communis*, between its tendons, the tibia, and ligament of the ankle.
4. *A large bursa*, common to the tendons of the peronei muscles.
5. *A bursa of the peroneus brevis*, proper to its tendon.
6. *The calcaneal bursa*, between the tendo Achillis and os calcis.

In the Sole of the Foot.

1. *A bursa for the tendon of the peroneus longus.*
2. *A bursa* common to the tendon of the flexor pollicis pedis longus, and the tendon of the flexor digitorum pedis communis longus profundus.
3. *A bursa of the tibialis posticus*, between its tendon, the tibia, and astragalus.
4. *Five bursæ for the flexor tendons*, which begin a little above the first joint of each toe, and extend to the root of the third phalanx, or insertion of the tendons.

BURSA'LIS. From its resemblance to a bursa, or purse. See *Obturator externus et internus*.

BURSA'LOGY. (*Bursalogia;* from βυρσα, a bag, and λογος, a discourse.) The doctrine of the bursæ mucosæ.

BUSELI'NUM. (From βου, great, and σελινον, parsley.) A large species of parsley.

Bu'ssii spiritus bezoardicus. The bezoardic spirit of Bussius, an eminent physician at Dresden A distillation of ivory, sal-ammoniac, amber, &c.

BUTCHERSBROOM. See *Ruscus*.

Bu'tiga. Small red pimples on the face. Called also *gutta rosacea*.

Bu'tino. Turpentine.

Bu'tomon. See *Iris pseudacorus*.

BUTTER. (*Butyrum;* from βους, a cow, and τυρος, *coagulum*, or cream.) "The oily, inflammable part of milk, which is prepared in many countries as an article of food. The common mode of preserving it is by the addition of salt, which will keep it good a considerable time, if in sufficient quantity. Mr. Eaton informs us, in his Survey of the Turkish Empire, that most of the butter used at Constantinople is brought from the Crimea and Kirban, and that it is kept sweet by melting it while fresh over a very slow fire, and removing the scum as it rises. He adds, that by melting butter in the Tartarian manner, and then salting it in ours, he kept it good and fine-tasted for two years; and that this melting, if carefully done, injures neither the taste nor colour. Thenard, too, recommends the Tartarian method. He directs the melting to be done on a water-bath, or at a heat not exceeding 180° F.; and to be continued until all the caseous matter has subsided to the bottom, and the butter is transparent. It is then to be decanted, or strained through a cloth, and cooled in a mixture of pounded ice and salt, or at least in cold spring water, otherwise it will become lumpy by crystallizing, and likewise not resist the action of the air so well. Kept in a close vessel, and in a cool place, it will thus remain, six months or more nearly as good as at first, particularly after the top is taken off. If beaten up with one-sixth of its weight of the cheesy matter when used, it will in some degree resemble fresh butter in appearance. The taste of rancid butter, he adds, may be much corrected by melting and cooling in this manner.

Dr. Anderson has recommended another mode of curing butter, which is as follows: Take one part of sugar, one of nitre, and two of the best Spanish great salt, and rub them together into a fine powder. This composition is to be mixed thoroughly with the butter, as soon as it is completely freed from the milk, in the proportion of one ounce to sixteen; and the butter thus prepared is to be pressed tight into the vessel prepared for it, so as to leave no vacuities. This butter does not taste well till it has stood at least a fortnight; it then has a rich marrow flavour, that no other butter ever acquires; and with proper care may be kept for years in this climate, or carried to the East Indies, if packed so as not to melt.

In the interior parts of Africa, Mr. Park informs us, there is a tree much resembling the American oak, producing a nut in appearance somewhat like an olive. The kernel of this nut, by boiling in water, affords a kind of butter, which is whiter, firmer, and of a richer flavour, than any he ever tasted made from cow's milk, and will keep without salt the whole year. The natives call it *shea toulou*, or tree butter. Large quantities of it are made every season."

Fresh butter is nourishing and relaxing, but it readily becomes sour, and, in general, agrees with few stomachs. Rancid butter is one of the most unwholesome and indigestible of all foods.

Butter of antimony. See *Murias antimonii.*

Butter of cacao. An oily concrete white matter, of a firmer consistence than suet, obtained from the cacao nut, of which chocolate is made. The method of separating it consists in bruising the cacao and boiling it in water. The greater part of the superabundant and uncombined oil contained in the nut is by this means liquefied, and rises to the surface, where it swims, and is left to congeal, that it may be the more easily taken off. It is generally mixed with small pieces of the nut, from which it may be purified, by keeping it in fusion without water in a pretty deep vessel, until the several matters have arranged themselves according to their specific gravities. By this treatment it becomes very pure and white.

Butter of cacao is without smell, and has a very mild taste, when fresh; and in all its general properties and habitudes it resembles fat oils, among which it must therefore be classed. It is used as an ingredient in pomatums.

BUTTER-BUR. See *Tussilago petasites.*

BUTTER-FLOWER. See *Ranunculus.*

Butter-milk. The thin and sour milk which is separated from the cream by churning it into butter.

BUTTERWORT. See *Pinguicula.*

[Button snake-root. See *Eryngium aquaticum.* A.]

Butua. See *Cissampelos pariera.*

BUTYRIC ACID. We owe the discovery of this acid to M. Chevreul. Butter, he says, is composed of two fat bodies, analogous to those of hog's lard, of a colouring principle, and a remarkably odorous one, to which it owes the properties that distinguish it from the fats, properly so called. This principle, which he has called butyric acid, forms well characterized salts with barytes, strontian, lime, the oxides of copper, lead, &c.; 100 parts of it neutralize a quantity of base which contains about 10 of oxygen. M. Chevreul has not explained his method of separating this acid from the other constituents of butter. See *Journ. de Pharmacie*, iii 80.

BUTY'RUM. See *Butter.*

Butyrum antimonii. See *Murias antimonii.*

BUXTON. A village in Derbyshire in which there are warm mineral springs. *Buxtonienses aquæ.* They have been long celebrated for their medicinal properties. With respect to sensible properties, the Buxton water cannot be distinguished from common spring water, when heated to the same temperature. Its temperature, in the gentleman's bath, is invariably 82°. The principal peculiarity in the appearance of this spring, is a large quantity of elastic vapour, that rises and forms bubbles, which pass through the water, and break as soon as they reach the surface. The air of these bubbles was ascertained, by Dr. Pearson, to consist of azotic gas, mixed with a small proportion of atmospheric air. Buxton water is frequently employed both internally and externally: one of which methods often proves beneficial when the other would be injurious: but, as a bath alone, its virtues may not be superior to those of tepid common water. As the temperature of 82° is several degrees below that of the human body, a slight shock of cold is felt on the first immersion into the bath; but this is almost immediately succeeded by a pleasing glow over the whole system. It is therefore proper for very delicate and irritable habits. The cases which derive most benefit from the *external* use of Buxton waters, are those in which a loss of action, and sometimes of sensation, affects particular limbs, in consequence of long-continued or violent inflammation, or external injury. Hence the chronic rheumatism succeeding the acute, and where the inflammation has been seated in particular limbs, is often wonderfully relieved by this bath. The *internal* use of the water has been found to be of considerable service in symptoms of defective digestion and derangement of the alimentary organs. A judicious use of this simple remedy will often relieve the heartburn, flatulency, and sickness; it will increase the appetite, animate the spirits, and improve the health. At first, however, it sometimes occasions a diarrhœa, which is rather salutary than detrimental; but costiveness is a more usual effect, especially in sluggish habits. It also affords great relief when taken internally, in painful disorders of the bladders and kidneys; and has likewise been recommended in cases of gout; but when taken for these complaints, the addition of some aromatic tincture is recommended. In all cases of active inflammation, the use of these waters should be carefully avoided, on account of their supposed heating properties. A full course consists of two glasses, each containing one-third of a pint, before breakfast; which quantity should be repeated between breakfast and dinner. In chronic cases, a long residence on the spot is requisite to insure the desired effect.

BU'XUS. (From πυκαζω, to become hard.) The box-tree. 1. The name of a genus of plants in the Linnæan system. Class, *Monœcia;* Order, *Triandria.*

2. The pharmacopœial name of the box. See *Buxus sempervirens.*

Buxus sempervirens. The systematic name of the *buxus* of the pharmacopœias. The leaves possess a very strong, nauseous, bitter taste, and aperient virtues. They are occasionally exhibited, in form of decoction, among the lower orders of people, in cases of dropsy, and asthma, and worms. As much as will lie upon a shilling, of the common dwarf box, dried and powdered, may be given at bed-time, every night, to an infant.

By'arus. A plexus of blood vessels in the brain.

Byng. A Chinese name for green tea.

Byre'thrum (*Beretta*, Ital. or *barette*, Fr. a cap.) *Byrethrus.* An odoriferous cap, filled with cephalic drugs, for the head.

By'rsa. (Βυρσα, leather.) A leather skin, to spread plasters upon.

Bysau'chen. (From βυω, to hide, and αυχην, the neck.) Morbid stiffness of the neck.

BYSSOLITE. A massive mineral of an olive green colour, found at the foot of Mount Blanc and near Oisans in gneiss.

By'ssus. (Hebrew.) 1. A woolly kind of moss

2. The Pudendum muliebre.

3. A kind of fine linen.

[4. The fine silky threads by which the *Mytilu* and *Pinna*, both bivalve shells, fasten themselves, and thereby remain attached to logs or stones in the water.

The Pinna affords the most and finest quantity of this byssus; and, in the Mediterranean, it has been collected and spun into silk, of which various ornamental articles have been made. A.]

By'thos. (Βυθος, deep.) An epithet used by Hippocrates for the bottom of the stomach.

By'zen. (From βυω, to rush together.) In a heap; throngingly. Hippocrates uses this word to express the hurry in which the menses flow in an excessive discharge.

C

CABALI'STICA ARS. (It is derived from the Hebrew word signifying to receive by tradition.) *Cabala; Cabula; Kabala.* The cabalistic art. A term that hath been anciently used, in a very mysterious sense, among divines; and since, some enthusiastic philosophers and chemists transplanted it into medicine, importing by it somewhat magical; but such unmeaning terms are now justly rejected.

Cabalistic art. See *Cabalistica ars.*

CABALLINE. (*Caballinus;* from καβαλλος, a horse.) Of, or belonging to, a horse; applied to the coarsest aloes, because it is so drastic as to be fit only for horses.

Caballine aloes. See *Aloe.*

CABBAGE. See *Brassica.*

Cabbage tree. See *Geoffræya jamaicensis.*

CACAGO'GA. (From κακκη, excrement, and αγω, to expel.) 1. Cathartics.

2. Ointments which, being rubbed on the fundament, procure stools.—*Paulus Æginefa.*

CACA'LIA. (From κακον, bad, and λιαν, exceedingly; because it is mischievous to the soil on which it grows.) *Cacamum.* The herb wild chervil, or wild carraways.

CA'CAMUM. See *Cacalia.*

CA'CAO. See *Theobroma cacao.*

CACAPHO'NIA. (From κακος, bad, and φωνη, the voice.) Defective articulation.

CACATO'RIA. (From *caco*, to go to stool.) An epithet given by Sylvius to a kind of intermittent fever, attended with copious stools.

CACCIO'NDE. A pill recommended by Baglivi against dysenteries; its basis is catechu.

CACHE'XIA. (From κακος, bad, and ἑξις, a habit.) A bad habit of body, known by a depraved or vitiated state of the solids and fluids.

CACHE'XIÆ. (The plural of *cachexia.*) A class of diseases in Cullen's Nosology, embracing three orders; viz. *Marcores, Intumescentiæ,* and *Impetigines.*

CACHINNA'TIO. (From *cachinno*, to laugh aloud.) A tendency to immoderate laughter, as in some hysteric and maniacal affections.

CA'CHLEX. A little stone, or pebble. Galen says, that the cachleces, heated in the fire and quenched in whey, become astringents, and useful in dysenteries.

CACHOLONG. A variety of quartz.

CACHO'RE. A name of catechu.

CA'CHRYS. (Καχρυς: which is used in various senses.) 1. Galen says, it sometimes means parched barley.

2. The name of a genus of plants in the Linnæan system. Class, *Pentandria;* Order, *Digynia.*

CACHRYS ODONTALGICA. A plant, the root of which may be substituted for that of the pyrethrum against toothache.

CACHU. See *Acacia catechu.*

CACHU'NDE. A medicine highly celebrated among the Chinese and Indians, made of several aromatic ingredients, perfumes, medicinal earths, and precious stones. They make the whole into a stiff paste, and form out of it several figures, according to their fancy, which are dried for use. These are principally used in the East Indies, but are sometimes brought over to Portugal. In China, the principal persons usually carry a small piece in their mouths, which is a continued cordial, and gives their breath a very sweet smell. It is highly esteemed as a medicine in nervous complaints; and it is reckoned a prolonger of life and a provocative to venery; the two great intentions of most of the medicines used in the East.

CACHY'MIA. Κακυμια. An imperfect metal, or an immature metalline ore, according to Paracelsus.

CACOALEXITE'RIUM. (From κακος, bad, and αλεξιτηρεω, to preserve.) An antidote to poison or against infectious diseases.

CACOCHO'LIA. (From κακος, and χολη, bile.) A vitiated or unhealthy condition of the bile.

CACOCHY'LIA. (From κακος, bad, and χυλη, the chyle.) Indigestion, or depraved chylification.

CACOCHY'MIA. (From κακος, bad, and χυμος, juice, or humour.) A diseased or depraved state of the humours.

CACOCNE'MUS. (From κακος, bad, and κνημη, the leg.) Having a natural defect in the tibia.

CACOCORE'MA. (From κακος, bad, and κορεω, to purge, or cleanse.) A medicine which purges off the vitiated humours.

CACODÆ'MON. (From κακος, bad, and δαιμων, a spirit.) An evil spirit, or genius, which was supposed to preside over the bodies of men, and afflict them with certain disorders. The nightmare.

CACO'DIA. (From κακος, bad, and ωζω, to smell.) A defect in the sense of smelling.

CACOE'THES. (From κακος, ill, and ηθος, a word which, when applied to diseases, signifies a quality, or a disposition.) Hippocrates applied this word to malignant and difficult distempers. Galen, and some others, express by it an incurable ulcer, that is rendered so through the acrimony of the humours flowing to it. Linnæus and Vogel use this term much in the same sense with Galen, and describe the ulcer as superficial, spreading, weeping, and with callous edges.

CACOPA'THIA. (From κακος, bad, and παθος, affection.) An ill affection of the body, or part.

CACOPHO'NIA. (From κακος, bad, and φωνη, the voice.) 1. A defect in the organs of speech.

2. A bad pronunciation.

CACOPRA'GIA. (From κακος, bad, and πραττω, to perform.) Diseased viscera.

CACORRY'THMUS. (From κακος, bad, and ρυθμος order.) A disordered pulse.

CACO'SIS. (From κακος, bad.) A bad disposition of body.

CACOSI'TIA. (From κακος, and σιτιον, food.) An aversion to food, or nausea.

CACOSPHY'XIA. (From κακος, bad, and σφυξις, pulse.) A disorder of the pulse.

CACOSTO'MACHUS. (From κακος, bad, and στομαχος, the stomach.) A bad or disordered stomach; applied also to food which the stomach rejects.

CACO'STOMUS. (From κακος, bad, and στομα, a mouth.) Having a bad formed, or disordered mouth.

CACOTHY'MIA. (From κακος, ill, and θυμος, the mind.) Any vicious disposition of the mind; or a diseased mind.

CACOTRO'PHIA. (From κακος, ill, and τροφη, nutriment.) 1. A vitiated nourishment.

2. A wasting of the body, from want of nutrition.

CA'CTUS. (From κακτος, the Greek name of a plant described by Theophrasta.) The name of a genus of plants in the Linnæan system. Class, *Icosandria;* Order, *Monogynia.* The melon-thistle, or prickly-pear.

CACTUS OPUNTIA. The systematic name of the *opuntia* of the pharmacopœias. The prickly leaves of this plant abound with a mucilaginous matter, which is esteemed in its native countries an emollient, in the form of poultice.

CACU'BALUS. (From κακος, evil, and βαλλω, to cast out; so named because it was thought to be efficacious in expelling poisons.) See *Cucubalus bacciferum.*

CA'CULE. The Arabian for cardamoms.

CACU'MEN. (*Cacumen, minis.* neut.) The top or point.

CADA'VER. (*Cadaver, veris.* neut., from *cado*, to fall: because the body, when deprived of life, falls to the ground.) A carcass, or body deprived of life.

CA'DMIA. (Hebrew.) The lapis calaminaris. See *Zinc.*

CADMIA METALLICA. A name given, by the Germans, to cobalt.

CADMIUM. "A new metal, first discovered by M. Stromeyer, in the autumn of 1817, in some carbonate of zinc which he was examining in Hanover. It has been since found in the Derbyshire silicates of zinc.

The following is Dr. Wollaston's process for procuring cadmium. From the solution of the salt of zinc supposed to contain cadmium, precipitate all the other metallic impurities by iron; filter and immerse a cylinder of zinc into the clear solution. If cadmium be present, it will be thrown down in the metallic state, and when redissolved in muriatic acid, will exhibit its peculiar character on the application of the proper tests.

M. Stromeyer's process consists in dissolving the substance which contains cadmium in sulphuric acid, and passing through the acidulous solution a current of sulphuretted hydrogen gas. He washes this precipitate, dissolves it in concentrated muriatic acid, and expels the excess of acid by evaporation. The residue is then dissolved in water, and precipitated by carbonate of ammonia, of which an excess is added, to redissolve the zinc and the copper that may have been precipitated by the sulphuretted hydrogen gas. The carbonate of cadmium being well washed, is heated, to drive off the carbonic acid, and the remaining oxide is reduced by mixing it with lamp-black, and exposing it to a moderate red heat in a glass or earthen retort.

The colour of cadmium is a fine white, with a slight shade of bluish-gray, approaching much to that of tin; which metal it resembles in lustre and susceptibility of polish. Its texture is compact, and its fracture hackly. It crystallizes easily in octohedrons, and presents on its surface, when cooling, the appearance of leaves of fern. It is flexible, and yields readily to the knife. It is harder and more tenacious than tin; and, like it, stains paper, or the fingers. It is ductile and malleable, but when long hammered, it scales off in different places. Its sp. grav. before hammering, is 8.6040; and when hammered, it is 8.6944. It melts, and is volatilized under a red heat. Its vapour, which has no smell, may be condensed in drops like mercury, which, on congealing, present distinct traces of crystallization.

Cadmium is as little altered by exposure to the air as tin. When heated in the open air, it burns like that metal, passing into a smoke, which falls and forms a very fixed oxide, of a brownish-yellow colour. Nitric acid readily dissolves it cold; dilute sulphuric, muriatic, and even acetic acids, act feebly on it with the disengagement of hydrogen. The solutions are colourless, and are not precipitated by water.

Cadmium forms a single oxide, in which 100 parts of the metal are combined with 14.352 of oxygen. The prime equivalent of cadmium deduced from this compound seems to be very nearly 7, and that of the oxide 8. This oxide varies in its appearance according to circumstances, from a brownish-yellow to a dark brown, and even a blackish colour. With charcoal it is reduced with rapidity below a red heat. It gives a transparent colourless glass bead with borax. It is insoluble in water, but in some circumstances forms a white hydrate, which speedily attracts carbonic acid from the air, and gives out its water when exposed to heat."—*Ure's Chem. Dict.*

CADOGAN, William, graduated at Oxford in 1755. Five years before, he had published a small treatise on the management of children, which was very much approved. In 1764, his "Dissertation on the Gout and all Chronic Diseases" appeared, which attracted considerable attention, being written in a popular style. He referred the gout principally to indolence, vexation, and intemperance; and his plan of treatment is generally judicious. He was a fellow of the London College of Physicians, and died in 1797, at an advanced age.

Cadtchu. See *Acacia catechu.*

CADU'CA. (From *cado*, to fall down.) See *Decidua.*

Caduci. The name of a class in Linnæus's Methodus calycina.

CADU'CUS. (From *cado*, to fall.) 1. *In Botany,* The falling off before the unfolding of the flower or leaf; as the *perianthium* of Papaver, the *stipulæ* of *Prunus avium.* This term is expressive of the shortest period of duration, and has different acceptations, according to the different parts of the plant to which it is applied. A calyx is said to be caducous, which drops at the first opening of the petals, or even before, as in the poppy. Petals are caducous, which are scarcely unfolded before they fall off, as in *Thalictrum;* and such leaves as fall off before the end of summer, have obtained this denomination. See *Deciduus* and *Parasiticus.*

2. The epilepsy or falling sickness is called *morbus caducus.*

CÆ'CITAS. (From *cæcus*, blind.) Blindness. See *Caligo* and *Amaurosis.*

CÆ'CUM. (From *cæcus*, blind: so called from its being perforated at one end only.) The cæcum, or blind gut. The first portion of the large intestines, placed in the right iliac region, about four fingers' breadth in length It is in this intestine that the ileum terminates by a valve, called the valve of the cæcum. The *appendicula cæci vermiformis* is also attached to it. See *Intestines.*

CÆ'LIUS, Aurelianus, is supposed to have been born at Sicca, in Africa, and is referred by Le Clerc to the fifteenth century, from the harshness of his style. He has left a Latin translation of the writings of Soranus, with additional observations, partly collected from others, partly from his own experience. The work is in eight books, three on acute, the rest on chronic disorders. He treats of several diseases not mentioned by any earlier writers, and has some observations in surgery peculiar to himself; he appears, too, generally correct in his remarks on the opinions of others.

Cæ'ros. Καιρος. Hippocrates, by this word, means the opportunity or moment in which whatever is to be effected should be done.

CÆSALPI'NA. (Named in honour of Cæsalpinus, chief physician to Pope Clement VIII.) The name of a genus of plants in the Linnæan system. Class, *Decandria;* Order, *Monogynia.*

Cæsalpina crista. The systematic name of the tree that affords the Brazil wood. It is of the growth of the Brazils in South America, and also of the Isle of France, Japan, and elsewhere. It is chiefly used as a red dye. See *Brazil wood.*

CÆSALPI'NUS, Andrew, was born in Tuscany, in 1519. He graduated at Pisa, and became professor in anatomy and medicine there; and was afterward made physician to Pope Clement VIII. He died in 1603. His works are numerous, and evince much genius and learning. In 1571, he published a work, defending the philosophy of Aristotle against the doctrines of Galen, from some passages in which he appears to have approached very near to a knowledge of the circulation of the blood; having explained the use of the valves of the heart, and pointed out the course which these compelled the blood to take on both sides during the contraction and dilatation of that organ. In a treatise "De Plantis," he justly compared the seeds to the eggs of animals; and formed an arrangement of them according to the parts of fructification. On medical subjects also he offered many judicious remarks.

CÆ'SARES. *Cæsones.* Children who are brought into the world as Julius Cæsar is said to have been. See *Cæsarian operation.*

CÆSA'RIAN OPERATION. (So called because Julius Cæsar is said to have been extracted in this manner.) *Hysterotomia. Hysterotomatocia.* The operation for extracting the fœtus from the uterus, by dividing the integuments of the abdomen and the uterus.

There are three cases in which this operation may be necessary.—1. When the fœtus is perceived to be alive, and the mother dies, either in labour or in the last two months. 2. When the fœtus is dead, but cannot be delivered in the usual way, from the deformity of the mother, or the disproportionate size of the child. 3. When both the mother and the child are living, but delivery cannot take place, from the same causes as in the second instance. Both the mother and the child, if accounts can be credited, have often lived after the Cæsarian operation, and the mother even borne children afterward. Heister gives a relation of such success, in his Institutes of Surgery; and there are some others. In England, the Cæsarian operation has almost always failed. Mr. James Barlow, of Chorley, Lancashire, succeeded, however, in taking a fœtus out of the uterus by this bold proceeding, and the mother was perfectly restored to health

Cæ'tchu. See *Acacia catechu.*

Caf; *Cafa; Caffa.* Names given by the Arabians to camphire.

CAFFEIN. The name of a bitter principle procured from coffee by Chenevix, by adding muriate of tin to an infusion of unroasted coffee. From this he obtained a precipitate, which he washed and decomposed by sulphuretted hydrogen. The supernatant liquid contained this principle, which occasioned a green precipitate in concentrated solutions of iron. When the liquid was evaporated to dryness, it was yellow and transparent, like horn. It did not attract moisture from the air, but was soluble in water and alkohol. The solution had a pleasant bitter taste, and assumed with alkalies a garnet-red colour. It is almost as delicate a test of iron as infusion of galls is; yet gelantine occasions no precipitate with it.

[" Caffein is a new principle, which was discovered in coffee by Robiquet. It is white, volatile, and crystallizable; and is particularly distinguished by the large quantity of nitrogen which it contains, being greater than that in almost any other vegetable. According to Dumas and Pelletier, it consists of 27 14 oxygen, 4.81 hydrogen, 46.51 carbon, and 21.54 nitrogen.—*Webster's Man. of Chem.* A.]

CAGA'STRUM. A barbarous term used by Paracelsus, to express the morbific matter which generates diseases.

CAITCHU. See *Acacia catechu.*

CAIUS, JOHN, was born at Norwich, in 1510. After studying at Cambridge, and in different parts of Italy, and distinguishing himself by his interpretations of Hippocrates, Galen, and other ancient authors, he graduated at Bologna. In 1544, he returned to this country, and for some time read lectures in anatomy to the corporation of surgeons in London. He afterward practised at Shrewsbury, having been admitted a fellow of the College of Physicians; and published a popular account of the memorable sweating sickness, which prevailed in 1551, subsequently reprinted, much improved, in Latin. He was made physician to Edward VI., to Mary, and to Elizabeth. On the death of Linacre, he was chosen President of the College of Physicians, and during the seven years for which he held that office, performed many important services. He was also a signal benefactor to Gonvil Hall, where he studied at Cambridge, having obtained permission to erect it into a college, considerably enlarging the building, and assigning provision for three fellows and twenty scholars. He was chosen master on the completion of the improvements, and retained that office till near the period of his death, which happened in 1573. He published a dissertation "De Canibus Britannicis," which Mr. Pennant has entirely followed in his British Zoology and some other learned works besides those already mentioned.

CA'JAN. See *Phascolus creticus.*

Ca'jeput oil. See *Melaleuca.*

CALA'BA. See *Catophyllum inophyllum.*

CALAGUA'LÆ RADIX. *Calaguelæ radix.* The root so called is knotty, and somewhat like that of the polypody tribe. It has been exhibited internally at Rome, with success, in dropsy; and it is said to be efficacious in pleurisy, contusions, abscesses, &c. It was first used in America, where it is obtained; and Italian physicians have since written concerning it, in terms of approbation.

CALAMA'CORUS. Indian reed.

CALAMAGRO'STIS. (From καλαμος, a reed, and αγρωστις, a sort of grass.) Reed grass. *Gramen Arundinacum.* The *Arundo calamagrostis* of Linnæus; the root of which is said to be diuretic and emmenagogue.

CALAMARIÆ. (From *calamus*, a reed.) The name of an order of Linnæus's fragments of a natural method, which embraces the reed-plants.

CALA'MBAC. An Indian name for agallochum. See *Lignum Aloes.*

CALAME'DON. (From καλαμος, a reed.) A sort of fracture which runs along the bone, in a straight line, like a reed, but is lunated in the extremity.

CA'LAMINA. See *Calamine.*

CALAMINA PRÆPARATA. Prepared calamine. Burn the calamine, and reduce it to powder; then let it be brought into the state of a very fine powder, in the same manner that chalk is directed to be prepared. See *Calamine.*

CA'LAMINE. (*Calamina;* from *calamus*, a reed: so called from its reed-like appearance.) *Cadmia; Cathmia; Cadmia lapidosa ærosa; Cadmia fossilis; Calamina; Lapis calaminaris.* A native carbonate of zinc. A mineral, containing oxide of zinc and carbonic acid, united with a portion of iron, and sometimes other substances. It is very heavy, moderately hard and brittle, of a gray, yellowish, red, or blackish brown; found in quarries of considerable extent, in several parts of Europe, and particularly in this country, in Derbyshire, Gloucestershire, Nottinghamshire, and Somersetshire; as also in Wales. The calamine of England is by the best judges, allowed to be superior in quality to that of most other countries. It seldom lies very deep, being chiefly found in clayey grounds near the surface. In some places it is mixed with lead ores. This mineral is an article in the materia medica; but, before it comes to the shops, it is usually roasted, or calcined, to separate some arsenical or sulphureous particles which, in its crude state, it is supposed to contain, and in order to render it more easily reducible into a fine powder. In this state, it is employed in collyria, for weak eyes, for promoting the cicatrization of ulcers, and healing excoriations of the skin. It is the basis of an officinal cerate, called Ceratum calaminæ by the London College, formerly called ceratum lapidis caliminaris, ceratum epuloticum; and ceratum carbonatis zinci impuri by the Edinburgh College. These compositions form the cerate which Turner strongly recommends for healing ulcerations and excoriations, and which have been popularly distinguished by his name. The collyria in which the prepared calamine has been employed, have consisted simply of that substance added to rose-water, or elder-flower water.

CALAMINT. See *Melissa calamintha.*

Calamint, mountain. See *Melissa grandiflora.*

CALAMI'NTHA. (From καλος, beautiful, or καλαμος, a reed, and μινθη, mint.) Common calamint. See *Melissa.*

CALAMINTHA ANGLICA. See *Melissa nepeta.*

CALAMINTHA HUMILIOR. The ground-ivy. See *Glecoma hederacea.*

CALAMINTHA MAGNA FLORE. See *Melissa grandiflora.*

CALAMINTHA MONTANA. See *Melissa Calamintha.*

CA'LAMUS. (From *Kalam*, an Arabian word.) 1. A general name denoting the stalk of any plant.

2. The name of a genus of plants in the Linnæan system. Class, *Hexandria;* Order, *Monogynia.*

CALAMUS AROMATICUS. See *Acorus calamus.*

[CALAMUS. Sweet flag-root. Acorus calamus, or calamus aromaticus. "The Acorus calamus is found in Europe, Asia, and North America. With us it grows in wet meadows, commonly in beds or bunches. The root has a strong aromatic odour, and a bitter spicy taste. Its properties depend upon a volatile oil, and a bitter matter soluble in water. Medicinally considered, it is stimulant, heating and tonic; and is given in flatulent colic, cramp of the stomach, &c., in the dose of a scruple and upwards."—*Big. Mat. Med.* A.]

CALAMUS AROMATICUS ASIATICUS. See *Acorus calamus.*

CALAMUS ODORATUS. The sweet-scented rush. See *Acorus calamus.*

CALAMUS ROTANG. The systematic name of the plant from which we obtain the Dragon's blood. *Cinnabaris græcorum; Draconthæma; Asegen; Asegon.* Dragon's blood. The red resinous juice which is obtained by wounding the bark of the *Calamus rotang;—caudice densissime aculeata, aculeis erectis, spadice erecto.* The *Petrocarpus draco* and *Dracæna draco* also afford this resin. It is chiefly obtained from the Molucca islands, Java, and other parts of the East Indies. It is generally much adulterated, and varied in goodness and purity. The best kind is of a dark red colour, which, when powdered, changes to crimson: it is insoluble in water, but soluble in a great measure in alkohol; it readily melts and catches flame, has no smell, but to the taste discovers some degree of warmth and pungency. The ancient Greeks were well acquainted with the adstringent power of this drug; in which character it has since been much employed in hæmorrhages, and in alvine fluxes. At present, however, it is not used internally, being superseded by more certain and effectual remedies of this numerous class.

CALAMUS SCRIPTORIUS. A furrow or kind of canal at the bottom of the fourth ventricle of the brain, so called from its resemblance to a writing pen.

CALAMUS VULGARIS. See *Acorus calamus.*

CALATHIANA. (From καλαθος, a twig basket; so called from the shape of its flowers.) The herb marsh-gentian. See *Gentiana pneumonanthe.*

CALBI'ANUM. The name of a plaster in Myrepsus.

CALCA'DINUM. Vitriol.

CALCA'DIS. An Arabian name for white vitriol and alkali.

CALCA'NEUM. (From *calx*, the heel.) *Calcar pterna; Os calcis.* The largest bone of the tarsus, which forms the heel. It is situated posteriorly under the astragalus, is very regular, and divided into a body and processes. It has a large *tuberosity* or knob, projecting behind to form the heel. A *sinuous cavity*, as its fore-part, which, in the fresh subject, is filled with fat, and gives origin to several ligaments. Two *prominences*, at the inner and fore-part of the bone, with a pit between them, for the articulation of the under and fore-part of the astragalus. A *depression*, in the external surface of the bone near its fore-part, where the tendon of the peronæus longus runs. A large *cavity*, at the inner side of the bone, for lodging the long flexors of the toes, together with the vessels and nerves of the sole. There are two *prominences*, at the under and back part of this bone, that give origin to the aponeurosis, and several muscles of the sole. The anterior surface of the os calcis is concave, for its articulation with the os cuboides, and it is articulated to the astragalus by ligaments.

CALCAN'THUM. (From χαλκος, brass, and ανθος, a flower; i. e. flowers of brass.) *Calcanthos.* Copperas; Vitriol.

CALCAR. (*Calcar, aris.* n. From *calx*, the heel; also from *caleo*, to heat.) 1. The heel-bone.

2. The furnace of a laboratory.

3. A spur. In botany, applied to a part of the ringent and personate corolla of plants. It is a tube forming an obtuse or acute sac, at the side of the receptacle. It is of rare occurrence.

CALCARATUS. Spurred; applied to the corols and nectaries of plants; as *Calcarata corolla, Nectarium calcaratum;* as in *Aquilegia* and *Antirrhinum linaria.*

CALCAREOUS. (*Calcarius;* from *calx*, lime.) That which partakes somewhat of the nature and qualities of *calx*.

Calcareous earth. See *Calx and Lime.*

CALCAREOUS SPAR. Crystallized carbonate of lime, which occurs in more than 600 different forms. It is found in veins in all rocks from granite to alluvial strata. The rarest and most beautiful crystals are found in Derbyshire, but it exists in every part of the world.

CALCA'RIS FLOS. The larkspur.

CALCA'RIUS. See *Calcareous.*

CALCARIUS LAPIS. Limestone.

CA'LCATAR. A name of vitriol.

CALCATRI'PPA. See *Ajuga pyramidalis.*

CALCEDONY. A mineral, so called from Calcedon, in Asia Minor, where it was found in ancient times. There are several sub-species, common calcedony, heliotrope, crysoprase, plasma, onyx, sand, and sardonyx.

Common calcedony occurs of various colours; it is regarded as pure silica with a little water. Very fine stalactical specimens have been found in Cornwall and Scotland.

CA'LCEUM EQUINUM. (From *calceus*, a shoe, and *equus*, a horse; so called from the figure of its leaf.) The herb colt's-foot. See *Tussilago farfara.*

CALCHANTRUM. Pliny's name for copperas.

CALCHI'THEOS. (From καλχιον, purple.) Verdigris.

CALCI'FRAGA. (From *calx*, a stone, and *frango*, to break; so named from its supposed property of breaking the human calculus.) Breakstone. In *Scribonius Largus*, it means, the herb spleenwort, or *scolopendrium;* others mean by it the *Pimpinella saxifraga* of Linnæus.

CALCINA'TION. Oxidation. The fixed residues of such matters as have undergone combustion are called cinders, in common language, and calces, but now more commonly oxides, by chemists; and the operation, when considered with regard to these residues, is termed calcination. In this general way, it has likewise been applied to bodies not really combustible, but only deprived of some of their principles by heat. Thus we hear of the calcination of chalk, to convert it into lime by driving off its carbonic acid and water; of gypsum, or plaster-stone, of alum, of borax, and other saline bodies, by which they are deprived of their water of crystallization; of bones which lose their volatile parts by this treatment, and of various other bodies.

CALCINA'TUS. Calcined.

CALCINATUM MAJUS. Whatever is dulcified by the chemical art, which was not so by nature; such as dulcified mercury, lead, and the like substances, which are very speedily consolidated.

CALCINATUM MAJUS POTERII. Mercury dissolved in aqua fortis, and precipitated with salt water. Poterius used it in the cure of ulcers.

CALCINATUM MINUS. Any thing which is sweet by nature, and speedily cures, as sugar, manna, tamarinds, &c.

CALCINO'NIA. See *Calcena.*

CA'LCIS AQUA. See *Calcis liquor.*

CA'LCIS LIQUOR. Solution of lime, formerly called *aqua calcis.* Lime-water. Take of lime, half a pound; boiling distilled water, twelve pints. Pour the water upon the lime, and stir them together; next cover the vessel immediately, and let it stand for three hours; then keep the solution upon the remaining lime in stopped glass bottles, and pour off the clear liquor when it is wanted for use.

Lime is soluble in about 450 times its weight of water, or little more than one grain in one fluid ounce It is given internally, in doses of two ounces and upwards, in cardialgia, spasms, diarrhœa, &c. and in proportionate doses in convulsions of children, arising from acidity, or ulcerated intestines, intermittent fevers, &c. Externally it is applied to burns and ulcers.

CALCIS MURIAS. *Calx solita; Sal ammoniacus fixus.* Muriate of lime. Take of the salt remaining after the sublimation of subcarbonate of ammonia two pounds, water a pint; mix and filter through paper. Evaporate the salt to dryness; and preserve it in a closely-stopped vessel. This preparation is exhibited with the same views as the muriate of barytes. It possesses deobstruent, diuretic, and cathartic virtues, and is much used by the celebrated Fourcroy against scrophula, and other analogous diseases. Six, twelve, and twenty grains, are given to children, three times a day, and a drachm to adults.

CALCIS MURIATIS LIQUOR. Take of muriate of lime two ounces, distilled water three fluid ounces; dissolve the salt in the water, and filter it through paper.

CA'LCIS OS. See *Calcaneum.*

CALCIS VIVI FLORES. The pellicle on the surface of lime water.

CALCITRA'PA. (An old botanical term of similar meaning to *tribulus*, compounded of *calco*, to tread or kick, and τρεπω, to turn, because the caltrops are continually kicked over, if they fail of their intended mischief. See *Trapa.*) See *Centaurea calcitrapa.*

CALCITRAPA OFFICINALIS. See *Centaurea solstitiales.*

CALCIUM. The metallic basis of lime. Sir H. Davy, the discoverer of this metal, procured it by the process which he used for obtaining *barium.* It was in such small quantities, that little could be said concerning its nature. It appeared brighter and whiter than either barium or strontium; and burned when gently heated, producing dry lime.

There is only one known combination of calcium and oxygen, which is the important substance called lime. The nature of this substance is proved by the phenomena of the combustion of calcium; the metal changing into the earth with the absorption of oxygen gas. When the amalgam of calcium is thrown into water, hydrogen gas is disengaged, and the water becomes a solution of lime. From the quantity of hydrogen evolved, compared with the quantity of lime formed in experiments of this kind, M. Berzelius endeavoured to ascertain the proportion of oxygen in lime. The nature of lime may also be proved by analysis. When potassium in vapour is sent through the earth ignited to whiteness, the potassium was found by Sir H. Davy to become potassa, while a dark gray substance of metallic splendour, which is calcium, either wholly or partially deprived of oxygen, is found imbedded in the potassa; for it effervesces violently, and forms a solution of lime by the action of water.

CALCSINTER. Stalactitical carbonate of lime, which is continually forming by the infiltration of carbonated lime water through the crevices of the roofs of caverns. The irregular masses on the bottoms of caves have been called *stalagmites.*

CALCTUFF. An alluvial formation of carbonate of lime, probably deposited from calcareous springs of a yellowish dull gray colour, containing impressions of vegetable matter.

CALCULI'FRAGUS. (From *calculus*, a stone, and *frango*, to break.) Stone-breaker, having the power to break stone in the human body. 1. A synonym of lithontriptic. See *Lithontriptic.*

2. The scolopendrium, and pimpernel. See *Calcifraga*

CA'LCULUS. (Diminutive of *calx*, a lime-stone. *Calculus humanus; Bezoar microcosmicum.* Gravel; Stone. In English we understand by *gravel*, small sand-like concretions, or stones, which pass from the kidneys through the ureters in a few days; and by *stone*, a calculous concretion in the kidneys, or bladder, of too large a size to pass, without great difficulty. Similar concretions are found occasionally in other cavities or passages. When a disposition to form minute calculi or gravel exists, we often find nephritic paroxysms, as they are called, (see *Nephritis*) which consist of pain in the back, shooting down through the pelvis to the thighs; sometimes a numbness in one leg, and a retraction of either testicle in men, symptoms arising from the irritation of a stone passing through the ureters, as these cross the spermatic cord, on the nerves passing to the lower extremities. These pains, often violent, are terminated by the painful discharge of small stones through the urethra, and the patient is for a time easy. What, however, is meant by the stone is a more serious and violent disease. It is singular that these discharges of small gravel do not usually terminate in stone. Many have experienced them during a long life, without any more serious inconvenience: while the latter is a disease chiefly of the young, and depending on circumstances not easily explained. If the stone attacks persons more advanced in age, it is often the consequence of paroxysms of gout, long protracted, and terminating imperfectly.

When once a stone has acquired a moderate size, it usually occasions the following symptoms:—frequent inclination to make water, excessive pain in voiding it drop by drop, and sometimes a sudden stoppage of it, if discharged in a stream; after making water, great torture in the glans penis, which lasts one, two, or three minutes; and, in most constitutions, the violent straining makes the rectum contract and expel its excrements; or, if it be empty, occasions a tenesmus, which is sometimes accompanied with a prolapsus ani. The urine is often tinctured with blood, from a rupture of the vessels, and sometimes pure blood itself is discharged. Sometimes the urine is very clear, but frequently there are great quantities of slimy sediment deposited at the bottom of it, which is only a preternatural separation of the mucilage of the bladder, but has often been mistaken for pus. The stone is a disease to which both sexes and all ages are liable; and calculi have even been found in the bladders of very young children, nay, of infants only six months old.

Women seem less subject to this complaint than men, either owing to constitutional causes, or to the capaciousness, shortness, and straightness of their urethræ, allowing the calculi to be discharged while small, together with the urine.

The Seat and Physical Properties of Urinary Calculi.

Calculi are found in different parts of the urinary system, in the pelvis of the kidney, in the ureters, in the bladder and urethra; but as they, for the most part, originate in the kidney, the calculi renales make the nucleus of the greatest number of urinary stones. The *calculi renales* differ greatly with respect to their external qualities; for the most part, however, they consist of small, concrete, roundish, smooth, glossy, and crystalline bodies, of a red-yellow colour, like that of wood, and so hard as to admit of polishing. On account of their minuteness, they easily pass through the urinary passages in form of gravel, which being sometimes of a rough surface, cause several complaints on their passage. But in some instances they are of too great a size to be able to pass along the ureters; in which case they increase in the kidneys, sometimes to a great size. Calculi renales of this kind are generally of a brown, dark red, or black colour, and surrounded with several strata of coagulated blood and pus; they have also been observed of a yellow, reddish, and lighter colour; and some consisting of a homogeneous stony mass, but white or gray calculi renales are very rarely to be met with. Among the great number that were examined, one or two only were found of a gray or blackish colour, and of a composition similar to those which generally bear the name of mulberry-like stones.

The stones in the ureters, which, on passing into the ureters, are prevented by their size from descending into the bladder, frequently increase very much: they however, rarely occur; their colour is white, and they consist of phosphate of lime.

The stones in the bladder are the most frequent urinary concrements that have been principally examined; they draw their first origin from the kidneys, whence they descend into the bladder, where they increase; or they immediately originate and increase in the bladder; or they arise from a foreign body that by chance has got into the bladder, which not unfrequently happens, particularly in the female sex. Concretions of this kind differ greatly in their respective physical qualities and external form, which, however, is generally spherical, oval, or compressed on both sides; and sometimes, when there are several stones in the bladder, they have a polyhedrous or cubical form; their extremities are frequently pointed or roundish, but they are very seldom found cylindrical, and more rarely with cylindrical ends.

There is a great variety in the size of the calculi, and likewise in their colour, which is materially different, according to their respective nature and composition. They occur, 1. of a yellowish colour, approaching nearly to red, or brown; such stones consist of lithic acid. 2. Gray, or more or less white; these stones always contain phosphates of earths. 3. Dark gray, or blackish; stones of this colour have oxalates of earths. Many stones show brown or gray spots, on a yellow or white ground, generally raised on the surface, and consisting of oxalate of lime, which is enclosed in lithic acid, when the ground colour of the stone is of a wood colour, or in phosphate of lime, when it is white. These spots are, in general, only to be observed in the middle of the stone, or at one of its extremities.

All that is here stated, is the result of observations on more than 600 calculi; and different other colours, that are said to have been observed, either arise from heterogeneous substances, or are merely variations of the above colours. Their surface is smooth and polished in some; in others, only smooth; and in others uneven, and covered with rough or smooth corpuscles, which are always of a yellow colour; in some, the surface is partly smooth and partly rough. The white ones are frequently even and smooth, half transparent, and covered with shining crystals, that generally indicate phosphate of ammonia, with magnesia; or they are faint, and consist of minute grains; or rough, in which case they consist of phosphate of lime. The brown and dark gray stones are, from their similarity to mulberries, called mulberry-stones, and being frequently very rugged, they cause the most pain of all.

On examining the specific weight of urinary calculi in more than 500 specimens, it was found to be, in the lightest, as 1213.1000, in the heaviest, as 1976.1000. Their smell is partly strong, like urine or ammonia, partly insipid, and terreous; especially the white ones, which are like sawed ivory, or rasped bone.

The internal texture of calculi is but seldom guessed from their external appearance, particularly when they exceed the size of a pigeon's egg. On breaking them, they generally separate into two or three strata, more or less thick and even, which prove that they are formed by different precipitations, at different times. In the middle, a nucleus is generally seen, of the same mass as the rest. When the place they are broken at is finely streaked, and of a yellow or reddish colour, the lithic acid predominates; but when they are half transparent, luminous like spar, they have ammoniacal phosphate of magnesia in them, and phosphate of lime, and then they are brittle and friable; but when they are so hard as to resist the instrument, of a smooth surface, and a smell like ivory, they contain oxalate of lime. It frequently happens, that the exterior stratum consists of white phosphate of earth, while the nucleus is yellow lithic acid, or oxalate of lime, covered sometimes with a yellow stratum of lithic acid, in which case the nucleus appears radiant; but when it consists of lithic acid, and is covered with white phosphate of earth, it is roundish, oval, and somewhat crooked. These concretions have very seldom three strata; namely, on the outside a phosphate, towards the inside lithic acid, and quite withinside an oxalate of lime; but still rarer these substances occur in more strata, or in another order, as before-mentioned.

Stones of the urethra are seldom generated in the urethra itself; however, there are instances of their having been formed in the fossa navicularis, by means of foreign bodies that have got into the urethra. We also very frequently observe stony concretements deposited between the glans and prepuce. All the concretions produced in the inside and outside the urethra consist of phosphate of earths, which are easily precipitated from the urine. There are likewise stones in the urethra which have come out of the bladder, having been produced there, or in the kidneys; and they generally possess the properties of stones of the kidneys.

The different constituents of Urinary Calculi.

"If we except Scheele's original observation concerning the uric or lithic acid, all the discoveries relating to urinary concretions are due to Dr. Wollaston; discoveries so curious and important, as alone are sufficient to entitle him to the admiration and gratitude of mankind. They have been fully verified by the subsequent researches of Fourcroy, Vauquelin, and Brande, Drs. Henry, Marcet, and Prout. Dr. Marcet, in his late valuable essay on the chemical history and medical treatment of calculous disorders, arranges the concretions into nine species.

1. The lithic acid calculus.
2. The ammonia-magnesian phosphate calculus.
3. The bone earth calculus, or phosphate of lime.
4. The fusible calculus, a mixture of the 2d and 3d species.
5. The mulberry calculus, or oxalate of lime.
6. The cystic calculus; cystic oxide of Dr. Wollaston.
7. The alternating calculus, composed of alternate layers of different species.
8. The compound calculus, whose ingredients are so intimately mixed, as to be separable only by chemical analysis.
9. Calculus from the prostate gland, which, by Dr. Wollaston's researches, is proved to be phosphate of lime, not distinctly stratified, and tinged by the secretion of the prostate gland.

To the above Dr. Marcet has added two new sub-species. The first seems to have some resemblance to the cystic oxide, but it possesses also some marks of distinction. It forms a bright lemon yellow residuum on evaporating its nitric acid solution, and is composed of laminæ. But the cystic oxide is not laminated, and it leaves a white residuum from the nitric acid solution. Though they are both soluble in acids as well as alkalies, yet the oxide is more so in acids than the new calculus, which has been called by Dr. Marcet, from its yellow residuum, *xanthic* oxide. Dr. Marcet's other new calculus was found to possess the properties of the fibrin of the blood, of which it seems to be a deposite. He terms it *fibrinous* calculus.

Species 1. *Uric acid calculi.* Dr. Henry says, in his instructive paper on urinary and other morbid concretions, read before the Medical Society of London, March 2, 1819, that it has never yet occurred to him to examine calculi composed of this acid in a state of absolute purity. They contain about 9-10ths of the pure acid, along with urea, and an animal matter which is not gelatin, but of an albuminous nature. This must not, however, be regarded as a cement. The calculus is aggregated by the cohesive attraction of the lithic acid itself. The colour of lithic acid calculi is yellowish or reddish-brown, resembling the appearance of wood. They have commonly a smooth, polished surface, a lamellar or radiated structure, and consist of fine particles well compacted. Their specific gravity varies from 1.3 to 1.8. They dissolve in alkaline lixivia, without evolving an ammoniacal odour, and exhale the smell of horn before the blowpipe. The relative frequency of lithic acid calculi will be seen from the following statement. Of 150 examined by Mr. Brande, 16 were composed wholly of this acid, and almost all contained more or less of it. Fourcroy and Vauquelin found it in the greater number of 500 which they analyzed. All those examined by Scheele consisted of it alone; and 300 analyzed by Dr. Pearson, contained it in greater or smaller proportion. According to Dr. Henry's experience, it constitutes 10 urinary concretions out of 26, exclusive of the alternating calculi. And Mr. Brande lately states, that out of 58 cases of *kidney* calculi, 51 were lithic acid, 6 oxalic and 1 cystic.

Species 2. *Ammonia-magnesian phosphate.* This calculus is white like chalk, is friable between the fingers, is often covered with dog-tooth crystals, and contains semi-crystalline layers. It is *insoluble* in alkalies, but soluble in nitric, muriatic, and acetic acids. According to Dr. Henry, the earthy phosphates, comprehending the 2d and 3d species, were to the whole number of concretions, in the ratio of 10 to 85. Mr. Brande justly observes, in the 16th number of his Journal, that the urine has at all times a tendency to deposite the triple phosphate upon any body over which it passes. Hence drains by which urine is carried off, are often incrusted with its regular crystals; and in cases where extraneous bodies have got into the bladder, they have often in a very short time become considerably enlarged by deposition of the same substance. When this calculus, or those incrusted with its semi-crystalline particles, are strongly heated before the blowpipe, ammonia is evolved, and an imperfect fusion takes place. When a little of the calcareous phosphate is present, however, the concretion readily fuses. Calculi composed *entirely* of the ammonia-magnesian phosphate are very rare. Mr. Brande has seen only two. They were crystallized upon the surface, and their fracture was somewhat foliated. In its pure state, it is even rare as an incrustation. The powder of the ammonia-phosphate calculus has a brilliant white colour, a faint sweetish taste, and is somewhat soluble in water. Fourcroy and Vauquelin suppose the above deposites to result from incipient putrefaction of urine in the bladder. It is certain that the triple phosphate is copiously precipitated from urine in such circumstances out of the body.

Species 3. The *bone earth calculus.* Its surface, according to Dr. Wollaston, is generally pale brown, smooth, and when sawed through it appears of a laminated texture, easily separable into concentric crusts. Sometimes, also, each lamina is striated in a direction perpendicular to the surface, as from an assemblage of crystalline needles. It is difficult to fuse this calculus by the blowpipe, but it dissolves readily in dilute muriatic acid, from which it is precipitable by ammonia. This species, as described by Fourcroy and Vauquelin, was white, without lustre, friable, staining the hands, paper, and cloth. It had much of a chalky appearance, and broke under the forceps, and was intimately mixed with a gelatinous matter, which is left in a membraneous form, when the earthy salt is withdrawn by dilute muriatic acid. Dr. Henry says, that he has never been able to recognise a calculus of pure phosphate of lime in any of the collections which he has examined; nor did he ever find the preceding species in a pure state, though a calculus in Mr. White's collection contained more than 90 per cent. of ammonia-magnesian phosphate.

Species 4. The *fusible calculus.* This is a very friable concretion, of a white colour, resembling chalk in appearance and texture; it often breaks into layers, and exhibits a glittering appearance internally, from intermixture of the crystals of triple phosphate. Sp. grav. from 1.14 to 1.47. Soluble in dilute muriatic and nitric acids, but not in alkaline lixivia. The nucleus is generally lithic acid. In 4 instances only out of 187, did Dr. Henry find the calculus composed throughout of the earthy phosphates. The analysis of fusible calculus is easily performed by distilled vinegar, which at a gentle heat dissolves the ammonia-magnesian phosphate, but not the phosphate of lime; the latter may be taken up by dilute muriatic acid. The lithic acid present will remain, and may be recognised by its solubility in the water of pure potassa or soda. Or the lithic acid may, in the first instance, be removed by the alkali, which expels the ammonia, and leaves the phosphate of magnesia and lime.

Species 5. The *mulberry calculus.* Its surface is rough and tuberculated; colour deep reddish-brown. Sometimes it is pale brown, of a crystalline texture, and covered with flat octohedral crystals. This calculus has commonly the density and hardness of ivory, a sp. grav. from 1.4 to 1.98, and exhales the odour of semen when sawed. A moderate red heat converts it into carbonate of lime. It does not dissolve in alkaline lixivia, but slowly and with difficulty in acids. When the oxalate of lime is voided directly after leaving the kidney, it is of a grayish-brown colour.

composed of small cohering spherules, sometimes with a polished surface resembling hempseed. They are easily recognised by their insolubility in muriatic acid, and their swelling up and passing into pure lime before the blowpipe. Mulberry calculi contain always an admixture of other substances besides oxalate of lime. These are, uric acid, phosphate of lime, and animal matter in dark flocculi. The colouring matter of these calculi is probably effused blood. Dr. Henry rates the frequency of this species at 1 in 17 of the whole which he has compared; and out of 187 calculi, he found that 17 were formed round *nuclei* of oxalate of lime.

Species 6. The *cystic-oxide calculus.* It resembles a little the triple phosphate, or more exactly magnesian limestone. It is somewhat tough when cut, and has a peculiar greasy lustre. Its usual colour is pale brown, bordering on straw yellow; and its texture is irregularly crystalline. It unites in solution with acids and alkalies, crystallizing with both. Alkohol precipitates it with nitric acid. It does not become red with nitric acid; and it has no effect upon vegetable blues. Neither water, alkohol, nor ether dissolves it. It is decomposed by heat into carbonate of ammonia and oil, leaving a minute residuum of phosphate of lime. This concretion is of very rare occurrence. Dr. Henry states its frequency to the whole as 10 to 985. In two which he examined, the nucleus was the same substance with the rest of the concretion; and in a third, the nucleus of a uric acid calculus was a small spherule of cystic oxide. Hence, as Dr. Marcet has remarked, this oxide appears to be in reality the production of the kidneys, and not, as its name would import, to be generated in the bladder. It might be called with propriety *renal* oxide, if its eminent discoverer should think fit.

Species 7. The *alternating calculus.* The surface of this calculus is usually white like chalk, and friable or semicrystalline, according as the exterior coat is the calcareous or ammonia-magnesian phosphate. They are frequently of a large size, and contain a nucleus of lithic acid. Sometimes the two phosphates form alternate layers round the nucleus. The above are the most common alternating calculi; next are those of oxalate of lime with phosphates; then oxalate of lime with lithic acid; and lastly, those in which the three substances alternate. The alternating, taken all together, occur in 10 out of 25, in Dr. Henry's list; lithic acid with phosphates, as 10 to 48; the oxalate of lime with phosphates, as 10 to 116; the oxalate of lime with lithic acid, as 10 to 170; the oxalate of lime with lithic acid and phosphates, as 10 to 265.

Species 8. The *compound calculus.* This consists of a mixture of lithic acid with the phosphates in variable proportions, and is consequently variable in its appearance. Sometimes the alternating layers are so thin as to be undistinguishable by the eye, when their nature can be determined only by chemical analysis. This species, in Dr. Henry's list, forms 10 in 235. About 1-40th of the calculi examined by Fourcroy and Vauquelin were compound.

Species 9 has been already described.

In almost all calculi, a central nucleus may be discovered, sufficiently small to have descended through the ureters into the bladder. The disease of stone is to be considered, therefore, essentially and originally as belonging to the kidneys. Its increase in the bladder may be occasioned, either by exposure to urine that contains an excess of the same ingredient as that composing the nucleus, in which case it will be uniformly constituted throughout; or if the morbid nucleus deposite should cease, the concretion will then acquire a coating of the earthy phosphates. It becomes, therefore, highly important to ascertain the nature of the most predominate nucleus. Out of 187 calculi examined by Dr. Henry, 17 were formed round nuclei of oxalate of lime; 3 round nuclei of cystic oxide; 4 round nuclei of the earthy phosphates; 2 round extraneous substances; and in 3 the nucleus was replaced by a small cavity, occasioned, probably, by the shrinking of some animal matter, round which the ingredients of the calculi (fusible) had been deposited. Rau has shown by experiment, that pus may form the nucleus of a urinary concretion. The remaining 158 calculi of Dr. Henry's list, had central nuclei composed chiefly of lithic acid. It appears also, that in a very great majority of the cases referred to by him, the disposition to secrete an excess of lithic acid has been the essential cause of the origin of stone. Hence it becomes a matter of great importance to inquire, what are the circumstances which contribute to its excessive production, and to ascertain by what plan of diet and medicine this morbid action of the kidney may best be obviated or removed. A calculus in Mr. White's collection had for its nucleus a fragment of a bougie, that had slipped into the bladder. It belonged to the fusible species, consisting of,

20 phosphate of lime,
60 ammonia-magnesian phosphate,
10 lithic acid,
10 animal matter.
—
100

In some instances, though these are comparatively very few, a morbid secretion of the earthy phosphates in excess, is the cause of the formation of stone. Dr. Henry relates the case of a gentleman, who, during paroxysms of gravel, preceded by severe sickness and vomiting, voided urine as opaque as milk, which deposited a great quantity of an impalpable powder, consisting of the calcareous and triple phosphate in nearly equal proportions. The weight of the body was rapidly reduced from 188 to 100 pounds, apparently by the abstraction of the earth of his bones; for there was no emaciation of the muscles corresponding to the above diminution.

The first rational views on the treatment of calculous disorders, were given by Dr. Wollaston. These have been followed up lately by some very judicious observations of Mr. Brande, in the 12th, 15th, and 16th numbers of his Journal; and also by Dr. Marcet, in his excellent treatise already referred to. Of the many substances contained in human urine, there are rarely more than three which constitute gravel; viz. calcareous phosphate, ammonia-magnesian phosphate, and lithic acid. The former two form a white sediment; the latter, a red or brown. The urine is always an acidulous secretion. Since by this excess of acid, the earthy salts, or white matter, are held in solution, whatever disorder of the system, or impropriety of food and medicine, diminishes that acid excess, favours the formation of the white deposite. The internal use of acids was shown by Dr. Wollaston to be the appropriate remedy in this case.

White gravel is frequently symptomatic of disordered digestion, arising from excess in eating or drinking; and it is often produced by too farinaceous a diet. It is also occasioned by the indiscreet use of magnesia, soda water, or alkaline medicines in general. Medical practitioners, as well as their patients, ignorant of chemistry, have often committed fatal mistakes, by considering the white gravel, passed on the administration of alkaline medicines, as the dissolution of the calculus itself; and have hence pushed a practice, which has rapidly increased the size of the stone. Magnesia, in many cases, acts more injuriously than alkali, in precipitating insoluble phosphate from the urine. The acids of urine, which, by their excess, hold the earths in solution, are the phosphoric, lithic, and carbonic. Mr. Brande has uniformly obtained the latter acid, by placing urine under an exhausted receiver; and he has formed carbonate of barytes, by dropping barytes water into urine recently voided.

The appearance of white sand does not seem deserving of much attention, where it is merely occasional, following indigestion brought on by an accidental excess. But if it invariably follows meals, and if it be observed in the urine, not as a mere deposite, but at the time the last drops are voided, it becomes a matter of importance, as the forerunner of other and serious forms of the disorder. It has been sometimes viewed as the *effect* of irritable bladder, where it was in reality the *cause.* Acids are the proper remedy, and unless some peculiar tonic effect be sought for in sulphuric acid, the vegetable acids ought to be preferred. Tartar, or its acid, may be prescribed with advantage, but the best medicine is citric acid, in daily doses from 5 to 30 grains. Persons returning from warm climates, with dyspeptic and hepatic disorders, often void this white gravel, for which they have recourse to empyrical solvents, for the most part alkaline, and are deeply injured. They ought to adopt an acidulous diet, abstaining from soda water, alkalies, malt liquor, madeira, and port; to eat salads, with acid fruits; and if habit requires it, a glass of cider, champagne, or claret, but the less of these fermented liquors the better. An effervescing draught is often very beneficial, made by dissolving 30 grains of bicarbonate of potassa, and 20 of citric acid, in separate teacups of water, mixing the solution in a large tumbler, and drinking the whole during the effervescence. This dose may be repeated 3 or 4 times a-day. The carbonic acid of the above medicine enters the circulation, and passing off by the bladder, is useful in retaining, particularly, the triple phosphate in solution, as was first pointed out by Dr. Wollaston. The bowels should be kept regular by medicine and moderate exercise. The febrile affections of children are frequently attended by an apparently formidable deposite of white sand in the urine. A dose of calomel will generally carry off both the fever and the sand. Air, exercise, bark, bitters, mineral tonics, are in like manner often successful in removing the urinary complaints of grown-up persons.

In considering the red gravel, it is necessary to distinguish between those cases in which the sand is actually voided, and those in which it is deposited, after some hours, from originally limpid urine. In the first, the sabulous appearance is an alarming indication of a tendency to form calculi; in the second, it is often merely a fleeting symptom of indigestion. Should it frequently recur, however, it is not to be disregarded.

Bicarbonate of potassa or soda is the proper remedy for the red sand, or lithic acid deposite. The alkali may often be beneficially combined with opium. Ammonia, or its crystallized carbonate, may be resorted to with advantage, where symptoms of indigestion are brought on by the other alkalies; and particularly in red gravel connected with gout, in which the joints and kidneys are affected by turns. Where potassa and soda have been so long employed as to disagree with the stomach, to create nausea, flatulency, a sense of weight, pain, and other symptoms of indigestion, magnesia may be prescribed with the best effects. The tendency which it has to accumulate in dangerous quantities in the intestines, and to form a white sediment in urine, calls on the practitioner to look minutely after its administration. It should be occasionally alternated with other laxative medicines. Magnesia dissolved in carbonic acid, as Mr. Scheweppe used to prepare it many years ago, by the direction of Mr. Brande, is an elegant form of exhibiting this remedy.

Care must be had not to push the alkaline medicines too far, lest they give rise to the deposition of earthy phosphates in the urine.

Cases occur in which the sabulous deposite consists of a mixture of lithic acid with the phosphates. The sediment of urine in inflammatory disorders is sometimes of this nature; and of those persons who habitually indulge in excess of wine; as also of those who, labouring under hepatic affections, secrete much albumen in their urine. Purges, tonics, and nitric acid, which is the solvent of both the above sabulous matters, are the appropriate remedies. The best diet for patients labouring under the lithic deposite, is a vegetable. Dr. Wollaston's fine observation, that the excrement of birds fed solely upon animal matter, is in a great measure lithic acid, and the curious fact since ascertained, that the excrement of the boa constrictor, fed also entirely on animals, is pure lithic acid, concur in giving force to the above dietetic prescription. A week's abstinence from animal food has been known to relieve a fit of lithic acid gravel, where the alkalies were of little avail. But we must not carry the vegetable system so far as to produce flatulency and indigestion.

Such are the principal circumstances connected with the disease of gravel in its incipient or sabulous state. The calculi formed in the kidneys are, as we have said above, either lithic, oxalic, or cystic; and very rarely indeed of the phosphate species. An aqueous regimen, moderate exercise on horseback, when not accompanied with much irritation, cold bathing, and mild aperients, along with the appropriate ch mical medicines, must be prescribed in kidney cases. These are particularly requisite immediately after acute pain in the region of the ureter, and inflammatory symptoms have led to the belief that a nucleus has descended into the bladder. Purges, diuretics, and diluents, ought to be liberally enjoined A large quantity of mucus streaked with blood, or of a purulent aspect, and hæmorrhagy, are frequent symptoms of the passage of the stone into the bladder.

When a stone has once lodged in the bladder, and increased there to such a size as no longer to be capable of passing through the urethra, it is generally allowed by all who have candidly considered the subject, and who are qualified by experience to be judges, that the stone can never again be dissolved; and although it is possible that it may become so loosened in its texture as to be voided piecemeal, or gradually to crumble away, the event is so rare as to be barely probable.

By examining collections of calculi we learn, that in by far the greater number of cases, a nucleus of lithic acid is enveloped in a crust of the phosphates. Our endeavours must therefore be directed towards reducing the excess of lithic acid in the urine to its natural standard; or, on the other hand, to lessen the tendency to the deposition of the phosphates. The urine must be submitted to chemical examination, and a suitable course of diet and medicines prescribed. But the chemical remedies must be regulated nicely, so as to hit the happy equilibrium, in which no deposite will be formed. Here is a powerful call on the physicians and surgeons to make themselves thoroughly versant in chemical science; for they will otherwise commit the most dangerous blunders in calculous complaints.

'The idea of dissolving a calculus of uric acid in the bladder, by the internal use of the caustic alkalies,' says Mr. Brande, 'appears too absurd to merit serious refutation.' In respect to the phosphates, it seems possible, by keeping up an unusual acidity in the urine, so far to soften a crust of the calculus, as to make it crumble down, or admit of being abraded by the sound; but this is the utmost that can be looked for; and the lithic nucleus will still remain. 'These considerations,' adds Mr. Brande, 'independent of more urgent reasons, show the futility of attempting the solution of a stone of the bladder by the injection of acid and alkaline solutions. In respect to the alkalies, if sufficiently strong to act upon the uric crust of the calculus, they would certainly injure the coats of the bladder; they would otherwise become inactive by combination with the acids of the urine, and they would form a dangerous precipitate from the same cause.'—'It therefore appears to me, that Fourcroy and others, who have advised the plan of injection, have thought little of all these obstacles to success, and have regarded the bladder as a lifeless receptacle, into which, as into an India rubber bottle, almost any solvent might be injected with impunity.'—*Journal of Science*, vol. viii. p. 216.

It does not appear that the peculiarities of water in different districts, have any influence upon the production of calculous disorders. Dr. Wollaston's discovery of the analogy between urinary and gouty concretions has led to the trial in gravel of the *vinum colchici*, the specific for gout. By a note to Mr. Brande's dissertation we learn, that benefit has been derived from it in a case of red gravel.

Dr. Henry confirms the above precepts in the following decided language. 'These cases, and others of the same kind, which I think it unnecessary to mention, tend to discourage all attempts to dissolve a stone supposed to consist of uric acid, after it has attained considerable size in the bladder; all that can be effected under such circumstances by alkaline medicines appears, as Mr. Brande has remarked, to be the precipitating upon it a coating of the earthy phosphates from the urine, a sort of concretion which, as has been observed by various practical writers, increases much more rapidly than that consisting of uric acid only. The same unfavourable inference may be drawn also from the dissections of those persons in whom a stone was supposed to be dissolved by alkaline medicines; for in these instances it has been found either encysted, or placed out of the reach of the sound by an enlargement of the prostate gland.'

The urinary calculus of a dog, examined by Dr. Pearson, was found to consist principally of the phosphates of lime and ammonia, with animal matter. Several taken from horses, were of a similar composi tion. One of a rabbit consisted chiefly of carbonate of lime and animal matter, with perhaps a little phos phoric acid. A quantity of sabulous matter, neither crystallized nor concrete, is sometimes found in the bladder of the horse: in one instance there were nearly 45 pounds. These appear to consist of carbonate of lime and animal matter. A calculus of a cat gave Fourcroy three parts of carbonate, and one of the phosphate of lime. That of a pig, according to Berthollet, was phosphate of lime.

The renal calculus in man appears to be of the same nature as the urinary. In that of the horse, Fourcroy found 3 parts of carbonate, and one of phosphate of lime. Dr. Pearson, in one instance, carbonate of lime, and animal matter; in two others, phosphates of lime and ammonia, with animal matter.

Arthritic calculi, or those formed in the joints of gouty persons, were once supposed to be carbonate of lime, whence they were called chalkstones; afterward it was supposed that they were phosphate of lime; but Dr. Wollaston has shown that they are lithate of soda. The calculi found sometimes in the pineal, prostate, salivary, and bronchial glands, in the pancreas, in the corpora cavernosa penis, and between the muscles, as well as the tartar, as it is called, that incrusts the teeth, appear to be phosphate of lime. Dr. Crompton, however, examined a calculus taken from the lungs of a deceased soldier, which consisted of lime 45, carbonic acid 37, albumen and water 18. It was very hard, irregularly spheroidal, and measured about 6¼ inches in circumference.

It has been observed, that the lithic acid, which constitutes the chief part of most human urinary calculi, and abounds in the arthritic, has been found in no phytivorous animal; and hence has been deduced a practical inference, that abstinence from animal food would prevent their formation. But we are inclined to think this conclusion too hasty. The cat is carnivorous; but it appeared above, that the calculus of that animal is equally destitute of lithic acid. If, therefore, we would form any deduction with respect to regimen, we must look for something used by man, exclusively of all other animals; and this is obviously found in fermented liquors, but apparently in nothing else: and this practical inference is sanctioned by the most respectable medical authorities.

The following valuable *criteria* of the different kinds of urinary calculi, have been given by M. Berzelius in his treatise on the use of the blowpipe:

'1. We may recognise *calculi* formed of *uric acid*, from their being carbonized and smoking with an animal odour, when heated by themselves on charcoal or platinum-foil. They dwindle away at the blowpipe flame. Towards the end, they burn with an increase of light; and leave a small quantity of very white alkaline ashes.

'To distinguish these concretions from other substances, which comport themselves in the above manner, we must try a portion of the calculus by the humid way. Thus a tenth of a grain of this calculus being put on a thin plate of glass or platinum, along with a drop of nitric acid, we must heat it at the flame of the lamp. The uric acid dissolves with effervescence. The matter, when dried with precaution to prevent it from charring, is obtained in a fine red colour. If the calculus contains but little uric acid, the substance sometimes blackens by this process. We must then take a new portion of the concretion, and after having dissolved it in nitric acid, remove it from the heat: the solution, when nearly dry, is to be allowed to cool and become dry. We then expose it, sticking to its support, to the warm vapour of caustic ammonia. (From water of ammonia heated in a tea-spoon.) This ammoniacal vapour developes a beautiful red colour in it. We may also moisten the dried matter with a little weak water of ammonia.

'If the concretions are a mixture of uric acid and earthy phosphate, they carbonize and consume like the above, but their residuum is more bulky; it is not alkaline, nor soluble in water. They exhibit with nitric acid and ammonia, the fine red colour of uric acid. Their ashes contain phosphate of lime, or of lime and magnesia.

'2. *The calculi of urate of soda* are hardly met with except in the concretions round the articulations of gouty patients. When heated alone upon charcoal, they blacken, exhaling an empyreumatic animal odour; they are with difficulty reduced into ashes, which are strongly alkaline, and are capable of vitrifying silica. When there are earthy salts (phosphates) in these concretions they afford a whitish or opaque gray glass.

'3. *The calculi of urate of ammonia* comport themselves at the blowpipe like those of uric acid. A drop of caustic potassa makes them exhale, at a moderate heat, much ammonia. We must not confound this odour with the slight ammoniaco-lixivial smell, which potassa disengages from the greater part of animal substances. Urate of soda is likewise found in these calculi.

'4. *Calculi of phosphate of lime.* They blacken, with the exhalation of an empyreumatic animal odour, without melting of themselves at the blowpipe, but whiten into an evident calcareous phosphate. With soda they swell up without vitrifying. Dissolved in boracic acid, and fused along with a little iron, they yield a bead of phosphuret of iron.

'5. *Calculi of ammoniaco-magnesian phosphate*, heated alone on a plate of platinum, exhale the empyreumatic animal odour, at the same time blackening, swelling up, and becoming finally grayish white. A kind of grayish-white enamel is in this manner obtained. With borax they melt into a glass, which is transparent, or which becomes of a milky-white on cooling. Soda in small quantity causes them to fuse into a frothy white slag; a larger quantity of soda makes them infusible. They yield, with iron and boracic acid, a bead of phosphuret of iron; with nitrate of cobalt, a glass of a deep red or brown. If salts of lime exist in these concretions, the mixture of them is less fusible.

'6. *Calculi of oxalate of lime*, exposed to the blowpipe, exhale at first the urinous smell; they become first of a dull colour at the flame, and afterward their colour brightens. What remains after a moderate ignition, effervesces with nitric acid. After a smart jet of the flame, there remains quicklime on the charcoal, which reacts like an alkali on the colour of litmus, wild mallow flower, or cabbage, and slakes with water. But this does not happen when the residuum consists of calcareous phosphate.

'7. *The siliceous calculus*, heated alone, leaves subcoriaceous or infusible ashes. Treated with a little soda, these dissolve with effervescence, but slowly, leaving a bead of glass of a gray colour, or of little transparency.

'8. Lastly, *the cystic oxyde calculi* afford nearly the same results as uric acid at the blowpipe. They readily take fire, burning with a bluish green flame, without melting, with the disengagement of a lively and very peculiar acid odour, which has some affinity to that of cyanogen. Their ashes, which are not alkaline, redissolve by a jet of the flame, into a grayish-white mass. They do not yield a red colour in their treatment with nitric acid, like the uric acid concretions.' "

The Causes of the Generation of Urinary Calculi.

To inquire into the causes by which urinary concretions are produced, is both interesting and useful, however attended with the greatest difficulties. The writings of medical authors are full of conjectures and hypotheses with regard to this subject, on which nothing could be ascertained before we had acquired an accurate knowledge of the nature of urinary concretions. It is owing to this circumstance that the most enlightened physicians acquiesced in ascribing the immediate cause of them to a superabundance of terreous matter in the urine; and Boerhaave, as well as, particularly, Van Swieten, imagined that the urine of all men contained calculous matter in the natural state, and that, for the generation of stones, a nucleus was only required, to attract it. That this may be the case, in some instances, is proved by frequent experience; but stones produced by foreign bodies, that have accidentally got into the urethra or bladder, are always white, and composed of phosphates of earths, and seldom or never covered with lithic acid, a substance which is observed to form the stones that most frequently occur; but even in these the nucleus consists of a substance formed in the body itself, as a particle descended from the kidneys, &c. which must, therefore, have necessarily originated in a peculiar internal cause. A superabundance of uric acid in stony patients, and its more copious generation than in a sound state, though it seems to be one of the principal and most certain causes, is by no means satisfactory, as it only explains the precipitation of stony matter from the urine, but not why it unites in strata. A coagulating substance is required for separating, attracting, and, as it were, agglutinating the condensible particles that are precipitated. This substance is undoubtedly the animal matter which we have constantly found in all calculous masses, and which seems to constitute the basis of stones, like the membraneous gelatina that of bones. It is known that the urine of calculous patients is generally muddy, ductile, in threads, slimy, and as if mixed with albumen, which quality it obtains at the moment when the ammonia is disengaged, or on the addition of potassa that separates it from the acid in which it was dissolved; and in all cases of superabundance of lithic acid the urine contains a great quantity of that animal matter, which promotes the precipitation of it, and attracts, and unites the particles thus separated. Hence it appears, that every thing capable of increasing the quantity of that pituitous gluten in the urine, may be considered as the remote cause of the formation of calculi. And the old ideas on pituitous temperaments, or superabundant pituita, &c. which were thought to dispose people to a calculus, seem to be connected with the late discoveries on the nature of urinary stones. Though the animal matter appears to be different in different calculi, yet it is certain, that every calculous substance contains an animal gluten, from which its concrete and solid state arises; whence we may fairly state the superabundance of that substance as the chief and principal cause of the formation of calculi.

There are, however, other causes which seem to have a particular influence on the nature of urinary stones, and the strata in which they are formed; but it is extremely difficult to penetrate and to explain them. We are, for instance, entirely ignorant of the manner in which urinary stones are formed from the oxalate of lime; though, from their occurring more frequently in children than in adults, we might be entitled to ascribe them to a disposition to acor, a cause considered by Boerhaave as the general source of a great number of diseases incident to the infantile age. This opinion seems to be proved by the ideas of Bonhomme, physician at Avignon, on the oxalic or saccharic acid, as the cause of mollities ossium in the rickets; by this acid being discovered in a species of saliva by Brugnatelli; and, lastly, by an observation of Turgais, who found this acid in the urine of a child diseased with worms. We but rarely observe saccharic acid in the human body, which appears to be mostly adventitious, and by which the animal matter is rendered coagulable, and deposited, or precipitated, with the oxalate of lime; or the oxalic acid decomposes the phosphate of lime, and forms an insoluble combination, incapable of being any longer kept dissolved in the urine. It is, however, extremely difficult to determine how far the constitution of the body is connected with that particular disposition in the urine, of precipitating sometimes phosphate of lime mixed with oxalate of lime, sometimes phosphate of ammoniacal magnesia, either by itself or mixed with lithic acid, &c. &c. Who can explain the reason why, of 600 stones, there were only two in which siliceous earth could be traced? Still more difficult is it to explain the causes why the above substances precipitate either at once or in different strata; but it may suffice to have shown how many observations and experiments are required, and what accurate attention and perseverance are necessary, in order to throw light on so difficult a subject.

The means to be employed in calculous complaints must vary according to circumstances. Permanent relief can be obtained only by the removal of the morbid concretion: and where this is of too large a size to be passed by the natural outlet, the operation of lithotomy becomes necessary. Various remedies indeed have been proposed as capable of dissolving urinary calculi; and some of them are certainly useful in palliating the symptoms, and perhaps preventing the formation of fresh calculous matter: but experience has not sanctioned their efficacy as actual lithontriptics; and by delaying the operation, we not only incur the risk of organic disease being produced, but the concretion may also become friable externally, so as to be with more difficulty removed. Sometimes, however, the advanced age of the patient, the complication with organic disease, or the exhausted state of the system, may render an operation inexpedient; or he may not be willing to submit to it; we shall then find some advantage from the use of chemical remedies, according to the morbid quality of the urine; that is generally from alkaline or earthy preparations, where a red deposite appears, and from acids where there is a white sediment. Tonic medicines may also be useful, and some of the mild astringents, especially uva ursi, and occasional narcotics, where violent pain attends: sometimes an inflammatory tendency may require fomentations, the local abstraction of blood, and other antiphlogistic measures. The most likely plan of effecting a solution of the calculus must certainly be that proposed by Fourcroy, namely, injecting suitable liquids into the bladder. The most common calculi, containing uric acid, are readily soluble in a solution of potassa, or soda, weak enough to be held in the mouth, or even swallowed without inconvenience; those which consist of phosphoric acid neutralized by lime, or other base, the next in frequency, dissolve in nitric or muriatic acid of no greater strength; the most rare variety, made up mostly of oxalate of lime, may be dissolved, but very slowly, in nitric acid, or solutions of the fixed alkaline carbonates, weak enough not to irritate the bladder. However, it is not easy to ascertain which of these solvents is proper in a particular case, for most calculi are not uniform throughout, owing probably to the urine having varied during their formation, so that the examination of this secretion will not certainly indicate the injection required. The plan recommended, therefore, is, the bladder having been evacuated, and washed out with tepid water, to inject first the alkaline solution, heated to the temperature of the body, and direct it to be retained for half an hour, or longer, if the person can bear it; then, to the liquor voided and filtered, add a little muriatic acid, which will cause a white precipitate, if there be any uric acid dissolved; and so long as this happens, the same injection should be used, otherwise diluted muriatic acid is to be thrown in, and ammonia added to it when discharged; whereby phosphate of lime, if there be any, is precipitated: and when neither of these succeeds, diluted nitric acid is to be tried; in each case varying the injection from time to time, as that previously used loses its efficacy. However, there appears one source of error in this method; namely, that the urine secreted, while the liquid is retained, may give rise to a precipitate, though none of the calculus may have been dissolved; it would therefore be proper to examine the urine previously, as well as occasionally during the use of injections, and, if necessary, correct its quality by the exhibition of proper internal medicines. See *Lithontriptics* and *Lithotomy*.

CALCULUS BILIARIS. See *Gall-stone*.

CALDA'RIUM. (From *caleo*, to make hot.) A vessel in the baths of the ancients, to hold hot water.

CALEFA'CIENT. (*Calefaciens*; from *calidus*, warm, and *facio*, to make.) A medicine, or other substance, which excites a degree of warmth in the parts to which it is applied: as *piper*, *spiritus vini*, &c. They belong to the class of stimulants.

CALE'NDULA. (*Quad singulis calendis*, i. e. *mensibus*, *florescat*; so called because it flowers every month.) 1. The name of a genus of plants in the Linnæan system. Class, *Syngenesia*; Order, *Polygamia necessaria*.

2. The pharmacopœial name of the single marigold. See *Calendula officinalis*.

CALENDULA ALPINA. The mountain arnica. See *Arnica montana*.

CALENDULA ARVENSIS. The wild marigold. See *Caltha palustris*.

CALENDULA OFFICINALIS. The garden marigold *Calendula sativa*; *Chrysanthemum*; *Sponsa solis*; *Caltha vulgaris*. The flowers and leaves of this plant, *Calendula*:—*seminibus cymbiformibus*, *muricatis*, *incurvatis omnibus*, of Linnæus, have been exhibited medicinally: the former, as aperients in uterine obstructions and icteric disorders, and as diaphoretics in exanthematous fevers; the latter, as gentle aperients, and to promote the secretions in general.

CALENDULA PALUSTRIS. Common single marsh-marigold. See *Caltha palustris*.

CA'LENTURE. A febrile delirium, said to be peculiar to sailors, wherein they imagine the sea to be green fields, and will throw themselves into it if not restrained. Bonetus, Dr. Oliver, and Dr. Stubbs, give an account of it.

CALE'SIUM The Indian name of a tree which grows in Malabar, the bark of which made into an ointment with butter, cures convulsions from wounds, and heals ulcers. The juice of the bark cures the aphthæ, and, taken inwardly, the dysentery.—*Ray.*

Calf's snout. See *Antirrhinum.*

CA'LI. (Arabian.) The same as kali

CALICHA'PA. The white-thorn.

CA'LIDUS. In medical language, it is commonly used for animal heat, or the vis vitæ· thus, *calidum animale innatum.*

CALIDÆ PLANTÆ. (From *calor*, heat.) Plants that are natives of warm climates.

CALIE'TA. (From καλιης, a nest, which it somewhat resembles.) *Calliette.* A fungus growing on the juniper-tree.

CALI'GO. (*Caligo, ginis.* fœm.) A disease of the eye, known by diminished or destroyed sight; and by the interposition of a dark body between the object and the retina. It is arranged by Cullen in the class *Locales*, and order *dysæsthesiæ.* The species of caligo are distinguished according to the situation of the interposed body: thus *caligo lentis*, *caligo corneæ*, *caligo pupillæ*, *caligo humorum*, and *caligo palpebrarum.*

CALIHA'CHA. The cassia-lignea, or cassia-tree of Malabar.

CALI'MIA. The lapis calaminaris.

CA'LIX. (*Calix, icis.* m.; from καλυπτω, to cover.) See *Calyx.*

CALLÆ'UM. (From καλλυνω, to adorn.) *Callæon.* The gills of a cock, which Galen says, is food not to be praised or condemned.

CALLE'NA. A kind of saltpetre.

CA'LLI. Nodes in the gout.—*Galen.*

CA'LLIA. (From καλος, beautiful.) A name of the chamomile.

CALLIBLE'PHARA. (From καλος, good, and βλεφαρον, the eyelid.) Medicines, or compositions, appropriated to the eyelids.

CALLICO'CCA. The name of a genus of plants in the Linnæan system. Class, *Pentandria*, Order, *Monogynia.*

CALLICOCCA IPECACUANHA. The plant from which ipecacuan root is obtained was long unknown; it was said by some writers to be the *Psychotria emetica:* Class, *Pentandria;* Order, *Monogynia;* by others, the *Viola ipecacuanha*, a syngenesious plant of the order *Monogynia.* It is now ascertained to be neither, but a small plant called *Callicocca ipecacuanha.* There are three sorts of ipecacuan to be met with in our shops, viz. the ash-coloured or gray, the brown, and the white.

The ash-coloured is brought from Peru, and is a small wrinkled root, bent and contorted into a great variety of figures, brought over in short pieces, full of wrinkles, and deep circular fissures, down to a small white woody fibre that runs in the middle of each piece: the cortical part is compact, brittle, looks smooth and resinous upon breaking: it has very little smell; the taste is bitterish and subacrid, covering the tongue, as it were, with a kind of mucilage.

The brown is small, somewhat more wrinkled than the foregoing; of a brown or blackish colour without, and white within; this is brought from Brazil.

The white sort is woody, and has no wrinkles, nor any perceptible bitterness in taste. The first, the ash-coloured or gray ipecacuan, is that usually preferred for medicinal use. The brown has been sometimes observed, even in a small dose, to produce violent effects. The white, though taken in a large one, has scarcely any effect at all. Experience has proved that this medicine is the safest emetic with which we are acquainted, having this peculiar advantage, that, if it does not operate by vomit, it readily passes off by the other emunctories. Ipecacuan was first introduced as an infallible remedy against dysenteries, and other inveterate fluxes, as diarrhœa, menorrhagia, leucorrhœa, &c. and also in disorders proceeding from obstructions of long standing; nor has it lost much of its reputation by time: its utility in these cases is thought to depend upon its restoring perspiration. It has also been successfully employed in spasmodic asthma, catarrhal and consumptive cases. Nevertheless, its chief use is as a vomit, and in small doses, joined with opium, as a diaphoretic. The officinal preparations are the *pulvis ipecacuanhæ compositus*, and the *vinum ipecacuanhæ.*

CALLI'CREAS. (From καλος, good, and κρεας, meat, so named from its delicacy as food.) Sweet bread See *Pancreas.*

CALLI'GONUM. (From καλος, beautiful, and γονυ, a knot, or joint; so named from its being handsomely jointed, like a cane.) The polygonum, or knot-grass

CALLIOMA'RCHUS. The Gaullic name, in Marcellus Empiricus, of colt's-foot.

CA'LLION. A kind of night-shade

CALLIPHY'LLUM. From καλλος, beauty, and φυλλον, a leaf.) See *Adianthum.*

CALLISTRU'THIA. (From καλος, good, and ςρυθος, a sparrow; because it was said to fatten sparrows.) A fig mentioned by Pliny, of a good taste.

CALLITRI'CHE. (From καλλος, beauty, and θριξ, hair; so named because it has the appearance of long, beautiful hair; or, according to Littleton, because it nourishes the hair, and makes it beautiful.) 1. The name of a genus of plants in the Linnæan system. Class, *Monandria;* Order, *Digynia.* Water starwort. Water chickweed.

2. The herb maidenhair. See *Adianthum.*

CALLO'NE. (From καλος, fair.) Hippocrates used this word, to signify that decency and gravity of character and deportment which it is necessary that all medical men should be possessed of.

CALLO'SITAS. Callosity, or preternatural hardness.

CALLOSITY. *Callositas.* Hardness.

CALLOSUS. Hard. Applied in surgery to parts which are morbidly hard; and, in botany, to seeds which are hard; as those of the *Citrus medica.*

CA'LLOUS. *Callosus.* Hardened or indurated, as the callous edges of ulcers.

CA'LLUS. (*Callus, i.* m.; and *Callum, i.* n.) 1. The bony matter deposited between the divided ends of broken bones, about the fourteenth day after the fracture. It is in reality nothing more than the new ossific substance formed by a process of nature, very similar to the growth of any other part of the body.

2. A preternatural hardness, or induration, of any fleshy part.

3. This term is applied in Good's Nosology to that species of ecphyma, which is characterized by callous extuberant thickening of the cuticle; insensible to the touch.

CALOCA'TANUS. (From καλος, beautiful, and καταvov, a cup; so called from the beauty of its flower and shape.) The wild poppy. See *Papaver rhœas.*

CALO'MELAS. (From καλος, good, and μελας, black; from its virtues and colour.) 1. The preparation called Æthiops mineral, or *hydrargyrus cum sulphure*, was formerly so named.

2. The chloride of mercury. See *Hydrargyri submurias.*

CALO'RIC. (*Caloricum;* from *calor*, heat.) Heat; Igneous fluid.

Heat and cold are perceptions of which we acquire the ideas from the senses; they indicate only a certain state in which we find ourselves, independent of any exterior object. But as these sensations are for the most part produced by bodies around us, we consider them as causes, and judging by appearances, we apply the terms *hot*, or *cold*, to the substances themselves; calling those bodies *hot*, which produce in us the sensation of heat, and those *cold*, which communicate the contrary sensation.

This ambiguity, though of little consequence in the common affairs of human life, has led unavoidably to confusion and perplexity in philosophical discussions. It was to prevent this, that the framers of the new nomenclature adopted the word *caloric*, which denotes that which produces the sensation of heat.

Theories of Heat.

Two opinions have long divided the philosophical world concerning the nature of heat.

1. The one is; that the cause which produces the sensation of heat, is a real, or distinct substance, universally pervading nature, penetrating the particles or pores of all bodies, with more or less facility, and in different quantities.

This substance, if applied to our system in a greater proportion than it already contains, warms it, as we call it, or produces the sensation of heat; and hence it has been called *caloric* or *calorific.*

2. The other theory concerning heat is; that the cause which produces that sensation is *not* a separate

or self-existing substance; but that it is merely like gravity, a property of matter; and that it consists in a specific or *peculiar motion*, or *vibration* of the particles of bodies.

The arguments in favour of the first theory have been principally deduced from the evolution and absorption of heat during chemical combinations; those of the latter are chiefly founded on the production of heat by friction For it has been observed, that whatever is capable of producing motion in the particles of any mass of matter, excites heat. Count Rumford and Professor Davy have paid uncommon attention to this fact, and proved, that heat continues to be evolved from a body subjected to friction, so long as it is applied, and the texture or form of the body not altered.

All the effects of heat, according to this theory, depend therefore entirely upon the vibratory motion of the particles of bodies. According as this is more or less intense, a higher or lower temperature is produced; and as it predominates over, is nearly equal or inferior to the attraction of cohesion, bodies exist in the gaseous, fluid, or solid state.

Different bodies are susceptible of it in different degrees, and receive and communicate it with different celerity. From the generation, communication, and attraction of this repulsive motion, under these laws, all the phenomena ascribed to heat are explicable.

Each of these theories has been supported by the most able philosophers, and given occasion to the most important disputes in which chemists have been engaged: which has contributed in a very particular manner to the advancement of the science. The obscurity of the subject, however, is such, that both parties have been able to advance most plausible arguments.

Setting aside all inquiries concerning the merits of these different doctrines, we shall confine ourselves to the general effects which heat produces on different bodies. For the phenomena which heat presents, and their relation to each other, may be investigated with sufficient precision, though the materiality, or immateriality of it, may remain unknown to us.

Nature of Heat.

Those who consider heat as matter, assert that caloric exists in two states, namely, in combination, or at liberty.

In the first state it is not sensible to our organs, nor indicated by the thermometer; it forms a constituent part of the body; but it may be brought back to the state of sensible heat. In this state it affects animals with the sensation of heat. It therefore has been called sensible or free heat, or fire; and is synonymous with uncombined caloric, thermometrical caloric, caloric of temperature, interposed caloric, &c. expressions now pretty generally superseded.

From the diversity of opinions among chemists respecting the nature of caloric, several other expressions have been introduced, which it is proper to notice. For instance, by *specific heat* is understood, the relatitive quantities of caloric contained in equal weights of different bodies at the same temperature. *Latent heat* is the expression used to denote that quantity of caloric which a body absorbs when changing its form. It is, however, more properly called *caloric of fluidity*. The disposition, or property, by which different bodies contain certain quantities of caloric, at any temperature, is termed their *capacity for heat*. By the expression of *absolute heat*, is understood the whole quantity of caloric which any body contains.

Methods of exciting and collecting Heat.

Of the different methods of exciting heat, the following are the most usual:

I. *Percussion or Collision.* This method of producing heat is the simplest, and therefore it is generally made use of in the common purposes of life for obtaining fire.

When a piece of hardened steel is struck with a flint, some particles of the metal are scraped away from the mass, and so violent is the heat which follows the stroke, that it melts and vitrifies them. If the fragments of steel are caught upon paper, and viewed with a microscope, most of them will be found perfect spherules, and very highly polished. Their sphericity demonstrates that they have been in a fluid state, and the polish upon their surface, shows them to be vitrified.

No heat, however has been observed to follow the percussion of liquids, nor of the softer kind of bodies which yield to a slight impulse.

2. *Friction.* Heat may likewise be excited by mere friction. This practice is still retained in some parts of the world. The natives of New Holland are said to produce fire in this manner, with great facility, and spread it in a wonderful manner. For that purpose, they take two pieces of dry wood; one is a stick, about eight or nine inches long, and the other piece is flat; the stick they bring to an obtuse point at one end, and pressing it upon the other piece, they turn it very nimbly, by holding it between both hands, as we do a chocolate-mill, often shifting their hands up, and then moving down upon it, in order to increase the pressure as much as possible. By this method they get fire in a few minutes, and from the smallest spark they increase it with great speed and dexterity.

If the irons at the axis of a coach-wheel are applied to each other, without the interposition of some unctuous matter to keep them from immediate contact, they will become so hot when the carriage runs swiftly along, as to set the wood on fire; and the fore-wheels, being smallest, and making most revolutions in a given time, will be most in danger.

The same will happen to mill-work, or to any other machinery.

It is no uncommon practice in this country, for blacksmiths to use a plate of iron as an extemporaneous substitute for a tinder-box; for it may be hammered on an anvil till it becomes red-hot, and will fire a brimstone match. A strong man who strikes quick, and keeps turning the iron so that both sides may be equally exposed to the force of the hammer, will perform this in less time than would be expected.

If, in the coldest season, one dense iron plate be laid on another, and pressed together by a weight, and then rubbed upon each other by reciprocal motions, they will gradually grow so hot as, in a short time, to emit sparks, and at last become ignited.

It is not necessary that the substances should be very hard; a cord rubbed backwards and forwards swiftly against a post or a tree will take fire.

Count Rumford and Professor Pictet have made some very ingenious and valuable experiments concerning the heat evolved by friction.

3. *Chemical Action.* To this belongs the heat produced by combustion. There are, besides this, many chemical processes wherein rapid chemical action takes place, accompanied with a developement of heat, or fire, and flame.

4. *Solar heat.* It is well known that the solar rays, when collected by a mirror, or lens, into a focus, produce the most astonishing effects.

Dr. Herschel has discovered that there are rays emitted from the sun, which have not the power of illuminating or producing vision: and that these are the rays which produce the heat of the solar light.

Consequently, heat is emitted from the sun in rays, but these rays are not the same with the rays of light.

5. *The Electric Spark, and Galvanism.* The effects of electricity are two well known in this point of view to need any description.

Galvanism has of late become a powerful instrument for the purpose of exciting heat. Not only easily inflammable substances, such as phosphorus, sulphur, &c. have been fired, but likewise, gold, silver, copper, tin, and the rest of the metals, have been burnt by means of galvanism.

General Effects of Heat.

The first and most obvious effect which heat produces on bodies, is its expansive property. Experience has taught us that, at all times, when bodies become hot, they increase in bulk. The bodies experience a dilatation which is greater in proportion to the accumulation of coloric, or in other words, to the intensity of the heat. This is a general law, which holds good as long as the bodies have suffered no change either in their combination or in the quantity of their chemical principles.

This power, which heat possesses, consists, therefore, in a constant tendency to separate the particles of bodies. Hence philosophers consider heat as the *repulsive power* which acts upon all bodies whatever, and which is in constant opposition to the power of attraction.

The phenomena which result from these mutual actions, seem, as it were, the secret springs of nature

Heat, however, does not expand all bodies equally, and we are still ignorant of the laws which it follows.

1. *Expansion of Fluid Bodies.* Take a glass globe, with a long slender neck (called a bold heat); fill it up to the neck with water, ardent spirit, or any other fluid which may be coloured with red or black ink, in order to be more visible, and then immerse the globe of the instrument in a vessel of hot water; the included fluid will instantly begin to mount into the neck. If it be taken out of the water and brought near the fire, it will ascend more and more, in proportion as it becomes heated; but, upon removing it from the source of heat, it will sink again: a clear proof that caloric dilates it, so as to make it occupy more space when hot than when cold. These experiments may, therefore, serve as a demonstration that heat expands *fluid* bodies.

2. *Expansion of Aëriform Bodies.* Take a bladder partly filled with air, the neck of which is closely tied, so as to prevent the enclosed air from escaping, and let it be held near a fire. The air will soon begin to occupy more space, and the bladder will become gradually distended; on continuing the expansion of the air, by increasing the heat, the bladder will burst with a loud report.

3. *Expansion of Solid Bodies.* If we take a bar of iron, six inches long, and put it into a fire till it becomes red-hot; and then measure it in this state accurately, it will be found 1-20th of an inch longer than it was before; that is, about 120th part of the whole. That the metal is proportionally expanded in breadth, will be seen by trying to pass it through an aperture which is fitted exactly when cold, but which will not admit it when red-hot. The bar is, therefore, increased in length and diameter.

To discover the minutest changes of expansion by heat, and the relative proportions thereof, instruments have been contrived, called *Pyrometers*, the sensibility of which is so delicate as to show an expansion of 1-100,000th of an inch.

It is owing to this expansion of metals, that the motion of time-pieces is rendered erroneous; but the ingenuity of artists has discovered methods of obviating this inaccuracy, by employing the greater expansion of one metal, to counteract the expansion of another; this is effected in what is called the grid-iron pendulum. Upon the same principle, a particular construction of watches has been contrived.

The expansion of metals is likewise one of the principal reasons that clocks and watches vary in winter and summer, when worn in the pocket, or exposed to the open air, or when carried into a hotter or a colder climate. For the number of the vibrations of the pendulum is always in the sub-duplicate ratio of its length, and as the length is changed by heat and cold, the times of vibration will be also changed. The quantity of alteration, when considered in a single vibration, is exceedingly small, but when they are often repeated, it will be very sensible. An alteration of one-thousandth part in the time of a single vibration of a pendulum which beats seconds, will make a change of eighty-six whole vibrations in twenty-four hours.

As different metals expand differently with the same degree of heat; those musical instruments, whose parts are to maintain a constant true proportion, should never be strung with different metals. It is on this account that harpsichords, &c. are out of tune by a change of temperature.

Bodies which are brittle, or which want flexibility, crack or break, if suddenly heated. This likewise depends upon the expansive force of heat, stretching the surface to which it is applied, while the other parts, not being equally heated, do not expand in the same ratio, and are therefore torn asunder or break. Hence thin vessels stand heat better than thick ones. The same holds, when they are suddenly cooled.

Measurement of Heat.

Upon the expansive property of heat, which we have considered before, is founded its artificial measurement. Various means have been employed to assist the imperfection of our sensations in judging of the different degrees of heat; for our feelings, unaided, afford but very inaccurate information concerning this matter; they indicate the presence of *heat*, only when the bodies presented to them are *hotter* than the actual temperature of our organs of feeling. When these bodies are precisely of the same temperature with our body, which we make the standard of comparison, we then are not sensible of the presence of heat in them. When their temperature is less than that of our bodies, their contact gives us what is called the sensation of cold.

The effects of heat upon material bodies in general, which are easily visible to us, afford more precise and determinate indications of the intensity, than can be derived from our feelings alone. The ingenuity of the philosopher and artist has therefore furnished us with instruments of measuring the relative heat or temperature of bodies. These instruments are called *Thermometers* and *Pyrometers*. By these, all degrees are measurable, from the slightest to that of the most intense heat. See *Thermometer* and *Pyrometer*.

Exceptions to the Expansion by Heat.

Philosophers have noticed a few exceptions to the law of heat expanding bodies. For instance; water, when cooled down within about 7° of the freezing point, instead of contracting on the farther deprivation of heat, actually expands.

Another seeming exception is manifested in alumine, or clay; others occur in the case of cast-iron, and a few other metals. Alumine contracts on being heated, and cast-iron, bismuth, &c. when fully fused, are more dense than when solid; for, as soon as they become so, they decrease in density, they expand in the act of cooling, and hence the sharpness of figures upon iron which has been cast in moulds, compared to that of many other metals.

Some philosophers have persuaded themselves that these exceptions are only *apparent*, but not really true. They say, when water freezes, it assumes a crystalline form, the crystals cross each other and cause numerous vacuities, and thus the ice occupies more space The same is the case with fused iron, bismuth, and antimony. The contraction of clay is considered owing to the loss of water, of which it loses a part at every increased degree of temperature hitherto tried; there is, therefore, a loss of matter; and a reduction of volume must follow: but others assert, that this only happens to a certain extent.

Mr. Tilloch has published a brief examination of the received doctrines respecting heat and caloric, in which these truths are more fully considered, together with many other interesting facts relative to the received notions of heat.

Equal Distribution of Heat.

If a number of bodies of different temperatures are placed in contact with each other, they will all at a certain time acquire a temperature, which is intermediate; the caloric of the hottest body will diffuse itself among those which are heated in a less degree, till they have all acquired a certain mean temperature. Thus, if a bar of iron, which has been made red-hot, be kept in the open air, it does not retain the heat which it had received, but becomes gradually colder and colder, till it arrives at the temperature of the bodies in its neighbourhood. On the other hand, if we cool down the iron bar by keeping it for some time covered with snow, and then carry it into a warm room, it does not retain its low temperature, but becomes gradually hotter, till it acquires the temperature of the room. It is therefore obvious, that in the one instance the temperature is lowered, and in the other it is raised.

These changes of temperature occupy a longer or a shorter time, according to the nature of the body, but they always take place at last. This law itself is, indeed, familiar to every one: when we wish to heat a body, we carry it towards the fire: when we wish to cool it, we surround it by cold bodies.

Propagation of Heat.

We have seen, that when bodies of higher temperature than others are brought into contact with each other, the heat is propagated from the first to the second, or the colder body deprives the warmer of its excess of heat. We shall now see that some bodies do so much more quickly than others. Through some bodies caloric passes with undiminished velocity, through others its passage is prodigiously retarded.

This disposition of bodies, of admitting, under equal circumstances, the refrigeration of a heated body within a shorter or a longer time, is called *the power of conducting heat;* and a body is said to be a *better* or *worse conductor of heat*, as it allows the refrigeration to go on quicker or slower. Those bodies, therefore, which possess the property of letting heat pass with facility, are called *good conductors*, those through which it passes with difficulty are called *bad conductors*, and those through which it is supposed not to pass at all, are called *non-conductors;* thus we say, in common language, some bodies are *warm*, or capable of preserving warmth, and from this arises the great difference in the sensation excited by different bodies, when applied at the same temperature to our organs of feeling. Hence, if we immerse our hand in mercury, we feel a greater sensation of cold than when we immerse it in water, and a piece of metal appears to be much colder than a piece of wood, though their temperatures, when examined by means of the thermometer, are precisely the same.

It is probable that all solids conduct heat in some degree, though they differ very much in their conducting power. Metals are the best conductors of heat; but the conducting powers of these substances are by no means equal. Stones seem to be the next best conductors. Glass conducts heat very slowly; wood and charcoal still slower; and feathers, silk, wool, and hair, are still worse conductors than any of the substances yet mentioned.

The best conductors of electricity and galvanism are also the best conductors of heat.

Experiment.—Take a number of straight wires, of equal diameters and lengths, but of different metals; for instance, gold, silver, copper, iron, &c.; cover each of them with a thin coat of wax, or tallow, and plunge their extremities into water, kept boiling, or into melted lead. The melting of the coat of wax will show that caloric is more quickly transmitted through some metals than others.

It is on this account also, that the end of a glass rod may be kept red-hot for a long time, or even melted, without any inconvenience to the hand which holds the other extremity; though a similar metallic rod, heated in the same manner, would very soon become too hot to be held.

Liquid and Aëriform Bodies convey Heat by an actual Change in the Situation of their Particles.

Count Rumford was the first who proved that fluids in general, and aëriform bodies, convey heat on a different principle from that observed in the solids. This opinion is pretty generally admitted, though various ingenious experiments have been made, by different philosophers, to prove the contrary. In water, for instance, the count has proved that caloric is propagated principally in consequence of the motion which is occasioned in the particles of that fluid.

All fluids are considered by him, strictly speaking, in a similar respect as *non-conductors* of caloric. They can receive it, indeed, from other substances, and can give it to other substances, but no particle can either receive it from or give it to another particle of the same kind. Before a fluid, therefore, can be heated or cooled, every particle must go individually to the substance from which it receives or to which it gives out caloric. Heat being, therefore, only propagated in fluids, in consequence of the internal motion of their particles, which transport the heat; the more rapid these motions are, the more rapid is the communication of heat. The cause of these motions is the change in the specific gravity of the fluid, occasioned by the change of temperature, and the rapidity is in proportion to the change of the specific gravity of the liquid by any given change of temperature. The following experiment may serve to illustrate this theory:

Take a thin glass tube, eight or ten inches long, and about an inch in diameter. Pour into the bottom part, for about the depth of one inch, a little water coloured with Brazil-wood, or litmus, and then fill up the tube with common water, extremely gently, so as to keep the two *strata* quite distinct from each other. Having done this, heat the bottom part of the tube over a lamp; the coloured infusion will then ascend, and gradually tinge the whole fluid; on the contrary, if the heat be applied above, the water in the upper part of the tube may be made to boil, but the colouring matter will remain at the bottom undisturbed. The heat cannot act downwards to make it ascend.

By thus being able to make the upper part of a fluid boil without heating the bottom part, water may be kept boiling for a considerable time in a glass tube over ice, without melting it

Other experiments, illustrating the same principle, may be found in count Rumford's excellent essays, especially in Essay the 7th; 1797.

To this indefatigable philosopher we are wholly indebted for the above facts: he was the first who taught us that air and water were nearly non-conductors. The results of his experiments, which are contained in the above essay, are highly interesting; they also show that the conducting power of fluids is impaired by the admixture of fibrous and glutinous matter.

Count Rumford proved that ice melted more than 80 times slower, when boiling hot water stood on its surface, than when the ice was placed to swim on the surface of the hot water. Other experiments showed that water, only eight degrees of Fahrenheit above the freezing point, or at the temperature of forty degrees, melts as much ice, in any given time, as an equal volume of that fluid at any higher temperature, provided the water stands on the surface of the ice. Water, at the temperature of 41°, is found to melt more ice, when standing on its surface, than boiling water. It appears, however, that liquids are not, as he supposes, complete non-conductors of caloric; because, if heat be applied at top, it is capable of making its way downwards, through water, for example, though very imperfectly and slowly.

It becomes farther evident, from the Count's ingenious experiments, that of the different substances used in clothing, hares' fur and eider-down are the warmest; next to these, beavers' fur, raw silk, sheep's wool, cotton wool, and lastly, lint, or the scrapings of fine linen. In fur, the air interposed among its particles is so engaged as not to be driven away by the heat communicated thereto by the animal body; not being easily displaced, it becomes a barrier to defend the animal body from the external cold. Hence it is obvious that those skins are warmest which have the finest, longest, and thickest fur; and that the furs of the beaver, otter, and other like quadrupeds, which live much in the water, and the feathers of water-fowl, are capable of confining the heat of those animals in winter, notwithstanding the coldness of the water which they frequent. Bears, and various other animals, inhabitants of cold climates, which do not often take the water, have their fur much thicker on their backs than on their bellies.

The snow which covers the surface of the earth in winter, in high latitudes, is doubtless designed as a garment to defend it against the piercing winds from the polar regions, which prevail during the cold season.

Without dwelling farther upon the philosophy of this truth, we must briefly remark that the happy application of this law, satisfactorily elucidates some of the most interesting facts of the economy of nature.

Theory of Caloric of Fluidity, or Latent Heat.

There are some bodies which, when submitted to the action of caloric, dilate to such a degree, and the power of aggregation subsisting among their particles is so much destroyed and removed to such a distance by the interposition of caloric, that they slide over each other in every direction, and therefore appear in a fluid state. This phenomenon is called *fusion.* Bodies thus rendered fluid by means of caloric, are said to be *fused*, or *melted;* and those that are subject to it, are called *fusible.*

The greater number of solid bodies may, by the application of heat, be converted into fluids. Thus metals may be fused; sulphur, resin, phosphorus, may be melted; ice may be converted into water, &c.

Those bodies which cannot be rendered fluid by any degree of heat hitherto known, are called *infusible.*

If the effects of heat, under certain circumstances, be carried still farther than is necessary to render bodies fluid, vaporization begins; the bodies then become converted into the vaporous or *gaseous state.* Vaporization, however, does not always require a previous fusion. Some bodies are capable of being converted into the vaporous state, without previously becoming fluid, and others cannot be volatilized at any temperature hitherto known: the latter are termed fixed.

Fluidity is, therefore, by no means essential to any species of matter, but always depends on the presence of a quantity of caloric. Solidity is the natural state of all bodies, and there can be no doubt that every fluid is capable of being rendered solid by a due reduction of temperature; and every solid may be fused by the agency of caloric, if the latter does not decompose them at a temperature inferior to that which would be necessary for their fusion.

Caloric of Fluidity.

Dr. Black was the first who proved that, whenever caloric combines with a solid body, the body becomes heated only, until it is rendered fluid: and that, while it is acquiring the fluid state, its temperature remains stationary, though caloric is continued to be added to it. The same is the case when fluids are converted into the aëriform or vaporous state.

From these facts, the laws of latent heat have been inferred. The theory may be illustrated by means of the following experiments:

If a lump of ice, at a low temperature, suppose at 22°, be brought into a warm room, it will become gradually less cold, as may be discovered by means of the thermometer. After a very short time, it will reach the temperature of 32° (the freezing point); but there it stops. The ice then begins to melt; but the process goes on very slowly. During the whole of that time its temperature continues at 32°; and as it is constantly surrounded by warm air, we have reason to believe that caloric is constantly entering into it; yet it does not become hotter till it is changed into water. Ice, therefore, is converted into water by a quantity of caloric uniting with it.

It has been found by calculation, that ice in melting absorbs 140° of caloric, the temperature of the water produced still remaining at 32°.

This fact may be proved in a direct manner.

Take one pound of ice, at 32°, reduced to a coarse powder; put it into a wooden bowl, and pour over it one pound of water, heated to 172°; all the ice will become melted, and the temperature of the whole fluid, if examined by a thermometer, will be 32°; 140° of caloric are therefore lost, and it is this quantity which was requisite to convert the ice into water. This experiment succeeds better, if, instead of ice, fresh-fallen snow be employed.

This caloric has been called *latent caloric*, because its presence is not measurable by the thermometer: also more properly caloric of fluidity.

Dr. Black has also ascertained by experiment, that the fluidity of melted wax, tallow, spermaceti, metals, &c. is owing to the same cause; and Landriani proved, that this is the case with sulphur, alum, nitrate of potassa, &c.

We consider it therefore as a general law, that whenever a solid is converted into a fluid, it combines with caloric, and that is the cause of fluidity.

Conversion of Solids and Fluids into the Aëriform or Gaseous State.

We have seen before, that, in order to render solids fluid, a certain quantity of caloric is necessary, which combines with the body, and therefore cannot be measured by the thermometer; we shall now endeavour to prove that the same holds good in respect to the conversion of solids or fluids into the vaporous or gaseous state.

Take a small quantity of carbonate of ammonia, introduce it into a retort, the neck of which is directed under a cylinder filled with mercury, and inverted in a basin of the same fluid. On applying heat to the body of the retort, the carbonate of ammonia will be volatilized, it will expel the mercury out of the cylinder, and become an invisible gas, and would remain so, if its temperature was not lowered.

The same is the case with benzoic acid, camphire, and various other substances.

All fluids may, by the application of heat, be converted into an aëriform elastic state.

When we consider water in a boiling state, we find that this fluid, when examined by the thermometer, is not hotter after boiling several hours, than when it began to boil, though to maintain it boiling a brisk fire must necessarily be kept up. What then, we may ask, becomes of the wasted caloric? It is not perceptible in the water, nor is it manifested by the steam; for the steam, if not compressed, upon examination, is found not to be hotter than boiling water. The caloric is therefore absorbed by the steam, and although what is so absorbed, is absolutely necessary for the conversion of water into the form of steam; it does not increase its temperature, and is therefore not appreciable by the thermometer.

The conclusion is farther strengthened by the heat given out by steam on its being condensed by cold. This is particularly manifested in the condensation of this fluid in the process of distilling, where, upon examining the refrigeratory, it will be found that a much greater quantity of caloric is communicated to it, than could possibly have been transmitted by the caloric which was sensibly acting before the condensation. This may be easily ascertained by observing the quantity of caloric communicated to the water in the refrigeratory of a still, by any given quantity of liquid that passes over.

1. The boiling point, or the temperature at which the conversion of fluids into gases takes place, is different in different fluids, but constant in each, provided the pressure of the atmosphere be the same.

Put any quantity of sulphuric æther into a Florence flask, suspend a thermometer in it, and hold the flask over an Argand's lamp, the æther will immediately begin to boil, and the thermometer will indicate 98° if the æther has been highly rectified.

If highly rectified ardent spirit is heated in a similar manner, the thermometer will rise to 176°, and there remain stationary.

If water is substituted, it will rise to 212°.

If strong nitrous acid of commerce be made use of, it will be found to boil at 248°; sulphuric acid and linseed-oil at 600°; mercury at 656°, &c.

2. The boiling point of fluids is raised by pressure.

Mr. Watt heated water under a strong pressure to 400°. Yet still, when the pressure was removed, only part of the water was converted into vapour, and the temperature of this vapour, as well as that of the remaining fluid, was no more than 212°. There was, therefore, 188° of caloric suddenly lost. This caloric was carried off by the steam. Now as only about one-fifth of the water was converted into steam, that steam must contain not only its own 188°, but also the 188° lost by each of the other four parts; that is to say, it must contain 188°×5, or about 940°. Steam, therefore, is water combined with at least 940° of caloric, the presence of which is not indicated by the thermometer.

3. When pressure is removed from the surface of bodies, their conversion into the gaseous state is greatly facilitated, or their boiling point is lowered.

In proof of this the following experiments may serve:

Let a small bottle be filled with highly rectified sulphuric æther, and a piece of wetted bladder be tied over its orifice around its neck. Transfer it under the receiver of an air-pump, and take away the superincumbent pressure of the air in the receiver. When the exhaustion is complete, pierce the bladder by means of a pointed sliding wire, passing through a collar of leather which covers the upper opening of the receiver. Having done this, the æther will instantly begin to boil, and become converted into an invisible gaseous fluid.

Take a small retort or Florence flask, fill it one half or less with water, and make it boil over a lamp; when kept briskly boiling for about five minutes, cork the mouth of the retort as expeditiously as possible, and remove it from the lamp.

The water, on being removed from the source of heat, will keep boiling for a few minutes, and when the ebullition begins to slacken, it may be renewed by dipping the retort into cold water, or pouring cold water upon it.

The water, during boiling, becomes converted into vapour; this vapour expels the air of the vessel, and occupies its place; on diminishing the heat, it condenses; when the retort is stopped, a partial vacuum is formed; the pressure becomes diminished, and a less degree of heat is sufficient to cause an ebullition.

For the same reason, water may be made to boil under the exhausted receiver at 94° Fahr., or even at a lower degree; alkohol at 56°; and æther at —20°.

On the conversion of fluids into gases is founded the following experiment, by which water is frozen by means of sulphuric æther.

Take a thin glass tube four or five inches long and about two or three-eighths of an inch in diameter, and a two-ounce bottle furnished with a capillary tube fitted to its neck. In order to make ice, pour a little water into the tube, taking care not to wet the outside, nor to leave it moist. Having done this, let a stream of sulphuric æther fall through the capillary tube upon that part of it containing the water, which by this means will be converted into ice in a few minutes, and this it will do even near a fire, or in the midst of summer.

If the glass tube, containing the water, be exposed to the brisk thorough air, or free draught of an open window, a large quantity of water may be frozen in a shorter time; and if a thin spire of wire be introduced previous to the congelation of the water, the ice will adhere to it, and may thus be drawn out conveniently.

A person might be easily frozen to death during very warm weather, by merely pouring upon his body for some time sulphuric æther, and keeping him exposed to a thorough draught of air.

Artificial Refrigeration.

The cooling or refrigeration of rooms in the summer season by sprinkling them with water, is on the principle of evaporation.

The method of making ice artificially in the East Indies depends on the same principle. The ice-makers at Benares dig pits in large open plains, the bottom of which they strew with sugar-canes or dried stems of maize or Indian-corn. Upon this bed they place a number of unglazed pans, made of so porous an earth that the water penetrates through their whole substance. These pans are filled toward evening in the winter season with water that has boiled, and left in that situation till morning, when more or less ice is found in them, according to the temperature and other qualities of the air; there being more formed in dry and warm weather, than in that which is cloudy, though it may be colder to the human body.

Every thing in this process is calculated to produce cold by evaporation; the beds on which the pans are placed, suffer the air to have a free passage to their bottoms; and the pans constantly oozing out water to their external surface, are cooled by the evaporation of it.

In Spain, they use a kind of earthen jars, called buxaros, which are only half-baked, the earth of which is so porous, that the outside is kept moist by the water which filters through it, and though placed in the sun, the water in the jar becomes as cold as ice.

It is a common practice in China to cool wine or other liquors by wrapping the bottle in a wet cloth, and hanging it up in the sun. The water in the cloth becomes converted into vapour, and thus cold is produced.

The blacks in Senegambia have a similar method of cooling water by filling tanned leather bags with it, which they hang up in the sun; the water oozes, more or less through the leather so as to keep the outer surface wet, which by its quick and continued evaporation cools the water remarkably.

The winds on the borders of the Persian gulf are often so scorching, that travellers are suddenly suffocated unless they cover their heads with a wet cloth; if this be too wet, they immediately feel an intolerable cold, which would prove fatal if the moisture was not speedily dissipated by the heat.

Condensation of Vapour.

If a cold vessel is brought into a warm room, particularly where many people are assembled, the outside of it will soon become covered with a sort of dew.

Before some changes of weather, the stone pavements, the walls of a house, the balustrades of staircases, and other solid objects, feel clammy and damp.

In frosty nights, when the air abroad is colder than the air within, the dampness of this air, for the same reason, settles on the glass panes of the windows, and is there frozen into curious and beautiful figures.

Thus *fogs* and *dews* take place, and in the higher regions clouds are formed from the condensed vapour. The still greater condensation produces *mists* and *rain*.

Capacity of Bodies for containing Heat.

The property which different bodies possess, of containing at the same temperature, and in equal quantities, either of mass or bulk, unequal quantities of heat, is called their capacity for heat. The capacities of bodies for heat are therefore considered as great or small in proportion as their temperatures are either raised by the addition, or diminished by the deprivation, of equal quantities of heat, in a less or greater degree.

In homogeneous bodies, the quantities of caloric which they contain are in the ratio of their temperature and mass: when, therefore, equal quantities of water, of oil, or of mercury, of unequal temperatures are mingled together, the temperature of the whole will be the *arithmetical* mean between the temperatures of the two quantities that had been mixed together. It is a self-evident truth that this should be the case, for the particles of different portions of the same substance being alike, their effects must be equal. For instance:

Mix a pound of water at 172° with a pound at 32°, half the excess of heat in hot water will quit it to go over into the colder portion; thus the hot water will be cooled 70°, and the cold will receive 70° of temperature; therefore 172—70, or $32 + 70 = 102$, will give the heat of the mixture. To attain the arithmetical mean very exactly, several precautions, however, are necessary.

When heterogeneous bodies of different temperatures are mixed together, the temperature produced is never the arithmetical mean of the two original temperatures.

In order to ascertain the comparative quantities of heat of different bodies, equal weights of them are mingled together; the experiments for this purpose being in general more easily executed than those by which they are compared from equal bulks.

Thus, if one pound of mercury heated to 410° Fahr., be added to one pound of water of 44°, the temperature of the blended fluids will not be changed to 77°, as it would be if the surplus of heat were divided among those fluids in the proportion of their quantities. It will be found, on examination, to be only 47°.

On the contrary, if the pound of mercury be heated to 44°, and the water to 110°, then, on stirring them together, the common temperature will be 107°.

Hence, if the quicksilver loses by this distribution 63° of caloric, an equal weight of water gains only 3° from this loss of 63° of heat. And, on the contrary, if the water loses 3°, the mercury gains 63°.

When, instead of comparing the quantities of caloric which equal *weights* of different bodies contain, we compare the quantities contained in equal *volumes*, we still find that an obvious difference takes place. Thus it is found by experiment, that the quantity of caloric necessary to raise the temperature of a given volume of water any number of degrees, is, to that necessary to raise an equal volume of mercury, the same number of degrees as 2 to 1. This is, therefore, the proportion between the comparative quantities of caloric which these two bodies contain, estimated by their volumes; and similar differences exist with respect to every other kind of matter.

From the nature of the experiments by which the quantities of caloric which bodies contain are ascertained, it is evident that we discover merely the *comparative*, not the *absolute* quantities. Hence water has been chosen as a standard, to which other bodies may be referred; its capacity is stated as the arbitrary term of 1000, and with this the capacities of other bodies are compared.

It need not be told that pains have been taken to estimate on these experiments that portion of heat which diffuses itself into the air, or into the vessel where the mercury and water are blended together. As however such valuations cannot be made with complete accuracy, the numbers stated above are only an approximation to truth.

Radiation of Caloric.

Caloric is thrown off or radiates from heated bodies in right lines, and moves through space with inconceivable velocity. It is retarded in its passage by atmospheric air, by colourless fluids, glass, and other transparent bodies.

If a glass mirror be placed before a fire, the mirror transmits the rays of light, but not the rays of heat.

If a plate of glass, talc, or a glass vessel filled with water, be suddenly interposed between the fire and the eye, the rays of light pass through it, but the rays of caloric are considerably retarded in its passage; for no heat is perceived until the interposed substance is saturated with heat, or has reached its *maximum*. It then ceases to intercept the rays of caloric, and allows them to pass as freely as the rays of light.

It has been lately shown by Dr. Herschel, that the rays of caloric are refrangible, but less so than the rays of light; and the same philosopher has also proved by experiment, that it is not only the rays of caloric emitted by the sun, which are refrangible, but likewise, the rays emitted by common fires, by candles, by heated iron, and even by hot water.

Whether the rays of caloric are differently refracted, in different mediums, has not yet been ascertained. We are certain, however, that they are refracted by all transparent bodies which have been employed as burning glasses.

The rays of caloric are also reflected by polished surfaces in the same manner as the rays of light.

This was long ago noticed by Lambert, Saussure, Scheele, Pictet, and lately by Dr. Herschel.

Professor Pictet placed two concave metallic mirrors opposite to each other, at the distance of about twelve feet. When a hot body, an iron bullet for instance, was placed in the focus of the one, and a mercurial thermometer in that of the other, a substance radiated from the bullet; it passed with incalculable velocity through the air, it was reflected from the mirrors, it became concentrated, and influenced the thermometer placed in the focus, according to the degree of its concentration.

An iron ball two inches in diameter, heated so that it was not luminous in the dark, raised the thermometer not less than ten and a half degrees of Reaumur's scale, in six minutes.

A lighted candle occasioned a rise in the thermometer nearly the same.

A Florence flask containing two ounces and three drachms of boiling water, raised Fahrenheit's thermometer three degrees. He blackened the bulb of his thermometer, and found that it was more speedily influenced by the radiation than before, and that it rose to a greater height.

M. Pictet discovered another very singular fact; namely, the *apparent radiation of cold*. When, instead of a heated body, a Florence flask full of ice or snow is placed in the focus of one of the mirrors, the thermometer placed in the focus of the other immediately descends, and ascends again whenever the cold body is removed.

This phenomenon may be explained on the supposition, that from every body at every temperature caloric radiates, but in less quantity as the temperature is low; so that in the above experiment, the thermometer gives out more caloric by radiation, than it receives from the body in the opposite focus, and therefore its temperature is lowered. Or, as Pictet has supposed, when a number of bodies near to each other have the same temperature, there is no radiation of caloric, because in all of them it exists in a state of equal tension; but as soon as a body at an inferior temperature is introduced, the balance of tension is broken, and caloric begins to radiate from all of them, till the temperature of that body is raised to an equality with theirs. In the above experiment, therefore, the placing the snow or ice in the focus of the mirror causes the radiation of caloric *from* the thermometer, and hence the diminution of temperature which it suffers.

These experiments have been since repeated by Dr. Young and Professor Davy, at the theatre of the Royal Institution. These gentlemen inflamed phosphorus by reflected caloric; and proved that the heat thus excited, was very sensible to the organs of feeling.

It is therefore evident, that caloric is thrown off from bodies in rays, which are invisible, or incapable of exciting vision, but which are capable of exciting heat.

These invisible rays of caloric are propagated in right lines, with extreme velocity; and are capable of the laws of reflection and refraction.

The heating agency however is different in the different coloured rays of the prismatic spectrum. According to Dr. Herschel's experiments, it follows inversely the order of the refrangibility of the rays of light. The least refrangible, possessing it in the greatest degree.

Sir Henry Englefield has lately made a series of experiments on the same subject, from which we learn, that a thermometer having its ball blackened, rose when placed in the *blue* ray of the prismatic spectrum in 3′ from 55° to 56°; in the *green*, in 3′ from 54° to 58°; in the *yellow*, in 3′ from 56° to 62°; in the *full red*, in 2 1-2′ from 56° to 72°; in the *confines of the red*, in 2 1-2′ from 58° to 73 1-2°; and *quite out of the visible light*, in 2 1-2′ from 61° to 79°.

Between each of the observations, the thermometer was placed in the shade so long as to sink it below the heat to which it had risen in the preceding observation; of course, its rise above that point could only be the effect of the ray to which it was exposed. It was continued in the focus long after it had ceased to rise; therefore the heats given are the greatest effects of the several rays on the thermometer in each observation. A thermometer placed constantly in the shade near the apparatus, was found scarcely to vary during the experiments.

Sir Henry made other experiments with thermometers with naked balls, and with others whose balls were painted white, for which we refer the reader to the interesting paper of the Baronet, from which the above experiments are transcribed.

Production of Artificial Cold, by means of Frigorific Mixtures.

A number of experiments have been lately made by different philosophers, especially by Pepys, Walker, and Lowitz, in order to produce artificial cold. And as these methods are often employed in chemistry, with a view to expose bodies to the influence of very low temperatures, we shall enumerate in a tabular form the different substances which may be made use of for that purpose, and the degrees of cold which they are capable of producing.

To produce the effects stated in the table, the salts must be reduced to powder, and contain their full quantity of water of crystallization. The vessel in which the freezing mixture is made, should be very thin, and just large enough to hold it, and the materials should be mixed together as expeditiously as possible, taking care to stir the mixture at the same time with a rod of glass or wood.

In order to obtain the full effect, the materials ought to be first cooled to the temperature marked in *the table*, by introducing them into some of the other frigorific mixtures, and then mingling them together in a similar mixture. If, for instance, we wish to produce —46°, the snow and diluted nitric acid ought to be cooled down to 0°, by putting the vessel which contains each of them into the fifth freezing mixture in the above table, before they are mingled together. If a more intense cold be required, the materials to produce it are to be brought to the proper temperature by being previously placed in the second freezing mixture

This process is to be continued till the required degree of cold has been procured.

A TABLE OF FREEZING MIXTURES.

Mixtures.		Thermometer sinks
Muriate of ammonia Nitrate of potassa Water	5 parts 5 16	From 50° to 10°.
Muriate of ammonia Nitrate of potassa Sulphate of soda Water	5 parts 5 8 16	From 50° to 4°.
Sulphate of soda Diluted nitric acid	3 parts 2	From 50° to —3°
Sulphate of soda Muriatic acid	8 parts 5	From 50° to 0°.
Snow Muriate of soda	1 part 1	From 32° to 0°.
Snow, or pounded ice Muriate of soda	2 parts 1 part	From 0° to —5°.
Snow, or pounded ice Muriate of soda Muriate of ammonia and nitrate of potassa	12 parts 5 5	From —5° to —18°.
Snow, or pounded ice Muriate of soda Nitrate of ammonia	12 parts 5 5	From —18° to —25°.
Snow Diluted nitric acid	3 parts 2	From 0° to —46°.
Muriate of lime Snow	3 parts 2	From 32° —50°.
Potassa Snow	4 parts 3	From 32° to —51°.
Snow Diluted sulphuric acid Diluted nitric acid	8 parts 3 3	From —10° to —56°
Snow Diluted sulphuric acid	1 part 1	From 20° to —60°.
Muriate of lime Snow	2 parts 1	From 0° to —66°.
Muriate of lime Snow	3 parts 1	From —40° to —73°.
Diluted sulphuric acid Snow	10 parts 8	From —68° to —91°.
Nitrate of ammonia Water	1 part 1	From 50° to 4°.
Nitrate of ammonia Carbonate of soda Water	1 part 1 1	From 50° to —7°.
Sulphate of soda Muriate of ammonia Nitrate of potassa Diluted nitric acid	6 parts 4 2 4	From 50° to —10°.
Sulphate of soda Nitrate of ammonia Diluted nitric acid	6 parts 5 4	From 50° to —14°.
Phosphate of soda Diluted nitric acid	9 parts 4	From 50° to —12°.
Phosphate of soda Nitrate of ammonia Diluted nitric acid	9 parts 6 4	From 50° to —21°.
Sulphate of soda Diluted sulphuric acid	5 parts 4	From 50° to 3°.

CALORI'METER. An instrument by which the whole quantity of absolute heat existing in a body in chemical union can be ascertained.

CALP. An argillo-ferruginous limestone.

CA'LTHA. (Καλθα, corrupted from χαλχα, yellow; from whence, says Vossius, come *calthula*, *caldula*, *caledula*, *calendula*.) The marigold. 1. The name of a genus of plants in the Linnæan system. Class, *Polyandria*; Order, *Polygynia*.

2. The pharmacopœial name of the herb wild marigold, so called from its colour.

CALTHA ARVENSIS. *Calendula arvensis; Caltha vulgaris*. The wild marigold is sometimes preferred to the garden marigold. Its juice is given, from one to four ounces, in jaundice and cachexia; and the leaves are commended as a salad for children afflicted with scrofulous humours.

CALTHA PALUSTRIS. *Populago*. Common single marsh marigold. It is said to be caustic and deleterious: but this may be questioned. The young buds of this plant make, when properly pickled, very good substitutes for capers.

Caltha vulgaris. See *Caltha arvensis.*

Ca'lthula. The caltha is so called.

CALTROPS. See *Trapa natans.*

CALU'MBA. The name now adopted by the London college of physicians for the root of the *Cocculus palmatus* of De Candolles, in his *Systema naturæ.* It was formerly called *Colombo; Calomba;* and *Colamba.* This root is imported from Colomba, in Ceylon, in circular, brown knobs, wrinkled on their outer surface, yellowish within, and consisting of cortical, woody, and medullary laminæ. Its smell is aromatic; its taste pungent, and very bitter. From Dr. Percival's experiments on the root, it appears that rectified spirit of wine extracts its virtues in the greatest perfection. The watery infusion is more perishable than that of other bitters. An ounce of the powdered root, half an ounce of orange-peel, two ounces of brandy, and four teen ounces of water, macerated twelve h urs without heat, and then filtered through paper, afford a sufficiently strong and tolerably pleasant infusion. The extract made first by spirit and then with water, and reduced by evaporation to a pillular consistence, is found to be equal, if not superior in efficacy, to the powder. As an antiseptic, Calumba root is inferior to the bark; but, as a corrector of putrid bile, it is much superior to the bark; whence also it is probable, that it would be of service in the West-India yellow fever. It also restrains alimentary fermentation, without impairing digestion; in which property it resembles mustard. It does not appear to have the least heating quality, and therefore may be used in phthisis pulmonalis, and in hectic cases, to strengthen digestion. It occasions no disturbance, and agrees very well with a milk diet, as it abates flatulence, and is indisposed to acidity. The London, Edinburgh, and Dublin colleges, direct a tincture of Calumba root. The dose of the powdered root is as far as half a drachm, which, in urgent cases, may be repeated every third or fourth hour.

[Calumbo. See *American Columbo.* A.]

CA'LVA. (From *calvus,* bald.) The scalp or upper part of the cranium or top of the head; so called because it often grows bald first.

CALVA'RIA. (From *calvus,* bald.) The upper part or the cranium which becomes soon bald. It comprehends all above the orbits, temples, ears, and occipital eminence.

CALVI'TIES. (From *calvus,* bald.) *Calvitium.* Baldness; want or loss of hair, particularly upon the sinciput.

This name is applied by Dr. Good to a species of his *trichosis athrix,* or baldness.

CALX. (*Calx, cis.* fœm; from *kalah,* to burn. Arabian.) 1. Chalk. Limestone.

2. Lime. *Calx viva.* The London College directs it to be prepared thus:—Take of limestone one pound: break it into small pieces, and heat it in a crucible, in a strong fire, for an hour, or until the carbonic acid is entirely driven off, so that on the addition of acetic acid, no bubbles of gas shall be extricated. Lime may be made by the same process from oyster-shells previously washed in boiling water, and cleared from extraneous matters. See *Lime*

Calx antimonii. See *Antimonii oxydum.*

Calx cum kali puro. See *Potassa cum calce.*

Calx hydrargyri alba. See *Hydrargyrum præcipitatum album.*

Calx metallic. A metal which has undergone the process of calcination, or combustion, or any other equivalent operation.

Calx viva. See *Calx.*

Calycanthemæ. (From *calyx,* the flower-cup, and ανθος, the flower.) The name of an order in Linnæus's fragments of a natural method, consisting of plants, which, among other characteristics, have the corolla and stamina inserted into the calyx.

CALYCIFLORÆ. (From *calyx,* and *flos,* a flower.) The name of an order in Linnæus's fragments of a natural method, consisting of plants which have the stamina inserted into the Calyx.

CALYCINUS. (From *calyx,* the flower-cup.) *Calycinalis.* Belonging to the calyx of a flower; applied to the nectary, *nectarium calycinum,* it being a production of the calyx; as in *Tropæolum majus,* the garden nasturtium.

CALYCULATUS. (From *calyculus,* a small calyx.) Calyculate. Applied to a *perianthium* when there are less ones, like scales, about its base; as in *Dianthus caryophyllus. Semina calyculata* are those which are enclosed in a hard bone-like calyx, as those of the *Coix lachryma,* or Job's tears.

CALYCULUS. (Diminutive of *calyx.*) A little calyx. A botanical term for

I. The membranaceous margin surrounding the apex of a seed.

The *varieties* are,

1. *Calyculus integer,* the margin perfect not incised; as in *Tanacetum vulgare,* and *Dipsacus laciniatus.*
2. *Calyculus palyaceus,* with chaffy scales; as in *Helianthus annuus.*
3. *Calyculus aristatus,* having two or three awns at the top; as in *Tagetes patula,* and *Bidens tripartita.*
4. *Calyculus rostratus,* the style of the germ remaining; as in *Sinapis,* and *Scandix cerefolium.*
5. *Calyculus cornutas,* horned, the rostrum bent; as in *Nigella damascena.*
6. *Calyculus cristatus,* a dentate, or incised membrane on the top of the seed; as in *Hedysarum crista galli.*

II. A little calyx exterior to another proper one.

Caly'pter. (From καλυπτω, to hide.) A carneous excrescence covering the hæmorrhoidal vein.

CALYPTRA. (From καλυπτω, to cover.) I. The veil, or covering of mosses. A kind of membraneous hood placed, on their capsule or fructification, like an extinguisher on a candle, well seen in *Bryum cæspitosum.* Linnæus considered it as a calyx, but other botanists, especially Schreber and Smith, reckon it to be a sort of corolla. It is either,

1. *Acuminate,* pointed; as in *Minium* and *Bryum.*
2. *Caducous,* falling off yearly; as in *Bauxbaumia.*
3. *Conical;* as in most mosses.
4. *Smooth;* as in *Hypnum.*
5. *Lævis,* without any inequalities; as in *Splanchnum.*
6. *Oblong;* as in *Minium.*
7. *Villous;* as in *Polytrichum.*
8. *Complete,* surrounding the whole of the top of the capsule.
9. *Dimidiate,* covering only half the capsule; as in *Bryum androgynum.*
10. *Dentate,* toothed in the margin; as in *Eucalypta ciliata.*

In many genera it is wanting.

II. The name in Tournefort, and writings of former botanists, for the proper exterior covering or coat of the seed, which falls off spontaneously.

CALYPTRATUS. (From *calyptra,* the veil, or covering of mosses.) Calyptrate: having a covering like the calyptra of mosses.

CALYX. (*Calyx, icis.* f.; καλυξ; from καλυπτω, to cover.) *Calix.* I. The flower-cup, or, more correctly, the external covering of the flower, for the most part green, and surrounding the corolla, or gaudy part.

There are five *genera* of calyces, or flower-cups.

1. *Perianthium.* 2. *Involucrum.*
3. *Amentum* 4. *Spatha.*
5. *Gluma.* 6. *Perichælium*
7. *Volva.*

II. The membrane which covers the papillæ in the pelvis of the human kidney.

CA'MARA. (From καμαρα, a vault.) *Camarium.* 1. The fornix of the brain.

2. The vaulted part of the auricle of the heart.

Cama'rium. (From καμαρα, a vault.) A vault. See *Camara.*

CAMARO'MA. (From καμαρα, a vault.) *Camarosis; Camaratio.* A fracture of the skull, in the shape of an arch or vault.

Cambirea. So Paracelsus calls the venereal bubo.

CA'MBIUM The gelatinous substance, or matter of organization which Du Hamel and Mirbel suppose produces the young bark, and new wood of plants

Cambium. (From *cambio,* to exchange.) The nutritious humour which is changed into the mater als of which the body is composed.

Cambo'dia. See *Stalagmitis.*

CAMBO'GIA. (From the province of *Cambaya,* in the East Indies;) *Cambodja* and *Cambogia; Cambodia; Cambogium; Gambogia; Gambogium.* See *Stalagmitis.*

Cambogia gutta. See *Stalagmitis.*

CAMBO'GIUM. See *Cambogia* and *Stalagmitis.*

Cambro-britannica. See *Rubus Chamæmorus.*

Cambu'ca. *Cambuta membrata.* So Paracelsus calls the venereal cancer. By some it is described as a bubo, an ulcer, an abscess on the pudenda; also a boil in the groin.

Ca'mbui. The wild American myrtle of Piso and Margrave, which is said to be astringent.

Camel's hay. See *Andropogon Schænanthus.*

CAMELEON MINERAL. When pure potassa and black oxide of manganese are fused together in a crucible, a compound is formed, whose solution in water, at first green, passes spontaneously through the whole series of coloured rays to the red. From this latter tint, the solution may be made to retrograde in colour to the original green, by the addition of potassa; or it may be rendered altogether colourless, by adding either sulphureous acid or chlorine to the solution, in which case there may or may not be a precipitate, according to circumstances.

CA'MERA. A chamber or cavity. The chambers of the eye are termed *cameræ.*

Camera'tio. See *Camaroma.*

Ca'mes. *Camet.* Silver.

Cami'nga. See *Canella alba.*

Ca'minus. A furnace and its chimney. In Rulandus it signifies a bell.

Cami'sia fœtus. (From the Arabic term *kamisah,* an under garment.) The shirt of the fœtus. See *Chorion.*

Camomile. See *Chamomile.*

Camomi'lla. Corrupted from *chamæmelum.*

CA'MMORUM. (Καμμορον, *quia homines, κακῳ μορῳ, perimat;* because if eaten, it brings men to a miserable end.) A species of monkshood. See *Aconitum napellus.*

CAMPA'NA. A bell. In chemistry, a receptacle like a bell, for making sulphuric acid; thus the oleum sulphuris per campanum.

CAMPANACEÆ. Bell-shaped flowers. The name of an order of Linnæus's natural method.

CAMPANIFORMIS. *Campanaceus; Campanulatus.* Bell-shaped; applied to the corolla and nectaries of plants.

CAMPA'NULA. (From *campana,* a bell; named from its shape.) The name of a genus of plants in the Linnæan system. Class, *Pentandria;* Order, *Monogynia.* The Bell-flower.

Campanula trachelium. *Cervicaria.* The Great Throat-wort: by some recommended against inflammatory affections of the throat and mouth.

CAMPAN'ULATUS. (From *Campanula,* a little bell.) Bell-shaped: applied to the corolla and nectary of plants, as in *Campanula.* See *Corolla* and *Nectarium.*

Ca'mpe. (From καμπτω, to bend.) A flexure or bending. It is also used for the ham, and a joint, or articulation.

Campeachy wood. See *Hæmatoxylon Campechianum.*

Campechense, lignum. See *Hæmatoxylon Campechianum,* or *Logwood.*

CAMPER, Peter, was born at Leyden in 1722, where he studied under Boerhaave, and took his degree in medicine. He then travelled for some years, and was afterward appointed a professor successively at Franeker, Amsterdam, and Groningen. He was subsequently occupied in prosecuting his favourite studies, in visiting various parts of Europe, by the different societies of which he was honourably distinguished, and in performing many public duties in his own country, being at length chosen one of the council of state. He died in 1789 of a pleurisy. He published some improvements in midwifery and surgery, but anatomy appears to have been his favourite pursuit. He finished two parts of a work of considerable magnitude and importance, in which the healthy and morbid structure of the arm, and of the pelvis, are exhibited in very accurate plates, from drawings made by himself: which he appears to have purposed extending to the other parts of the body. There are also some posthumous works of Camper possessing great merit, partly on subjects of natural history, partly evincing the connexion between anatomy and painting; in which latter judicious rules are laid down for exhibiting the diversity of features in persons of various countries and ages, and representing the different emotions of the mind in the countenance; also for delineating the general forms of other animals, which he shows to be modified according to their economy.

CAMPESTRIS. Of or belonging to the field; applied as a trivial name to many plants, which are common in the fields.

CAMPHIRE. See *Laurus camphora.*

Camphor. See *Laurus camphora.*

CA'MPHORA. (*Camphura.* Arabian. The ancients meant by camphor what now is called asphaltum, or Jews' pitch; καφουρα.) See *Laurus camphora.*

Ca'mphoræ flores. The subtle substance which first ascends in subliming camphor. It is nothing more than the camphor.

Camphoræ flores compositi. Camphor sublimed with benzoin.

CA'MPHORAS. A camphorate. A salt formed by the union of the camphoric acid with a salifiable base, thus, *camphorate of alumine, camphorate of ammonia,* &c.

CAMPHORA'SMA. (From *camphora;* so called from its camphor-like smell.) Turkey balsam. See *Dracocephalum.*

CAMPHORA'TA. See *Camphorosma.*

Camphora'tum oleum. See *Linimentum camphoræ.*

CAMPHORIC ACID. *Acidum camphoricum.* An acid with peculiar properties is obtained, by distilling nitric acid eight times following from camphor; and the following is the account Bouillon Lagrange gives of its preparation and properties.

One part of camphor being introduced into a glass retort, four parts of nitric acid of the strength of 36 degrees are to be poured on it, a receiver adapted to the retort, and all the joints well luted. The retort is then to be placed on a sand-heat, and gradually heated. During the process a considerable quantity of nitrous gas, and of carbonic acid gas, is evolved; and part of the camphor is volatilized, while another part seizes the oxygen of the nitric acid. When no more vapours are extricated, the vessels are to be separated, and the sublimed camphor added to the acid that remains in the retort. A like quantity of nitric acid is again to be poured on this, and the distillation repeated. This operation must be reiterated till the camphor is completely acidified. Twenty parts of nitric acid at 36 are sufficient to acidify one of camphor.

When the whole of the camphor is acidified, it crystallizes in the remaining liquor. The whole is then to be poured out upon a filter, and washed with distilled water, to carry off the nitric acid it may have retained. The most certain indication of the acidification of the camphor is its crystallizing on the cooling of the liquor remaining in the retort. To purify this acid it must be dissolved in hot distilled water, and the solution, after being filtered, evaporated nearly to half, or till a slight pellicle forms; when the camphoric acid will be obtained in crystals on cooling.

The camphoric acid has a slightly acid, bitter taste, and reddens infusion of litmus.

It crystallizes; and the crystals upon the whole resemble those of muriate of ammonia. It effloresces on exposure to the atmosphere; is not very soluble in cold water; when placed on burning coals, it gives out a thick aromatic smoke, and is entirely dissipated; and with a gentle heat melts, and is sublimed. The mineral acids dissolve it entirely. It decomposes the sulphate and muriate of iron. The fixed and volatile oils dissolve it. It is likewise soluble in alkohol, and is not precipitated from it by water; a property that distinguishes it from the benzoic acid. It unites easily with the earths and alkalies, and forms camphoratis.

To prepare the *camphorates of lime, magnesia,* and *alumina,* these earths must be diffused in water, and crystallized camphoric acid added. The mixture must then be boiled, filtered while hot, and the solution concentrated by evaporation.

The *camphorate of barytes* is prepared by dissolving the pure earth in water, and then adding crystallized camphoric acid.

Those of *potassa, soda,* and *ammonia,* should be prepared with their carbonates dissolved in water; these solutions are to be saturated with crystallized camphoric acid, heated, filtered, evaporated, and cooled; by which means the camphorates will be obtained.

If the camphoric acid be very pure, they have no smell; if it be not, they have always a slight smell of camphor.

The *camphorates of alumina* and *barytes* leave a little acidity on the tongue; the rest have a slightly bitterish taste.

They are all decomposed by heat; the acid being separated and sublimed, and the base remaining pure; that of ammonia excepted, which is entirely volatilized.

If they be exposed to the blowpipe, the acid burns with a blue flame: that of ammonia gives first a blue flame; but toward the end it becomes red.

The *camphorates of lime* and *magnesia* are little soluble, the others dissolve more easily.

The mineral acids decompose them all. The alkalies and earths act in the order of their affinity for the camphoric acid; which is, lime, potassa, soda, barytes, ammonia, alumina, magnesia.

Several metallic solutions, and several neutral salts, decompose the camphorates; such as the nitrate of barytes, most of the calcareous salts, &c.

The camphorates of lime, magnesia, and barytes, part with their acid to alkohol.—*Lagrange's Manuel d'un Cours de Chimie.*

CAMPHORO'SMA. (From *camphora*, and οσμη, smell; so called from its smelling of camphire.) The camphor-smelling plant.

1. The name of a genus of plants in the Linnæan system. Class, *Tetrandria*, Order, *Monogynia*.

2. The pharmacopœial name of the camphorata. See *Camphorosma Monspeliensis.*

CAMPHOROSMA MONSPELIENSIS. The systematic name of the plant called *camphorata* in the pharmacopœias. *Chamæpeuce—Camphorata hirsuta—Camphorosma Monspeliaca.* Stinking ground-pine. This plant, *Camphorosma—foliis hirsutis linearibus*, of Linnæus, took its name from its smell resembling so strongly that of camphor: it has been exhibited internally, in form of decoction, in dropsical and asthmatic complaints, and by some is esteemed in fomentations against pain. It is rarely, if ever, used in modern practice.

CA'MPTER. (From καμπτω, to bend.) An inflexion or incurvation.

CA'MPULUM. (From καμπτω, to twist about.) A distortion of the eyelids or other parts.

CAMPYLO'TIS. (From καμπυλος, bent.) A preternatural incurvation, or recurvation of a part; also a distortion of the eyelids.

CA'MPYLUM. See *Campylotis.*

CA'NABIL. A sort of medicinal earth.

CANABI'NA AQUATICA. See *Bidens.*

CA'NABIS INDICA. See *Bangue* and *Cannabis.*

CANABIS PEREGRINA. See *Caunabis.*

Ca'nada balsam. See *Pinus balsamea.*

Canada maidenhair. See *Adianthum pedatum.*

CANADE'NSIS. (Brought from *Canada.*) Canadian. A name of a balsam. See *Pinus balsamea.*

CANALICULATUS. Channelled; having a long furrow; applied to leaves, pods, &c. See *Leaf* and *Legumen.*

CANALI'CULUS. (Diminutive of *canalis*, a channel.) A little canal. See *Canalis arteriosus.*

CANA'LIS. (From χανος, an aperture, or rather from *canna*, a reed.) A canal.

1. Specifically applied to many parts of the body; as *canalis nasalis*, &c.

2. The hollow of the spine.

3. A hollow round instrument like a reed, for embracing and holding a broken limb.

CANALIS ARTERIOSUS. *Canaliculus arteriosus; Canalis botalii.* A blood-vessel peculiar to the fœtus, disappearing after birth; through which the blood passes from the pulmonary artery into the aorta.

CANALIS NASALIS. A canal going from the internal canthus of the eye downwards into the nose; it is situated in the superior maxillary bone, and is lined with the pituitary membrane continued from the nose.

CANALIS PETITIANUS. A triangular cavity, naturally containing a moisture between the two laminæ of the hyaloid membrane of the eye, in the anterior part, formed by the separation of the anterior lamina from the posterior. It is named after its discoverer, M. Petit.

CANALIS SEMICIRCULARIS. Semicircular canal. There are three in each ear placed in the posterior part of the labyrinth. They open by five orifices into the vestibulum. See *Ear.*

CANALIS SEMISPETROS. The half bony canal of the ear.

CANALIS VENOSUS. A canal peculiar to the fœtus, disappearing after birth, that conveys the maternal blood from the *porta* of the liver to the ascending *vena cava.*

Cana'ry balm. See *Dracocephalum.*

CA'NCAMUM GRÆCORUM. See *Hymenæa courbaril*

CANCELLA'TUS. Having the reticulated appearance of the *cancelli* of bones.

CANCE'LLI. Lattice-work; applied to the reticular substance in bones.

CANCE'LLUS. (From *cancer*, a crab.) A species of cray-fish, called Bernard the hermit and the wrong heir; the *Cancer cancellus* of Linnæus; supposed to cure rheumatism, if rubbed on the part.

CA'NCER. 1. The common name of the crab-fish. See *Cancer Astacus.*

2. The name of a disease, from καρκινος, a crab; so called by the ancients, because it exhibited large blue veins like crab's claws: likewise called *Carcinoma, Carcinos*, by the Greeks, *Lupus* by the Romans, because it eats away the flesh like a wolf. Dr. Cullen places this genus of disease in the class *Locales*, and order *Tumores.* He defines it a painful scirrhous tumour, terminating in a fatal ulcer. Any part of the body may be the seat of cancer, though the glands are most subject to it. It is distinguished according to its stages, into *occult* and *open;* by the former is meant its scirrhous state, which is a hard tumour that sometimes remains in a quiet state for many years. When the cancerous action commences in it, it is attended with frequent shooting pains: the skin that covers it becomes discoloured, and ulceration sooner or later takes place: when the disease is denominated *open* cancer. Mr. Pearson says, "When a malignant scirrhus or a watery excrescence hath proceeded to a period of ulceration, attended with a constant sense of ardent and occasionally shooting pains, is irregular in its figure, and presents an unequal surface; if it discharges sordid, sanious, or fœtid matter; if the edges of the sore be thick, indurated, and often exquisitely painful, sometimes inverted, at other times retorted, and exhibit a serrated appearance; and should the ulcer in its progress be frequently attended with hæmorrhage, in consequence of the erosion of blood-vessels; there will be little hazard of mistake in calling it a cancerous ulcer." In men, a cancer most frequently seizes the tongue, mouth, or penis; in women, the breasts or the uterus, particularly about the cessation of their periodical discharges; and in children, the eyes. The following description of Scirrhus and Cancer, from the above writer, will serve to elucidate the subject. A hard unequal tumour that is indolent, and without any discoloration in the skin, is called a scirrhus; but when an itching is perceived in it, which is followed by a pricking, shooting, or lancinating pain, and a change of colour in the skin, it is usually denominated a cancer. It generally is small in the beginning, and increases gradually; but though the skin changes to a red or livid appearance, and the state of the tumour from an indolent to a painful one, it is sometimes very difficult to say when the scirrhus really becomes a cancer, the progress being quick or slow according to concurring causes. When the tumour is attended with a peculiar kind of burning, shooting pains, and the skin hath acquired the dusky purple or livid hue, it may then be deemed the malignant scirrhus or *confirmed cancer.* When thus far advanced in women's breasts, the tumour sometimes increases speedily to a great size, having a knotty unequal surface, more glands becoming obstructed, the nipple sinks in, turgid veins are conspicuous, ramifying around, and resembling a crab's claws. These are the characteristics of an occult cancer on the external parts; and we may suspect the existence of one internally, when such pain and heat as has been described, succeed in parts where the patient hath before been sensible of a weight and pressure, attended with obtuse pain. A cancerous tumour never melts down in suppuration like an inflammatory one; but when it is ready to break open, especially in the breast, it generally becomes prominent in some minute point, attended with an increase of the peculiar kind of burning, shooting pain, felt before at intervals, in a less degree and deeper in the body of the gland. In the prominent part of the tumour, in this state, a corroding ichor sometimes transudes through the skin, soon forming an ulcer: at other times a considerable quantity of a thin lymphatic fluid tinged with blood from

eroded vessels is found on it. Ulcers of the cancerous nature discharge a thin, fœtid, acrid sanies, which corrodes the parts, having thick, dark-coloured retorted lips; and fungous excrescences frequently rise from these ulcers, notwithstanding the corrosiveness of the discharge. In this state they are often attended with excruciating, pungent, lancinating, burning pains, and sometimes with bleeding.

Though a scirrhus may truly be deemed a cancer, as soon as pain is perceived in it, yet every painful tumour is not a cancer; nor is it always easy to say whether a cancer is the disorder or not. Irregular hard lumps may be perceived in the breast; but on examining the other breast, where no uneasiness is perceived, the same kind of tumours are sometimes found, which renders the diagnostic uncertain. Yet in every case after the cessation of the catamenia, hard, unequal tumours in the breast are suspicious; nor, though without pain, are they to be supposed indolent or innoxious.

In the treatment of this disease, our chief reliance must be on extirpating the part affected. Some have attempted to dispel the scirrhous tumour by leeches and various discutient applications, to destroy it by caustics, or to check its progress by narcotics; but without material success. Certainly before the disease is confirmed, should any inflammatory tendency appear, antiphlogistic means may be employed with propriety; but afterward the operation should not be delayed: nay, where the nature of the tumour is doubtful, it will be better to remove it, than incur the risk of this dreadful disease. Some surgeons, indeed, have contested the utility of the operation; and no doubt the disease will sometimes appear again; from constitutional tendency, or from the whole not having been removed: but the balance of evidence is in favour of the operation being successful, if performed early, and to an adequate extent. The plan of destroying the part by caustic is much more tedious, painful, and uncertain. When the disease has arisen from some accident, not spontaneously, when the patient is otherwise healthy, when no symptoms of malignancy in the cancer have appeared, and the adjacent glands and absorbents seem unaffected, we have stronger expectation of success: but unless all the morbid parts can be removed without the risk of dividing important nerves or arteries, it should scarcely be attempted. In operating it is advisable, 1. To make the external wound sufficiently large, and nearly in the direction of the subjacent muscular fibres. 2. To save skin enough to cover it, unless diseased. 3. To tie every vessel which might endanger subsequent hæmorrhage. 4. To keep the lips of the wound in contact, not interposing any dressing, &c. 5. To preserve the parts in an easy and steady position for some days, before they are inspected. 6. To use only mild and cooling applications during the cure. Supposing, however, the patient will not consent to an operation, or circumstances render it inadmissible, the uterus, for example, being affected, internal remedies may somewhat retard its progress, or alleviate the sufferings of the patient; those, which have appeared most beneficial, are, 1. Arsenic, in very small doses long continued. 2. Conium, in doses progressively increased to a considerable extent. 3. Opium. 4. Belladonna. 5. Solanum. 6. Ferrum ammoniatum. 7. Hydrargyri oxymurias. 8. The juice of the galium aparine. When the part is external, topical applications may be useful to alleviate pain, cleanse the sore, or correct the fœtor; especially, 1 Fresh-bruised hemlock leaves. 2. Scraped young carrots. 3. The fermenting poultice. 4. Finely levigated chalk. 5. Powdered charcoal. 6. Carbonic acid gas, introduced into a bladder confined round the part. 7. A watery solution of opium. 8. Liquid tar, or tar-water. But none of these means can be relied upon for effecting a cure.

3. See *Carcinus.*

Cancer astacus. The systematic name of the crab-fish, from which the claws are selected for medical use. Crab's claws and crab's eyes, as they are called, which are concretions found in the stomach, are of a calcareous quality, and possess antacid virtues. They are exhibited with their compounds in pyrosis, diarrhœa, and infantile convulsions from acidity.

Cancer cancellus. See *Cancellus.*

Cancer gammarus. The systematic name of the lobster

Cancer munditorium. A peculiar ulceration of the scrotum of chimney-sweepers.

Ca'nchrys. Parched barley.—*Galen.*

Cancre'na. Paracelsus uses this word instead of gangræna.

Cancro'rum chelæ. Crab's claws. See *Carbonas calcis*, and *Cancer astacus.*

Cancrorum oculi. See *Carbonas calcis*, and *Cancer astacus.*

CA'NCRUM. (From *cancer*, a spreading ulcer.) The canker.

Cancrum oris. Canker of the mouth; a fretted ulceration of the gums.

CANDE'LA. (From *candeo*, to shine.) A candle.

Candela fumalis. A candle made of odoriferous powders and resinous matters, to purify the air and excite the spirits.

Candela regia. See *Verbascum.*

Candela'ria. (From *candela*, a candle; so called from the resemblance of its stalks to a candle.) Mullein. See *Verbascum.*

Candy carrot. See *Athamanta cretensis.*

Cane'la. Sometimes used by the ancients for cinnamon, or rather cassia.

CANE'LLA. (*Canella*, diminutive of *canna*, a reed; so named because the pieces of bark are rolled up in the form of a reed.) The name of a genus of plants in the Linnæan system. Class, *Dodecandria;* Order, *Monogynia.* The canella-tree.

Canella alba. The pharmacopœial name of the laurel-leaved canella. See *Winteria aromatica.*

Canella cubana. See *Canella alba.*

Canellæ malabaricæ cortex. See *Laurus cassia.*

Canelli'fera malabarica. See *Laurus cassia.*

Caneon. (From καννη, because it was made of split cane.) A sort of tube or instrument, mentioned by Hippocrates, for conveying the fumes of antihysteric drugs into the womb.

Ca'nicæ. (From *canis*, a dog, so called by the ancients, because it was food for dogs.) Coarse meal Hence *panis caniceus* means very coarse bread.

CANICI'DA. (From *canis*, a dog, and *cædo*, to kill, so called because dogs are destroyed by eating it.) Dog's bane. See *Aconitum.*

CANICI'DIUM. (From *canis*, a dog, and *cædo*, to kill.) The anatomical dissection of living dogs; for the purpose of illustrating the physiology of parts.

Canina lingua. See *Cynoglossum.*

Canina malus. The mandragora.

Canina rabies. See *Hydrophobia.*

CANINE. Whatever partakes of, or has any relation to, the nature of a dog.

Canine appetite. See *Bulimia.*

Canine madness. See *Hydrophobia.*

Canine teeth. *Dentes canini; Cynodontes; Cuspidati* of Mr. John Hunter; because they have the two sides of their edge sloped off to a point, and this point is very sharp or cuspidated; *columellares* of Varo and Pliny. The four eye-teeth are so called from their resemblance to those of the dog. See *Teeth.*

CANI'NUS. (From *canis*, a dog.) 1. a tooth is so called, because it resembles that of a dog. See *Teeth.*

2. The name of a muscle, because it is near the canine tooth. See *Levator anguli oris.*

3. A disease to which dogs are subject is called *Rabies canina.* See *Hydrophobia.*

Caninus sentis. See *Rosa canina.*

Caniru'bus. (From *canis*, and *rubus*, a bramble.) See *Rosa canina.*

CA'NIS. 1. A dog. The white dung of this animal, called *album græcum*, was formerly in esteem, but now disused.

2. The frænum of the penis.

Canus interfector. Indian barley. See *Veratrum sabadilla.*

Canis ponticus. See *Castor.*

CANNA. (Hebrew.) 1. A reed or hollow cane.

2. The fibula, from its resemblance to a reed.

Canna fistula. See *Cassia fistula.*

Canna indica. See *Sagittaria alexipharmica.*

Canna major. The tibia.

Canna minor cruris. The fibula.

Cannabi'na. (From *canna*, a reed, named from its reed-like stalk.) So Tournefort named his *datisca.*

CA'NNABIS. (From καννα, a reed. Καvvαβοι are foul springs, wherein hemp, &c. grow naturally. Or from *kanaba*, from *kanah*, to mow. Arabian.) Hemp 1. The name of a genus of plants in the Linnæan system. Class, *Diœcia;* Order, *Pentandria*.

2. The pharmacopœial name of the hemp-plant. See *Cannabis sativa*.

Cannabis sativa. The systematic name of the hemp-plant. It has a rank smell of a narcotic kind. The effluvia from the fresh herb are said to affect the eyes and head, and that the water in which it has been long steeped is a sudden poison. Hemp-seeds, when fresh, afford a considerable quantity of oil. Decoctions and emulsions of them have been recommended against coughs, ardor urinæ, &c. Their use, in general, depends on their emollient and demulcent qualities. The leaves of an oriental hemp, called *bang* or *bangue*, and by the Egyptians *assis*, are said to be used in eastern countries, as a narcotic and aphrodisiac. See *Bangue*.

CA'NNULA. (Diminutive of *canna*, a reed.) The name of a surgical instrument. See *Canula*.

CA'NON. Κανων. A rule or canon, by which medicines are compounded.

Cano'nial. Κανονιαι. Hippocrates in his book De Aëre, &c. calls those persons thus, who have straight, and not prominent bellies. He would intimate that they are disposed, as it were, by a straight rule.

Cano picon. (From κανωποι, the flower of the elder.) 1. A sort of spurge, so named from its resemblance

2. A collyrium, of which the chief ingredient was elder flowers.

Canopi'te. The name of a collyrium mentioned by Celsus.

Cano'pum. Κανωπον. The flower or bark of the elder-tree, in Paulus Ægineta.

Canta'brica. See *Convolvulus*.

Canta'brum. (From *kanta*, Hebrew.) In Cœlius Aurelianus it signifies bran.

Ca'ntacon. Garden saffron.

Ca'ntara. The plant which bears the St. Ignatius's bean. See *Ignaria amara*.

CANTERBURY. The name in history of a much celebrated town in Kent, in which there is a mineral water, *Cantuariensis aqua*, strongly impregnated with iron, sulphur, and carbonic acid gas; it is recommended in disorders of the stomach, in gouty complaints, jaundice, diseases of the skin, and chlorosis.

Ca'nthari figulini. Earthen cucurbits.

CA'NTHARIS. (*Cantharis*, pl. *cantharides:* from κανθαρος, a beetle, to which tribe it belongs.) *Musca Hispanica; Lytta vesicatoria;* The blistering fly; Spanish fly. These flies have a green shining gold body, and are common in Spain, Italy, France, and Germany. The largest come from Italy, but the Spanish cantharides are generally preferred. The importance of these flies, by their stimulant, corrosive, and epispastic qualities, in the practice of physic and surgery, is very considerable; indeed, so much so, as to induce many to consider them as the most powerful medicine in the materia medica. When applied on the skin, in the form of a plaster, it soon raises a blister full of serous matter, and thus relieves inflammatory diseases, as phrenitis, pleuritis, hepatitis, phlegmon, bubo, myositis, arthritis, &c. The tincture of these flies is also of great utility in several cutaneous diseases, rheumatic affections, sciatic pains, &c. but ought to be used with much caution. See *Blister*, and *Tinctura cantharidis*. This insect is two-thirds of an inch in length, one-fourth in breadth, oblong, and of a gold shining colour, with soft elytera or wing sheaths, marked with three longitudinal raised stripes, and covering brown membraneous wings. An insect of a square form, with black feet, but possessed of no vesicating property, is sometimes mixed with the cantharides. They have a heavy disagreeable odour, and acrid taste

If the inspissated watery decoction of these insects be treated with pure alkohol, a solution of a resinous matter is obtained, which being separated by gentle evaporation to dryness, and submitted for some time to the action of sulphuric æther, forms a yellow solution. By spontaneous evaporation, crystalline plates are deposited, which may be freed from some adhering colouring matter by alkohol. Their appearance is like spermaceti. They are soluble in boiling alkohol, but precipitate as it cools. They do not dissolve in water. According to Robiquet, who first discovered them, these plates form the true blistering principle. They might be called *Vesicatoria*. Besides the above peculiar body, cantharides contain, according to Robiquet, a green bland oil, insoluble in water, soluble in alkohol; a black matter, soluble in water, insoluble in alkohol, without blistering properties; a yellow viscid matter, mild, soluble in water and alkohol; the crystalline plates; a fatty bland matter; phosphates of lime and magnesia; a little acetic acid, and much lithic or uric acid. The blistering fly taken into the stomach in doses of a few grains, acts as a poison, occasioning horrible satyriasis, delirium, convulsions, and death. Some frightful cases are related by Orfila, vol. i. part second. Oils, milk, syrups, frictions on the spine, with volatile liniment and laudanum, and draughts containing musk, opium, and camphorated emulsion, are the best antidotes.

["Cantharides Vittatæ. Potato flies. The *Cantharis vittata* of Olivier, called *Lytta vittata* by Fabricius, inhabits the United States and South America. It is also given by Pallas among his insects of Siberia. It feeds on different plants, but chiefly on the potato vine, and is easily caught in the morning and towards night. It agrees with the Spanish fly in its generic character, but is a smaller insect, having its elytra or wing cases black with a yellow stripe and margin, its head reddish yellow, and its abdomen and legs black. This fly is found by abundant experience to possess all the vesicating powers of the European cantharis, and to exert the same effect, when internally administered, upon the bladder and urethra. The potato fly might well supersede the Spanish, were it not that its visits in different years vary greatly as to certainty and numbers. It is probable that many insects of the coleopterous class possess vesicating powers. Recently a fly possessing this quality was sent from the country to a physician in Boston. It proved to be the meloe proscarabeus of Linnæus. The discovery of the epispastic property in any native insect, is an object of interest. But that such insects may become extensively useful, they must be abundant and easy of collection."—*Big. Mat. Med.* A.]

Ca'nthum. Sugar-candy.

CA'NTHUS. (Κανθος, the tire or iron binding of a cart-wheel. Dr. Turton, in his glossary, supposes from its etymology, that it originally signified the circular extremity of the eyelid.) The angle or corner of the eye, where the upper and under eyelids meet. That next the nose is termed the internal or greater canthus; and the other, the external or less canthus.

Cantion. Sugar.

CA'NULA. (Diminutive of *canna*, a reed.) *Cannula*. A small tube. The term is generally applied to a tube adapted to a sharp instrument, with which it is thrust into a cavity or tumour, containing a fluid; the perforation being made, the sharp instrument is withdrawn, and the canula left, in order that the fluid may pass through it.

Canusa. Crystal.

CAOUTCHOU'C. The substance so called is obtained from the vegetable kingdom, and exists also in the mineral.

1. The first, known by the names Indian rubber, Elastic gum, Cayenne resin, Cautchuc, and Caoutchouc, is prepared principally from the juice of the *Siphonia elastica;—foliis ternatis ellipticis integerrimis subtis canis longe petiolatis*, (Suppl. Plant.) and also from the *Jatropha elastica* and *Unceola elastica* The manner of obtaining this juice is by making incisions through the bark of the lower part of the trunk of the tree, from which the fluid resin issues in great abundance, appearing of a milky whiteness as it flows into the vessel placed to receive it, and into which it is conducted by means of a tube or leaf fixed in the incision, and supported with clay. On exposure to the air, this milky juice gradually inspissates into a soft, reddish, elastic, resin. It is formed by the Indians in South America into various figures, but is commonly brought to Europe in that of pear-shaped bottles, which are said to be formed by spreading the juice of the Siphonia over a proper mould of clay; as soon as one layer is dry, another is added, until the bottle be of the thickness desired. It is then exposed to a thick dense smoke, or to a fire, until it becomes so dry as not to stick to the fingers, when, by means of

certain instruments of iron, or wood, it is ornamented on the outside with various figures. This being done, it remains only to pick out the mould, which is easily effected by softening it with water.

"The elasticity of this substance is its most remarkable property: when warmed, as by immersion in hot water, slips of it may be drawn out to seven or eight times their original length, and will return to their former dimensions nearly. Cold renders it stiff and rigid, but warmth restores its original elasticity. Exposed to the fire it softens, swells up, and burns with a bright flame. In Cayenne it is used to give light as a candle. Its solvents are æther, volatile oils, and petroleum. The æther, however, requires to be washed with water repeatedly, and in this state it dissolves it completely. Pelletier recommends to boil the caoutchouc in water for an hour; then to cut it into slender threads; to boil it again about an hour; and then to put it into rectified sulphuric æther in a vessel close stopped. In this way he says it will be totally dissolved in a few days, without heat, except the impurities, which will fall to the bottom if æther enough be employed. Berniard says, the nitrous æther dissolves it better than the sulphuric. If this solution be spread on any substance, the æther evaporates very quickly, and leaves a coating of caoutchouc unaltered in its properties. Naphtha, or petroleum, rectified into a colourless liquid, dissolves it, and likewise leaves it unchanged by evaporation. Oil of turpentine softens it, and forms a pasty mass, that may be spread as a varnish, but is very long in drying. A solution of caoutchouc in five times its weight of oil of turpentine, and this solution dissolved in eight times its weight of dry ing linseed oil by boiling, is said to form the varnish of air-balloons. Alkalies act upon it so as in time to destroy its elasticity. Sulphuric acid is decomposed by it; sulphurous acid being evolved, and the caoutchouc converted into charcoal. Nitric acid acts upon it with heat; nitrous gas being given out, and oxalic acid crystallizing from the residuum. On distillation it gives out ammonia, and carburetted hydrogen.

Caoutchouc may be formed into various articles without undergoing the process of solution. If it be cut into a uniform slip of a proper thickness, and wound spirally round a glass or metal rod, so that the edges shall be in close contact, and in this state be boiled for some time, the edges will adhere so as to form a tube. Pieces of it may be readily joined by touching the edges with the solution in æther; but this is not absolutely necessary, for, if they be merely softened by heat, and then pressed together, they will unite very firmly.

If linseed oil be rendered very drying by digesting it upon an oxide of lead, and afterward applied with a small brush on any surface, and dried by the sun or in the smoke, it will afford a pellicle of considerable firmness, transparent, burning like caoutchouc, and wonderfully elastic. A pound of this oil, spread upon a stone, and exposed to the air for six or seven months, acquired almost all the properties of caoutchouc; it was used to make catheters and bougies, to varnish balloons, and for other purposes.

Of the mineral caoutchouc there are several varieties:—1. Of a blackish-brown, inclining to olive, soft, exceedingly compressible, unctuous, with a slightly aromatic smell. It burns with a bright flame, leaving a black oily residuum, which does not become dry. 2. Black, dry, and cracked on the surface, but, when cut into, of a yellowish-white. A fluid resembling pyrolignic acid exudes from it when recently cut. It is pellucid on the edges, and nearly of a hyacinthine red colour. 3. Similar to the preceding, but of a somewhat firmer texture, and ligneous appearance, from having acquired consistency in repeated layers. 4. Resembling the first variety, but of a darker colour, and adhering to gray calcareous spar, with some grains of galæna. 5. Of a liver-brown colour, having the aspect of the vegetable caoutchouc, but passing by gradual transition into a brittle bitumen, of vitreous lustre, and a yellowish colour. 6. Dull reddish-brown, of a spongy or cork-like texture, containing blackish-gray nuclei of impure caoutchouc. Many more varieties are enumerated.

One specimen of this caoutchouc has been found in a petrified marine shell enclosed in a rock, and another enclosed in a crystallized fluor spar.

The mineral caoutchouc resists the action of solvents still more than the vegetable The rectified oil of petroleum affects it most, particularly when by partial burning it is resolved into a pitchy viscous substance. A hundred grains of a specimen analyzed in the dry way by Klaproth, afforded carburetted hydrogen gas 38 cubic inches, carbonic acid gas 4, bituminous oil 73 grains, acidulous phlegm 1.5, charcoal 6.25, lime 2, silex 1.5, oxide of iron .75, sulphate of lime .5, alumina .25.

CAPAIBA. See *Copaifera officinalis.*

CAPAIVA. See *Copaifera officinalis.*

CAPELI'NA. (From *capeline*, French, a woman's hat, or bandage.) A double-headed roller, put round the head.

CAPE'LLA. A cupel or test. Also a name for a goat.

CAPER. See *Capparis.*

Caper-bush. See *Capparis.*

CA'PETUS. (Καπετος, *per aphæresin*, pro σκαπετος; from σκαπτω, to dig.) Hippocrates means by this word a foramen, which is impervious, and needs the use of a chirurgical instrument to make an opening; as the anus of some new-born infants.

CA'PHORA. (Arabian.) Camphire.

CA'PHURA BAROS INDORUM. A name for camphire.

CAPHURÆ OLEUM. An aromatic oil distilled from the root of the cinnamon-tree.

CAPILLACEUS. Capillary.

CAPILLARIS. See *Capillary.*

CAPILLARES PLANTÆ. Capillary, or hair-shaped plants.

CAPILLARIS VERMICULUS. See *Crinones* and *Dracunculus.*

CAPI'LLARY. (*Capillaris;* from *capillus*, a little hair: so called from the resemblance to hair or fine thread.) 1. Capillary vessels. The very small ramifications of the arteries, which terminate upon the external surface of the body, or on the surface of internal cavities, are called capillary.

2. Capillary attraction. See *Attraction.*

3. Applied to parts of plants, which are, or resemble, hairs: thus, a capillary root is one which consists of many very fine fibres, as that of *Festuca ovina*, and most grasses.

CAPILLA'TIO. (From *capillus*, a hair.) A capillary fracture of the cranium.

CAPI'LLUS. (Quasi *capitis pilus*, the hair of the head.) The hair. Small, cylindrical, transparent, insensible, and elastic filaments, which arise from the skin, and are fastened in it by means of small roots. The human hair is composed of a spongy, cellular texture, containing a coloured liquid, and a proper covering. Hair is divided into two kinds; *long*, which arises on the scalp, cheek, chin, breasts of men, the anterior parts of the arms and legs, the arm-pits, groins, and pelvis: and *short*, which is softer than the long, and is present over the whole body, except only the palm of the hand and sole of the foot. The hair originates in the adipose membrane from an oblong membraneous bulb, which has vessels peculiar to it. The hair is distinguished by different names in certain parts; as, *capillus*, on the top of the head: *crinis*, on the back of the head; *circrinnus*, on the temples; *cilium*, on the eyelids; *supercilium*, on the eyebrows; *vibrissa*, in the nostrils; *barba*, on the chin; *pappus*, on the middle of the chin; *mystax*, on the upper lip; *pilus*, on the body.

From numerous experiments Vauquelin infers, that black hair is formed of nine different substances, namely:—

1. An animal matter, which constitutes the greater part. 2. A white concrete oil, in small quantity 3. Another oil of a grayish-green colour, more abundant than the former. 4. Iron, the state of which in the hair is uncertain. 5. A few particles of oxide of manganese 6. Phosphate of lime. 7. Carbonate of lime, in very small quantity. 8. Silex, in a conspicuous quantity. 9. Lastly, a considerable quantity of sulphur.

The same experiments show, that red hair differs from black only in containing a red oil instead of a blackish-green oil, and that white hair differs from both these only in the oil being nearly colourless, and in containing phosphate of magnesia, which is not found in them.

CAPILLUS VENERIS. See *Adianthum.*

CAPILLUS VENERIS CANADENSIS. See *Adianthum canadense.*

CAPIPLE'NIUM. (From *caput*, the head, and *plenus*, full; a barbarous word: but Baglivi uses it to signify that continual heaviness or disorder in the head, which the Greeks call καρηβαρια.) A catarrh.

CAPISTRA'TIO. (From *capistrum*, a bridle: so called because the præpuce is restrained as, it were with a bridle.) See *Phimosis*.

CAPI'STRUM. (From *caput*, the head.)

1. A bandage for the head is so called.

2. In Vogel's Nosology it is the same as *Trismus*.

CA'PITAL. *Capitalis*. 1. Belonging to the caput, or head.

2. The head or upper part of an alembic.

CAPITA'LIA. (From *caput*, the head.) Medicines which relieve pains of the head.

CAPITATUS. (From *caput*, the head.) Headed. See *Capitulum*.

CAPITE'LLUM. The head or seed vessels, frequently applied to mosses, &c.

CAPITILU'VIUM. (From *caput*, the head, and *lavo*, to wash.) A lotion for the head.

CA'PITIS OBLIQUUS INFERIOR ET MAJOR. See *Obliquus inferior capitis*.

CAPITIS PAR TERTIUM FALLOPII. See *Trachelo-mastoideus*.

CAPITIS POSTICUS. See *Rectus capitis posticus major*.

CAPITIS RECTUS. See *Rectus capitis posticus minor*.

CAPI'TULUM. (Diminutive of *caput*, the head.)

1. A small head.

2. A protuberance of a bone, received into the concavity of another bone.

3. An alembic.

In botany, the term for a species of inflorescence, called a head or tuft, formed of many flowers, in a globular form, upon a common peduncle.

From the insertion of the flowers, it is called,

1. *Pedunculated*; as in *Astragalus syriacus*, and *Eryngium maritimum*.

2. *Sessile*; as in *Trifolium tomentosum*.

3. *Terminal*; as in *Monarda fistulosa*.

4. *Axillary*; as in *Gomphrena sessilis*.

From the figure, it is said to be,

1. *Globose*; as in *Gomphrena globosa*.

2. *Subrotund*; as in *Trifolium pratense*.

3. *Conic*; as in *Trifolium montanum*.

4. *Dimidiate*, flat on one side, round on the other; as in *Trifolium lupinaster*.

From its covering,

1. *Naked*; as in *Illecebrum polygonoides*.

2. *Foliose*; as in *Plantago indica*.

A capitulum that is very small, and is mostly in the axilla, is called *Glomerulus*.

CAPI'VI. See *Copaifera officinalis*.

CAPNELÆ'UM. (From καπνος, smoke, and ελαιον, oil; so named from its smoky exhalations when exposed to heat.) In Galen's works it means a resin.

CA'PNIAS. (From καπνος, a smoke.) 1. A jasper of a smoky colour.

2. A vine which bears white and part black grapes.

CAPNI'STON. (From καπνος, smoke.) A preparation of spice and oil, made by kindling the spices, and fumigating the oil.

CAPNI'TIS. (From καπνος, smoke; so called from its smoky colour.) Tutty.

CAPNOI'DES. (From καπνος, fumitory, and ειδος, likeness.) Resembling fumitory.

CA'PNOS. (Καπνος, smoke; so called, says Blanchard, because its juice, if applied to the eyes, produces the same effect and sensations as smoke.) *Capnus*. The herb fumitory. See *Fumaria*.

CAPNUS. See *Capnos*.

CA'PPA. (*À capite*, from the head: so called from its supposed resemblance.) The herb monkshood. See *Aconitum*.

CA'PPARIS. (From *cabar*, Arab. or παρα το καππανειν αραν, from its curing madness and melancholy.) The caper plant.

1. The name of a genus of plants in the Linnæan system. Class, *Polyandria*; Order, *Monogynia*.

2. The pharmacopœial name of the caper plant. See *Capparis spinosa*.

CAPPARIS SPINOSA. The systematic name of the caper plant. *Capparis:—pedunculis solitariis unifloris, stipulis spinosis, foliis annuis, capsulis ovalibus* of Linnæus. The buds, or unexpanded flowers of this plant are in common use as a pickle, which is said to possess antiscorbutic virtues. The bark of the root was formerly in high esteem as a deobstruent.

CAPREOLA'RIS. (From *capreolus*, a tendril.) *Capreolatus*. Resembling in its contortions, or other appearance, the tendrils of a vine; applied to the spermatic vessels.

CAPREOLA'TUS. See *Capreolaris*.

CAPRE'OLUS. (Dim. of *caprea*, a tendril. Dr. Turton suggests its derivation from *caper*, a goat, the horn of which its contortions somewhat resemble.)

1. The helix or circle of the ear, from its tendril-like contortion.

2. A Tendril. See *Cirrus*.

CAPRICO'RNUS. Lead.

CAPRIFICATION. (*Caprificatio*; from *caprificus*, a wild fig.) The very singular husbandry, or management of fig-trees.

CAPRIFI'CUS. (From *caper*, a goat, and *ficus*, a fig; because they are a chief food of goats.) The wild fig-tree. See *Ficus*.

CAPRIMULGUS. A species of bird, the goat-sucker, to which belong the night-hawk and the whip-poor-will.

CAPRI'ZANS. Galen and others used this word to express an inequality in the pulse, when it leaps, and, as it were, dances in uncertain strokes and periods.

CAPSE'LLA. (Diminutive of *capsa*, a chest, from its resemblance.) A name in Marcellus Empiricus for viper's bugloss; the *Echium Italicum*, of Linnæus.

CA'PSICUM. (From καπτω, to bite; on account of its effect on the mouth.)

1. The name of a genus of plants in the Linnæan system. Class, *Pentandria*; Order, *Monogynia*.

2. The pharmacopœial name of the capsicum. See *Capsicum annuum*.

CAPSICUM ANNUUM. The systematic name of the plant from which we obtain Cayenne pepper. Guinea pepper. *Piper indicum; Lada chilli; Capo Molago; Solanum urens; Siliquastrum Plinii; Piper Brazilianum; Piper Guineense; Piper Calecuticum; Piper Hispanicum; Piper Lusitanicum.* Cayenne pepper. This species of pepper is obtained from the *Capsicum; caule herbaceo, pedunculus solitariis* of Linnæus. What is generally used under the name of Cayenne pepper, however, is an indiscriminate mixture of the powder of the dried pods of many species of capsicum, but especially of the capsicum minimum, or bird pepper, which is the hottest of all. These peppers have been chiefly used as condiments. They prevent flatulence from vegetable food, and give warmth to the stomach, possessing all the virtues of the oriental spices, without producing those complaints of the head which the latter are apt to occasion. An abuse of them, however, gives rise to visceral obstructions, especially of the liver. In the practice of medicine, there can be little doubt that they furnish us with one of the purest and strongest stimulants which can be introduced into the stomach, and may be very useful in some paralytic and gouty cases. Dr. Adair, who first introduced them into practice, found them useful in the cachexia Africana, which he considers as a most frequent and fatal predisposition to disease among the slaves. Dr. Wright says, that in dropsical and other complaints where chalybeates are indicated, a minute portion of powdered capsicum forms an excellent addition, and recommends its use in lethargic affections. This pepper has also been successfully employed in a species of cynanche maligna, which proved very fatal in the West Indies, resisting the use of Peruvian bark, wine, and other remedies commonly employed. In tropical fevers, coma and delirium are common attendants; and, in such cases, cataplasms of capsicum have a speedy and happy effect. They redden the parts, but seldom blister unless when kept on too long. In ophthalmia from relaxation, the diluted juice of capsicum is found to be a valuable remedy. Dr. Adair gave six or eight grains for a dose, made into pills; or else he prepared a tincture by digesting half an ounce of the pepper in a pound of alkohol, the dose of which was one or two drachms, diluted with a sufficient quantity of water. A *tinctura capsici* is now for the first time introduced into the London pharmacopœia.

["This article is well known for its excessively pungent and biting acrimony, exceeding that of any other article used with food. The principle on which its pungency depends is soluble in both water and alkohol, and is not dissipated by boiling. Its solutions are disturbed by various reagents, which, however, are of no consequence in practical use. It is found to contain cinchonin, resin, mucilage, and an acrid principle said to be alkaline. It is sometimes adulterated with red-lead to increase its weight.

Capsicum is a warm, powerful stimulant, promoting digestion, and obviating flatulence. Its abuse, however, produces visceral obstructions, and an inflammatory disposition in the system. It is never of service to the healthy. In disease it is administered to stimulate the stomach when in a torpid state, and to excite the nerves of the paralytic and lethargic. In the West Indies it has been employed both externally and internally in ulcerated sore throat. It is applied as a gargle in this disease, and in paralysis of the tongue. Its chief use, however, is as a rubefacient to the skin, upon which it acts with great power. The *dose* internally is from five to ten grains. The rubefacient cataplasm is made of meal and vinegar heated, and its surface covered with pulverized capsicum."—*Big. Mat. Med.* A.]

CA'PSULA. (Diminutive of *capsa*, a chest or case.) A capsule. 1. A membraneous production enclosing a part of the body like a bag; as the capsular ligaments, the capsule of the crystalline lens, &c.

2. In botany, a dry, woody, coriaceous, or membraneous pericarpium, or seed-vessel, generally splitting into several valves.

The parts of a capsule, are,

1. The *valves*, or external shell, into which the capsule splits.

2. The *sutures*, or the external surface in which the valves are joined.

3. The *dissepimenta*, or partitions by which the capsule is divided into several cells.

4. The *loculamenta*, or cells, the spaces between the partitions and valves.

5. The *columella*, or central column, or filament, which unites the partitions, and to which the seeds are usually attached.

From the number of the valves, a capsule is said to be,

1. *Bivalved;* as in *Magnolia*, and *Capraria*.

2. *Three-valved;* as in *Canna indica*.

3. *Four-valved;* as in *Datura stramonium* and *Œnothera biennis*.

4. *Five-valved;* as in *Illecebrum*, and *Coris*.

5. *Manyvalved;* as in *Hura crepitans*.

6. *Operculate*, or *circumcised*, the operculum splitting horizontally; as in *Hyosciamus niger*, and *Lecythis ollaria*.

From the number of *cells*,

1. *Unilocular*, when there is no partition; as in *Parnassia palustris*, and *Agrostema*.

2. *Bilocular*, two-celled; as *Hyosciamus niger*, and *Datura stramonium*.

3. *Trilocular*, three-celled; as in *Æsculus hypocastanum*, and *Iris germanica*.

4. *Quinquelocular*, five-celled; as in *Hibiscus syriacus*, and *Azalea procumbens*.

5. *Novemlocular*, nine-celled; as in *Punica granatum*.

6. *Submultilocular*, when there are many cells, and the partitions do not reach the middle of the capsule; as in *Papaver somniferum*.

From the appearance of the external surface, a capsule is called,

1. *Glabrous;* as in *Papaver somniferum*.

2. *Aculeate;* as in *Datura stramonium*.

3. *Muricate;* as in *Canna indica*.

From the number of tubercles on the external surface,

1. *Capsula dicocca*, or *didyma;* as in *Spigelia*.

2. *C. tricocca;* as in *Euphorbia lathyrus*, and *Cneorum tricoccum*.

3. *C. tetracocca;* as in *Paururus cernuus*, and *Evonymus europeus*.

From the number of contiguous capsules,

1. *C. simplex*, if solitary.

2. *C. duplex*, two aggregated; as in *Pæonia officinalis*.

3. *C. triplex;* as in *Veratrum album*.

4. *C. quintuplex;* as in *Aquilegia vulgaris*, and *Nigella*.

5. *C. multiplex;* as in *Sempervivum tectorum*.

From the substance, a capsule is called,

1 *Membranaceous;* as in *Datura stramonium*.

2. *Corticated*, the external fungous membrane receding from the capsule; as in *Ricinus communis*.

3. *Woody*, very hard, yet splitting; as in *Hura crepitans*.

4. *Baccated*, when the seed is surrounded by a pulp, as *Evonymus europeus*, and *Samyda*.

5. *Spurious*, if the calyx, capsule-like, surrounding the seed, splits; as in *Fagus sylvatica*.

The number of seeds contained in the capsule, gives rise to the following distinctions.

1. *Capsula monosperma*, one-seeded; as in *Gomphrenia*, *Herniaria*, and *Salsola*.

2. *C. disperma*, two-seeded; as in *Hebenstratia*, and *Buffonia*.

3. *C. Trisperma*, three-seeded; as in *Glaux*, and *Hudsonia*.

4. *C. polysperma*, many-seeded; as in *Papaver somniferum*.

CAPSULA ATRABILARIS. See *Renal Glands*.

CAPSULA RENALIS. See *Renal Glands*.

CA'PSULAR. (*Capsularis;* from *capsa*, a bag.) Surrounding a part, like a bag: applied to a ligament which surrounds every moveable articulation, and contains the synovia like a bag.

CA'PSULE. See *Capsula*.

CAPSULE OF GLISSON. *Capsula Glissonii. Vagina portæ; Vagina Glissonii.* A strong tunic, formed of cellular texture, which accompanies the vena portæ, and its most minute ramifications, throughout the whole liver.

CA'PULUM. (From καμπτω, to bend.) A contortion of the eyelids, or other parts.

CA'PUR. (Arabian.) Camphire.

CA'PUT. (*Caput, itis.* neut.; from *capio*, to take; because from it, according to Varro, the senses take their origin.) 1. The head, cranium, or skull. It is situated above or upon the trunk, and united to the cervical vertebræ. It is distinguished into skull and face. On the skull are observed *vertex*, or crown; *sinciput*, or foreparts; *occiput*, or hinder part; and the *temples*. The parts distinguished on the face are well known; as the forehead, nose, eyes, &c. The arteries of the head are branches of the carotids; and the veins empty themselves into the jugulars. See *Skull* and *Face*.

2. The upper extremity of a bone; as the head of the humerus or femur.

3. The origin of a muscle; as the long head of the biceps.

4. A protuberance like the head of any thing; as caput gallinaginis.

5. The beginning of a part; as caput cœci.

6. The remains of any thing after its destruction by fire, or other means: hence caput mortuum, or ashes.

CAPUT GALLINAGINIS. *Verumontanum.* A cutaneous eminence in the urethra of men, before the neck of the bladder, somewhat like the head of a woodcock in miniature, around which the seminal ducts, and the ducts of the prostate gland, open.

CAPUT MORTUUM. A fanciful term, much used by the old chemists, but now entirely rejected. It denoted the fixed residue of operations. As the earlier chemists did not examine these, they did not find any inconvenience in one general term to denote them: but the most slender acquaintance with modern chemistry must show, that it is utterly impracticable to denote, by one general term, all the various matters that remain fixed in certain degrees of heat. The term is obsolete, but spoken of fancifully.

CAPUT OBSTIPUM. The wry neck. Mostly a spasmodic complaint.

CAPUT PURGIA. (A barbarous word, from *caput*, the head, and *purgo*, to purge.) Medicines which, by causing a defluxion from the nose, purge, as it were, the head, as some errhines do.

CAPYRI'DION. (From καπυρος, burnt.) *Capyrion.* A medicated cake, much baked.

CAPY'RION. See *Capyridion*.

CA'RABUS. A genus of insects of the beetle kind. Two species, the *chrysocephalus* and *ferrugineus*, have been recommended for the toothache. They must be pressed between the fingers, and then rubbed on the gum and tooth affected.

CAROCO'SMOS. A name of the sour mare's milk, so much admired by the Tartars.

CARAGUA'TA. The aloe of Brazil.

CARA'NNA. (Spanish.) *Caragna. Caranna*

gummi. Bresilis. A concrete resinous juice, that exudes from a large tree, of which we have no particular account. It is brought from New Spain and America, in little masses, rolled up in leaves of flags; externally and internally it is of a brownish colour, variegated with irregular white streaks. When fresh, it is soft and tenacious; but becomes dry and friable by keeping. Pure caranna has an agreeable aromatic smell, especially when heated, and a bitterish slightly pungent taste. It was formerly employed as an ingredient in vulnerary balsams, strengthening, discutient, and suppurating plasters; but its scarcity has caused it to be forgotten.

CARAWAY. See *Carum.*

CA'RBASUS. Καρβασος. Scribonius Largus uses this word for lint.

["CARBAZOTIC ACID. By the action of nitric acid upon indigo, a substance is obtained in yellow brilliant crystalline plates, which exhibits acid properties, and has been called by Dr. Liebig, *carbazotic acid*, a name derived from its composition, which is as follows:

Carbon, ...13.043 or 15 atoms.
Azote, ...16.167 or 3 ——
Oxygen, ...48.790 or 15 ——

To obtain carbazotic acid, the following process has been given by Dr. Liebig:

A portion of the best indigo is to be broken into small fragments, and moderately heated with eight or ten times its weight of nitric acid, of moderate strength. It will dissolve, evolving nitrous vapours and swelling up in the vessel; after the scum has fallen, the liquid is to be boiled, and nitric acid is added as long as any red vapours are disengaged. When the liquid has become cold, a large quantity of semi-transparent yellow crystals will be formed, and if the operation has been well conducted, no artificial tannin or resin will be obtained. The crystals are to be washed with cold water, and then boiled in water sufficient to dissolve them. If any oily drops of tannin form on the surface of the solution, they must be carefully removed by touching them with filtering paper. Then filtering the fluid, and allowing it to cool, yellow brilliant crystalline plates will be obtained, which will not lose their lustre by washing. To obtain the substance perfectly pure, the crystals must be redissolved in boiling water, and neutralized by carbonate of potassa. Upon cooling, a salt of potassa will crystallize, which should be purified by repeated crystallizations.

When the substance is heated, it fuses, and is volatilized without decomposition; when subjected to a strong heat, it inflames without explosion, its vapours burning with a yellow flame, and a carbonaceous residue remaining. It is but little soluble in cold water, but much more so in boiling water; the solution has a bright yellow colour, reddens litmus, has an extremely bitter taste, and acts like a strong acid on metallic oxides, dissolving them, and forming peculiar crystallizable salts. Ether and alkohol dissolve it readily.

Carbazotic acid combines with bases, and forms salts called *carbazotates.*" (Of which the following have been determined:)

Carbazotate of Potassa, crystallizes in long, yellow, semi-transparent, and very brilliant needles; it dissolves in 260 parts of water at 59° Fah. Strong acids decompose it. When a little is gradually heated in a glass tube, it first fuses, and then suddenly explodes, breaking the tube to atoms; traces of charcoal are observed on the fragments. The slight solubility of this salt supplies an easy method of testing and separating potassa in a fluid. Even the potassa in tincture of litmus may be discovered by it; on the addition of a few drops of carbazotic acid dissolved in alkohol, to infusion of litmus, crystals of the salt gradually separate. The salt contains no water of crystallization. Its composition is potassa 16.21, acid 83.79.

Carbazotate of Soda crystallizes in fine silky yellow needles, having the general properties of the salt of potassa, but soluble in from 20 to 24 parts of water at 59° F.

Carbazotate of Ammonia forms very long, flattened, brilliant, yellow crystals, very soluble in water. Heated carefully in a glass tube, it fuses, and is volatilized without decomposition; heated suddenly, it inflames without explosion, and leaves much carbonaceous residue.

Carbazotate of Baryta, obtained by heating carbonate of baryta, and carbazotic acid with water, crystallizes in quadrangular prisms of a deep colour, and dissolves easily in water. When heated it fuses, and is decomposed with very powerful explosion, producing a vivid yellow flame: 100 parts lose at 212° F. 125 parts of water; 100 parts of the anhydrous salt contain 75.72 acid, and 24.28 baryta.

Carbazotate of Lime obtained like the salt of baryta, forms flattened, quadrangular prisms, very soluble in water, and detonating like the salt of potassa.

Carbazotate of Magnesia forms very long indistinct needles, of a clear yellow colour, is very soluble and detones violently.

Carbazotate of Copper, prepared by decomposing sulphate of copper by carbazotate of baryta: it crystallizes with difficulty; the crystals being of a fine green colour: it is deliquescent; when heated it is decomposed without explosion.

Carbazotate of Silver. Carbazotic acid readily dissolves oxide of silver, when heated with it and water; and the solution, gradually evaporated, yields starry groups of fine acicular crystals of the colour and lustre of gold; the salt dissolves readily in water; when heated to a certain degree; it does not detonate, but fuses like gunpowder.

Proto-carbazotate of Mercury, obtained in small yellow triangular crystals, by mixing boiling solutions of the carbazotate of potassa or soda, and protonitrate of mercury. It requires more than 1200 parts of water for its solution; it consists of 53.79 acid, and 46.21 protoxide of mercury per cent.

Carbazotate of Lead may be formed by decomposing a salt of lead by carbazotate of potassa or soda: it is a yellow powder, but slightly soluble, and detonating by heat.

All these salts detonate much more powerfully when heated in close vessels, than when heated in the air, and what is remarkable, those bases yielding oxygen most readily are those which explode with least force."—From Webster, as taken from *Ann. de Chim* xxv. 72, and *Quart. Jour.* N. S. iii. A.]

CA'RBO. (*Charbah*, Hebrew, burnt or dried.) Coal.

1. In medicine and chemistry, it is commonly understood to mean charcoal, and receives its name from its mode of preparation, which is by burning pieces of light wood into a dry, black coal.

2. A carbuncle. See *Anthrax.*

CARBO LIGNA. Charcoal. As an external application, powdered charcoal has been recommended in the cure of gangrene, from external causes, and all descriptions of fœtid ulcers. Meat which has acquired a mawkish or even putrid smell, is found to be rendered perfectly sweet, by rubbing it with powdered charcoal. It is also used as tooth-powder.

CA'RBON. (From *carbo*, coal.) Chemists apply this term to the diamond, and what is commonly called charcoal. The diamond is the purest form of it.

1. When vegetable matter, particularly the more solid, as wood, is exposed to heat in close vessels, the volatile parts fly off, and leave behind a black porous substance, which is charcoal. If this be suffered to undergo combustion in contact with oxygen, or with atmospheric air, much the greater part of it will combine with the oxygen, and escape in the form of gas; leaving about a two-hundredth part, which consists chiefly of different saline and metallic substances. This pure inflammable part of the charcoal is what is commonly called *carbon;* and if the gas be received into proper vessels, the carbon will be found to have been converted by the oxygen into an acid, called the carbonic. See *Carbonic acid.*

From the circumstance, that inflammable substances refract light in a ratio greater than that of their densities, Newton inferred, that the diamond was inflammable. The quantity of the inflammable part of charcoal, requisite to form a hundred parts of carbonic acid, was calculated by Lavoisier to be twenty-eight parts. From a careful experiment of Mr. Tennant, 27.6 parts of diamond, and 72.4 of oxygen, formed 100 of carbonic acid; and hence he inferred the identity of diamond and the inflammable part of charcoal.

Well-burned charcoal is a conductor of electricity, though wood simply deprived of its moisture by baking is a non-conductor; but it is a very bad conductor of caloric, a property of considerable use on many occasions, as in lining crucibles.

It is insoluble in water, and hence the utility of charring the surface of wood exposed to that liquid, in order to preserve it, a circumstance not unknown to the ancients. This preparation of timber has been proposed as an effectual preventive of what is commonly called the dry rot. It has an attraction, however, for a certain portion of water, which it retains very forcibly. Heated red-hot, or nearly so, it decomposes water; forming with its oxygen carbonic acid, or carbonic oxide, according to the quantity present; and with the hydrogen a gaseous carburet, called carburetted hydrogen, or heavy inflammable air.

Charcoal is infusible by any heat. If exposed to a very high temperature in close vessels, it loses little or nothing of its weight, but shrinks, becomes more compact, and acquires a deeper black colour.

Recently prepared charcoal has a remarkable property of absorbing different gases, and condensing them in its pores, without any alteration of their properties or its own.

Very light charcoal, such as that of cork, absorbs scarcely any air; while the pit-coal of Rastiberg, sp. gr. 1.326, absorbs ten times and a half its volume. The absorption was always completed in 24 hours. This curious faculty, which is common to all porous bodies, resembles the action of capillary tubes on liquids. When a piece of charcoal, charged with one gas, is transferred into another, it absorbs some of it, and parts with a portion of that first condensed. In the experiments of Messrs. Allen and Pepys, charcoal was found to imbibe from the atmosphere in a day about one-eighth of its weight in water. For a general view of absorption, see *Gas*.

When oxygen is condensed by charcoal, carbonic acid is observed to form at the end of several months. But the most remarkable property displayed by charcoals impregnated with gas, is that with sulphuretted hydrogen when exposed to the air or oxygen gas. The sulphuretted hydrogen is speedily destroyed, and water and sulphur result, with the disengagement of considerable heat. Hydrogen alone has no such effects. When charcoal was exposed by Sir Humphrey Davy to intense ignition *in vacuo*, and in condensed azot, by means of Mr. Children's magnificent voltaic battery, it slowly volatilized, and gave out a little hydrogen. The remaining part was always much harder than before; and in one case so hard as to scratch glass, while its lustre was increased. This fine experiment may be regarded as a near approach to the production of diamond.

Charcoal has a powerful affinity for oxygen; whence its use in disoxygenating metallic oxides, and restoring their base to its original metallic state, or reviving the the metal. Thus too it decomposes several of the acids, as the phosphoric and sulphuric, from which it abstracts their oxygen, and leaves the phosphorus and sulphur free.

Carbon is capable of combining with sulphur, and with hydrógen. With iron it forms steel; and it unites with copper into a carburet, as observed by Dr. Priestley.

A singular and important property of charcoal is that of destroying the smell, colour, and taste of various substances: for the first accurate experiments on which we are chiefly indebted to Mr. Lowitz, of Petersburgh, though it had been long before recommended to correct the fœtor of foul ulcers, and as an antiseptic. On this account it is certainly the best dentifrice. Water that has become putrid by long keeping in wooden casks, is rendered sweet by filtering through charcoal powder, or by agitation with it; particularly if a few drops of sulphuric acid be added. Common vinegar boiled with charcoal powder becomes perfectly limpid. Saline solutions, that are tinged yellow or brown, are rendered colourless in the same way, so as to afford perfectly white crystals. The impure carbonate of ammonia obtained from bones, is deprived both of its colour and fœtid smell by sublimation with an equal weight of charcoal powder. Malt spirit is freed from its disagreeable flavour by distillation from charcoal; but if too much be used, part of the spirit is decomposed. Simple maceration, for eight or ten days, in the proportion of about 1-150th of the weight of the spirit, improves the flavour much. It is necessary that the charcoal be well burned, brought to a red heat before it is used, and used as soon as may be, or at least be carefully excluded from the air. The proper proportion too should be ascertained by experiment on a small scale. The charcoal may be used repeatedly, by exposing it for some time to a red heat before it is again employed.

Charcoal is used on particular occasions as fuel, on account of its giving a strong and steady heat without smoke. It is employed to convert iron into steel by cementation. It enters into the composition of gunpowder. In its finer states, as in ivory-black, lamp-black, &c. it forms the basis of black paints, Indian ink, and printers' ink.

The purest carbon for chemical purposes is obtained by strongly igniting lamp-black in a covered crucible. This yields, like the diamond, unmixed carbonic acid by combustion in oxygen.

Carbon unites with all the common simple combustibles, and with azot, forming a series of most important compounds. With sulphur it forms a curious limpid liquid, called carburet of sulphur, or sulphuret of carbon. With phosphorus it forms a species of compound, whose properties are imperfectly ascertained. It unites with hydrogen in two definite proportions, constituting subcarburetted and carburetted hydrogen gases. With azot it forms prussic gas, the cyanogen of Gay Lussac. Steel and plumbago are two different compounds of carbon with iron. In black chalk we find this combustible intimately associated with silica and alumina. The primitive combining proportion, or prime equivalent of carbon, is 0.75 on the oxygen scale.

2. *Carbon mineral.* This is of a gray blackish colour. It is charcoal with various proportions of earth and iron, without bitumen. It has a silky lustre, and the fibrous texture of wood. It is found in small quantities, stratified with brown coal, slate coal, and pitch coal.

Carbon, gaseous oxide of. Gaseous oxide of carbon was first described by Dr. Priestley, who mistook it for a hydrocarbonate. With the true nature of it, we have been only lately acquainted. It was first proved to be a peculiar gas, by Mr. Cruikshank, of Woolwich, who made it known to us as such, in April, 1801, through the medium of Nicholson's Journal for that month. Several additional properties of this gas were soon afterward noticed by Desormes, Clement, and others. Gaseous oxide of carbon forms an intermediate substance between the pure hydrocarbonates and carbonic acid gas; but not being possessed of acid properties, Mr. Cruikshank called it, conformably to the rules of the chemical nomenclature, *gaseous oxide of carbon*, for it consists of oxygen and carbon rendered gaseous by caloric. See *Carbonic oxide*.

Carbonaceous acid. See *Carbonic acid.*

CARBO'NAS. (*Carbonas, atis.* m.; from carbonic acid being one of its constituents.) A carbonate. A salt formed by the union of carbonic acid with a salifiable basis. The carbonates employed in medicine are:

1. The potassæ carbonas.
2. The sodæ carbonas.
3. The creta præparata, and the testæ præparatæ, which are varieties of carbonate of lime.

When the base is imperfectly neutralized by the carbonic acid, the salt is termed a subcarbonate; of which kind are employed medicinally,

1. The potassæ subcarbonas.
2. The sodæ subcarbonas, and the sodæ subcarbonas exsiccata.
3. The ammoniæ subcarbonas, and the liquor ammoniæ subcarbonatis.
4. The plumbi subcarbonas.
5. The ferri subcarbonas.
6. The magnesiæ subcarbonas.

Carbonas ammoniæ. See *Ammoniæ subcarbonas*

Carbonas calcis. Carbonate of lime. Several varieties of this are used in medicine: the purest and best are the creta præparata, testæ preparatæ, chelæ cancrorum, testæ ovorum, and oculi cancrorum.

Carbonas ferri. See *Ferri subcarbonas.*

Carbonas magnesiæ. See *Magnesiæ subcarbonas*

Carbonas plumbi. See *Plumbi subcarbonas.*

Carbonas potassæ. See *Potassæ carbonas*

Carbonas sodæ. See *Sodæ carbonas.*

CARBONATE. See *Carbonas.*

Carbonate of barytes. See *Heavy spar.*

Carbonated hydrogen gas. See *Carburetted hydrogen gas.*

CA'RBONIC ACID. *Acidum carbonicum.* Fixed air; Carbonaceous acid; Calcareous acid; Aërial acid. "This acid, being a compound of carbon and oxygen, may be formed by burning charcoal; but as it exists in great abundance ready formed, it is not necessary to have recourse to this expedient. All that is necessary is to pour sulphuric acid, diluted with five or six times its weight of water, on common chalk, which is a compound of carbonic acid and lime. An effervescence ensues; carbonic acid is evolved in the state of gas, and may be received in the usual manner.

Carbonic acid abounds in great quantities in nature, and appears to be produced in a variety of circumstances. It composes 44-100th of the weight of limestone, marble, calcareous spar, and other natural specimens of calcareous earth, from which it may be extricated, either by the simple application of heat, or by the superior affinity of some other acid; most acids having a stronger action on bodies than this. This last process does not require heat, because fixed air is strongly disposed to assume the elastic state. Water, under the common pressure of the atmosphere, and at a low temperature, absorbs somewhat more than its bulk of fixed air, and then constitutes a weak acid. If the pressure be greater, the absorption is augmented. It is to be observed, likewise, that more gas than water will absorb should be present. Heated water absorbs less; and if water impregnated with this acid be exposed on a brisk fire, the rapid escape of the aërial bubbles affords an appearance as if the water were at the point of boiling, when the heat is not greater than the hand can bear. Congelation separates it readily and completely from water; but no degree of cold or pressure has yet exhibited this acid in a dense or concentrated state of fluidity.

Carbonic acid gas is much denser than common air, and for this reason occupies the lower parts of such mines or caverns as contain materials which afford it by decomposition. The miners call it choke damp. The Grotto del Cano, in the kingdom of Naples, has been famous for ages on account of the effects of a stratum of fixed air which covers its bottom. It is a cave or hole in the side of a mountain, near the lake Agnano, measuring not more than eighteen feet from its entrance to the inner extremity; where if a dog or other animal that holds down its head be thrust, it is immediately killed by inhaling this noxious fluid.

Carbonic acid gas is emitted in large quantities by bodies in the state of the vinous fermentation, and on account of its great weight, it occupies the apparently empty space or upper part of the vessels in which the fermenting process is going on. A variety of striking experiments may be made in this stratum of elastic fluid. Lighted paper, or a candle dipped into it, is immediately extinguished; and the smoke remaining in the carbonic acid gas renders its surface visible, which may be thrown into waves by agitation like water. If a dish of water be immersed in this gas, and briskly agitated, it soon becomes impregnated, and obtains the pungent taste of Pyrmont water. In consequence of the weight of the carbonic acid gas, it may be lifted out in a pitcher, or bottle, which, if well corked, may be used to convey it to great distances, or it may be drawn out of a vessel by a cock like a liquid. The effects produced by pouring this invisible fluid from one vessel to another, have a very singular appearance: if a candle or small animal be placed in a deep vessel, the former becomes extinct, and the latter expires in a few seconds, after the carbonic acid gas is poured upon them, though the eye is incapable of distinguishing any thing that is poured. If, however, it be poured into a vessel full of air, in the sunshine, its density being so much greater than that of the air, renders it slightly visible by the undulations and streaks it forms in this fluid, as it descends through it.

Carbonic acid reddens infusion of litmus; but the redness vanishes by exposure to the air, as the acid flies off. It has a peculiar sharp taste, which may be perceived over vats in which wine or beer is fermenting, as also in sparkling Champaign, and the brisker kinds of cider. Light passing through it is refracted by it, but does not effect any sensible alteration in it, though it appears, from experiment, that it favours the separation of its principles by other substances. It will not unite with an overdose of oxygen, of which it contains 72 parts in 100, the other 28 being pure carbon. It not only destroys life, but the heart and muscle of animals killed by it lose all their irritability, so as to be insensible to the stimulus of galvanism.

Carbonic acid is dilated by heat, but not otherwise altered by it. It is not acted upon by oxygen, or any of the simple combustibles. Charcoal absorbs it, but gives it out again unchanged, at ordinary temperatures; but when this gaseous acid is made to traverse charcoal ignited in a tube, it is converted into carbonic oxide. Phosphorus is insoluble in carbonic acid gas; but, as already observed, is capable of decomposing it by compound affinity, when assisted by sufficient heat; and Priestley and Cruikshank have shown that iron, zinc, and several other metals, are capable of producing the same effect. If carbonic acid be mixed with sulphuretted, phosphuretted, or carburetted gas, it renders them less combustible, or destroys their combustibility entirely, but produces no other sensible change. Such mixtures occur in various analyses, and particularly in the products of the decomposition of vegetable and animal substances. The inflammable air of marshes is frequently carburetted hydrogen intimately mixed with carbonic acid gas, and the sulphuretted hydrogen gas obtained from mineral waters is very often mixed with it.

Carbonic acid appears from various experiments of Ingenhuosz to be of considerable utility in promoting vegetation. It is probably decomposed by the organs of plants, its base furnishing part at least of the carbon that is so abundant in the vegetable kingdom, and its oxygen contributing to replenish the atmosphere with that necessary support of life, which is continually diminished by the respiration of animals and other causes.

The most exact experiments on the neutral carbonates concur to prove, that the prime equivalent of carbonic acid is 2.75; and that it consists of one prime of carbon=0.75+2.0 oxygen.

Water absorbs about its volume of this acid gas, and thereby acquires a specific gravity of 1.0015. On freezing it, the gas is as completely expelled as by boiling. By artificial pressure with forcing pumps, water may be made to absorb two or three times its bulk of carbonic acid. When there is also added a little potassa or soda, it becomes the *aërated* or *carbonated alkaline water*, a pleasant beverage, and a not inactive remedy in several complaints, particularly dyspepsia, hiccup, and disorders of the kidneys. Alkohol condenses twice its volume of carbonic acid. The most beautiful analytical experiment with carbonic acid, is the combustion of potassium in it, the formation of potassa, and the deposition of charcoal.

In point of affinity for the earths and alkalies, carbonic acid stands apparently low in the scale. Before its true nature was known, its compounds with them were not considered as salts, but as the earths and alkalies themselves, only distinguished by the names of *mild, or effervescent*, from their qualities of effervescing with acids, and wanting causticity.

The *carbonates* are characterized by effervescing with almost all the acids, even the acetic, when they evolve their gaseous acid, which, passed into lime water by a tube, deprives it of its taste, and converts it into chalk and pure water.

The carbonate of barytes, found native in Cumberland, by Dr. Withering. From this circumstance it has been termed Witherite. It has been likewise called *aërated heavy spar*, *aërated baroselenite*, *aërated heavy earth* or *barytes*, *barolite*, &c.

Carbonate of strontian, found native in Scotland, at Strontian in Argyllshire, and at Leadhills.

Carbonate of lime exists in great abundance in nature, variously mixed with other bodies, under the names of *marble*, *chalk*, *limestone*, *stalactites*, &c. in which it is of more important and extensive use than any other of the salts, except perhaps the muriate of soda.

The carbonate, or rather *sub-carbonate* of *potassa*, was long known by the name of *vegetable alkali*. It was also called *fixed nitre*, *salt of tartar*, *salt of wormwood*, &c. according to the different modes in which it was procured; and was supposed to retain something of the virtues of the substance from which it was extracted. This error has been sometime exploded, but the knowledge of its true nature is of more recent date.

As water at the usual temperature of the air dissolves rather more than its weight of this salt, we have thus a ready mode of detecting its adulterations in general; and as it is often of consequence to know how much alkali a particular specimen contains, this may be ascertained by the quantity of sulphuric acid it will saturate. This salt is deliquescent. It consists of 6 potassa+2.75 carbonic acid=8.75.

The bi-carbonate of potassa crystallizes in square prisms, the apices of which are quadrangular pyramids. It has a urinous but not caustic taste; changes the syrup of violets green: boiling water dissolves five-sixths of its weight, and cold water one-fourth; alkohol, even when hot, will not dissolve more than 1-1200th. Its specific gravity is 2.012. When it is very pure and well crystallized it effloresces on exposure to a dry atmosphere, though it was formerly considered as deliquescent. It was thought that the common salt of tartar of the shops was a compound of this carbonate and pure potassa; the latter of which, being very deliquescent, attracts the moisture of the air till the whole is dissolved. From its smooth feel, and the manner in which it was prepared, the old chemists called this solution *oil of tartar per deliquium*.

The bi-carbonate of potassa melts with a gentle heat, loses its water of crystallization, amounting to 9-100th, and gives out a portion of its carbonic acid; though no degree of heat will expel the whole of the acid. Thus, as the carbonate of potassa is always prepared by incineration of vegetable substances, and lixiviation, it must be in the intermediate state; or that of a carbonate with excess of alkali: and to obtain the true carbonate we must saturate this salt with carbonic acid, which is best done by passing the acid in the state of gas through a solution of the salt in twice its weight of water; or, if we want the potassa pure, we must have recourse to lime, to separate that portion of acid which fire will not expel.

The bi-carbonate, usually called *super-carbonate* by the apothecaries, consists of 2 primes of carbonic acid =5.500, 1 of potassa=6, and 1 of water=1.125, in all 12.625.

The carbonate of soda has likewise been long known, and distinguished from the preceding by the name of *mineral alkali*. In commerce it is usually called *barilla*, or *soda;* in which state, however, it always contains a mixture of earthy bodies, and usually common salt. It may be purified by dissolving it in a small portion of water, filtering the solution, evaporating at a low heat, and skimming off the crystals of muriate of soda as they form on its surface. When these cease to form, the solution may be suffered to cool, and the carbonate of soda will crystallize.

It is found abundantly in nature. In Egypt, where it is collected from the surface of the earth, particularly after the desiccation of temporary lakes, it has been known from time immemorial by the name of *nitrum, natron*, or *natrum*. A great deal is prepared in Spain by incinerating the maritime plant of salsola; and it is manufactured in this country, as well as in France, from different species of sea-weeds. It is likewise found in mineral water, and also in some animal fluids.

It crystallizes in irregular or rhomboidal decaëdrons, formed by two quadrangular pyramids, truncated very near their bases. Frequently it exhibits only rhomboidal laminæ. Its specific gravity is 1.3591. Its taste is urinous, and slightly acrid, without being caustic. It changes blue vegetable colours to a green. It is soluble in less than its weight of boiling water, and twice its weight of cold. It is one of the most efflorescent salts known, falling completely to powder in no long time. On the application of heat it is soon rendered fluid from the great quantity of its water of crystallization; but is dried by a continuance of the heat, and then melts. It is somewhat more fusible than the carbonate of potassa, promotes the fusion of earths in a greater degree, and forms a glass of better quality. Like that, it is very tenacious of a certain portion of its carbonic acid. It consists in its dry state of 4 soda, +2.75 acid, =6.75.

But the crystals contain 10 prime proportions of water. They are composed of 22 soda, +15.3 carbonic acid, +62.7 water in 100 parts, or of 1 prime of soda =4.1 of carbonic acid =2.75, and 10 of water =11.25, in whole 18.

The *bi-carbonate of soda* may be prepared by saturating the solution of the preceding salt with carbonic acid gas, and then evaporating with a very gentle heat to dryness, when a white irregular saline mass is obtained. The salt is not crystallizable. Its constituents are 4 soda, +5.50 carb. acid, +1.125 water, =10.625; or in 100 parts 37.4 soda, +52 acid, +10.6 water.

The carbonate of magnesia, in a state of imperfect saturation with the acid, has been used in medicine for some time under the simple name of magnesia. It is prepared by precipitation from the sulphate of magnesia by means of carbonate of potassa. Equal parts of sulphate of magnesia and carbonate of potassa, each dissolved in its own weight of boiling water, are filtered and mixed together hot; the sulphate of potassa is separated by copious washing with water; and the carbonate of magnesia is then left to drain, and afterward spread thin on paper, and carried to the drying stove. When once dried it will be in friable white cakes, or a fine powder.

To obtain carbonate of magnesia saturated with acid, a solution of sulphate of magnesia may be mixed cold with a solution of carbonate of potassa; and at the expiration of a few hours, as the superfluous carbonic acid that held it in solution flies off, the carbonate of magnesia will crystallize in very regular transparent prisms of six equal sides. It may be equally obtained by dissolving magnesia in water impregnated with carbonic acid, and exposing the solution to the open air.

These crystals soon lose their transparency, and become covered with a white powder. Exposed to the fire in a crucible, they decrepitate slightly, lose their water and acid, fall to powder, and are reduced to one-fourth of the original weight. When the common carbonate is calcined in the grate, it appears as if boiling, from the extrication of carbonic acid; a small portion ascends like a vapour, and is deposited in a white powder on the cold bodies with which it comes into contact; and in a dark place, toward the end of the operation, it shines with a bluish phosphoric light. It thus loses half its weight, and the magnesia is left quite pure.

As the magnesia of the shops is sometimes adulterated with chalk, this may be detected by the addition of a little sulphuric acid diluted with eight or ten times its weight of water, as this will form with the magnesia a very soluble salt, while the sulphate of lime will remain undissolved. Calcined magnesia should dissolve in this dilute acid without any effervescence.

The crystallized carbonate dissolves in forty-eight times its weight of cold water; the common carbonate requires at least ten times as much, and first forms a paste with a small quantity of the fluid.

The carbonate of ammonia, once vulgarly known by the name of *volatile sal ammoniac*, and abroad by that of *English volatile salt*, because it was first prepared in this country, was commonly called *mild volatile alkali*, before its true nature was known.

When very pure it is in a crystalline form, but seldom very regular Its crystals are so small, that it is difficult to determine their figure. The taste and smell of this salt are the same with those of pure ammonia, but much weaker. It turns the colour of violets green, and that of tumeric brown. It is soluble in rather more than twice its weight of cold water, and in its own weight of hot water; but a boiling heat volatilizes it. When pure, and thoroughly saturated, it is not perceptibly alterable in the air; but when it has an excess of ammonia, it softens and grows moist. It cannot be doubted, however, that it is soluble in air; for if left in an open vessel, it gradually diminishes in weight, and its peculiar smell is diffused to a certain distance. Heat readily sublimes, but does not decompose it.

It has been prepared by the destructive distillation of animal substances, and some others, in large iron pots, with a fire increased by degrees to a strong red-heat, the aqueous liquor that first comes over being removed, that the salt might not be dissolved in it Thus we had the *salt of hartshorn, salt of soot, essential salt of vipers*, &c. If the salt were dissolved in the water, it was called *spirit* of the substance from which it was obtained. Thus, however, it was much contaminated by a fœtid animal oil, from which it required to be subsequently purified, and is much better fabricated by mixing one part of muriate of ammonia and two of carbonate of lime, both as dry as possible, and subliming in an earthen retort.

Sir H. Davy has shown that its component parts

vary, according to the manner of preparing it. The lower the temperature at which it is formed, the greater the proportion of acid and water. Thus, if formed at the temperature of 300°, it contains more than fifty per cent. of alkali; if at 60°, not more than twenty per cent.

There are three or four definite compounds of carbonic acid and *ammonia.*

The first is the solid *sub-carbonate* of the shops. It consists of 55 carbonic acid, 30 ammonia, and 15 water; or probably of 3 primes carbonic acid, 5 ammonia, and 2 water; in all 14.7 for its equivalent.

2d, Gay Lussac has shown that when 100 volumes of ammoniacal gas are mixed with 50 of carbonic acid, the two gases precipitate in a solid salt, which must consist by weight of 56 1-3 acid +43 2-3 alkali, being in the ratio of a prime equivalent of each.

3d, When the pungent sub-carbonate is exposed in powder to the air, it becomes scentless by the evaporation of a definite portion of this ammonia. It is then a compound of about 55 or 56 carbonic acid, 21.5 ammonia, and 22.5 water. It may be represented by 2 primes of acid, 1 of ammonia, and 2 of water, =9.875.

Another compound, it has been supposed, may be prepared by passing carbonic acid through a solution of the sub-carbonate till it be saturated. This, however, may be supposed to yield the same product as the last salt. Lussac infers the neutral carbonate to consist of equal volumes of the two gases, though they will not directly combine in these proportions. This would give 18.1 to 46.5; the very proportions in the scentless salt. For 46.5: 18.1: : 55: 21.42.

It is well known as a stimulant usually put into smelling-bottles, frequently with the addition of some odoriferous oil.

Fourcroy has found, that an *ammoniaco-magnesian carbonate* is formed on some occasions. Thus, if carbonate of ammonia be decomposed by magnesia in the moist way, leaving these two substances in contact with each other in a bottle closely stopped, a complete decomposition will not take place, but a portion of this trisalt will be formed. The same will take place if a solution of carbonate of magnesia in water, impregnated with carbonic acid, be precipitated by pure ammonia; or if ammoniaco-magnesian sulphate, nitrate, or muriate, be precipitated by carbonate of potassa or of soda.

The properties of this triple salt are not much known, but it crystallizes differently from the carbonate of either of its bases, and has its own laws of solubility and decomposition.

The carbonate of glucine is in a white, dull, clotty powder, never dry, but greasy, and soft to the feel. It is not sweet, like the other salts of glucine, but insipid. It is very light, insoluble in water, perfectly unalterable by the air, but very readily decomposed by fire. A saturated solution of carbonate of ammonia takes up a certain portion of this carbonate, and forms with it a triple salt.

Carbonic acid does not appear to be much disposed to unite with *argillaceous earth.* Most clays, however, afford a small quantity of this acid by heat. The snowy white substance, resembling chalk, and known by the name of *lac lunæ,* is found to consist almost wholly of alumina, saturated with carbonic acid. A saline substance, consisting of two six-sided pyramids, joined at one common base, weighing five or six grains, and of a taste somewhat resembling alum, was produced by leaving an ounce phial of water impregnated with carbonic acid, and a redundancy of alumina, exposed to spontaneous evaporation for some months.

Vauquelin has found, that *carbonate of zircone* may be formed by evaporating muriate of zircone, redissolving it in water, and precipitating by the alkaline carbonate. He also adds, that it very readily combines, so as to form a triple salt, with either of the three alkaline carbonates."—*Ure's Chem. Dict.*

This gas is much esteemed in the cure of typhus fevers, and of irritability and weakness of stomach, producing vomiting. Against the former diseases it is given by administering yest, bottled porter, and the like; and for the latter it is disengaged from the carbonated alkali by lemon juice, in a draught given while effervescing.

CARBONIC OXIDE. Gaseous oxide of carbon. "A gaseous compound of one prime equivalent of carbon, and one of oxygen, consisting by weight of 0.75 of the former, and 1.00 of the latter. Hence the prime of the compound is 1.75, the same as that of azote. This gas cannot be formed by the chemist by the direct combination of its constituents; for at the temperature requisite for effecting a union, the carbon attracts its full dose of oxygen, and thus generates carbonic acid. It may be procured by exposing charcoal to a long continued heat. The last products consist chiefly of carbonic oxide.

To obtain it pure, however, our only plan is to abstract one proportion of oxygen from carbonic acid, either in its gaseous state, or as condensed in the carbonates.

If we subject to a strong heat, in a gun barrel or retort, a mixture of any dry earthy carbonate, such as chalk, or carbonate of strontites, with metallic filings or charcoal, the combined acid is resolved into the gaseous oxide of carbon. The most convenient mixture is equal parts of dried chalk and iron, or zinc filings.

The specific gravity of this gas is stated by Gay Lussac and Thenard, from theoretical considerations, to be 0.96782, though Mr. Cruikshanks's experimental estimate was 0.9569.

This gas burns with a dark blue flame. Sir H. Davy has shown, that though carbonic oxide, in its combustion, produces less heat than other inflammable gases, it may be kindled at a much lower temperature. It inflames in the atmosphere, when brought into contact with an iron wire heated to dull redness, whereas carburetted hydrogen is not inflammable by a similar wire, unless it is heated to whiteness, so as to burn with sparks. It requires, for its combustion, half its volume of oxygen gas, producing one volume of carbonic acid. It is not decomposable by any of the simple combustibles, except potassium and sodium. When potassium is heated in a portion of the gas, potassa is formed with the precipitation of charcoal, and the disengagement of heat and light. Perhaps iron, at a high temperature, would condense the oxygen and carbon by its strong affinity for these substances. Water condenses 1-50th of its bulk of the gas. The above processes are those usually prescribed in our systematic works, for procuring the oxide of carbon. In some of them, a portion of carbonic acid is evolved, which may be withdrawn by washing the gaseous product with weak solution of potassa, or milk of lime. We avoid the chance of this impurity by extricating the gas from a mixture of dry carbonate of barytes and iron filings, or of oxide of zinc, and previously calcined charcoal. The gaseous product from the first mixture, is pure oxide of carbon. Oxide of iron, and pure barytes, remain in the retort. Carbonic oxide, when respired, is fatal to animal life. Sir H. Davy took three inspirations of it, mixed with about one-fourth of common air; the effect was a temporary loss of sensation, which was succeeded by giddiness, sickness, acute pains in different parts of the body, and extreme debility. Some days elapsed before he entirely recovered. Since then, Mr. Witter of Dublin was struck down in an apoplectic condition, by breathing this gas; but he was speedily restored by the inhalation of oxygen. See an interesting account of this experiment, by Mr. Witter, in the Phil. Mag. vol. 43.

When a mixture of it and chlorine is exposed to sunshine, a curious compound, discovered by Dr. John Davy, is formed, to which he gave the name of phosgene gas. It has been called chlorocarbonic acid, though chlorocarbonous acid seems a more appropriate name."—*Ure's Chem. Dict.*

CARBUNCLE. 1. The name of a gem highly prized by the ancients, probably the *alamandine,* a variety of noble garnet.

2. The name of a disease. See *Anthrax.*

CARBU'NCULUS. (Diminutive of *carbo,* a burning coal.) A carbuncle. See *Anthrax.*

CARBURET. *Carburetum.* A combination of charcoal with any other substance: thus carburetted hydrogen is hydrogen holding carbon in solution; carburetted iron is steel, &c.

CARBURET OF SULPHUR. Sulphuret of carbon Alkohol of sulphur. "This interesting liquid was originally obtained by Lampadius in distilling a mixture of pulverized pyrites and charcoal in an earthen retort, and was considered by him as a peculiar compound of sulphur and hydrogen. But Clement and

Desormes first ascertained its true constitution to be carburetted sulphur; and they invented a process of great simplicity, for at once preparing it, and proving its nature. Thoroughly calcined charcoal is to be put into a porcelain tube, that traverses a furnace at a slight angle of inclination. To the higher end of the tube, a retort of glass, containing sulphur, is luted; and to the lower end is attached an adopter tube, which enters into a bottle with two tubulures, half full of water, and surrounded with very cold water or ice. From the other aperture of the bottle, a bent tube proceeds into the pneumatic trough. When the porcelain tube is brought into a state of ignition, heat is applied to the sulphur, which subliming into the tube, combines with the charcoal, forming the liquid carburet.

The carburet of sulphur dissolves camphor. It does not unite with water; but very readily with alkohol and æther. With chloride of azot it forms a non-detonating compound. The waters of potassa, barytes, and lime, slowly decompose it, with the evolution of carbonic acid gas. It combines with ammonia and lime, forming carbo-sulphurets. The carburet, saturated with ammoniacal gas, forms a yellow pulverulent substance, which sublimes unaltered in close vessels, but is so deliquescent that it cannot be passed from one vessel to another without absorbing moisture. When heated in that state, crystals of hydrosulphuret of ammonia form. The compound with lime is made by heating some quicklime in a tube, and causing the vapour of carburet to pass through it. The lime becomes incandescent at the instant of combination.

When the carburet is left for some weeks in contact with nitro-muriatic acid, it is converted into a substance having very much the appearance and physical properties of camphor; being soluble in alkohol and oil, and insoluble in water. This substance is, according to Berzelius, a triple acid, composed of two atoms of muriatic acid, one atom of sulphurous acid, and one atom of carbonic acid. He calls it, muriatico-sulphurous-carbonic acid.

When potassium is heated in the vapour of the carburet, it burns with a reddish flame, and a black film appears on the surface. On admitting water, a greenish solution of sulphuret of potassa is obtained, containing a mixture of charcoal. From its vapour passing through ignited muriate of silver, without occasioning any reduction of the metal, it is demonstrated that this carburet is destitute of hydrogen.

When the compound of potassa, water, and carburet of sulphur, is added to metallic solutions, precipitates of a peculiar kind, called carbo-sulphurets, are obtained.

Carburet of sulphur was found by Dr. Brewster to exceed all fluid bodies in refractive power, and even the solids, flint-glass, topaz, and tourmaline. In dispersive power it exceeds every fluid substance except oil of cassia, holding an intermediate place between phosphorus and balsam of Tolu."—*Ure.*

Carburetted hydrogen gas. *Carbonated hydrogen gas; Heavy inflammable air; Hydro-carbonate. Olefiant gas. Hydroguret of carbon.* "Of this compound gas we have two species, differing in the proportions of the constituents. The first, consisting of 1 prime equivalent of each, is carburetted hydrogen; the second, of 1 prime of carbon, and 2 of hydrogen, is subcarburetted hydrogen.

1. *Carburetted hydrogen,* the percarburetted of the French chemists, is, according to Mr. Brande, the only definite compound of these two elements. To prepare it, we mix, in a glass retort, 1 part of alkohol and 4 of sulphuric acid, and expose the retort to a moderate heat. The gas is usually received over water; though De Saussure states, that this liquid absorbs more than 1-7th of its volume of the gas. It is destructive of animal life. Its specific gravity is 0.978, according to Saussure. 100 cubic inches weigh 28.80 gr. It possesses all the mechanical properties of air. It is invisible, and void of taste and smell, when it has been washed from a little æthereous vapour. The effect of heat on this gas is curious. When passed through a porcelain tube, heated to a cherry-red, it lets fall a portion of charcoal, and nearly doubles its volume. At a higher temperature it deposites more charcoal, and augments in bulk; till finally, at the greatest heat to which we can expose it, it lets fall almost the whole of its carbon, and assumes a volume 3½ times greater than it had at first These remarkable results, observed with great care, have induced the illustrious Berthollet to conclude, with much plausibility, that hydrogen and carbon combine in many successive proportions. The transmission of a series of electric sparks through this gas, produces a similar effect with that of simple heat.

Carburetted hydrogen burns with a splendid white flame. When mixed with three times its bulk of oxygen, and kindled by a taper or the electric spark, it explodes with great violence.

When this gas is mixed with its own bulk of chlorine, the gaseous mixture is condensed over water into a peculiar oily-looking compound. Hence this carburetted hydrogen was called by its discoverers, the associated Dutch chemists, *olefiant gas.* Robiquet and Colin formed this liquid in considerable quantities, by making two currents of its constituent gases meet in a glass globe. The olefiant gas should be in rather larger quantity than the chlorine, otherwise the liquid becomes of a green colour, and acquires acid properties. When it is washed with water, and distilled off dry muriate of lime, it may be regarded as pure. It is then a limpid colourless essence of a pleasant flavour, and a sharp, sweet, and not disagreeable taste. At 45° its specific gravity is 2.2201. Dr. Thompson calls this fluid *chloric æther,* and it may with propriety, Mr. Brande thinks, be termed *hydro chloride of carbon.*

Olefiant gas is elegantly analyzed by heating sulphur in it over mercury. One cubic inch of it, with 2 grains of sulphur, yields 2 cubic inches of sulphuretted hydrogen, and charcoal is deposited. Now we know that the latter gas contains just its own volume of hydrogen.

2. *Subcarburetted hydrogen.* This gas is supposed to be procured in a state of definite composition, from the mud or stagnant pools or ditches. We have only to fill a wide-mouthed goblet with water, and inverting it in the ditch-water, stir the bottom with a stick. Gas rises into the goblet.

The fire-damp of mines is a similar gas to that of ditches. There is in both cases an admixture of carbonic acid, which lime or potassa-water will remove. A proportion of air is also present, the quantity of which can be ascertained by analysis. By igniting acetate of potassa in a gun-barrel, an analogous species of gas is obtained.

Subcarburetted hydrogen is destitute of colour, taste, and smell. It burns with a yellow flame, like that of a candle.

As the gas of ditches and the choke-damp of mines is evidently derived from the action of water on decaying vegetable or carbonaceous matter, we can understand that a similar product will be obtained by passing water over ignited charcoal, or by heating moistened charcoal or vegetable matter in retorts. The gases are here, however, a somewhat complex mixture, as well as what we obtain by igniting pit coal and wood in iron retorts. The combustion of subcarburetted hydrogen with common air takes place only when they are mixed in certain proportions. If from 6 to 12 parts of air be mixed with one of carburetted hydrogen, we have explosive mixtures. Proportions beyond these limits will not explode. In like manner, from 1 to 2½ of oxygen must be mixed with one of the combustible gas, otherwise we have no explosion. Sir H. Davy says, that this gas has a disagreeable empyreumatic smell, and that water absorbs 1-30th of its volume of it."—*Ure.*

CA'RCARUS. (From καρκαιρω, to resound.) *Carcaros.* A fever in which the patient has a continual horror and trembling, with an unceasing sounding in his ears.

Ca'rcax. (From καρα, a head.) A species of poppy, with a very large head.

Ca'rcer. A remedy, according to Paracelsus, for restraining the motions of body, the extravagant and libidinous conversation in some disorders; as in *Chorea Sancti Viti,* &c.

Carche'sius. (Καρχησιος. The openings at the top of a ship's mast through which the rope passes.) A name of some bandages noticed by Galen, and described by Oribasius.

CARCINO'MA. (*Carcinoma, atis.* n. From καρκινος, a cancer.) See *Cancer.*

CARCINUS. (Καρκινος, a cancer.) *Carcinos.* See *Cancer.*

Cardama'ntica. (From καρδαμον, the nasturtium A species of sciatica cresses

Cardamele'um. A medicine of no note, mentioned by Galen.

CARDAMI'NE. (*Cardamine es.* f.; from καρδια, the heart; because it acts as a cordial and strengthener, or from its having the taste of cardamum, that is, nasturtium, or cress.) Cuckoo-flower. 1. The name of a genus of plants in the Linnæan system. Class, *Tetradynamia;* Order, *Siliquosa.*

2. The pharmacopœial name of the cuckoo-flower. See *Cardamine pratensis.*

Cardamine pratensis. The systematic name of the common ladies' smock, or cuckoo-flower, called *cardamine* in the pharmacopœias. *Cardamantica; Nasturtium; aquaticum; Culi flos; Iberis sophia; Cardamine:—foliis pinnatis, foliolis, radicalibus subrotundis, caulinis lanceolatis* of Linnæus. The flower has a place in the materia medica, upon the authority of Sir George Baker, who has published five cases, two of Chorea Sancti Viti, one of spasmodic asthma, one of hemiplegia, and a case of spasmodic affections of the lower limbs, wherein the *flores cardamines* were supposed to have been successfully used. A variety of virtues have been given to this plant, but it does not deserve the attention of practitioners.

CARDAMO'MUM. (From καρδαμον and αμωμον: because it partakes of the nature, and is like both the cardamum and amomum.) The cardamom. See *Amomum*, *Elettaria*, and *Illicium.*

Cardamomum majus. See *Amomum granum paradisi.*

Cardamomum medium. The seeds correspond, in every respect, with the less, except in being twice as long, but no thicker than the *Cardamomum minus.*

Cardamomum minus. See *Elettaria cardamomum.*

Cardamomum piperatum. See *Amomum granum paradisi.*

Cardamomum siberiense. See *Illicium stellatum.*

CA'RDAMUM. (From καρδια, the heart; because it comforts and strengthens the heart.) The cardamum. See *Amomum*, *Elettaria*, and *Illicium.*

CA'RDIA. (From κεαρ, the heart.) 1. This term was applied by the Greeks to the heart.

2. The superior opening of the stomach.

CARDI'AC. (*Cardiacus;* from καρδια, the heart.) A cordial. See *Cordial.*

Cardiaca confectio. See *Confectio aromatica.*

Cardiaca herba. So named from the supposed relief it gives in faintings and disorders of the stomach. The pharmacopœial name of the plant called Motherwort. See *Leonurus cardiaca.*

Cardiaca passio. The cardiac passion. Ancient writers frequently mention a disorder under this name, which consists of that oppression and distress which often accompanies fainting.

Cardiacus morbus. A name by which the ancients called the typus fever.

CARDIA'LGIA. (From καρδια, the cardia, and αλγος, pain.) Pain at the stomach. The heartburn. Dr. Cullen ranks it as a symptom of dyspepsia. Heartburn is an uneasy sensation in the stomach, with anxiety, a heat more or less violent, and sometimes attended with oppression, faintness, an inclination to vomit, or a plentiful discharge of clear lymph, like saliva. This pain may arise from various and different causes; such as *flatus;* from *sharp humours*, either acid, bilious, or rancid; from *worms* gnawing and vellicating the coats of the stomach; from *acrid* and *pungent food*, such as spices, aromatics, &c.; as also from *rheumatic* and *gouty humours*, or *surfeits;* from too free a use of tea, or watery fluids relaxing the stomach, &c.; *from the natural mucus* being abraded, particularly in the upper orifice of the stomach.

Cardialgia sputatoria. See *Pyrosis.*

Cardime'lech. (From καρδια, the heart, and *meleck*, Heb. a governor.) A fictitious term in Dolæus's Encyclopedia, by which he would express a particular active principle in the heart, appointed to what we call the vital functions.

Cardimo'na. Pain at the stomach.

Cardinal flowers. See *Lobelia.*

Cardiname'ntum. (From *cardo*, a hinge.) An articulation like a hinge.

CARDIO'GMUS. (From καρδιωσσω, to have a pain in the stomach.) 1. A distressing pain at the præcordia or stomach.

2. An aneurism in or near the heart, which occasions pain in the præcordia.

3. A variety of the *Exangia aneurisma* of Good's nosological arrangement.

CARDIO'NCHUS. (From καρδια, the heart, and ογκος, a tumour.) An aneurism in the heart, or in the aorta near the heart.

Cardiotro'tus. (From καρδια, the heart, and τιτρωσκω, to wound.) One who hath a wound in his heart.

CARDI'TIS. (From καρδια, the heart.) *Empresma carditis* of Good. Inflammation of the heart. It is a genus of disease arranged by Cullen in the class *Pyrexiæ*, and order *Phlegmasiæ*. It is known by pyrexia, pain in the region of the heart, great anxiety, difficulty of breathing, cough, irregular pulse, palpitation, and fainting, and the other symptoms of inflammation.

The treatment of carditis is, in a great measure, similar to that of pneumonia. It is necessary to take blood freely, as well generally as locally, and apply a blister near the part. Purging may be carried to a greater extent than in pneumonia; and the use of digitalis is more important, to lessen the irritability of the heart. It is equally desirable to promote diaphoresis, but expectoration is not so much to be looked for, unless indeed, as very often happens, the inflammation should have extended, in some degree, to the lungs.

Cardite. See *organic relics.*

CA'RDO. A hinge. 1. The articulation called *Ginglymus.*

2. The second vertebra of the neck.

Cardo'nium. Wine medicated with herbs.—*Paracelsus.*

Cardopa'tium. The low carline thistle. Most probably the *Carlina acaulis* of Linnæus, said to be diaphoretic.

CA'RDUUS. (*A carere, quasi aptus carendæ lanæ*, being fit to tease wool; or from κειρω, to abrade; so named from its roughness, which abrades and tears whatever it meets with.) The thistle or teasel. The name of a genus of plants in the Linnæan system. Class, *Syngenesia;* Order, *Polygamia æqualis.*

Carduus acanthus. The bear's breech.

Carduus altilis. The artichoke.

Carduus arvensis. The way-thistle. See *Serratula arvensis.*

Carduus benedictus. See *Centaurea.*

Carduus hæmorrhoidalis. The common creeping way-thistle. *Serratula arvensis* of Linnæus.

Carduus lacteus. See *Carduus marianus*

Carduus mariæ. See *Carduus marianus.*

Carduus marianus. The systematic name of the officinal *Carduus mariæ.* Common milk-thistle, or Lady's thistle. *Carduus: foliis amplexicaulibus, hastato-pinnatifidis, spinosis; calycibus aphyllis; spinis caliculatis, duplicato-spinosis*, of Linnæus. The seeds of this plant, and the herb, have been employed medicinally. The former contain a bitter oil, and are recommended as relaxants. The juice of the latter is said to be salutary in dropsies, in the dose of four ounces; and, according to Miller, to be efficacious against pungent pains. The leaves when young surpass, when boiled, the finest cabbage, and in that state are diuretic.

Carduus sativus. The artichoke.

Carduus solstitialis. The *Calcitrapa officinalis* of Linnæus.

Carduus tomentosus. The woolly thistle. See *Onopordium acanthium.*

CAREBA'RIA. (From καρη, the head, and βαρος, weight.) A painful and uneasy heaviness of the head

CARE'NUM. (From καρη, the head.) Galen uses this word for the head.

Carenum vinum. Strong wine.

Careum. (From *Caria*, the country whence they were brought.) The caraway.

CA'REX. (*Carex, icis*, fœm. from *careo*, not *quia viribus careat*, but because, from its roughness, it is fit *ad carendum*, to card, tease, or pull.) Sedge The name of a genus of plants in the Linnæan system Class, *Monœcia;* Order, *Triandria.*

Carex arenaria. The systematic name of the officinal *sarsaparilla germanica*, which grows plentifully on the sea coast. The root has been found serviceable in some mucal affections of the trachea, in rheumatic pains, and gouty affections. These roots, and those of the *carex hirta*, are mixed with the true sarsaparilla, which they much resemble.

CA'RICA. (From *Caria*, the place where they were cultivated.) The fig. See *Ficus carica*.

CARICA PATAYA. Papaw-tree. This is a native of both Indies, and the Guinea coast of Africa. When the roundish fruit are nearly ripe, the inhabitants of India boil and eat them with their meat, as we do turnips. They have somewhat the flavour of a pompion. Previous to boiling, they soak them for some time in salt and water, to extract the corrosive juice, unless the meat they are to be boiled with should be very salt and old, and then this juice being in them, will make them as tender as a chicken. But they mostly pickle the long fruit, and thus they make no bad succedaneum for mango. The buds of the female flowers are gathered, and made into a sweetmeat; and the inhabitants are such good husbands of the produce of this tree, that they boil the shells of the ripe fruit into a repast, and the insides are eaten with sugar in the manner of melons. Every part of the papaw-tree, except the ripe fruit, affords a milky juice, which is used, in the isle of France, as an effectual remedy for the tape-worm. In Europe, however, whither it has been sent in the concrete state, it has not answered, perhaps from some change it had undergone, or not having been given in a sufficient dose.

A very remarkable circumstance regarding the papaw-tree, is the extraction from its juice of a matter exactly resembling the flesh or fibre of animals, and hence called vegetable fibrin.

CARICUM. (From *Caricus*, its inventor.) *Carycum*. An ointment for cleansing ulcers, composed of hellebore, lead, and cantharides.

CA'RIES. (From *carah*, Chald.) *Gangrena Caries* of Good. Rottenness, mortification of the bones

[Cooper derives caries from κειρω, to abrade. "It is a disease of the bones, supposed to be very analogous to ulceration of the soft parts; and this comparison is one of great antiquity, having been made by Galen. However, by the generality of the ancients, caries was not discriminated from necrosis.

"It was from the surgeons of the eighteenth century that more correct opinions were derived respecting caries. Until this period, writers had done little more than mentioning the complaint, and the methods of treating it. Some new light was thrown upon the subject by J. L. Petit, in his remarks upon exostosis and caries. But, as he only spoke of the disorder as one of the terminations of exostosis, he has not entered far into the consideration of it. The best observations on caries were first made by Dr. A. Monro, *primus*. This memoir contains the earliest correct ideas of *dry caries*, or necrosis, which is rightly compared to mortification of the soft parts, and named *gangrenous aries*.

"The bones, like other parts of the body, are composed of arteries, veins, absorbent vessels, nerves, and a cellular texture; they are endued with vitality; they are nourished, they grow, waste, are repaired, and undergo various mutations, according to the age of the individual; and they are subject to diseases analogous to those of the soft parts. To the phosphate of lime, which is more or less distributed in their texture, they owe all their solidity; and, perhaps, it is to the same earthy substance that the difference in their vital properties, and in their diseases, from those of the rest of the body, is to be referred. In fact, this particular organization, and inferior vitality of the bones, are generally supposed to account for the small number, peculiar character, and general slow progress of their diseases."—*Cooper's Surg. Dict.* A.]

CARI'MA. The cassada bread.

CARI'NA. The keel of a ship. 1. A name formerly applied to the back bone.

2. In botany, the keel, or that part of the petals which compose a papilionaceous flower, consisting of two, united or separate, which embrace the internal or genital organs. See *Corolla*.

CARINATUS. Keel-shaped; applied to leaves and petals when the back is longitudinally prominent like the keel of a boat; as in the leaf of the *Allium carinatum*, and the petals of the *Allium ampellprasum Carum carui*.

CARINTHINE. A subspecies of mineral augite found in Carinthia.

CARIOUS. When a part of a bone is deprived of its vitality, it is said to be carious, dead, or rotten: hence carious tooth, &c.

CA'RIUM TERRA. Lime.

CARIVILLA'NDI. Sarsaparilla root.

CARLI'NA. (From *Carolus*, Charles the Great, or Charlemagne; because it was believed that an angel showed it to him, and that, by the use of it, his army was preserved from the plague.) Carline thistle. The name of a genus of plants in the Linnæan system. Class, *Syngenesia*; Order, *Polygamia æqualis*. The officinal name of two kinds of plants.

CARLINA ACAULIS. The systematic name of the *chamæleon album*. *Carlina*; *Cardopatium*. Carline thistle. Star thistle. *Carlina—caule unifloro, flore breviore*, of Linnæus. The root of this plant is bitter, and said to possess diaphoretic and anthelmintic virtues. It is also extolled by foreign physicians in the cure of acute, malignant, and chronic disorders, particularly gravel and jaundice.

CARLINA GUMMIFERA. *Carduus pinea*; *Ixine*. Pine thistle. This plant is the *Atractylis gummifera* of Linnæus. The root, when wounded, yields a milky, viscous juice, which concretes into tenaceous masses, at first whitish, resembling wax, when much handled growing black; it is said to be chewed with the same views as mastich.

Carline thistle. See *Carlina acaulis*.

CA'RLO SANCTO RADIX. St. Charles's root, so called by the Spaniards, on account of its great virtues. It is found in Mechoachan, a province in America. Its bark hath an aromatic flavour, with a bitter acrid taste. The root itself consists of slender fibres. The bark is sudorific, and strengthens the gums and stomach.

CA'RMEN. (*Carmen, inis*. neut. A verse; because charms usually consisted of a verse.) A charm; an amulet.

CARMES. (The Carmelite friars, Fr.) Carmelite water; so named from its inventors; composed of baum, lemon-peel, &c.

CARMINA'NTIA. See *Carminative*.

CARMI'NATIVE. (*Carminativus*; from *carmen*, a verse, or charm; because practitioners, in ancient times, ascribed their operation to a charm or enchantment.) That which allays pain and dispels flatulencies of the primæ viæ. The principal carminatives are the semina cardamomi, anisi et carui; olea essentialia carui, anisi et juniperi; confectio aromatica; pulvis aromaticus; tinctura cardamomi; tinctura cinnamomi composita; zingiber; stimulants; tonics; bitters; and astringents.

CARMINE. A red pigment prepared from cochineal.

CARMINIUM. The name given by the French chemists to the colouring matter of cochineal. See *Coccus cacti*.

CARNABA'DIUM. Caraway-seed.

CA'RNEA COLUMNA. A fleshy pillar or column. The name of some fleshy fasciculi in the ventricles of the heart. See *Heart*.

CARNELIAN. A subspecies of calcedony.

CARNICULA. (Diminutive of *caro, carnis*, flesh.) A small fleshy substance; applied to the substance which surrounds the gums.

CARNIFO'RMIS. (From *caro*, flesh, and *forma*, likeness.) Having the appearance of flesh. It is commonly applied to an abscess, where the flesh surrounding the orifice is hardened, and of a firm consistence.

CARNOSUS. Fleshy; applied to loaves, pods, &c. of a thick pulpy substance; as in the leaves of all those plants called succulent, especially *cedum crassula*, &c.

CA'RO. (*Caro, carnis*. fœm.) 1. Flesh. The red part or belly of a muscle.

2. The pulp of fruit.

CAROLI'NA. See *Carlina*.

CAROMEL. The smell exhaled from sugar at the calcining heat.

CARO'PI. The *Amomum verum*.

CARO'RA. A chemical vessel that resembles a urinal.

CARO'SIS. See *Carus*.

CARO'TA. See *Daucus*.

CAROTID. (From καροω, to cause to sleep; because, if tied with a ligature, the animal becomes comatose, and has the appearance of being asleep.) An artery of the neck. See *Carotid artery*.

CAROTID ARTERY. *Arteria carotidea.* The carotids are two considerable arteries that proceed, one on each side of the cervical vertebræ, to the head, to supply it with blood. The right carotid does not arise immediately from the arch of the aorta, but is given off from the arteria innominata. The left arises from the arch of the aorta. Each carotid is divided into external and internal, or that portion without and that within the cranium. The external gives off eight branches, to the neck and face, viz. *anteriorly*, the superior thyroideal, the sublingual, the inferior maxillary, the external maxillary; *posteriorly*, the internal maxillary, the occipital, the external auditory, and the temporal. The internal carotid or cerebral artery, gives off four branches within the cavity of the cranium; the anterior cerebral, the posterior, the central artery of the optic nerve, and the internal orbital.

CARO'UM. The caraway-seed.

CA'RPASUS. (So named ϖαρα το καρον ποιησαι: because it makes the person who eats it appear as if he was asleep.) An herb, the juice of which was formerly called *opocarpason*, *opocarpathon*, or *opocalpason;* according to Galen, it resembles myrrh; but is esteemed highly poisonous.

CARPA'THICUM BALSAMUM. See *Pinus Cembra.*

CARPENTA'RIA. (From *carpentarius*, a carpenter; and so named from its virtues in healing cuts and wounds made by a tool.) A vulnerary herb; not properly known what it is, but believed to be the common milfoil or yarrow, the *Achillæa millifolium* of Linnæus.

CARPHA'LEUS. (From καρφω, to exsiccate.) Hippocrates uses this word to mean *dry*, opposed to *moist.*

CARPHOLO'GIA. (From καρφος, the nap of clothes, and λεγω, to pluck.) *Carpologia.* A delirious picking of the bed-clothes, a symptom of great danger in diseases. See *Floccilatio.*

CA'RPHUS. (From καρφη, a straw.) 1. In Hippocrates it signifies a mote, or any small substance.

2. A pustule of the smallest kind.

3. The herb fenugreek.

CA'RPIA. (From *carpo*, to pluck, as lint is made from linen cloth.) Lint.

CARPI'SMUS. The wrist.

CARPOBA'LSAMUM. (From καρπος, fruit, and βαλσαμον, balsam.) See *Amyris gileadensis.*

CARPOLO'GIA. See *Carphologia.*

CARPOTICA. (*Carpoticus;* from καρπωσις, *fruitio*, from καρπως, *fructus.*) The name of an order of diseases in the class *Genetica* of Good's Nosology; diseases afflicting the impregnation. It embraces four genera. 1. *Paracyesis*, morbid pregnancy. 2. *Parodynia*, morbid labour. 3. *Eccyesis*, extra uterine fœtation. 4. *Pseudocyesis*, spurious pregnancy.

CA'RPUS. (Καρπος, the wrist.) The wrist, or carpus. It is situated between the forearm and hand. See *Bone.*

CARROT. See *Daucus carota.*

Carrot, candy. See *Athamanta Cretensis.*

Carrot poultice. See *Cataplasma dauci.*

CA'RTHAMUS. (From καθαιρω, to purge.) 1. The name of a genus of plants in the Linnæan system. Class, *Syngenesia;* Order, *Polygamia æqualis.*

2. The pharmacopœial name of the saffron flower. See *Carthamus tinctorius.*

CARTHAMUS TINCTORIUS. The systematic name of the saffron flower, or bastard saffron, called also *Cnicus; Crocus saracenicus; Carthamum officinarum; Carduus sativus. Carthamus—foliis ovatis, integris, serrato-aculeatis* of Linnæus. The seeds, freed from their shells, have been celebrated as a gentle cathartic, in the dose of one or two drachms. They are also supposed to be diuretic and expectorant; particularly useful in humoral asthma, and similar complaints. The *carthamus lanatus* is considered in France as a febrifuge and sudorific. The dried flowers are frequently mixed with saffron, to adulterate it. The plant is cultivated in many places on account of its flowers, which are used as a dye.

"In some of the deep reddish, yellow, or orange-coloured flowers, the yellow matter seems to be of the same kind with that of the pure yellow flowers; but the red to be of a different kind from the pure red ones. Watery menstrua take up only the yellow, and leave the red, which may afterward be extracted by alkohol, or by a weak solution of alkali. Such particularly are the saffron-coloured flowers of carthamus. These, after the yellow matter has been extracted by water, are said to give a tincture to ley; from which, on standing at rest for some time, a deep red fecula subsides called safflower, and from the countries whence it is commonly brought to us, Spanish red and China lake. This pigment impregnates alkohol with a beautiful red tincture; but communicates no colour to water.

Rouge is prepared from carthamus. For this purpose the red colour is extracted by a solution of the subcarbonate of soda, and precipitated by lemon juice previously depurated by standing. This precipitate is dried on earthen plates, mixed with talc, or French chalk, reduced to a powder by means of the leaves of shave-grass, triturated with it till they are both very fine, and then sifted. The fineness of the powder and proportion of the precipitate constitute the difference between the finer and cheaper rouge. It is likewise spread very thin on saucers, and sold in this state for dying.

Carthamus is used for dying silk of a poppy, cherry, rose, or bright orange-red. After the yellow matter is extracted as above, and the cakes opened, it is put into a deal trough, and sprinkled at different times with pearl ashes, or rather soda, well powdered and sifted, in the proportion of six pounds to a hundred, mixing the alkali well as it is put in. The alkali should be saturated with carbonic acid. The carthamus is then put on a cloth in a trough with a grated bottom, placed on a larger trough, and cold water poured on, till the large trough is filled. And this is repeated, with the addition of a little more alkali toward the end, till the carthamus is exhausted and become yellow. Lemon juice is then poured into the bath, till it is turned of a fine cherry colour, and after it is well stirred, the silk is immersed in it. The silk is wrung, drained, and passed through fresh baths, washing and drying after every operation, till it is of a proper colour; when it is brightened in hot water, and lemon juice. For a poppy or fire colour a slight annotto ground is first given; but the silk should not be alumed. For a pale carnation a little soap should be put into the bath. All these baths must be used as soon as they are made; and cold, because heat destroys the colour of the red feculæ."

CARTHEUSER, JOHN FREDERICK, a professor of medicine at Francfort, on the Oder, acquired considerable reputation about the middle of the last century, by several luminous works on botany and pharmacy; especially his "Rudimenta Materiæ Medicæ Rationalis," and "De Genericis quibusdam Plantarum Principiis." He had two sons, Frederick Augustus and William, also of the medical profession, and authors of some less important works.

CARTHUSIA'NUS. (From the monks of that order, who first invented it.) A name of the precipitated sulphur of antimony.

CARTILAGE. See *Cartilago.*

CARTILAGINEUS. Cartilaginous. 1. Applied, in anatomy, to parts which naturally, or from disease, have a cartilaginous consistence.

2. In botany, to leaves which have a hard or horny leaf-edge, as in several species of saxifrage. See *Leaf.*

CARTILA'GO. (*Cartilago, inis.* fœm. Quasi *carnilago;* from *caro, carnis*, flesh.) A white elastic, glistening substance, growing to bones, and commonly called *gristle.* Cartilages are divided, by anatomists, into *obducent*, which cover the moveable articulations of bones; *inter-articular*, which are situated between the articulations, and *uniting* cartilages, which unite one bone with another. Their use is to facilitate the motions of bones, or to connect them together.

The chemical analysis of cartilage affords one-third the weight of the bones, when the calcareous salts are removed by digestion in dilute muriatic acid. It resembles coagulated albumen. Nitric acid converts it into gelatin. With alkalies it forms an animal soap. Cartilage is the primitive paste, into which the calcareous salts are deposited in the young animal. In the disease rickets, the earthy matter is withdrawn by morbid absorption, and the bones return into the state nearly of flexible cartilage. Hence arise the distortions characteristic of this disease.

CARTILAGO ANNULARIS. See *Cartilago cricoidea.*

CARTILAGO ARYTÆNOIDEA. See *Larynx.*

CARTILAGO CRICOIDEA. The cricoid cartilage belongs to the larynx, and is situated between the thyroid and arytenoid cartilages and the trachea; it constitutes, as it were, the basis of the many annular cartilages of the trachea.

Cartilago ensiformis. *Cartilago xiphoidea.* Ensiform cartilage. A cartilage shaped somewhat like a sword or dagger, attached to the lowermost part of the sternum, just at the pit of the stomach.

Cartilago scutiformis. See *Thyroid cartilage.*

Cartilago thyroidea. See *Thyroid cartilage.*

Cartilago xiphoidea. See *Cartilago ensiformis.*

CA'RUI. (*Caruia.* Arabian.) The caraway. See *Carum.*

CA'RUM. (Καρος; so named from *Caria*, a province of Asia.) The Caraway. 1. The name of a genus of plants in the Linnæan system. Class, *Pentandria;* Order, *Monogynia.*

2. The pharmacopœial name of the caraway plant. See *Carum carui.*

Carum carui. The systematic name for the plant, the seeds of which are called caraways. It is also called *Carvi; Cuminum pratense; Carus; Caruon.* The seeds are well known to have a pleasant spicy smell, and a warm aromatic taste; and, on this account, are used for various economical purposes. They are esteemed to be carminative, cordial, and stomachic, and recommended in dyspepsia, flatulencies, and other symptoms attending hysterical and hypochondriacal disorders. An essential oil and distilled water are directed to be prepared from them by the London College.

CA'RUNCLE. (*Caruncula;* diminutive of *caro*, flesh.) *Ecphynia caruncula* of Good. A little fleshy excrescence; as the carunculæ myrtiformes, carunculæ lachrymales, &c.

CARUNCULA. See *Caruncle.*

Caruncula lachrymalis. A long conoidal gland, red externally, situated in the internal canthus of each eye, before the union of the eyelids. It appears to be formed of numerous sebaceous glands, from which many small hairs grow. The hardened smegma observable in this part of the eye in the morning, is separated by this caruncle.

Carunculæ mamillares. The extremities of the tubes in the nipple.

Carunculæ myrtiformes. When the hymen has been lacerated by attrition, there remain in its place two, three, or four caruncles, which have received the name of myrtiform.

Carunculæ papillares. The protuberances within the pelvis of the kidney, formed by the papillous substance of the kidney.

Ca'ruon. See *Carum.*

CA'RUS. (Καρος; from καρα, the head, as being the part affected.) *Caros; Carosis.* 1. Insensibility and sleepiness, as in apoplexy, attended with quiet respiration.

2. A lethargy, or a profound sleep, without fever.

3. Dr. Good gives this name to a genus in his Nosology, embracing those diseases characterized by muscular immobility; mental or corporeal torpitude, or both. It has six species; *Carus asphyxia; ecstasis; catalepsia; lethargus; apoplexia; paralysis.*

4. The caraway seed.

Ca'rva. The cassia lignea.

Cary'don. See *Caryedon.*

Carye'don. (From καρυα, a nut.) *Carydon.* A sort of fracture, where the bone is broken into small pieces, like the shell of a cracked nut.

Caryocosti'num. An electuary; so named from two of its ingredients, the clove and costus.

CARYOPHYLLA'TA. (From καρυοφυλλον, the caryophyllus; so named, because it smells like the caryophyllus, or clove July flower.) See *Geum urbanum.*

Caryophylloi'des cortex. See *Laurus culilawan.*

CARYOPHY'LLUM. (Καρυοφυλλον; from καρυον, a nut, and φυλλον, a leaf; so named because it was supposed to be the leaf of the Indian nut.) The clove. See *Eugenia caryophyllata.*

Caryophyllum aromaticum. See *Eugenia caryophyllata.*

Caryophillum rubrum. The clove pink. See *Dianthus caryophyllus.*

CARYOPHY'LLUS. The clove-tree. The name of a genus of plants in the Linnæan system. Class, *Polyandria;* Order, *Monogynia.* See *Eugenia carophyllata.*

Caryophyllus aromaticus americanus. See *Myrtus pimenta.*

Caryophyllus hortensis. See *Dianthus caryophyllus.*

Caryophyllus vulgaris. See *Geum urbanum.*

Caryo'tis. (From καρυον, a nut.) *Caryota.* Galen gives this name to a superior sort of date, of the shape of a nut.

CASCARI'LLA. (Diminutive of *cascara*, the bark, or shell. Spanish.) A name given originally to small specimens of cinchona; but now applied to another bark. See *Croton cascarilla.*

Cas'chu. See *Acacia catechu.*

Cashew-nut. See *Anacardium occidentale.*

Cashow. See *Acacia catechu.*

CASEIC ACID. *Acidum caseicum.* The name given by Proust to an acid formed in cheeses, to which he ascribes their flavour.

Ca'sia. See *Cassia.*

Casmina'ris. See *Cassumuniar.*

Ca'ssa. (Arabian.) The breast.

CASSA'DA. See *Jatropha manihot.*

Ca'ssamum. The fruit of the balsam of Gilead-tree, or *Amyrus opobalsamum.*

Ca'ssava. See *Jatropha manihot.*

CASSEBOHM, Frederic, a professor of anatomy at Halle in Saxony, published, in 1730, a treatise on the difference between the Fœtus and Adult, in which he notices the descent of the testicle from the abdomen, and, four years after, a very minute and exact description of the ear. He likewise explained, in subsequent publications, the manner of dissecting the muscles and the viscera; but an early death prevented his completing his design of elucidating the anatomy of the whole body in the same way.

CASSERIUS, Julius, was born of humble parents at Placentia, in 1545. He became servant to Fabricius at Padua, who, observing his talent, first taught him anatomy, then made him his assistant, and finally coadjutor in the professorship in 1609. He pursued the study with uncommon zeal, expending almost all his profits in procuring subjects, and in having drawings and prints made of the parts, which he discovered, or traced more accurately than his predecessors. He employed comparative anatomy, not as a substitute for, but only as a clue to that of the human subject. He published an account of the organs of voice and hearing, which he afterward extended to the other senses, explaining also the uses of these parts. Some years after his death, in 1616, the rest of his plates, amounting to 78, with the explanations, were published with the works of Spigelius.

CA'SSIA. (From the Arabic *katsia*, which is from *katsa*, to tear off; so called from the act of stripping the bark from the tree.) The name of a genus of plants in the Linnæan system. Class, *Decandria;* Order, *Monogynia.*

Cassia bark. See *Laurus cassia.*

Cassia caryophyllata. The clove bark tree. See *Myrtus caryophyllata.*

Cassia fistula. *Cassia nigra; Cassia fistularis; Alexandrina; Chaiarxambar; Canna; Cassia solutiva; Tlai Xiem.* The purging cassia. This tree, *Cassia—foliis quinquejugis ovatis acuminatis glabris, petiolis eglandulatis* of Linnæus, is a native of both Indies. The pods of the East India cassia are of a less diameter, smoother, and afford a blacker, sweeter, and more grateful pulp, than those which are brought from the West Indies. Those pods which are the heaviest, and in which the seeds do not rattle on being shaken, are commonly the best, and contain the most pulp, which is the part medicinally employed, and to be obtained in the manner described in the pharmacopœias. The best pulp is of a bright shining black colour, and of a sweet taste, with a slight degree of acidity. It has been long used as a laxative medicine, and being gentle in its operation, and seldom disturbing the bowels, is well adapted to children, and to delicate or pregnant women. Adults, however, find it of little effect, unless taken in a very large dose, as an ounce or more; and, therefore, to them this pulp is rarely given, but usually conjoined with some of the brisker purgatives. The officinal preparation of this drug is the confectio cassiæ; it is also an ingredient in the confectio sennæ.

Cassia fistularis. See *Cassia fistula.*

Cassia latinorum. See *Osyris.*

CASSIA LIGNEA. See *Laurus cassia.*

CASSIA MONSPELIENSIUM. See *Osyris.*

CASSIA NIGRA. See *Cassia fistula.*

CASSIA POETICA. Poet's rosemary; a plant which grows in the south of Europe, and is said to be astringent. See *Osyris.*

Cassia, purging. See *Cassia fistula.*

CASSIA SENNA. The systematic name of the plant which affords senna. *Senna alexandrina; Senna italica.* Senna, or Egyptian cassia. *Cassia—foliis sejugis subovatis, petiolis eglandulatis* of Linnæus. The leaves of senna, which are imported here from Alexandria, for medicinal use, have rather a disagreeable smell, and a subacrid, bitterish, nauseous taste. They are in common use as a purgative. The formulæ given of the senna by the colleges, are in infusion, a compound powder, a tincture, and an electuary. See *Infusum sennæ,* &c.

CASSIA SOLUTIVA. See *Cassia fistula.*

CASSIA MARYLANDICA. See *American senna.*

CASSIÆ ARAMENTUM. The pulp of cassia.

CASSIÆ FLORES. What are called cassia flowers in the shops, are the flowers of the true cinnamon-tree, *Laurus cinnamomum* of Linnæus. They possess aromatic and adstringent virtues, and may be successfully employed in decoctions, &c. in all cases where cinnamon is recommended. See *Laurus cinnamomum.*

CASSIÆ PULPA. See *Cassia fistula*

Cassius's Precipitate. The purple powder, which forms on a plate of tin immersed in a solution of gold. It is used to paint in enamel.

CA'SSOB. An obsolete term for kali.

CASSOLETA. Warm fumigations described by Marcellus.

CASSONADA. Sugar.

CASSUMMU'NIAR. (Of uncertain derivation; perhaps Indian.) *Casamunar; Casmina; Risagon; Bengale Indorum.* The root, occasionally exhibited under one of these names, is brought from the East Indies. It comes over in irregular slices of various forms, some cut transversely, others longitudinally. The cortical part is marked with circles of a dusky brown colour: the internal part is paler, and unequally yellow. It possesses moderately warm, bitter, and aromatic qualities, and a smell like ginger. It is recommended in hysterical, epilectic, and paralytic affections.

CASTA'NEA. (Καςανον; from *Castana,* a city in Thessaly, whence they were brought.) See *Fagus castanea.*

CASTANEA EQUINA. The horse-chesnut. See *Æsculus hippocastanum.*

CASTELLANUS, PETER, or DU CHATEL, was born at Grammont, in Flanders, in 1585. His rapid improvement in the Greek language procured him the professorship, at Lovain, in 1609; but he did not graduate in medicine till nine years after. At the same period, he published the lives of eminent physicians in Latin, written in a concise but very entertaining manner, with useful references to the original authorities. He died in 1632.

CASTELLUS, BARTHOLOMEW, an Italian physician, who practised at Messina about the end of the 16th century. He was author of two works, both for a long time extremely popular, a Synopsis of Medicine, and "Lexicon Medicum Græco-Latinum," in which great learning and judgment are conspicuous.

CASTJOE. See *Acacia catechu.*

CASTLE-LEOD. The name of a place in Ross-shire, in Scotland, where there is a sulphureous spring, celebrated for the cure of cutaneous diseases and foul ulcers.

CASTOR. (*Castor:* from καςωρ, the beaver, *quasi* γαςωρ; from γαςηρ, the belly: because of the largeness of its belly; or *a castrando,* because he was said to castrate himself in order to escape the hunters.)

1. The name of a genus of animals.

2. The English name of the *Castoreum* of the pharmacopœias, a peculiar concrete substance obtained from the Castor fiber of Linnæus. See *Castor fiber.*

CASTOR FIBER. The systematic name of the beaver, an amphibious quadruped inhabiting some parts of Prussia, Russia, Germany, &c.; but the greatest number of these animals is met with in Canada. The name of *castoreum,* or castor, is given to two bags, situated in the inguinal regions of the beaver, which contain a very odorous substance, soft, and almost fluid when recently cut from the animal, but which dries, and assumes a resinous consistence in process of time. The best comes from Russia. It is of a grayish yellow, or light brown colour. It consists of a mucilage, a bitter extract, a resin, an essential oil, in which the peculiar smell appears to reside, and a flaky crystalline matter, much resembling the adipocire of biliary calculi. Castor has an acrid, bitter, and nauseous taste; its smell is strong and aromatic, yet at the same time fœtid. It is used medicinally, as a powerful antispasmodic in hysterica and hypochondriacal affections, and in convulsions, in doses of from 10 to 30 grains. It has also been successfully administered in epilepsy and tetanus. It is occasionally adulterated with dried blood, gum-ammoniacum, or galbanum, mixed with a little of the powder of castor, and some quantity of the fat of the beaver.

Castor oil. See *Ricinus.*

Castor, Russian. See *Castor fiber.*

CASTOREUM. See *Castor fiber.*

CASTORI'UM. See *Castoreum.*

CASTRATION. (*Castratio, onis.* f.; from *castro* to emasculate, *quia castrando vis libidinis extinguitur.*) 1. A chirurgical operation, by which a testicle is removed from the body.

2. Botanists apply this term to the removal of the anthera of a flower, and to a plant naturally wanting this organ.

CASTRE'NSIS. (From *castra,* a camp.) Belonging to a camp: applied to those diseases with which soldiers, encamped in marshy places, are afflicted.

CATA'BASIS. (From καπαβαινω, to descend) An operation downwards.

CATABI'BASIS. (From καταβιβαζω, to cause to descend.) An expulsion of the humours downwards

CATABLACEU'SIS. (From καταβλακευω, to be useless.) Hippocrates uses this word to signify carelessness and negligence in the attendance on and administration to the sick.

CATABLE'MA. (From καταβαλλω, to throw round.) The outermost fillet, which secures the rest of the bandages.

CATABRONCHE'SIS. (From κατα, and βρογχος, the throat; or καταβρογχιζω, to swallow.) The act of swallowing.

CATACAU'MA. (From κατακαιω, to burn.) A burn or scald.

CATACAU'SIS. (From κατακαιω, to burn.) 1. The act of combustion, or burning.

2. The name of a genus of diseases in Dr. Good's Nosology: general combustibility of the body. It has only one species, *Catacausis ebriosa.*

CATACECLI'MENUS. (From κατακλινομαι, to lie down.) Keeping the bed, from the violence of a disease.

CATACECRA'MENUS. (From κατακεραννομι, to reduce to small particles.) Broken into small pieces: applied to fractures.

CATACERA'STICA. (From κατακεραννυμι, to mix together.) Medicines which obtund the acrimony of humours, by mixing with them and reducing them.

CATACLIDE'SIS. (From καταχλιδαω, to indulge in delicacies.) A gluttonous indulgence in sloth and delicacies, to the generation of diseases.

CATACHRI'SMA. An ointment.

CATACHRI'STON. (From καταχριω, to anoint.) An ointment.

CATA'CLASIS. (From κατακλαω, to break, or distort.) Distorted eyelids.

CA'TACLEIS. (From κατα, beneath, and κλεις, the clavicle.) *Catacleis.* The subclavicle, or first rib, which is placed immediately under the clavicle.

CATACLI'NES. (From κατακλινω, to lie down.) One who, by disease, is fixed to his bed.

CATA'CLISIS. (From κατακλινω, to lie down.) A lying down. Also incurvation.

CATACLY'SMA. (From κατακλυζω, to wash.) A clyster.

CATACLY'SMUS. (From κατακλυζω, to wash.) 1. An embrocation.

2. A dashing of water upon any part.

CATACRE'MNOS. (From κατα, and κρημνος, a precipice.) Hippocrates means, by this word, a swoln and inflamed throat, from the exuberance of the parts.

CATACRU'SIS. (From κατακρουω, to drive back.) A revulsion of humours.

CATADOULE'SIS. (From καταδουλοω, to enslave.) The subduing of passions, as in a phrensy, or fever.

CATÆGIZE'SIS. (From καταιγιζω, to repel.) A revulsion or rushing back of humours, or wind in the intestines.

CATÆONE'SIS. (From καταιονεω, to irrigate.) Irrigation by a plentiful affusion of liquor on some part of the body.

CATA'GMA. (From κατα, and αγω, to break.) A fracture. Galen says a solution of the bone is called *catagma*, and *elcos* is a solution of the continuity of the flesh: that when it happens to a cartilage, it has no name, though Hippocrates calls it *catagma*.

CATAGMA'TICA. (From καταγμα, a fracture.) Catagmatics. Remedies which promote the formation of callus.

CATAGO'GE. (From καταγομαι, to abide.) The seat or region of a disease or part.

CATAGYIO'SIS. (From καταγυιοω, to debilitate.) An imbecility and enervation of the strength and limbs.

CATALE'PSIS. (From καταλαμβανω, to seize, to hold.) *Catoche; Catochus; Congelatio; Detentio; Encatalepsis;* by Hippocrates, *Aphonia;* by Antigenes, *Anaudia;* by Cælius Aurelianus, *Apprehensio, Oppressio; Comprehensio; Carus catalepsia* of Good; *Apoplexia cataleptica* of Cullen. Catalepsy. A sudden suppression of motion and sensation, the body remaining in the same posture that it was in when seized.

Dr. Cullen says, he has never seen the catalepsy except when counterfeited; and is of opinion, that many of those cases related by other authors, have also been counterfeited. It is said to come on suddenly, being only preceded by some languor of body and mind, and to return by paroxysms. The patients are said to be for some minutes, sometimes (though rarely) for some hours, deprived of their senses, and all power of voluntary motion; but constantly retaining the position in which they were first seized, whether lying or sitting; and if the limbs be put into any other posture during the fit, they will keep the posture in which they are placed. When they recover from the paroxysm, they remember nothing of what passed during the time of it, but are like persons awakened out of a sleep.

CATALO'TICA. (From καταλοαω, to grind down.) Medicines to soften and make smooth the rough edges and crust of cicatrices.

CATA'LYSIS. (Καταλυσις: from καταλυω, to dissolve or destroy.) It signifies a palsy, or such a resolution as happens before the death of the patient; also that dissolution which constitutes death.

CATAMARA'SMUS. (From καταμαραινω, to grow thin.) 1. An emaciation of the body.

2. The resolution of tumours.

CATAMASSE'SIS. (From καταμασσομαι, to manducate.) The grinding of the teeth, and biting of the tongue; common in epilepsy.

CATAME'NIA. (*Catamenia, orum,* neut. pleur.; from κατα, according to, and μην, the month.) *Menses.* The monthly discharge from the uterus of females, between the ages of 14 and 45. Many have questioned whether this discharge arose from a mere rupture of vessels, or whether it was owing to a secretory action. There can be little doubt of the truth of the latter. The secretory organ is composed of the arterial vessels situated in the fundus of the uterus. The dissection of women, who have died during the time of their menstruating, proves this. Sometimes, though very rarely, women, during pregnancy, menstruate; and when this happens, the discharge takes place from the arterial vessels of the vagina. During pregnancy and lactation, when the person is in good health, the catamenia, for the most part, cease to flow. The quantity a female menstruates at each time is very various; depending on climate, and a variety of other circumstances. It is commonly in England from five to six ounces; it rarely exceeds eight. Its duration is from three to four, and sometimes, though rarely, five days With respect to the nature of the discharge, it differs very much from pure blood; it never coagulates; but is sometimes grumous, and membranes like the decidua are formed in difficult menstruations: in some women it always smells rank and peculiar; in others it is inodorous. The use of this monthly secretion is said to be to render the uterus fit for the conception and nutrition of the fœtus; therefore girls rarely conceive before the catamenia appear, and women rarely after their entire cessation; but very easily soon after menstruation.

CATANA'NCE. Succory.

CATANI'PHTHIS. (From κατανιπτω, to wash. Washed, or scoured. Used by Hippocrates of a diarrhœa washed and cleansed by boiled milk.

CATANTLE'MA. (From καταντλαω, to pour upon.) A lotion by infusion of water, or medicated fluids.

CATANTLE'SIS. A medicated fluid.

CATAPA'SMA. (From καταπασσω, to sprinkle., *Catapastum; Conspersio; Epipaston; Pasma; Sympasma; Aspersio; Aspergo.* The ancient Greek physicians meant by this, any dry medicine reduced to powder, to be sprinkled on the body. Their various forms and uses may be seen in Paul of Egina, lib. vii. cap. xiii.

CATAPAU'SIS. (From καταπαυω, to rest, or cease.) That rest or cessation from pain which proceeds from the resolution of uneasy tumours.

CATAPE'LTES. (From κατα, against, and πελτη, a shield.) 1. This word means a sling, a granado, or battery.

2. It was formerly used to signify the medicine which heals the wounds and bruises made by such an instrument.

CATA'PHORA. (From καταφερω, to make sleepy.) A preternatural propensity to sleep; a mild apoplexy; a species of Dr. Good's *Carus Lethargus;* remissive lethargy.

CATAPHRA'CTA. (From καταφρασσω, to fortify.) A bandage on the thorax.

CATAPLA'SMA. (*Cataplasma, matis.* neut.; from καταπλασσω, to spread like a plaster.) A poultice. The following are among the most useful:—

CATAPLASMA ACETOSÆ. Sorrel poultice. The leaves are to be beaten in a mortar into a pulp. A good application to scorbutic ulcers.

CATAPLASMA AERATUM. See *Cataplasma fermenti.*

CATAPLASMA ALUMINIS. This application was formerly used to inflammation of the eyes, which was kept up from weakness of the vessels; it is now seldom used, a solution of alum being mostly substituted.

CATAPLASMA CONII. Hemlock poultice. ℞. Conii foliorum exsiccatorum ℥j. Aquæ fontanæ, ℔ij. To be boiled till only a pint remains, when as much linseed-meal as necessary is to be added. This is an excellent application to many cancerous and scrofulous ulcers, and other malignant ones; frequently producing great diminution of the pain of such diseases, and improving their appearance. Justamond preferred the fresh herb bruised.

CATAPLASMA CUMINI. Take of cumin seeds, one pound; bay-berries, the leaves of water germander dried, Virginia snake-root, of each three ounces; cloves, one ounce; with honey equal to thrice the weight of the powder formed: of these make a cataplasm. It was formerly called Theriaca Londinensis. This is a warm and stimulating poultice, and was formerly much used as an irritating antiseptic application to gangrenous ulcers, and the like. It is now seldom ordered.

CATAPLASMA DAUCI. Carrot poultice. ℞. Radicis dauci recentis, ℔j. Bruise it in a mortar into a pulp. Some, perhaps, with reason, recommend the carrots to be first boiled. The carrot poultice is employed as an application to ulcerated cancers, scrofulous sores of an irritable kind, and various inveterate malignant ulcers.

CATAPLASMA FERMENTI. Yest cataplasm. Take of flour a pound; yest half a pint. Mix and expose to a gentle heat, until the mixture begins to rise. This is a celebrated application in cases of sloughing and mortification.

CATAPLASMA FUCI. This is prepared by bruising a quantity of the marine plant, commonly called sea tang, which is afterward to be applied by way of a poultice. Its chief use is in cases of scrofula, white swellings, and glandular tumours more especially. When this vegetable cannot be obtained in its recent state, a common poultice of sea-water and oatmeal has been subtituted by the late Mr. Hunter, and other surgeons of eminence.

CATAPLASMA LINI. Linseed poultice. ℞. Farinæ lini, ℔ss. Aquæ ferventis, ℔jss. The powder is to be gradually sprinkled into the water, while they are quickly blended together with a spoon. This is the best and most convenient of all emollient poultices for common cases, and has, in a great measure, superceded the bread and milk one, so much in use formerly.

CATAPLASMA PLUMBI ACETATIS. ℞. Liquoris plumbi acetatis, ʒj. Aquæ distill. ℔j. Micæ panis, q. s. Misce. Practitioners, who place much confidence in the virtues of lead, often use this poultice in cases of inflammation.

CATAPLASMA SINAPEOS. See *Cataplasma sinapis.*

CATAPLASMA SINAPIS. Mustard cataplasm. Take of mustard-seed, linseed, of each powdered half a pound; boiling vinegar, as much as is sufficient. Mix until it acquires the consistence of a cataplasm.

CATAPLE'XIS. (From κατα, and πγησσω, to strike.) Any sudden stupefaction, or deprivation of sensation, in any of the members, or organs.

CATAPO'SIS. (From καταπινω, to swallow down.) According to Aretæus, it signifies the instruments of deglutition.

CATAPO'TIUM. (Καταποτιον; from καταπινω, to swallow down.) A pill.

CATAPSY'XIS. (From ψυχω, to refrigerate.) A coldness, or chillness, without shivering, either universal, or of some particular part.

CATAPTO'SIS. (From καταπιπτω, to fall down.) A falling down. 1. Such as happens in apoplexy.

2. The falling down of a limb from palsy.

CATAPU'TIA. (From κaταπυθω, to have an ill savour; or from the Italian, *cacapuzza*, which has the same meaning; so named from its fœtid smell.) Spurge.

CATAPUTIA MAJOR. See *Ricinus.*

CATAPUTIA MINOR. See *Euphorbia Lathyris.*

CA'TARACTA. (From καταρασσω, to confound or disturb: because the sense of vision is confounded, if not destroyed.) A cataract; a disease of the eye. *Paropsis cataracta* of Good. The *Caligo lentis* of Cullen. Hippocrates calls it γλαυκωμα. Galen, υποχυμα. The Arabians, *gutta opaca.* Celsus, *suffusio.* It is a species of blindness, arising almost always from an opacity of the crystalline lens, or its capsule, preventing the rays of light passing to the optic nerve. It commonly begins with a dimness of sight; and this generally continues a considerable time before any opacity can be observed in the lens. As the disease advances, the opacity becomes sensible, and the patient imagines there are particles of dust, or motes, upon the eye, or in the air, which are called *muscæ volitantes.* This opacity gradually increases till the person either becomes entirely blind, or can merely distinguish light from darkness. The disease commonly comes on rapidly, though sometimes its progress is slow and gradual. From a transparent state, it changes to a perfectly white, or light gray colour. In some very rare instances, a black cataract is found. The consistence also varies, being at one time hard, at another entirely dissolved. When the opaque lens is either more indurated than in the natural state, or retains a tolerable degree of firmness, the case is termed a *firm* or hard cataract. When the substance of the lens seems to be converted into a whitish or other kind of fluid, lodged in the capsule, the case is denominated a *milky* or *fluid cataract.* When the substance is of a middling consistence, neither hard nor fluid, but about as consistent as a thick jelly, or curds, the case is named a *soft* or caseous cataract. When the anterior or posterior layer of the crystalline capsule becomes opaque, after the lens itself has been removed from this little membraneous sac, by a previous operation, the affection is named a *secondary membraneous cataract.* There are many other distinctions made by authors. Cataract is seldom attended with pain; sometimes, however, every exposure to light creates uneasiness, owing probably to the inflammation at the bottom of the eye. The real cause of cataract is not yet well understood. Numbers of authors consider it as proceeding from a preternatural contraction of the vessels of the lens, arising from some external violence, though more commonly from some internal and occult cause. The cataracta is distinguished from gutta serena, by the pupils in the latter being never affected with light, and from no opacity being observed in the lens. It is distinguished from hypopyon, staphyloma, or any other disease in the forepart of the eye, by the evident marks which these affections produce, as well as by the pain attending their beginning. But it is difficult to determine when the opacity is in the lens, or in its capsule. If the retina (which is an expansion of the optic nerve in the inside of the eye) be not diseased, vision may, in most cases, be restored, by either depressing the diseased lens, which is termed couching, or extracting it.

CATARRHEU'MA. (From καταρρεω, to flow from.) A defluxion of humours from the air-passages.

CATARRHE'XIS. (From καταρρηγνυω, to burst out.) A violent and copious eruption or effusion; joined with κοιλιας, it is a copious evacuation from the belly, and sometimes alone it is of the same signification. Vogel applies it to a discharge of pure blood from the intestines, such as takes place in dysentery.

CATARRHŒCUS. (From καταρρεω, to flow from.) A disease proceeding from a dischaige of phlegm.

CATA'RRHOPA. (From καταρρεω, to flow down.) Tubercles tending downward; or, as Galen states, those that have their apex on a depending part have received this appellation.

CATA'RRHOPOS. (Καταρροπος νουσος.) A remission of the disease, or its decline, opposed to the paroxysm.

CATA'RRHUS. (From καταρρεω, to flow down.) *Coryza.* A catarrh. An increased secretion of mucus from the membranes of the nose, fauces, and bronchia, with fever, and attended with sneezing, cough, thirst, lassitude, and want of appetite. It is a genus of disease in the class *Pyrexiæ*, and order *Profluvia* of Cullen. There are two species of catarrh viz. *catarrhus à frigore*, which is very common, and is called a cold in the head; and *catarrhus à contagio*, the influenza, or epidemic catarrh, which sometimes seizes a whole city. Catarrh is also symptomatic of several other diseases. Hence we have the *catarrhus rubeolosus; tussis variolosa, verminosa, calculosa, phthisica, hysterica, à dentitione, gravidarum, metalli colarum*, &c.

Catarrh is seldom fatal, except in scrofulous habits, by laying the foundation of phthisis; or where it is aggravated by improper treatment, or repeated exposure to cold, into some degree of peripneumony; when there is hazard of the patient, particularly if advanced in life, being suffocated by the copious effusion of viscid matter into the air-passages. The epidemic is generally, but not invariably, more severe than the common form of the disease. The latter is usually left to subside spontaneously, which will commonly happen in a few days, by observing the antiphlogistic regimen. If there should be fixed pain of the chest, with any hardness of the pulse, a little blood may be taken from the arm, or topically, followed by a blister: the bowels must be kept regular, and diaphoretics exhibited, with demulcents and mild opiates to quiet the cough. When the disease hangs about the patient in a chronic form, gentle tonics and expectorants are required, as myrrh, squill, &c. In the epidemic catarrh more active evacuations are often required, the lungs being more seriously affected; but though these should be promptly employed, they must not be carried too far, the disease being apt to assume the typhoid character in its progress; and as the chief danger appears to be of suffocation happening from the cause abovementioned, it is especially important to promote expectoration, first by antimonials, afterward by squill, the inhalation of steam, &c. not neglecting to support the strength of the patient as the disease advances.

CATARRHUS A FRIGORE. The common defluxion from the head from cold.

CATARRHUS A CONTAGIO. The influenza.

CATARRHUS BELLINSULANUS. Mumps. See *Cynanche parotidæa.*

CATARRHUS SUFFOCATIVUS. The croup. See *Cynanche trachealis.*

CATARRHUS VESICÆ. A discharge of mucus from the bladder.

CATARRTI'SMUS. (From καταρτιζω, to make perfect. According to Galen, it is a translation of a bone from a preternatural to its natural situation.

CATASA'RCA. (From κατα and σαρξ, flesh.) See *Anasarca.*

CATASBE'STIS. (From κατα and σβεννυμι, to extinguish.) The resolution of tumours without suppuration.

CATASCHA'SMUS. (From κατασχαζω, to scarify.) Scarification.

CATASEI'SIS. (From κατα, and σειω, to shake.) A concussion.

CATASPA'SMA. (From $\kappa\alpha\tau\alpha\sigma\pi\alpha\omega$, to draw backwards.) A revulsion or retraction of humours, or parts

CATASTA'GMOS. (From $\kappa\alpha\tau\alpha$, and $\sigma\tau\alpha\zeta\omega$, to distil.) The name which the Greeks, in the time of Celsus, had for distillation.

CATASTA'LTICUS. (From $\kappa\alpha\tau\alpha\sigma\tau\epsilon\lambda\lambda\omega$, to restrain, or contract.) Styptic, astringent, repressing.

CATA'STASIS. Καταστασις. The constitution, state, or condition of any thing.

CATA'TASIS. (From $\kappa\alpha\tau\alpha\tau\epsilon\iota\nu\omega$, to extend.) In Hippocrates it means the extension of a fractured limb, or a dislocated one, in order to replace it. Also the actual replacing it in a proper situation.

CATA'XIS. (From $\kappa\alpha\tau\alpha\gamma\omega$, to break.) A fracture. Also a division of parts by an instrument.

CATE. See *Acacia catechu.*

CATECHO'MENUS. (From $\kappa\alpha\tau\epsilon\chi\omega$, to resist.) Resisting and making ineffectual the remedies which have been applied or given.

CA'TECHU. (It is said, that, in the Japanese language, *kate* signifies a tree, and *chu*, juice.) See *Acacia Catechu.*

CATEIA'DION. (From $\kappa\alpha\tau\alpha$, and $\epsilon\iota\alpha$, a blade of grass.) An instrument mentioned by Aretæus, having at the end a blade of grass, or made like a blade of grass, which was thrust into the nostrils to provoke a hæmorrhage when the head ached.

CATE'LLUS. (Dim. of *catulus*, a whelp.) 1. A young whelp.

2. Also a chemical instrument called a cupel, which was formerly in the shape of a dog's head.

CATHÆ'RESIS. (From $\kappa\alpha\theta\alpha\iota\rho\omega$, to take away.) 1. The subtraction or taking away any part or thing from the body.

2. Sometimes it means an evacuation, and Hippocrates uses it for such.

3. A consumption of the body, as happens without manifest evacuation.

CATHÆRE'TICA. (From $\kappa\alpha\theta\alpha\iota\rho\omega$, to take away.) Medicines which consume or remove superfluous flesh.

CATHA'RMA. (From $\kappa\alpha\theta\alpha\iota\rho\omega$, to remove.) The excrements, or humours, purged off from the body.

CATHA'RMUS. (From $\kappa\alpha\theta\alpha\iota\rho\omega$, to remove.) 1. A purgation of the excrements, or humours.

2 A cure by incantation, or the royal touch.

CATHA'RSIA. (From $\kappa\alpha\theta\alpha\iota\rho\omega$, to purge.) Medicines which have a purging property.

CATHA'RSIS. (From $\kappa\alpha\theta\alpha\iota\rho\omega$, to take away.) Purgation of the excrements, or humours, either medically or naturally.

CATHA'RTIC. (*Catharticus;* from $\kappa\alpha\theta\alpha\iota\rho\omega$, to purge.) That which, taken internally, increases the number of alvine evacuations. These medicines have received many appellations: *purgantia; catocathartica; catoretica; catoteretica; dejectoria; alviduca.* The different articles referred to this class are divided into five orders.

1. *Stimulating cathartics*, as jalap, aloes, bitter apple, and croton oil, which are well calculated to discharge accumulations of serum, and are mostly selected for indolent and phlegmatic habits, and those who are hard to purge.

2. *Refrigerating cathartics*, as sulphate of soda, supertartrate of potassa, &c. These are better adapted for plethoric habits, and those with an inflammatory diathesis.

3. *Adstringent cathartics*, as rhubarb and damask roses, which are mostly given to those whose bowels are weak and irritable, and subject to diarrhœa.

4. *Emollient cathartics*, as manna, malva, castor oil, and olive oil, which may be given in preference to other cathartics, to infants and the very aged.

5. *Narcotic cathartics*, as tobacco, hyoscyamus, and digitalis. This order is never given but to the very strong and indolent, and to maniacal patients, as their operation is very powerful.

Murray, in his Materia Medica, considers the different cathartics under the two divisions of laxatives and purgatives; the former being mild in their operation, and merely evacuating the contents of the intestines; the latter being more powerful, and even extending their stimulant operation to the neighbouring parts. The following he enumerates among the principal laxatives:—manna, Cassia fistula, Tamarindus indica, Ricinus communis, Sulphur, Magnesia. Under the head of purgatives, he names Cassia senna, Rheum palmatum, Convolvulus jalapa, Helleborus niger, Bryonia alba, Cucumis colocynthis, Momordica elaterium, Rhamnus catharticus, Aloe perfoliata, Convolvulus scammonia, Gambogia, Submurias hydrargyri, Sulphas magnesia, Sulphas sodæ, Sulphas potassæ, Supertartras potassæ, Tartras potassæ, Tartras potassæ et sodæ, Phosphas sodæ, Murias sodæ Terebinthina veneta, Nicotiana tabacum.

Cathartic Glaubers salt. See *Sodæ sulphas.*

Cathartic Salt. See *Sulphas magnesia*, and *Sulphas soda.*

CATHARTINE. A substance of a reddish colour, a peculiar smell, and a bitter nauseous taste, soluble in water and alkohol, but insoluble in æther; obtained by Lassaigne and Fenuelle from the leaves of senna.

CATHE'DRA. (From $\kappa\alpha\theta\epsilon\zeta o\mu\alpha\iota$, to sit.) The anus, or rather, the whole of the buttocks, as being the part on which we sit.

CATHERE'TICA. (From $\kappa\alpha\theta\alpha\iota\rho\omega$, to remove.) Corrosives. Applications which, by corrosion, remove superfluous flesh.

CA'THETER. (*Catheter, teris.* m. Καθετηρ; from $\kappa\alpha\theta\iota\eta\mu\iota$, to thrust into.) A long and hollow tube, that is introduced by surgeons into the urinary bladder, to remove the urine, when the person is unable to pass it. Catheters are either made of silver or of the elastic gum. That for the male urethra is much longer than that for the female, and so curved, if made of silver, as to adapt itself to the urethra.

CATHETERI'SMUS. (From $\kappa\alpha\theta\epsilon\tau\eta\rho$, a catheter.) The operation of introducing the catheter.

CATHI'DRYSIS. (From $\kappa\alpha\theta\iota\delta\rho\upsilon\omega$, to place together.) The reduction of a fracture, or operation of setting a broken bone.

CA'THMA. A name for litharge.

CA'THODOS. (From $\kappa\alpha\tau\alpha$, and $o\delta o\varsigma$.) A descent of humours.

CATHO'LCEUS. (From $\kappa\alpha\tau\alpha$, and $o\lambda\kappa\epsilon\omega$, to draw over.) An oblong fillet, made to draw over and cover the whole bandage of the head.

CATHO'LICON. (From $\kappa\alpha\tau\alpha$, and $o\lambda\iota\kappa o\varsigma$, universal.) A universal medicine: formerly applied to a medicine, that was supposed to purge all the humours.

[" CATHRAL, ISAAC, M. D., was a native of Philadelphia, and studied medicine under the direction of the late Dr. John Redman, the preceptor of Rush and Wistar. After acquiring all the instruction in his profession, which the opportunities of Philadelphia offered, aided by a diligent attention on his part, he visited Europe, and attended the practice of the London hospitals, and the lectures of the most distinguished professors in that city. During the prevalence of the widely destroying epidemic fevers of 1793, '97, '98, and '99, he remained in the city, instead of seeking safety by flying, and was a severe sufferer by the disease of the first of those years. Previously to his illness, and after his recovery, besides attending to practice, he lost no opportunity of investigating every phenomenon connected with that pestilential epidemic, which could in any manner tend to illustrate its pathology, or the peculiarities it exhibited. In the year 1794, he published his remarks thereon, and the mode of treatment he pursued. In conjunction with Dr. Physick, he dissected the bodies of some subjects of the fever of 1793, in order to discover the morbid effects produced by it on the system, and in particular reference to the nature of that singular and generally fatal symptom, the dark-coloured ejection from the stomach, in some cases of the disease. The result of their joint labours was published by them, with their individual signatures, and he afterward continued his dissections alone, with unabating zeal, whenever opportunity offered, during the subsequent epidemics and occasional appearance of the disease, which more or less occurred for several years, until he obtained all the light which he thought dissection and experiment could throw upon its production and nature. In the year 1800, he read to the American Philosophical Society, of which he had been elected a member, an interesting paper on that subject. This paper affords ample evidence of the patient and accurate manner in which he investigated that hitherto inexplicable and supposed pestilential appearance, and of his fearless zeal in the prosecution of medical science. It is inserted in the 5th vol. of the Transactions of the Society, and was also published in pamphlet form, of 32 pages. A full account of it may be found in the 4th volume of the New-York Medical Repository. He died on the 22d

February, 1819, in the 56th year of his age, by a stroke of the apoplexy

"Dr. Cathrall was educated in the religious principles of the Society of Friends, and naturally possessed a grave turn of mind, and a serious deportment. Retired in his habits, he was shy in making acquaintances, but firm in his friendships, and a well-bred gentleman in his manners. In the important and endearing relations of a son, husband, and father, he was truly estimable. As a member of society, he set an example of rigid morality and inflexible integrity, attributes which every medical man ought to be proud to have annexed to his character, however distinguished his literary acquirements may be."—*Thacher's Med. Biog.* A.]

CATHY'PNIA. (From κατα, and υπνος, sleep.) A profound but unhealthy sleep.

CA'TIAS. (From καθιημι, to place in.) An incision knife, formerly used for opening an abscess in the uterus, and for extracting a dead fœtus.

CATI'LLUS. See *Catellus.*

CA'TINUM ALUMEN. A name given to potassa.

CA'TINUS. Κατανον. A crucible.

CAT-KIN. See *Amentum.*

CA'TMINT. (So called, because cats are very fond of it.) See *Nepeta.*

CATOCATHA'RTICA. (From κατω, downward, and καθαιρω, to purge.) Medicines that operate by stool.

CATO'CHE. (From κατεχω, to detain.) See *Catalepsis.*

CATOCHEI'LUM. (From κατω, beneath, and χειλος, the lip.) The lower lip.

CA'TOCHUS. (From κατεχω, to detain.) A spasmodic disease in which the body is rigidly held in an upright posture.

CATOMI'SMUS. (From κατω, below, and ωμος, the shoulder.) By this word, P. Ægineta expresses a method of reducing a luxated shoulder, by raising the patient over the shoulder of a strong man, that by the weight of the body, the dislocation may be reduced.

CATO'PSIS. (From κατοπτομαι, to see clearly.) An acute and quick perception. The acuteness of the faculties which accompanies the latter stages of consumption.

CATOPHYLLUM INOPHYLLUM. *Calaba.* The Indian mastich-tree. A native of America, where the whole plant is considered as a resolvent and anodyne.

CATO'PTER. (From κατα, and οπτομαι, to see; by metaphor, a probe.) An instrument called a speculum ani.

CATORCHI'TES. (From κατα, and ορχις, the orchis.) A wine in which the orchis root has been infused.

CATORE'TICA. (From κατω, downwards, and ρεω, to flow.) *Catoteretica; Catoterica.* Medicines which purge by stool.

CATOTERE'TICA. See *Catoretica.*

CATOTICA. (*Catoticus;* from κατω, below; whence κατωτερος, and κατωτατος, *inferior,* and *infernus.*) The name of an order of the class *Eccritica,* in Good's Nosology; diseases affecting internal surfaces; defined, pravity of the fluids, or emunctories that open into the internal surfaces of organs. It embraces *hydropsis, emphysema, paruria,* and *lithia.*

CATS-EYE. A mineral, much valued as a precious stone, brought from Ceylon.

CATULO'TICA. (From κατουλοω, to cicatrize.) Medicines that cicatrize wounds.

CATUTRI'PALI. A name of the *Piper longum.*

CATULUS. See *Amentum.*

CAU'CALIS. (From καυκιον, a cup; or from δαυκαλις, the daucus.) 1. The name of a family, or genus of plants. Class *Pentandria;* Order, *Monogynia.*

2. Bastard parsley; so named from the shape of its flower.

3. The wild carrot.

CAUCALOI'DES. (From *caucalis,* and ειδος, a likeness, from its likeness to the flower of the caucalis.) Like unto the caucalis. The patella is sometimes so called.

CAU'DA. (From *cado,* to fall; because it hangs or falls down behind.) A tail.

1. The tail of animals.

2. A name formerly given to the os coccygis, that being in tailed animals the beginning of the tail.

3. A fleshy substance, projecting from the lips of the vagina, and resembling a tail, according to Aetius.

4. Many herbs are called cauda, with the affixed name of some animal, the tail of which the herb is supposed to be like; as *cauda equina,* horse-tail; *cauda muris,* mouse-tail; and in many other instances.

CAUDA EQUINA. 1. The spinal marrow, at its termination about the second lumbar vertebra, gives off a large number of nerves, which, when unravelled, resemble the horse's tail; hence the name. See *Medulla spinalis.*

2. See *Hippuris vulgaris.*

CAUDA SEMINIS. The tail, or elongated, generally feathery appendage to a seed, formed of the permanent style. It is simple, in *Geranium zonale;* hairy, in *Clematis* and *Pulsatilla;* and geniculate in *Tormentilla.*

CAUDA'TIO. (From *cauda,* a tail.) An elongation of the clitoris.

CAUDATUS. (From *cauda,* a tail.) Tailed: applied to seeds which have a tail-like appendage; as those of the *Clematis vitalba,* and *Anemone sulphurea.*

CAUDEX. (*Caudex, icis.* m.) The body of the root of a plant. See *Radix.*

CAUL. 1. The English name for the omentum See *Omentum.*

2. The amnion, which is sometimes torn by the child's head, passing from the uterus, and comes away with it wholly separated from the placenta.

CAULE'DON. (From καυλος, a stalk.) A transverse fracture, when the bone is broken, like the stump of a tree.

CAU'LIFLOWER. A species of brassica, the flower of which is cut before the fructification expands. The observations which have been made concerning cabbages are applicable here. Cauliflower is, however, a far more delicious vegetable. See *Brassica capitata.*

CAULINUS. Cauline. Belonging to the stem Leaves and peduncles are so called, which grow on or come immediately from, the stem.

CAU'LIS. (*Caulis, is.* m. Καυλος; from *kalab,* a Chaldean word.) The stalk or stem of herbaceous plants. The characters of the stalk are, that it is rarely ligneous, and lives but one or two years in the natural state of the plant.

A plant is said to be

Caulescent, when furnished with a stem.

Acauline, when without a stem; as in Caulina acaulis.

From its *duration,* the stem is distinguished into,

1. *Caulus herbaceus,* which perishes every year; as Melissa officinalis.

2. *Caulis suffruticosus,* which perishes half way down every year; as Cheiranthus incanus.

3. *Caulis fruticosus,* shrubby, having many stems, which do not perish in the winter; as Melissa fruticosa.

4. *Caulis arboreus;* as the trunk of trees.

From the substance, it is distinguished into,

5. *Caulis fistulosus,* hollow internally; as in Anethum graveolens, and Allium fistulosum.

6. *Caulis loculamentosus,* hollow and divided into cells; as in Angelica, Archangelica, and Phellandrum aquaticum.

7. *Caulis inanis,* or *medullosus,* empty or pithy; as in Sambucus nigra.

8. *Caulis solidus,* solid; as in Mentha and Melissa.

9. *Caulis ligneus,* woody; as Prunus spinosa.

10. *Caulis carnosus,* fleshy; as in Sedum arboreum, and Stapelia hirsuta.

11. *Caulis pulposus,* pulpy; as in Mesembryanthemum crystallinum.

12. *Caulis fibrosus,* separable into long fibres; as Cocos nucifera.

13. *Caulis succosus,* full of a juice; as in the Euphorbias, and Chelidonium majus.

From the difference of the surface, the *caulis* is said to be

14. *Glaber,* or *lævis,* smooth, without any hairiness, or roughness, or inequality; as Lepedium latifolium.

15. *Scaber,* or *asper,* when it has hard inequalities; as in Galium aperine, and Lithospermum arvense.

16. *Suberosus,* corky, as Passiflora suberosa, and Quercus suber.

17. *Rimosus,* cracky; as in Ulmus campestris.

18. *Tuberculatus,* with rough nobs; as in Cissus tuberculata.

19. *Tunicatus,* the cuticle peeling off spontaneously

in large portions; as in Betula alba, and some of the Spiræas.
20. *Striatus*, having superficial longitudinal lines; as in Chærophyllum sylvestre, Aster sibiricus, and Daphne mezereon.
21. *Sulcatus*, furrowed, fluted, when longitudinally indented with long and deep hollows; as in Celosia coccynea, Selinum carvifolia, Pimpinella sanguisarba, Doronicum pardalianches.
22. *Perfoliatus*, perfoliate; as in Bupleurum perfoliatum.
The *figure* affords the following distinctions:
23. *Caulis teres*, or *cylindricus*, round, without angles; as Sinapis arvensis.
24. *Semiteres*, half-rounded, flat on one side; as Hyacinthus orientalis, Allium descendens.
25. *Caulis compressus*, which implies that two sides of the stem are flat, and approach each other; as in Poa compressa, Lathyrus latifolius, Pancratium declinatum.
26. *Caulis anceps*, two-edged; as Iris graminea, Hypericum androsemum.
27. *Caulis angulatus*, presenting several acute angles in its circumference.
a. *Triangulatus*, three-cornered; as in Cactus triangularis.
b. *Quadrangulatus*, four-cornered; as Cactus teragonus.
c. *Quinqueangulatus;* as in Cactus pentagonus.
d. *Sexangulatus*, six-cornered; as Cactus hexagonus.
e. *Multangulatus*, many cornered; as Cactus cereus.
28. *Caulis obtusangulatus*, obtuse-angled; as in Scrophularia nodosa.
29. *Caulis acutangulatus*, acute-angled; as in Scrophularia aquatica.
30. *Caulis triquetrus*, three-sided, when there are three flat sides, forming acute angles; as Hedysarum triquetrum, Viola mirabilis, Carex acuta.
31. *Caulis tetraquetrus*, four-sided; as in Hypericum quadrangulare, Monarda fistulosa, Mentha officinalis.
32. *Caulis membranaceus*, leaf-like; as in Cactus phyllanthus.
33. *Caulis alatus*, when the edges or angles expand into leaf-like borders; as in Onopordium acanthium, and Lathyrus latifolius.
34 *Caulus articulatus*, jointed; as Cactus flagelliformis, and Lathyrus sylvestris.
35. *Caulis nodosus*, knotty, divided at intervals by swellings; as in Scandix nodosa, Geranium nodosum.
36. *Caulis enodus*, without knot.
From the directions, a stem is called
37. *Rectus*, erect, when it ascends almost perpendicularly; as the firs, Chenopodium scoparium, &c.
38. *Strictus*, straight, perfectly perpendicular; as Alcea Rosea.
39. *Obliquus*, oblique; as the Solidago Mexicana.
40. *Ascendens*, ascending, when its lower portion forms a curve, the convexity of which is towards the earth, or rests upon it, and the summit rises; as exemplified in many grasses, Trifolium pratense, Hedysarum onobrychis.
41. *Descendens*, or *Declinatus*, the reverse of the former, forming an arch, towards the ground; as in Pancratium declinatum, Ficus carica.
42. *Nutans*, or *cernuus*, nodding, when bent towards the summit; as Polygonatum multiflora.
43. *Procumbens*, or *Prostatus*, lying on the earth; as Veronica officinalis.
44. *Decumbens*, rising a little, and returning to the earth; as Thymus serphyllum.
45. *Repens*, creeping and sending radicles into the ground; as Trifolium repens, Gnaphalium repens.
46. *Flexuosis*, zigzag; as in Celestrus buxifolius, and solidago flexicaulis.
47. *Radicans*, sending fibres which take root in the earth; as Ficus Indica.
48. *Sarmentosus*, trailing, or sending off a runner, which fixes on neighbouring bodies; as the Hedera helix.
49 *Stoloniferus*, sending off radicating stolos; as Agrostis stolonifera, and Fragaria vesca.
50. *Scandens*, climbing, furnished with tendrils; as Solanum dulcamara, Cobœa scandens.
51. *Volubilis*, twining, winding itself spirally round any other plant or body.
a. *Dextrorsum*, when from right to left; as Phaseolus multiflorus, and Convolvulus.
b. *Sinistrorsum*, in the opposite direction, or following the apparent motion of the sun; as the Lonicera periclemimum, and Humulus lupulus.
52. *Laxus*, bent by the lightest wind; as Secale sereale, and Juncus bufonius.
53. *Rigidus*, breaking when lightly bent; as Boerhaavia scandens.
When *clothed* with any kind of appendage, the stem is designated by a term expressive of this; thus,
54. *Caulis foliosus*, when leafy; as Melissa officinalis.
55. *Caulus aphyllus*, when without leaves; as Asphodelus fistulosus.
56. *Caulus squamosus*, scaly; as the Orobranche major.
57. *Caulis stipulatus*, when furnished with stipulæ; as Cystus helianthemum, and Geranium terebinthinaceum.
58. *Caulis imbricatus*, tiled or covered with little leaves or scales; as Crassula imbricata, Aloe viscosa.
59. *Caulus vaginatus*, sheathed, embraced by the base of a leaf as by a sheath; as Canna indica, Arundo donax.
60. *Caulis bulbiferus*, bulb-bearing, when studded with bulbs in the axilla of the leaves; as Lilium bulbiferum.
61. *Caulis nudus*, naked, without leaf, scale, or other covering; as Cuscuta europea.
From its mode of *branching*, into
62. *Caulis simplex*, having few branches; as Campanula perfoliata, Verbascum thapsus.
63. *Caulis simplicissimus*, without branches; as Orobanche americana and major, Campanula barbata.
64. *Caulis prolifer*, giving off branches only from the tops of the former; as the Dracena draco.
65. *Caulis dichotomus*, forked, always divided into pairs; as in Horanthus europæus and Valeriana locusta.
66. *Caulis ramosus*, branched; as Rosmarinus officinalis.
67. *Caulis ramossissimus*, having many branches; as Chenopodium scoparia, Ulmus, Grossularia, &c.
68. *Caulis paniculatus*, paniculate; as in Crambe tataria.
From the *pubescence* and *armature*, or defences, into
69. *Caulis spinosus*, when furnished with sharp spines; as Prunus spinosa, and Mespilus oxyacantha
70. *Caulis aculeatus*, prickly, when covered with sharp-pointed bodies; as Rosa centifolia and eleganterea.
71. *Caulis cetaceus*, bristly, when the armature consists of brushes of minute bristles; as Cactus flagelliformis.
72. *Caulis ramentaceus*, ramentaceous; as in Erica ramentacea.
73. *Caulis pilosus*, hairy, the pubescence consisting of long hairs; as Hieraccum pilocella, Salvia pratensis.
74. *Caulis muricatus*, or *hispidus*, when the hairs are stiff or bristly; as Borago officinalis, and Echium vulgare.
75. *Caulis tomentosus*, downy, soft to the touch, like down; as Verbascum thapsus, and Geranium rotundifolium.
76. *Caulis villosus*, shaggy; as Stachys germanica, and Veronica villosa.
77. *Caulis lanatus*, woolly, when the hairs are long and matted; as in Stachys lanata, and Ballota lanata.
78. *Caulis sericus*, silky, when the hairs are shining and silky.
Instead of pubescence, the covering is in some instances either a dry powdery, or a moist, excretion; and hence, the stem is denominated either
79. *Incanus*, or *pruinosus*, when covered with a fine white dust; as the Artiplex portulacoidis.
80. *Farinosus*, mealy; as the Primula farinosa.
81. *Glaucus*, of a sea-green colour; as Ricinus officinalis.
82. *Viscidus*, viscid, covered with a resinous exudation; as Siline viscosa.
83. *Glutinosus*, glutinous, when the exudation is adhesive and soluble in water; as in Primula glutinosa.
The primary division of a stem is into *lateral stems* or *branches*. These are variously denominated

From their *situation*, into

84. *Opposite*, when one branch stands on the opposite side of the stem to another, and their bases are nearly on the same plane; as in Mentha arvensis.

85. *Alternate*, one opposite to another, alternately; as Althæa officinalis.

86. *Verticillated*, when more than two proceed from a centre, like the spokes of a wheel; as Pinus abies.

87. *Scattered*, when given off from the stem in any indeterminate manner.

From their *direction*, the branches, or rami, are termed,

88. *Patentes*, spreading, when the angle formed by the branch and the upper part of the stem is obtuse; as in Galium mollugo, and Cestus italicus.

89. *Patentissimi*, proceeding at a right angle from the stem, or horizontally; as Ammania ramosior, and Asparagus officinalis.

90. *Brachiati*, brachiate, spread in four directions, crossing each other alternately in pairs; as Syringa vulgaris, and Pānisteria brachiata.

91. *Deflexi*, bending downward from the stem, in an arched or curved direction; as Pinus larix.

92. *Reflexi*, hanging almost perpendicularly from the stem; as Salix babylonica.

93. *Retroflexi*, turned backward; as in Solanum dulcamara.

94. *Introflexi*, bent inward, when the tops bend towards the stem; as Populus dilatata.

95. *Fastigiati*, when the tops of the branches, from whatever part of the stem they spring, rise nearly to the same height; as Chrysanthemum corymbosum, and Dianthus barbatus.

96. *Vigati*, weak and long; as Salix viminalis.

97. *Appressi*, approximated, when nearly parallel and close to the stem; as Genista tinctoria.

98. *Fulcrate*, supported, when they project nearly horizontally, and give out root-like shoots from the under side, which, extending until they reach the ground, take root, and serve as props to the branches; as in the banyan-tree, or Ficus religiosus.

Caulis florida. Cauliflower.

Caulo'des. (From καυλος, a stem.) The white or green cabbage.

Caulo'tom. (From καυλος, a stem; because it grows upon a stalk.) A name given to the beet.

CAU'MA. (Καυμα, heat; from καιω, to burn.) The heat of the body in a fever.

2. The heat of the atmosphere, in a fever.

3. The name given by Good and Young, to an inflammatory fever.

Cau'nga. A name of the areca.

CAU'SIS. (From καιω, to burn.) A burn; or rather, the act of combustion, or burning.

CAUSO'DES. (From καιω, to burn.) A term applied by Celsus to a burning fever.

CAUSO'MA. (From καιω, to burn.) An ardent or burning heat and inflammation. A term used by Hippocrates.

CAUSTIC. See *Causticum*.

Caustic alkali. The pure alkalies are so called. See *Alkali*.

Caustic barley. See *Cevadilla*.

Caustic lunar. See *Argenti nitras*.

Caustic volatile alkali. See *Ammonia*.

CAU'STICUM. (From καιω, to burn; because it always produces a burning sensation.) A caustic. A substance which has so strong a tendency to combine with organized substances, as to destroy their texture. See *Escharotic*.

Causticum americanum. The cevadilla. See *Veratrum sabadilla*.

Causticum antimoniale. Muriate of antimony.

Causticum arsenicale. See *Arsenical caustic*.

Causticum commune fortius. See *Potassa cum calce*.

Causticum lunare. See *Argenti nitras*.

CAU'SUS. (From καιω, to burn.) A highly ardent fever. According to Hippocrates, a fiery heat, insatiable thirst, a rough and black tongue, complexion yellowish, and the saliva bilious, are its pecular characteristics. Others also are particular in describing it; but, whether ancients or moderns, from what they relate, this fever is no other than a continued *ardent fever* in a bilious constitution. In it the heat of the body is intense; the breath is particularly fiery; the extremities are cold; the pulse is frequent and small the heat is more violent internally than externally and the whole soon ends in recovery or death.

CAUTERY. (*Cauterium*, from καιω, to burn.) Cauteries were divided, by the ancients, into *actual* and *potential;* but the term is now given only to the red-hot iron, or *actual cautery*. This was formerly the only means of preventing hœmorrhages from divided arteries, till the invention of the ligature. It was also used in diseases, with the same view as we employ a blister. *Potential* cautery was the name by which kali purum, or potassa, was distinguished in former dispensatories. Surgeons of the present day understand, by this term, any caustic application.

CA'VA. See *Cavus*.

CAVE'RNA. (From *cavus*, hollow.) A cavern The pudendum muliebre.

CAVIARE. *Caviarium*. A food made of the hard roes of sturgeon, formed into a soft mass, or into cakes, and much esteemed by the Russians.

Cavi'cula. (Diminutive of *cavilla*.) See *Cavilla*.

Cavi'lla. (From *cavus*.) The ankle, or hollow of the foot.

CA'VITY. (*Cavitas*, from *cavus*, hollow.) 1. Any cavity, or hollowness.

2. The auricle of the heart was formerly called *cavitas innominata*, the hollow without a name.

CAVUS. Hollow. 1. The name of a vein, *vena cava*. See *Veins*.

2. Applied to the roots of plants; as that of the *Fumaria cava*.

Cawk. A term by which the miners distinguish the opaque specimens of sulphate of barytes.

Cayenne pepper. See *Capsicum*.

Cazabi. See *Jatropha*.

CEANO'THUS. (From κεανωθος, quia κεει ανωθεν, because it pricks at the extreme part.) A genus of plants in the Linnæan system. Class, *Pentandria*, Order, *Monogynia*.

Ceanothus americanus. *Celastrus; Celastus* Some noted Indians depend more on this plant, than on the lobelia, for the cure of syphilis, and use it in the same manner as lobelia.

Cea'sma. (From κεω, to split, or divide.) *Ceasmus* A fissure, or fragment.

Ce'ber. (Arabian.) The Lignum aloes. Also the capparis.

Ceripi'ra. (Indian.) A tree which grows in Brazil, decoctions of the bark of which are used in baths and fomentations, to relieve pains in the limbs, and cutaneous diseases.

CE'DAR. See *Pinus cedrus*.

Ce'dma. (From κεδαω, to disperse.) A defluxion, or rheumatic affection, of the parts about the hips.

Ce'drinum lignum. See *Pinus cedrus*.

Cedri'tes. (From κεδρος, the cedar-tree.) Wine in which the resin which distils from the cedar-tree has been steeped.

CE'DRIUM. 1. Cedar, or cedar-tree

2. Common tar, in old writings.

Cedrome'la. The fruit of the citron-tree.

Cedrone'lla. Turkey baum.

Cedro'stis. (From κεδρος, the cedar-tree.) A name of the white bryony, which smells like the cedar, See *Bryonia alba*.

CE'DRUS. (From *Kedron*, a valley where this tree grows abundantly.) See *Pinus cedrus*.

Cedrus americana. The arbor vitæ.

Cedrus baccifera. The savine.

Cei'ria. (From κειρω, to abrade.) The tape worm; so called from its excoriating and abrading the intestines.

CE'LANDINE. See *Chelidonium majus*.

Cela'strus. (From κελα, a dart, which it represents. See *Ceanothus americanus*.

Celastus. See *Ceanothus americanus*.

CE'LE. (From κηλη.) A tumour caused by the protrusion of any soft part. Hence the compound terms *hydrocele*, *bubonocele*, &c.

CE'LERY. The English name for a variety of the apium graveolens.

CELESTINE. So called from its occasional delicate blue colour. A native sulphate of strontites. See *Heavy spar*.

Ce'lis. (From καιω, to burn.) A spot or blemish upon the skin, particularly that which is occasioned by a burn.

CELLA TURCICA. See *Sella turcica.*

CE'LLULA. (Diminutive of *cella*, a cell.) A little cell, or cavity.

CELLULÆ MASTOIDÆ. See *Temporal bones.*

CE'LLULAR. *Cellularis.* Having little cells.

CELLULAR MEMBRANE. *Membrana cellulosa: Tela cellulosa; Panniculus adiposus; Membrana adiposa, pinguedinosa* et *reticularis.* Cellular tissue. The cellular tissue of the body, composed of laminæ and fibres variously joined together, which is the connecting medium of every part of the body. It is by means of the communication of the cells of this membrane, that the butchers blow up their veal. The cellular membrane is, by some anatomists, distinguished into the reticular and adipose membrane. The former is evidently dispersed throughout the whole body, except the substance of the brain. It makes a bed for the other solids of the body, covers them all, and unites them one to another. The adipose membrane consists of the reticular substance, and a particular apparatus for the secretion of oil, and is mostly found immediately under the skin of many parts, and about the kidneys.

CELOTO'MIA. (From κηλη, hernia, and τεμνω, to cut.) The operation for hernia.

CE'LSA. A term of Paracelsus, to signify what is called the live blood in any particular part

CE'LSUS, AURELIUS CORNELIUS. It is commonly supposed, that this esteemed ancient author was a Roman of the Cornelian family, born towards the end of the reign of Augustus, and still living in the time of Caligula. But these points are not established upon certain testimony, and it is even disputed whether he practised medicine; though his perfect acquaintance with the doctrines of his predecessors, his accurate descriptions of diseases, and his judicious rules of treatment, appear to leave little room for doubt on that head. At any rate, his eight books, "De Medicina," have gained him deserved celebrity in modern times, containing a large fund of valuable information; detailed in remarkably elegant and concise language. In surgery particularly he has been greatly admired, for the methods of practice laid down, and for describing several operations as they are still performed. There have been numerous editions of his work, and translations of it into the several modern languages.

CEMENT. Chemists call by this name whatever they employ to unite or cement things together; as lutes, glues, solders of every kind.

CEMENTATION. A chemical process, which consists in surrounding a body in the solid state with the powder of some other bodies, and exposing the whole for a time in a closed vessel, to a degree of heat not sufficient to fuse the contents. Thus iron is converted into steel by cementation with charcoal; green bottle glass is converted into porcelain by cementation with sand, &c.

CEME'NTERIUM. A crucible.

CE'NCHRAMIS. (From κεγχρος, millet.) A grain or seed of the fig.

CE'NCHRIUS. A species of herpes that resembles κεγχρος, or millet.

CENEANGEI'A. (From κενος, empty, and αγγος, a vessel.) A deficiency of blood, or other fluids in the vessels; so that they have not their proper quantity.

CENI'GDAM. *Ceniplam; Cenigotam; Cenipolam.* An instrument anciently used for opening the head in epilepsies.

CENIOTE'MIUM. A purging remedy, formerly of use in the venereal disease, supposed to be mercurial.

CENO'SIS. (From κενος, empty.) Evacuation. It imports a general evacuation. *Catharsis* was applied to the *evacuation* of a particular humour, which offends with respect to quality.

CENOTICA. (*Cenoticus;* from κενωσις, *evacuatio, exinanitio*, emptiness.) The name of an order in the class *Genetica* of Good's Nosology: diseases affecting the fluids, and embracing *paramenia, leucorrhœa, blenorrhœa, spermorrhœa*, and *galactea.*

CENTAU'REA. (So called from *Chiron*, the centaur, who is said to have employed one of its species to cure himself of a wound accidentally received, by letting one of the arrows of Hercules fall upon his foot.) The name of a genus of plants in the Linnæan system, of the Order, *Polygamia frustanea;* Class, *Syngenesia.*

CENTAUREA BEHEN. The systematic name of the officinal *behen album; Jacea orientalis patula; Rhaponticoides lutea.* The true white behen of the ancients. The root possesses astringent virtues.

CENTAUREA BENEDICTA. The systematic name of the blessed or holy thistle. *Carduus benedictus; Cnicus sylvestris; Centaurea benedicta—calycibus duplicato-spinosis lanatis involucratis, foliis semidecurrentibus denticulato-spinosis* of Linnæus. This exotic plant, a native of Spain, and some of the Archipelago islands, obtained the name of Benedictus, from its being supposed to possess extraordinary medicinal virtues. In loss of appetite, where the stomach was injured by irregularities, its good effects have been frequently experienced. It is a powerful bitter tonic and adstringent. Bergius considers it as antacid, corroborant, stomachic, sudorific, diuretic, and eccoprotic. Chamomile flowers are now generally substituted for the *Carduus benedictus*, and are thought to be of at least equal value.

CENTAUREA CALCITRAPA. The systematic name of the common star-thistle. Star-knapweed. *Calcitrapa; Carduus stellatus; Jacea ramosissima, stellata, rupina.* The plant thus called in the pharmacopœias, is the *Centaurea—calycibus subduplicato-spinosis, sessilibus; foliis pinnatifidis, linearibus dentatis; caule piloso*, of Linnæus, every part of which is bitter. The juice, or extract, or infusion, is said to cure intermittents; and the bark of the root, and the seeds, have been recommended in nephritic disorders, and in suppression of urine. It scarcely differs, in its effects, from other bitters, and is now little used.

CENTAUREA CENTAURIUM. *Rhaponticum vulgare: Centaurium magnum; Centaurium majus.* Greater centaury. The root of this plant was formerly used as an aperient and corroborant in alvine fluxes. It is now totally discarded from the Materia Medica of this country.

CENTAUREA CYANUS. The systematic name of the blue-bottle, or corn-flower plant. *Cyani. Cyanus.* The flowers of this plant, *Centaurea—calycibus serratis: foliis linearibus, integerrimis, infimis dentatis*, of Linnæus, were formerly in frequent use; but their antiphlogistic, antispasmodic, cordial, aperient, diuretic, and other properties, are now, with great propriety, forgotten.

CENTAUREA SOLSTITIALIS. *Calcitrapa officinalis; Carduus stellatus luteus; Carduus solstitialis; Jacea stellata; Jacea lutea capite spinoso minori; Leucanthe veterum.* St. Barnaby's thistle. It is commended as an anticteric, anticachectic, and lithontriptic, but is, in reality, only a weak tonic.

CENTAURIOI'DES. The gratiola.

CENTAU'RIUM. (From κενταυρος, a centaur: so called, because it was feigned that Chiron cured Hercules's foot, which he had wounded with a poisonous arrow, with it.) Centaury. See *Chironia centaurium.*

CENTAURIUM MAGNUM. See *Centaurea Centaurium.*

CENTAURIUM MAJUS. See *Centaurea Centaurium.*

CENTAURIUM MINUS. See *Chironia centaurium.*

CENTAU'RY. See *Chironia.*

CENTIMOR'BIA. (From *centum*, a hundred, and *morbus*, a disease.) The *Lysimachia nummularia*, or moneywort, was so named, from its supposed efficacy in the cure of a multitude of disorders.

CENTINO'DIA. See *Centum nodia.*

CENTI'PES. (From *centum*, a hundred, and *pes*, a foot.) The woodlouse, so named from the multitude of its feet.

CENTRA'TIO. (From *centrum*, a centre.) The concentration and affinity of certain substances to each other. Paracelsus expresses by it the degenerating of a saline principle, and contracting a corrosive and exulcerating quality. Hence *Centrum salis* is said to be the principle and cause of ulcers.

CE'NTRIUM. (From κεντεω, to prick.) A plaster recommended by Galen against stitches and pains in the side.

CE'NTRUM. (From κεντεω, to point or prick.) 1. The middle point of a circle.

2. In chemistry, it is the residence or foundation of matter.

3. In medicine, it is the point in which its virtue resides.

4. In anatomy, the middle point of some parts is so named, as *centrum nerveum*, the middle or tendinous part of the diaphragm

Centrum nerveum. The centre of the diaphragm. See *Diaphragm.*

Centrum ovale. When the two hemispheres of the brain are removed on a line with a level of the *corpus callosum*, the internal medullary part presents a somewhat oval centre, which is called *centrum ovale.* Vieussenius supposed all the medullary fibres met at this place.

Centrum tendinosum. The tendinous centre of the diaphragm. See *Diapragm.*

CENTUMNO'DIA. (From *centum*, a hundred, and *nodus*, a knot; so called from its many knots or joints.) *Centinodia.* Common knot-grass. See *Polygonum aviculare.*

Centu'nculus. Bastard pimpernel.

CE'PA. (From κηπος, a wool-card, from the likeness of its roots.) The onion. See *Allium cepa.*

Cepæ'a. A species of onion.

CEPHALÆ'A. (From κεφαλη, the head.) 1. The flesh of the head which covers the skull.

2. A headache. Dr. Good makes this a genus of disease in his Order, *Systatica;* Class, *Neurotica.* It has five species, *Cephalæa graverus, intensa, hemicrania, pulsatilis, nauscosa.*

CEPHA'LALGIA. (From κεφαλη, the head, and αλγος, pain.) *Cephalæa.* The headache. It is symptomatic of very many diseases, but is rarely an original disease itself. When mild, it is called cephalalgia; when inveterate, cephalæa. When one side of the head only is affected, it takes the names of *hemicrania, migrana, hemipagia,* and *megrim;* in one of the temples only, *crotaphos;* and that which is fixed to a point, generally in the crown of the head, is distinguished by the name of *clavus.*

Cephala'rtica. (From κεφαλη, the head, and αρτιζω, to make pure.) Medicines which purge the head.

CE'PHALE. Κεφαλη. The head.

CEPHALIC. (From κεφαλη, the head.) Pertaining to the head. 1. A variety of external and internal medicines are so called, as being adapted for the cure of disorders of the head. Of this class are the snuffs, which produce a discharge from the mucous membrane of the nose, &c.

2. Nerves, arteries, veins, muscles, &c. are so called, which are situated on the head.

3. The name of a vein of the arm, which it was supposed went to the head.

Cephalic vein. (*Vena cephalica;* so called because the head was supposed to be relieved by opening it.) The anterior or outermost vein of the arm, that receives the cephalic of the thumb.

Cephalicus pulvis. A powder prepared from asarum.

CEPHALI'TIS. (From κεφαλη, the head.) Inflammation of the head. *Empresma cephalitis* of Good. See *Phrenitis.*

CEPHALO. This term is joined to others to denote the connexion of the muscle, artery, nerve, &c. to the head.

CEPHALONO'SUS. (From κεφαλη, the head and νοσος, a disease.) Any disease of the head. Applied to the febris hungarica, in which the head is principally affected.

Cephalo-pharyngeus. (From κεφαλη, the head, and φαρυγξ, the throat.) A muscle of the pharynx. See *Constrictor pharyngis inferior.*

CEPHALOPONIA. (From κεφαλη, the head, and πονος, pain.) Headache.

Cepi'ni. Vinegar.

Cepula. Large myrobalans.

CERA. Wax. Bees' wax. A solid concrete substance, collected from vegetables by bees, and extracted from their combs after the honey is got out, by heating and pressing them.

It was long considered as a resin, from some properties common to it with resins. Like them it furnishes an oil and an acid by distillation, and is soluble in all oils; but in several respects it differs sensibly from resins. Like these, wax has not a strong aromatic taste and smell, but a very weak smell, and when pure, no taste. With the heat of boiling water, no principles are distilled from it; whereas, with that heat, some essential oil, or at least a spiritus rector, is obtained from every resin. Farther, wax is less soluble in alkohol. If wax be distilled with a heat greater than that of boiling water, it may be decomposed, but not so easily as resins can. By this distillation, a small quantity of water is first separated from the wax, and then some very volatile and very penetrating acid accompanied with a small quantity of a very fluid and very odoriferous oil. As the distillation advances, the acid becomes more and more strong, and the oil more and more thick, till its consistence is such that it becomes solid in the receiver, and is then called butter of wax. When the distillation is finished, nothing remains but a small quantity of coal, which is almost incombustible.

Wax cannot be kindled, unless it is previously heated and reduced into vapours; in which respect it resembles fat oils. The oil of butter of wax may, by repeated distillations, be attenuated and rendered more and more fluid, because some portion of acid is thereby separated from these substances; which effect is similar to what happens in the distillation of other oils and oily concretes: but this remarkable effect attends the repeated distillation of oil and butter of wax, that they become more and more soluble in alkohol; and that they never acquire greater consistence by evaporation of their more fluid parts. Boerhaave kept butter of wax in a glass vessel, open, or carelessly closed, during twenty years, without acquiring a more solid consistence. It may be remarked, that wax, its butter, and its oil, differ entirely from essential oils and resins in all the above-mentioned properties, and that in all these they perfectly resemble sweet oils. Hence Maquer concludes, that wax resembles resins only in being an oil rendered concrete by an acid; but that it differs essentially from these in the kind of the oil, which in resins is of the nature of essential oils, while in wax and in other analogous oily concretions (as butter of milk, butter of cocoa, fat of animals, spermaceti, and myrtle-wax) it is of the nature of mild unctuous oils, that are not aromatic, and not volatile, and are obtained from vegetables by expression. It seems probable, that the acidifying principle, or oxygen, and not an actual acid, may be the leading cause of the solidity, or low fusibility of wax.

In the state in which it is obtained from the combs, it is called yellow wax, *cera flava;* and this, when new, is of a lively yellow colour, somewhat tough, yet easy to break: by age, it loses its fine colour, and becomes harder and more brittle. Yellow wax, after being reduced into thin cakes, and bleached by a long exposure to the sun and open air, is again melted, and formed into round cakes, called virgin wax, or white wax, *cera alba.* The chief medicinal use of wax, is in plasters, unguents, and other like external applications, partly for giving the requisite consistence to other ingredients, and partly on account of its own emollient quality.

Cera alba. See *Cera.*

Cera dicardo. The carduus pinea.

Cera flava. Yellow wax. See *Cera.*

[Cera vegetabilis. Vegetable wax, or natural wax. Wax seems to abound in some plants more than in others, and is easily collected from them. The bayberry (*Myrica cerifera*) abounds on the sandy shores of the United States, and in the autumn the wax is scraped from the plants, and, when melted and run into cakes, forms a beautiful green vegetable wax, which is made into wax tapers, or sometimes melted with a portion of tallow, and made into candles, which partake of the green colour of the wax, and are called *bayberry candles*, the vegetable *cera* giving hardness and consistence to the candles, and therefore more useful in the heat of summer. We recollect seeing a large specimen of white vegetable wax in the possession of Dr. S. L. Mitchill, received by him from South America, and exhibited to his class when he lectured on Materia Medica, in the College of Physicians and Surgeons of New-York. On inquiry, since, he informs us, that he never could ascertain the botanical name of the plant, though it was said to be a tree. A.]

Ceræ'æ. (From κερας, a horn.) So Rufus Ephesius calls the cornua or appendages of the uterus.

Cerani'tes. (From κεραννυμι, to temper together.) A name formerly applied to a pastil, or troch, by Galen.

Ce'ras. (Κερας, a horn.) A wild sort of parsnip is so named from its shape.

CE'RASA. (Κερασος, the cherry-tree; from Κερασουντη, a town in Pontus, whence Lucullus first brought them to Rome: or from κηρ, the heart; from the fruit having a resemblance to it in shape and colour.) The cherry. See *Prunus*.

CERASA NIGRA. See *Prunus avium*.

CERASA RUBRA. See *Prunus cerasus*.

CERASIA'TUM. (From *cerasus*, a cherry; so called because cherries are an ingredient.) A purging medicine in Libavius.

CE'RASIN. The name given by Dr. John of Berlin, to those gummy substances which swell in cold water, but do not readily dissolve in it. Cerasin is soluble in boiling water, but separates in a jelly when the water cools. Water, acidulated with sulphuric, nitric, or muriatic acid, by the aid of a gentle heat, forms a permanent solution of cerasin. Gum tragacanth is the best example of this species of vegetable product.

CERA'SIUS. (From *cerasus*, a cherry.) *Crasios.* The name of two ointments in Mesue.

CERA'SMA. (From κεραννυμι, to mix.) A mixture of cold and warm water, when the warm is poured into the cold.

CE'RASUS. The cherry and cherry-tree. See *Prunus cerasus*.

CE'RATE. *Ceratum.* A composition of wax, oil, or lard, with or without other ingredients. The obsolete synonymes are, *cerelæum*, *ceroma*, *ceronium*, *cerotum*, *ceratomalagma.* Cerates take their name from the wax which enters into their composition, and to which they owe their consistence, which is intermediate between that of plasters and that of ointments; though no very definite rule for this consistence is, in fact, either given or observed.

CERA'TIA. (From κερας, a horn, which its fruit resembles.) See *Ceratonia siliqua*.

CERATIA DIPHYLLUS. See *Courbaril*

CERA'TICUM. See *Ceratonia siliqua*.

CERA'TO. (From κερας, a horn.) Some muscles have this word as a part of their names, from their shape.

CERATO-GLOSSUS. (From κερας, a horn, and γλωσσα, a tongue.) A muscle, so named from its shape and insertion into the tongue. See *Hyoglossus*.

CERATO-HYOIDEUS. See *Stylo-hyoideus*.

CERATO MALAGMA. A cerate.

CERATOI'DES. (From κερατος, the genitive of κερας, horn, and ειδος, appearance.) See *Cornea*.

CERATO'NIA. (Κερατωνια of Galen and Paulus Ægineta; so called from its horn-like pod.) The name of a genus of plants. Class, *Polygamia;* Order, *Triœcia*.

CERATONIA SILIQUA. The systematic name of the plant which affords the sweet pod. *Ceratium; Ceratia; Siliqua dulcis.* The pods are about four inches in length, and as thick as one's finger, compressed and unequal, and mostly bent; they contain a sweet brown pulp, which is given in the form of decoction, as a pectoral in asthmatic complaints and coughs.

CERA'TUM. (*Ceratum; i.* m.; from *cera*, wax, because its principal ingredient is wax.) See *Cerate*.

CERATUM ALBUM. See *Ceratum cetacei*.

CERATUM CALAMINÆ. *Ceratum lapidis calaminaris; Ceratum epuloticum.* Calamine cerate. Take of prepared calamine, yellow wax, of each half a pound; olive oil, a pint. Mix the oil with the melted wax; then remove it from the fire, and, as soon as it begins to thicken, add the calamine, and stir it constantly until the mixture becomes cold A composition of this kind was first introduced under the name of Turner's cerate. It is well calculated to promote the cicatrization of ulcers.

CERATUM CANTHARIDIS. *Ceratum Lyttæ.* Cerate of blistering fly. Take of spermaceti cerate, six drachms; blistering flies, in very fine powder, a drachm. Having softened the cerate by heat, add the flies, and mix them together.

CERATUM CETACEI. *Cratum spermatis ceti Ceratum album.* Spermaceti cerate. Take of spermaceti, half an ounce; white wax, two ounces; olive oil, 4 fluid-ounces. Add the oil to the spermaceti and wax, previously melted together, and stir them until the mixture becomes cold. This cerate is cooling and emollient, and applied to excoriations, &c.: it may be used with advantage in all ulcers, where no stimulating substance can be applied, being extremely mild and unctuous.

CERATUM CITRINUM. See *Ceratum resinæ*.

CERATUM CONII. Hemlock cerate. ℞ unguenti conii, ℔j. Spermatis ceti, ℥ ij. Ceræ albæ, ℥ iij. Misce. One of the formulæ of St. Bartholomew's hospital occasionally applied to cancerous, scrofulous, phagedenic, herpetic, and other inveterate sores.

CERATUM EPULOTICUM. See *Ceratum calaminæ*.

CERATUM LAPIDIS CALAMINARIS. See *Ceratum calaminæ*.

CERATUM LITHARGYRI ACETATI COMPOSITUM. See *Ceratum plumbi compositum*.

CERATUM PLUMBI ACETATIS. *Unguentum cerussæ acetatæ* Cerate of acetate of lead. Take of acetate of lead, powdered, two drachms; white wax, two ounces; olive oil, half a pint. Dissolve the wax in seven fluid-ounces of oil; then gradually add thereto the acetate of lead, separately rubbed down with the remaining oil, and stir the mixture with a wooden slice, until the whole has united. This cerate is cooling and desiccative.

CERATUM PLUMBI COMPOSITUM. *Ceratum lithargyri acetati compositum.* Compound cerate of lead. Take of solution of acetate of lead, two fluid-ounces and a half; yellow wax, four ounces; olive oil, nine fluid-ounces; camphor, half a drachm. Mix the wax previously melted, with eight fluid-ounces of oil; then remove it from the fire, and, when it begins to thicken, add gradually the solution of acetate of lead, and constantly stir the mixture with a wooden slice until it gets cold. Lastly, mix in the camphor, previously dissolved in the remainder of the oil. Its virtues are cooling, desiccative, resolvent against chronic rheumatism, &c. &c.; and as a proper application to superficial ulcers, which are inflamed.

CERATUM RESINÆ. *Ceratum resinæ flavæ; Ceratum citrinum.* Resin cerate. Take of yellow resin, yellow wax, of each a pound; olive oil, a pint. Melt the resin and wax together, over a slow fire; then add the oil, and strain the cerate, while hot, through a linen cloth. Digestive.

CERATUM SABINÆ. Savine cerate. Take of fresh leaves of savine, bruised, a pound; yellow wax, half a pound; prepared lard, two pounds. Having melted together the wax and lard, boil therein the savine leaves, and strain through a linen cloth. This article is of late introduction, for the purpose of keeping up a discharge from blistered surfaces. It was first described by Mr. Crowther, and has since been received into extensive use, because it does not produce the inconveniences that follow the constant application of the common blistering cerate. A thick white layer forms daily upon the part, which requires to be removed, that the cerate may be applied immediately to the surface from which the discharge is to be made.

CERATUM SAPONIS. Soap cerate. Take of hard soap, eight ounces: yellow wax, ten ounces; semivitreous oxide of lead, powdered, a pound; olive oil, a pint; vinegar, a gallon. Boil the vinegar, with the oxide of lead, over a slow fire, constantly stirring, until the union is complete; then add the soap, and boil it again in a similar manner, until the moisture is entirely evaporated; then mix in the wax, previously melted with the oil. Resolvent; against scrofulous tumours, &c. It is a convenient application in fractures, and may be used as an external dressing for ulcers.

CERATUM SIMPLEX. *Ceratum.* Simple cerate. Take of olive oil, four fluid-ounces; yellow wax, four ounces: having melted the wax, mix the oil with it.

CERATUM SPERMATIS CETI. See *Ceratum cetacei*.

CE'RBERUS. (Κερβερος; because, like the dog Cerberus, it has three heads, or principal ingredients, each of which is eminently active.) A fanciful name given to the compound powder of scammony.

CERCHNA'LEUM. (From κερχω, to make a noise.) A wheezing, or bubbling noise, made by the trachea, in breathing.

CE'RCHNOS. (From κερχω, to wheeze.) *Cerchnus.* Wheezing. Dr. Good applies it to a species of his genus *Rhonchus*, to designate a primary evil or disease; *rhonchus cerchnus*, or wheezing.

CERCHNO'DES. (From κερχω, to wheeze.) *Cerchodes.* One who labours under a dense breathing, accompanied with a wheezing noise.

CERCHO'DES. See *Cerchnodes*.

CE'RCIS. (Κερκις literally means the spoke of a wheel, and has its name from the noise which wheels often make; from κρεκω, to shriek.) The radial bone of the fore-arm was formerly so called from its shape, like a spoke Also a pestle from its shape.

CERCO'SIS. (From κερκος, a tail.) 1. A polypus of the uterus.

2. An enlargement of the clitoris.

CE'REA. (From *cera*, wax.) The cerumen aurium, or wax of the ear.

CEREA'LIA. (Solemn feasts to the goddess Ceres.) All sorts of corn, of which bread or any nutritious substance is made, come under the head of *cerealia*, which term is applied by bromatologists as a genus.

CEREBE'LLA URINA. Paracelsus thus distinguishes urine which is whitish, of the colour of the brain, and from which he pretended to judge of some of its disorders.

CEREBE'LLUM. (Diminutive of *cerebrum.*) The little brain. A somewhat round viscus, of the same use as the brain; composed, like the brain, of a cortical and medullary substance, divided by a septum into a right and left lobe, and situated under the tentorium, in the inferior occipital fossæ. In the cerebellum are to be observed the *crura cerebelli*, the fourth ventricle, the *valvula magna cerebri*, and the *protuberantiæ vermiformes*.

CE'REBRUM. (*Quasi cerebrum;* from καρα, the head.) The brain. A large round viscus, divided superiorly into a *right* and *left hemisphere*, and inferiorly into *six lobes*, two anterior, two middle, and two posterior; situated within the cranium, and surrounded by the dura and pia mater, and tunica arachnoides. It is composed of a *cortical substance*, which is external; and a *medullary*, which is internal. It has three *cavities*, called *ventricles;* two anterior, or lateral, which are divided from each other by the *septum lucidum*, and in each of which is the *choroid plexus*, formed of blood-vessels; the third ventricle is a space between the thalami nervorum opticorum. The principal prominences of the brain are, the *corpus callosum*, a medullary eminence, conspicuous upon laying aside the hemispheres of the brain; the *corpora striata*, two striated protuberances, one in the anterior part of each lateral ventricle; the *thalami nervorum opticorum*, two whitish eminences behind the former, which terminate in the optic nerves; the *corpora quadrigemina*, four medullary projections, called by the ancients *nates* and *testes;* a little cerebrine tubercle lying upon the nates, called the *pineal gland;* and, lastly, the *crura cerebri*, two medullary columns, which proceed from the basis of the brain to the *medulla oblongata*. The cerebral arteries are branches of the carotid and vertebral arteries. The veins terminate in *sinuses*, which return their blood into the internal jugulars. The use of the brain is to give off nine pairs of nerves, and the spinal marrow, from which thirty-one more pairs proceed, through whose means the various senses are performed, and muscular motion excited. It is also considered as the organ of the intellectual functions.

Vauquelin's analysis of the brain is in 100 parts; 80 water, 4.53 white fatty matter, 0.7 reddish fatty matter, 7 albumen, 1.12 osmazome, 1.5 phosphorus, 5.15 acids, salts, and sulphur.

CEREBRUM ELONGATUM. The medulla oblongata, and medulla spinalis.

CEREFO'LIUM. A corruption of *chærophyllum.* See *Scandix cerefolium.*

CEREFOLIUM HISPANICUM. Sweet-cicely. See *Scandix odorata.*

CEREFOLIUM SYLVESTRE. See *Chærophyllum sylvestre.*

CERELÆ'UM. (From κηρος, wax, and ελαιον, oil.) A cerate, or liniment, composed of wax and oil. Also the oil of tar.

CEREOLUS. A wax bougie.

CE'REUS MEDICATUS. See *Bougie.*

CEREVI'SIA. (From *ceres*, corn, of which it is made.) Any liquor made from corn, especially ale and strong beer.

CEREVISIÆ CATAPLASMA. Into the grounds of strong beer, stir as much oatmeal as will make it of a suitable consistence. This is sometimes employed as a stimulant and an antiseptic to mortified parts.

CEREVISIÆ FERMENTUM. See *Fermentum Cerevisiæ.*

CE'RIA. (From *cereus*, soft, pliant.) The flat worms which breed in the intestines. See *Tænia.*

CERIN. 1. Subercerin. A peculiar substance which precipitates on evaporation from alkohol, which has been digested on cork.

2. The name given by Dr. John to the part of common wax which dissolves in alkohol.

3. The name of a variety of the mineral *allanite.*

CE'RION. (From κηριον, a honey-comb.) An eruptive disorder of the head. See *Achor.*

CERITE. The siliciferous oxide of cerium. A rare mineral of a rose-red colour, found only in the copper mine of Bastnacs, in Sweden. It consists of silica, oxide of cerium, and oxide of iron, lime, and carbonic acid.

CERIUM. The name of the metal, the oxide of which exists in the mineral cerite.

To obtain the oxide of the new metal, the cerite is calcined, pulverized, and dissolved in nitromuriatic acid. The filtered solution being neutralized with pure potassa, is to be precipitated by tartrate of potassa; and the precipitate, well washed, and afterwards calcined, is oxide of cerium.

Cerium is susceptible of two stages of oxidation; in the first it is white, and this by calcination becomes of a fallow-red.

The white oxide exposed to the blowpipe soon becomes red, but does not melt, or even agglutinate. With a large proportion of borax it fuses into a transparent globule.

The white oxide becomes yellowish in the open air, but never so red as by calcination, because it absorbs carbonic acid, which prevents its saturating itself with oxygen, and retains a portion of water, which diminishes its colour.

Alkalies do not act on it; but caustic potassa in the dry way, takes part of the oxygen from the red oxide so as to convert it into the white without altering its nature.

The protoxide of cerium is composed by Hisinger of 85.17 metal + 14.83 oxygen, and the peroxide of 79.3 metal + 20.7. The protoxide has been supposed a binary compound of cerium 5.75 + oxygen 1, and the peroxide a compound of 5.75 × 2 of cerium + 3 oxygen. An alloy of this metal with iron was obtained by Vauquelin.

The salts of cerium are white or yellow-coloured, have a sweet taste, yield a white precipitate with hydrosulphuret of potassa, but none with sulpheretted hydrogen; a milk-white precipitate, soluble in nitric and muriatic acids, with ferroprussiate of potassa, and oxalate of ammonia; none with infusion of galls, and a white one with arseniate of potassa.

CERO'MA. (From κηρος, wax.) *Ceronium.* Terms used by the ancient physicians for an unguent, or cerate, though originally applied to a particular composition which the wrestlers used in their exercises.

CEROPI'SSUS. (From κηρος, wax, and πισσα, pitch.) A plaster composed of pitch and wax.

CEROTUM. Κηρωτον. A cerate.

[CERULIN. "By the action of sulphuric acid on indigo, two new substances are obtained, termed, by Mr Crum, *Cerulin* and *Phenicin.* To prepare the former, the indigo is digested in the acid, the mixture is dissolved in a large quantity of sulphuric acid, and the filtered solution is precipitated by potassa. The precipitate consists of *cerulin*, in combination with the sulphate of potassa, and has been called *Ceruleo-sulphate of potassa.* It requires about 120 parts of water for its solution, and forms a very deep blue-coloured liquid. In its property of forming insoluble compounds with neutral salts, cerulin is analogous to tan. From its ultimate analysis, it appears to consist of 1 atom of indigo + 4 atoms of water."—*Webster's Man. of Chem.* A.]

CERU'MEN. (*Cerumen;* diminutive of *cera*, wax.) Wax. See *Cera.*

CERUMEN AURIUM. *Cerea; Aurium sordes; Marmorata aurium; Cypsele; Cypselis; Fugile.* The waxy secretion of the ear, situated in the meatus auditorius externus.

["CERUMEN AURIS. A degree of deafness is frequently produced by the lodgment of hard dry pellets of this substance in the meatus auditorius. The best plan, in such cases, is to syringe the ear with warm water, which should be injected with moderate force. In some instances, deafness seems to depend on a defective secretion of the cerumen, and a consequent dryness of the meatus. Here, a drop or two of sweet oil may now and then be introduced into the ear, and fomentations applied."—*Cooper's Surg. Dict.* A.]

CERU'SSA. (Arabian.) Cerusse. See *Plumbi subcarbonas.*

CERUSSA ACETATA. See *Plumbi acetas.*

CERVI SPINA. See *Rhamnus catharticus.*

CERVI'CAL. (*Cervicalis*; from *cervix*, the neck.) Belonging to the neck; as cervical nerves, cervical muscles, &c.

Cervical artery. Arteria cervicalis. A branch of the subclavian.

Cervical vertebræ. The seven uppermost of the vertebræ, which form the spine. See *Vertebræ.*

CERVICA'RIA. (From *cervic*, the neck; so named because it was supposed to be efficacious in disorders and ailments of the throat and neck.) The herb throatwort.

CE'RVIX. (*Cervix, vicis.* f.; quasi *cerebri via*; as being the channel of the spinal marrow.) 1. The neck. That part of the body which is between the head and shoulders.

2. Applied also to organs, or parts which have some extent, to distinguish their parts; as the *cervix uteri*, neck of the uterus; *cervix vesicæ*, neck of the bladder, neck of a bone, &c.

CESPITITIÆ PLANTÆ. (From *cespes*, a sod, or turf.) The name of a class of plants in Sauvages' Methodus Foliorum, consisting of plants which have only radical leaves; as primrose, &c.

CESPITOSUS. (From *cespes*, a sod, or turf.) A plant is so called which produces many stems from one root, thereby forming a close thick carpet on the surface of the earth.

CESPITOSÆ PALUDES. Turf-bogs.

CESTRI'TES. (From κεϛρον, betony.) Wine impregnated with betony.

CE'STRUM. (From κεϛρα, a dart; so called from the shape of its flowers, which resemble a dart; or because it was used to extract the broken ends of darts from wounds.) See *Betonica officinalis.*

CETA'CEUM. Spermaceti. See *Physeter macrocephalus.*

CE'TERACH. (Blanchard says this word is corrupted from *Pteryga*, πτηρυξ, q. v. as peteryga, ceteryga, and ceterach.) See *Asplenium ceterach.*

CETIC ACID. *Acidum ceticum.* The name given by Chevreuil to a supposed peculiar principle of spermaceti, which he has lately found to be the substance he has called *margarine*, combined with a fatty matter.

CETINE. The name given by Chevreuil to spermaceti. See *Fat.*

CEVADIC ACID. By the action of potassa on the fat matter of the cevadilla, a plant that comes from Senegal, called by the French *petite orge*, there is obtained in the same way as the delphinic acid, an acid which is called the cevadic.

CEVADATE. A salt formed by the combination of the cevadic acid, with earthy, alkaline, and metallic bases.

CEVADILLA. (Dim. of *ceveda*, barley. Spanish.) See *Veratrum sabatilla.*

Ceyenne pepper. See *Capsicum.*

CEYLANITE. The name of the mineral called pleonaste, by Haüy, which comes from Ceylon, commonly in round pieces, but occasionally in crystals. It is of an indigo blue colour, and splendent internally.

CHABASITE. The name of a mineral found in the quarry of Alteberg, near Oberstein, in crystals, the primitive form of which is nearly a cube. It is white, or with a tinge of rose colour, and sometimes transparent.

CHACARI'LLÆ CORTEX. See *Croton Cascarilla.*

CHÆROFO'LIUM. See *Scandix.*

CHÆROPHY'LLUM. (Χαιροφυλλον; from χαιρω, to rejoice, and φυλλον, a leaf; so called from the abundance of its leaves.) Chervil. 1. The name of a genus of plants in the Linnæan system. Class, *Pentandria*; Order, *Digynia.*

2. The pharmacopœial name of some plants. See *Scandix*, and *Chærophyllum sylvestre.*

CHÆROPHYLLUM SYLVESTRE. The systematic name of the *Cicutaria*, or bastard hemlock. *Chærophyllum; caule lævi striato; geniculis tumidiusculis*, of Linnæus. It is often mistaken for the true hemlock. It may with great propriety be banished from the list of officinals, as it possesses no remarkable property.

CHÆ'TA. (From χεω, to be diffused.) An obsolete name of the human hair.

CHALA'SIS. (From χαλαω, to relax.) Relaxation.

CHALA'STICA. (From χαλαω, to relax.) Medicines which relax

CHALA'ZION. (From χαλαζα, a hailstone.) *Chalaza; Chalazium; Granado.* An indolent moveable tubercle on the margin of the eyelid, like a hail-stone. A species of hordeolum. It is that well-known affection of the eye, called a stye, or stian. It is white, hard, and encysted, and differs from the *crithe*, another species, only in being moveable. Writers mention a division of Chalazion into scirrhous, cancerous, cystic, and earthy.

CHA'LBANE. Καλβανη. Galbanum.

CHALCA'NTHUM. (From χαλκος, brass, and ανθος, a flower.) Vitriol; or rather, vitriol calcined red. The flowers of brass.

CHALCEI'ON. A species of pimpinella.

CHALCOI'DEUM OS. The os cuneiforme of the tarsus. See *Cuneiform bone.*

CHALKITIS. See *Colcothar.*

CHALI CRATUM. (From χαλις, an old word that signifies pure wine, and κεραννυμι, to mix.) Wine mixed with water.

CHALI'NOS. *Chalinus.* That part of the checks, which, on each side, is contiguous to the angles of the mouth.

CHALK. A very common species of calcareous earth, or carbonate of lime, of a white colour. See *Creta.*

CHALK, BLACK. Drawing slate, found in primitive mountains, and used in crayon drawing, whence its name.

CHALK, RED. A clay coloured with oxide of iron.

CHALK-STONE. A name given to the concretions in the hands and feet of people violently afflicted with the gout, from their resembling chalk, though chemically different. Dr. Wollaston first demonstrated their true composition to be uric acid combined with ammonia, and thus explained the mysterious pathological relation between gout and gravel.

Gouty concretions are soft and friable. They are insoluble in cold, but slightly in boiling water. An acid being added to this solution, seizes the soda, and the uric acid is deposited in small crystals. These concretions dissolve readily in water of potassa. An artificial compound may be made by triturating uric acid and soda with warm water, which exactly resembles gouty concretions in its chemical constitution.

CHALY'BEATE. (*Chalybeatus*; *chalybs*, from iron, or steel.) Of or belonging to iron. A term given to any medicine into which iron enters; as chalybeate mixture, pills, waters, &c.

CHALYBEATE WATER. Any mineral water which abounds with iron; such as the water of Tunbridge, Spa, Prymont, Cheltenham, Scarborough, and Hartfel; and many others.

[*Chalybeate waters* are so numerous in the United States as to attract little or no attention unless connected with some peculiarity of circumstance, besides the mere solution of iron. The Ballston and Saratoga waters, of New-York, although they contain iron, are not ranked among the chalybeates, having other and more powerful ingredients in their composition. Of the pure chalybeate waters, containing nothing but iron in solution, those most resorted to for health and pleasure are the Stafford Springs, in Connecticut, and Orange and Schooley's Mountain Springs in New-Jersey. The Stafford Springs are at the foot of a sand stone ridge, (old red sand-stone formation of Werner.) Orange Springs are in the same sand-stone formation, in the beautiful town of Orange, in New-Jersey, about 20 miles from New-York. There is an excellent house of entertainment at the springs, and there is a salubrious and well-cultivated country surrounding it. Adjacent to the springs is a considerable elevation, from which an extensive prospect is obtained. The city and bay of New-York are plainly visible, with other and more distant prospects. The water of the springs is strongly impregnated, is not very palatable, and is only drunk by invalids, whose physicians recommend them.

Schooley's Mountain Spring is about 60 miles from New-York, and about the same distance from Philadelphia, and is resorted to in summer by the inhabitants of both cities, and other places. It is on the side of a mountain nearly 1500 feet above tide water. The water runs in a constant stream from the crack of a rock by the side of the road leading down a ravine of the mountain, which from its elevation is cool and salubrious. On the top of the mountain is an extensive plain, crossed by good roads. There are several public houses in the neighbourhood of the spring. The water is a simple chalybeate, without being aërated. The iron is deposited in an ochreous sediment as the water passes over the rock. The mountain appears to be a vast deposite of iron ore, much of which is magnetic, affecting the surveyor's compass. Loose specimens of magnet are occasionally picked up on the mountain. A.]

CHALYBIS RUBIGO PRÆPARATA. See *Ferri subcarbonas.*

CHA'LYBS. (From *Chalybes*, a people in Pontus, who dug iron out of the earth.) *Acies.* Steel. The best, hardest, finest, and the closest-grained forged iron. As a medicine, steel differs not from iron. See *Iron.*

CHALYBS TARTARIZATUS. See *Ferrum tartarizatum.*

CHAMÆBA'LANUS. (From χαμαι, on the ground, and βαλανος, a nut.) Wood pea; Earth nut.

CHAMÆBU'XUS. (From χαμαι, on the ground, and πυξος, the box-tree.) The dwarf box-tree.

CHAMÆCE'DRUS. (From χαμαι, on the ground, and κεδρος, the cedar-tree.) *Chamæcedrys.* A species of dwarf abrotanum.

CHAMÆCI'SSUS. (From χαμαι, on the ground, and κισσος, ivy.) Ground-ivy.

CHAMÆCLE'MA. (From χαμαι, on the ground, and κλημα, ivy.) The ground-ivy.

CHAMÆCRISTA. The *Cassia chamæcrista* of Linnæus, a decoction of which drank liberally is said to be serviceable against the poison of the night-shade.

CHAMÆ'DRYS. (From χαμαι, on the ground, and δρυς, the oak; so called from its leaves resembling those of the oak.) See *Teucrium chamædrys*

CHAMÆDRYS FRUTESCENS. A name for teucrium.

CHAMÆDRYS INCANA MARITIMA. See *Teucrium marum.*

CHAMÆDRYS PALUSTRIS. See *Teucrium scordium.*

CHAMÆDRYS SPURIA. See *Veronica officinalis.*

CHAMÆDRYS SYLVESTRIS. Wild germander. The *Veronica chamædrys.*

CHAMÆLE'A. (From χαμαι, on the ground, and ελαια, the olive-tree.) See *Daphne alpina.*

CHAMÆLÆA'GNUS. (From χαμαι, on the ground, and ελαιαγνος, the wild olive.) See *Myrica gale.*

CHAMÆ'LEON. (From χαμαι, on the ground, and λεων, a lion, *i. e.* dwarf lion.) 1. The chamæleon, an animal supposed to be able to change his colour at pleasure.

2. The name of many thistles, so named from the variety and uncertainty of their colours.

CHAMÆLEON ALBUM. See *Carlina acaulis.*

CHAMÆLEON VERUM. See *Cnicus.*

CHAMÆLEU'CE. (From χαμαι, on the ground, and λευκη, the herb colt's-foot.) See *Tussilago farfara.*

CHAMÆLI'NUM. (From χαμαι, on the ground, and λινον, flax.) Purging flax. See *Linum catharticum.*

CHAMÆME'LUM. (From χαμαι, on the ground, and μηλον, an apple; because it grows upon the ground, and has the smell of an apple.) See *Anthemis nobilis.*

CHAMÆMELUM CANARIENSE. The *Chrysanthemum frutescens* of Linnæus.

CHAMÆMELUM CHRYSANTHEMUM. The *Bupthalmum germanicum* of Linnæus.

CHAMÆMELUM FŒTIDUM. The *Anthemis cotula* of Linnæus.

CHAMÆMELUM NOBILE. See *Anthemis nobilis.*

CHAMÆMELUM VULGARE. See *Matricaria chamomilla.*

CHAMÆ'MORUS. (Χαμαιμορεα; from χαμαι, on the ground, and μορεα, the mulberry-tree.) See *Rubus chamæmorus.*

CHAMÆPEU'CE. (From χαμαι, on the ground, and πευκη, the pine-tree.) See *Camphorosma Monspeliensis.*

CHAMÆ'PITYS. (*Chamæpitys, yos.* f.; from χαμαι, the ground, and πιτυς, the pine-tree.) See *Teucrium chamæpitys.*

CHAMÆPITYS MOSCHATA. The French ground pine. See *Teucrium iva.*

CHAMÆ'PLION. See *Erysimum alliaria.*

CHAMÆRA'PHANUS. (From χαμαι, on the ground, and ραφανος, the radish.) 1. The upper part of the root of apium, according to P. Ægineta The smal age, or parsley.

2. The dwarf radish.

CHAMÆ'RIPHES. The *Chamærops humilis*, or dwarf palm. The fruit called wild dates, are adstringent.

CHAMÆRODODE'NDRON. (From χαμαι, on the ground, and ροδοδενδρον, the rose laurel.) The *Azalæa pontica* of Linnæus.

CHAMÆRUBUS. (From χαμαι, on the ground, and *rubus*, the bramble.) See *Rubus chamæmorus.*

CHAMÆSPA'RTIUM. (From χαμαι, on the ground, and σπαρτιον, Spanish broom.) See *Genista tinctoria.*

CHAMBER. *Camara.* The space between the capsule of the crystalline lens and the corner of the eye, is divided by the iris into two spaces, called chambers; the space before the iris is termed the anterior chamber; and that behind it, the posterior. They are filled with an aqueous fluid.

CHAMBERLEN, HUGH, a native of London, about the middle of the 17th century. He succeeded his father as a practitioner in midwifery, and had also two brothers in the same profession. They invented among them an instrument, the obstetric forceps, which greatly facilitated delivery in many cases, and often saved the child: but to him alone, as most distinguished, the merit has been usually ascribed. In 1683, he published a translation of Mauriceau's Observations, which was much sought after. The instrument procured him great celebrity in this, as well as other countries; and, with successive improvements by Smellie, &c. still continues to be esteemed one of the most valuable adjuvants in the obstetric art. The period of his death is not ascertained.

[CHAMITE. See *organic relics.* A.]

CHAMOMILE. See *Anthemis nobilis.*

Chamomile, stinking. See *Anthemis cotula.*

CHAMOMI'LLA. From χαμαι, on the ground, and μηλον, an apple.) See *Anthemis nobilis.*

CHAMOMILLA NOSTRAS. See *Matricaria Chamomilla.*

CHAMOMILLA ROMANA. See *Anthemis.*

CHAMPIGNION. See *Agaricus pratensis.*

CHA'NCRE. (French. From καρκινος, cancer.) A sore which arises from the direct application of the venereal poison to any part of the body. Of course it mostly occurs on the genitals. Such venereal sores as break out from a general contamination of the system, in consequence of absorption, never have the term chancre applied to them.

Channelled leaf. See *Leaf.*

CHAOMA'NTIA SIGNA. So Paracelsus calls those prognostics that are taken from observations of the air; and the skill of doing this, he calls *Chaomancia.*

CHAO'SDA. Paracelsus uses this word as an epithet for the plague.

CHAPMAN, EDMUND, was born about the end of the 17th century; and, after becoming properly instructed as a surgeon and accoucheur, settled in London, and soon distinguished himself by his success in difficult labours. His plan consisted chiefly in turning the child, and delivering by the feet when any part but the head presented; also in often availing himself of the forceps of Chamberlen, much improved by himself, and of which he had the merit of first giving an account to the public in his treatise on Midwifery, in 1732. He also ably defended the cause of the men-midwives against the attack of Douglas, in a small work, in 1737.

CHA'RABE. An Arabian name for amber.

CHA'RADRA. (From χαρασσω, to excavate.) The bowels, or sink of the body.

CHARAMAIS. The purging hazel-nut.

CHARANTIA. See *Momordica elaterium.*

CHARCOAL. When vegetable substances are exposed to a strong heat in the apparatus for distillation, the fixed residue is called charcoal. For general purposes, wood is converted into charcoal by building it up in a pyramidal form, covering the pile with clay or earth, and leaving a few air holes, which are closed as soon as the mass is well lighted; and by this means the combustion is carried on in an imperfect manner.

In charring wood it has been conjectured, that a portion of it is sometimes converted into a pyrophorus, and that the explosions that happen in powder-mills are sometimes owing to this.

Charcoal is made on the great scale, by igniting wood in iron cylinders. When the resulting charcoal is to be used in the manufacture of gunpowder, it is essential that the last portion of vinegar and tar be suffered to escape, and that the reabsorption of the crude vapours be prevented, by cutting off the communication between the interior of the cylinders and the apparatus for condensing the pyrolignous acid, whenever the fire is withdrawn from the furnace. If this precaution be not observed, the gunpowder made with the charcoal would be of inferior quality.

In the third volume of Tilloch's magazine, we have some valuable facts on charcoal, by Mr. Mushet. He justly observes, that the produce of charcoal in the small way, differs from that on the large scale, in which the quantity of char depends more upon the hardness and compactness of the texture of wood, and the skill of the workman in managing the pyramid of fagots, than on the absolute quantity of carbon it contains.

Clement and Desormes say, that wood contains one-half its weight of charcoal. Proust says, that good pit-coals afford 70, 75, or 80 per cent. of charcoal or coke; from which only two or three parts in the hundred of ashes remain after combustion.—*Tilloch's Mag.* vol. viii.

Charcoal is black, sonorous, and brittle, and in general retains the figure of the vegetable it was obtained from. If, however, the vegetable consist for the most part of water or other fluids, these in their extrication will destroy the connexion of the more fixed parts. In this case the quantity of charcoal is much less than in the former. The charcoal of oily or bituminous substances is of a light pulverulent form, and rises in soot. This charcoal of oils is called lamp-black. A very fine kind is obtained from burning alkohol. See *Carbon.*

CHA'RDONE. The artichoke.

CHARISTOLO'CHIA. (From χαρις, joy, and λοχια, the lochia; so named from its supposed usefulness to women in childbirth.) The plant mugwort. See *Artemisia vulgaris.*

CHARLTON, WALTER, was born in Somersetshire, 1619. After graduating at Oxford, where he distinguished himself by his learning, he was appointed physician to Charles I., and admitted a fellow of the Royal College of Physicians, in London. He had afterward the honour of attending Charles II., and was one of the first members of the Royal Society. He was author of several publications, on medical and other subjects; the former of which contained little original matter, but had the merit of spreading the knowledge of the many improvements made about that period, particularly in anatomy and physiology; the principal of them are his "Exercitationes Pathologicæ," and his "Natural History of Nutrition, Life, and Voluntary Motion." In 1689, he was chosen president of the College, and held that office two years He afterward retired to Jersey, and died in 1707.

CHA'RME. (From χαιρω, to rejoice.) *Charmis.* A cordial mentioned by Galen.

CHA'RPIE. The French. For scraped linen, or lint.

CHA'RTA. (Chaldean.) 1. Paper.

2. The amnios, or interior fœtal membrane, was called the *charta virginea*, from its likeness to a piece of fine paper.

CHA'RTREUX, POUDRE DE. (So called because it was said to have been invented by some friars of the Carthusian order.) A name of the kermes mineral, or hydrosulphuret of antimony.

CHA'SME. (From χαινω, to gape.) *Chasmus.* Oscitation, or gaping.

CHASTE TREE. See *Agnus castus.*

CHA'TE. The *Cucumus ægyptia.*

["CHAUNCEY, CHARLES, M.D. second President of Harvard College, was born in England in 1589. He had his grammar education at Westminster, and was at the school when the gunpowder plot was to have taken effect, and must have perished if the parliament-house had been blown up. At the university of Cambridge he commenced Bachelor of Divinity, and took the degree of M.D. Being intimately acquainted with Archbishop Usher, one of the finest scholars in Europe, he had more than common advantages to expand his mind, and make improvements in literature. A more learned man than Mr. Chauncey was not to be found among the fathers of New-England. He had been chosen Hebrew professor at Cambridge, by the heads of both houses, and exchanged this branch of instruction to oblige Dr. Williams, Vice-Chancellor of the university. He was well skilled in many oriental languages, but especially the Hebrew, which he knew by very close study, and by conversing with a Jew, who resided in the same house. He was also an accurate Greek scholar, and was made professor of this language when he left the other professorship. This uncommon scholar became a preacher, and was settled at Ware. He displeased archbishop Laud, by opposing the book of sports, and reflecting upon the discipline of the church, which caused him to emigrate to Plymouth, in Massachusetts, in 1638.

President Chauncey is said to have been an eminent physician; but we are not informed to what extent he devoted himself to the practice. He left six sons, all of whom were educated at Harvard college, and were preachers. Some of them were learned divines. Dr. Mather says they were all eminent physicians, as their father was before them."—*Thach. Med. Biog.* A.]

Chay. See *Oldenlandia umbellata.*

Chaya. See *Oldenlandia umbellata.*

CHEEK-BONE. See *Jugale os.*

CHEESE. *Caseus.* The coagulum of milk. When prepared from rich milk, and well made, it is very nutritious in small quantities; but mostly indigestible when hard and ill prepared, especially to weak stomachs. If any vegetable or mineral acid be mixed with milk, the cheese separates, and, if assisted by heat, coagulates into a mass. The quantity of cheese is less when a mineral acid is used. Neutral salts, and likewise all earthy and metallic salts, separate the cheese from the whey. Sugar and gum-arabic produce the same effect. Caustic alkalies will dissolve the curd by the assistance of a boiling heat, and acids occasion a precipitation again. Vegetable acids have very little solvent power upon curd. This accounts for a greater quantity of curd being obtained when a vegetable acid is used. But what answers best is rennet, which is made by macerating in water a piece of the last stomach of a calf, salted and dried for this purpose.

Scheele observed, that cheese has a considerable analogy to albumen, which it resembles in being coagulable by fire and acids, soluble in ammonia, and affording the same products by distillation or treatment with nitric acid. There are, however, certain differences between them. Rouelle observed, likewise, a striking analogy between cheese and the gluten of wheat, and that found in the feculæ of green vegetables. By kneading the gluten of wheat with a little salt and a small portion of a solution of starch, he gave it the taste, smell, and unctuosity of cheese; so that after it had been kept a certain time, it was not to be distinguished from the celebrated Rochefort cheese, of which it had all the pungency. This caseous substance from gluten, as well as the cheese of milk, appears to contain acetate of ammonia, after it has been kept long enough to have undergone the requisite fermentation, as may be proved by examining it with sulphuric acid, and with potassa. The pungency of strong cheese too, is destroyed by alkohol.

In the 11th volume of Tilloch's Magazine, there is an excellent account of the mode of making Cheshire cheese, taken from the Agricultural Report of the county. "If the milk," says the reporter, "be set together very warm, the curd will be firm; in this case, the usual mode is to take a common case-knife, and make incisions across it, to the full depth of the knife's blade, at the distance of about one inch; and again crossways in the same manner, the incisions intersecting each other at right angles. The whey rising through these incisions is of a fine pale-green colour. The cheese-maker and two assistants then proceed to break the curd: this is performed by their repeatedly putting their hands down into the tub; the cheese-maker, with the skimming-dish in one hand, breaking every part of it as they catch it, raising the curd from the bottom, and still breaking it. This part of the business is continued till the whole is broken uniformly small; it generally takes up about forty minutes, and the curd is then left covered over with a cloth for about half an hour, to subside. If the milk has been set cool together, the curd will be much more tender, the whey will not be so green, but rather of a milky appearance.

CHEILOCA'CE. (From χειλος, a lip, and κακον, an evil.) A swelling of the lips, or canker in the mouth.

Cheime'lton. (From χειμα, winter.) A chilblain. See *Pernio.*

CHEIRA'NTHUS. (From χειρ, a hand, and ανθος, a flower; so named from the likeness of its blossoms to the fingers of the hand.) The name of a genus of plants in the Linnæan system. Class, *Tetradynamia*, Order, *Siliquosa*. The wall-flower.

Cheiranthus cheiri. The systematic name of the wall-flower. *Leucoium luteum: Viola lutea.* Common yellow wall-flower. The flowers of this plant, *Cheiranthus; foliis lanceolatis, acutis, glabris; ramis angulatis; caule fruticoso*, of Linnæus, are recommended as possessing nervine and deobstruent virtues. They have a moderately strong, pleasant smell, and a nauseous, bitter, somewhat pungent taste

[Cheiranthodendron. A tree growing in Mexico, so called from the appearance of the flower representing the human hand and fingers. (From χειρ, a hand, ανθος, a flower, and δενδρον, a tree.) It is a large tree, bearing a flower resembling a human hand. The part producing this resemblance is the pistillum, which rises above the calyx, and is divided into five parts, analogous to the thumb and fingers. The resemblance is very striking, but the digits are sharp and pointed, more like claws. We have seen preserved specimens of the flowers in very good order. A.]

CHEIRA'PSIA. (From χειρ, the hand, and απτομαι, to touch.) The act of scratching; particularly the scratching one hand with another, as in the itch.

CHEI'RI. (*Cheiri*, Arabian.) See *Cheiranthus Cheiri.*

CHEIRIA'TER. (From χειρ, the hand, and ιατρος, a physician.) A surgeon whose office it is to remove maladies by operations of the hand.

CHEIRI'SMA. (From χειριζομαι, to labour with the hand.) Handling. Also a manual operation.

CHEIRI'XIS. (From χειριζομαι, to labour with the hand.) The art of surgery.

CHEIRONO'MIA. (From χειρονομεω, to exercise with the hands.) An exercise mentioned by Hippocrates, which consisted of gesticulations with the hands, like our dumb-bells.

CHE'LA. (Χηλη, *forceps;* from χεω, to take.) 1. A forked probe, for drawing a polypus out of the nose.

2. A fissure in the feet, or other places.

3. The claw of crabs, which lays hold like forceps.

Chelæ cancrorum. See *Cancer.*

Cheli'don. The bend of the arm.

CHELIDO'NIUM. (From χελιδων, the swallow. It is so named from an opinion, that it was pointed out as useful for the eyes by swallows, who are said to open the eyes of their young by it; or because it blossoms about the time when swallows appear.) Celandine. A genus of plants in the Linnæan system. Class, *Polyandria;* Order, *Monogynia.* There is only one species used in medicine, and that rarely.

Chelidonium majus. *Papaver corniculatum, luteum; Curcum.* Tetterwort, and great celandine. The herb and root of this plant, *Chelidonium—pedunculis umbellatus*, of Linnæus, have a faint, unpleasant smell, and a bitter, acrid, durable taste, which is stronger in the roots than the leaves. They are aperient and diuretic, and recommended in icterus, when not accompanied with inflammatory symptoms. The chelidonium should be administered with caution, as it is liable to irritate the stomach and bowels. Of the dried root, from ʒ ss to ʒ j is a dose; of the fresh root, infused in water, or wine, the dose may be about ℥ ss. The decoction of the fresh root is used in dropsy, cachexy, and cutaneous complaints. The fresh juice is used to destroy warts, and films in the eyes; but, for the latter purpose, it is diluted with milk.

Chelidonium minus. The pill-wort. See *Ranunculus ficaria.*

CHELO'NE. Χελωνη. 1. The tortoise.

2. An instrument for extending a limb, and so called because, in its slow motions, it represents a tortoise. This instrument is mentioned in Oribasius.

Chelo'nion. (From χελωνη, the tortoise; so called from its resemblance to the shell of a tortoise.) A hump or gibbosity in the back.

CHELTENHAM. The name of a village, now become a large and populous town, in Gloucestershire. It is celebrated for its purging waters, the reputation of which is daily increasing, as it possesses both a saline and chalybeate principle. When first drawn, it is clear and colourless, but somewhat brisk; has a saline, bitterish, chalybeate taste. It does not keep, nor bear transporting to any distance; the chalybeate part being lost by precipitation of the iron, and in the open air it even turns fœtid. The salts, however, remain. Its heat, in summer, was from 50° to 55° or 59°, when the medium heat of the atmosphere was nearly 15° higher. On evaporation, it is found to contain a calcareous earth, mixed with ochre and a purging salt. A general survey of the component parts of this water, according to a variety of analyses, shows that it is decidedly saline, and contains much more salt than most mineral waters. By far the greater part of the salts are of a purgative kind, and therefore an action on the bowels is a constant effect, notwithstanding the considerable quantity of selenite and earthy carbonates, which may be supposed to have a contrary tendency. Cheltenham water is, besides, one of the strongest chalybeates we are acquainted with. The iron is suspended entirely by the carbonic acid, of which gas the water contains about an eighth of its bulk; but, from the abundance of earthy carbonates, and oxide of iron, not much of it is uncombined. It has, besides, a slight impregnation of sulphur, but so little as to be scarcely appreciable, except by very delicate tests. The sensible effects produced by this water, are generally, on first taking it, a degree of drowsiness, and sometimes headache, but which soon go off spontaneously, even previous to the operation on the bowels. A moderate dose acts powerfully, and speedily, as a cathartic, without occasioning griping, or leaving that faintness and languor which often follow the action of the rougher cathartics. It is principally on this account, but partly too from the salutary operation of the chalybeate, and perhaps the carbonic acid, that the Cheltenham water may be, in most cases, persevered in, for a considerable length of time, uninterruptedly, without producing any inconvenience to the body; and during its use, the appetite will be improved, the digestive organs strengthened, and the whole constitution invigorated. A dose of this water, too small to operate directly on the bowels, will generally determine pretty powerfully to the kidneys. As a purge, this water is drank from one to three pints; in general, from half a pint to a quart is sufficient. Half a pint will contain half a drachm of neutral purging salts, four grains of earthy carbonates, and selenite, about one-third of a grain of oxide of iron; together with an ounce in bulk of carbonic acid and half an ounce of common air, with a little sulphuretted hydrogen. Cheltenham water is used, with considerable benefit, in a number of diseases, especially of the chronic kind, and particularly those called bilious: hence it has been found of essential service in the cure of glandular obstructions, and especially those that affect the liver, and the other organs connected with the functions of the alimentary canal. Persons who have injured their biliary organs, by a long residence in hot climates, and who are suffering under the symptoms, either of excess of bile or deficiency of bile, and an irregularity in its secretion, receive remarkable benefit from a course of this water, judiciously exhibited. Its use may be here continued, even during a considerable degree of debility; and from the great determination to the bowels, it may be employed with advantage to check the incipient symptoms of dropsy, and general anasarca, which so often proceed from an obstruction of the liver. In scrofulous affections, the sea has the decided preference; in painful affections of the skin, called scorbutic eruptions, which make their appearance at stated intervals, producing a copious discharge of lymph, and an abundant desquamation, in common with other saline purgative springs, this is found to bring relief; but it requires to be persevered in for a considerable time, keeping up a constant determination to the bowels, and making use of warm bathing. The season for drinking the Cheltenham water is during the whole of the summer months.

CHE'LYS. (Χελυς, a shell.) The breast is so called, as resembling, in shape and office, the shell of some fishes.

Chely'scion. (From χελυς, the breast.) A dry, short cough, in which the muscles of the breast are very sore.

Che'ma. A measure mentioned by the Greek physicians, supposed to contain two small spoonfuls.

CHE'MIA. See *Chemistry.*

CHE'MICAL. Of or belonging to chemistry.

CHEMISTRY. (Χυμια, and sometimes χημια: *Chamia*, from *chama*, to burn, Arab. this science being the examination of all substances by fire.) *Chemia; Chimia; Chymia.* The learned are not yet agreed as to the most proper definition of chemistry. Boerhaave seems to have ranked it among the arts. According to Macquer, it is a science, the object of which is to discover the nature and properties of all bodies by their analyses and combinations. Dr. Black says, it is a science which teaches, by experiments, the effects of heat and mixture on bodies; and Fourcroy defines it a science which teaches the mutual actions of all natural bodies on each other. "Chemistry," says Jacquin, "is that branch of natural philosophy which unfolds the nature of all material bodies, determines the number and properties of their component parts, and teaches us how those parts are united, and by what means they may be separated and recombined." Mr. Heron defines it, "That science which investigates and explains the laws of that attraction which takes place between the minute component particles of natural bodies." Dr. Ure's definition is, "the science which investigates the composition of material substances, and the permanent changes of constitution which their mutual actions produce." The objects to which the attention of chemists is directed, comprehend the whole of the substances that compose the globe.

CHEMO'SIS. (From χαινω, to gape; because it gives the appearance of a gap, or aperture.) Inflammation of the conjunctive membrane of the eye, in which the white of the eye is distended with blood, and elevated above the margin of the transparent cornea. In Cullen's Nosology, it is a variety of the ophthalmia membranarum, or an inflammation of the membranes of the eye.

Chenopodio-morus. (From *chenopodium* and *morus*, the mulberry; so called because it is a sort of chenopodium, with leaves like a mulberry.) The herb mulberry-blight. The *Blitum capitatum* of Linnæus.

CHENOPO'DIUM. (From χην, a goose, and πους, a foot; so called from its supposed resemblance to a goose's foot.) The name of a genus of plants in the Linnæan system. Class, *Pentandria;* Order, *Digynia.* The herb chenopody: goose's foot.

Chenopodium ambrosioides. The systematic name of the Mexican tea-plant. *Botrys Mexicana; Botrys ambrosioides Mexicana; Chenopodium Mexicanum; Botrys Americana.* Mexico tea; Spanish tea and Artemisian botrys. *Chenopodium—foliis lanceolatis dentatis, racemis foliatis simplicibus*, of Linnæus. A decoction of this plant is recommended in paralytic cases. Formerly the infusion was drank instead of Chinese tea.

Chenopodium anthelminticum. The seeds of this plant, *Chenopodium—foliis ovato-oblongis dentatis, racemis aphyllis*, of Linnæus, though in great esteem in America, for the cure of worms, are seldom exhibited in this country. They are powdered and made into an electuary, with any proper syrup, or conserve.

["The *Chenopodium anthelminticum*, is a native plant, found in the middle and southern states, usually known by the names of *wormseed* and *Jerusalem oak.* The name wormseed is applied in Europe to the *Artemisia santonica*, a very different plant. The chenopodium is accounted a good vermifuge, especially in the lumbrici of children. The expressed juice of the whole plant is sometimes given in the *dose* of a table-spoonful to a child two or three years old. More frequently the powdered seeds are employed, mixed with treacle or syrup. The seeds yield a volatile oil on distillation, which is prescribed in *doses* of six or eight drops, in sugar or some suitable vehicle."—*Big. Mat. Med.* A.]

Chenopodium bonus Henricus. The systematic name of the English mercury. *Bonus Henricus; Tota bona; Lapathum unctuosum; Chenopodium; Chenopodium—foliis triangulari-sagittatis, integerrimis, spicis compositis aphyllis axillaribus*, of Linnæus. The plant to which these names are given, is a native of this country, and common in waste grounds from June to August. It differs little from spinach when cultivated; and in many places the young shoots are eaten in spring like asparagus. The leaves are accounted emollient, and have been made an ingredient in decoctions for clysters. They are applied by the common people to flesh wounds and sores under the notion of drawing and healing.

Chenopodium botrys. The systematic name of the Jerusalem oak. *Botrys vulgaris; Botrys; Ambrosia; Artemisia chenopodium; Atriplex odorata; Atriplex suaveolens; Chenopodium—foliis oblongis sinuatis, racemis nudis multifidis*, of Linnæus. This plant was formerly administered in form of decoction in some diseases of the chest; as humoral asthma, coughs, and catarrhs. It is now fallen into disuse.

Chenopodium fœtidum. See *Chenopodium vulvaria.*

Chenopodium vulvaria. The systematic name for the stinking orach. *Atriplex fœtida; Atriplex olida; Vulvaria; Garosmum; Raphex; Chenopodium fœtidum; Blitum fœtidum.* The very fœtid smell of this plant, *Chenopodium—foliis integerrimis rhombeo ovatis, floribus conglomeratis axillaribus*, of Linnæus, induced physicians to exhibit it in hysterical diseases. It is now superseded by more active preparations. Messrs. Chevalier and Lasseigne have detected ammonia in this plant in an uncombined state, which is probably the vehicle of the remarkably nauseous odour which it exhales, strongly resembling that of putrid fish. When the plant is bruised with water, and the liquor expressed and afterward distilled, we procure a fluid which contains the subcarbonate of ammonia, and an oily matter, which gives the fluid a milky appearance. If the expressed juice of the chenopodium be evaporated to the consistence of an extract, it is found to be alkaline; there seems to be acetic acid in it. Its basis is said to be of an albuminous nature. It is stated also to contain a small quantity of the substance which the French call osmazome, a little of an aromatic resin, and a bitter matter, soluble both in alkohol and water, as well as several saline bodies.

Che'ras. (From χεω, to pour out.) An obsolete name of struma, or scrofula.

Cherefo'lium. See *Scandix cerefolium.*

CHE'RMES. (Arabian.) A small berry, full of insects like worms: the juice of which was formerly made into a confection, called confectio alkermes, which has been long disused. The worm itself was also so called.

Chermes mineralis. Hydro-sulphuret of antimony.

Cherni'bium. *Chernibion.* In Hippocrates it signifies a urinal.

Chero'nia. (From Χειρων, the Centaur.) See *Chironia centaurium.*

CHERRY. See *Cerasa nigra*, and *Cerasa rubra.*

Cherry bay. The *Lauro-cerasus.*

Cherry-laurel. The *Lauro-cerasus.*

Cherry, winter. The *Alkekengi.*

CHERVI'LLUM. See *Scandix cerefolium.*

CHESELDEN, William, was born in Leicestershire, 1688. After serving his apprenticeship to a surgeon at Leicester, he came to study at St. Thomas's hospital, to which he afterward became surgeon. He began to give lectures at the early age of 22, and about the same period was elected Fellow of the Royal Society Two years after, he published his "Anatomical Description of the Human Body," with some select cases in surgery, which passed through several editions; in one of which he detailed his success in the operation of lithotomy by the lateral method, as it is termed, which he found not so liable to failure as the high operation. He also gave, in the Philosophical Transactions, an interesting account of a grown person whom he restored to sight after being blind from infancy; and furnished some other contributions to the same work. Besides being honourably distinguished by some of the French societies, he was appointed principal surgeon to Queen Caroline, to whom he dedicated his splendid work on the bones in 1733. He was four years after chosen surgeon to Chelsea Hospital, and retired from public practice, and lived to the age of 64.

CHESNUT. See *Æsculus* and *Fagus.*

Chesnut, horse. See *Æsculus Hippocastanum.*

Chesnut, sweet. See *Fagus castanea.*

Cheu'sis. (From χεω, to pour out.) Liquation Infusion.

Cheva'stre. A double-headed roller, applied by

its middle below the chin; then running on each side, it is crossed on the top of the head; then passing to the nape of the neck, is there crossed: it then passes under the chin, where crossing, it is carried to the top of the head, &c. until it is all taken up.

CHEYNE, George, was born in Scotland, 1670. After graduating in medicine, he came to London, at the age of 30, and published a Theory of Fevers, and five years after a work on Fluxions, which procured his election into the Royal Society; and this was soon followed by his "Philosophical Principles of Natural Religion." Being naturally inclined to corpulency, and indulging in free living, he became, when only of a middle age, perfectly unwieldy, with other marks of an impaired constitution; against which, finding medicines of little avail, he determined to abstain from all fermented liquors, and confine himself to a milk and vegetable diet. This plan speedily relieved the most distressing symptoms, which led him after a while to resume his luxuries; but finding his complaints presently returning, he resorted again to the abstemious plan; by a steady perseverance in which he retained a tolerable share of health to the advanced age of 72. In 1722, in a treatise on the gout, &c. he first inculcated this plan; and two years after greatly enlarged on the same subject, in his celebrated "Essay on Health and Long Life." His "English Malady, or Treatise on Nervous Diseases," which he regarded as especially prevalent in this country, a very popular work, published 1733, contains a candid and judicious narrative of his own case.

CHEZANAN'CE. (From χεζω, to go to stool, and αναγκη, necessity.) 1. Any thing that creates a necessity to go to stool.

2. In P. Ægineta, it is the name of an ointment, with which the anus is to be rubbed for promoting stools.

CHI'A. (From Χιος, an island where they were formerly propagated.) 1. A sweet fig of the island of Cyprus, Chio, or Scio.

2. An earth from the island of Chio, formerly used in fevers.

3. A species of turpentine. See *Pistacia terebinthus.*

Chi'acus. (From Χιος, the island of Scio.) An epithet of a collyrium, the chief ingredient of which was wine of Chios.

Chi'adus. In Paracelsus it signifies the same as furunculus.

Chian turpentine. See *Pistacia terebinthus.*

Chia'smus. (From χιαζω, to form like the letter X, chi.) The name of a bandage, the shape of which is like the Greek letter X, *chi.*

CHIASTOLITE. The name of a mineral found in Britany and Spain, somewhat like steatite.

Chia'stos. The name of a crucial bandage in Oribasius; so called from its resembling the letter X, *chi*

Chia'stre. The name of a bandage for the temporal artery. It is a double-headed roller, the middle of which is applied to the side of the head, opposite to that in which the artery is opened, and, when brought round to the part affected, it is crossed upon the compress that is laid upon the wound, and then, the continuation is over the coronal suture, and under the chin; then crossing on the compress, the course is, as at the first, round the head, &c. till the whole roller is taken up.

Chi'bou. A spurious species of gum-elemi, spoken of by the faculty of Paris, but not known in England.

Chichi'na. Contracted from China Chinæ. See *Cinchona.*

CHICKEN. The young of the gallinaceous order of birds, especially of the domestic fowl. See *Phasianus gallus.*

CHICKEN POX. See *Varicella.*

CHICKWEED. See *Alsine media.*

CHICOYNEAU, Francis, was born at Montpelier in 1672, the second son of a professor there, who becoming blind, he was appointed to discharge his duties, after taking his degrees in medicine. Having acquitted himself very creditably, he was deputed with other physicians to Marseilles in 1720, to devise measures for arresting the progress of the plague, which in the end almost depopulated that city. The zeal which he evinced on that occasion was rewarded by a pension; and on the death of his father-in law, M. Chirac, in 1731, he was appointed to succeed him as first physician to the king; and received also other honours previously to his death in 1752. He published in 1721, in conjunction with the other physicians, an account of the plague at Marseilles, in which the opinion is advanced, that the disease was not contagious: and having received orders from the king to collect all the observations that had been made concerning that disease, he drew up an enlarged treatise with much candour, and containing a number of useful facts, which was made public in 1744.

[Chigoe, or *gigger.* A small insect so called in the West India islands, infesting the feet of those who go barefoot, and particularly the negroes. It is a very minute insect, and, when magnified, has very much the appearance of a flea. It penetrates the skin of the feet without producing pain, and there forms its nidus. As it increases in growth in its new situation, it produces little swellings and intolerable itching. The female negroes carefully extract them with a needle. When they are not extracted, the parent deposites its eggs, and as these hatch, the irritation causes increased swellings and ulceration, which sometimes cause the loss of limbs, and even death to the sufferers. Poultices of Indian meal are the only applications to heal the ulcerations and abscesses caused by the chigoes. A.]

CHILBLAIN. See *Pernio.*

[" CHILDS, Timothy, M.D., was born at Deerfield, Massachusetts, February, 1748. He was entered as a member of Harvard College in 1764, but was under the necessity of taking a dismission at the close of his junior year, by the failure of the funds on which he had relied to carry him through the regular course of that seminary. From Cambridge he returned to Deerfield, where he studied physic and surgery with Dr. Williams; and from whence, in 1771, at the age of twenty-three, he removed to practise in Pittsfield.

An ardent and decided friend of civil liberty, he took a deep interest in those great political questions which at that period were agitated between Great Britain and her American colonies. No young man, perhaps, was more zealously opposed to the arbitrary encroachment of the British parliament than Dr. Childs, and as a proof of the confidence reposed in him by the fathers of the town, it need only be mentioned that in 1774, when the crisis of open hostility was approaching, he was appointed chairman of a committee to draw a petition to his Majesty's Justices of Common Pleas in the county of Berkshire, remonstrating against certain acts of parliament which had just been promulgated, and praying them to stay all proceedings till those unjust and oppressive acts should be repealed.

In the same year, (1774,) Dr. Childs took a commission in a company of minute-men, which, in compliance with a recommendation from the convention of the New-England states, was organized in that town. When the news of the battle of Lexington in 1775 was received, he marched with his company to Boston, where he was soon after appointed a surgeon of Colonel Patterson's regiment. From Boston he went with the army to New-York, and from thence accompanied the expedition to Montreal. In 1777 he left the army, and resumed his practice in the town of Pittsfield, and continued in it till less than a week before his death, at the advanced age of seventy-three.

In 1792, Dr. Childs was elected a representative to the General Court, and for several years received the same pledge of public confidence. He also held a seat in the senate for a number of years, by the suffrages of the county in which he lived and died. But it was in his profession he was most highly honoured and extensively useful. He was early elected a member of the Massachusetts Medical Society, and held the office of counsellor of that society to the time of his death. In the year 1811, the University of Cambridge conferred on him the degree of Doctor of Medicine When the district society, composed of the fellows of the state society, was established in the county in which he lived, he was appointed censor, and elected to the office of president.

As a practitioner, Dr. Childs stood high in public estimation, both at home and abroad. For more than thirty years he was the only physician of note in the town; and this single fact strongly testifies to the uncommon estimation in which he was held by those who were most competent to judge of his professional skill and success. He died on the 25th Feb. 1821, as he lived, honoured, respected, and lamented."—*Th. Med. Biog.* A.]

CHI'LI, BALSAMUM DE. Salmon speaks, but without any proof, of its being brought from Chili. The Barbadoes tar, in which are mixed a few drops of the oil of aniseed, is usually sold for it.

CHILIODY'NAMON. (From χιλιοι, a thousand, and δυναμις, virtue.) In Dioscorides, this name is given on account of its many virtues. An epithet of the herb *Polemonium.* Most probably the wood sage, *Teucrium scorodonia* of Linnæus.

CHILIOPHYLLON. (From χιλιοι, a thousand, and φυλλον, a leaf, because of the great number of leaflets.) A name of the milfoil. See *Achillea millefolium.*

CHI'LON. Χειλων. An inflamed and swelled lip.

CHILPELA'GUA. A variety of capsicum.

CHIME'THLON. A chilblain.

CHI'MIA. See *Chemistry.*

CHIMIA'TER. (From χυμια, chemistry, and ιατρος, a physician.) A physician who makes the science of chemistry subservient to the purposes of medicine.

CHIMO'LEA LAXA. Paracelsus means, by this word, the sublimed powder which is separated from the flowers of saline ores.

CHI'NA. (So named from the country of China, from whence it was brought.) See *Smilax China.*

CHINA CHINÆ. A name given to the Peruvian bark.

CHINA OCCIDENTALIS. *China spuria nodosa; Smilax pseudo-China; Smilax Indica spinosa;* American or West-Indian China. This root is chiefly brought from Jamaica, in large round pieces full of knots. In scrofulous disorders, it has been preferred to the oriental kind. In other cases it is of similar but inferior virtue.

CHINA SUPPOSITA. See *Senesio pseudochina.*

CHINCHI'NA. See *Cinchona.*

CHINCHI'NA CARIBÆA. See *Cinchona Caribæa.*

CHINCHINA DE SANTA FE'. There are several species of bark sent from Santa Fé; but neither their particular natures, nor the trees which afford them, are yet accurately determined.

CHINCHINA JAMAICENSIS. See *Cinchona Caribæa.*

CHINCHINA RUBRA. See *Cinchona oblongifolia.*

CHINCHINA DE ST. LUCIA. St. Lucia bark. See *Cinchona floribunda.*

CHINCOUGH. See *Pertussis.*

CHINE'NSIS. See *Citrus aurantium.*

Chinese Smilax. See *Smilax China.*

Chio turpentine. See *Pistacia terebinthus.*

CHI'OLI. In Paracelsus it is synonymous with furunculus.

CHIRA'GRA. (From χειρ, the hand, and αγρα, a seizure.) The gout in the joints of the hand. See *Arthritis.*

CHIRO'NES. (From χειρ, the hand.) Small pustules on the hands and feet, enclosed in which is a troublesome worm.

CHIRO'NIA. (From *Chiron,* the Centaur, who discovered its use.) 1. The name of a genus of plants in the Linnæan system. Class, *Pentandria;* Order, *Monogynia.*

2. (From χειρ, the hand.) An affection of the hand, where it is troubled with chirones.

CHIRONIA CENTAURIUM. The systematic name of the officinal centaury. *Centaurium minus vulgare; Centaurium parvum; Centaurium minus; Libadium; Chironia—corollis quinquefidis infundibuliformibus, caule dichotomo, pistillo simplici,* of Linnæus. This plant is justly esteemed to be the most efficacious bitter of all the medicinal plants indigenous to this country. It has been recommended, by Cullen, as a substitute for gentian, and by several is thought to be a more useful medicine. The tops of the centaury plant are directed for use by the colleges of London and Edinburgh, and are most commonly given in infusion; but they may also be taken in powder, or prepared into an extract.

[CHIRONIA ANGULARIS. See *American centaury.* A.]

CHIRO'NIUM. (From Χειρων, the Centaur, who is said to have been the first who healed them.) A malignant ulcer, callous on its edges, and difficult to cure.

CHIROTHE'CA. (From χειρ, the hand, and τιθημι, to put.) A glove of the scarfskin, with the nails, which is brought off from the dead subject, after the cuticle is loosened by putrefaction, from the parts under it.

CHIR'URGIA. (From χειρ, the hand, and εργον, a work; because surgical operations are performed by the hand.) Chirurgery, or surgery.

CHI'TON. Χιτον. A coat, or membrane.

[CHITONITE. See *Organic relics.* A.]

CHI'UM. (From Χιος, the island where it was produced.) An epithet of a wine made at Scio.

CHLIA'SMA. (From χλιαινω, to make warm.) A warm fomentation.

CHLORA'SMA. (From χλωρος, green.) See *Chlorosis.*

CHLORATE. A compound of chloric acid with a salifiable basis.

CHLORIC ACID. *Acidum chloricum.* "It was first eliminated from salts containing it by Gay Lussac, and described by him in his admirable memoir on iodine, published in the 91st volume of the *Annales de Chimie.* When a current of chlorine is passed for some time through a solution of barytic earth in warm water, a substance called hyperoxymuriate of barytes by its first discoverer, Chenevix, is formed, as well as some common muriate. The latter is separated, by boiling phosphate of silver in the compound solution. The former may then be obtained by evaporation, in fine rhomboidal prisms. Into a dilute solution of this salt, Gay Lussac poured weak sulphuric acid. Though he added only a few drops of acid, not nearly enough to saturate the barytes, the liquid became sensibly acid, and not a bubble of oxygen escaped. By continuing to add sulphuric acid with caution, he succeeded in obtaining an acid liquid entirely free from sulphuric acid and barytes, and not precipitating nitrate of silver. It was chloric acid dissolved in water. Its characters are the following.

This acid has no sensible smell. Its solution in water is perfectly colourless. Its taste is very acid and it reddens litmus without destroying the colour It produces no alteration on solution of indigo in sulphuric acid. Light does not decompose it. It may be concentrated by a gentle heat, without undergoing decomposition, or without evaporating. It was kept a long time exposed to the air without sensible diminution of its quantity. When concentrated, it has something of an oily consistency. When exposed to heat, it is partly decomposed into oxygen and chlorine, and partly volatilized without alteration. Muriatic acid decomposes it in the same way, at the common temperature. Sulphurous acid, and sulphuretted hydrogen, have the same property; but nitric acid produces no change upon it. Combined with ammonia, it forms a fulminating salt, formerly described by M. Chenevix. It does not precipitate any metallic solution. It readily dissolves zinc, disengaging hydrogen; but it acts slowly on mercury. It cannot be obtained in the gaseous state. It is composed of 1 volume chlorine + 2.5 oxygen, or, by weight, of 100 chlorine, 111.70 oxygen, if we consider the specific gravity of chlorine to be 2.4866.

To the preceding account of the properties of chloric acid, M. Vauquelin has added the following. Its taste is not only acid, but astringent, and its odour, when concentrated, is somewhat pungent. It differs from chlorine, in not precipitating gelatine. When paper stained with litmus is left for some time in contact with it, the colour is destroyed. Mixed with muriatic acid, water is formed, and both acids are converted into chlorine. Sulphurous acid is converted into sulphuric, by taking oxygen from the chloric acid, which is consequently converted into chlorine.

Chloric acid combines with the bases, and forms the *chlorates,* a set of salts formerly known by the name of the *hyperoxygenated muriates.* They may be formed either directly by saturating the alkali or earth with the chloric acid, or by the old process of transmitting chlorine through the solutions of the bases, in Woolfe's bottles. In this case the water is decomposed. Its oxygen unites to one portion of the chlorine, forming chloric acid, while its hydrogen unites to another portion of chlorine, forming muriatic acid, and hence, chlorates and muriates must be contemporaneously generated, and must be afterward separated by crystallization, or peculiar methods.

The *chlorate of potassa* or *hyperoxymuriate,* has been long known, and may be procured by receiving chlorine, as it is formed, into a solution of potassa. When the solution is saturated, it may be evaporated gently, and the first crystals produced will be the salt desired, this crystallizing before the simple muriate, which is produced at the same time with it. Its crystals are in shining hexaëdral laminæ, or rhomboidal plates. It is soluble in 17 parts of cold water; and, but very sparingly, in alkohol. Its taste is cooling, and rather unpleasant. Its specific gravity is 2.0. 16 parts of water, at 60°, dissolve one of it, and 2½ of boiling water. The purest oxygen is extracted from this salt, by exposing it to a gentle red heat. One hundred grains yield about 115 cubic inches of gas. It consists of 9.5 chloric acid+6 potassa=15.5, which is the prime equivalent of the salt.

The effects of this salt on inflammable bodies are very powerful. Rub two grains into powder in a mortar, add a grain of sulphur, mix them well by gentle trituration, then collect the powder into a heap, and press upon it suddenly and forcibly with the pestle, a loud detonation will ensue. If the mixture be wrapped in strong paper, and struck with a hammer, the report will be still louder. Five grains of the salt, mixed in the same manner with two and a half of charcoal, will be inflamed by strong trituration, especially if a grain or two of sulphur be added, but without much noise. If a little sugar be mixed with half its weight of the chlorate, and a little strong sulphuric acid poured on it, a sudden and vehement inflammation will ensue; but this experiment requires caution, as well as the following. To one grain of the powdered salt in a mortar, add half a grain of phosphorus; it will detonate, with a loud report, on the gentlest trituration. In this experiment the hand should be defended by a glove, and great care should be taken that none of the phosphorus get into the eyes. Phosphorus may be inflamed by it under water, putting into a wine-glass one part of phosphorus and two of the chlorate, nearly filling the glass with water, and then pouring in, through a glass tube reaching to the bottom, three or four parts of sulphuric acid. This experiment, too, is very hazardous to the eyes. If olive or linseed oil be taken instead of phosphorus, it may be inflamed by similar means on the surface of the water. This salt should not be kept mixed with sulphur, or perhaps any inflammable substance, as in this state it has been known to detonate spontaneously. As it is the common effect of mixtures of this salt with inflammable substances of every kind, to take fire on being projected into the stronger acids, Chenevix tried the experiment with it mixed with diamond powder in various proportions, but without success.

Chlorate of soda may be prepared in the same manner as the preceding, by substituting soda for potassa; but it is not easy to obtain it separate, as it is nearly as soluble as the muriate of soda, requiring only 3 parts of cold water. Vauquelin formed it, by saturating chloric acid with soda; 500 parts of the dry carbonate yielding 1100 parts of crystallized chlorate. It consists of 4 soda, 9.5 acid=13.5, which is its prime equivalent. It crystallizes in square plates, produces a sensation of cold in the mouth, and a saline taste; is slightly deliquescent, and in its other properties resembles the chlorate of potassa.

Barytes appears to be the next base in order of affinity for *this acid.* The best method of forming it is to pour hot water on a large quantity of this earth, and to pass a current of chlorine through the liquid kept warm, so that a fresh portion of barytes may be taken up as the former is saturated. This salt is soluble in about four parts of cold water, and less of warm, and crystallizes like the simple muriate. It may be obtained, however, by the agency of double affinity; for phosphate of silver boiled in the solution will decompose the simple muriate, and the muriate of silver and phosphate of barytes being insoluble, will both fall down and leave the chlorate in solution alone. The phosphate of silver employed in this process must be perfectly pure, and not the least contaminated with copper.

The *chlorate of strontites* may be obtained in the same manner. It is deliquescent, melts immediately in the mouth, and produces cold; is more soluble in alkohol than the simple muriate, and crystallizes in needles.

The *chlorate of lime*, obtained in a similar way, is extremely deliquescent, liquefies at a low heat, is very soluble in alkohol, produces much cold in solution, and has a sharp bitter taste.

Chlorate of ammonia is formed by double affinity, the carbonate of ammonia decomposing the earthy salts of this genus, giving up its carbonic acid to their base, and combining with their acid into chlorate of ammonia, which may be obtained by evaporation. It is very soluble both in water and alkohol, and decomposed by a moderate heat.

The *chlorate of magnesia* much resembles that of lime.

To obtain *chlorate of alumina*, Chenevix put some alumina, precipitated from the muriate, and well washed, but still moist, into a Woolfe's apparatus, and treated it as the other earths. The alumina shortly disappeared; and on pouring sulphuric acid into the liquor, a strong smell of chloric acid was perceivable; but on attempting to obtain the salt pure by means of phosphate of silver, the whole was decomposed, and nothing but chlorate of silver was found in the solution."

CHLORIC OXIDE. Deutoxide of chlorine. When sulphuric acid is poured upon hyper-oxymuriate of potassa in a wine-glass, very little effervescence takes place, but the acid gradually acquires an orange colour, and a dense yellow vapour, of a peculiar and not disagreeable smell, floats on the surface. These phenomena led Sir H. Davy to believe, that the substance extricated from the salt is held in solution by the acid. After various unsuccessful attempts to obtain this substance in a separate state, he at last succeeded by the following method: About 60 grains of the salt are triturated with a little sulphuric acid, just sufficient to convert them into a very solid paste. This is put into a retort, which is heated by means of hot water. The water must never be allowed to become boiling hot, for fear of explosion. The heat drives off the new gas, which may be received over mercury. This new gas has a much more intense colour than euchlorine It does not act on mercury. Water absorbs more of it than euchlorine. Its taste is astringent. It destroys vegetable blues without reddening them. When phosphorus is introduced into it, an explosion takes place. When heat is applied, the gas explodes with more violence, and producing more light than euchlorine. When thus exploded, two measures of it are converted into nearly three measures, which consist of a mixture of one measure chlorine, and two measures oxygen. Hence, it is composed of one atom chlorine and four atoms oxygen.

Deutoxide of chlorine has a peculiar aromatic odour, unmixed with any smell of chlorine. A little chlorine is always absorbed by the mercury during the explosion of the gas. Hence the small deficiency of the resulting measure is accounted for. At common temperatures none of the simple combustibles which Sir H. Davy tried, decomposed the gas, except phosphorus. The taste of the aqueous solution is extremely astringent and corroding, leaving for a long while a very disagreeable sensation. The action of liquid nitric acid on the chlorate of potassa affords the same gas, and a much larger quantity of this acid may be safely employed than of the sulphuric. But as the gas must be procured by solution of the salt, it is always mixed with about one-fifth of oxygen."

CHLORIDE. A compound of chlorine with different bodies.

Chloride of azot. See *Nitrogen.*

CHLO'RINE. (So called from χλωρος, green, because it is of a green colour.) Oxygenated muriatic acid. "The introduction of this term, marks an era in chemical science. It originated from the masterly researches of Sir H. Davy on the oxymuriatic acid gas of the French school; a substance which, after resisting the most powerful means of decomposition which his sagacity could invent, or his ingenuity apply, he declared to be, according to the true logic of chemistry, an elementary body, and not a compound of muriatic acid and oxygen, as was previously imagined, and as its name seemed to denote. He accordingly assigned to it the term chlorine, descriptive of its colour; a name now generally used. The chloridic theory of combustion, though more limited in its applications to the chemical phenomena of nature, than the antiphlogistic of Lavoisier, may justly be regarded as of equal importance to the advancement of the science it self When we now survey the Transactions of the

Royal Society for 1808, 1809, 1810, and 1811, we feel overwhelmed with astonishment at the unparalleled skill, labour, and sagacity, by which the great English chemist, in so short a space, prodigiously multiplied the objects and resources of the science, while he promulgated a new code of laws, flowing from views of elementary action, equally profound, original, and sublime. The importance of the revolution produced by his researches on chlorine, will justify us in presenting a detailed account of the steps by which it has been effected. How entirely the glory of this great work belongs to Sir H. Davy, notwithstanding some invidious attempts in this country to tear the well-earned laurel from his brow, and transfer it to the French chemists, we may readily judge by the following decisive facts.

The second part of the Phil. Trans. for 1809, contains researches on oxymuriatic acid, its nature and combinations, by Sir H. Davy, from which the following interesting extracts are taken.

'In the Bakerian lecture for 1808,' says he, 'I have given an account of the action of potassium upon muriatic acid gas, by which more than one-third of its volume of hydrogen is produced; and I have stated, that muriatic acid can in no instance be procured from oxymuriatic acid, or from dry muriates, unless water or its elements be present.

'In the second volume of the *Mémoires* D'Arcueil, Gay Lussac and Thenard have detailed an extensive series of facts, upon muriatic acid, and oxymuriatic acid. Some of their experiments are similar to those I have detailed in the paper just referred to; others are peculiarly their own, and of a very curious kind; their general conclusion is, that muriatic acid gas contains about one quarter of its weight of water; and that oxymuriatic acid is not decomposable by any substances but hydrogen, or such as can form triple combinations with it.

'One of the most singular facts that I have observed on this subject, and which I have before referred to, is, that charcoal, even when ignited to whiteness in oxymuriatic or muriatic acid gases, by the voltaic battery, effects no change in them, if it has been previously freed from hydrogen, by intense ignition *in vacuo*.

'This experiment, which I have several times repeated, led me to doubt of the existence of oxygen in that substance, which has been supposed to contain it, above all others, in a loose and active state; and to make a more rigorous investigation, than had hitherto been attempted for its detection.'

He then proceeds to interrogate nature, with every artifice of experiment and reasoning, till he finally extorts a confession of the true constitution of this mysterious muriatic essence. The above paper, and his Bakerian lecture, read before the Royal Society in Nov. and Dec. 1810, and published in the first part of their Transactions for 1811, present the whole body of evidence for the undecompounded nature of oxymuriatic acid gas, thenceforward styled chlorine; and they will be studied in every enlightened age and country, as a just and splendid pattern of inductive Baconian logic. These views were slowly and reluctantly admitted by the chemical philosophers of Europe.

In 1812, Sir H. Davy published his Elements of Chemical Philosophy, containing a systematic account of his new doctrines concerning the combination of simple bodies. Chlorine is there placed in the same rank with oxygen, and finally removed from the class of acids. In 1813, Thenard published the first volume of his *Traité de Chimie Elémentaire Théorique et Pratique*. This distinguished chemist, the fellow-labourer of Gay Lussac in those able researches on the alkalies and oxymuriatic acid, which form the distinguished rivalry of the French school, to the brilliant career of Sir H. Davy, states, at p. 584, of the above volume, the composition of oxymuriatic acid as follows:

'*Composition.* The oxygenated muriatic gas contains the half of its volume of oxygen gas, not including that which we may suppose in muriatic acid. It thence follows, that it is formed of 1.9183 of muriatic acid, and 0.5517 of oxygen; for the specific gravity of oxygenated muriatic gas is 2.47, and that of oxygen gas 1.1034.'— 'Chenevix first determined the proportion of its constituent principles. Gay Lussac and Thenard determined it more exactly, and showed that we could not decompose the oxygenated muriatic gas, but by putting it in contact with a body capable of uniting with the *two* elements of this gas, or with muriatic acid. They announced at the same time that they could explain all the phenomena which it presents, by considering it as a simple or as a compound body. However, this last opinion appeared more probable to them. Davy, on the contrary, embraced the first, admitted it exclusively, and sought to fortify it by experiments which are peculiar to him.' P. 585.

In the second volume of Thenard's work, published in 1814, he explains the mutual action of chlorine and ammonia gases, solely on the oxygenous theory. 'On peut démontrer par ce dernier procédé, que le gas muriatique oxigéné, doit contenir la moitié de son volume d'origène, uni à l'acide muriatique.' P. 147.— In the 4th volume, which appeared in 1816, we find the following passages: '*Oxygenated muriatic gas.*— Oxygenated muriatic gas, in combining with the metals, gives rise to the neutral muriates. Now, 107.6 of oxide of silver, contain 7.6 of oxygen, and absorb 26.4 of muriatic acid, to pass to the state of neutral muriate. Of consequence, 348 of this last acid supposed dry, and 100 of oxygen, form this gas. But the sp. gr. of oxygen is 1.1034, and that of oxygenated muriatic gas is 2.47; hence, this contains the half of its volume of oxygen.' P. 52.

The force of Sir H. Davy's demonstrations, pressing for six years on the public mind of the French philosophers, now begins to transpire in a note to the above passage.—'We reason here,' says Thenard, 'obviously on the hypothesis, which consists in regarding oxygenated muriatic gas as a compound body.' This pressure of public opinion becomes conspicuous at the end of the volume. Among the additions, we have the following decisive evidence of the lingering attachment to the old theory of Lavoisier and Berthollet.—'A pretty considerable number of persons who have subscribed for this work, desiring a detailed explanation of the phenomena which oxygenated muriatic gas presents, on the supposition that this gas is a simple body, we are now going to explain these phenomena, on this supposition, by considering them attentively. The oxygenated muriatic gas will take the name of *chlorine;* its combinations with phosphorus, sulphur, azot, metals, will be called *chlorures;* the muriatic acid, which results from equal parts in volume of hydrogen and oxygenated muriatic gases, will be *hydrochloric acid;* the superoxygenated muriatic acid, will be *chlorous acid;* and the hyperoxygenated muriatic, *chloric acid;* the first, comparable to the hydriodic acid, and the last to the iodic acid.' In fact, therefore, we evidently see, that so far from the *chloridic* theory originating in France, as has been more than insinuated, it was only the researches on iodine, so admirably conducted by Gay Lussac, that, by their auxiliary attack on the oxygen hypothesis, eventually opened the minds of its adherents to the evidence long ago advanced by Sir H. Davy. It will be peculiarly instructive, to give a general outline of that evidence, which has been mutilated in some systematic works on chemistry, or frittered away into fragments.

Sir H. Davy subjected oxymuriatic gas to the action of many simple combustibles, as well as metals, and from the compounds formed, endeavoured to eliminate oxygen, by the most energetic powers of affinity and voltaic electricity, but without success, as the following abstract will show.

If oxymuriatic acid gas be introduced into a vessel exhausted of air, containing tin, and the tin be gently heated, and the gas in sufficient quantity, the tin and the gas disappear, and a limpid fluid, precisely the same as Libavius's liquor, is formed: If this substance is a combination of muriatic acid and oxide of tin, oxide of tin ought to be separated from it by means of ammonia. He admitted ammoniacal gas over mercury to a small quantity of the liquor of Libavius; it was absorbed with great heat, and no gas was generated; a solid result was obtained, which was of a dull white colour; some of it was heated, to ascertain if it contained oxide of tin; but the whole volatilized, producing dense pungent fumes.

Another experiment of the same kind, made with great care, and in which the ammonia was used in great excess, proved that the liquor of Libavius cannot be decompounded by ammonia; but that it forms a new combination with this substance.

He made a considerable quantity of the solid compound of oxymuriatic acid and phosphorus by combustion, and saturated it with ammonia, by heating it in a proper receiver filled with ammoniacal gas, on which it acted with great energy, producing much heat; and they formed a white opaque powder. Supposing that this substance was composed of the dry muriates and phosphates of ammonia; as muriate of ammonia is very volatile, and as ammonia is driven off from phosphoric acid by a heat below redness, he conceived that, by igniting the product obtained, he should procure phosphoric acid; he therefore introduced some of the powder into a tube of green glass, and heated it to redness, out of the contact of air, by a spirit lamp; but found, to his great surprise, that it was not at all volatile, nor decomposable at this degree of heat, and that it gave off no gaseous matter.

The circumstance, that a substance composed principally of oxymuriatic acid, and ammonia, should resist decomposition or change at so high a temperature, induced him to pay particular attention to the properties of this new body.

It has been said, and taken for granted by many chemists, that when oxymuriatic acid and ammonia act upon each other, water is formed: he several times made the experiment, and was convinced that this is not the case.

He mixed together sulphurated hydrogen in a high degree of purity, and oxymuriatic acid gas, both dried, in equal volumes. In this instance the condensation was not 1-40th.; sulphur, which seemed to contain a little oxymuriatic acid, was formed on the sides of the vessel; no vapour was deposited, and the residual gas contained about 19-20ths of muriatic acid gas, and the remainder was inflammable.

When oxymuriatic acid is acted upon by nearly an equal volume of hydrogen, a combination takes place between them, and muriatic acid gas results. When muriatic acid gas is acted on by mercury, or any other metal, the oxymuriatic acid is attracted from the hydrogen by the stronger affinity of the metal, and an oxymuriate, exactly similar to that formed by combustion, is produced.

The action of water upon those compounds which have been usually considered as muriates, or as dry muriates, but which are properly combinations of oxymuriatic acid with inflammable bases, may be easily explained, according to these views of the subject. When water is added in certain quantities to Libavius's liquor, a solid crystallized mass is obtained, from which oxide of tin and muriate of ammonia can be procured by ammonia. In this case, oxygen may be conceived to be supplied to the tin, and hydrogen to the oxymuriatic acid.

The compound formed by burning phosphorus in oxymuriatic acid, is in a similar relation to water. If that substance be added to it, it is resolved into two powerful acids; oxygen, it may be supposed, is furnished to the phosphorus to form phosphoric acid, hydrogen to the oxymuriatic acid to form common muriatic acid gas.

He caused strong explosions from an electrical jar to pass through oxymuriatic gas, by means of points of platina, for several hours in succession; but it seemed not to undergo the slightest change.

He electrized the oxymuriates of phosphorus and sulphur for some hours, by the power of the voltaic apparatus of 1000 double plates. No gas separated, but a minute quantity of hydrogen, which he was inclined to attribute to the presence of moisture in the apparatus employed; for he once obtained hydrogen from Libavius's liquor by a similar operation. But he ascertained that this was owing to the decomposition of water adhering to the mercury: and in some late experiments made with 2000 double plates, in which the discharge was from platina wires, and in which the mercury used for confining the liquor was carefully boiled, there was no production of any permanent elastic matter.

Few substances, perhaps, have less claim to be considered as acid, than oxymuriatic acid. As yet we have no right to say that it has been decompounded; and as its tendency of combination is with pure inflammable matters, it may possibly belong to the same class of bodies as oxygen.

May it not in fact be a *peculiar* acidifying and dissolving principle, forming compounds with combustible bodies, analogous to acids containing oxygen or oxides, in their properties and powers of combination; but differing from them, in being for the most part decomposable by water? On this idea, muriatic acid may be considered as having hydrogen for its basis, and oxymuriatic acid for its acidifying principle; and the phosphoric sublimate as having phosphorus for its basis, and oxymuriatic acid for its acidifying matter; and Libavius's liquor, and the compounds of arsenic with oxymuriatic acid, may be regarded as analogous bodies. The combinations of oxymuriatic acid with lead, silver, mercury, potassium, and sodium, in this view, would be considered as a class of bodies related more to oxides than acids, in their powers of attraction. —*Bak. Lec.* 1809.

On the Combinations of the Common Metals with Oxygen and Oxymuriatic Gas.

Sir H. used in all cases small retorts of green glass, containing from three to six cubical inches, furnished with stop-cocks. The metallic substances were introduced, the retort exhausted and filled with the gas to be acted upon, heat was applied by means of a spirit lamp, and after cooling, the results were examined, and the residual gas analyzed.

All the metals that he tried, except silver, lead, nickel, cobalt, and gold, when heated, burnt in the oxymuriatic gas, and the volatile metals with flame Arsenic, antimony, tellurium, and zinc, with a white flame, mercury with a red flame. Tin became ignited to whiteness, and iron and copper to redness; tungsten and manganese to dull redness; platina was scarcely acted upon at the heat of fusion of the glass.

The product from mercury was corrosive sublimate. That from zinc was similar in colour to that from antimony, but was much less volatile.

Silver and lead produced horn-silver and horn-lead; and bismuth, butter of bismuth.

In acting upon metallic oxides by oxymuriatic gas, he found that those of lead, silver, tin, copper, antimony, bismuth, and tellurium, were decomposed in a heat below redness, but the oxides of the volatile metals more readily than those of the fixed ones. The oxides of cobalt and nickel were scarcely acted upon at a dull red heat. The red oxide of iron was not affected at a strong red heat, while the black oxide was readily decomposed at a much lower temperature; arsenical acid underwent no change at the greatest heat that could be given it in the glass retort, while the white oxide readily decomposed.

In cases where oxygen was given off, it was found exactly the same in quantity as that which had been absorbed by the metal. Thus, two grains of red oxide of mercury absorbed 9-10ths of a cubical inch of oxymuriatic gas, and afforded 0.45 of oxygen. Two grains of dark olive oxide from calomel decomposed by potassa, absorbed about 94-100ths of oxymuriatic gas, and afforded 24-100ths of oxygen, and corrosive sublimate was produced in both cases.

In the decomposition of the white oxide of zinc, oxygen was expelled exactly equal to half the volume of the oxymuriatic acid absorbed. In the case of the decomposition of the black oxide of iron, and the white oxide of arsenic, the changes that occurred were of a very beautiful kind; no oxygen was given off in either case, but butter of arsenic and arsenical acid formed in one instance, and the ferruginous sublimate and red oxide of iron in the other.

General Conclusions and Observations, illustrated by Experiments.

Oxymuriatic gas combines with inflammable bodies, to form simple binary compounds; and in these cases, when it acts upon oxides, it either produces the expulsion of their oxygen, or causes it to enter into new combinations.

If it be said that the oxygen arises from the decomposition of the oxymuriatic gas, and not from the oxides, it may be asked, why it is always the quantity contained in the oxide? and why in some cases, as those of the peroxides of potassium and sodium, it bears no relation to the quantity of gas?

If there existed any acid matter in oxymuriatic gas, combined with oxygen, it ought to be exhibited in the fluid compound of one proportion of phosphorus, and two of oxymuriatic gas; for this, on such an assumption, should consist of muriatic acid (on the old hypothesis, free from water) and phosphorous acid; but this substance has no effect on litmus paper, and does not act under common circumstances, on fixed alkaline bases, such as dry lime or magnesia. Oxymuriatic gas, like oxygen, must be combined in large quantity with peculiar inflammable matter, to form acid matter. In its union with hydrogen, it instantly reddens the driest litmus paper, though a gaseous body. Contrary to acids, it expels oxygen from protoxides, and combines with peroxides.

When potassium is burnt in oxymuriatic gas, a dry compound is obtained. If potassium combined with oxygen is employed, the whole of the oxygen is expelled, and the same compound formed. It is contrary to sound logic to say, that this exact quantity of oxygen is given off from a body not known to be compound, when we are certain of its existence in another; and all the cases are parallel.

Scheele explained the bleaching powers of the oxymuriatic gas, by supposing that it destroyed colours by combining with phlogiston. Berthollet considered it as acting by supplying oxygen. He made an experiment, which seems to prove that the pure gas is incapable of altering vegetable colours, and that its operation in bleaching depends entirely upon its property of decomposing water, and liberating its oxygen.

He filled a glass globe, containing dry powdered muriate of lime, with oxymuriatic gas. He introduced some dry paper tinged with litmus that had been just heated, into another globe containing dry muriate of lime: after some time this globe was exhausted, and then connected with the globe containing the oxymuriatic gas, and by an appropriate set of stop-cocks, the paper was exposed to the action of the gas. No change of colour took place, and after two days there was scarcely a perceptible alteration.

Some similar paper dried, introduced into gas that had not been exposed to muriate of lime, was instantly rendered white.

It is generally stated in chemical books, that oxymuriatic gas is capable of being condensed and crystallized at a low temperature. He found by several experiments that this is not the case. The solution of oxymuriatic gas in water freezes more readily than pure water, but the pure gas dried by muriate of lime undergoes no change whatever, at a temperature of 40 below 0° of Fahrenheit. The mistake seems to have arisen from the exposure of the gas to cold in bottles containing moisture.

He attempted to decompose boracic and phosphoric acids by oxymuriatic gas, but without success; from which it seems probable, that the attractions of boracium and phosphorus for oxygen are stronger than for oxymuriatic gas. And from the experiments already detailed, iron and arsenic are analogous in this respect, and probably some other metals.

Potassium, sodium, calcium, strontium, barium, zinc, mercury, tin, lead, and probably silver, antimony, and gold, seem to have a stronger attraction for oxymuriatic gas than for oxygen.

'To call a body which is not known to contain oxygen, and which cannot contain muriatic acid, oxymuriatic acid, is contrary to the principles of that nomenclature in which it is adopted; and an alteration of it seems necessary to assist the progress of discussion, and to diffuse just ideas on the subject. If the great discoverer of this substance had signified it by any simple name, it would have been proper to have recurred to it; but dephlogisticated marine acid is a term which can hardly be adopted in the present advanced era of the science.

'After consulting some of the most eminent chemical philosophers in this country, it has been judged most proper to suggest a name founded upon one of its obvious and characteristic properties—its colour, and to call it *chlorine* or *chloric* gas.

'Should it hereafter be discovered to be compound, and even to contain oxygen, this name can imply no error, and cannot necessarily require a change.

'Most of the salts which have been called muriates, are not known to contain any muriatic acid, or any oxygen. Thus Libavius's liquor, though converted into a muriate by water, contains only tin and oxymuriatic gas, and horn-silver seems incapable of being converted into a true muriate.'—*Bak. Lec.* 1811.

We shall now exhibit a summary view of the preparation and properties of chlorine.

Mix in a mortar 3 parts of common salt and 1 of black oxide of manganese. Introduce them into a glass retort, and add 2 parts of sulphuric acid. Gas will issue, which must be collected in the water-pneumatic trough. A gentle heat will favour its extrication. In practice, the above pasty-consistenced mixture is apt to boil over into the neck. A mixture of liquid muriatic acid and manganese is therefore more convenient for the production of chlorine. A very slight heat is adequate to its expulsion from the retort. Instead of manganese, red oxide of mercury, or puce-coloured oxide of lead, may be employed.

This gas, as we have already remarked, is of a greenish yellow-colour, easily recognised by daylight, but scarcely distinguishable by that of candles. Its odour and taste are disagreeable, strong, and so characteristic, that it is impossible to mistake it for any other gas. When we breathe it, even much diluted with air, it occasions a sense of strangulation, constriction of the *thorax*, and a copious discharge from the nostrils. If respired in larger quantity, its excites violent coughing, with spitting of blood, and would speedily destroy the individual, amid violent distress. Its specific gravity is 2.4733. This is better inferred from the specific gravities of hydrogen and muriatic acid gases, than from the direct weight of chlorine, from the impossibility of confining it over mercury. On volume of hydrogen, added to one of chlorine, form two of the acid gas. Hence, if from twice the specific gravity of muriatic gas=2.5427, we subtract that of hydrogen=0.0694, the difference 2.4733 is the sp. gr. of chlorine. 100 cubic inches at mean pressure and temperature weigh 75½ grains. See *Gas*.

In its perfectly dry state, it has no effect on dry vegetable colours. With the aid of a little moisture, it bleaches them into a yellowish-white. Scheele first remarked this bleaching property; Berthollet applied it to the art of bleaching in France; and from him Mr. Watt introduced its use into Great Britain.

If a lighted wax taper be immersed rapidly into this gas, it consumes very fast, with a dull reddish flame, and much smoke. The taper will not burn at the surface of the gas. Hence, if slowly introduced, it is apt to be extinguished. The alkaline metals, as well as copper, tin, arsenic, zinc, antimony, in fine laminæ or filings, spontaneously burn in chlorine. Metallic chlorides result. Phosphorus also takes fire at ordinary temperatures, and is converted into a chloride. Sulphur may be melted in the gas without taking fire. It forms a liquid chloride, of a reddish colour. When dry, it is not altered by any change of temperature. Enclosed in a phial with a little moisture, it concretes into crystalline needles, at 40° Fahr.

According to Thenard, water condenses, at the temperature of 68° F. and at 29.92 barom. 1 1-2 times its volume of chlorine, and forms *aqueous* chlorine, formerly called liquid oxymuriatic acid. This combination is best made in the second bottle of a Woolfe's apparatus, the first being charged with a little water, to intercept the muriatic acid gas, while the third bottle may contain potassa-water or milk of lime, to condense the superfluous gas. Thenard says, that a kilogramme of salt is sufficient for saturating from 10 to 12 litres of water. These measures correspond to 2 1-3 lbs. avoirdupois, and to from 21 to 25 pints English. There is an ingenious apparatus for making aqueous chlorine, described in Berthollet's Elements of Dying, vol. i.; which, however, the happy substitution of slacked lime for water, by Mr. Charles Tennant, of Glasgow, has superseded, for the purposes of manufacture. It congeals by cold at 40° Fahr. and affords crystallized plates, of a deep yellow, containing a less proportion of water than the liquid combination. Hence when chlorine is passed into water at temperatures under 40°, the liquid finally becomes a concrete mass, which at a gentle heat liquefies with effervescence, from the escape of the excess of chlorine. When steam and chlorine are passed together through a red-hot porcelain tube, they are converted into muriatic acid and oxygen. A like result is obtained by exposing aqueous chlorine to the solar rays; with this difference, that a little chloric acid is formed. Hence aqueous chlorine should be kept in a dark place. Aqueous chlorine attacks almost all the metals at an ordinary temperature, forming muriates or chlorides, and heat is evolved. It has the smell, taste, and colour of chlorine; and acts, like it, on vegetable and animal colours. Its taste is somewhat astringent, but not in the least degree acidulous.

When we put in a perfectly dark place, at the ordi

nary temperature, a mixture of chlorine and hydrogen it experiences no kind of alteration, even in the space of a great many days. But if, at the same low temperature, we expose the mixture to the diffuse light of day, by degrees the two gases enter into chemical combination, and form muriatic acid gas. There is no change in the *volume* of the mixture, but the change of its *nature* may be proved, by its rapid absorbability by water, its not exploding by the lighted taper, and the disappearance of the chlorine hue. To produce the complete discoloration, we must expose the mixture finally for a few minutes to the sunbeam. If exposed at first to this intensity of light, it explodes with great violence, and instantly forms muriatic acid gas. The same explosive combination is produced by the electric spark and the lighted taper. Thenard says, a heat of 392° is sufficient to cause the explosion. The proper proportion is an equal volume of each gas. Chlorine and nitrogen combine into a remarkable detonating compound, by exposing the former gas to a solution of an ammoniacal salt. Chlorine is the most powerful agent for destroying contagious *miasmata*. The disinfecting phials of Morveau evolve this gas."—*Ure.*

CHLORITE. A mineral usually friable or very easy to pulverize, composed of a multitude of little spangles, or shining small grains, falling to powder under the pressure of the fingers There are four sub-species.

1. *Chlorite earth.* In green, glimmering, and somewhat pearly scales, with a shining green streak.

2. *Common chlorite.* A massive mineral of a blackish-green colour, a shining lustre, and a foliated fracture passing into earthy.

3. *Chlorite slate.* A massive, blackish-green mineral, with a resinous lustre, and curve slaty or scaly-foliated fracture.

4. *Foliated chlorite.* Colour between mountain and blackish-green.

CHLORIODATE. A compound of the chloriodic acid with a salifiable basis.

CHLORIODE ACID. *Acidum chloriodicum.* See *Chloriodic acid.*

CHLORIODIC ACID. *Acidum chloriodicum. Chloriode acid.* Sir H. Davy formed it, by admitting chlorine in excess to known quantities of iodine, in vessels exhausted of air, and repeatedly heating the sublimate. Operating in this way, he found that iodine absorbs less than one-third of its weight of chlorine.

Chloriodic acid is a very volatile substance, formed by the sublimation of iodine in a great excess of chlorine, is of a bright yellow colour; when fused it becomes of a deep orange, and when rendered elastic, it forms a deep orange-coloured gas. It is capable of combining with much iodine when they are heated together; its colour becomes, in consequence, deeper, and the chloriodic acid and the iodine rise together in the elastic state. The solution of the chloriodic acid in water, likewise dissolves large quantities of iodine, so that it is possible to obtain a fluid containing very different proportions of iodine and chlorine.

When two bodies so similar in their characters, and in the compounds they form, as iodine and chlorine, act upon substances at the same time, it is difficult, Sir H. observes, to form a judgment of the different parts that they play in the new chemical arrangement produced. It appears most probable, that the acid property of the chloriodic compound depends upon the combination of the two bodies; and its action upon solutions of the alkalies and the earths may be easily explained, when it is considered that chlorine has a greater tendency than iodine to form double compounds with the metals, and that iodine has a greater tendency than chlorine to form triple compounds with oxygen and the metals.

A triple compound of this kind with sodium may exist in sea water, and would be separated with the first crystals that are formed by its evaporation. Hence, it may exist in common salt. Sir H. Davy ascertained, by feeding birds with bread soaked with water, holding some of it in solution, that it is not poisonous like iodine itself.—*Ure's Ch. Dict.*

CHLORO-CARBONOUS ACID. "The term chloro-carbonic which has been given to this compound is incorrect, leading to the belief of its being a compound of chlorine and acidified charcoal, instead of being a compound of chlorine and the protoxide of charcoal. Chlorine has no immediate action on carbonic oxide, when they are exposed to each other in common daylight over mercury: not even when the electric spark is passed through them. Experiments made by Dr. John Davy, in the presence of his brother Sir H. Davy, prove that they combine rapidly when exposed to the direct solar beams, and one volume of each is condensed into one volume of the compound. The resulting gas possesses very curious properties, approaching to those of an acid. From the peculiar potency of the sunbeam in effecting this combination, Dr. Davy called it *phosgene gas.* The constituent gases, dried over muriate of lime, ought to be introduced from separate reservoirs into an exhausted globe, perfectly dry, and exposed for fifteen minutes to bright sunshine, or for twelve hours to daylight. The colour of the chlorine disappears, and on opening the stop-cock belonging to the globe under mercury recently boiled, an absorption of one-half the gaseous volume is indicated. The resulting gas possesses properties perfectly distinct from those belonging to either carbonic oxide or chlorine.

It does not fume in the atmosphere. Its odour is different from that of chlorine, something like that which might be imagined to result from the smell of chlorine combined with that of ammonia. It is in fact more intolerable and suffocating than chlorine itself, and affects the eyes in a peculiar manner, producing a rapid flow of tears, and occasioning painful sensations.

It reddens dry litmus paper; and condenses four volumes of ammonia into a white salt, while heat is evolved. This ammoniacal compound is neutral, has no odour, but a pungent saline taste; is deliquescent, decomposable by the liquid mineral acids, dissolves without effervescing in vinegar, and sublimes unaltered in muriatic, carbonic, and sulphurous acid gases. Sulphuric acid resolves itself into carbonic and muriatic acids, in the proportion of two in volume of the latter, and one of the former. Tin, zinc, antimony, and arsenic, heated in chloro-carbonous acid abstract the chlorine, and leave the carbonic oxide expanded to its original volume. There is neither ignition nor explosion takes place, though the action of the metals is rapid. Potassium acting on the compound gas produces a solid chloride and charcoal. White oxide of zinc, with chloro-carbonous acid, gives a metallic chloride, and carbonic acid. Neither sulphur, phosphorus, oxygen, nor hydrogen, though aided by heat, produce any change on the acid gas. But oxygen and hydrogen together, in due proportions, explode in it; or mere exposure to water converts it into muriatic and carbonic acid gases.

From its completely neutralizing ammonia, which carbonic acid does not; from its separating carbonic acid from the subcarbonate of this alkali, while itself is not separable by the acid gases or acetic acid, and its reddening vegetable blues, there can be no hesitation in pronouncing the chloro-carbonous compound to be an acid. Its saturating powers indeed surpass every other substance. None condenses so large a proportion of ammonia.

One measure of alkohol condenses twelve of chloro-carbonous gas without decomposing it; and acquires the peculiar odour and power of affecting the eyes.

To prepare the gas in a pure state, a good air-pump is required, perfectly tight stop-cocks, dry gases, and dry vessels. Its specific gravity may be inferred from the specific gravities of its constituents, of which it is the sum. Hence $2.4733 + 0.9722 = 3.4455$, is the specific gravity of chloro-carbonous gas; and 100 cubic inches weigh 105.15 grains. It appears that when hydrogen, carbonic oxide, and chlorine, mixed in equal volumes, are exposed to light, muriatic and chloro-carbonous acids are formed, in equal proportions, indicating an equality of affinity.

The paper in the Phil. Trans. for 1812, from which the preceding facts are taken, does honour to the school of Sir H. Davy. Gay Lussac and Thenard, as well as Dr. Murray, made controversial investigations on the subject at the same time, but without success. Thenard has, however, recognised its distinct existence and properties, by the name of *carbo-muriatic* acid, in the 2d volume of his System, published in 1814, where he considers it as a compound of muriatic and carbonic acids, resulting from the mutual actions of the *oxygenated muriatic acid* and carbonic oxide."—*Ure.*

CHLOROCYANIC ACID. *Acidum chloro-cyanicum.* Chloroprussic acid. "When hydrocyanic acid is mixed with chlorine, it acquires new properties. Its odour is much increased. It no longer forms prussian blue with solutions of iron, but a green precipitate, which becomes blue by the addition of sulphurous acid. Hydrocyanic acid, thus altered, had acquired the name of *oxyprussic*, because it was supposed to have acquired oxygen. Gay Lussac subjected it to a minute examination, and found that it was a compound of equal volumes of chlorine and cyanogen, whence he proposed to distinguish it by the name of chlorocyanic acid. To prepare this compound, he passed a current of chlorine into solution of hydrocyanic acid, till it destroyed the colour of sulphate of indigo; and by agitating the liquid with mercury, he deprived it of the excess of chlorine. By distillation, afterward, in a moderate heat, an elastic fluid is disengaged, which possesses the properties formerly assigned to *oxyprussic* acid. This, however, is not pure chlorocyanic acid, but a mixture of it with carbonic acid, in proportions which vary so much as to make it difficult to determine them.

When hydrocyanic acid is supersaturated with chlorine, and the excess of this last is removed by mercury, the liquid contains chlorocyanic and muriatic acids. Having put mercury into a glass jar until it was 3-4ths full, he filled it completely with that acid liquid, and inverted the jar in a vessel of mercury. On exhausting the receiver of an air-pump, containing this vessel, the mercury sunk in the jar, in consequence of the elastic fluid disengaged. By degrees, the liquid itself was entirely expelled, and swam on the mercury on the outside. On admitting the air, the liquid could not enter the tube, but only the mercury, and the whole elastic fluid condensed, except a small bubble. Hence it was concluded, that chlorocyanic acid was not a permanent gas, and that, in order to remain gaseous under the pressure of the air, it must be mixed with another gaseous substance.

The mixture of chlorocyanic and carbonic acids has the following properties. It is colourless. Its smell is very strong. A very small quantity of it irritates the pituitory membrane, and occasions tears. It reddens litmus, is not inflammable, and does not detonate when mixed with twice its bulk of oxygen or hydrogen. Its density, determined by calculation, is 2.111. Its aqueous solution does not precipitate nitrate of silver nor barytes water. The alkalies absorb it rapidly, but an excess of them is necessary to destroy its odour. If we then add an acid, a strong effervescence of carbonic acid is produced, and the odour of chlorocyanic acid is no longer perceived. If we add an excess of lime to the acid solution, ammonia is disengaged in abundance. To obtain the green precipitate from solution of iron, we must begin by mixing chlorocyanic acid with that solution. We then add a little potassa, and at last a little acid. If we add the alkali before the iron, we obtain no green precipitate.

Chlorocyanic acid exhibits with potassium almost the same phenomena as cyanogen. The inflammation is equally slow, and the gas diminishes as much in volume."—*Ure.*

CHLOROPHANE. A violet fluor spar, found in Siberia.

CHLOROPHILE. The name lately given by Pelletier and Caventou to the green matter of the leaves of plants. They obtain it by pressing, and then washing in water, the substance of many leaves, and afterward treating it with alkohol. A matter was dissolved, which, when separated by evaporation, and purified by washing in hot water, appeared as a deep-green resinous substance. It dissolves entirely in alkohol, æther, oils, or alkalies; it is not altered by exposure to air; it is softened by heat, but does not melt; it burns with flame, and leaves a bulky coal. Hot water slightly dissolves it. Acetic acid is the only acid that dissolves it in great quantity. If an earthy or metallic salt be mixed with the alkoholic solution, and then alkali or alkaline subcarbonate be added, the oxide or earth is thrown down in combination with much of the green substance, forming a lake. These lakes appear moderately permanent when exposed to the air. It is supposed to be a peculiar proximate principle.

CHLOROPRUSSIC ACID. See *Chlorocyanic acid.*

CHLORO'SIS. (From χλωρος, green, pale; from χλοα, or χλοη, *herba virens*: and hence χλωρασμα and χλωριασις, *viror, pallor;* so called from the yellow-greenish look those have who are affected with it.) *Febris alba; Febris amatoria; Icterus albus; Chlorasma.* The green-sickness. A genus of disease in the class *Cachexiæ*, and order *Impetigines* of Cullen. It is a disease which affects young females who labour under a retention or suppression of the menses. Heaviness, listlessness to motion, fatigue on the least exercise, palpitations of the heart, pains in the back, loins, and hips, flatulency, and acidities in the stomach and bowels, a preternatural appetite for chalk, lime, and various other absorbents, together with many dyspeptic symptoms, usually attend on this disease. As it advances in its progress, the face becomes pale, or assumes a yellowish hue; the whole body is flaccid, and likewise pale; the feet are affected with œdematous swellings; the breathing is much hurried by any considerable exertion of the body; the pulse is quick, but small; and the person is apt to be affected with many of the symptoms of hysteria. To procure a flow of the menses, proves in some cases a very difficult matter; and where the disease has been of long standing, various morbid affections of the viscera are often brought on, which at length prove fatal. Dissections of those who have died of chlorosis, have usually shown the ovaria to be in a scirrhous, or dropsical state. In some cases, the liver, spleen, and mesenteric glands, have likewise been found in a diseased state

The cure is to be attempted by increasing the tone of the system, and exciting the action of the uterine vessels. The first may be effected by a generous nutritive diet, with the moderate use of wine; by gentle and daily exercise, particularly on horseback; by agreeable company, to amuse and quiet the mind; and by tonic medicines, especially the preparations of iron, joined with myrrh, &c. Bathing will likewise help much to strengthen them, if the temperature of the bath be made gradually lower, as the patient bears it; and sometimes drinking the mineral chalybeate waters may assist. The bowels must be kept regular, and occasionally a gentle emetic will prepare for the tonic plan. The other object of stimulating the uterine vessels may be attained by the exercises of walking and dancing; by frequent friction of the lower extremities; by the pediluvium, hip-bath, &c.; by electric shocks, passed through the region of the uterus; by active purgatives, especially those formula containing aloes, which acts particularly on the rectum. These means may be resorted to with more probability of success, when there appear efforts of the system to produce the discharge, the general health having been previously improved. Various remedies have been dignified with the title of emmenagogues, though mostly little to be depended on, as madder, &c. In obstinate cases, the tinctura lyttæ, or savine, may be tried, but with proper caution, as the most likely to avail.

CHLOROUS ACID. *Acidum chlorosum.* See *Chlorous oxide.*

CHLOROUS OXIDE. Euchorine. Protoxide of chlorine. "To prepare it, put chlorate of potassa into a small retort, and pour in twice as much muriatic acid as will cover it, diluted with an equal volume of water. By the application of a gentle heat, the gas is evolved. It must be collected over mercury.

Its tint is much more lively, and more yellow than chlorine, and hence its discoverer named it *euchlorine* Its smell is peculiar, and approaches to that of burnt sugar. It is not respirable. It is soluble in water, to which it gives a lemon colour. Water absorbs 8 or 10 times its volume of this gas. Its specific gravity is to that of common air nearly as 2.40 to 1; for 100 cubic inches weigh, according to Sir H. Davy, between 74 and 75 grains. If the compound gas result from 4 volumes of chlorine + 2 of oxygen, weighing 12.1154, which undergo a condensation of one-sixth, then the specific gravity comes out 2.423, in accordance with Sir H. Davy's experiments. He found that 50 measures detonated in a glass tube over pure mercury, lost their brilliant colour, and became 60 measures, of which 40 were chlorine and 20 oxygen.

This gas must be collected and examined with much prudence, and in very small quantities. A gentle heat, even that of the hand, will cause its explosion, with such force as to burst thin glass. From this facility of decomposition, it is not easy to ascertain the action of combustible bodies upon it. None of the metals that burn in chlorine act upon this gas at common temperatures; but when the oxygen is separated, they then inflame in the clorine. This may be readily exhibited, by first introducing into the protoxide a little Dutch foil, which will not be even tarnished; but on applying a heated glass tube to the gas in the neck of the bottle, decomposition instantly takes place, and the foil burns with brilliancy. When already in chemical union, therefore, chlorine has a stronger attraction for oxygen than for metals; but when insulated, its affinity for the latter is predominant. Protoxide of chlorine has no action on mercury, but chlorine is rapidly condensed by this metal into calomel. Thus, the two gases may be completely separated. When phosphorus is introduced into the protoxide, it instantly burns, as it would do in a mixture of two volumes of chlorine and one of oxygen; and a chloride and acid of phosphorus result. Lighted taper and burning sulphur likewise instantly decompose it. When the protoxide, freed from water, is made to act on dry vegetable colours, it gradually destroys them, but first gives to the blues a tint of red; from which, from its absorbability by water, and the strongly acrid taste of the solution approaching to sour, it may be considered as approximating to an acid in its nature."—*Ure.*

Chlorure of iodine. The chloriodic acid.

CHNUS. (From χναυω, to grind, or rasp.) 1. Chaff; Bran.

2. Fine wool, or lint, which is, as it were, rasped from lint.

CHO'ANA. (Χοανα, a funnel; from χεω, to pour out.) 1. A funnel.

2. The infundibulum of the kidney and brain.

CHO'ANUS. A furnace made like a funnel, for melting metals.

CHO'COLATE. (Dr. Alston says this word is compounded of two Indian words, *choco*, sound, and *atte*, water; because of the noise made in its preparation.) An article of diet prepared from the cacao-nut; highly nourishing, particularly when boiled with milk and eggs. It is frequently recommended as a restorative in cases of emaciation and consumption. See *Theobroma cacao.*

Chocolate tree. See *Theobroma cacao.*

CHŒ'NICIS. (From χοινικις, the nave of a wheel.) The trepan; so called by Galen and P. Ægineta.

CHŒ'RADES. (From χοιρος, a swine.) The same as scrofula.

CHŒRADOLE'THRON. (From χοιρος, a swine, and ολεθρος, destruction; so named from its being dangerous if eaten by hogs.) Hogbane. A name in Aëtius for the *Xanthium*, or louse-bur.

CHOI'RAS. (From χοιρος, a swine; so called because hogs are diseased with it.) See *Scrofula.*

Choke damp. The name given by miners to a noxious air, which is now known to be *carbonic acid gas*, found in mines, wells, and mineral springs. See *Carbonic acid.*

CHO'LADES. (From χολη, the bile.) So the smaller intestines are called, because they contain bile.

CHOLÆUS. (Χολαιος, bilious.) Biliary.

CHOLA'GO. See *Cholas.*

CHOLAGO'GA. (From χολη, bile, and αγω, to evacuate.) *Chologon.* By cholagogues, the ancients meant only such purging medicines as expelled the internal fæces, which resembled the cystic bile in their yellow colour, and other properties.

CHO'LAS. (From χολη, the bile.) *Cholago.* All the cavity of the right hypochondrium, and part of the neighbourhood, is so called because it contains the liver which is the strainer of the gall.

CHO'LE. Χολη. The bile.

CHOLE'DOCHUS. (From χολη, bile, and δεχομαι, to receive; receiving or retaining the gall.) The receptacle of bile.

CHOLEDOCHUS DUCTUS. *Ductus communis choledochus.* The common biliary duct, which conveys both cystic and hepatic bile into the intestinum duodenum.

CHOLE'GON. See *Cholagoga.*

CHOLERA. (Celsus derives it from χολη, and ρεω, literally a flow of bile, and Trallian, from χολας, and ρεω, intestinal flux.) *Diarrhœa cholerica; Felliflua passio.* A genus of disease arranged by Cullen in the class *Neuroses*, and order *Spasmi.* It is a purging and vomiting of bile, with anxiety, painful gripings, spasms of the abdominal muscles, and those of the calves of the legs. There are two species of this genus:—1. *Cholera spontanea*, which happens, in hot seasons, without any manifest cause. 2. *Cholera accidentalis*, which occurs after the use of food that digests slowly, and irritates. In warm climates it is met with at all seasons of the year, and its occurrence is very frequent; but in England, and other cold climates, it is apt to be most prevalent in the middle of summer, particularly in the month of August; and the violence of the disease has usually been observed to be greater in proportion to the intenseness of the heat. It usually comes on with soreness, pain, distension, and flatulency in the stomach and intestines, succeeded quickly by a severe and frequent vomiting, and purging of bilious matter, heat, thirst, a hurried respiration, and frequent but weak and fluttering pulse. When the disease is not violent, these symptoms, after continuing for a day or two, cease gradually, leaving the patient in a debilitated and exhausted state; but where the disease proceeds with much violence, there arises great depression of strength, with cold clammy sweats, considerable anxiety, a hurried and short respiration, and hiccups, with a sinking, and irregularity of the pulse, which quickly terminate in death; an event that not unfrequently happens within the space of twenty-four hours.

The appearances generally observed on dissection are, a quantity of bilious matter in the primæ viæ, the ducts of the liver relaxed and distended; and several of the viscera have been found displaced, probably by the violent vomiting. In the early period of the disease, when the strength is not much exhausted, the object is to lessen the irritation, and facilitate the discharge of the bile, by tepid demulcent liquids, frequently exhibited. It will likewise be useful to procure a determination to the surface by fomentations to the abdomen, the pediluvium, or even the warm bath. But where the symptoms are urgent, and the patient appears rapidly sinking from the continued vomiting, violent pain, &c. it is necessary to give opium freely, but in a small bulk; from one to three grains, or even more, in a table spoonful of linseed infusion, or with an effervescing saline draught; which must be repeated at short intervals, every hour perhaps, till relief be obtained. Sometimes, where the stomach could not be got to retain the opium, it has answered in the form of clyster; or a liniment containing it may be rubbed into the abdomen; or a blister, applied over the stomach, may lessen the irritability of that organ. Afterward the bile may be allowed to evacuate itself downwards; or mild aperients, or clysters, given, if necessary, to promote its discharge. When the urgent symptoms are relieved, the strength must be restored by gentle tonics, as the aromatic bitters, calumba, and the like, with a light nutritious diet: strong toast and water is the best drink, or a little burnt brandy may be added if there is much langour. Exposure to cold must be carefully avoided, particularly keeping the abdomen and the feet warm; and great attention is necessary to regulate the bowels, and procure a regular discharge of bile, lest a relapse should happen. It will also be proper to examine the state of the abdomen, whether pressure give pain at any part, because inflammation in the primæ viæ is very liable to supervene, often in an insidious manner; should that be the case, leeches, blistering the part, and other suitable means, must be promptly resorted to.

CHOLE'RICA. (From χολερα, the cholera.) Medicines which relieve the cholera.

CHOLESTERIC ACID. "When the fat matter of the human biliary calculi is treated with nitric acid, which Chevreuil proposed to call cholesterine, there is formed a peculiar acid, which is called the cholesteric. To obtain it, the cholesterine is heated with its weight of concentrated nitric acid, by which it is speedily attacked and dissolved. There is disengaged, at the same time, much oxide of azot; and the liquor, on cooling, and especially on the addition of water, lets fall a yellow matter, which is the cholesteric acid impure, or impregnated with nitric acid. It may be purified by repeated washings in boiling water. However, after having washed it, it is better to effect its fusion in the midst of hot water; to add to it a small quantity of carbonate of lead; to let the whole boil for some hours, decanting and renewing the water from time to time; then to put the remaining dried mass in contact with alkohol, and to evaporate the alkoholic solution. The residuum now obtained is the purest possible cholesteric acid.

This acid has an orange-yellow colour when it is in mass; but it appears in white needles, when dissolved in alkohol, and left to spontaneous evaporation. Its taste is very feeble, and slightly styptic; its taste resembles that of butter; and its specific gravity is intermediate between that of alkohol and water. It fuses at 58° C. and is not decomposed till the temperature be raised much above that of boiling water. It then affords oil, water, carbonic acid, and carburetted hydrogen, but no trace of ammonia. It is very soluble in alkohol, sulphuric and acetic æther, in the volatile oils of lavender, rosemary, turpentine, bergamot, &c. It is, on the other hand, insoluble in the fixed oils of olives, sweet almonds, and castor oil. It is equally so in the vegetable acids, and almost entirely insoluble in water, which takes up merely enough to make it redden litmus. Both in the cold, and with heat, nitric acid dissolves without altering it. Concentrated sulphuric acid acting on it for a considerable time, only carbonizes it.

It appears that the cholesteric acid is capable of uniting with the greater part of the salifiable bases. All the resulting salts are coloured, some yellow, others orange, and others red. The cholesterates of potassa, soda, ammonia, and probably of morphia, are very soluble and deliquescent; almost all the others are insoluble, or nearly so. There is none of them which cannot be decomposed by all the mineral acids, except the carbonic, and by the greater part of the vegetable acids; so that on pouring one of these acids into a solution of the cholesterate, the cholesteric acid is instantly separated in flocks. The soluble cholesterates form precipitates in all the metallic solutions, whose base has the property of forming an insoluble or slightly soluble salt with cholesteric acid.

Pelletier and Caventou found the cholesterate of barytes to consist of 100 of acid, and 56.259 base; whence the prime equivalent of the former appears to be about 17.35. Yet they observed, on the other hand, that on treating the cholesterate of lead with sulphuric acid, they obtained as much sulphate of lead as of cholesterate. From this experiment, the equivalent of the dry acid would seem to be 5; hence we may imagine, that when the cholesteric acid unites to the oxide of lead, and in general to all the oxides which have a slight affinity for oxygen, there takes place something similar to what happens in the reaction of oxide of lead and oxalic acid."—*Journ. de Phar.* iii. 292.

CHOLESTERINE. The name given by Chevreuil to the pearly substance of human biliary calculi. It consists of 72 carbon, 6.66 oxygen, and 21.33 hydrogen, by Berard.

CHOLICE'LE. (From χολη, bile, and κηλη, a tumour.) A swelling formed by the bile accumulated in the gall-bladder.

CHOLOLITHUS. (From χολη, bile, and λιθος, a stone, gall-stone.) A name of a genus of disease in the Class, *Cœliaca*; Order, *Splanchnica*, of Good's Nosology, characterized by pain about the region of the liver, catenating with pain at the pit of the stomach; the pulse unchanged; sickness; dyspepsy; inactivity; bilious concretion in the gall bladder, or bile ducts. It has two species, *Chololithus quiescens*, the quiescent gall-stone, and *C. means*, the passing of gall-stones.

CHOLOLITHICUS. Of or belonging to gall-stone.

CHOLO'MA. (From χωλος, lame, or maimed.) 1. A halting, or lameness in the leg.

2. Galen says that, in Hippocrates, it signifies any distortion of a limb.

CHONDRO. Some muscles have this word forming a part of their name, because they are connected with a particular cartilage.

CHONDROGLO'SSUS. (From χονδρον, a cartilage, and γλωσση, the tongue.) A muscle so named from its insertion, which is in the basis or cartilaginous part of the tongue. See *Hyoglossus*.

CHONDRO'LOGY. (*Chondrologia*; from χονδρος, a cartilage, and λογος, a discourse.) A discourse on cartilages.

CHONDRO-PHARYNGÆUS. (From χονδρος, a cartilage, and φαρυγξ, the upper part of the fauces.) A muscle so named because it rises in the cartilaginous part of the tongue, and is inserted in the pharynx.

CHO'NDROS. Χονδρος. 1. A cartilage.

2. A food of the ancients, the same as alica.

3. Any grumous concretion.

CHONDROSYNDE'SMUS. (From χονδρος, a cartilage, and συνδεω, to tie together.) A cartilaginous ligament.

CHO'NDRUS. A cartilage.

CHO'NE. Χωνη. The infundibulum.

CHO'RA. Χωρα. A region. Galen, in his book De Usu Partium, expresses by it particularly the cavities of the eyes; but, in others of his writings, he intimates by it any void space.

CHO'RDA. (From χορδη, which properly signifies an intestine, or gut, of which a chord may be made.) 1. A cord, or assemblage of fibres.

2. A tendon.

3. A painful tension of the penis in the venerea disease.

4. Sometimes the intestines are called chordæ.

CHORDA MAGNA. A name of the *tendo Achillis*

CHORDA TYMPANI. A branch of the seventh pair of nerves. The portio dura of the seventh pair of nerves, having entered the tympanum, sends a small branch to the stapes, and another more considerable one, which runs across the tympanum from behind forwards, passes between the long leg of the incus and the handle of the malleus, then goes out at the same place where the tendon of the anterior muscle of the malleus enters. It is called chorda tympani, because it crosses the tympanum as a cord crosses the bottom of a drum. Dr. Monro thinks, that the chorda tympani is formed by the second branch of the fifth pair, as well as by the portio dura of the seventh.

CHORDA TENDINEA. The tendinous and cord-like substances which connect the *carneæ columnæ* of the ventricles of the heart to the auricular valves.

CHORDA WILLISII. The small fibres which cross the sinuses of the dura mater. They are so termed, because Willis first described them.

CHORDA'PSUS. (From χορδη, a cord, and απτω, to knit.) A sort of painful colic, where the intestines appear to be twisted into knots.

CHORDEE'. (*Chordé*. French.) A spasmodic contraction of the penis, that sometimes attends gonorrhœa, and is often followed by a hæmorrhage.

CHO'REA. (Χορεια; from χορος, a chorus, which of old accompanied dancing. It is called St. Vitus's dance, because some devotees of St. Vitus exercised themselves so long in dancing, that their intellects were disordered, and could only be restored by dancing again at the anniversary of St. Vitus.) *Chorea Sancti Viti. Synclonus chorea* of Good. St. Vitus's dance. Convulsive motions of the limbs, as if the person were dancing. It is a genus of disease, arranged by Cullen in the class *Neuroses*; and order *Spasmi*. These convulsive motions, most generally, are confined to one side, and affect principally the arm and leg. When any motion is attempted to be made, various fibres of other muscles act which ought not; and thus a contrary effect is produced from what the patient intended. It is chiefly incident to young persons of both sexes, and makes its attack between the age of ten and fifteen, occurring but seldom after that of puberty.

By some practitioners it has been considered rather as a paralytic affection than as a convulsive disorder, and has been thought to arise from a relaxation of the muscles, which, being unable to perform their functions in moving the limbs, shake them irregularly by jerks. Chorea Sancti Viti is occasioned by various irritations, as teething, worms, offensive smells, poisons, &c. It arises likewise in consequence of violent affections of the mind, as horror, fear, and anger. In many cases it is produced by general weakness; and, in a few, it takes place from sympathy, at seeing the disease in others.

The fits are sometimes preceded by a coldness of the feet and limbs, or a kind of tingling sensation, that ascends like cold air up the spine, and there is a flatulent pain in the left hypochondrium, with obstinate costiveness. At other times, the accession begins with yawning, stretching, anxiety about the heart, palpitations, nausea, difficulty of swallowing, noise in the ears, giddiness, and pains in the head and teeth; and then come on the convulsive motions.

These discover themselves at first by a kind of lameness, or instability of one of the legs, which the person draws after him in an odd and ridiculous manner; nor can he hold the arm of the same side still for a moment: for if he lays it on his breast, or any other part of his body, it is forced quickly from thence by an involuntary motion. If he is desirous of drinking, he uses many singular gesticulations before he can carry the cup to his head, and it is forced in various directions, till at length he gets it to his mouth; when he pours the liquor down his throat in great haste, as if he meant to afford amusement to the by-standers. Sometimes various attempts at running and leaping take place; and at others, the head and trunk of the body are affected with convulsive motions. In many instances, the mind is affected with some degree of fatuity, and often shows the same causeless emotions (such as weeping and laughing) which occur in hysteria. When this disease arises in children, it usually ceases about the age of puberty; and in adults, is often carried off by a change from the former mode of living. Unless it passes into some other disease, such as epilepsy, it is hardly attended with danger.

The leading indications in the treatment of this complaint are, 1. To obviate the several exciting causes; 2. To correct any faulty state of the constitution, which may appear to give a predisposition; 3. To use those means which experience has shown best calculated to allay irregular muscular action. Among the sources of irritation, the most common is the state of the bowels; and the steady, but moderate, use of active cathartics has often a great effect upon the disease, improving the appetite and strength at the same time. Senna, scammony, jalap, &c. may be exhibited according to circumstances, often in conjunction with calomel, particularly where the liver is torpid. The general debility usually attending indicates the employment of tonics, as the cinchona, chalybeates, or sulphate of zinc, which is particularly useful; and with these, cold bathing, not too long continued, may be advantageously conjoined; also requiring the patient to use muscular exertion, as much as they can readily, will assist materially in the cure. Sometimes in violent cases, and in irritable constitutions, the occasional exhibition of opium, or other sedative, may be required, taking care, however, that the bowels are not confined thereby. Occasionally too, where the above means are not successful, the more powerful antispasmodics may be tried, as æther, camphor, musk, &c. Electricity also has been by some recommended.

CHO'RION. (From χωρεω, to escape; because it always escapes from the uterus with the fœtus.) Shaggy chorion. The external membrane of the fœtus in utero.

CHO'ROID. (*Choroidea;* from χοριον, the chorion, and ειδος, resemblance.) Resembling the chorion, a membrane of the fœtal ovum.

CHOROID MEMBRANE. *Membrana choroides.* The second tunic of the eye, lying immediately under the sclerotica, to which it is connected by vessels. The true knowledge of this membrane is necessary to a perfect idea of the iris and uvea. The tunica choroidea commences at the optic nerve, and passes forwards, with the sclerotic coat, to the beginning of the cornea transparens, where it adheres very firmly to the sclerotic membrane, by means of a cellular membrane, in the form of a white fringe, called the *ciliary circle.* It then recedes from the sclerotica and cornea and ciliary circle, directly downwards and inwards, forming a round disk, which is variously coloured; hence, blue, black eyes, &c. This coloured portion, reflected inwards, is termed the *iris*, and its posterior surface is termed *uvea.* The choroid membrane is highly vascular, and its external vessels are disposed like stars, and termed *vasa vorticosa.* The internal surface of this membrane is covered with a black pigment, called the pigment of the choroid membrane.

CHOROID PLEXUS. *Plexus choroideus.* A plexus of blood-vessels, situated in the lateral ventricles of the brain.

Choroid tunic. See *Choroid membrane.*

CHRI'SIS. (From χριω, to anoint.) An inunction, or anointing of any part.

Christmas rose. See *Helleborus niger.*

CHRIS'TUM. (From χριω, to anoint.) An unguent, or ointment of any kind.

CHRO'MAS. A chromate, or salt, formed by the union of chromic acid with salifiable bases; as chromate of lead, &c.

["*Chromate of iron*, is found in large quantities, at the bare hills, near Baltimore, (Maryland,) massive and granular, in veins and masses disseminated through a serpentine rock. Perhaps in no part of the world has so much been discovered at one place. it furnishes the means of preparing the beautiful paint called the chromic yellow, with which carriages and furniture are now painted in the United States. Chromate of iron, in octaedral crystals, very small and magnetic, is found at the same place, and has nowhere else been discovered, as far as we can learn from the writings of mineralogists. The crystals are found in the ravines, and on the sand of the rivulets of the bare-hills, mixed with granular chromate of iron. The *green oxide of chrome* is also found there, colouring the talc, as well as the *ruby* or *violet coloured ore.*"—*Bruce's Min. Jour.* A.]

CHROMATI'SMUS. (From χρωματιζω, to colour.) The morbid discoloration of any of the secretions, as of the urine, or blood.

CHRO'MIC ACID. *Acidum chromicum.* "This acid was extracted from the red lead ore of Siberia, by treating this ore with carbonate of potassa, and separating the alkali by means of a more powerful acid. In this state it is a red or orange-coloured powder, of a peculiar rough metallic taste, which is more sensible in it than in any other metallic acid. If this powder be exposed to the action of light and heat, it loses its acidity, and is converted into green oxide of chrome, giving out pure oxygen gas. The chromic acid is the first that has been found to deoxygenate itself easily by the action of heat, and afford oxygen gas by this simple operation. It appears that several of its properties are owing to the weak adhesion of a part at least of its oxygen. The green oxide of chrome cannot be brought back to the state of an acid, unless its oxygen be restored by treating it with some other acid.

The chromic acid is soluble in *water*, and crystallizes, by cooling and evaporation, in longish prisms of a ruby red. Its taste is acrid and styptic. Its specific gravity is not exactly known; but it always exceeds that of water. It powerfully reddens the tincture of turnsole.

Its action on *combustible substances* is little known If it be strongly heated with charcoal, it grows black, and passes to the metallic state without melting

Of the *acids*, the action of the muriatic on it is the most remarkable. If this be distilled with the chromic acid, by a gentle heat, it is readily converted into chlorine. It likewise imparts to it by mixture the property of dissolving gold; in which the chromic resembles the nitric acid. This is owing to the weak adhesion of its oxygen, and it is the only one of the metallic acids that possesses this property.

The extraction of chromic acid from the French ore, is performed by igniting it with its own weight of nitre in a crucible. The residue is lixiviated with water which being then filtered, contains the chromate of potassa. On pouring into this a little nitric acid and muriate of barytes, an instantaneous precipitate of the chromate of barytes takes place. After having procured a certain quantity of this salt, it must be put in its moist state into a capsule, and dissolved in the smallest possible quantity of weak nitric acid. The barytes is to be then precipitated by very dilute sulphuric acid, taking care not to add an excess of it. When the liquid is found by trial to contain neither sulphuric acid nor barytes, it must be filtered. It now consists of water, with nitric and chromic acids. The whole is to be evaporated to dryness, conducting the heat at the end so as not to endanger the decomposition of the chromic acid, which will remain in the capsule under the form of a reddish matter. It must be kept in a glass phial well corked.

Chromic acid, heated with a powerful acid, becomes *chromic oxide;* while the latter, heated with the hydrate of an alkali, becomes chromic acid. As the solution of the oxide is green, and that of the acid yellow, these transmutations become very remarkable to the eye. From Berzelius's experiments on the combinations of the chromic acid with barytes, and oxide of lead, its prime equivalent seems to be 6.5; consisting of 3.5 chromium, and 3.0 oxygen.

It readily unites with *alkalies*, and is the only acid that has the property of colouring its salts, whence the name of chromic has been given it. If two parts of the red lead ore of Siberia in fine powder be boiled with one of an alkali saturated with carbonic acid, in forty parts of water, a carbonate of lead will be precipitated, and the *chromate* remain dissolved. The solutions are of a lemon colour, and afford crystals of a somewhat deeper hue. Those of *chromate of ammonia* are in yellow laminæ, having the metallic lustre of gold.

The *chromate of barytes* is very little soluble, and that of lime still less. They are both of a pale yellow, and when heated give out oxygen gas, as do the alkaline chromates.

If the chromic acid be mixed with filings of tin and the muriatic acid, it becomes at first yellowish-brown, and afterward assumes a bluish-green colour, which preserves the same shade after desiccation. Æther alone gives it the same dark colour. With a solution of nitrate of mercury, it gives a precipitate of a dark cinnabar colour. With a solution of nitrate of silver, it gives a precipitate, which, the moment it is formed, appears of a beautiful carmine colour, but becomes purple by exposure to the light. This combination, exposed to the heat of the blow-pipe, melts before the charcoal is inflamed, and assumes a blackish and metallic appearance. If it be then pulverized, the powder is still purple; but after the blue flame of the lamp is brought into contact with this powder, it assumes a green colour, and the silver appears in globules disseminated through its substance.

With nitrate of copper it gives a chesnut-red precipitate. With the solution of sulphate of zinc, muriate of bismuth, muriate of antimony, nitrate of nickel, and muriate of platina, it produces yellowish precipitates, when the solutions do not contain an excess of acid. With muriate of gold it produces a greenish precipitate.

When melted with borax, or glass, or acid of phosphorus, it communicates to it a beautiful emerald-green colour.

If paper be impregnated with it, and exposed to the sun a few days, it acquires a green colour, which remains permanent in the dark.

A slip of iron, or tin, put into its solution, imparts to it the same colour.

The aqueous solution of tannin produces a flocculent precipitate of a brown fawn colour.

Sulphuric acid, when cold, produces no effect on it; but when warm it makes it assume a bluish-green colour."—*Ure's Dict.*

CHROMIUM. (*Chromium, ii.* n.; from χρωμα, colour: because it is remarkable for giving colour to its combinations.) The name of a metal which may be extracted either from the native chromate of lead or of iron. The latter being cheapest and most abundant, is usually employed.

The brown chromate of iron is not acted upon by nitric acid, but most readily by nitrate of potassa, with the aid of a red heat. A chromate of potassa, soluble in water, is thus formed. The iron oxide thrown out of combination may be removed from the residual part of the ore by a short digestion in dilute muriatic acid. A second fusion with ¼ of nitre, will give rise to a new portion of chromate of potassa. Having decomposed the whole of the ore, we saturate the alkaline excess with nitric acid, evaporate and crystallize. The pure crystals, dissolved in water, are to be added to a solution of neutral nitrate of mercury; whence, by complex affinity, red chromate of mercury precipitates. Moderate ignition expels the mercury from the chromate, and the remaining chromic acid may be reduced to the metallic state, by being exposed in contact of the charcoal from sugar, to a violent heat.

Chromium thus procured, is a porous mass of agglutinated grains. It is very brittle, and of a grayish-white, intermediate between tin and steel. It is sometimes obtained in needleform crystals, which cross each other in all directions. Its sp. gravity is 5.9. It is susceptible of a feeble magnetism. It resists all the acids except nitromuriatic, which, at a boiling heat, oxidizes it and forms a muriate. Thenard describes only one oxide of chromium; but there are probably two, besides the acid already described.

1. The *protoxide* is green, infusible, indecomposable by heat, reducible by voltaic electricity, and not acted on by oxygen or air. When heated to dull redness with the half of its weight of potassium or sodium, it forms a brown matter, which, cooled and exposed to the air, burns with flame, and is transformed into chromate of potassa or soda, of a canary-yellow colour. It is this oxide which is obtained by calcining the chromate of mercury in a small earthen retort about ¾ of an hour. The beak of the retort is to be surrounded with a tube of wet linen, and plunged into water, to facilitate the condensation of the mercury. The oxide, newly precipitated from acids, has a dark-green colour, and is easily redissolved; but exposure to a dull-red heat ignites it, and renders it denser, insoluble, and of a light-green colour. This change arises solely from the closer aggregation of the particles, for the weight is not altered.

2. The *deutoxide* is procured by exposing the protonitrate to heat, till the fumes of nitrous gas cease to issue. A brilliant brown powder, insoluble in acids, and scarcely soluble in alkalies, remains. Muriatic acid digested on it exhales chlorine, showing the increased proportion of oxygen in this oxide.

3. The *tritoxide* has been already described among the acids. It may be directly procured by adding nitrate of lead to the above nitrochromate of potassa, and digesting the beautiful orange precipitate of chromate of lead with moderately strong muriatic acid, till its power of action be exhausted. The fluid produced is to be passed through a filter, and a little oxide of silver very gradually added, till the whole solution becomes of a deep red tint. This liquor, by slow evaporation, deposites small ruby-red crystals, which are the hydrated chromic acid. The prime equivalent of chromic acid deduced from the chromates of barytes and lead by Berzelius, is 6.544, if we suppose them to be neutral salts. According to this chemist, the acid contains double the oxygen that the green oxide does. But if those chromates be regarded as subsalts, then the acid prime would be 13.088, consisting of 6 oxygen = 7.088 metal; while the protoxide would consist of 3 oxyxen + 7.088 metal; and the deutoxide of an intermediate proportion.

CHRO'NIC. (*Chronicus;* from χρονος, time.) A term applied to diseases which are of long continuance, and mostly without fever. It is used in opposition to the term acute. See *Acute.*

CHRU'PSIA. (From χροα, colour, and οψις, sight.) *Visus coloratus.* A disease of the eyes, in which the person perceives objects of a different colour from their natural one.

CHRYSA'NTHEMUM. (From χρυσος, gold, and ανθεμον, a flower.) 1. The name of a genus of plants in the Linnæan system. Class, *Syngenesia*; Order. *Polygamia.* Sun-flower, or marigold.

2. Many herbs are so called, the flowers of which are of a bright yellow colour.

Chrysanthemum leucanthemum. The systematic name of the great ox-eye daisy. Maudlin-wort *Bellis-major; Buphthalmum majus; Leucanthemum vulgare; Bellidioides; Consolida media; Oculus bovis.* The *Chrysanthemum;—foliis amplexicaulibus, oblongis, supernè serratis, infernè dentatis*, of Linnæus. The flowers and herb were formerly esteemed in asthmatic and phthisical diseases, but have now deservedly fallen into disuse.

Chry'se. (From χρυσος, gold.) The name of a yellow plaster.

Chysele'ctrum. (From χρυσος, gold, and ηλεκτρον, amber.) Amber of a golden yellow colour.

Chrysi'ppea. (From *Chrysippus*, its discoverer.) An herb enumerated by Pliny.

Chrysi'tis. (From χρυσος, gold.) 1. Litharge.

2. The yellow foam of lead.

3. The herb yarrow, from the golden colour of its flower.

CHRYSOBA'LANUS. (From χρυσος, gold, and βαλανος, a nut; so named because of its colour, which, before it is dried, is yellow.) The nutmeg.

CHRYSOBERYL. Cymophane of Haüy. A mineral of an asparagus green colour and vitreous lustre, found in the Brazil, and Ceylon.

[Chrysoberyl is found in the United States, and is sometimes employed in jewelry. In the township of Haddam, on the Connecticut river, and in the State of Connecticut, it occurs in granite in six-sided prisms and six-sided tables; its colour varies from greenish yellow to yellowish green. A.]

CHRYSOCO'LLA. (From χρυσος, gold, and κολλη, cement.) Gold solder; Borax.

CHYSO'COMA. (From χρυσος, gold, and κομη, hair; so called from its golden, hair like appearance.) The herb milfoil, or yarrow. See *Achillea millefolium.*

Chrysogo'nia. (From χρυσος, gold, and γινομαι, to become.) A tincture of gold.

Chrysola'chanon. (From χρυσος, gold, and λαχανον, a pot-herb; so named from its having a yellow leaf.) The herb orach; a species of atriplex.

CHRYSOLITE. Peridot of Haüy. Topaz of the ancients, while our topaz is their chrysolite. The hardest of all gems of a pistachio-green colour. It comes from Egypt and Bohemia.

CHRYSOSPLE'NIUM. (From χρυσος, gold, and ασπλενιον, spleenwort.) The name of a genus of plants in the Linnæan system. Class, *Decandria*; Order, *Digynia*. Golden saxifrage.

CHRYSOPRASE. A variety of calcedony.

Chrysu'lcus. (From χρυσος, gold, and ελκω, to take away.) The aqua regia which has the property of dissolving gold.

[CHURCH, Dr. Benjamin, was graduated at Howard College in 1754. He established himself as a physician in the town of Boston, where he rose to very considerable eminence in his profession. As a skilful and dexterous operator in surgery, he was inferior to no one of his contemporaries in New-England; and as a physician, he was in a career of distinguished reputation. He possessed a brilliant genius, a lively poetic fancy, and was an excellent writer. For several years preceding the American revolution, he was a conspicuous character, and had great influence among the leading whigs and patriots of the day. When the war commenced in 1775, his character was so high that he was appointed physician-general to the army.

But while he was performing the duties assigned him, circumstances occurred which led to a suspicion that he held a treacherous correspondence with the enemy. Certain letters in cipher were intercepted, which he had written to a relation in Boston. He was immediately arrested, imprisoned, and tried before a military tribunal appointed to investigate his conduct, and was pronounced guilty of a criminal correspondence with the enemy. It appears that the only evidence by which he was convicted, rested on an intercepted letter directed to a friend in Boston. This letter was written in cipher, and when it was deciphered and examined, its contents seemed in a considerable degree to justify the plea which he had made, that it was designed as an innocent stratagem to deceive and draw from the enemy some information for the benefit of the public. Dr. C. was, at the same time, a member of the House of Representatives, from which he would have been expelled had he not resigned his seat. He was, however, arraigned before the House, subjected to a rigid examination, and his letter was read by himself by paragraphs, and commented upon, and explained. His defence before the House may be considered as a specimen of brilliant talents and great ingenuity. "Confirmed," said he, in assured innocence, "I stand prepared for your keenest searchings. The warmest bosom here does not flame with a brighter zeal for the security, happiness, and liberties of America, than mine." So high was party zeal, and such the jealousy and prejudice of the day, that a torrent of indignation was ever at hand to sweep from the land every guilty or suspected character. In the instance of Dr. C., there were not a few among the most respectable and intelligent of the community, who expressed strong doubts of a criminal design in his conduct. It was, however, his hard fate to pine in prison until the following year, when he obtained permission to depart for the West Indies. The vessel in which he sailed was supposed to have foundered at sea, as no tidings respecting her were ever obtained. A.]

CHUSITE. A yellowish-green translucent mineral, found by Saussure in the cavities of porphyries, in the environs of Limbourg.

CHYAZIC ACID. See *Prussic acid*.

Chyla'ria. (From χυλος, chyle.) A discharge of a whitish mucous urine, of the colour and consistence of chyle.

CHYLE. *Chylus*. The milk-like liquor observed some hours after eating, in the lacteal vessels of the mesentery, and in the thoracic duct. It is separated by digestion from the chyme, and is that fluid substance from which the blood is formed. See *Digestion*.

"The chyle may be studied under two different forms:

1st, When it is mixed with chyme in the small intestine.

2d, Under the liquid form, circulating in the chyliferous vessels, and the thoracic duct.

No person having particularly engaged in the examination of the chyle during its stay in the small intestine, our knowledge on this point is little. The liquid chyle contained in the chyliferous vessels has been examined with great care.

In order to procure it, the best manner consists in giving food to an animal, and, when the digestion is supposed to be in full activity, to strangle it, or to cut the spinal marrow behind the occipital bone. The whole length of the breast is cut open; the hand is thrust in so as to pass a ligature which embraces the aorta, the œsophagus, and the thoracic duct, the nearest to the neck possible; the ribs of the left side are then twisted or broken, and the thoracic duct is seen, closely adhering to the œsophagus. The upper part is detached, and carefully wiped, to absorb the blood; it is cut, and the chyle flows into the vessel intended to receive it.

The ancients were acquainted with the existence of the chyle, but their ideas of it were very inexact; it was observed anew at the beginning of the seventeenth century; and being, in certain conditions, of an opaque white, it was compared to milk: the vessels that contain it were even named *lacteal vessels*, a very improper expression, since there is very little other similarity between chyle and milk except the colour.

It is only in modern times, and by the labours of Dupuytren, Vauquelin, Emmert, and Marcet, that positive notions concerning the chyle have been acquired.

We shall give the observations of these learned men, with the addition of our own.

If the animal from which the chyle is extracted has eaten animal or vegetable substances of a fatty nature, the liquid drawn from the thoracic duct is of a milky white, a little heavier than distilled water, of a strong spermatic odour, of a salt taste, slightly adhering to the tongue, and sensibly alkaline.

Chyle, very soon after it has passed out of the vesse that contained it, becomes firm, and almost solid: after some time, it separates into three parts; the one solid that remains at the bottom, another liquid at the top, and a third that forms a very thin layer at the surface of the liquids. The chyle, at the same time, assumes a vivid rose colour.

When the chyle proceeds from food that contains no fat substance, it presents the same sort of properties, but instead of being opaque white, it is opaline, and almost transparent; the layer which forms at the top is less marked than in the former sort of chyle.

Chyle never takes the hue of the colouring substances mixed in the food, as many authors have pretended.

Animals that were made to eat indigo, saffron, and madder, furnished a chyle, the colour of which had no relation to that of the substances.

Of the three substances into which the chyle separates when abandoned to itself, that of the surface, of an opaque white colour, is a fatty body; the solid part is formed of fibrin and a little colouring matter; the liquid is like the serum of the blood.

The proportion of these three parts is variable according to the nature of the food. There are species of chyle, such as that the sugar, which contain very little fibrin; others, such as that of flesh, contain more. The same thing happens with the fat matter, which is very abundant when the food contains grease or oil, while there is scarcely any seen when the food is nearly deprived of fatty bodies.

The absorption of the chyle has been attributed to the capillarity of the lacteal radicles, to the compression of the chyle by the sides of the small intestine, &c. Latterly, it has been pretended that it takes place by virtue of the proper sensibility of the absorbing mouths, and of the insensible organic contractility that they are supposed to possess. It first enters the threads of the lacteal vessels, it then traverses the mesenteric glands, it arrives at the thoracic duct, and at last enters the subclavian vein.

The causes that determine its motion are the contractility proper to the chyliferous vessels, the unknown cause of its absorption, the pressure of the abdominal muscles, particularly in the motions of respiration, and, perhaps, the pulsation of the arteries of the abdomen.

If we wish to have a correct idea of the velocity with which the chyle flows into the thoracic duct, we must open this canal in a living animal, at the place where it opens into the subclavian vein. We find that this rapidity is not very great, and that it increases every time that the animal compresses the viscera of the abdomen, by the abdominal muscles; a similar effect is produced by compressing the belly with the hand.

However, the rapidity of the circulation of the chyle appears to me to be in proportion to the quantity formed in the small intestine; this last is in proportion to the quantity of the chyme: so that if the food is in great abundance, and of easy digestion, the chyle will flow quickly; if, on the contrary, the food is in small quantity, or, which is the same thing, if it is of difficult digestion, as less chyle will be formed, so its progress will be more slow.

It would be difficult to appreciate the quantity of chyle that would be formed during a given digestion, though it ought to be considerable. In a dog of ordinary size, that had eaten animal food at discretion, an incision into the thoracic duct of the neck (the dog being alive) gave about half an ounce of liquid in five minutes, and the running was not suspended during the whole continuance of the formation of the chyle, that is, during several hours.

It is not known whether there is any variation in the rapidity of the motion of the chyle during the same digestion; but, supposing it uniform, there would enter six ounces of chyle per hour into the venous system. We may presume that the proportion of chyle is more considerable in man, whose chyliferous organs are more voluminous, and in whom the digestion is, in general, more rapid than in the dog."—*Magendie's Physiology.*

The chyle is mixed with the albuminous and gelatinous lymph in the thoracic duct, which receives them from the lymphatics.

The uses of the chyle are, 1. To supply the matter from which the blood and other fluids of our body are prepared; from which fluids the solid parts are formed. 2. By its acescent nature, it somewhat restrains the putrescent tendency of the blood: hence the dreadful putridity of the humours from starving; and thus milk is an excellent remedy against scurvy. 3. By its very copious aqueous latex, it prevents the thickening of the fluids, and thus renders them fit for the various secretions. 4. The chyle secreted in the breasts of puerperal women, under the name of milk, forms the most excellent nutriment of all aliments for new-born infants.

CHYLIFICA'TION. (*Chylificatio;* from *chylus,* and *fio,* to become.) *Chylifactio.* The process carried on in the small intestines, and principally in the duodenum, by which the chyle is separated from the chyme.

CHYLI'SMA. (From χυλος, juice.) An expressed juice.

CHYLOPOIE'TIC. (*Chylopoieticus;* from χυλος, chyle, and ποιεω, to make.) Chylopoietic. Any thing connected with the formation of chyle; thus chylopoietic viscera, chylopoietic vessels, &c.

CHYLO'SIS. (From χυλος, juice.) Chylification, or the changing the food into chyle.

CHYLOSTA'GMA. (From χυλος, juice, and ςαζω, to distil.) The distillation or expression of any juice, or humid part from the rest.

CHYLOSTAGMA DIAPHORETICUM. A name given by Mindererus to a distillation of Venice treacle and mithridate.

CHYLUS. (Χυλος, *succus,* from χυω, juice.) See *Chyle.*

CHYME. (*Chymus;* from χυμος, which signifies humour or juice.) The ingested mass of food that passes from the stomach into the duodenum, and from which the chyle is prepared in the small intestines by the admixture of the bile, &c. See *Digestion*

CHY'MIA. Chemistry.

CHYMIA'TER. A chemical physician.

CHYMIA'TRIA. (From χυμια, chemistry, and ιαομαι, to heal.) The art of curing diseases by the application of chemistry to the uses of medicine.

CHYMO'SIS. See *Chemosis.*

CHY'NLEN RADIX. A cylindrical root, of the thickness of a goose-quill, brought from China. It has a bitterish taste, and imparts a yellow tinge to the saliva. The Chinese hold it in great estimation as a stomachic, infused in wine.

CHY'SIS. (From χυω, to pour out.) Fusion, or the reduction of solid bodies into fluid by heat.

CHY'TLON. (From χυω, to pour out.) An anointing with oil and water.

CIBA'LIS. (From *cibus,* food.) Of or belonging to food.

CIBALIS FISTULA. An obsolete term for the œsophagus

CIBA'TIO. (From *cibus,* food.) The taking of food.

CI'BUR. An obsolete term for sulphur.

CICATRISANT. (*Cicatrisans;* from *cicatrico,* to skin over.) Such applications as dispose wounds and ulcers to dry up and heal, and to be covered with a skin.

CICA'TRIX. (From *cicatrico,* to heal up or skin over.) A seam or scar upon the skin, after the healing of a sore or ulcer.

Cicely, sweet. See *Scandix odorata.*

CI'CER. (A plant so called. The *Cicerones* had their name from this pulse, as the *Pisones* had from the pisum or pea, and the *Lentuli* from the lens or lentil.) 1. The name of a genus of plants in the Linnæan system. Class, *Diadelphia;* Order, *Decandria.* The vetch.

2. The pharmacopœial name of the common cich or ciches.

CICER ARIETINUM. The systematic name of the *cicer* plant. *Erebinthus; Cicer—foliis serratis,* of Linnæus. The seeds have been employed medicinally, but are now fallen into disuse. In some places they are toasted, and used as coffee; and in others, ground into a flour for bread. The colour of the arillus of the seed is sometimes white, red, or black; hence the distinction into *cicer album, rubrum,* and *nigrum.*

CI'CERA. (From *cicer,* the vetch.) A small pill of the size of a vetch.

CICERA TARTARI. Small pills composed of turpentine and cream of tartar, of the size of a vetch.

CICHO'RIUM. (Originally, according to Pliny, an Egyptian name, and adopted by the Greeks. It is written sometimes Κιχορειον: whence Horace has *cichoreæ, levesque malvæ:* sometimes Κιχοριον or Κιχωριον. It is supposed by some to have this name, παρα το δια των χωριων κιειν, from its creeping through the fields. Others derive it from κιχεω, *invenio;* on account of its being so readily found, or so common.) Succory. 1. The name of a genus of plants in the Linnæan system. Class, *Syngenesia;* Order, *Polygamia æqualis.*

2. The pharmacopœial name of the wild cichory. See *Cichorium intybus.*

CICHORIUM ENDIVIA. The systematic name of the endive. *Endivia; Endiva; Cichorium;—floribus solitariis, pendunculatis, foliis integris; crenatis,* of Linnæus, is an extremely wholesome salad, possessing bitter and anodyne qualities.

CICHORIUM INTYBUS. The systematic name of the wild succory. *Cichorium; Cichoreum; Cichorium sylvestre vel officinarum, Cichorium;—floribus geminis, sessilibus; foliis runcinatis,* of Linnæus. It belongs to the same family with the garden endive, and by some botanists has been supposed to be the same plant in its uncultivated state; but the endive commonly used as salad is an annual, or at most a biennial plant, and its parent is now known to be the *cichorium endivia.* Wild succory or cichory, abounds with a milky juice, of a penetrating bitterish taste, and of no remarkable smell, or particular flavour: the roots are more bitter than the leaves or stalks, and these much more so than the flowers. By culture in gardens, and by blanching, it loses its bitterness, and may be eaten early in the spring in salads. The roots, if gathered before the stem shoots up, are also eatable, and when dried may be made into bread. The roots and leaves of this plant are stated by Lewis to be very useful aperients, acting mildly and without irritation, tending rather to abate than to increase heat, and which may therefore be given with safety in hectic and inflammatory cases. Taken freely, they keep the belly open, or produce a gentle diarrhœa; and when thus continued for some time, they have often proved salutary in the beginning obstructions of the viscera, in jaundices, cachexies, hypochondriacal and other chronical disorders. A decoction of this herb, with others of the like kind, in whey, and rendered purgative by a suitable addition of polychrest salt, was found a useful remedy in cases of biliary calculi, and promises advantage in many complaints requiring what have been termed attenuants and resolvents. The virtues of succory, like those of dandelion, reside in its milky juice; and we are warranted, says Dr. Woodville, in asserting, that the expressed juice of both these plants, taken in large doses frequently repeated, has been found an efficacious remedy in phthisis pulmonalis, as well as the various other affections above mentioned. The milky juice may be extracted by boiling in water, or by pressure. The wild and the garden sorts are used indifferently. If the root is cut into small pieces, dried, and roasted, it resembles coffee, and is sometimes a good substitute for it.

CI'CHORY. See *Cichorium intybus*.

Cichory, wild. See *Cichorium intybus*.

CICINDE'LA. (A dim. of *candela*: i. e. a little candle; so called from its light.) The glowworm. By some thought to be anodyne, lithontriptic, though probably neither. Not used in the present day.

CICI'NUM OLEUM. (From κικι, the ricinus.) An oil, obtained by boiling the bruised seeds of the *Jatropha curcas* of Linnæus. It is somewhat similar in its properties to castor oil.

CI'CLA. A name for the white beet.

CICU'TA. (*Quasi cæcuta*, blind; because it destroys the sight of those who use it. Cicuta signifies also the internode, or space between two joints of a reed; or the hollow stem of any plant which the shepherds used for making their rural pipes. *Est mihi disparibus septem conjuncta cicutis fistula.* Virgil.) Hemlock. 1. The name of a genus of plants in the Linnæan system. Class, *Pentandria*; Order, *Digynia*.

2. The name, in most pharmacopœias, of the common hemlock. See *Conium*.

CICUTA AQUATICA. See *Cicuta virosa*.

CICUTA VIROSA. The systematic name of the *Cicuta aquatica*; *Cicutaria virosa*; *Sium majus alterum angustifolium*; *Sium erucæ folio*; long-leaved water hemlock and cow-bane. This plant, *Cicuta—umbellis oppositifoliis; petiolis marginatis obtusis*, of Linnæus, is seldom employed medicinally in the present day. It is an active poison, and often eaten by mistake for the wild smallage, the *Apium graveolens*, of Linnæus; when it produces tremors, vertigo, a violent burning at the stomach, epilepsy, convulsions, spasms of the jaw, a flowing of blood from the ears, tumefaction of the abdomen, and death.

CICUTA'RIA. (From *cicuta*, hemlock.) Bastard hemlock. See *Chærophyllum sylvestre*.

CICUTARIA AQUATICA. See *Phellandrium aquaticum*.

CICUTARIA VIROSA. See *Cicuta virosa*.

CIDO'NIUM. See *Pyrus cydonia*.

CILIA. (The plural of *cilium*.) A species of pubescence of plants which consists of hairs on the margin of a leaf or petal, giving it a fringed appearance.

CI'LIAR. (*Ciliaris*; from *cilium*, the eyelid.) Belonging to the eyelid.

CILIAR LIGAMENT. *Ligamentum ciliare*. The circular portion that divides the chroid membrane from the iris, and which adheres to the sclerotic membrane. It appears like a white circular ring. See *Choroid membrane*.

CILIARE LIGAMENTUM See *Choroid membrane*.

CILIARIS MUSCULUS. That part of the musculus orbicularis palpebrarum which lies nearest the cilia, considered by Riolan as a distinct muscle.

CILIATUS. Bordered, fringed: applied to leaves, corolla, petals, &c.: hence *folium ciliatum*, *anthodium ciliatum*, and *petala ciliata*. See *Leaf*, *Corolla*, *Anthodium*, *Petalum*.

CI'LIUM. (From *cilleo*, to move about.) The eyelid or eyelash. See also *Cilia*.

CILIARY PROCESSES. The white folds at the margin of the uvea in the eye, covered with a black matter, which proceed from the uvea to the crystalline lens, upon which they lie.

CI'LLO. (From *cilium*, the eyelid.) One who is affected with a spasm or trembling of the eyelids.

CILLO'SIS. (From *cilium*, the eyelid.) A spasmodic trembling of the eyelids.

Cimeter shaped. See *Leaf*.

CIMEX. (From κειμαι, to inhabit; so called because they infest houses.) The name of a genus of insects in the Linnæan system. The wall-louse or bug.

CIMEX DOMESTICUS. Six or seven are given inwardly to cure the ague, just before the fits come on, and have the same effect with every thing nauseous and disgusting.

[CIMICIFUGA. *Black snake root.* This is the root of *Actæa racemosa* of Wildenow, an American plant. According to the late Dr. Barton, a decoction of it forms a useful astringent gargle in sore throats, and also cures psora. We are told that the Indians made great use of it in rheumatism; also as an agent *ad partum accelerandum*. Dr. Tully acquaints me, that he has found it diaphoretic, diuretic, and moderately tonic, forming a useful auxiliary in the treatment of acute and chronic rheumatism, and of dropsy; likewise operating very beneficially in hysteria. It is usually given in the form of decoction.—*Big. Mat. Med.* A.]

CIMO'LIA ALBA. (From Κιμωλος, Cimolus, an island in the Cretan sea, where it is procured.) See *Cimolite*.

CIMOLIA PURPURESCENS. Fullers-earth.

CIMOLITE. Cimolian earth. The *Cimolia* of Pliny. An earth of a grayish white colour, which consists of silex, alumina, oxide of iron, and water.

CI'NA CINÆ. See *Cinchona*.

CI'NÆ SEMEN. See *Artemisia santonica*.

CI'NARA. (From κινεω, to move; *quasi movet ad venerem vel urinam*.) Artichoke. 1. The name of a genus of plants in the Linnæan system. Class, *Syngenesia*; Order, *Polygamia æqualis*.

2. The pharmacopœial name for the common artichoke. See *Cinara scolymus*.

CINARA SCOLYMUS. The systematic name of the artichoke, called in the pharmacopœias *Alcocalum*; *Agriocinara*; *Articoculus*; *Artischocas lævis*; *Costus nigra*; *Carduus sativus non spinosus*; *Cinara hortensis*; *Scolymus sativus*; *Carduus domesticus capite majore*; *Carduus altilis*. The *Cinara—foliis subspinosis pinnatis indivisique, calycinis squamis ovatis*, of Linnæus. A native of the southern parts of Europe, but cultivated here for culinary purposes. The leaves are bitter, and afford, by expression, a considerable quantity of juice, which, when strained, and mixed with an equal quantity of white wine, has been given successfully in dropsies, in the dose of 3 or 4 tablespoonfuls night and morning, but it is very uncertain in the operation.

CINCHO'NA. (Geoffroy states that the use of this bark was first learned from the following circumstance:—Some cinchona trees being thrown by the winds into a pool of water, lay there till the water became so bitter, that every body refused to drink it. However, one of the neighbouring inhabitants being seized with a violent paroxysm of fever, and finding no other water to quench his thirst, was forced to drink of this, by which he was perfectly cured. He afterward related the circumstance to others, and prevailed upon some of his friends, who were ill of fevers, to make use of the same remedy, with whom it proved equally successful. The use of this excellent remedy, however, was very little known till about the year 1638, when a signal cure having been performed by it on the Spanish viceroy's lady, the Countess del Cinchon, at Lima, it came into general use, and hence it was distinguished by the appellation of *cortex cinchonæ*, and *pulvis comitissæ*, or the Countess's powder. On the recovery of the Countess, she distributed a large quantity of the bark to the Jesuits, in whose hands it acquired still greater reputation, and by them it was first introduced into Europe, and thence called *cortex*, or *pulvis jesuiticus*, *pulvis patrum*; and also Cardinal del Lugo's powder, because that charitable prelate bought a large quantity of it at great expense for the use of the religious poor at Rome.) 1. The name of a genus of plants in the Linnæan system. Class, *Pentandria*; Order, *Monogynia*. Cinchona, or Peruvian bark-tree.

2. The pharmacopœial name of several kinds of barks; called also *Cortex*. *Cortex china*; *China*; *Chinchina*; *Kina kina*, *Kinkina*; *Quina quina*, *Quinquina*; the trees affording which, grow wild in the hilly parts of Peru; the bark is stripped from the branches, trunk, and root, and dried. Three kinds of it are now in use.

1. *Cortex cinchonæ cordifoliæ*.—The plant which affords this species is the *Cinchona cordifolia*, of Zea

the *Cinchona officinalis*, of Linnæus; the *Cinchona macrocarpa*, of Wildenow. Heart-leaved cinchona. The bark of this tree is called *yellow bark*, because it approaches more to that colour than either of the others does. It is in flat pieces, not convoluted like the pale, nor dark-coloured like the red; externally smooth, internally of a light cinnamon colour, friable and fibrous, has no peculiar odour different from the others, but a taste incomparably more bitter, with some degree of astringency.

2. *Cortex cinchonæ lancifoliæ.*—This species is obtained from the *Cinchona lancifolia* of Zea. Lance-leaved cinchona. This is the *quilled bark*, which comes in small quilled twigs, breaking close and smooth, friable between the teeth, covered with a rough coat of a brownish colour, internally smooth, and of a light brown; its taste is bitter, and slightly astringent; flavour slightly aromatic, with some degree of mustiness.

3. *Cortex cinchonæ oblongifolia.*—This kind is procured from *Cinchona oblongifolia* of Zea. Oblong-leaved cinchona. This is the *red bark:* it is in large thick pieces, externally covered with a brown rugged coat, internally more smooth and compact, but fibrous, of a dark red colour; taste and smell similar to that of the *cinchonæ lancifoliæ cortex*, but the taste rather stronger.

From the general analysis of bark, it appears to consist, besides the woody matter which composes the greater part of it, of gum, resin, gallic acid, of very small portions of tannin and essential oil, and of several salts having principally lime for their basis. Seguin also supposed the existence of gelatin in it, but without sufficient proof. Cold water infused on pale bark for some hours, acquires a bitter taste, with some share of its odour; when assisted by a moderate heat, the water takes up more of the active matter; by decoction, a fluid, deep coloured, of a bitter styptic taste, is obtained, which, when cold, deposites a precipitate of resinous matter and gallic acid. By long decoction, the virtues of the bark are nearly destroyed, owing to the oxygenation of its active matter. Magnesia enables water to dissolve a larger portion of the principles of bark, as does lime, though in an inferior degree. Alkohol is the most powerful solvent of its active matter. Brandy and other spirits and wines, afford also strong solutions, in proportion to the quantity of alkohol they contain. A saturated solution of ammonia is also a powerful solvent; vinegar is less so even than water. By distillation, water is slightly impregnated with the flavour of bark; it is doubtful whether any essential oil can be obtained.

The action of menstrua on the red bark is nearly the same, the solutions only being considerably stronger, or containing a larger quantity of resinous matter, and of the astringent principle.

The analysis of the yellow bark shows that its active principles are more concentrated than in either of the others, affording to water, alkohol, &c. tinctures, much stronger both in bitterness and astringency, especially in the former principle.

Vauquelin made infusions of all the varieties of cinchona he could procure, using the same quantities of the barks and water, and leaving the powders infused for the same time. He observed, 1. That certain infusions were precipitated abundantly by infusion of galls, by solution of glue and tartar emetic. 2. That some were precipitated by glue, but not by the two other reagents; and, 3. That others were, on the contrary, by nutgalls, and tartar emetic, without being affected by glue. 4. And that there were some which yielded no precipitate by nutgalls, tannin, or emetic tartar. The cinchonas that furnished the first infusion were of excellent quality; those that afforded the fourth were not febrifuge; while those that gave the second and third were febrifuge, but in a smaller degree than the first. Besides mucilage, kinate of lime, and woody fibre, he obtained in his analyses a resinous substance, which appears not to be identic in all the species of bark. It is very bitter, very soluble in alkohol, in acids, and alkalies; scarcely soluble in cold water, but more soluble in hot. It is this body which gives to infusions of cinchona the property of yielding precipitates by emetic tartar, galls, gelatin; and in it the febrifuge virtue seems to reside. It is this substance in part which falls down on cooling decoctions of cinchona, and from concentrated infusions. A table of precipitations by glue, tannin, and tartar emetic, from infusions of different barks, has been given by Vauquelin.

Pelletier and Caventou analyzed the *Cinchona condaminæa*, gray bark, and found it composed of, 1. cinchonina, united to kinic acid; 2. green fatty matter; 3. red colouring matter, slightly soluble; 4. tannin; 5. yellow colouring matter; 6. kinite of lime; 7. gum; 8. starch; 9. lignine.

The red bark has been considered as superior to the pale, the yellow is represented, apparently with justice, as being more active than either of the others.

The effects of Peruvian bark are those of a powerful and permanent tonic, so slow in its operation, that its stimulating property is scarcely perceptible by any alteration in the state of the pulse, or of the temperature of the body. In a large dose, it occasions nausea and headache; in some habits it operates as a laxative; in others it occasions costiveness. It is one of those medicines, the efficacy of which, in removing disease, is much greater than could be expected, *à priori*, from its effects on the system in a healthy state.

Intermittent fever is the disease, for the cure of which bark was introduced into practice, and there is still no remedy which equals it in power. The disputes respecting the mode of administering it are now settled. It is given as early as possible, after clearing the stomach and bowels, in the dose of from one scruple to a drachm every second or third hour, during the interval of the paroxysm; and it may even be given during the hot fit, but it is then more apt to excite nausea.

In remittent fever it is given with equal freedom, even though the remission of the fever may be obscure.

In some forms of continued fever which are connected with debility, as in typhus, cynanche maligna, confluent small-pox, &c. it is regarded as one of the most valuable remedies. It may be prejudicial, however, in those diseases where the brain or its membranes are inflamed, or where there is much irritation, marked by subsultus tendinum, and convulsive motions of the extremities; and in pure typhus it appears to be less useful in the beginning of the disease than in the convalescent stage.

Even in fevers of an opposite type, where there are marks of inflammatory action, particularly in acute rheumatism, bark has been found useful after blood-letting. In erysipelas, in grangrene, in extensive suppuration, and venereal ulceration, the freeuse of bark is of the greatest advantage.

In the various forms of passive hæmorrhagy, in many other diseases of chronic debility, dyspepsia, hypochondriasis, paralysis, rickets, scrofula, dropsy, and in a variety of spasmodic affections, epilepsy, chorea, and hysteria, it is administered as a powerful and permanent tonic, either alone, or combined with other remedies suited to the particular case.

The officinal preparations of bark are an infusion, decoction, an extract, a resinous extract, a simple tincture, an ammoniated and a compound tincture. The usual dose is half a drachm of the powder. The only inconvenience of a larger dose is its sitting uneasy on the stomach. It may therefore, if necessary, be frequently repeated, and in urgent cases may be taken to the extent of an ounce, or even two ounces, in twenty-four hours.

The powder is more effectual than any of the preparations; it is given in wine, in anyspirituous liquor; or, if it excite nausea, combined with an aromatic. The cold infusion is the least powerful, but most grateful; the decoction contains much more of the active matter of the bark, and is the preparation generally used when the powder is rejected; its dose is from two to four ounces. The spirituous tincture, though containing still more of the bark, cannot be extensively used on account of the menstruum, but is principally employed, occasionally, and in small doses of two or three drachms, as a stomachic. The extract is a preparation of considerable power, when properly prepared, and is adapted to those cases where the remedy requires to be continued for some time. It is then given in the form of pill, in doses of from five to fifteen grains.

Bark is likewise sometimes given in the form of enema; one scruple of the extract, or two drachms of the powder, being diffused in four ounces of starch mucilage. The decoction is also sometimes applied as a fomentation to ulcers.

CINCHONA CARIBÆA. The systematic name of the Caribæan bark-tree. It grows in Jamaica, where it is called the sea-side beech. According to Dr. Wright, the bark of this tree is not less efficacious than that of the cinchona of Peru, for which it will prove a useful substitute; but by the experiments of Dr. Skeete, it appears to have less astringent power.

CINCHONA CONDAMINŒA. See *Cinchona* and *Cinchonina.*

CINCHONA CORDIFOLIA. See *Cinchona.*

CINCHONA FLAVA. See *Cinchona.*

CINCHONA FLORIBUNDA. The systematic name of the plant which affords the Saint Luc bark. *Cinchona—floribus paniculatis glabris, capsulis turbinatis lævibus, foliis ellipticis acuminatis glabris*, of Linnæus. It has an adstringent, bitter taste, somewhat like gentian. It is recommended in intermittents, putrid dysentery, and dyspepsia; it should always be joined with some aromatic. Dr. Withering considers this bark as greatly inferior to that of the other species of this genus. In its recent state it is considerably emetic and cathartic, properties which in some degree it retains on being dried; so that the stomach does not bear this bark in large doses, and in small ones its effects are not such as to give it any peculiar recommendation.

CINCHONA LANCIFOLIA. See *Cinchona.*

CINCHONA OBLONGIFOLIA. See *Cinchona.*

CINCHONA OFFICINALIS. The name of the officinal Peruvian bark. See *Cinchona.*

CINCHONA RUBRA. See *Cinchona.*

CINCHONA SANCTA FE'. Several species of cinchona have been lately discovered at Sancta Fé, yielding barks both of the pale and red kind; and which, from their sensible qualities, are likely upon trial to become equally useful with those produced in the kingdom of Peru.

CINCHONIA. See *Cinchonina.*

CINCHONINA. *Cinchonia; Quinia; Quinina.* Cinchonine or Quinine is the salifiable base, or vegetable alkali, discovered in the Cinchona condaminœa, by Pelletier and Caventou. The person, however, who first recognised its existence, though he did not ascertain its alkaline nature, or study its combinations with acids, was Gornis of Lisbon.

The following process for extracting cinchonina is that of Henry, the younger, which the above chemists approve. A kilogramme of bark reduced into a fine powder, is to be acted on twice with heat, by a dilute sulphuric acid, consisting of 50 or 60 grammes, diluted with 8 kilogrammes of water for each time. The filtered decoctions are very bitter, have a reddish colour, which assumes on cooling a yellowish tint. To discolour (blanch) these liquors, and saturate the acid, either pulverized quicklime or magnesia may be employed. The liquors, entirely deprived of colour, are to be passed through a cloth, and the precipitate which forms is to be washed with a small quantity of water, to separate the excess of lime (if this earth has been used). The deposite on the cloth, well drained and almost completely deprived of moisture for twelve hours, after having been put three successive times to digest in alkohol of 36° (0.837), will furnish, by distilling of the liquid alkohol, a brown viscid matter, becoming brittle on cooling. It is to be acted on with water sharpened with sulphuric acid, and the refrigerated liquor will afford about thirty grammes of white crystals, entirely soluble in alkohol, scarcely soluble in cold water, but more in boiling water, particularly if this be slightly acidulated. They consist of pure sulphate of cinchonina. They ought to be brilliant, crystallized in parallelopipeds, very hard, and of a glassy-white. It should burn without leaving any residuum. Other processes have been given, of which a full account will be found in the 12th volume of the Journal of Science, p. 325. From a solution of the above salt, the cinchonina may be easily obtained by the addition of any alkali. The cinchonina falls down, and may be afterward dissolved in alkohol, and crystallized by evaporation. Its form is a rhomboidal prism, of 108° and 72°, terminated by a bevelment. It has but little taste, requiring 7000 parts of water for its solution; but when dissolved in alkohol, or an acid, it has the bitter taste of bark. When heated it does not fuse before decomposition. It consists of oxygen, hydrogen, and carbon, the latter being predominant. It dissolves in only very small quantities in the oils, and in sulphuric ether.

The sulphate is composed of cinchonina	100
Sulphuric acid	13

whence the prime equivalent would appear to be 38.5. The muriate is more soluble. It consists of

Cinchonina	100
Muriatic acid	7.9

The nitrate is uncrystallizable. Gallic, oxalic, and tartaric acids, form neutral salts with cinchonina, which are soluble only with excess of acid. Hence infusion of nut-galls gives, with a decoction of good cinchona, an abundant precipitate of gallate of cinchonina.

Robiquet gives as the composition of a subsulphate of cinchonina of the first crystallization,

Sulphuric acid	11.3
Cinchonina	79.0

The alkaline base found in yellow barks is called *Quinina.* It is extracted in exactly the same way. Red bark contains a mixture of these two alkalies The febrifuge virtue of the sulphates is considered to be very great.

CINCI'NNUS. The hair on the temples.

CINCLE'SIS. (From κιγκλιζω, to move.) *Cinclismus.* An involuntary nictitation or winking. *Vogel.*

CINERA'RIUM (From *cinis*, ashes.) The ash-hole of a chemical instrument.

CI'NERES. (Plural of *cinis*, ashes.) Ashes.

CINERES CLAVELLATA. See *Potassa impura.*

CINERES RUSSICI. See *Potassa impura.*

CINERI'TIOUS. (*Cineritius;* from *cinis*, ashes.) Of the colour of ashes. A name applied to the cortical substance of the brain, from its resemblance to an ash-colour.

CINERI'TIUM. (From *cinis*, ashes.) A cupel or test; so named from its being commonly made of the ashes of vegetables or bones.

CINE'RULAM. A name for spodium.

CINETICA. (Κινη7ικος, having the power of motion.) The name of an order in the class *Neuroses* of Good's Nosology. Diseases affecting the muscles, and embracing *Entasia*, *Clonus*, and *Synclonus.*

CINE'TUS. The diaphragm.

CINGULA'RIA. (From *cingulum*, a girdle; because it grows in that shape.) The lycopodium.

CI'NGULUM. (From *cingo*, to bind.) A girdle or belt about the loins.

CINGULUM MERCURIALE. A mercurial girdle, called also *cingulum sapientiæ*, and *singulum stultitiæ.* It was an invention of Rulandus's: different directions are given for making it, but the following is one of the neatest:—"Take three drachms of quicksilver; shake it with two ounces of lemon-juice until the globules disappear; then separate the juice, and mix with the extinguished quicksilver, half the white of an egg; gum-dragon, finely powdered, a scruple; and spread the whole on a belt of flannel."

CINGULUM SANCTI JOHANNIS. A name of the artemisia.

CINIFICA'TUM. A name for calcinatum.

CINIS. (*Cinis*, *eris.* m., in the plural *cineres.*) The ash which remains after burning any thing.

CI'NNABAR. (*Cinnabaris*, *ris.* f. Pliny says the Indians call by this name a mixture of the blood of the dragon and elephant, and also many substances which resemble it in colour, particularly the minium; but it now denotes the red sulphuret of mercury.)

1. An ore of mercury, consisting of that mineral united to sulphur. A native sulphuret of mercury See *Hydrargyri sulphuretum rubrum.*

2. An artificial compound of mercury and sulphur, called factitious cinnabar, red sulphuret of mercury, and vermilion. See *Hydrargyri sulphuretum rubrum.*

CINNABARIS FACTITIA. Factitious cinnabar. See *Hydrargyri sulphuretum rubrum.*

CINNABARIS GRÆCORUM. The sanguis draconis and cinnabar.

CINNABARIS NATIVA. Native cinnabar. See *Hydrargyri sulphuretum rubrum.*

CINNAMO'MUM. (From *kinamon*, Arabian.) Cinnamon. See *Laurus cinnamomum.*

CINNAMON. 1. The name of a tree. See *Laurus cinnamomum.*

2. The name of a stone, which is a rare mineral

found in the sand of rivers in Ceylon, of a blood and hyacinth red, passing into orange yellow.

CINQUEFOIL. See *Potentilla reptans*.

CI'ON. (Κιων, a column; from κιω, to go.)

1. The uvula was formerly so named from its pyramidal shape.

2. An enlargement of the uvula.

CIO'NIS. (From κιων, the uvula.) An enlargement and painful swelling of the uvula.

CIPOLIN. A marble from Rome and Autun.

CIRCÆ'A. (From *Circe*, the enchantress: so named from the opinion that it was used by Circe in her enchanted preparations.) 1. The name of a genus of plants in the Linnæan system. Class, *Diandria;* Order, *Monogynia*. Enchanter's nightshade.

2. The name in some pharmacopœias for the *Circæa lutetiana*, which is now fallen wholly into disuse.

CIRCOCE'LE. (Κιρσοκηλη; from κιρσος, *varix*, or a dilatation of a vein, and κηλη, a tumour.) *Varicocele*. A morbid or varicose distention and enlargement of the spermatic veins; it is frequently mistaken for a descent of a small portion of omentum. The uneasiness which it occasions is a kind of pain in the back, generally relieved by suspension of the scrotum; and whether considered on account of the pain, or on account of the wasting of the testicle, which now and then follows, it may truly be called a disease. It has been resembled to a collection of earth-worms. It is most frequently confined to that part of the spermatic process, which is below the opening in the abdominal tendon; and the vessels generally become rather larger as they approach the testes. There is one sure method of distinguishing between a circocele and omental hernia; place the patient in a horizontal posture, and empty the swelling by pressure upon the scrotum; then put the fingers firmly upon the upper part of the abdominal ring, and desire the patient to rise; if it is a hernia, the tumour cannot reappear, as long as the pressure is continued at the ring; but if a circocele, the swelling returns with increased size, on account of the return of blood into the abdomen being prevented by the pressure.

CI'RCOS. (From κιρκος, a circle.) A ring. It is sometimes used for the sphincter muscle which is round like a ring.

CIRCULA'TION. (*Circulatio;* from *circulo*, to compass about.) *Circulatio sanguinis*. Circulation of the blood. A vital action performed by the heart in the following manner: the blood is returned by the descending and ascending venæ cavæ into the right auricle of the heart, which, when distended, contracts, and sends its blood into the right ventricle; from the right ventricle it is propelled through the pulmonary artery to circulate through, and undergo a change in the lungs, being prevented from returning into the right auricle by the closing of the valves, which are situated there for that purpose. Having undergone this change in the lungs, it is brought to the left auricle of the heart by the four pulmonary veins, and from thence it is evacuated into the left ventricle. The left ventricle, when distended, contracts, and throws the blood through the aorta to every part of the body, to be returned by the veins into the two venæ cavæ. It is prevented from passing back from the left ventricle into the auricle by a valvular apparatus; and the pulmonary artery and aorta at their origin are also furnished with similar organs, to prevent its returning into the ventricles. This is a brief outline of the circulation, the particulars of which we shall now describe.

"The best informed physiologists avow that the circulation of the venous blood is still very little understood. We shall describe here only its most apparent phenomena, leaving the most delicate questions until we treat of the relation of the flowing of the blood in the veins, with that in the arteries. We will then speak of the cause that determines the entrance of blood into the venous radicles.

To have a general, but just idea of the course of the blood in the veins, we must consider that the sum of the small veins forms a cavity much larger than that of the larger but less numerous veins, into which they pass; that these bear the same relation to the trunks in which *they* terminate: consequently, the blood which flows in the veins from branches towards the trunks, passes always from a larger to a smaller cavity; now, the following principle of hydro-dynamics may here be perfectly applied:

When a liquid flows in a tube which it fills completely, the quantity of this liquid which traverses the different sections of the tube in a given time ought to be every where the same: consequently, when the tube increases, the velocity diminishes; when the tube diminishes, the velocity increases in rapidity.

Experience confirms this principle, and its just application to the current of venous blood. If a very small vein is cut, the blood flows from it very slowly; it flows quicker from a larger vein, and it flows with considerable rapidity from an open venous trunk.

Generally there are several veins to transport the blood that has traversed an organ towards the larger trunks. On account of their anastomoses, the compressure or ligature of one or several of these veins does not prevent or diminish the quantity of blood that returns to the heart; it merely acquires a greater rapidity in the veins which remain free.

This happens when a ligature is placed on the arm for the purpose of bleeding. In the ordinary state, the blood, which is carried to the fore-arm and the hand, returns to the heart by four deep veins, and at least as many superficial ones; but as soon as the ligature is tightened, the blood passes no longer by the subcutaneous veins, and it traverses with difficulty those which are deeper seated. If one of the veins is then opened at the bend of the arm, it passes out in form of a continued jet, which continues as long as the ligature remains firm, and stops as soon as it is removed.

Except in particular cases, the veins are not much distended by the blood; however, those in which it moves with the greatest rapidity are much more so: the small veins are scarcely distended at all. For a reason very easy to be understood, all the circumstances that accelerate the rapidity of the blood in a vein, produce also an augmentation in the distention of the vessel.

The introduction of blood into the veins taking place in a continued manner, every cause which arrests its course produces distention of the vein, and the stagnation of a greater or less quantity of blood in its cavity, below the obstacle.

The sides of the veins seem to have but a small influence upon the motion of the blood; they easily give way when the quantity augments, and return to their usual form when it diminishes; but their contraction is limited; it is not sufficiently strong to expel the blood completely from the vein, and therefore those of dead bodies always contain some.

A great number of veins, such as those of the bones, of the sinuses of the *dura mater*, of the testicles, of the liver, &c., the sides of which adhere to an inflexible canal, can have evidently no influence upon the motion of the blood that flows in their cavity.

However, it is to the elasticity of the sides of the veins, and not to a contraction similar to that of the muscles that we must attribute the faculty which they possess of diminishing the size when the column of blood diminishes: this diminution is also much more marked in those that have the thickest sides, such as the superficial veins.

If the veins have themselves very little influence upon the motion of the blood, many other necessary causes exert a very evident effect. Every continued or alternate pressure upon a vein, when strong enough to flatten it, may prevent the passage of the blood; if it is not so strong, it will oppose the dilatation of the vein by the blood, and consequently favour its motion. The constant pressure which the skin of the members exert upon the veins that are below it, renders the flow of the blood more easy and rapid in these vessels. We cannot doubt this, for all the circumstances that diminish the contractility of the tissue of the skin, are sooner or later followed by a considerable dilatation of the veins, and in certain cases by varix; we know also that mechanical compression, exerted by a proper bandage, reduces the veins again to their ordinary dimensions, and also regulates the motion of the blood within them.

In the abdomen, the veins are subject to the alternate pressure of the diaphragm, and of the abdominal muscles, and this cause is equally favourable to the flow of the venous blood in this part.

The veins of the brain support also a considerable pressure, which must produce the same result.

Whenever the blood runs in the direction of its weight it flows with greater facility; the contrary takes place when it flows against the direction of its gravity.

We must not neglect to notice the relations of these accessory causes with the disposition of the veins. Where they are very marked, the veins present no valves, and their sides are very thin, as is seen in the abdomen, the chest, the cavity of the skull, &c.; where these have less influence, the veins present valves, and have thicker sides; lastly, where they are very weak, as in the subcutaneous veins, the valves are numerous, and the sides have a considerable thickness.

We must take care, however, not to confound among the circumstances favourable to the motion of the blood in the veins, causes which act in another manner.

For example, it is generally known that the contraction of the muscles of the fore-arm and the hand during bleeding, accelerate the motion of the blood which passes through the opening of the vein; physiologists say that the contraction of the muscles compresses the deep veins, and expels the blood from them, which then passes into the superficial veins. Were it thus, the acceleration would be only instantaneous, or at least of short duration, while it generally continues as long as the contraction. We shall see, farther on, how this phenomenon ought to be explained.

When the feet are plunged some time in hot water, the subcutaneous veins swell, which is generally attributed to the rarefaction of the blood; though the true cause is the augmentation of the quantity of blood in the feet, but particularly at the skin, an augmentation which ought naturally to accelerate the motion of the blood in the veins, since they are in a given time traversed by a greater quantity of blood.

After what has preceded, we can easily suppose that the venous blood must be frequently stopped or hindered in its course, either by the veins suffering too strong a pressure in the different positions of the body, or by other bodies pressing upon it, &c.: *hence the necessity* of the numerous anastomoses that exist not only in the small veins, but among the large, and even among the largest trunks. By these frequent communications, one or several of the veins being compressed in such a way, that they cannot permit the passage of the blood, this fluid turns and arrives at the heart by other directions.—one of the uses of the azygos vein appears to be to establish an easy communication between the superior and inferior vena cava. Its principal utility, however, seems to consist in its being the common termination of most of the intercostal veins.

There is no obscurity in the action of the valves of the veins; they are real valves, which prevent the return of the blood towards the venous radicles, and which do this so much better in proportion as they are large, that is to say, more suitably disposed to stop entirely the cavity of the vein.

The friction of the blood against the sides of the veins; its adhesion to these same sides, and the want of fluidity, must modify the motion of the blood in the veins, and tend to retard it; but in the present state of physiology and hydrodynamics, it is impossible to assign the precise effect of each of these particular causes.

We ought to perceive, by what has been said upon the motion of the venous blood, that it must undergo great modifications, according to an infinity of circumstances.

At any rate, the venous blood of every part of the body arrives at the right auricle of the heart by the trunks that we have already named; viz. two very large, the venæ cavæ, and one very small, the coronary vein.

The blood probably flows in each of these veins with different rapidity: what is certain, is, that the three columns of liquid make an effort to pass into the auricle, and that the effort must be considerable. If it is contracted, this effort has no effect: but, as soon as it dilates, the blood enters its cavity, fills it completely, and even distends the sides a little; it would immediately enter the ventricle, if it did not contract itself at this instant. The blood then confines itself to filling up exactly the cavity of the auricle; but this very soon contracts, compresses the blood, which escapes into the place where there is least compression. Now it has only two issues: 1st, by the vena cava; 2dly, by the opening which conducts into the ventricle. The columns of blood which are coming to the auricle present a certain resistance to its passage into the cavæ or coronary veins. On the contrary, it finds every facility to enter the ventricle, since the latter dilates itself with force, tends to produce a vacuum, and consequently draws on the blood instead of repulsing it.

However, all the blood that passes out of the auricle does not enter the ventricle; it has been long observed that, at each contraction of the auricle, a certain quantity of blood flows back into the superior and inferior venæ cavæ; the undulation produced by this cause is sometimes felt as far as the external iliac veins, and into the jugulars; it has a sensible influence, as we will see, upon the flowing of the blood in several organs, and particularly in the brain.

The quantity of blood which flows back in this manner, varies according to the facility with which this liquid enters the ventricle. If at the instant of its dilatation, the ventricle still contains much blood, which has not passed into the pulmonary artery, it can only receive a small quantity of that of the auricle, and then the reflux will be of greater extent.

This happens when the flowing of the blood in the pulmonary artery is retarded, either by obstacles in the lungs, or by the want of sufficient force in the ventricle. This reflux, of which we speak, is the cause of the beating which is seen in the veins of certain sick persons, and which bears the name of *venous pulse.* Nothing similar can take place in the coronary vein, for its opening is furnished with a valve, which shuts on the instant of the contraction of the auricle.

The instant in which the auricle ceases to contract, the ventricle enters into contraction, the blood it contains is strongly pressed, and tends to escape in every direction: it would return so much more easily into the auricle, that, as we have already frequently said, it dilates just at this instant; but the tricuspid valve which shuts the *auriculo-ventricular* opening prevents this reflux. Being raised by the liquid introduced below it, and which tends to pass into the auricle, it gives way until it has become perpendicular to the axis of the ventricle; its three divisions then shut almost completely the opening, and as the tendons of the *columnæ carneæ* do not permit them to go farther, the valve resists the effort of the blood, and thus prevents it from passing into the auricle.

It is not the same with the blood, which, during the dilatation of the ventricle, corresponded to the auricular surface of the valve; it is evident that in the motion of the ventricle it is carried forward into the auricle, where it mixes with that which comes from the *venæ cavæ* and coronary veins.

Not being able to overcome the resistance of the tricuspid valve, the blood of the ventricle has no other issue than the pulmonary artery, into which it enters by raising the three sigmoid valves that supported the column of blood contained in the artery during the dilatation of the ventricle.

Suppose the artery full of blood, and left to itself, the liquid will be pressed in the whole extent of the vessel, by the sides which tend to contract upon the cavity; the blood, being thus pressed, will endeavour to escape in every direction; now it has only two ways to pass, by the cardiac orifice, and by the numerous small vessels that terminate the artery in the tissue of the lungs.

The orifice of the pulmonary artery in the heart being very large, the blood would easily pass into the ventricle, if there were not a particular apparatus at this orifice, intended to prevent this; the three sigmoid valves. Being pressed against the sides of the artery, at the instant that the ventricle sends a wave of blood that way, these folds become perpendicular to its axis; as soon as the blood tends to flow back into the ventricle, they place themselves so as to shut up the cavity of this vessel completely.

On account of the bag-like form of the sigmoid valves, they are swelled by the blood that enters into their cavity, and their margin tends to assume a circular figure. Now, three circular portions, placed upon each other, necessarily leave a space between them.

When the valves, therefore, of the pulmonary artery are lowered by the blood, there ought to remain an opening by which this liquid may flow back into the ventricle.

If each valve were alone, it would undoubtedly take a semicircular form; but there are three of them;

being pressed by the blood, they lie all close together: and, as they cannot extend as far as their fibres permit them, they press upon each other, on account of the small space in which they are contained, and which does not permit their extending themselves. The valves then assume the figure of three triangles, whose summit is in the centre of the artery, and the sides are in *juxta position*, so as completely to intercept the cavity of the artery. Perhaps the *knots*, or *buttons*, which are upon the summit of some of the triangles, are intended to shut more perfectly the centre of the artery.

Finding no passage into the ventricle, the blood will pass into the radicles of the pulmonary veins, with which the small arteries that terminate the pulmonary artery form a continuation, and this passage will continue as long as the sides of the artery press the contained blood with sufficient force; and, except in the trunk and the principal branches, this effect continues until the whole of the blood is expelled.

We might suppose the smallness of the vessels that terminate the pulmonary artery an obstacle to the flowing of the blood: that might be, if they were not numerous, or if the capacity of the whole were less, or even equal to that of the trunk; but as they are innumerable, and their capacity is much greater than that of the trunk, there is no difficulty in the motion. It is true that the distention or subsidence of the lungs renders this passage more or less easy.

In order that this flowing may take place with facility, the force of contraction of the different divisions of the artery ought to be every where in relation to their size; if, on the contrary, that of the small were greater than that of the large, as soon as the first had expelled the blood by which they were filled, they would not be sufficiently distended by the blood coming from the second, and the flowing of the blood would be retarded: now, what takes place is quite the contrary of this supposition. If the pulmonary artery of a living animal were tied immediately above the heart, almost all the blood contained in the artery at the instant of the ligature, would pass quickly into the pulmonary veins, and arrive at the heart.

This is what happens when the blood contained in the pulmonary artery is exposed to the single action of this vessel; but in the common state, at each contraction of the right ventricle, a certain quantity of blood is thrown with force into the artery; the valves are immediately raised; the artery, and almost all its divisions, are so much more distended, in proportion as the heart is more forcibly contracted, and as the quantity of blood injected into the artery is greater. The ventricle dilates immediately after its contraction, and at this instant the sides of the artery contract also; the sigmoid valves descend and shut the pulmonary artery, until they are raised by a new contraction of the ventricle.

Such is the second cause of the motion of the blood in the artery that goes towards the lungs: we see it is intermittent; let us endeavour to appreciate its effects: for which purpose, let us consider the most apparent phenomena of the flow of the blood in the pulmonary artery.

It has been just observed, that in the instant the ventricle injects the blood into the artery, the trunk, and all the divisions of a certain size, undergo an evident dilatation. This phenomenon is called the *pulsation* of the artery. The pulsation is very sensible near the heart; it becomes feeble in proportion to its distance from it; when the artery, by being divided, has become very small, it ceases.

Another phenomenon, which is only the consequence of the preceding, is observed when the artery is opened.

If it be near the heart, and in a place where the beating is sensible, the blood spouts out by jerks; if the opening be made far from the heart, and in a small division, the jet is continued and uniform; lastly, if one of the very small vessels that terminate the artery be opened, the blood flows, but without forming any jet: it flows uniformly in a sheet.

We see at first, in these phenomena, a new application of the principle of hydro-dynamics, as already mentioned, with regard to the influence of the size of the tube upon the liquid that flows in it: the greater the tube is, the rapidity is the less. This capacity of the vessel increasing according as it advances towards the lungs, the quickness of the blood necessarily diminishes.

With regard to the pulsation of the artery, and the jet of blood that escapes from it when it is open, we see plainly that these two effects depend on the contraction of the right ventricle, and the introduction of a certain quantity of blood into the artery, which takes place by this means while flowing through the small vessels that terminate the artery, and that give commencement to the pulmonary veins; the venous blood changes its nature by the effect of the contact of the air; it acquires the qualities of arterial blood: it is this change in the properties of the blood which essentially constitutes respiration.

At the instant in which the venous blood traverses the small vessels of the pulmonary lobules, it assumes a scarlet colour; its odour becomes stronger, and its taste more distinct, its temperature rises about a degree; a part of its serum disappears in the form of vapour in the tissue of the lobules, and mixes with the air. Its tendency to coagulate augments considerably which is expressed by saying that its *plasticity* becomes stronger, its specific gravity diminishes, as well as its capacity for caloric. The venous blood, having acquired these characters, now becomes arterial blood, and enters the radicles of the pulmonary veins, which have their origin, like the veins properly so called, in the tissue of the lungs; that is, they form at first an infinite number of radicles, which appear to be the continuation of the pulmonary artery. These radicles unite to form thicker roots, which become still thicker. Lastly, they all terminate in four vessels, which open, after a short passage, into the left auricle. The pulmonary veins are different from the other veins, in their not anastomosing after they have acquired a certain thickness; a similar disposition has been seen in the divisions of the artery which is distributed to the lungs.

The pulmonary veins have no valves, and their structure is similar to that of the other veins; their middle membrane is, however, a little thicker, and it appears to possess more elasticity. The blood passes into the radicles of the pulmonary veins, and very soon reaches the trunk of these veins: in this passage it presents a gradually accelerated motion, in proportion as it passes from the small veins into the larger: finally, it does not at all flow by jerks, and it appears nearly equally rapid in the four pulmonary veins. From the pulmonary veins the left auricle receives the blood.

The mechanism by which the blood traverses the left auricle and ventricle is the same as that by which the venous blood traverses the right cavities.

When the left auricle dilates, the blood of the four pulmonary veins enters and fills it; when it contracts, part of the blood passes into the ventricle, and part flows back into the pulmonary veins; when the ventricle dilates, it receives the blood which comes from the auricle, and a small quantity of that of the *aorta;* when it contracts, the mitral valve is raised, it shuts the *auriculo-ventricular* opening, and the blood, not being able to return into the auricle, it enters into the aorta by raising the three sigmoid valves, which were shut during the dilatation of the ventricle.

It is necessary to remark, however, that the fleshy columns having no existence in the auricle, their influence cannot exist as in the right, and the arterial ventricle being much thicker than the venous, it compresses the blood with a much greater force than the right, which was indispensable on account of the distance to which it has to send this liquid.

Course of the blood in the aorta, and its divisions.—Notwithstanding the differences which exist between this and the pulmonary artery, the phenomena of the motion of the blood are nearly the same in both: thus a ligature being applied upon this vessel, near the heart, in a living animal, it contracts in its whole length, and, except a small quantity that remains in the principal arteries, the blood passes immediately into the veins.

Some authors doubt the fact of the contraction of the arteries; the following experiment may be made to convince them: uncover the carotid artery of a living animal the length of several inches; take the transverse dimension of the vessel with compasses, tie it at two different points at the same time, and you may then have any length whatever of artery full of blood; make a small opening in the sides of this portion of the artery, you will immediately see almost the whole of the blood pass out, and it will even spout to a certain distance. Then measure the breadth with the compasses, and there will be no doubt of the artery being much contracted, if the rapid expulsion of the blood has not already convinced you. This experiment also proves that the force with which the artery contracts is sufficient to expel the blood that it contains.

Passage of the blood of the arteries into the veins.—When, in the dead body, an injection is thrown into an artery, it immediately returns by the corresponding vein: the same thing takes place, and with still more facility, if the injection is thrown into the artery of a living animal. In cold-blooded animals, the blood can be seen, by the aid of a microscope, passing from the arteries into the veins. The communication between these vessels is then direct, and very easy; it is natural to suppose that the heart, after having forced the blood to the last arterial twigs, continues to make it move into the venous radicles, and even into the veins. Harvey, and a great number of celebrated anatomists, thought so. Lately, Bichât has been strongly against this doctrine: he has limited the influence of the blood; he pretends that it ceases entirely in the place where the arterial is changed into venous blood, that is, in the numerous small vessels that terminate the arteries and commence the veins. In this place, according to him, the *action of the small vessels alone* is the cause of the motion of the blood.

Remarks on the Movements of the Heart.—A. The right auricle and ventricle, and the left auricle and ventricle, the action of which we have studied separately, in reality form only one organ, which is the heart.

The auricles contract and dilate together; the same thing takes place with the ventricles, whose movements are simultaneous.

When the contraction of the heart is spoken of, that of the ventricle is understood. Their contraction is called *systole*, their dilatation *diastole*.

B. Every time that the ventricles contract, the whole of the heart is rapidly carried forward, and the point of this organ strikes the left lateral side of the chest, opposite the internal of the sixth and seventh true ribs.

C. The number of the pulsations of the heart is considerable; it is generally greater in proportion as the person is younger.

At birth it is from 130 to 140 in a minute.
At one year...... 120 to 130.
At two years..... 100 to 110.
At three years.... 90 to 100.
At seven years.... 85 to 90.
At fourteen years 80 to 85.
At adult age.. ... 75 to 80.
At first old age.... 65 to 75.
At confirmed old age 60 to 65.

But these numbers vary according to an infinity of circumstances, sex, temperament, individual disposition, &c.

The affections of the mind have a great influence upon the rapidity of the contractions of the heart; every one knows that even a slight emotion immediately modifies the contractions, and generally accelerates them. In this respect great changes take place also by diseases.

D. Many researches have been made to determine with what force the ventricles contract. In order to appreciate that of the left ventricle, an experiment has been made, which consists in crossing the legs, and placing upon one knee the ham of the other leg, with a weight of 55 pounds appended to the extremity of the foot. This considerable weight, though placed at the extremity of such a long lever, is raised at each contraction of the ventricle, on account of the tendency to straighten the accidental curvature of the popliteal artery, when the legs are crossed in this manner.

This experiment shows that the force of contraction of the heart is very great; but it cannot give the exact value of it. Mechanical physiologists have made great efforts to express it in numbers. Borelli compares the force which keeps up the circulation to that which would be necessary to raise 180,000 pounds; Hales believes it to be 51 pounds 5 ounces; and Keil reduces it to from 15 to 8 ounces. Where shall we find the truth in these contradictions?

It seems impossible to know exactly the force developed by the heart in its contraction; it very probably varies according to numerous causes, such as age, the volume of the organ, the size of the individual, the particular disposition, the quantity of blood, the state of the nervous system, the action of the organs, the state of health or of sickness, &c.

All that has been said of the force of the heart relates only to its contraction, its dilatation having been considered as a passive state, a sort of repose of the fibres; however, when the ventricles dilate, it is with a very great force, for example, capable of raising a weight of twenty pounds, as may be observed in animals recently dead. When the heart of a living animal is taken hold of by the hand, however small it may be, it is impossible by any effort to prevent the dilatation of the ventricles. The dilatation of the heart, then, cannot be considered as a state of inaction or repose.

E. The heart moves from the first days of existence of the embryo to the instant of death by decrepitude.

Why does it move? This question has been asked by ancient and modern philosophers and physiologists. The *wherefore* of phenomena is not easy to be given in physiology; almost always what is taken for such is only in other terms the expression of the phenomena; but it is remarkable how easily we deceive ourselves in this respect; one of the strongest proofs of it is afforded by the different explanations of the motion of the heart.

The ancients said that there was a *pulsific virtue* in the heart, a *concentrated fire*, that gave motion to this organ. Descartes imagined that *an explosion as sudden as that of gunpowder* took place in the heart. The motion of the heart was afterward attributed to the *animal spirits*, to the *nervous fluid*, to the *soul*, to the *process of the nervous system*, to the *archea:* Haller considers it as an effect of irritability. Lately, Legallois has endeavoured to prove, by experiments, that the principle or cause of the motion of the heart has its seat in the spinal marrow.

Remarks upon the circular Motion of the Blood, or the Circulation.—We now know all the links of the circular chain that the sanguiferous system represents; we know how the blood is carried from the lungs toward all the other parts of the body, and how it returns from these parts to the heart. Let us examine these phenomena in a general manner, in order to show the most important.

A. The quantity of blood contained in the system is very considerable. It has been estimated by several authors at from 24 to 30 pounds. This value cannot be at all exact, for the quantity of blood varies according to numerous causes.

The relation of the mass of the arterial with that of the venous blood, is somewhat better known. This last, contained in vessels larger than that of the arteries, is necessarily in greater quantity, though we cannot say exactly how much greater its mass is than that of the arterial blood.

B. The circulatory path of the blood being continuous, and the capacity of the canal variable, the rapidity of this fluid must be variable also; for the same quantity must pass through all the points in a given time: observation confirms this. The rapidity is great in the trunk, and the principal divisions of the pulmonary artery and aorta: it diminishes much in the secondary divisions; it diminishes still more at the instant of the passage from the arteries into the veins; it continues to augment in proportion as the blood passes from the roots of the veins into larger roots, and lastly into the large veins; but the rapidity is never so great in the venæ cavæ as in the aorta. In the trunks and the principal arterial divisions, the course of the blood is not only continued under the influence of the contraction of the arteries, but, besides, it flows in jerks by the effect of the contraction of the ventricles. This jerking manifests itself in the arteries by a simple dilatation in those that are straight, and by a dilatation and tendency to straighten in those which are flexuous.

The pulse is formed by the first of these phenomena, to which the second is sometimes joined. It is not easy to study, in man or in the animals, except where the arteries are laid close upon a bone, because they do not then retire from under the finger when it is placed upon them, as happens to arteries in soft parts.

In general, the pulse makes known the principal modification of the contraction of the left ventricle, its quickness, its intensity, its weakness, its regularity, its irregularity. The quantity of the blood is also known by the pulse. If it is great, the artery is round, thick, and resisting. If the blood is in small quantity, the artery is small and easily flattened. Certain dispositions in the arteries have an influence also upon the pulse, and may render it different in the principal arteries.

C. The beating of the arteries is necessarily felt in the organs which are next them, and so much more in proportion as the arteries are more voluminous, and as the organs give way with less facility. The jerk which they undergo is generally considered as favourable to their action, though no positive proof of it exists.

In this respect none of the organs ought to be more affected than the brain. The four cerebral arteries unite in circles at the base of the skull, and raise the brain at each contraction of the ventricle, as it is easy to be convinced of by laying bare the brain of an animal, or by observing this organ in wounds of the head. Probably, the numerous angular bendings of the internal carotid arteries, and of the vertebrals before their entrance into the skull, are useful for moderating this shaking; these bendings must also necessarily retard the course of the blood in these vessels.

When the arteries penetrate in a voluminous state into the parenchyma of the organs, as the liver, the kidneys, &c., the organ must also receive a jerk at each contraction of the heart. The organs into which the vessels enter, after being divided and subdivided, can suffer nothing similar.

D. From the lungs to the left auricle the blood is of the same nature; however, it sometimes happens that it is not the same in the four pulmonary veins. For instance, if the lungs are so changed that the air cannot penetrate into the lobules, the blood which traverses them will not be changed from venous to arterial blood; it will arrive at the heart without having undergone this change; but in its passage through the left cavities it will be intimately mixed with that of the lungs opposite. The blood is necessarily homogeneous from the left ventricle to the last divisions of the aorta; but, being arrived at these small divisions, its elements separate; at least there exists a great number of parts, such as the serous membranes, the cellular tissue, the tendons, the aponeuroses, the fibrous membranes, &c., into which the red part of the blood is never seen to penetrate, and the capillaries of which contain only serum.

This separation of the elements of the blood takes place only in a state of health; when the parts that I have mentioned become diseased, it often happens that their small vessels contain blood, possessed of all its characteristic properties.

There have been endeavours to explain this particular analysis of the blood by the small vessels. Boerhaave, who admitted several sorts of globules of different sizes in the blood, said, that globules of a certain largeness could only pass into vessels of an appropriate size: we have seen that globules, such as they were admitted by Boerhaave, do not exist.

Bichât believed that there existed in the small vessels a particular sensibility, by which they admitted only the part of the blood suitable to them. We have already frequently contested ideas of this kind; neither can they be admitted here; for the most irritating liquids, introduced into the arteries, pass immediately into the veins, without any opposition to their passage by the capillaries.

E. The elements of the blood separate in traversing the small vessels; sometimes the serum escapes, and spreads upon the surface of the membrane: sometimes the fatty matter is deposited in cells; here the mucus, there the fibrine; elsewhere are the foreign substances, which were accidentally mixed with the arterial blood. In losing these different elements, the blood assumes the qualities of venous blood. At the same time that the arterial blood supplies these losses, the small veins absorb the substances with which they are in contact. In the intestinal canal, for example, they absorb the drinks; on the other hand, the lymphatic trunks pour the lymph and the chyle into the venous system; it is certain, then, that the venous blood cannot be homogeneous, and that its composition must be variable in the different veins; but, having reached the heart, by the motions of the right auricle and ventricle, and the disposition of the fleshy columns, the elements all mix together, and when they are completely mixed, they pass into the pulmonary artery.

F. A general law of the economy is, that no organ continues to act without receiving arterial blood; from this results, that all the other functions are dependent on the circulation; but the circulation, in its turn, cannot continue without the respiration by which the arterial blood is formed, and without the action of the nervous system, which has a great influence upon the rapidity of the flowing of the blood, and upon its distribution in the organs. Indeed, under the action of the nervous system, the motions of the heart, and consequently the general quickness of the course of the blood, are quickened or retarded. Thus, when the organs act voluntarily or involuntarily, we learn from observation, that they receive a greater quantity of blood without the motion of the general circulation being accelerated on that account; and if their action predominates, the arteries which are directed there, increase considerably. If, on the contrary, the action diminishes, or ceases entirely, the arteries become smaller, and permit only a small quantity to reach the organ. These phenomena are manifest in the muscles: the circulation becomes more rapid in them when they contract; if they are often contracted, the volume of their arteries increases; if they are paralyzed, the arteries become very small, and the pulse is scarcely felt.

The circulation, then, may be influenced by the nervous system in three ways: 1st, By modifying the motions of the heart; 2dly, By modifying the capillaries of the organs, so as to accelerate the flowing of the blood in them; 3dly, By producing the same effects in the lungs, that is, by rendering the course of the blood more or less easy through this organ.

The acceleration of the motions of the heart becomes sensible to us by the manner in which the point of the organ strikes the walls of the chest. The difficulty of the capillary circulation is discovered by a feeling of numbness and a particular prickling; and when the pulmonary circulation is difficult, we are informed of it by an oppression or sense of suffocation, more or less strong.

Probably the distribution of the filaments of the great sympathetic on the sides of the arteries, has some important use; but this use is entirely unknown; we have received no light on the point by any experiment."—*Magendie's Elements of Physiology.*

Circula'tor. (From *circulo*, to compass about.) A wandering practiser in medicine. A quack; a mountebank.

Circulato'rium. (From *circulo*, to move round.) A chemical digesting vessel in which the fluid performs a circulatory motion.

CI'RCULUS. (Dim. of *circus*, a circle.) 1. A circle or ring.

2. Any part of the body which is round or annular, as *circulus oculi.*

3. A round chemical instrument sometimes called abbreviatorium by the old chemists.

Circulus arteriosus iridis. The artery which runs round the iris and forms a circle, is so termed.

Circulus quadruplex. A bandage.

Circumcaula'lis. A name of the adnata of the eye.

CIRCUMCI'SION. (*Circumcisio*, from *circumcido*, to cut about.) The cutting off the prepuce from the glans penis; an ancient custom, still practised among the Jews, and rendered necessary by the heat of the climate in which it was first practised, to prevent collections and a vitiated state of the sebaceous secretion from the odoriferous glands of the part.

CIRCUMFLE'XUS. (*Circumflexus*, sc. *musculus.*) A muscle of the palate. *Tensor palati* of Innes. *Circumflexus palati mollis* of Albinus. *Spheno-salpingo-staphilinus, seu staphilinus externus* of Winslow. *Musculus tubæ novæ* of Valsalva. *Palato-salpingeus* of Douglas. *Pterigo-staphylinus* of Cowper, and *Petrosalpingo staphilin* of Dumas. It arises from the spinous process of the sphenoid bone, behind the foramen ovale, which transmits the third branch of the fifth pair of nerves, and from the Eustachian tube, not far from its osseous part; it then runs down along the pterygoideus internus, passes over the hook of the internal plate of the pterygoid process by a round tendon, which soon spreads into a broad membrane. It is inserted into the velum pendulum palati, and the semilunar edge of the os palati, and extends as far as the suture which joins the two bones. Generally some of its posterior fibres join with the constrictor pharyngis superior, and palato-pharyngæus. Its use is to stretch the velum, to draw it downwards, and to the side towards the hook. It hath little effect upon the tube, being chiefly connected to its osseous part.

CIRCUMGYRA'TIO. (From *circumgyro*, to turn round.) Circumgyration, or the turning a limb round in its socket.

CIRCUMLI'TIO. (From *circumlino*, to anoint all over.) A medicine used as a general unction or liniment to the part.

CIRCUMOSSA'LIS. (From *circum*, about, and *os*, a bone.) Surrounding a bone as the periosteum does; or surrounded by a bone.

CIRCUMSCISUS. Circumcised. Applied to a membranous capsule, separating into two parts by a complete circular fissure.

CI'RCUS. (Κιρκος; from *carka*, a Chaldean word, to surround.) 1. A circle or ring.

2. A circular bandage.

CIRNE'SIS. (From κιρναω, to mix.) A union of separate things.

CIRRUS. (From κερας, a horn, because it has the appearance of a horn) *Cirrhus*. A clasper or tendril. One of the *fulcra* or props of plants. A long, cylindrical, slender, spiral body, issuing from various parts of plants.

From their *origin*, Cirri are distinguished into,

1. *Foliar*, when they are a continuation of the midrib of a simple leaf; as in *Fumaria claviculata*, *Mimosa scandens*, and *Gloriosa superba*.

2. *Petiolar*, when terminating the common petiole of a compound leaf; as in *Pisum sativum*. This is sometimes distinguished by the number of leaflets which grow under it: hence *cirri diphylli*, *tetraphylli*, and *polyphylli*.

3. *Peduncular*, when they proceed from the peduncle; as in *Vitis vinifera*.

4. *Axillary*, which arise from the stem or branches in the axillæ of the leaves; as in *Passiflora incarnata*.

5. *Subaxillary*, when they originate below the leaf.

6. *Lateral*, when at the side of it; as in *Bryonia*.

From the division of its apex, a Cirrus is,

1. *Simple*, consisting of one undivided piece; as in *Momordica balsaminea*, *Passiflora quadrangularis*, and *Bryonia dioica*.

2. *Compound*, consisting of a stalk variously branched or divided.

3. *Bifid*, when it has two divisions; as in *Vitis vinifera*, *Lathyrus palustris*, *Ervum tetraspermum*, &c.

4. *Trifid*, when there are three; as in *Bignonia unguis*, and *Lathyrus hirsutus*.

5. *Multifid*, or *branched*, when the divisions are more numerous; as in *Lathyrus latifolius*, and *Cobea scandens*.

From its *convolution* into,

1. *Convolute*, when all the gyrations are regular in the same direction; as in *Hedera quinquefolia*.

2. *Revolute*, winding itself irregularly, sometimes on one side, sometimes on the other; as in *Passiflora incarnata*.

CIRROSUS. Having a cirrus or tendril. Applied to a leaf tipped with a tendril; as in *Gloriosa* and *Flagellaria*, two Indian plants.

CI'RSIUM ARVENSE. (From κιρσος, a vein, or swelling of a vein, which this herb was supposed to heal.) The common way thistle, or *Serratula arvensis* of Linnæus.

CIRSOCE'LE. See *Circocele*.

CIRSOI'DES. (From κιρσος, a varix, and ειδος, likeness.) Resembling a varix: an epithet applied by Rufus Ephesius to the upper part of the brain.

CI'RSOS. (Κιρσος; from κιρσοω, to dilate.) A preternatural distention of any part of a vein. See *Varix*.

CI'SSA. (From κισσα, a gluttonous bird.) A depraved appetite, proceeding from previous gluttony and voracity.

CISSA'MPELOS. (From κισσος, ivy, and αμπελος, the vine.) The name of a genus of plants in the Linnæan system. Class, *Diœcia*; Order, *Monadelphia*. The wild vine with leaves like ivy

CISSAMPELOS PAREIRA. The systematic name of the *Pareira brava; Pareyra; Ambutua; Butua; Overo butua*. The root of this plant, *Cissampelos—foliis peltatis cordatis emarginatis*, of Linnæus; a native of South America and the West Indies, has no remarkable smell, but to the taste it manifests a notable sweetness of the liquorice kind, together with a considerable bitterness, and a slight roughness covered by the sweet matter. The facts adduced on the utility of the *radix pareiræ bravæ* in nephritic and calculous complaints, are principally by foreigners, and no remarkable instances of its efficacy are recorded by English practitioners.

CISSA'RUS. See *Cistus Creticus*.

CISSI'NUM. (From κισσος, ivy.) The name of a plaster mentioned by Ægineta.

CI'STA. (From κειμαι, to lie.) A cyst.

CISTE'RNA. (From *cista*, a cyst.) The fourth ventricle of the brain is so called from its cavity; also the lacteal vessels in the breasts of women.

CI'STHORUS. See *Cistus Creticus*.

CISTIC. See *Cystic*.

CISTIC OXIDE. See *Calculus*.

CI'STUS. (Κισ7ος, the derivation of which is uncertain; perhaps from *kis*, Heb.) The name of a genus of plants in the Linnæan system. Class, *Polyandria*; Order, *Monogynia*. The Cistus.

CISTUS CRETICUS. The systematic name of the plant from which the ladanum of the shops is obtained, called also *Cistus ladanifera*, *Cisthorus; Cissarus; Dorycinium*. *Cistus—arborescens extipulatus, foliis spatulato-ovatis petiolatis enerviis scabris calycinis lanceolatis*, of Linnæus. The resinous juice called ladanum exudes upon the leaves of this plant in Candia, where the inhabitants collect it by lightly rubbing the leaves with leather, and afterward scraping it off, and forming it into irregular masses for exportation. Three sorts of ladanum have been described by authors, but only two are to be met with in the shops. The best, which is very rare, is in dark-coloured masses, of the consistence of a soft plaster, and growing still softer on being handled; the other is in long rolls, coiled up, much harder than the preceding, and not so dark. The first has commonly a small, and the last a large admixture of fine sand, without which they cannot be collected pure, independently of designed abuses: the dust blown on the plant by winds, from the loose sands among which it grows, being retained by the tenacious juice. The soft kind has an agreeable smell, and a lightly pungent bitterish taste: the hard is much weaker. Ladanum was formerly much employed internally as a pectoral and adstringent in catarrhal affections, dysenteries, and several other diseases; at present, however, it is wholly confined to external use, and is an ingredient in the stomachic plaster, *emplastrum ladani*.

CISTUS HUMILIS. A name most probably of the *Lichen caninus* of Linnæus.

CISTUS LADANIFERA. See *Cistus creticus*

CISTUS LEDON. See *Ledum palustre*.

CITE'SIUS (CITOIS), FRANCIS, of Poitiers, in France, who, after graduating at Montpelier in 1596, and practising a few years in his native city, went to Paris, and acquired great celebrity, being made physician to Cardinal Richelieu. He published a treatise on the Colica Pictonum, which was much esteemed, noticing its termination in paralysis of the extremities. He also gave an account of a girl who had fasted for three years; in which case he appears to have been imposed upon. In another publication he advocates repeated bleeding, as well as purging, in small-pox, and other fevers of an inflammatory type. He died in 1652, at the advanced age of 80.

CI'THARUS. (From κιθαρα, a harp.) The breast is sometimes so named from its shape.

CITRA'GO. (From *citrus*, a citron; so called from its citron-like smell.) *Citraria*. Baum. See *Melissa*.

CI'TRAS. (*Citras, atis*. fœm.: from *citrus*, the lemon.) A citrate. A salt formed by the union of the citric acid, or acid of lemons, with the salifiable bases; as *citrate of ammonia*, *citrate of potassa*.

CITRATE. See *Citras*.

CI'TREA. See *Citrus medica*.

CI'TREUM. (From *citrus*.) The citron-tree. See *Citrus medica*.

CI'TRIC ACID. *Acidum citricum* "The juice of

lemons, or limes, has all the characters of an acid of considerable strength; but on account of the mucilaginous matter with which it is mixed, it is very soon altered by spontaneous decomposition. Various methods have been contrived to prevent this effect from taking place, in order that this wholesome and agreeable acid might be preserved for use in long voyages, or other domestic occasions. The juice may be kept in bottles under a thin stratum of oil, which indeed prevents, or greatly retards, its total decomposition; though the original fresh taste soon gives place to one which is much less grateful. In the East Indies it is evaporated to the consistence of a thick extract. If this operation be carefully performed by a very gentle heat, it is found to be very effectual. When the juice is thus heated, the mucilage thickens, and separates in the form of flocks, part of which subside, and part rise to the surface: these must be taken out. The vapours which arise are not acid. If the evaporation be not carried so far as to deprive the liquid of its fluidity, it may be long preserved in well closed bottles; in which, after some weeks standing, a farther portion of mucilage is separated, without any perceptible change in the acid.

Of all the methods of preserving lemon-juice, that of concentrating it by frost appears to be the best, though in the warmer climates it cannot conveniently be practised. Lemon-juice, exposed to the air in a temperature between 50° and 60°, deposites in a few hours a white semi-transparent mucilaginous matter, which leaves the fluid, after decantation and filtration, much less alterable than before. This mucilage is not of a gummy nature, but resembles the gluten of wheat in its properties: it is not soluble in water when dried. More mucilage is separated from lemon-juice by standing in closed vessels. If this depurated lemon-juice be exposed to a degree of cold of about seven or eight degrees below the freezing point, the aqueous part will freeze, and the ice may be taken away as it forms; and if the process be continued until the ice begins to exhibit signs of acidity, the remaining acid will be found to be reduced to about one-eighth of its original quantity, at the same time that its acidity will be eight times as intense, as is proved by its requiring eight times the quantity of alkali to saturate an equal portion of it. This concentrated acid may be kept for use, or, if preferred, it may be made into a dry lemonade, by adding six times its weight of fine loaf sugar in powder.

The above processes may be used when the acid of lemons is wanted for domestic purposes, because they leave it in possession of the oils, or other principles, on which its flavour peculiarly depends; but in chemical researches, where the acid itself is required to be had in the utmost purity, a more elaborate process must be used. Boiling lemon-juice is to be saturated with powdered chalk, the weight of which is to be noted, and the powder must be stirred up from the bottom, or the vessel shaken from time to time. The neutral saline compound is scarcely more soluble in water than selenite; it therefore falls to the bottom, while the mucilage remains suspended in the watery fluid, which must be decanted off; the remaining precipitate must then be washed with warm water until it comes off clear. To the powder thus edulcorated, a quantity of sulphuric acid, equal the chalk in weight, and diluted with ten parts of water, must be added, and the mixture boiled a few minutes. The sulphuric acid combines with the earth, and forms sulphate of lime, which remains behind when the cold liquor is filtered, while the disengaged acid of lemons remains dissolved in the fluid. This last must be evaporated to the consistence of a thin syrup, which yields the pure citric acid in little needle-like crystals. It is necessary that the sulphuric acid should be rather in excess, because the presence of a small quantity of lime will prevent the crystallization. This excess is allowed for above.

Its taste is extremely sharp, so as to appear caustic. It is among the vegetable acids the one which most powerfully resists decomposition by fire.

In a dry and warm air it seems to effloresce; but it absorbs moisture when the air is damp, and at length loses its crystalline form. A hundred parts of this acid are soluble in seventy-five of water at 60°. Though it is less alterable than most other solutions of vegetable acids, it will undergo decomposition when long kept.

It is not altered by any combustible substance, charcoal alone appears to be capable of whitening it. The most powerful acids decompose it less easily than they do other vegetable acids; the sulphuric evidently converts it into acetic acid. The nitric acid likewise, if employed in large quantity, and heated on it a long time, converts the greater part of it into acetic acid, and a small portion into oxalic.

The *citrate of lime* has been mentioned already in treating of the mode of purifying the acid.

The *citrate of potassa* is very soluble and deliquescent.

The *citrate of soda* has a dull saline taste; dissolves in less than twice its weight of water, crystallizes in six-sided prisms with flat summits; effloresces slightly, but does not fall to powder; boils up, swells, and is reduced to a coal on the fire. Lime water decomposes it, but does not render the solution turbid, notwithstanding the little solubility of citrate of lime.

Citrate of ammonia is very soluble; does not crystallize unless its solution be greatly concentrated; and forms elongated prisms.

Citrate of magnesia does not crystallize. When its solution had been boiled down, and it had stood some days, on being slightly shaken it fixed in one white opaque mass, which remained soft, separating from the sides of the vessel, contracting its dimensions, and rising in the middle like a kind of mushroom.

All the citrates are decomposed by the powerful acids, which do not form a precipitate with them, as with the oxalates and tartrates. The oxalic and tartaric acids decompose them, and form crystallized or insoluble precipitates in their solutions. All afford traces of acetic acid, or a product of the same nature, on being exposed to distillation: this character exists particularly in the metallic citrates. Placed on burning coals they melt, swell up, emit an empyreumatic smell of acetic acid, and leave a light coal. All of them, if dissolved in water, and left to stand for a time, undergo decomposition, deposite a flocculent mucus which grows black, and leaves their bases combined with carbonic acid, one of the products of the decomposition. Before they are completely decomposed, they appear to pass to the state of acetates.

The affinities of the citric acid are arranged by Vauquelin in the following order: barytes, lime, potassa, soda, strontian, magnesia, ammonia, alumina. Those for zircone, glucine, and the metallic oxides, are not ascertained.

The citric acid is found in many fruits united with the malic acid.

Citric acid being more costly than tartaric, may be occasionally *adulterated* with it. This fraud is discovered, by adding slowly to the acid dissolved in water a solution of subcarbonate of potassa, which will give a white pulverulent precipitate of tartar, if the citric be contaminated with the tartaric acid. When one part of citric acid is dissolved in 19 of water, the solution may be used as a substitute for lemon-juice. If before solution the crystals be triturated with a little sugar and a few drops of the oil of lemons, the resemblance to the native juice will be complete. It is an antidote against sea scurvy; but the admixture of mucilage and other vegetable matter in the recent fruit of the lemon, has been supposed to render it preferable to the pure acid of the chemist."—*Ure's Chem. Dict*

CITRINA'TIO. Complete digestion.

CITRI'NULA. (A diminutive of *citrus*.) A small citron or lemon.

CITRON. See *Citrus medica*.

Citrul, Sicilian. See *Cucurbita citrullus*.

CITRU'LLUS. See *Cucurbita citrullus*.

CI'TRUS. 1. The name of a genus of plants in the Linnæan system. Class, *Polyadelphia*; Order, *Icosandria*.

2. The name of the lemon. See *Citrus medica*.

CITRUS AURANTIUM. The systematic name of the orange tree and fruit. *Aurantium*; *Aurantium Hispalense*; *Aurantium Chinense*; *Malus aurantia major*; *Malus aurantia*; *Aurantium vulgare*; *Malus aurantia vulgaris*; *Mala aurea*; *Chrysomelia*; *Nerantia*; *Martianum pomum*; *Poma aurantia*. The China and Seville orange are both only varieties of the same species: *Citrus:—petiolis alatis, foliis acuminatis*, of Linnæus. The latter is specified in our pharmacopœias; and the *flowers*, *leaves*, *yellow rind*, and *juice*, are made use of for different medical purposes.

The flowers, *flores naphæ*, are highly odoriferous, and are used as a perfume; they are bitter to the taste; they give their taste and smell both to water and to spirit, but most perfectly to rectified spirit of wine. The water which is distilled from these flowers, is called *aqua florum naphæ*. In distillation, they yield a small quantity of essential oil, which is called *oleum* vel *essentia neroli:* they are brought from Italy and France. Orange flowers were, at one time, said to be a useful remedy in convulsive diseases; but experience has not confirmed the virtues attributed to them.

The *leaves* have a bitterish taste, and yield, by distillation, an essential oil; indeed, by rubbing them between the fingers and the thumb, they manifest considerable fragrance. They have been applied for the same purposes as the flowers, but without success.

The *yellow rind* of the fruit, freed from the white fungous part, has a grateful aromatic flavour, and a warm, bitterish taste. Infused in boiling water, it gives out nearly all its smell and taste: cold water extracts the bitter, but very little of the flavour. In distillation, a light, fragrant, essential oil rises, without the bitter. Its qualities are those of an aromatic and bitter. It has been employed to restore the tone of the stomach, and is a very common addition to combinations of bitters, used in dyspepsia. It has likewise been given in intermittents, in doses of a drachm, twice or thrice a day. It is also much celebrated as a powerful remedy, in menorrhagia, and immoderate uterine evacuations.

The *juice* of Seville oranges is a grateful acid, which, by allaying heat, quenching thirst, promoting various excretions, and diminishing the action of the sanguiferous system, proves extremely useful in both ardent and putrid fevers; though the China orange juice, as impregnated with a larger proportion of sugar, becomes more agreeable, and may be taken in larger quantities. The Seville orange juice is particularly serviceable as an antiscorbutic, and alone will prevent or cure scurvy in the most apparently desperate circumstances. In dyspepsia, from putrid bile in the stomach, both lemon and orange juice are highly useful.

CITRUS MEDICA. The systematic name of the lemon-tree. *Limon; Limonia mala; Malus medica; Malus limonia acida; Citrea malus; Citrus.* The tree which affords the lemon is the *Citrus:—petiolis linearibus*, of Linnæus: a native of the upper part of Asia, but cultivated in Spain, Portugal, and France. The juice, which is much more acid than that of the orange, possesses similar virtues. It is always preferred where a strong vegetable acid is required. Saturated with the fixed vegetable alkali, it forms the citrate of potassa, which is in frequent extemporaneous use in febrile diseases, and by promoting the secretions, especially that of the skin, proves of considerable service in abating the violence of fever. This medicine is also often employed to restrain vomiting. As an antiscorbutic, lemon juice has been often taken on board ships destined for long voyages; but even when well depurated of its mucilaginous parts, it is found to spoil by long keeping. To preserve it in purity for a considerable length of time, it is necessary that it should be brought to a highly concentrated state, and for this purpose it has been recommended to expose the juice to a degree of cold sufficient to congeal the aqueous and mucilaginous parts. After a crust of ice is formed, the juice is poured into another vessel; and, by repeating this process several times, the remaining juice, it is said, has been concentrated to eight times its original strength, and kept without suffering any material change for several years. Whytt found the juice of lemon to allay hysterical palpitations of the heart, after various other medicines had been experienced ineffectual; and this juice, or that of oranges, taken to the quantity of four or six ounces in a day, has sometimes been found a remedy in the jaundice. The exterior rind of the lemon is a very grateful aromatic bitter, not so hot as orange peel, and yielding in distillation a less quantity of oil, which is extremely light, almost colourless, and generally brought from the southern parts of Europe, under the name of Essence of Lemons. The lemon-peel, though less warm, is similar in its qualities to that of the orange, and is employed with the same intentions. The pharmacopœias direct a syrup of the juice, *syrupus limonis*, and the peel enters into some vinous and aqueous bitter infusions; it is also ordered to be candied; and the essential oil is an ingredient in some formulæ.

The citron-tree is also considered as belonging to the same species, the *Citrus medica* of Linnæus. Its fruit is called *Cedromela*, which is larger and less succulent than the lemon; but in all other respects the citron and lemon trees agree. The citron juice, when sweetened with sugar, is called by the Italians *Agro di cedro*. The *Citrus mella rosa* of Lamarck, is another variety of the *Citrus medica* of Linnæus. It was produced, at first, casually, by an Italian's grafting a citron on a stock of a bergamot pear-tree; whence the fruit produced by this union participated both of the citron-tree and the pear-tree. The essence prepared from this fruit is called essence of bergamote and essentia de cedra.

CI'TTA. A voracious appetite.

CITTO'SIS. See *Chlorosis*.

CIVET-CAT. See *Zibethum*.

CIVE'TTA. (From *sebet*, Arabian.) *Zibethum* Civet; an unctuous odoriferous drug used by perfumers, collected between the anus and the organs of generation of a fierce carnivorous quadruped met with in China and the East and West Indies, called a civet-cat, the *Viverra Zibethum* of Linnæus, but bearing a greater resemblance to a fox or marten than a cat.

Several of these animals have been brought into Holland, and afford a considerable branch of commerce, particularly at Amsterdam. The civet is squeezed out in summer every other day, in winter twice a-week: the quantity procured at once is from two scruples to a drachm or more. The juice thus collected is much purer and finer than that which the animal sheds against shrubs or stones in its native climates.

Good civet is of a clear yellowish or brownish colour, not fluid nor hard, but about the consistence of butter or honey, and uniform throughout; of a very strong smell; quite offensive when undiluted; but agreeable when only a small portion of civet is mixed with a large one of other substances.

Civet unites with oils, but not with alkohol. Its nature is therefore not resinous.

CLAP. See *Gonorrhœa*.

CLA'RET. (*Claretum;* from *clareo*, to be clear.) A French wine, that may be given with great advantage, as a tonic and antiseptic, where red port wine disagrees with the patient; and in typhoid fevers of children, and delicate females, it is far preferable, as a common drink.

CLARE'TUM. 1. The wine called *claret*. See *Claret*.

2. A wine impregnated with spices and sugar, called by some *Vinum Hippocraticum*.

3. A *Claretum purgatorium*, composed of a vinous infusion of glass of antimony with cinnamon water and sugar, is mentioned by Schrœder.

CLARIFICA'TIO. The depuration of any thing, or process of freeing a fluid from heterogeneous matter, or feculencies.

["CLARK, JOHN. The name of John Clark has been, for a longer succession of years than any other in our country, distinguished in the ranks of medical practitioners. Of the earliest physician of that name, who probably came from England in 1631 or 1632, and after living a few years in Boston, removed to Rhode Island, where he died April 20th, 1676, filling a long course of service in administering to the religious as well as natural wants of his neighbours" He was succeeded by several individuals of the same name, who were all conspicuous members of the medical profession.—*Thach. Med. Biog.* A.]

CLASS. (*Classis;* from καλεω, *congrego*, a class being nothing more than a multitude assembled apart.) The name of a primary division of bodies in natural history.

CLARY. See *Salvia*.

CLA'SIS. (From κλαω, to break.) *Clasma.* A fracture.

CLAU'STRUM. (From *claudo*, to shut.) *Cleithrum gutturis.* Any aperture which has a power of contracting itself, or closing its orifice by any means; as the passage of the throat.

CLAUSTRUM VIRGINITATIS. The hymen.

CLAUSU'RA. (From *claudo*, to shut.) An imperforation of any canal or cavity in the body. Thus *clausura uteri* is a preternatural imperforation of the uterus; *clausura tubarum Fallopiarum*, a morbid imperforation of the Fallopian tubes, mentioned by Ruysch as one cause of infecundity.

CLAVA RUGOSA. See *Acorus calamus*.

CLAVARIA. (From *clava*, a club.) The name of a genus of plants, Class, *Cryptogamia;* Order, *Fungi*. Club-shaped fungus.

CLAVARIA COROLLOIDES. The systematic name of the *Fungus corolloides* of old writers; called also *crotelus*. It was once used as a strengthener and astringent.

CLAVA'TIO. (From *clava*, a club.) A sort of articulation without motion, where the parts are, as it were, driven in with a hammer, like the teeth in the sockets. See *Gomphosis*.

CLAVATUS. Clubbed. Applied to parts of plants, as the stigma of the Genipi.

CLAVELLATUS. (From *clavus*, a wedge. The name cineres clavellati originated from the little wedges or billets, into which the wood was cut to burn for potassa.) See *Potassa impura*.

CLA'VICLE. (*Clavicula*, diminutive of *clavis;* so called from its resemblance to an ancient key.) Collar-bone. The clavicle is placed at the root of the neck, and at the upper part of the breast. It extends across, from the tip of the shoulder to the upper part of the sternum; it is a round bone, a little flattened towards the end, which joins the scapula; it is curved like an Italic *S*, having one curve turned out towards the breast: it is useful as an arch, supporting the shoulders, preventing them from falling forwards upon the breast, and making the hands strong antagonists to each other; which, without this steadying, they could not have been.

1. The thoracic end, that next the sternum, or what may be called the inner head of the clavicle, is round and flat, or button-like; and it is received into a suitable hollow on the upper piece of the sternum. It is not only, like other joints, surrounded by a capsule or purse; it is further provided with a small moveable cartilage, which, like a friction wheel in machinery, saves the parts and facilitates the motions, and moves continually as the clavicle moves.

2. But the outward end of the clavicle is flattened, as it approaches the scapula, and the edge of that flatness is turned to the edge of the flattened acromion, so that they touch but in one single point. This outer end of the clavicle, and the corresponding point of the acromion, are flattened and covered with a crust of cartilage; but the motion here is very slight and quite insensible; they are tied firmly by strong ligaments; and we may consider this as almost a fixed point, for there is little motion of the scapula upon the clavicle; but there is much motion of the clavicle upon the breast, for the clavicle serves as a shaft, or axis, firmly tied to the scapula, upon which the scapula moves and turns, being connected with the trunk only by this single point, viz. the articulation of the clavicle with the breast-bone.

CLAVI'CULA. See *Clavicle*.

CLAVI'CULUS. See *Clavicle*.

CLA'VIS. (From *claudo*, to shut.) The clavicle.

CLA'VUS. (A nail.) 1. A corn called *clavus*, from its resemblance to the head of a nail; *Ecphyma clavus* of Good. A roundish, horny, cutaneous extuberance, with a central nucleus, sensible at its base; found chiefly on the toes, from the pressure of tight shoes.

2. A painful and often an intermitting affection of the head, and mostly a severe pulsating pain in the forehead, which may be covered by one's thumb, giving a sensation like as if a nail were driven into the part. When connected with hysterics, it is called *Clavus hystericus*.

3. An artificial palate.

4. Diseased uterus.

CLAVUS HYSTERICUS. See *Clavus*.

CLAVUS OCULORUM. A staphyloma, or tumour on the eyelids.

CLAY. *Argilla*. Argillaceous earth, of which there are many kinds, and being opaque and noncrystallized bodies, of dull fracture, afford no good principle for determining their species; yet as they are extensively distributed in nature, and are used in many arts, they deserve particular attention. The argillaceous minerals are all sufficiently soft to be scratched by iron; they have a dull or even earthy fracture; they exhale, when breathed on, a peculiar smell called argillaceous. The clays form with water a plastic paste, possessing considerable tenacity, which hardens with heat, so as to strike fire with steel. Marles and chalks also soften in water, but their paste is not tenaceous, nor does it acquire a siliceous hardness in the fire. The affinity of the clays for moisture is manifested by their sticking to the tongue, and by the intense heat necessary to make them perfectly dry. The odour ascribed to clays breathed upon, is due to the oxide of iron mixed with them Absolutely pure clays emit no smell.

1. *Porcelain earth*, the kaolin of the Chinese.—This mineral is friable, meagre to the touch, and, when pure, forms with difficulty a paste with water.

2. *Potter's clay*, or *plastic clay*.—The clays of this variety are compact, smooth, and almost unctuous to the touch, and may be polished by the finger when they are dry. They have a great affinity to water, form a tenacious paste, and adhere strongly to the tongue.

3. *Loam*.—This is an impure potter's clay, mixed with mica and iron ochre.

4. *Variegated clay*.—Is striped or spotted with white, red, or yellow colours.

5. *Slate clay*.—Colour, gray or grayish-yellow.

6. *Claystone*.—Colour, gray, of various shades, sometimes red, and spotted, or striped.

7. *Adhesive slate*.—Colour, light-greenish gray.

8. *Polishing slate* of Werner.—Colour, cream-yellow, in alternate stripes.

9. *Common clay* may be considered to be the same as *loam*.

CLAY, PURE. See *Alumina*.

CLAY-SLATE. Argillaceous slate. Argillite of Kirwan. A mineral which is extensively distributed, forming a part of both primitive and transition mountains of slate, is found in many countries.

["CLAYTON, DR. JOHN, an eminent botanist and physician, of Virginia, was born in England in 1685, and came to Virginia in 1705, and resided near Williamsburg. He was elected a member of several of the first literary societies of Europe, and corresponded with many of the most learned naturalists of that period. As a practical botanist, he was, probably, not inferior to any one of the age. He passed a long life in exploring and describing the plants of his country, and is supposed to have enlarged the botanical catalogue as much as any man who ever lived. He is the author of "Flora Virginica," a work published by Gronovius at Leyden, 8vo. in 1739, 1743, and 1762. He published in the philosophical transactions several communications, treating of the culture of the different species of tobacco, and an ample account of the medicinal plants which he had discovered in Virginia. He also left behind him two volumes of manuscript neatly prepared for the press, and a Hortus Siccus with marginal notes and references for the engraver who should prepare the plates for his proposed work. He died December 15th, 1773, in the 88th year of his age. During the year preceding his decease, such was the vigour of his constitution, even at this advanced period, and such was his zeal in botanical researches, that he made a botanical tour through Orange County; and it is believed that he had visited most of the settled parts of Virginia. His character stands very high as a man of integrity, and as a good citizen."—*Thach. Med. Biog.* A.]

["CLAYTON, DR. JOSHUA, was Governor of the State of Delaware, and a member of the United States Senate; he died in 1799. He was highly respectable in the medical profession, in which he practised for many years.

In 1792, he addressed a friend as follows: "During the late war, the Peruvian bark was very scarce and dear. I was at that time engaged in considerable practice, and was under the necessity of seeking a substitute for the Peruvian bark. I conceived that the poplar, Liriodendron tulipifera, had more aromatic and bitter than the Peruvian, and less astringency. To correct and amend those qualities, I added to it nearly an equal quantity of the bark of the root of dogwood, cornus florida, and half the quantity of the inside bark of the white-oak tree. This remedy I prescribed for several years, in every case in which I conceived the Peruvian bark necessary or proper, with a least equal if not superior success. I used it in every species of intermittent, gangrenes, mortifications, and in short, every case of debility."—*Thach. Med. Biog.* A.]

CLEAVAGE. This term is applied to the mechanical division of crystals, by showing the direction in which their *laminæ* can separate, enables us to determine the mutual inclination of these *laminæ*: Werner called it *durchgang*, but he attended only to the number of directions in which this mechanical division of the plates, or cleavage, could be effected. In the interior of many minerals, the direction of the cleavage may be frequently seen, without using any mechanical violence.

CLEAVERS. See *Galium aparine.*

CLEGHORN, GEORGE, was born near Edinburgh, in 1716, and, after studying in that city, went at the age of twenty to Minorca, as a regimental surgeon. During the thirteen years that he spent there, he sedulously studied the natural productions of the island. In 1750, coming to London, he published his "Treatise on the Diseases of Minorca," which displays great observation and ability. He then went to Dublin, and gave lectures on anatomy with such success, that he was soon after appointed public professor; and, in 1774, an honorary member of the College of Physicians there. He died in 1789.

CLEI'DION. *Clidion.* The epithet of a pastil, described by Galen and Paulus Ægineta; and it is the name also of an epithem described by Aëtius.

CLEIDO'MA. (From κλειδοω, to close.) A pastil, or troch. Also the clavicle.

CLEIDOMASTOIDE'US. (From κλεις, the clavicle, and μαςοειδης, the mastoid process.) See *Sterno-cleido-mastoideus.*

CLEISA'GRA. (From κλεις, the clavicle, and αγρα, a prey.) The gout in the articulation of the clavicles.

CLEI'THRON. (From κλειδω, to shut.) See *Claustrum.*

CLE'MATIS. (From κλημα, a tendril; so named from its climbing up trees, or any thing it can fasten upon with its tendrils.) The name of a genus of plants in the Linnæan system. Class, *Polyandria;* Order, *Polygynia.*

CLEMATIS RECTA. The systematic name of the upright virgin's-bower. *Flammula Jovis. Clematis—foliis pinnatis, foliolis ovato lanceolatis integerrimis, caule erecto, floribus pentapetalis tetrapetalisque* of Linnæus. More praises have been bestowed upon the virtue which the leaves of this plant are said to possess, when exhibited internally, as antivenereal, by foreign physicians, than its trials in this country can justify. The powdered leaves are sometimes applied externally to ulcers, as an escharotic.

CLEMATIS VITALBA. The systematic name of the traveller's-joy. *Vitalba; Atragene; Viorna; Clematis arthragene* of Theophrastus. This plant is common in our hedges, and is the *Clematis—foliis pinnatius, foliolis cordatis scandentibus,* of Linnæus. Its leaves, when fresh, produce a warmth on the tongue, and if the chewing is continued, blisters arise. The same effect follows their being rubbed on the skin. The plant has been administered internally to cure lues venerea, scrofula, and rheumatism. In France, the young sprouts are eaten, when boiled, as hoptops are in this country.

CLEMATI'TIS. The same as clematis.

CLEO'NIS COLLYRIUM. The name of a collyrium described by Celsus.

CLEONIS GLUTEN. An astringent formula of myrrh, frankincense, and white of egg mixed together.

CLE'PSYDRA. (From κλεπτω, to conceal, and υδωρ, water.) Properly, an instrument to measure time by the dropping of water through a hole, from one vessel to another; but it is used to express a chemical vessel, perforated in the same manner. It is also an instrument mentioned by Paracelsus, contrived to convey suffumigations to the uterus in hysterical cases.

CLEYER, ANDREW, was born at Cassel, in the beginning of the 17th century. After studying medicine, he went as physician to Batavia, where he resided many years. He transmitted several interesting communications to the Imperial Academy, of which he had been chosen a member, particularly "An Account of Hydatids found in a Human Stomach," and "Of the Custom of the Indians of taking Opium;" also descriptions and drawings of the plants indigenous in Java, especially the moxa, ginseng, and tea-plant. He likewise published, in 1680, a curious specimen of Chinese medicine.

CLI'BANUS. (Quasi καλιβανος; from καλυπτω, to conceal.) A portable furnace, or still, in which the materials to be wrought on are shut up.

CLIFTON, FRANCIS, after studying at Oxford, came to London, and was admitted Fellow of the College of Physicians, as well as of the Royal Society, about the year 1730. Two years after, he published on "The State of Physic, ancient and modern, with a Plan for improving it;" in which a law is proposed, to compel practitioners to send to a public institution descriptions of the several cases which come under their care. He was also author of "A plain and sure Way of practising Physic;" and translated some parts of Hippocrates into English, with notes.

CLIMA'CTER. (From κλιμαζω, to proceed gradually.) The progression of the life of man. It is usually divided into periods of seven years.

Climacteric. See *Septenary.*

CLIMATE. The prevailing constitution of the atmosphere, relative to heat, wind, and moisture, peculiar to any region. This depends chiefly on the latitude of the place, its elevation above the level of the sea, and its insular or continental position. Springs which issue from a considerable depth, and caves about 50 feet under the surface, preserve a uniform temperature through all the vicissitudes of the season This is the mean temperature of that country.

It appears very probable, that the climates of European countries were more severe in ancient times than they are at present. Cæsar says, that the vine could not be cultivated in Gaul, on account of its winter-cold. The rein-deer, now found only in the zone of Lapland, was then an inhabitant of the Pyrenees. The Tiber was frequently frozen over, and the ground about Rome covered with snow for several weeks together, which almost never happens in our times. The Rhine and the Danube, in the reign of Augustus, were generally frozen over for several months of winter. The barbarians, who overran the Roman empire a few centuries afterward, transported their armies and wagons across the ice of these rivers. The improvement that is continually taking place in the climate of America, proves, that the power of man extends to phenomena, which, from the magnitude and variety of their causes, seemed entirely beyond his control. At Guiana, in South America, within five degrees of the line, the inhabitants living amid immense forests, a century ago, were obliged to alleviate the severity of the cold by evening fires. Even the duration of the rainy season has been shortened by the clearing of the country, and the warmth is so increased, that a fire now would be deemed an annoyance. It thunders continually in the woods, rarely in the cultivated parts.

Drainage of the ground, and removal of forests, however, cannot be reckoned among the sources of the increased warmth of the Italian winters. Chemical writers have omitted to notice an astronomical cause of the progressive amelioration of the climates of the northern hemisphere. In consequence of the apogee portion of the terrestrial orbit being contained between our vernal and autumnal equinox, our summer half of the year, or the interval which elapses between the sun's crossing the equator in spring, and in autumn, is about *seven* days longer than our winter half year. Hence also, one reason for the relative coldness of the southern hemisphere.

[While Dr. Priestley was engaged, during the month of July, 1801, in making experiments with a double convex lens upon some metallic substances at Northumberland, in Pennsylvania, he wrote thus to Dr. Mitchill: "If I have a few days more sunshine, I shall finish what I am about, and write the next post. Happily we are never long without sunshine, whereas in England I have often waited months; and the days in which I could use a burning lens have not, I am confident, exceeded one fortnight in some whole years, and I have often watched every gleam the year through. I think the climate of this country greatly preferable to that of England."—*Med. Repos.* A.]

CLI'MAX. (From κλιμαζω, to proceed.) A name of some antidotes, which, in regular proportion, increased or diminished the ingredients of which it was composed, e. g. ℞. *Chamædryos* ℥iij. *Centaurii* ℥ij. *Hyperici* ℥j.

Climbing birthwort. See *Aristolochia clematitis.*

Climbing stem. See *Caulis.*

CLI'NICAL. (*Clinicus;* from κλινη, a bed.) Any thing concerning a bed: thus clinical lectures, notes, a clinical physician, &c.; which mean lectures given at the bedside, observations taken from patients when in bed, a physician who visits his patients in their bed, &c.

CLINKSTONE. A stone of an imperfectly slaty nature, which rings like metal, when struck with a hammer.

CLI'NOID. (*Clinoideus;* from κλινη, a bed, and ειδος, resemblance.) Resembling a bed. The four processes surrounding the sella turcica of the sphenoid bone are so called, of which two are anterior, and two posterior.

CLINOMASTOIDE'US. A corruption of cleidomastoideus. See *Sterno-cleido-mastoideus.*

CLINOMETER. An instrument for measuring the dip of mineral strata.

CLI'SSUS. A chemical term denoting mineral compound spirits; but antimony is considered as the basis clyssi. See *Clyssus.*

CLITO'RIDIS MUSCULUS. See *Erector clitoridis.*

CLI'TORIS. (From κλειω, to enclose, or hide; because it is hid by the labia pudendorum.) *Columella.* A small glandiform body, like a penis in miniature, and, like it, covered with a prepuce, or fore-skin. It is situated above the nymphæ, and before the opening of the urinary passage of women. Anatomy has discovered, that the clitoris is composed, like the penis, of a cavernous substance, and of a glans, which has no perforation, but is like that of the penis, exquisitely sensible. The clitoris is the principal seat of pleasure: during coition it is distended with blood, and after the venereal orgasm it becomes flaccid and falls. Instances have occurred where the clitoris was so enlarged as to enable the female to have venereal commerce with others; and, in Paris, this fact was made a public exhibition of to the faculty. Women thus formed appear to partake, in their general form, less of the female character, and are termed hermaphrodites. The clitoris in children is larger, in proportion, than in full-grown women: it often projects beyond the external labia at birth.

CLITORI'SMUS. (From κλειτορις; the clitoris.) An enlargement of the clitoris.

CLO'NIC. (From κλονεω, to move to and fro.) See *Convulsion.*

CLONO'DES. (From κλονεω, to agitate.) A strong unequal pulse.

CLONUS. (From κλονεω, to agitate.) The name of a genus of disease in the Class, *Neuroses;* Order, *Lenetica,* of Good's Nosology. Clonic spasm, comprising six species: *Clonus singultus, sternutatio, palpitatio, nictitatio, subsultus,* and *pandiculatio.*

["CLOSSEY, SAMUEL, M.D. was an Irish physician, of very respectable attainments, who established himself in medical practice in New-York. He had, previously to his arrival in America, attained a high degree of eminence in the medical profession, both as a practitioner, and an author of an interesting volume on morbid anatomy; this was entitled "Observations on some of the Diseases of the Human Body, chiefly taken from the Dissections of Morbid Bodies;" it was published in London in 1763. He was for a short time chosen to the anatomical chair, and the professorship of Natural Philosophy in King's College, now Columbia College. Upon the organization of the first medical school in New-York, in 1768, Dr. Clossey was chosen the professor of Anatomy, and directed his labours with great assiduity to the establishment of that institution. Political difficulties in the American government, caused him to return to his own country, where he died a short time after his arrival."—*Thach. Med. Biog.* A.]

CLOVE. See *Eugenia caryophyllata.*

Clove-bark. See *Myrtus caryophyllata.*

Clove-gilliflower. See *Dianthus caryophyllus.*

Clove-pink. See *Dianthus caryophyllus.*

Cloven-leaf. See *Leaf.*

CLOWES, WILLIAM, an eminent English surgeon of the 16th century, received his education under George Keble, whose skill he strongly commends. After serving for some time professionally in the navy, he settled in London, and was made surgeon to Christ's and St. Bartholomew's hospitals, and appears to have had considerable practice. In 1586, he was sent Low Countries, to the assistance of the army under the Earl of Leicester; and on his return was appointed surgeon to the Queen. His works are in the English language, but evince much learning, as well as skill in his profession. The first which he published was on the lues venerea, in 1585; in which he notices the increasing frequency of that disease, and states that in five years he had cured above a thousand patients labouring under it at St. Bartholomew's hospital. But his most celebrated publication appeared three years after, on the method of treating wounds of various kinds, the result of extensive experience, sanctioned by references to the most approved writers. He appears to have possessed an enlarged understanding, and was very severe on all quacks and impostors; and he may justly be reckoned among the restorers and improvers of surgery in modern times.

CLUNE'SIA. (From *clunes,* the buttocks.) An inflammation of the buttocks.

CLU'PEA. The name of a genus of fishes, in the Linnæan system.

CLUPEA ALOSA. The Linnæan name for the shad or chad, the flesh of which is by some commended as a restorative.

[CLUPEA is the generic name for the herring tribe, to which the shad belongs, and which is the best and largest of them all. It is one of the most excellent eatable fish that frequents the waters of the United States. It is a migratory fish appearing on our coast in March and April, and disappearing by June. It comes from the Gulf of Mexico, and in its course northwardly, ascends our fresh water rivers to deposite its spawn. It is taken in immense numbers in the Delaware, the Hudson, and the Connecticut rivers, in April and May. After depositing its spawn in the upper and small branches of these fresh streams, the shad returns to the ocean, so altered in shape and size as hardly to be known for the same fish; and hence it is called *maugre shad,* not fit to eat, and not suffered to be sold in the New-York markets. A.]

CLUPEA ENCRASICOLUS. The anchovy, a little fish found in great abundance about the island of Gorgona, near Leghorn. It is prepared for sale, by salting and pickling. It is supposed the ancient Greeks and Romans prepared a kind of garum for the table from this fish. Its principal use is, as a sauce for seasoning.

CLU'SIA. (So called in memory of Charles Clusius, an eminent botanist.) The name of a genus of plants in the Linnæan system. Class, *Polygamia;* Order, *Monœcia.* Balsam-tree.

CLU'STER. See *Racemus.*

CLU'TIA. (Named after Cluyt, and sometimes spelled *cluytia.*) The name of a genus of plants in the Linnæan system. Class, *Diœcia;* Order, *Gynandria*

CLUTIA ELUTHERIA. The systematic name of the tree which is by some supposed to afford the cascarilla bark.

CLUY'TIA. See *Clutia.*

CLY'DON. Κλυδων. A fluctuation and flatulency in the stomach.

CLYPEA'LIS. (From *clypeus,* a shield.) Formed like a shield.

CLY'SMUS. (From κλυζω, to wash.) *Clysma.* A glyster.

CLY'SSUS. *Clissus.* A term anciently used by the chemists for medicines made by the reunion of different principles, as oil, salt, and spirit, by long digestion; but it is not now practised, and the term is almost lost.

CLYSSUS ANTIMONII. *Clyssus mineralis.* A weak acid of sulphur.

CLY'STER. (*Clysterium.* From κλυζω, to cleanse.) A glyster. See *Enema.*

CNE'MIA. (From κνημη, the tibia.) Any part connected with the tibia.

CNEMODACTYLÆ'US. (From κνημη, the tibia, and δακτυλος, a finger, or toe.) A muscle, the origin of which is in the tibia, and insertion in the toes. See *Extensor longus digitorum pedis.*

CNE'SIS. (From κναω, to scratch.) *Cnismos.* A painful itching.

CNICILÆ'ON. (From κνικος, cnicus, and ελαιον, oil.) Oil made of the seeds of cnicus. Its virtues are the same with those of the ricinus, but in an inferior degree.

CNI'CUS. (From κναω, to scratch.) The plant used by Hippocrates by this name, is supposed to be the carthamus; but modern botanists exclude it from the species of this plant.

CNICUS CERNUUS. The systematic name of the nodding cnicus, the tender stalks of which are, when boiled and peeled, eaten by the Siberians as a food.

CNICUS LANATUS. *Chamælim verum.* The distaff thistle. Formerly used as a depuration, but now forgotten.

CNICUS OLERACEUS. Round-leaved meadow thistle. The leaves of this plant are boiled in the northern parts of Europe, and eaten as we do cabbage.

CNICUS SYLVESTRIS. See *Centaurea benedicta.*

CNIDIA GRANA. See *Daphne mezereum.*

CNIDII COCCI. See *Daphne mezereum.*

CNIDII GRANA. See *Daphne mezereum.*

CNIDO'SIS. (From κνιδη, the nettle.)

1. An itching sensation, such as is perceived from the nettle.

2. A dry ophthalmy.

CNIPO'TES. An itching.

CNI'SMOS. See *Cnesis.*

CNY'MA. (From κναω, to scrape, or grate.) In Hippocrates it signifies a rasure, puncture, or vellication: also the same as cnesis.

COADUNATÆ. (From *coadunare*, to join or gather together.) The name of an order of plants, in Linnæus's Fragments of a Natural Method.

COA'GULABLE. Possessing the property of coagulation. See *Albumen.*

Coagulable lymph. See *Albumen.*

COAGULA'NT. (*Coagulans; from coagulo*, to incrassate, or curdle.) Having the power of coagulating the blood or juices flowing from it.

COAGULA'TION. (*Coagulatio; from con*, and *ago*, to drive together.) The separation of the coagulable particles, contained in any fluid, from the more thin and not coagulable particles: thus, when milk curdles, the coagulable particles form the curd; and when acids are thrown into any fluid containing coagulable particles, they form what is called a *coagulum.*

COA'GULUM. A term applied frequently to blood and other fluids, when they assume a jelly-like consistency.

COAGULUM ALUMINIS. This is made by beating the white of eggs with a little alum, until it forms a coagulum. It is recommended as an efficacious application to relaxations of the conjunctive membrane of the eye.

COAK. Charred coal.

["The substance called coke is light, spongy, and of a shining steel-gray colour. It burns less easily than coal, but produces a great heat, and does not cake nor smoke. The preparation of coke may be conducted in the same manner as that of charcoal from wood. By this process, from 700 to 1100 lbs. of coke are obtained from one ton of coal; but the volatile products, consisting of bitumen, or coal-tar, and ammonia, are lost. For collecting these, a plan has been contrived by Lord Dundonald, and successfully executed. The coke is prepared in ovens, or stoves, almost close; and from 120 tons of coal are collected about 3½ tons of tar, and a quantity of ammoniacal salt."—*Cleav. Min.*

In the modern process of making gas for burning from bituminous coal, the profit arises principally from preserving the coak and ammoniacal liquor, while most of the tar is decomposed and converted into gas. A.]

COAL. A combustible mineral, of which there are many species.

COALTE'RNÆ FEBRES. (From *con*, and *alternus*, alternate.) Fevers mentioned by Bellini, which he describes as two fevers affecting the same patient, and the paroxysm of one approaching as that of the other subsides.

COARCTA'TIO. (From *coarcto*, to straighten.) The contraction or diminution of any thing. Formerly applied to the pulse: it meant a lessening in number.

COARCTATUS. Crowded. A panicle is so called, which is dense or crowded; as in *Phleum paniculatum*, the inflorescence of which looks, at first sight, like a cylindrical spike; but when bent to either side, separates into branched lobes, constituting a real panicle.

COARTICULA'TIO. (From *con*, and *articulatio*, an articulation.) That sort of articulation which has manifest motion.

COBALT. A brittle, somewhat soft, but difficultly fusible metal, of a reddish-gray colour, of little lustre, and a sp. gr. of 8.6. Its melting point is said to be 130° Wedgewood. It is generally associated in its ores with nickel, arsenic, iron, and copper; and the cobalt of commerce usually contains a proportion of these metals. To separate them, calcine with four parts of nitre, and wash away, with hot water, the soluble arseniate of potassa. Dissolve the residuum in dilute nitric acid, and immerse a plate of iron in the solution, to precipitate the copper. Filter the liquid and evaporate to dryness. Digest the mass with water of ammonia, which will dissolve only the oxides of nickel and cobalt. Having expelled the excess of alkali by a gentle heat from the clear ammoniacal solution, add cautiously water of potassa, which will precipitate the oxide of nickel. Filter immediately, and boil the liquid, which will throw down the pure oxide of cobalt. It is reduced to the metallic state by ignition in contact with lamp-black and oil. Laugier treats the above ammoniacal solution with oxalic acid. He then redissolves the precipitated oxalates of nickel and cobalt in concentrated water of ammonia, and exposes the solution to the air. As the ammonia exhales, oxalate of nickel, mixed with ammonia, is deposited. The nickel is entirely separated from the liquid by repeated crystallizations. There remains a combination of oxalate of cobalt and ammonia, which is easily reduced by charcoal to the metallic state. The small quantity of cobalt remaining in the precipitated salt of nickel, is separated by digestion in water of ammonia.

Cobalt is susceptible of magnetism, but in a lower degree than steel and nickel.

Oxygen combines with cobalt in two proportions; forming the dark-blue protoxide, and the black deutoxide. The first dissolves in acids without effervescence. It is procured by igniting gently in a retort the oxide precipitated by potassa from the nitric solution. Prout says, the first oxide consists of 100 metal + 19.8 oxygen; and Rothoff makes the composition of the deutoxide 100 + 36.77. If we call the first 18.5, and the second 37; then the prime equivalent of cobalt will be 5.4; and the two oxides will consist of

Protox.	Cobalt, 5.4	100	84.38
	Oxygen, 1.0	18.5	15.62
			100.00
Deutox.	Cobalt, 5.4	100	73
	Oxygen, 2.0	37	27
			100

The precipitated oxide of cobalt, washed and gently heated in contact with air, passes into the state of black peroxide.

When cobalt is heated in chlorine, it takes fire, and forms the chloride. The iodide, phosphuret, and sulphuret of this metal, have not been much examined.

The salts of cobalt are interesting from the remarkable changes of colour which they can exhibit.

Their solution is red in the neutral state, but green with a slight excess of acid; the alkalies occasion a blue-coloured precipitate from the salts of pure cobalt, but reddish-brown when arsenic acid is present. sulphuretted hydrogen produces no precipitate, but hydrosulphurets throw down a black powder, soluble in excess of the precipitant; tincture of galls gives a yellowish-white precipitate; oxalic acid throws down the red oxalate. Zinc does not precipitate this metal.

COBALUS. The demon of mines, which obstructed and destroyed the miners.

COBHAM. The name of a town in Surrey, in the neighbourhood of which is a weak saline purging water.

CO'BRA DE CAPELLO. (From *cobra*, the head, or covering, Spanish. See *Crotalus horridus.*

Cocao, butter of. See *Butter of Cocao.*

Cocao-nut. See *Cocos nucifera.*

COCCA CNIDIA. See *Daphne mezereum.*

COCCA'RIUM. (From κοκκον, a berry.) A very small pill.

COCCINE'LLA. (Diminutive of *coccus*, a berry; from its resemblance to a berry.) See *Coccus cacti.*

COCCO-BALSAMUM. The fruit of the *Amyris gileadensis.*

COCCOGNI'DIA. See *Daphne mezereum*

COCCOLITE. A mineral of a green colour, of various shades, found with granular limestone, garnet, and magnetic iron-stone, in Norway, Sweden, and Spain.

CO'CCOS. See *Daphne mezereum.*

CO'CCULUS. (Diminutive of κοκκος, a berry.) 1. A little berry.

2. The name given by De Candolle, in his *Systema Naturæ*, to a new genus of plants.

3. COCCULUS INDICUS. See *Menispermum cocculus.*

4. COCCULUS PALMATUS. The systematic name of the plant, which affords the calumba root of the pharmacopœias. See *Calumba.*

CO'CCULUS INDI AROMATICUS. Jamaica pepper. See *Myrtus pimenta.*

CO'CCUM. A species of capsule, but separated from it by Gærtner, who defines it to be a dry seed-vessel, more or less aggregate, not solitary, the sides of which are elastic, projecting the seeds with great force; as in the *Euphorbia.*

COCCUM BAPHICUM. A name for chermes.

CO'CCUS. The name, in entomology, for a tribe of insects.

COCCUS CACTI. The systematic name of the cochineal animal, or insect. *Coccinella; Coccinilla; Ficus Indiæ grana; Scarabæolus hemisphæricus; Cochinelifera cochinilla; Coccus Americanus; Cochinella; Coccus indicus tinctorius.* Cochineal. That which is used is the female insect found on, and collected in South America from, the *Opuntia*, or Indian fig-tree. It possesses stimulating qualities, and is ordered by the College in the *tinctura cardamomi composita*, and *tinctura cinchonæ composita;* but, most probably, merely on account of the beautiful red colour which it imparts to them.

[The cochineal is not now used in this country as a medicine. It is principally employed in producing a beautiful scarlet colour, in dying calico, colouring morocco leather, &c. A.]

COCCYGE'US. (*Coccygeus;* from κοκκυξ: because it is inserted into the coccyx.) A muscle of the os coccygis, situated within the pelvis. *Ischio-cocigien* of Dumas. It arises tendinous and fleshy, from the spinous process of the ischium, and covers the inside of the sacro-ischiatic ligament; from this narrow beginning it gradually increases to form a thin fleshy belly, interspersed with tendinous fibres. It is inserted into the extremity of the os sacrum, and nearly the whole length of the os coccygis laterally. Its use is to support and move the os coccygis forwards, and to tie it more firmly to the sacrum.

CO'CCYGIS OS. (From κοκκυξ, the cuckoo, the bill of which bird it is said to represent.) *Cauda. Ossis sacri acumen. Coccyx.* This bone is a small appendage to the point of the sacrum, terminating this inverted column with an acute point, and found in very different conditions in the several stages of life. In the child, it is merely cartilage, and we can find no point of bone: during youth, it is ossifying into distinct bones, which continue moveable upon each other till manhood: then the separate bones gradually unite with each other, so as to form one conical bone, with bulgings and marks of the pieces of which it was originally composed; but still the last bone continues to move upon the joint of the sacrum, till, in advanced years, it is at last firmly united; later in women than in men, with whom it is often fixed at twenty or twenty-five. It is not, like the os sacrum, flat, but of a roundish form, convex without, and concave inwards; forming with the sacrum the lowest part of the pelvis behind. It has no holes like the sacrum; has no communication with the spinal canal, and transmits no nerves; but points forwards to support the lower parts of the rectum; thus it contracts the lower opening of the pelvis, so as to support effectually the rectum, bladder, and womb; and yet continues so moveable in women, as to recede in time of labour, allowing the head of the child to pass.

CO'CCYX. (Κοκκυξ, the cuckoo.) See *Coccygis os.* Also the part in which the os coccygis is placed.

CO'CHENILIN. *Carminium.* The name of the colouring principle of cochineal.

CO'CHIA. (From κοχαω, to turn or make round.) An ancient name of some officinal pills. The pill of cochia of the shops, in the present day, is the compound colocynth pill.

CO'CHINEAL. See *Coccus cacti.*

CO'CHLEA. (From κοχαζω, to turn round.) A cavity of the internal ear, resembling the shell of a snail, in which are the *modiolus*, or *nucleus*, extending from its basis to the *apex*, the *scala tympani*, *scala vestibuli*, and *spiral lamina.* See *Ear.*

COCHLEA TERRESTRIS. See *Limax.*

COCHLEA'RE. (Crom *cochlea*, a cockle, the shell of which its bowl represents.) A spoon. *Cochleare amplum* or *magnum* is a table-spoon, calculated to hold half a fluid ounce; *cochleare medium* is a dessert or pap spoon, supposed to hold two tea-spoonfuls; and *cochleare minimum*, a tea-spoon, which holds about one fluid drachm.

COCHLEA'RIA. (From *cochleare*, a spoon; so called from its resemblance.) The name of a genus of plants in the Linnæan system. Class, *Tetradynamia;* Order, *Siliculosa.*

COCHLEARIA ARMORACIA. The systematic name of the horse-radish; *Raphanus rusticanus; Armoracia; Raphanus marinus; Raphanus sylvestris; Cochlearia—foliis radicalibus lanceolatis crenatis caulinis incisis*, of Linnæus. The root of this plant has long been received into the materia medica, and is also well known at our tables. "It affects the organs both of taste and smell with a quick penetrating pungency; nevertheless it contains in certain vessels a sweet juice, which sometimes exudes in little drops upon the surface. Its pungent matter is of a very volatile kind, being totally dissipated in drying, and carried off in evaporation, or distillation by water; as the pungency exhales, the sweet matter of the root becomes more sensible, though this also is, in a great measure, dissipated or destroyed. It impregnates both water and spirit, by infusion, or by distillation, very richly with its active matters. In distillation with water, it yields a small quantity of essential oil, exceedingly penetrating and pungent."

Dr. Cullen has mentioned every thing necessary to be known respecting the medicinal virtues of horse-radish, we shall therefore transcribe all that the ingenious professor has written on this subject. "The root of this plant only is employed; and it affords one of the most acrid substances of this order (*Siliculosa*), and therefore proves a powerful stimulant, whether externally or internally employed. Externally, it readily inflames the skin, and proves a rubefacient that may be employed with advantage in palsy and rheumatism; and if its application be long continued, it produces blisters. Taken internally, it may be so managed as to relieve hoarseness, by acting on the fauces. Received into the stomach, it stimulates this, and promotes digestion; and therefore is properly employed as a condiment with our animal food. If it be infused in water, and a portion of this infusion be taken with a large draught of warm water, it readily proves emetic, and may either be employed by itself to excite vomiting, or to assist the operation of other emetics. Infused in water, and taken into the stomach, it proves stimulant to the nervous system, and is thereby useful in palsy, and, if employed in large quantity, it proves heating to the whole body; and thereby it proves often useful in chronic rheumatism, whether arising from scurvy or other causes. Bergius has given us a particular method of exhibiting this root, which is, by cutting it down, without bruising, into small pieces; and these, if swallowed without chewing, may be taken down in large quantities, to that of a table-spoonful And the author alleges, that, in this way, taken in the morning for a month together, this root has been extremely useful in arthritic cases; which, however, I suppose to have been of the rheumatic kind. It would seem, in this manner employed, analogous to the use of unbruised mustard-seed; it gives out in the stomach its subtile volatile parts, that stimulate considerably without inflaming. The matter of horse-radish like the same matter of the other siliquose plants carried into the blood-vessels, passes readily into the kidneys, and proves a powerful diuretic, and is therefore useful in dropsy; and we need not say, that, in this manner, by promoting both urine and perspiration, it has been long known as one of the most powerful antiscorbutics."

COCHLEARIA HORTENSIS. Lemon scurvy-grass See *Cochlearia officinalis.*

COCHLEARIA OFFICINALIS. The systematic name of the lemon scurvy-grass. *Cochlearia hortensis; Cochlearia—foliis radicalibus cordato subrotundis; caulinis oblongis subsinuatis*, of Linnæus. This indigenous plant is cultivated in gardens for its medicinal qualities. Its expressed juice has been long considered as the most effectual of the scorbutic plants.

COCHLEATUS. Spiral, like the winding of a shell. Applied in botany to leaves, leguminous seeds, &c.; as *legumen cochleatum*, seen in *Medicago polymorpha*, and the seeds of the *Salsola*.

Cocho'ne. (From κοχαω, to turn round.) Galen explains this to be the juncture of the ischium, near the seat or breech; whence, says he, all the adjacent parts about the seat are called by the same name. Hesychius says, that *cochone* is the part of the spine which is adjacent to the os sacrum.

["COCHRAN, John, M.D. This gentleman was born in 1730, in Chester county, state of Pennsylvania. About the time he finished his medical studies, the war of 1755 commenced in America, between England and France. The army then presented to the mind of Dr. Cochran a scene of usefulness and farther improvement. As there were not any great hospitals at that time in the provinces, he readily perceived that the army would be an excellent school for his improvement, especially in surgery, as well as in the medical treatment of many diseases. He soon obtained the appointment of Surgeon's Mate in the Hospital Department; and having continued with the northern army during the whole of that war, enjoying the friendship and advice of Dr. Munro, and other eminent surgeons and physicians, he quitted the service with the character of an able and experienced practitioner.

When (twenty years after) the war became serious between Great Britain and the United States, Dr. Cochran was too zealous a whig, and too much attached to the interests of his native country, to remain an idle spectator. Towards the last of the year 1776, he offered his services as a volunteer in the hospital department General Washington afterward recommended him to Congress. He was accordingly appointed, in April, 1777, Physician and Surgeon General in the middle department. In the month of October, 1781, Congress was pleased to give him the appointment of Director General of the hospitals of the United States; an appointment that was the more honourable because it was not solicited by him. A short time after the peace, Dr. Cochran removed with his family to New-York, where he attended to the duties of his profession until the adoption of the new Constitution, when his friend President Washington, retaining, to use his own words, "a cheerful recollection of his past services," nominated him to the office of Commissioner of Loans for the State of New-York. This office he held until a paralytic stroke disabled him in some measure from the discharge of its duties; upon which he gave in his resignation, and retired to Palatine, in the county of Montgomery, where he terminated a long and useful life, on the 6th of April, 1807, in the 77th year of his age."—*Thach. Med. Biog.* A.]

COCK. The male of the domestic fowl. See *Phasianus gallus*.

COCKBURN, William, was born in the latter part of the 17th century. After being some years physician to the navy, he settled in London; and soon distinguished himself so much, that he was admitted into the College, as well as the Royal Society, and made physician to King William. He published a "Treatise on Sea Diseases," which was often reprinted, and translated into French and German. He referred the scurvy principally to the diet of seamen, and considered fresh provisions as the chief remedy for it. He wrote also on Alvine Fluxes, on Gonorrhœa, (which he contends may exist independent of syphilis,) and on the Human Œconomy; which latter publication was much noticed at the time, but is since superseded by more accurate treatises.

CO'COS. (So called from the Portuguese *coco*, or *coquen*, the three holes at the end of the cocoa-nut shell, giving it the resemblance of a monkey's head.) The name of a genus of plants in the Linnæan system. Class, *Monœcia;* Order, *Hexandria*.

Cocos butyracea. The systematic name of the plant which affords the palm oil; *Cocos—inermis, frondibus, pennatis ; foliolis simplicibus*, of Linnæus. The *oleum palmæ* is produced chiefly by bruising and dissolving the kernels of the fruit in water, without the aid of heat, by which the oil is separated, and rises to the surface, and on being washed two or three times, is rendered fit for use. When brought into this country, it is of the consistence of an ointment, and of an orange-yellow colour, with little taste, and of a strong, though not disagreeable smell. Its use is confined to external applications in pains, tumours, and sprains; but it appears to possess very little, if any, advantage over other bland oils.

Cocos nucifera. The systematic name of the plant, the fruit of which is the cocoa-nut. Within the nut is found a kernel, as pleasant as an almond, and also a large quantity of liquor resembling milk, which the Indians greedily drink before the fruit is ripe, it being then pleasant, but when the nut is matured, the liquor becomes sour. Some full-grown nuts will contain a pint or more of this milk, the frequent drinking of which seems to have no bad effects upon the Indians; yet Europeans should be cautious of making too free with it at first, for when Lionel Wafer was at a small island in the South Sea, where the tree grew in plenty, some of his men were so delighted with it, that at parting they resolved to drink their fill, which they did; but their appetites had like to have cost them their lives, for though they were not drunk, yet they were so chilled and benumbed, that they could not stand, and were obliged to be carried aboard by those who had more prudence than themselves, and it was many days before they recovered. The shells of these nuts being hard, and capable of receiving a polish, they are often cut transversely, when, being mounted on stands, and having their edges silvered, or gilt, or otherwise ornamented, they serve the purpose of drinking-cups. The leaves of the tree are used for thatching, for brooms, baskets, and other utensils; and of the reticular web, growing at their base, the Indian women make cauls and aprons.

CO'CTION. (*Coctio;* from *coquo*, to boil.) Concoction. 1. The digestion of the food in the stomach. See *Digestion*.

2. A boiling or decoction. See *Decoction*.

3. It was formerly used in a medical sense, signifying that alteration, whatever it be, or however occasioned, which is made in the crude matter of a distemper, whereby it is either fitted for a discharge, or rendered harmless to the body. This is often brought about by nature; that is, by the vis vitæ, or the disposition or natural tendency of the matter itself, or else by proper remedies, which may so alter its bulk, figure cohesion, or give it a particular determination, so as to prevent any farther ill effects, or drive it quite out of the body. And that time of a disease wherein this action is performing, is called its state of coction. It is now fallen into disuse.

Cocu'stu. The name for courbaril.

Coda'ga pala. See *Nerium antidysentericum*.

Codegella. A name given by the Italians to the carbuncle. See *Anthrax*.

Codoce'le. (From κωδια, a bulb, and κηλη, a tumour.) A bubo.

CŒCA'LIS. (From *cæcum*, the blind gut, through which it runs.) A vein, being a branch from the concave side of the vena mesaraica.

Cœ'la. (From κοιλος, hollow.) Applied to depression, or hollow parts on the surface of the body, as the hollow pits above, and sometimes below the eyes: the hollow parts at the bottom of the feet.

CŒ'LIA. (From κοιλος, hollow.) A cavity in any part of the body; as the belly, the womb, &c.

CŒ'LIAC. (*Cœliacus*, belonging to the belly; from κοιλια, the belly.) Appertaining to the belly.

Cœliac artery. *Arteria cœliaca*. The first branch given off from the aorta in the cavity of the abdomen. It sends branches to the diaphragm, stomach, liver, pylorus, duodenum, omentum, and spleen.

Cœliac passion. (From κοιλια, the belly.) *Cœlica chylosa; Cœlica lactea*. There are very great differences among physicians concerning the nature of this disease. Sauvages says it is a chronic flux, in which the aliment is discharged half digested. Dr. Cullen considers it as a species of diarrhœa, and mentions it in his third and fourth species, under the terms mucosa, chylosa, lactea; making the purulenta only symptomatic. See *Diarrhœa*. It is attended with great pains in the stomach, resembling the pricking of pins; rumbling and flatus in the intestines; white stools, because deprived of bile; while the patient becomes weak and lean.

CŒLIACA. (*Cœliacus;* from κολαια, *alvus venter*.) Dr. Good selects this name for the first class of diseases in his Nosology; diseases of the digestive function. It contains two orders, *Enterica* and *Splanchnica*.

COELO'MA. (From κοιλος, hollow.) An ulcer in the tunica cornea of the eye.

COELOSTO'MIA. See *Coilostomia*.

CŒNOLO'GIA. (From κοινος, common, and λογος, discourse.) A consultation, or common consideration of a disease, by two or more physicians.

CŒNO'TES. (From κοινος, common.) The physicians of the methodic sect asserted that all diseases arose from relaxation, stricture, or a mixture of both. These were called *cœnotes*, viz. what diseases have in common.

CŒRU'LEUS LAPIS. The sulphate of copper. See *Cupri sulphas*.

CŒ'TE. (From κειμαι, to lie down.) A bed, or couch, for a sick person.

CO'FFEA. (From *kofuah*, a mixing together, Hebrew; so called from the pleasant potation which is made from its berry: others assert that the true name is *Caffe*, from *Caffa* a province in South America, where the tree grows spontaneously in great abundance.) The name of a genus of plants in the Linnæan system. Class, *Pentandria; Order, Monogynia*. The coffee-tree.

COFFEA ARABICA. The plant which affords coffee. *Jasminum Arabicam; Choava*. Coffee is the seed of the *Coffea—floribus quinquefidis, dispermis*, of Linnæus.

The coffee-tree is cultivated in Arabia, Persia, the East Indies, the Isle of Bourbon, and several parts of America. Good Turkey coffee is by far the most salutary of all liquors drunk at meal-time. It possesses nervine and adstringent qualities, and may be drunk with advantage at all times, except when there is bile in the stomach. It is said to be a good antidote against an over dose of opium, and to relieve obstinate spasmodic asthmas. For the latter purpose, the coffee ought to be of the best Mocco, newly burnt, and made very strong, immediately after grinding it. Sir John Pringle commonly ordered one ounce for a dose; which is to be repeated fresh, after the interval of a quarter or half an hour; and which he directed to be taken without milk or sugar.

Besides the peculiar bitter principle, which is described under the name *Caffein*, coffee contains several other vegetable products. According to Cadet, 64 parts of raw coffee consists of 8 gum, 1 resin, 1 extractive and bitter principle, 3.5 gallic acid, 0.14 albumen, 43.5 fibrous insoluble matter, and 6.86 loss. Herman found in 1920 grains of

	Levant Coffee,	Mart. Coffee,
Resin	74	68
Extractive	320	310
Gum	130	144
Fibrous matter	1335	1386
Loss	61	12
	1920	1920

The nature of the volatile fragment principle developed in coffee by roasting, has not been ascertained. The Dutch in Surinam improve the flavour of their coffee by suspending bags of it, for two years, in a dry atmosphere. They never use new coffee.

If coffee be drunk warm within an hour after dinner, it is of singular use to those who have headache, from weakness in the stomach, contracted by sedentary habits, close attention, or accidental drukenness. It is of service when the digestion is weak; and persons afflicted with the sick headache are much benefited by its use, in some instances, though this effect is by no means uniform. Coffee is often imitated by roasting rye with a few almonds.

["COFFIN, NATHANIEL, M.D., son of Dr. N. Coffin, one of the most eminent physicians in the state of Maine. The first ancestor of his family who came to this country was Tristram Coffin, who emigrated from England in 1642.

Dr. Nathaniel Coffin was born in Portland, on the 3d of May, 1744, in which place he always lived, and where he closed his long and useful life. The country at the time of his birth, for may miles round Casco bay, including the site of Portland, was called Falmouth; afterward, the part most thickly settled, lying on the harbour, was incorporated into a separate town by the name of Portland.

He completed his preparatory medical education under his father; but the limited means of scientific improvement then existing in this thinly peopled section of the country, induced the son, with the advice of his father, to embark for England at the age of eighteen. He there prosecuted his studies at Guy's and St. Thomas's hospitals, under the distinguished Hunter, Akenside, M'Kenzie, and others; and returned to commence the practice of his profession at the early age of twenty-one.

Possessing a constitution naturally healthy and vigorous, and a mind resolute and intelligent, there was no peril which he was not prepared to encounter, and no adversity which he could not endure; and he has well deserved the distinction awarded him by the public, for his constant and unremitted exertions during a period of more than sixty years.

Dr. Coffin was surrounded, in the early part of his career, by suffering friends and patients; but his life was closed amid the blessings of freedom and independence. In the peaceful evening of his days, all the enjoyments of prosperity and affection clustered around his dwelling; but it should not be forgotten that the respectability and happiness he had experienced, were the well earned reward of the virtues the talents, and the faithfulness of former years.

In his manners, he was a polished specimen of the state of American society existing before the Revolution; he was one of the most graceful gentlemen of the old school, and his deportment was marked by a uniform and captivating urbanity. He died on the 18th of October, 1826, aged 82 years."—*Thacher's Med. Biog.* A.]

COGAN, WILLIAM, was born in Somersetshire, about the middle of the 16th century. He studied, and took the degree of bachelor in medicine, at Oxford; soon after which he was appointed master of the school at Manchester, where he also practised in his profession till his death in 1607. He published a curious book, abounding in classical quotations, entitled "The Haven of Health," in which he strongly recommends temperance and exercise. There is added an account of the sweating sickness; and of a remarkable disorder, which prevailed at Oxford in July and August, 1575, before he left it, by which he states, that in thirty-seven days "there died 510 persons, all men, and no women."

COHE'SION. (*Cohæsio;* from *con*, and *hæreo*, to stick together.) *Vis cohæsionis; Vis adhæsionis; Vis attractionis*. That power by which the particles of bodies are held together. See *Attraction*.

COHOBA'TION. (A term invented by Paracelsus.) *Cohobatio; Cohobium; Cohoph*. The ancient chemists use this term to signify the distillation of a fluid poured afresh upon a substance of the same kind as that upon which it was before distilled, and repeating this operation several times to make it more efficacious.

CO'HOL. (*Cohol*, Hebrew.) Castellus says this word is used in Avicenna, to express dry collyria for the eyes, in fine powder.

COI'LIMA. (From κοιλια, the bowels.) A sudden swelling of the belly from wind.

COILOSTO'MIA. (From κοιλος, hollow, and ςομα, the mouth.) *Cœlostomia*. A defect of speaking, from the palate, or through the nose, the voice being so obscured as to sound as if it proceeded from a cavern.

COINDICA'NTIA. (From *con*, and *indico*, to indicate.) Signs, or symptoms, are called coindicant, when, besides the usual incidental appearances, there occur others, as age, habit, season, &c.

COI'RA. A name for catechu.

COITER, VOLCHER, was born at Groningen in 1534. After studying at the different universities in Italy, he attended as physician to the French army during one campaign, that he might have more opportunity for investigating human anatomy. He then settled at Nuremberg, where he continued till his death in 1576. He made considerable improvements in anatomy and surgery. He found that the brain had a motion communicated to it by the arteries; and that in some animals the organ might be removed without destroying life. He first described the corpora lutea in the ovaria; and noticed the order in which the parts of the chick are evolved. He described the frontal sinuses, and the organ of hearing, more accurately than any preceding author. He pointed out two muscles which depress the eyebrows, and two which perform the same office to the lips. He observed, that injuries to the brain are more dangerous when the dura mater remains entire; and therefore he boldly divided that membrane. He was also accustomed to pare down fungi arising from the brain. He published good plates of the cartilages, of the fœtal skeleton, and of those of various animals, &c.

CO'ITUS. (From *coeo*, to go together.) The conjunction of the male and female in the act of procreation.

[Coke. See *Coak*. A.]

CO'LA. (From κωλον, a joint.) The joints.

Colato'ria lactea. Astruc says they were formerly called glands, and are situated in the third and internal tunic of the uterus, and that they are vesiculo-vascular bodies.

COLATO'RIUM. (From *colo*, to strain.) A strainer of any kind.

COLATU'RA. (From *colo*, to strain.) A filtered or strained liquor.

COLBATCH, John, was born in the latter part of the 17th century. He practised in London, first as a surgeon and apothecary, afterward as a physician, and had considerable repute. He published several works: the first was "A New Light of Chirurgery," condemning the use of tents, and the injection of acrid substances into wounds; then a treatise, in which most diseases are ascribed to alkalescency, and acids strongly recommended; this, in a subsequent publication, he applied particularly to the gout; lastly, he highly extolled the misletoe, as a remedy for epilepsy and other nervous diseases.

COLCHESTER. The name of a seaport on the coast of Essex, near which is a mineral water, *aqua Colcestrensis*, which is of the bitter purging kind, similar to that of Epsom, but not so strong.

CO'LCHICUM. (From *Colchis*, a city of Armenia, where this plant is supposed to have been common.) 1. The name of a genus of plants in the Linnæan system. Class, *Hexandria;* Order, *Trigynia*. Meadow-saffron.

2. The pharmacopœial name of the meadow-saffron. See *Colchicum autumnale*.

Colchicum autumnale. The systematic name of the common meadow-saffron. *Colchicum—foliis planis lanceolatis erectis*, of Linnæus. A native of England. The sensible qualities of the fresh root are very various, according to the place of growth and season of the year. In autumn it is almost inert; but in the beginning of summer, highly acrid: hence some have found it to be a corrosive poison, while others have eaten it in considerable quantity, without experiencing any effect. When it is possessed of acrimony, this is of the same nature with that of garlic, and some other plants, and is entirely destroyed by drying. The German physicians have celebrated its virtues as a diuretic, in hydrothorax and other dropsies; and, in France, it continues to be a favourite remedy; but it is, nevertheless, in this country, unsuccessful, or at best a very uncertain remedy. The expressed juice is used, in Alsace, to destroy vermin in the heads of children. The officinal preparations of colchicum are, syrupus colchici autumnalis, Edin. Pharm. The oxymel colchici of the former London pharmacopœia is now omitted, and the acetum colchici ordered in its room; as the honey may easily be added extemporaneously, if it be thought requisite. The active ingredient of this plant has lately been ascertained to be an alkali, possessing peculiar properties. See *Veratria*.

["Colchicum is in large doses a deleterious, acrid narcotic; in small ones, a cathartic and diuretic; possessing, likewise, peculiar properties of a sedative kind. It appears to have been known to the ancients as a poison, and during the last century it has been occasionally employed as a medicine in dropsy, asthma, and some other chronic diseases. Recently it has excited much notice, especially in Great Britain, as a remedy in gout, and a sedative in various painful and inflammatory affections. The interest excited by a secret French specific, the Eau Medicinale, which was found to relieve the paroxysms of gout, led to various imitations and substitutes for that preparation. Among these, a various tincture of colchicum was found very nearly to resemble the foreign compound, both in its sensible qualities and medicinal effects. Accordingly, the Wine of Colchicum became a prevailing medicine for gout, and was used with various success in that disease by different practitioners. The use of colchicum was soon extended to chronic rheumatism, and other painful affections, and at length it was applied, by Mr. Haden and others, to the cure of acute inflammatory diseases, and the treatment of cases in which blood-letting is commonly employed. Sufficient evidence has been published to establish the fact, that this medicine, when possessed of its full activity, may be so managed, as to diminish morbid force and frequency of the pulse, to allay pain and other phenomena of inflammation, and in certain cases to fulfil the object of depletion by the lancet. The Messrs. Haden inform us, that in pure inflammations, if it be given every four hours until it produce an abundant purgative effect, the pulse will become nearly natural, from being either quick and hard, or slow and full; that in many cases, its use may be substituted for blood-letting, at least when inflammation does not exist to an alarming degree in a vital part; and that the patient is left in a state favourable to more rapid recovery, when fever and inflammation have been removed by colchicum, than when the same end has been effected by other means. In chronic rheumatism, it is said rarely to fail, if persevered in for a time sufficiently long; in habitual discharges of blood from plethora, it has been substituted for frequent venesections; and after accidents, it is said to have the power of averting the severe consequences which usually follow such cases.

In Boston, considerable attention has been bestowed upon the effects of colchicum in different diseases. The article employed has been the bulb, imported in a live state, packed in sand, and dried immediately after its arrival. The sprouting of the flower-bud, during transportation, did not appear to lessen its activity. Administered in powder, this medicine has been found, in a variety of instances, to relieve the symptoms of pulmonary and of peritoneal inflammation, in a manner not easily to be accounted for, except by the reduction of the inflammation. Its most frequent operation, I believe, when fairly tried, has been to allay pain, reduce the pulse, and diminish symptomatic fever; to move the bowels, generally within twenty-four hours, and to excite nausea and great disgust, if the dose be large. It has, nevertheless, sometimes failed to produce these effects. In rheumatic complaints, its success has been equivocal, but, on the whole, rather favourable to its reputation than otherwise.

Colchicum has, of late, been most frequently administered in powder. Five grains may be given, three times a day, to an adult, where the stomach is not particularly delicate. This quantity I have found to remain on the stomach, and to move the bowels, commonly on the second day. In important cases, the dose may be increased to eight or nine grains, if nausea does not prevent. In chronic cases, the *dose* of five or six grains may be given, according to Mr. Hayden, once a-day, in the morning, and continued for weeks together. This writer combined with it small quantities of sulphate and carbonate of potass, and gave it in a state of effervescence, with an acid.

It is prudent to begin the use of a new parcel, or specimen, with smaller doses than those above specified, and gradually to increase them, since the root is at some times more active than at others. The variable activity of the medicine is, indeed, a great impediment to its usefulness, and nothing can be more discordant than the statements of writers on this subject. Professor Murray has cited various instances in which this root has produced distressing, and even fatal effects; while, on the other hand, an author by the name of Kratochville asserts, that himself and others have eaten drachms of the root, both in spring and fall, with impunity; and Orfila tells us, that he had repeatedly given several bulbs to dogs, in the month of June, without causing them any inconvenience."—*Big. Mat. Med.* A.]

[Colchici semina. The seeds of Colchicum.—These have been proposed, by Dr. Williams, as a substitute for the bulb, possessing all the medicinal advantages of the plant, attended with greater mildness and uniformity of operation. Several practitioners have agreed in their accounts of the efficacy of these seeds, particularly in chronic rheumatism. Dr. Williams uses a *wine*, made by infusing two ounces of the seeds in a pint of sherry. From one to three drachms are given, once or twice a-day, in aromatic water. He also employs a tincture, made with the same proportions. In this country, colchicum seeds have been used with some benefit in rheumatic complaints. They apparently possess the advantage of being less liable than the root to alter by age. I have found two or three grains of the powder to produce vomiting and purging in a mild degree, and ten grains to bring on powerful vomiting and purging, with vertigo and impaired vision during twenty-four hours."—*Big. Mat. Med.* A.]

Colchicum illyricum. The plant supposed to afford the root called hermodactyl. See *Hermodactylus*.

Colchicum zeylanicum. See *Zedoaria*.

COLCOTHAR. *Chalcitis; Colcothar vitrioli.* The brown-red oxide of iron, which remains after the distillation of the acid from sulphate of iron.

Colcothar vitrioli. See *Colcothar*.

COLD. 1. A privation of heat. It is nothing positive, but somewhat of the negative kind. The human body contains within itself, as long as it is living, a principle of warmth: if any other body, being in contact with it, abstracts the heat with unusual rapidity, it is said to be cold; but if it carries off the heat more slowly than usual, or even communicates heat to our body, it is said to be hot.

2. A cold is a popular name also for a catarrh. See *Catarrhus*.

Cold Affusion. See *Affusion*.

["COLDEN, Cadwallader, Esq. This truly worthy and eminent character, who united in himself the several qualities we are accustomed to admire in the physician, naturalist, and philosopher, was the son of the Rev. Alexander Colden, of Dunse, in Scotland, and was born on the 17th day of February, 1688. After he had laid the foundation of a liberal education, under the immediate inspection of his father, he went to the University of Edinburgh, where, in 1705, he completed his course of collegiate studies. He now devoted his attention to medicine and mathematical science, until the year 1708, when, being allured by the fame of William Penn's colony, he came over to this country about two years after. He practised physic, with no small share of reputation, till 1715, when he returned to England. While in London, he was introduced to that eminent philosopher, Dr. Edmund Halley, who formed so favourable an opinion of a paper on Animal Secretion, written by Dr. Colden in early life, that he read it before the Royal Society, the notice of which learned body it greatly attracted. At this time he formed an acquaintance with some of the most distinguished literary and scientific characters, with whom he ever after maintained a regular correspondence. From London he went to Scotland, and married a young lady of a respectable Scotch family, by the name of Chrystie, with whom he returned to America in 1716.

In 1718, he settled in the city of New-York; but soon after relinquished the practice of physic, and became a public character; he held, in succession, the office of Surveyor General of the Province, Master in Chancery, Member of the Council, and Lieutenant Governor. Previous to his acceptance of this last station, he obtained a patent for a tract of land, designated by the name of Coldenham, near Newburgh, to which place he retired with his family, about the year 1755, and spent a great part of his life. Here he appears to have been occupied, without interruption, in the pursuit of knowledge, particularly in botanical and mathematical studies, at the same time that he continued his correspondence with learned men in Europe and America.

In 1761, he was appointed Lieutenant Governor of New-York, which commission he held until the time of his decease the administration of the government repeatedly falling on him, by the death or absence of several governors in chief. His political character was rendered very conspicuous by the firmness of his conduct, during the violent commotions which preceded the Revolution. His administration is also memorable for several charters of incorporation, for useful and benevolent purposes. After the return of Governor Tryon, in 1775, he was relieved from the cares of government. He then retired to a seat on Long Island, where a recollection of his former studies, and a few select friends, ever welcomed by a social and hospitable disposition, cheered him in his last days. He died in the 89th year of his age, on the memorable 28th of September, 1776, a few hours before the city of New-York was in flames, retaining his senses to the last, and expiring without a groan.

Dr. Colden began, at an early period of his life, to pay great attention to the vegetable productions of America, in which delightful study his daughter after ward became distinguished. In honour of Dr. Colden, Linnæus named a plant, of the tetandrous class, Coldenia. This plant, Miss Colden had first described. He was attentive to the physical constitution of the country, and left a long course of diurnal observations on the thermometer, barometer, and winds. He also wrote a history of the prevalent diseases of the climate, and, if he was not the first to recommend the cooling regimen in the cure of fevers, he was certainly one of its earliest and warmest advocates; and opposed, with great earnestness, the prevailing mode of treatment in the small-pox.

In the years 1741 and '42, a fever, which occasioned great mortality, prevailed in the city of New-York, and created much alarm. He communicated his thoughts to the public, on the most probable method of curing the calamity, in a small treatise, in which he enlarged on the pernicious effects of marshy exhalations, moist air, damp cellars, filthy stores, and dirty streets; showed how much these nuisances prevailed, in many parts of the city, and pointed out the remedies. The corporation of the city presented him their thanks, and established a plan for draining and clearing out the city, which was attended with the most salutary effects. He published a treatise "On the Cure of Cancer." Another essay of his, "On the Virtues of the Great Water Dock," introduced him to an acquaintance with Linnæus. In 1753, he published some observations on an epidemical sore throat, which appeared in Massachusetts, in 1735, and had spread over a great part of North America. These observations are to be found in Cary's American Museum.

When he became acquainted with Linnæus's system of botany, he applied himself with new delight to that study. His descriptions, of between three and four hundred American plants, were printed in the Acta Upsaliensia. He published the "History of the Five Indian Nations," in 2 vols. 12mo. But the subject which drew Dr. Colden, at one period of his life, from every other pursuit, was what he first published, under the title of "The Cause of Gravitation," which being much enlarged, was republished by Dodsley, in 1751, in 1 vol. 4to., entitled, "The Principles of Action in Matter, &c."

Though his principal attention, after the year 1760, was necessarily directed from philosophical to political matters, he maintaind, with great punctuality, his literary correspondence, particularly with Linnæus of Upsal, Gronovius of Leyden, Drs. Porterfield, and Whytte of Edinburgh, Dr. Fothergill, and Mr. Collinson, F.R.S. of London. There were also several communications on mathematical and astronomical subjects, between him and the Earl of Macclesfield. With most of the eminent men of our own country he held an almost uninterrupted epistolary correspondence. Among them we may mention the names of Dr. Garden, Mr. J. Bartram, Dr. Douglass, Dr. John Bard, Dr. Samuel Bard, James Alexander, Esq., and Dr. Franklin. With Dr. Franklin, in particular, he was a constant and intimate correspondent, and they regularly communicated to each other their philosophical and physical discoveries, especially on electricity. In their letters are to be observed the first dawnings of many of those discoveries which Dr. Franklin has communicated to the world, and which so much astonished and benefitted mankind. In a letter to one of his friends, Dr. Franklin gives an account of the organization of the American Philosophical Society, in which he mentions that Dr. Colden first suggested the idea and plan of that institution.

The numerous manuscript papers left by Dr. Colden at the time of his death, which for many years were supposed to have been lost, have been lately found, and are now in possession of his grandson, Cadwallader D. Colden, Esq. They are chiefly on historical and philosophical subjects, and many of them are of the greatest value. Among these are Observations on Smith's History of New-York, in a series of letters to his son, Alexander Colden: An Introduction to the Study of Philosophy: a correct copy of his Account of the Fever which prevailed in New-York in the years 1741-2. This production may be found in Hosack and Francis's Register, vol. i. An Inquiry into the Principles of Vital Motion: A Translation of the Letters of Cicero, with an Introduction by C. Colden: *Plantæ Coldenhamiæ in provincia Noveboracensi spontanea crescentes, quas ad methodum Linnæi Sexualem, anno 1742, observavit Cadwallader Colden:* A corrected and augmented copy of his Principles of Action in Matter: A Treatise on Electricity, &c. Besides these, there is a great mass of correspondence on medical, philosophical, and literary subjects, with many eminent physicians and philosophers in Europe and America. These letters carry his correspondence back to the year 1710, and bring it down, almost uninterruptedly, till the time of his death. There are, too, a great variety of papers on public affairs, which must be considered as documents of primary importance, as they necessarily contain numerous facts which throw light on the history of this State. Dr. Colden was unquestionably a man of various and extensive learning, of superior talents, of the most indefatigable industry, and, indeed, in many respects, his character will not suffer by a comparison with that of our illustrious countryman, Benjamin Franklin.—*Thacher's Med. Biography.* A.]

COLE, WILLIAM, studied at Oxford, and took his degree there in 1666. After practising some time in Bristol, he came to London, and distinguished himself by several publications on physiology and medicine, which, however, are too theoretical. The principal are on animal secretion, on apoplexy, on the cause of fever, on insensible perspiration, &c. He published also a case of epilepsy, cured, in his opinion, by the misletoe.

CO'LES. (From καυλος, a stalk.) *Colis.* The penis.

COLEWORT. See *Brassica.*

CO'LICA. (From κωλον, colon, the name of one of the intestines.) The colic. The appellation of colic is commonly given to all pains in the abdomen, almost indiscriminately; but, from the different causes and circumstances of this disorder, it is differently denominated. When the pain is accompanied with a vomiting of bile, or with obstinate costiveness, it is called a *bilious colic;* if flatus causes the pain, that is, if attended with temporary distention, relieved by the discharge of wind, it takes the name of *flatulent* or *windy colic;* when accompanied with heat and inflammation, it takes the name of *inflammatory colic,* or *enteritis.* When this disease arises to a violent height, and is attended with obstinate costiveness, and an evacuation of fæces by the mouth, it is called *passio iliaca,* or iliac passion.

Dr. Cullen places this genus of disease in the class *neuroses,* and order *spasmi;* and defines it pain of the abdomen, particularly around the umbilicus, attended with vomiting and costiveness. He enumerates seven species.

1. *Colica spasmodica,* with retraction of the navel, and spasm of the muscles of the belly.

2. *Colica pictonum.* This is called from the place where it is endemial, the Poictou, the Surinam, the Devonshire colic; from its victims, the plumbers' and the painters' colic; from its symptoms, the dry bellyache, the nervous and spasmodic colic. It has been attributed to the poison of lead, and this is undoubtedly the cause, when it occurs to glaziers, painters, and those employed in lead works; but, though this is one, it is by no means the only cause. In Devonshire, it certainly more often arises from the early cider. made of harsh, unripe fruit, and in the West Indies from new rum. The characteristics of this disease are, obstinate costiveness, with a vomiting of an acrid or porraceous bile, pains about the region of the navel, shooting from thence to each side with excessive violence, strong convulsive spasms in the intestines, and a tendency to a paralysis of the extremities. It is occasioned by a long-continued costiveness; by an accumulation of acrid bile; by cold, applied either to the extremities or to the belly itself; by a free use of unripe fruits, and by great irregularity in the mode of living. From its occurring frequently in Devonshire, and other cider countries, it has been supposed to arise from an impregnation of lead received into the stomach; but this seems to be a mistake, as it is a very prevalent disease in the West Indies likewise, where no cider is made, and where there is only a very small quantity of lead in the mills employed to extract the juice from the sugar-canes. One or other of the causes just enumerated, may justly be said always to give rise to this species of colic.

The disease comes on gradually, with a pain at the pit of the stomach, extending downwards to the intestines, accompanied with eructations, slight sickness at the stomach, thirst, anxiety, obstinate costiveness, and a quick contracted pulse. After a short time, the pains increase considerably in violence; the whole region of the belly is highly painful to the touch; the muscles of the abdomen are contracted into hard irregular knots or lumps; the intestines themselves exhibit symptoms of violent spasm, insomuch that a glyster can hardly be injected, from the powerful contraction of the sphincter ani; and there is constant restlessness, with a frequent vomiting of an acrid or porraceous matter, but more particularly after taking either food or medicine.

Upon a farther increase of the symptoms, or their not being quickly alleviated, the spasms become more frequent, as well as violent; the costiveness proves invincible, and an inflammation of the intestines ensues, which soon destroys the patient by gangrene. In an advanced stage of the disease, it is no uncommon occurrence for dysuria to take place, in a very high degree.

The dry bellyache is always attended with some degree of danger; but which is ever in proportion to the violence of the symptoms, and the duration of the disease. Even when it does not prove fatal, it is too apt to terminate in palsy, and to leave behind it contractions of the hands and feet, with an inability in their muscles to perform their office; and in this miserable state of existence, the patient lingers out many wretched years.

Dissections of this disease usually show the same morbid appearances as in common colic, only in a much higher degree; namely, irregular contractions and distentions of the intestines, often with marks of inflammation.

[Miners, and manufacturers of white-lead, red-lead, plumbers, pewterers, shot-casters, are all subject to the same forms of disease which attack painters. In making white-lead, in the old way, the most dangerous time is when the pots are uncovered, and during that operation, few or none of those engaged in the corroding house escape without a severe turn of the painters' cholic. In making red-lead, the persons who attend the furnace and stir the metal, never escape the operation with impunity, being attacked with weakness, loss of appetite, nervous trembling, or cholic. White and red-lead are the most extensively used, and produce the most mischief, but the other preparations of lead exert a similar injurious effect upon the human constitution.

Dr. James Mann, hospital-surgeon in the U. S. army during the late war, has related the ill effects arising from the use of the acetate of lead as an astringent. When the dysentery prevailed in the northern army on the frontiers of New-York and Canada, it was found that a few grains of acetate of lead was effectual in restraining the evacuations. In some cases, where it was necessary to continue the remedy, the disease was allayed; but the patients afterward died with torpor or paralysis of the intestines, or other fatal operation of the lead as a poison. A.]

3. *Colica stercorea,* which happens from obstinate and long continued costiveness.

4. *Colica accidentalis,* called also cholera sicca, from acrid undigested matters.

5. *Colica meconialis,* in infants, from a retention of meconium.

6. *Colica callosa,* with a sensation of a stricture in some part of the colon, and frequently of previous flatulence, gradually passing off; the habit costive, or fæces liquid, and in small quantity.

7. *Colica calculosa,* from calculi formed in the intestines, attended with a fixed hardness in some part of the abdomen. It is distinguished by the previous discharge of calculi.

8. *Colica flatulentia* may be added to these species. It is distinguished by a sudden fulness, with pain and constipation, relieved by a discharge of wind from the mouth, or anus.

The colic is distinguished from inflammation of the intestines by the pain being *wringing,* and not of a burning kind; by the *spasmodic contraction* of the abdominal muscles; by the *absence* or *trifling* degree of fever; by the *state* of the pulse, and by the *diminution* of pain upon pressure, which increases it in enteritis.

The flatulent and inflammatory colic are thus distinguished from each other:—In the flatulent colic, the pain comes on by fits, flies from one part of the bowels to another, and is much abated by a discharge of wind, either upwards or downwards; but in the inflammatory colic the pain remains equable, and fixed and settled in one spot; the vomitings are severe, and frequently bilious; the belly is obstinately bound, and the pulse quick and feverish.

The colic should be distinguished from a fit of the gravel; stones passing through the ureters; rheumatic pains in the muscles of the belly; a beginning dysentery; the blind piles; and from a stone passing through the gall-duct. Gravel in the kidneys produces often colic pains, not easily distinguishable; but when stones pass through the ureters, the testicle on that side is often retracted, the leg is benumbed, a pain shoots down the inside of the thigh; symptoms occasioned by the stone passing through the ureter over the spermatic chord, or the sacro-sciatic nerve. Rheumatic pains in the muscles of the belly rarely affect so accurately the umbilical region, but dart in various directions, to the chest, or to the pelvis, and are attended with soreness, not confined to the abdomen. A beginning dysentery differs little from colic. The pain from the blind piles is confined to the rectum: and that from a stone in the gall-duct, is felt in the pit of the stomach, occasionally shooting through the body to the back.

The treatment of this disease must vary according to its form: but the leading indications are, 1. To obviate inflammation. 2. To relax the spasm, and relieve the pain attending. 3. To remove local irritation, especially by evacuating the alvine contents. 4. By various prophylactic measures to guard against a relapse.

1. The chief danger arising from inflammation supervening, it may be prudent to anticipate this, where the habit and strength will allow, by taking away an adequate quantity of blood from the arm, or more generally by leeches to the abdomen, but especially where any sign of inflammation appears, this plan becomes necessary, followed by a hot bath, or fomentations, a blister to the abdomen, &c. as detailed under *enteritis*.

2. The means already noticed may serve to relax spasm also, though not requisite in slight cases, besides the various antispasmodic remedies, as æther, assafœtida, &c., likewise aromatics, or spirituous liquors, will often by their stimulus on the stomach afford relief in flatulent colic, though their use is sometimes hurtful; but by far the most powerful remedy is opium in adequate quantity, which is best regulated in severe attacks, by giving divided doses at short intervals till ease is obtained.

3. Local irritation may sometimes be relieved by chemical remedies, as antacids, particularly magnesia, &c.; but for the most part the evacuation of the intestines should be attempted, when the pain is relieved. To prepare for this, calomel may be given in conjunction with the opium, and when the patient has been some time at ease, this may be followed up by castor oil, sulphate of magnesia, or other mild laxative, repeated till the desired effect be produced; or where these do not presently operate, some more active cathartics, as the compound extract of colocynth, jalap, &c. should be tried. If the stomach be irritable, the effervescing saline draught may enable it to retain them; and clysters will often assist the articles taken by the mouth, particularly where there are indurated fæces. In very obstinate cases, an injection of tobacco smoke has often succeeded in procuring evacuations: also putting the feet for some time in cold water, or pouring this on the abdomen and lower extremities. Sometimes it has been necessary to remove fæcal accumulations mechanically per anum.

4. The great liability of this complaint to return renders it necessary for some time after carefully to regulate the diet, to attend to the state of the bowels, as well as of the liver, to avoid the several causes, especially cold, maintaining the functions of the skin by suitable clothing, exercise, &c In the colica pictonum, stimulant aperients, as the peruvian balsam, mustard, &c. steadily persisted in, will mostly effect a complete cure; and mercury has been by some highly extolled; by others, astringents, especially alum, though certainly somewhat objectionable, as liable to confine the bowels.

Colica accidentalis. Colic from crudities in the bowels.

Colica arteria sinistra. The lower mesenteric artery.

Colica arteria superior. The upper mesenteric artery.

Colica biliosa. Colic from excess of bile.

Colica calculosa. Colic from stony matters in the intestines.

Colica callosa. Colic from hardened and obstinate strictures.

Colica damnoniorum. Colic peculiar to Devonshire. See *Colica*.

Colica febricosa. Colic with fever.

Colica flatulenta. Colic from wind.

Colica gravidarum. Colic in pregnant women.

Colica hysterica. Hysteric colic.

Colica lactantium. Colic peculiar to nurses.

Colica lapsonica. Colic peculiar to Laplanders

Colica meconialis. Colic from meconium in infants.

Colica mesenterica. Colic from diseased mesentery.

Colica nervosa. The nervous colic.

Colica pancreatica. Colic from diseased pancreas.

Colica phlogistica. Colic with inflammation.

Colica pictonum. See *Colica*.

Colica pituitosa. The spasmodic colic.

Colica plethorica. The inflammatory colic.

Colica plumbariorum. The colic of lead-workers.

Colica pulsatilis. The inflammatory colic.

Colica saturnina. The Devonshire colic. See *Colica*.

Colica scirrhosa. The colic from scirrhous tumours.

Colica spasmodica. The spasmodic colic.

Colica stercorea. Colic from retained fæces.

Colica vena. A branch of the upper mesenteric vein.

Colica vena recta. The vein of the colon.

Colica verminosa. The colic from worms.

CO'LICE. The colic.

COLIFO'RMIS. (From *cola*, a strainer, and *forma*, a likeness; so called from its having many perforations, like a strainer.) *Califorme os*. A name formerly given to the ethmoid bone.

Coli'phium. (From κωλον, a limb, and ιφι, strongly.) A kind of bread given to wrestlers. It was made of flour and bran together, and was thought to make men athletic.

Co'lis. See *Coles*.

COLLA'PSUS. (From *collabor*, to shrink down.) A wasting or shrinking of the body, or strength.

Collate'nna. A specific vulnerary.

Collatera'les. So Spigelius calls the erectores penis from their collateral order of fibres.

Colle'tica. (From κολλα, glue.) Conglutinating medicines.

Colli'ciæ. (From *colligo*, to collect.) The union of the ducts, which convey the humours of the eyes from the puncta lachrymalia to the cavity of the nose.

COLLI'CULUM. (Diminutive of *collis*, a hill.) 1. A small eminence.

2. The nympha, or prominency, without the vagina of women.

COLLIGA'MEN. (From *colligo*, to tie together.) A ligament.

COLLINS, Samuel, was born in the early part of the 17th century. After studying at Cambridge and Oxford, he went to the Russian court as physician, and continued there nine years. On his return, he was made Fellow of the College of Physicians in London. He afterward published a History of the Court of Russia, and, in 1685, a system of anatomy, treating of the body of man, animals, and plants, with numerous plates. The comparative anatomy, to which Dr. Tyson greatly contributed, was much admired, though now superseded by other publications.

COLLIQUAME'NTUM. (From *colliqueo*, to melt.) A term first made use of by Dr. Harvey, in his appli cation of it to the first rudiments of an embryo, in generation.

COLLI'QUATIVE. (*Colliquativus*, from *colliqueo*, to melt.) Any excessive evacuation is so called which melts down, as it were, the strength of the body: hence colliquative perspiration, colliquative diarrhœa, &c.

COLLI'SIO. (From *collido*, to beat together.) A contusion.

Co'llix. (From κολον, food.) A troch, or lozenge.

COLLOBO'MA. (From κολλαω, to glue together.) *Colobroma*. 1. The growing together of the eyelids.

2. The want of any member of the body.

COLLO'DES. (From κολλα, glue.) Glutinous.

CO'LLUM. (From κωλον, a member, as being one of the chief; or diminutive of *columna*, as being the pillar and support of the head.) The Neck. See *Neck*.

COLLUTION. *Collutio*. The washing of the mouth, or any other part.

COLLUTO'RIUM. (From *colluo*, to wash.) A gargarism, or wash for the mouth.

COLLU'VIES. (From *colluo*, to cleanse.) Filth; Excrement. The discharge from an old ulcer.

CO'LLYRIS. (Κολλυρις. A little round cake; so called from its likeness to a cake.) A bump, or knob, which rises after a blow.

COLLY'RIUM. (From κωλυω, to check, and ῥους, a defluxion; because it stops the defluxion.) A medicine was formerly so called which was applied to check any discharge. The term is now only given to fluid applications for the eyes, or eye-waters.

[Collyria, the plural of *Collyrium*. "The Collyria of the Pharmacopœia are metallic lotions, prepared of such strength as to be applicable to the eyes in many cases of disease; also occasionally to mucous membranes of other parts, and to inflamed or excoriated surfaces.

Collyrium plumbi acetatis. *Collyrium of acetate of lead*. This is of use as a sedative and astringent lotion in some forms of chronic ophthalmia. It is also useful as a discutient in erysipelatous and other superficial inflammations. It is sometimes employed as an injection in gonorrhœa; but when this practice is adopted, a weaker solution is preferable.

Collyrium plumbi acetatis et opii. *Collyrium of opium and acetate of lead*. This resembles the preceding, but agrees better with irritable cases of chronic opthalmia.

Collyrium zinci acetatis. *Collyrium of acetate of zinc*. A double decomposition takes place during the preparation of this article; sulphate of lead is deposited, and acetate of zinc remains dissolved. It is a valuable astringent collyrium.

Collyrium zinci sulphatis. *Collyrium of sulphate of zinc*. This is one of the best astringent lotions for cases of ophthalmia, which requires remedies of that class. I have observed it to agree particularly well with the weak eyes of nursing women.—*Big. Mat. Med.* A.]

Coloboma. See *Colloboma*.

Colobo'mata. In Celsus this word is expressed by curta. Both the words signify a deficiency in some part of the body, particularly the ears, lips, or alæ of the nostrils.

Coloca'sia. (From κολον, food, and καζω, to adorn; so called from its use as a food, and the custom of wearing its flowers in wreaths.) The faba Ægyptia. See *Nymphæa nelumbo*.

COLOCY'NTHIS. (From κωλον, the colon, and κινεω, to move; because of its great purging powers.) *Coloquinteda*. See *Cucumis colocynthis*.

COLO'MBO. See *Calumba*.

CO'LON. (*Colon*, *i*. neut.; Κωλον, quasi κοιλον; from κοιλος, hollow: so called from its capacity, or from its generally being found empty, and full of wind in dissection.) The greater portion of the large intestine is so called. It proceeds towards the liver, by the name of the *ascending portion of the colon;* and having reached the liver, forms a *transverse arch* across to the other side. The colon then descends, forming what is termed its *sigmoid flexure*, into the pelvis, where the gut is called rectum. See *Intestine*.

COLOPHO'NIA. (Κολοφωνια, the city from whence it was first brought.) Colophony. 1. The black resin which remains in the retort, after distilling the common resin with a strong fire.

2. Paracelsus seems to mean by it what is now prescribed by the name of *terebinthina cocta*.

3. The ancients, and particularly Galen, seemed to understand by it a soft kind of mastich, from *Chio*, probably the same as our *Chio* turpentine.

COLOPHONITE. Resinous garnet of Haüy and Jameson. A mineral of a blackish or yellowish brown, or orange-red colour, and a resino-adamantine lustre, found in magnetic ironstone, in Norway and in Ceylon.

COLOQUINTIDA. See *Cucumis colocynthis*.

COLORATUS. Coloured: applied to leaves, calyces, seeds, &c. to express any colour besides green, as in *Arum bicolor;* or to any part thereof when of another colour than green, as in *Amaranthus tricolor;* and to a *perianthium*, when not of a green colour, as that of the *Gomphrena globosa:* and the seeds of *Chærophyllum aureum*.

COLO'STRUM. (From κολον, food, or κολλωμαι, to agglutinate; so called, either because it is the first food of the young, or from its being at that time peculiarly glutinous.) 1. The first milk in the breasts after delivery.

2. An emulsion made by the solution of turpentine with the yelk of an egg.

COLOT, Germain, a French surgeon of the 15th century, appears to have been the first of the profession who practised lithotomy, that operation having been previously in the hands of itinerant practitioners. He acquired great celebrity by his skill, and was much in favour with Lewis IX., who granted him a pension. Several of his descendants, in succession, enjoyed great reputation as lithotomists.

COLOT, Francis, the last of them, left a treatise, published in 1727, describing the method of operating with the greater apparatus, the invention whereof he ascribes to John de Romanis, an Italian physician, about two centuries before. But this has long been superseded by the less apparatus, which Mr. Sharp attributes to another French surgeon, Mons. Foubert.

Colotoi'des. (From κωλωτης, a lizard, and ειδος, likeness.) Variegated like the skin of a lizard. Hippocrates applied it to the excrements.

Coloured leaf. See *Leaf*.

COLPOCE'LE. (From κολπος, the vagina, and κηλη, a tumour.) A hernia forced into the vagina. See *Hernia vaginalis*.

COLPOPTO'SIS. (From κολπος, the vagina, and πιπτω, to fall down.) A bearing down of the vagina. See *Hernia vaginalis*.

COLT'S-FOOT. See *Tussilago*.

CO'LUBER. (*Quod colit umbram*, because it delighteth in the shade.) A genus of animals in the Linnæan arrangement, of which there are many species.

Coluber berus. The systematic name of the viper, which possesses the power of forming a poisonous fluid in little bags near its teeth. The flesh is perfectly innocent, and often taken by the common people against the king's evil, and a variety of disorders of the skin. Experience evinces it to be an inefficacious substance.

Colubri'na virginiana. See *Aristolochia serpentaria*.

Colubrinum lignum. (*Colubrinus;* from *coluber;* so called from the snake-like contortions of its roots.) This species of snake-wood is brought from America. It is solid, ponderous, acrid, extremely bitter, and inodorous; its bark is of a ferruginous colour, covered with cineritious spots.

COLU'MBA. See *Calumba*.

COLUMBIC ACID. *Acidum Columbicum*. "The experiments of Hatchett have proved, that a peculiar mineral from Massachusetts, deposited in the British Museum, consisted of one part of oxide of iron, and somewhat more than three parts of a white-coloured substance, possessing the properties of an acid. Its basis was metallic. Hence he named this Columblum, and the acid the Columbic. Dr. Wollaston, by very exact analytical comparisons, proved, that the acid of Hatchett was the oxide of the metal lately discovered in Sweden by Ekeberg, in the mineral yttrotantalite, and thence called tantalum. Dr. Wollaston's method of separating the acid from the mineral is peculiarly elegant. One part of tantalite, five parts of carbonate of potassa, and two parts of borax, are fused together in a platina crucible. The mass, after being softened in water, is acted on by muriatic acid. The iron and manganese dissolve, while the columbic acid remains at the bottom. It is in the form of a white powder, which is insoluble in nitric and sulphuric acids, but partially in muriatic. It forms with barytes an insoluble salt, of which the proportions, according to Berzelius, are 24.4 acid, and 9.75 barytes. By oxidizing a portion of the revived tantalum or columbium, Berzelius concludes the composition of the acid to be 100 metal, and 5.485 oxygen."

COLUMBINE. See *Aquilegia*.

COLU'MBIUM. Hatchett describes the ore, from which this metal is obtained, as being of a dark brownish gray externally, and more inclining to an iron-gray internally; the longitudinal fracture he found lamellated, and the cross fracture had a fine grain. Its lustre was vitreous, slightly inclining, in some parts, to metallic; moderately hard, and very brittle. The colour of the streak, or powder, was dark chocolate-brown. "If the oxide of columbium, described under *Columbic acid*, be mixed with charcoal, and exposed to a violent heat in a charcoal crucible, the metal columbium will be obtained. It has a dark gray colour; and when newly abraded, the lustre nearly of iron. Its sp. gr., when in agglutinated particles, was found by Dr. Wollaston to be 5.61. These metallic grains scratch glass, and are easily pulverized. Neither nitric, muriatic, nor nitro-muriatic acid, produces any change in this metal, though digested on it for several days. It has been alloyed with iron and tungsten."

[This metal, which was said to have been first discovered in a specimen found in Massachusetts, it appears (Med. Repos. vol. viii. p. 437,) was taken from a spring of water in the town of New-London, in Connecticut, and near the house in which Governor Winthrop used to live, about three miles distant from the margin of the salt water at the head of the harbour.

"Within a short time after the discovery of columbium by Mr. Hackett in 1801, a metallic substance was also discovered in Sweden, by Mr. Ekeberg, differing from every metal then known to him; and accordingly he described the properties by which it might be distinguished from those which it most nearly resembled. But although the Swedish metal has retained the name of *Tantalum*, given to it by Mr. Ekeberg, a reasonable degree of doubt has been entertained by chemists, whether these two authors had not, in fact, described the same substances; and it has been regretted that the discoverers themselves, who would have been most able to remove the uncertainty, had not had opportunities of comparing their respective minerals, or the products of their analyses."—*Min. Jour.*

The doubt, however, has been removed, as Dr. Wollaston had obtained portions of both metals, and upon examination and analysis has determined, that *Columbium* and *Tantalum* are one and the same metal. A.]

Columbo'be. See *Calumba*.

COLUME'LLA. (Diminutive of *columna*, a column.) 1. A column or little pillar.

2. The central column, or filament, which unites the partitions of the capsule of plants. The seeds are usually attached to it. See also *Uvula* and *Clitoris*.

Columella'ris. (From *columella*, a little column.) A name of the dens caninus.

COLU'MNA. A column, or pillar. Many parts of the body, which in their shape or office resemble columns, are so named; as columnæ carneæ, &c.

Columna carnea. See *Heart*.

Columna nasi. The lowest and fleshy part of the nose, which forms a part of the septum.

Columna oris. The uvula.

COLUMNIFERÆ. The name of an order of plants in Linnæus's Fragments of a Natural Method, consisting of plants, the stamina and pistil of which have the appearance of a pillar in the centre of the flower.

COLUMNULA. A little column. The name given by botanists to the filament which passes through the middle of the capsule of frondose mosses, to which the seeds are connected; also called *Sphrongidium*.

Colu'rium. (Παρα το κολλαν τον ρουν: because it prevents a defluxion.) A tent to thrust into a sore, to prevent a defluxion of humours.

CO'MA. (From κω, or κεω, to lie down.) In pathology, a propensity to sleep. This word anciently meant any total suppression of the powers of sense; but now it means a lethargic drowsiness.

In botany, 1. A fasciculus of leaves on the top of a stem or stipe. It is said to be,

a. *Foliose*, when formed of leaves; as in *Bromelia ananas*.

b. *Frondose*, when proceeding from the frond at the apex of the stipe; as in *Palms*.

c. *Bracteal*, formed of floral leaves; as in *Lavendula stœchas*.

2. Gœrtner applies this term to the feathery crown of seeds furnished with a capsule.

Coma somnolentum. Is when the patient continues in a profound sleep; and, when awakened, immediately relapses, without being able to keep open his eyes.

Coma vigil. A disease where the patients are continually inclined to sleep, but cannot.

CO'MATA. (*Comata*, the plural of *coma*.) An order of the class *Neuroses* of Cullen's Nosology, embracing diseases that are characterized by a diminution of the powers of voluntary motion, with sleep or the senses impaired.

COMATOSE. Having a strong propensity to sleep.

COMBINATION. The intimate union of the particles of different substances by chemical attraction, so as to form a compound possessed of new and peculiar properties.

COMBUSTIBLE. Having the property of burning. See *Combustion*.

COMBU'STIO. (From *comburo*, to burn.) A burn, or scald. See *Burn*.

COMBUSTION. (*Combustio; from comburo*, to burn.) Burning. Among the various operations of chemistry, none acts a more conspicuous part than combustion; and in proportion to its utility in the science, the necessity of thoroughly investigating its nature and mode of action, becomes more obvious to the philosophical chemist.

Lavoisier's Theory of Combustion.

Lavoisier's theory of combustion is founded upon the absorption of oxygen by a combustible body.

Taking this for granted, it follows that combustion is only the play of affinity between oxygen, the matter of heat, and a combustible body.

When an *incombustible* body (a brick for instance) is heated, it undergoes no change, except an augmentation of bulk and temperature; and when left to itself, it soon regains its former state. But when a *combustible* body is heated to a certain degree, in the open air, it becomes on a sudden intensely hot, and at last emits a copious stream of caloric and light to the surrounding bodies. During this emission, the burning body gradually wastes away. It either disappears entirely, or its physical properties become totally altered. The principal change it suffers, is that of being no longer capable of combustion. If either of these phenomena, namely, the emission of heat and light, and the waste of substance, be wanting, we do not say that a body is undergoing combustion, or that it is burning. It follows, therefore, that every theory of combustion ought to explain the following facts:

1. Why a burning body is consumed, and its individuality destroyed.

2. Why, during the progress of this alteration, heat and light are emitted.

For the elucidation of these objects, Lavoisier's theory has laid down the following laws:

1. Combustion cannot take place without the presence of oxygen, and is more rapid in proportion to the quantity of this agent, in contact with the inflamed body.

2. In every act of combustion, the oxygen present is consumed.

3. The weight of the products of every body after combustion, corresponds with the weight of the body before combustion, *plus* that of the oxygen consumed.

4. The oxygen absorbed by the combustible body may be recovered from the compound formed, and the weight regained will be equal to the weight which disappeared during the combustion.

5. In every instance of combustion, light and heat, or fire, are liberated.

6. In a limited quantity of air, only a certain quantity of the combustible body can be burnt.

7. The air, wherein a body has been burnt, is ren

tered unfit for continuing combustion, or supporting animal life.

Though every case of combustion requires that light and heat should be evolved, yet this process proceeds very differently in different circumstances; hence the terms *ignition;* or glowing heat; *inflammation*, or accension; and *detonation*, or explosion.

Ignition takes place when the combustible body is not in an aëriform state.

Charcoal, pyrophorous, &c. furnish instances of this kind.

It seems as if the phenomenon of glowing was peculiar to those bodies which require a considerable quantity of caloric, to become converted into the gaseous state.

The disengagement of caloric and light is rendered more evident to the senses in the act of

Inflammation, or accension. Here the combustible substances are more easily converted into an elastic or aëriform state. Flame, therefore, consists of the inflammable matter in the act of combustion in the gaseous state. When all circumstances are favourable to the complete combustion of the products, the flame is perfect; if this is not the case, part of the combustible body, capable of being converted into the gaseous state, passes through the luminous flame unburnt, and exhibits the appearance of smoke. Soot, therefore, always indicates an imperfect combustion. Hence a common lamp smokes, an Argand's lamp yields no smoke.

This degree of combustion is very accurately exemplified in the

Flame of candles.—When a candle is first lighted, which must be done by the application of actual flame, a degree of heat is given to the wick, sufficient to destroy the affinity of its constituent parts; part of the tallow is instantly melted, volatilized, and burnt. As this is destroyed by combustion, another portion melts, rises, and supplies its place, and undergoes a like change. In this way combustion is maintained. The tallow is liquefied as it comes into the vicinity of the flame, and is, by the capillary attraction of the wick, drawn up to supply the place of what is burnt; the unmelted tallow, by this means, forms a kind of cup.

The congeries of capilary tubes which form the wick is black, because the charcoal of the cotton becomes predominant, the circumambient air is defended by the flame from oxidising it; it therefore remains, for a considerable time, in its natural state; but when the wick, by the continual consumption of tallow, becomes too long to support itself in a perpendicular position, its upper extremity projects nearly out of the cone of the flame, and there forms a support for an accumulation of soot, which is produced by the imperfect combustion. A candle, in this situation, affords scarcely one-tenth of the light it can otherwise give, and tallow candles, on this account, require continual snuffing.

But if the candle be made of wax, the wick does not long occupy its place in the middle of the flame; its thinness makes it bend on one side, when its length is too great for its vertical position; its extremity comes then into contact with the air, and is completely burnt, or decomposed, except so much of it as is defended by the continual afflux of the melted wax. This small wick, therefore, performs the office of snuffing itself. The difficult fusibility of wax enables us to use a thinner wick for it than can be used for tallow, which is more fusible. But wax being a substance which contains much more oxygen than tallow or oil, the light it affords is not so luminous.

Detonation is an instantaneous combustion, accompanied with a loud report; it takes place in general when the compounds resulting from the union of two or more bodies, occupy much more or less space than the substances did before their union; a great impulse is therefore given to the surrounding air, or else a vacuum is formed, and the air rushing in from all sides to fill it up is the cause of the report.

A mixture of oxygen and hydrogen gases detonates very loud. Gunpowder, fulminating gold, silver, and mercury; oxygenated muriate of potassa; and various other explosive compounds, are capable of producing very loud detonations.

With respect to the disengagement of light and caloric.

By the older chemists, it was universally supposed that the light and heat emitted during combustion, proceeded from the inflammable body; and this opinion would indeed appear unquestionable, while the composition of the atmosphere was imperfectly known. The burning body appeared luminous and felt hot, and no other agent was supposed to be concerned; the conclusion that the light and heat were evolved from the burning substance, was, therefore, unavoidable. But when the nature of the asmosphere was ascertained, and when it became evident that part of the air was absorbed during combustion, the former conclusion fell to the ground; for when two bodies exert a mutual action on each other, it becomes *à priori* equally probable that the products may be derived from either of them; consequently, the light and heat evolved might proceed either from the one or the other. Whether they proceed fom the atmosphere, or from the combustible body, they must be separated at the part where the combination takes place; that is, upon the surface of the burning body itself; and consequently it appeared luminous and heated, while the air being invisible escaped observation.

When the laws of heat became known, at least when it was ascertained that bodies contain at the same temperature, and in equal quantities, either of mass or bulk, unequal quantities of heat, the conclusion became probable, that the caloric evolved in combustion proceeded rather from the oxygen gas of the atmosphere, than from the combustible body; since the former contains a much larger quantity than the latter. The caloric evolved was therefore supposed to be derived from the *condensation* of the oxygen gas in the new combination into which it entered.

Though *approaching* to the truth, this explanation is not strictly true. It is not merely from the oxygen gas being *condensed* that the caloric is evolved, because, in many cases of combustion, the product still exists in the gaseous state, and in others, the quantity of caloric evolved bears no proportion to the degree of condensation. Philosophers ascribed this to a change of capacity; for, in different bodies, the difference in the proportion of the capacities before and after combustion, is by no means uniform; and hence the difference in the quantities of caloric extricated in various cases of combustion.

This being premised, it remains to explain the origin of the light emitted during combustion; for although we take it for granted that the caloric is evolved from the oxygen gas, we cannot infer that the light has the same origin.

It is very probable that light is a constituent part of inflammable bodies; for it is frequently evolved in combinations when the oxygen is merely *transferred* from one inflammable substance to another. In those cases it must proceed from the inflammable body. The accension of oils by the affusion of acids, the combustion of metals in the same way, furnish instances of the kind.

It seems, therefore, probable, that the light is derived from the inflammable substance; and that the oxygen, combining with the bases of these substances, disengages the light.

It may be concluded then, that light enters into the composition of all combustible bodies; but as we are unable to separate the light, so as to obtain these bodies pure, we treat of them as simple bodies.

According to this theory, the combustion of phosphorous in oxygen gas, is, therefore, the effect of a double affinity. The basis of the oxygen gas unites with the phosphorus, to form phosphoric acid; and the light disengaged from the phosphorus, together with the heat of the oxygen gas, produces the vivid flame.

The quantity of light emitted by different bodies is supposed to depend on the quantity contained in them, and on the proportion in which it is united to caloric.

Such is the theory of combustion of Lavoisier, modified by Gren, Leonardi, and Richter.

Thomson's Theory of Combustion.

Though the preceding theory of combustion is simple and beautiful, it appears, from what we are now going to state, to be by no means completely satisfactory.

It has misled chemists, by confining the term combustion to the act of oxygenation, and considering that all bodies, during their combustion, combine with oxygen, without at the same time recollecting that this latter effect may take place without any of the phenomena usually attendant on combustion; and that, though certainly all combustion presupposes the combination of oxygen with a base, yet this combination may be, and repeatedly is, effected where no combustion can possibly take place. Nothing can be more evident than the difference which, in numberless instances, prevails between the act of oxygenation in bodies and that of combustion, inasmuch as neither the phenomena attending on, nor the results arising from them, are the same. That a distinction therefore should be made between these processes is obvious; and it is on this account that Dr. Thomson has offered a theory, which considers this subject in a new point of view, and which bids fair to enable us to estimate the phenomena of combustion much better than has hitherto been done.

According to Dr. Thomson's theory, all the bodies concerned in combustion are either, 1. *Combustibles.*—2. *Supporters of combustion.*—3. *Incombustibles.*

I. COMBUSTIBLE BODIES are those substances which are said, in common language, to *burn.* During the combustion, they appear to emit light and heat, and, at the same time, gradually waste away. When this change has reached its *maximum*, the process of combustion is at an end.

The class of combustibles is very numerous; but all the bodies belonging to it may be subdivided into three sets, namely:

1. Simple combustibles. 2. Compound combustibles. 3. Combustible oxides, &c.

Simple Combustibles.

1. Sulphur. 4. Hydrogen gas.
2. Phosphorus. 5. All the metals.
3. Diamond, or Carbon. 6. Boron.

Compound Combustibles.

The *compound combustibles* consist of compounds, formed by the simple combustibles uniting together, and are of course much more numerous than the simple combustibles. They may be arranged under the five following heads:

1. Sulphurets. 3. Carburets.
2. Phosphurets. 4. Alloys.
5. Sulphuretted, phosphuretted, and carburetted hydrogen.

The *combustible oxides* are either simple, having a single base, or compound, having more than one base. All the simple combustible oxides are by combustion converted into acids.

The compound combustible oxides are by far the most numerous.

II. The SUPPORTERS OF COMBUSTION are bodies which are not of themselves, strictly speaking, capable of undergoing combustion, but which are absolutely necessary for the process; for no combustible body can burn unless some one or other of them be present. Whenever they are excluded, combustion ceases. All the supporters of combustion known at present are oxygen, chlorine, iodine, and the compounds which these form with each other, and with azote.

There are indeed certain substances besides these, which possess nearly the same properties; these shall be afterward enumerated under the title of *partial supporters.*

III. The INCOMBUSTIBLE BODIES are neither capable of undergoing combustion themselves, nor of supporting the combustion of those bodies that are; they are therefore not immediately connected with combustion; though most of them appear to be the results of that process. Azot, the alkalies, earths, &c. come under this division.

Some of the alkalies and earths possess certain properties in common with combustibles, and are capable of exhibiting phenomena somewhat analogous to combustion; which will be described afterward under the title of *semi-combustion.*

In every case of combustion, there must therefore be present a *combustible* body, and a *supporter* of combustion. During combustion, the combustible always unites with the supporter. *It is this combination which occasions the apparent waste and alteration of the combustible.* The new compound thus formed is a *product of combustion.* Every product of combustion is either, 1. *an acid*, or, 2. *an oxide*, &c. It is true, indeed, that other bodies sometimes make their appearance during combustion, but these will be found, upon examination, not to be products, nor to have undergone combustion.

Thus one of the two characteristic marks which distinguish combustion, namely, the apparent *waste and alteration of the combustible body*, has been fully explained. For the explanation of it we are indebted to Lavoisier, as stated before.

But though the combination of the combustible with oxygen, or other supporter, be a constant part of combustion, yet the facility with which combustibles burn is not proportional to their apparent affinity for oxygen.

Phosphorus, for instance, burns more readily than charcoal; yet charcoal is capable of abstracting oxygen from phosphorus, and of course has a greater affinity for it. Some of the combustible oxides take fire more readily than some of the simple combustibles; alkohol, æther, and oils, are exceedingly combustible, whereas all the metals require very high temperature when the supporter is air.

This greater combustibility of combustible oxides is probably owing to the weaker affinity by which their particles are united. Hence they are more easily separated than homogeneous particles, and of course combine more readily with oxygen; those simple combustibles which melt easily, or which are in the state of lastic fluids, are also very combustible, because the cohesion between their particles is easily overcome.

It is owing to the same inferiority in the cohesion of heterogeneous particles, that some of the compound supporters occasion combustion in circumstances when the combustibles would not be acted on by simple supporters.

Thus phosphorus burns in air at the common temperature; but it does not burn in oxygen gas, unless its temperature be raised. Thus also oils burn rapidly when mixed with nitric acid. Nitrous gas and nitrous oxide constitute exceptions to this rule.

None of the *products* of combustion are combustible, according to the definition of combustion here given. This want of combustibility is not owing to their being saturated with oxygen; for several of them are capable of combining with an *additional dose* of it. But, during this combination, no caloric or light is ever emitted; and the compound formed differs essentially from a *product* of combustion; for by this additional dose of oxygen, the *product* is converted into a *supporter. Hence we see that combustion ought not to be confounded with the combination of a body with oxygen*, as was done formerly.

Combustion, indeed, cannot take place without the combination of oxygen or other supporter; but oxygen may combine with bodies in different proportions without the phenomena of combustion; and the *product obtained* by combustion is capable of becoming converted into a *supporter* of *combustion;* for instance, if lead be melted, and kept so for some time, it becomes covered with a gray pellicle, or *oxide of lead*, a product consisting of oxygen and lead; but if this oxide is suffered to be heated longer, it absorbs an additional quantity of oxygen, and becomes converted into a yellow powder, called *yellow oxide of lead.* If this yellow oxide be again exposed to heat, it absorbs still more oxygen, and becomes converted into *red oxide of lead.* When the *supporters* thus formed by the combination of oxygen with *products*, are made to support combustion, they do not lose all their oxygen, but only the additional dose which constituted them supporters. Of course they are again reduced to their original state of products of combustion. Hence it follows, that they owe their properties as supporters, not to the *whole* of the oxygen which they contain, but to the *additional dose* which constituted them supporters. We may therefore call them *partial supporters;* indicating by the term, that part only of their oxygen is capable of supporting combustion, and not the whole.

All the partial supporters with which we are acquainted, contain a metallic basis; for metallic oxides are the only products at present known, capable of combining with an additional dose of oxygen. It is a circumstance highly deserving attention, that when metals are capable of combining with several doses of oxygen, the product, or oxide formed by combustion, is seldom or never that which contains a *maximum* of oxygen.

Thus it is evident that several of the products of

combustion are capable of combining with oxygen. *The incombustibility of products, therefore, is not owing to their want of affinity for oxygen*, but to some other cause.

No product of combustion is capable of *supporting* combustion. This is not occasioned by any want of affinity to combustible bodies; for several of them are capable of combining with an additional dose of their basis. But by this combination, they *lose* their properties as products, and are converted into *combustibles*. The process, therefore, differs essentially from combustion. Thus phosphoric acid, a product of combustion, is capable of combining with an additional dose of phosphorus, and forming *phosphorous* acid, a combustible body. When this last acid is heated in contact with a supporter, it undergoes combustion; but it is only the additional dose of the combustible which burns, and the whole is converted into phosphoric acid. Hence we see that it is not the whole basis of these compounds which is combustible, but merely the additional dose. The compounds, therefore, formed by the union of a product and combustible, may be termed *partial combustibles;* indicating by the name, that a part only of the base is capable of undergoing combustion. Since the products of combustion are capable of combining with oxygen, but never exhibit the phenomena of combustion, except when they are in the state of partial combustibles, combustible bodies must contain a substance which they lose in burning, and to which they owe their combustibility; for, after they have lost it, they unite to oxygen *without* exhibiting the phenomena of combustion.

Though the products of combustion are not capable of supporting combustion, they not unfrequently part with their oxygen just as supporters do, give it out to combustibles, and convert them into products; but during this process, no heat or light is ever evolved. Water, for instance, gives out its oxygen to iron, and converts it into the *black oxide*, a product. Thus we see that the oxygen of products is capable of converting combustibles into products, just as the oxygen of supporters; but during the combination of the last only, are heat and light emitted. The oxygen of supporters then contain something which the oxygen of products wants.

Whenever the whole of the oxygen is abstracted from products, the combustibility of their base is restored as completely as before combustion; but no substance is capable of abstracting the whole of the oxygen, except a *combustible*, or a *partial combustible.* Water, for instance, is a product of combustion, whose base is hydrogen. To restore the combustibility of the hydrogen, we have only to mix water with iron or zinc filings, and an acid; the metal is oxidized, and the hydrogen gas is evolved as combustible as ever. But no substance, except a combustible, is capable of separating hydrogen gas from water, by combining with its oxygen. Thus we see that combustibles are capable of restoring the combustibility of the bases of products; but they themselves lose their combustibility by the process, and are converted into products. Combustibility, therefore, may be thrown at pleasure from one body to another.

From these facts it is obvious, that the products of combustion may be formed without combustion; but in these cases a new combustible is always evolved. The process is merely an interchange of combustibility; for the combustible is converted into a product only by means of a product. Both the oxygen and the base of the product having undergone combustion, have lost something which is essential to combustion. The process is merely a double decomposition. The product yields its oxygen to the combustible, while at the same time the combustible gives out something to the base of the product; the combustibility of that base then is restored by the loss of its oxygen, and by the restoration of something which it receives from the other combustible thus converted into a product.

There is indeed another method of forming the products of combustion without actual combustion in certain cases; but the phenomena are much more complicated. This method is to expose them to the action of some of the supporters dissolved in water; especially nitric acid. Thus most of the metallic oxides may be formed without combustion by the action of that acid on the metals. But, in that case, a new supporter is always evolved, namely, nitrous gas; ammonia, a new combustible, is also usually formed; and, not unfrequently, the *product* is converted into a *partial supporter*.

No *supporter* can be produced by combustion, or by any equivalent process. As several of the supporters consist of oxygen combined with a base, it follows as a consequence, that oxygen may combine with a base without losing that ingredient, which occasions combustion. The act of combination of oxygen with a base, therefore, is by no means the same with combustion. If we take a view of the different supporters, we shall find that all of them which can be obtained artificially, are procured either from other supporters, or by the agency of electricity.

I. Oxygen gas may be procured from nitric acid, and from several of the partial supporters, as the black oxide of manganese, the red oxides of lead and of mercury. The action of heat is always necessary; but the process is very different from combustion.

II. Air, as far as is known at present, cannot be formed artificially. The gas, indeed, which comes over during part of the usual distillation of nitrate of potassa and sulphuric acid, to obtain nitric acid, resembles air very closely. But it is obtained from a supporter.

III. Nitrous oxide has hitherto been only procured from nitrous gas and nitric acid, (in nitrate of ammonia,) both of which are supporters.

IV. Nitrous gas can only be procured by the decomposition of nitric acid, a supporter.

V. Oxymuriatic acid, or Chlorine, can be formed by the action of muriatic acid on the black oxide of manganese, the red oxides of lead, iron, or mercury; all of which are partial supporters.

VI. Nitric acid is formed spontaneously upon the surface of the earth, by processes with which we are but imperfectly acquainted; but which certainly have no resemblance to combustion. Its oxygen is probably furnished by the *air*, which is a supporter; at least, it has been observed, that nitrogen and oxygen, at high temperatures, are capable of forming nitric acid.

This formation of nitric acid by means of electricity, has been considered as a combustion, but for what reason it is not easy to say: the substance acted upon is not a combustible with a supporter, but a supporter alone. Electricity is so far from being equivalent to combustion, that it sometimes acts in a manner diametrically opposite; *unburning*, if we may use the expression, a substance which has already undergone combustion, and converting a *product* into a *combustible* and a *supporter*. Thus it decomposes water, and converts it into oxygen and hydrogen gas; therefore it must be capable of supplying the substances which the oxygen and combustible lose when they combine by combustion, and form a product.

Several of the supporters and partial supporters are capable of combining with combustibles, without undergoing decomposition, or exhibiting the phenomena of combustion. In this manner, the yellow oxide of gold combines with ammonia; the red oxide of mercury with oxalic acid; and oxymuriatic acid with ammonia. Thus also nitrate of potassa may be combined, or at least intimately mixed, with several combustible bodies, as in gunpowder, fulminating powder, &c. In all these compounds, the oxygen of the supporter and the combustible retain the ingredients which render them susceptible of combustion; hence the compound is still combustible. And in consequence of the intimate combination of the component parts, the least alteration is apt to destroy the equilibrium which subsists between them; the consequence is, combustion and the formation of a new compound. Hence these compounds burn with amazing facility not only when heated, but when triturated, or struck smartly with a hammer. They have therefore received the name of *detonating* or *fulminating* bodies. Thus we have fulminating gold, fulminating mercury, fulminating powder, &c.

Such are the properties of the combustibles, the supporters, and the products; and such the phenomena which they exhibit when made to act upon each other.

If we compare together the *supporters* and the *products*, we shall find that they resemble each other in many respects. Both of them contain oxygen, or other supporter, as an essential constituent part; both are capable of converting combustibles into products; and several of both combine with combustibles and with additional doses of oxygen. But they differ from each other in their effects on combustibles. The former only produce combustion; whereas the products convert combustibles into products without combustion. Now, as the ultimate change produced upon combustibles by both these sets of bodies is the same, and as the substance which combines with the combustibles is in both cases the same, oxygen, for instance, we must conclude that this oxygen in the supporters contains something which the oxygen of the products wants, something which separates during the passage of the oxygen from the product to the combustible, and occasions the combustion, or emission of fire, which accompanies this passage. The oxygen of supporters then contains some ingredient which the oxygen of products wants. Many circumstances concur to render it probable that this ingredient is *caloric*.

The *combustibles* and the *products* also resemble each other. Both of them contain the same or a similar base; both frequently combine with combustibles, and likewise with oxygen; but they differ essentially in the phenomena which accompany their combination with oxygen. In the one case, *fire is emitted;* in the other, not. If we recollect that no substance but a combustible is capable of restoring combustibility to the base of a product, and that at its doing so it always loses its own combustibility; and if we recollect farther, that the base of a product does not exhibit the phenomena of combustion even when it combines with oxygen, we cannot avoid concluding, that all combustibles contain an ingredient which they lose when converted into products, and that this loss contributes to the fire which makes its appearance during the conversion. Many circumstances contribute to render it probable that this ingredient is *light*.

If we suppose that the oxygen of supporters contains caloric as an essential ingredient, and that light is a component part of all combustibles, the phenomena of combustion above enumerated, numerous and intricate as they are, admit of an easy and obvious explanation. The component parts of the oxygen of supporters are two; namely, 1. a base, 2. caloric. The component parts of combustibles are likewise two; namely, 1. a base, 2. light. During combustion, the base of the oxygen combines with the base of the combustible, and forms the product; while, at the same time, the caloric of the oxygen combines with the light of the combustible, and the compound flies off in the form of fire. Thus combustion is a double decomposition: the oxygen and combustible divide themselves each into two portions, which combine in pairs; the one compound is the *product*, and the other the *fire*, which escapes.

Hence the reason that the oxygen of products is unfit for combustion. It wants its caloric. Hence the reason that combustion does not take place when oxygen combines with products, or with the base of supporters. These bodies contain no light. The caloric of the oxygen of course is not separated, and no fire appears. And this oxygen still retaining its caloric, is capable of producing combustion whenever a body is presented which contains light, and whose base has an affinity for oxygen. Hence also the reason why a combustible alone can restore combustibility to the base of a product. In all such cases, a double decomposition takes place. The oxygen of the product combines with the base of the combustible, while the light of the combustible combines with the base of the product.

But the application of this theory to all the different phenomena described above, is so obvious, that it is needless to give any more examples. Let us rather inquire, with the author, into the evidences which can be brought forward in its support.

As caloric and light are always emitted during combustion, it follows that they must have previously existed in the combustible, the supporter, or in both.

That the oxygen of the supporters contains either one or both of these substances, follows incontrovertibly from a fact already mentioned, namely, that the oxygen of products will not support combustion, while that of supporters will. Hence the oxygen of supporters must contain something which the oxygen of the products wants, and this something must be caloric, or light, or both.

That the oxygen of some of the supporters at least contains caloric, as an ingredient, has been proved, in a atisfactory manner, by the experiments of Crawford, Lavoisier, and La Place. Thus the temperature of hot-blooded animals is maintained by the decomposition of *air*. Now, if the oxygen of one supporter contains caloric, the same ingredient must exist in the oxygen of every supporter, because all of them are obviously in the same state. Hence we conclude that the oxygen of every supporter contains caloric as an essential ingredient.

The light emitted during combustion must either proceed from the combustible or the supporter. That it proceeds from the combustible, must appear pretty obvious, if we recollect that the colour of the light emitted during combustion varies, and that this variation usually depends, not upon the supporter, but upon the combustible. Thus charcoal burns with a red flame, sulphur with a blue or violet, zinc with a greenish white, &c.

The formation of combustibles in plants, obviously requires the presence and agency of light. The leaves of plants emit oxygen gas, when exposed to the sun's rays, but never in the shade, or in the dark.

Besides vegetation, we are acquainted with two other methods of *unburning* products, or of converting them into products and combustibles, by exposing them, in certain circumstances, to the agency of *fire*, or of *electricity*. The oxides of gold, mercury, &c. when heated to redness, are decomposed, oxygen gas is emitted, and the pure metal remains behind. In this case, the necessary caloric and light must be furnished by the fire; a circumstance which explains why such reductions always require a red heat. When carbonic acid is made to pass repeatedly over red-hot charcoal, it combines with a portion of charcoal, and is converted into gaseous oxide of carbon. If this gas be a combustible oxide, the base of the carbonic acid and its oxygen must have been supplied with light and caloric from the fire; but if it be a *partial combustible*, it is merely a compound of carbonic acid and charcoal: which of the two it is, remains still to be ascertained.

Electricity decomposes water, and converts it into oxygen gas and hydrogen gas; it must, therefore, supply the heat and the light which these bodies lost when converted into a product.

These facts, together with the exact correspondence of the theory given above with the phenomena of combustion, render it so probable, that Dr. Thompson has ventured to propose it as an additional step towards a full explanation of the theory of combustion. Every additional experiment has served to confirm it more and more. It even throws light upon the curious experiments of the accension of metals with sulphur, which succeed *in vacuo*, under mercury, in nitrogen gas, &c.

Dr. Thompson has noticed, that the same emission of caloric and light, or of *fire*, takes place when melted sulphur is made to combine with potassa, or with lime, in a crucible or glass tube, and likewise when melted phosphorus is made to combine with lime heated to redness. He supposes that, in all probability, barytes and strontia exhibit the same phenomenon when combined with melted sulphur or phosphorus; and perhaps some of the metals when combined with phosphorus.

The phenomena Dr. Thompson explains thus:—The sulphur and phosphorus are in the melted state, and therefore contain caloric as an ingredient; the alkalies, earths, and metals which produce the phenomenon in question, contain light as an essential ingredient. The sulphur, or phosphorus, combines with the base of the metal, earth, or alkali; while at the same time, the *caloric*, to which the sulphur or phosphorus owed its fluidity, combines with the *light* of the metal, earth, or alkali; and the compound flies off under the form of *fire*.

Thus the process is exactly the same with combustion, excepting as far as regards the product. The melted sulphur, or phosphorus, acts the part of the *supporter*, while the metal, earth, or alkali, occupies the place of the *combustible*. The first furnishes caloric, the second light, while the base of each combines together. Hence we see that the base of sulphurets and phosphurets resembles the base of products in being destitute of light; the formation of these bodies exhibiting the separation of fire like *combustion*, but the product differing from a product of combustion in being destitute of oxygen, Dr. Thompson distinguishes the process by the title of *semi-combustion;* indicating by the term, that it possesses one half of the characteristic marks of combustion, but is destitute of the other half.

The only part of this theory which requires proof is, that light is a component part of the earths and alkalies. But as potassa and lime are the only bodies of that nature, which we are certain to be capable of exhibiting the phenomena of semi-combustion, the proofs must of necessity be confined to them. That *lime* contains light as a component part, has been long known. Meyer and Pelletier observed long ago, that when water is poured upon lime, not only heat but light is emitted. Light is emitted also abundantly, when sulphuric acid is poured upon magnesia, or upon lime, potassa, or soda, freed from the water of crystallization. In all these cases, a *semi-combustion* takes place. The water and the acid being solidified, give out *caloric*, while the lime or potassa gives out *light*.

That lime, during its burning, combines with light, and that light is a component part of lime, is demonstrated by the following experiment, for which we are indebted to Scheele.

Fluor spar (fluate of lime) has the property of phosphorescing strongly when heated, but the experiment does not succeed twice with the same specimen. After it has been once heated sufficiently, no subsequent heat will cause it to phosphoresce. Now phosphorescence is merely the emission of light; light of course is a component part of fluor spar, and heat has the property of separating it. But the phosphorescing quality of the spar may be again recovered to it, or, which is the same thing, the light which the spar had lost may be restored by the following process:—

Decompose the fluate of lime by sulphuric acid, and preserve the fluoric acid separate. Boil the sulphate of lime thus formed, with a sufficient quantity of carbonate of soda; a double decomposition takes place; sulphate of soda remains in solution, and carbonate of lime precipitates. Ignite this precipitate in a crucible, till it is reduced to lime, and combine it with the fluoric acid to which it was formerly united. The fluor spar thus regenerated, phosphoresces as at first. Hence the lime, during its ignition, must have combined with light.

That potassa contains light, may be proved in the same manner as the existence of that body in lime. Now, as potassa is deprived of its carbonic acid by lime, the Doctor supposes that the process must be a double decomposition; namely, that the base of the lime combines with carbonic acid, while its light combines with the potassa.

These remarks on semi-combustion might easily be much enlarged upon: for it is obvious, that whenever a liquid combines with a solid containing light, and the product is a solid body, something analogous to semi-combustion must take place.

COMEDO. (From *comedo*, a glutton.) The comedones of old writers are a sort of worm which eats into the skin and devours the flesh.

CO'MFREY. See *Symphytum*.

Comi'sdi. The gum-arabic.

Comi'ste. The epilepsy. This name arose from the frequency of persons being seized with this disorder, while in the assemblies called Comitia.

Comiti'ssa. A countess. Some preparations are distinguished by this name; as *Pulvis Comitissæ de Cantia*, the Countess of Kent's powder. Also the Cinchona was called *Pulvis Comitissæ*.

Commage'num. (From *Commagene*, a place in Syria, whence it was brought.) Syrian ointment, mentioned by Galen.

COMMANDUCA'TIO. (From *commanduco*, to eat.) The act of mastication, or chewing.

Comma'nsum. (From *commando*, to eat.) A masticatory. A medicine put into the mouth and chewed, to promote a discharge of phlegm, or saliva.

Commendato'rius. (From *commendo*, to recommend.) An epithet of the traumatic balsam, *tinctura Benzoes composita*, from its singular virtues and usefulness.

Co'mmi. Gum. When alone it signifies gum-arabic. The κομμι λευκον, mentioned by Hippocrates in his De Morb. Mulieb., is gum-arabic.

COMMISSU'RA. (From *committo*, to join together.) A suture, juncture, or joint A term applied in anatomy to the corners of the lips, where they meet together; and also to certain parts of the brain which go across and join one hemisphere to the other.

Commissura anterior cerebri. The white nerve-like substance which crosses the anterior part of the third ventricle of the brain, immediately above the infundibulum, and between the anterior crura of the fornix; uniting one hemisphere of the brain with the other.

Commissura magna cerebri. The *corpus callosum* of the brain is so termed by some writers.

Commissura posterior cerebri. A white nerve-like substance, which passes from one hemisphere of the brain across to the other, immediately over the opening of the aqueduct of Sylvius, in the posterior part of the third ventricle of the brain, and above the *corpora quadrigemina*.

Commu'nicant. (From *communico*, to make partake.) A term applied by Bellini, to fevers of two kinds afflicting the same person, wherein as one goes off the other immediately succeeds.

Compa'ges. (From *compingo*, to put together.) A suture, or joint. A commissure.

COMPA'RATIVE. That which illustrates by comparing with the human body: applied to anatomy and physiology. See *Anatomy*.

Compeba. See *Piper Cubeba*.

Complete Flower. See *Flos*.

Completion. A term used by the ancient writers in various acceptations; but latterly it signifies only the same as *Plethora*.

COMPLE'XUS. (From *complector*, to comprise.) *Complexus seu biventer cervicis* of Albinus. *Dorso trachelon occipital* of Dumas. A muscle situated on the back part of the neck, that draws the head backwards, and to one side: and when both act, they draw the head directly backward. It arises from the transverse processes of the seven superior vertebræ of the back, and four inferior of the neck, by as many distinct tendinous origins; in its ascent, it receives a fleshy slip from the spinous process of the first vertebra of the back: from these different origins it runs upwards, and is every where intermixed with tendinous fibres. It is inserted, tendinous and fleshy, into the inferior edge of the protuberance in the middle of the os occipitis, and into a part of the curved line that runs forwards from that protuberance. It draws the head backwards.

Complexus minor. See *Trachelo-mastoideus*.

COMPOSITUS. Compound. The result or effect of a composition of different things; or that which arises from them. It stands opposed to simple. In botany, applied to leaves and flowers. See *Flos*, and *Folium*.

COMPOUND. See *Compositus*.

Compound affinity. See *Attraction*.

COMPRE'SSION. (*Compressio;* from *comprimo*, to press together.) A diseased state of the body, or of a part, the effect of something pressing upon it. The term is generally applied to the brain. Compression of the brain should be distinguished from concussion and inflammation. When the brain is compressed either by bone, extravasated blood, or any other fluid, there is a general insensibility, the eyes are half open, the pupils dilated and motionless, even when a candle is brought near the eye; the retina is insensible; the limbs relaxed; the breathing stertorous; the pulse slow, and, according to Abernethy, less subject to intermission than in cases of concussion. Nor is the patient ever sick, when the pressure on the brain, and the general insensibility, are considerable; for the very action of vomiting betrays an irritability in the stomach and œsophagus.

COMPRE'SSOR. (*Compressor;* from *comprimo*, to press together.) A name applied to those muscles which press together the parts on which they act.

Compressor naris. *Rinæus vel nasalis* of Douglas. *Transversalis vel myrtiformis* of Winslow. *Dilatores alarum nasi* of Cowper; and *Maxillo narinal* of Dumas. A muscle of the nose, that compresses the alæ towards the septum nasi, particularly when we want to smell acutely. It also corrugates the nose, and assists in expressing certain passions. It arises, by a narrow beginning, from the root of the ala nasi externally, and spreads into a number of thin separate fibres, which run up along the cartilage in an oblique manner towards the back of the nose, where it joins with its fellow, and is inserted into the narrow extremity of the os nasi, and nasal process of the superior maxillary bone.

COMPRESSUS. Compressed; flattened laterally; applied to leaves. See *Leaf*.

COMPTONITE. A new mineral first brought into this country by Lord Compton, and found in drusy cavities, in ejected masses, on Mount Vesuvius.

COMPU'NCTIO. (From *compungo*, to prick.) A puncture.

CONA'RIUM. (From κωνος: so named from its conical shape.) A cone. See *Pineal gland*.

CONCAU'SA. (From *con*, with, and *causa*, a cause.) A cause which co-operates with another in the production of a disease.

CONCAVUS. Hollow; depressed in the middle. Applied to leaves, petals, &c. depressed in their centre, owing, as it were, to a tightness in some part of the circumference; as in *Cyamus nelumbo*, and the petals of the *Galanthus nivalus*.

CONCENTRA'TION. (*Concentratio*; from *con*, and *centrum*, a centre.) The volatilizing of part of the water of fluids, in order to improve their strength. The matter to be concentrated, therefore, must be of superior fixity to water. This operation is performed on some acids, particularly the sulphuric and phosphoric. It is also employed in solutions of alkalies and neutral salts.

CONCENTRIO. *Bulbus concentricus*. A concentric bulb, is one of the laminated kind, well illustrated in the common onion, *Allium cepa*.

CONCEPTACULUM. A former name for what is now called in botany receptaculum.

CONCE'PTION. (*Conceptio*; from *concipio*, to conceive.) The impregnation of the ovulum in the female ovarium, by the subtile prolific aura of the semen virile. In order to have a fruitful coition, it is necessary that the semen be propelled into the uterus, or vagina, so that its fecundating vapour shall be conveyed through the Fallopian tube to the ovarium: it is also necessary that there be a certain state of the ovarium of the female in order to impregnate it; which is, that the ovum shall be mature, and embraced by the fimbriæ of the Fallopian tube, to convey that vivifying principle to the ovum. See *Generation*.

CO'NCHA. (*Concha*, κογχη, a liquid measure among the Athenians.) A term applied by anatomists to several parts of the body; as the hollow of the ear, the spongy bones of the nose, &c.

CONCHA AURICULÆ. See *Auricula*.

CONCHA AURIS. The hollow part of the cartilage of the outer ear.

CONCHA MARGARITIFERA. The shell from which pearls are obtained. See *Margarita*.

CONCHÆ NARIUM. The turbinated portion of the ethmoid bone, and the inferior spongy bones of the nose, which are covered by the Schneiderian membrane, are so termed.

CO'NCHUS. (From κογχη, a shell; so named from their likeness to a shell.) The cranium, and the cavity of the eye.

[CONCHOLITE. See *Organic relics*.]

CONCI'DENS. (From *concido*, to decay.) 1. A decrease of bulk in the whole or any part of the body.

2. A diminution of a tumour.

CONCOAGULA'TIO. (From *con*, and *coagulo*, to coagulate together.) The coagulation or crystallization of different salts, first dissolved together in the same fluid.

CONCO'CTIO. (From *concoquo*, to digest.) 1. Concoction; digestion. This term was formerly very generally used to express that operation of nature upon morbid matter, which renders it fit to be separated from the healthy fluid.

2. The alteration which the food undergoes in the primæ viæ.

CONCREMA'TIO. (From *con*, and *cremo*, to burn together.) Calcination.

CONCRE'TION. (*Concretio*; from *concresco*, to grow together.)

1. The condensation of any fluid substance into a more solid consistence.

2. The growing together of parts which, in a natural state, are separate.

CONCU'RSUS. (From *concurro*, to meet together.) The congeries or collection of symptoms which constitute and distinguish the particular disease.

CONCU'SSION. (From *concutio*, to shake together.) Concussion of the brain. Various alarming symptoms, followed sometimes by the most fatal consequences, are found to attend great violence offered to the head; and upon the strictest examination, both of the living and the dead, neither fissure, fracture, nor extravasation of any kind can be discovered. The same symptoms and the same events are met with when the head has received no injury at all *ab externo*, but has only been violently shaken; nay, when only the body, or general frame, has seemed to have sustained the violence. The symptoms attending a concussion, are generally in proportion to the degree of violence which the brain itself has sustained, and which, indeed, is cognizable only by the symptoms. If the concussion be very great, all sense and power of motion are immediately abolished, and death follows soon; but between this degree and that slight confusion (or stunning, as it is called,) which attends most violences done to the head, there are many shades. The following is Abernethy's description of the symptoms of concussion, which he is of opinion, may be divided into three stages.

The first is that state of insensibility and derangement of the bodily powers which immediately succeeds the accident. While it lasts, the patient scarcely feels any injury that may be inflicted on him. His breathing is difficult, but in general without stertor; his pulse intermitting, and his extremities cold. But such a state cannot last long; it goes off gradually, and is succeeded by another, which is considered as the *second* stage of concussion. In this, the pulse and respiration become better, and, though not regularly performed, are sufficient to maintain life, and to diffuse warmth over the extreme parts of the body. The feeling of the patient is now so far restored, that he is sensible of his skin being pinched; but he lies stupid and inattentive to slight external impressions. As the effects of concussion diminish, he becomes capable of replying to questions put to him in a loud tone of voice, especially when they refer to his chief suffering at the time, as pain in the head, &c.; otherwise he answers incoherently, and as if his attention was occupied by something else. As long as the stupor remains, the inflammation of the brain seems to be moderate; but as the former abates, the latter seldom fails to increase; and this constitutes the *third* stage, which is the most important of the series of effects proceeding from a concussion.

These several stages vary considerably in their degree and duration; but more or less of each will be found to take place in every instance where the brain has been violently shaken. Whether they bear any certain proportion to each other or not, is not known; indeed, this will depend upon such a variety of circumstances in the constitution, the injury, and the after treatment, that it must be difficult to determine.

To distinguish between an extravasation and a concussion by the symptoms only, Mr. Potts says, is frequently a very difficult matter; sometimes an impossible one. The similarity of the effects, in some cases, and the very small space of time which may intervene between the going off of the one and accession of the other, render this a very nice exercise of the judgment. The first stunning or deprivation of sense, whether total or partial, may be from either, and no man can tell from which; but when these first symptoms have been removed, or have spontaneously disappeared, if such patient is again oppressed with drowsiness, or stupidity, or total or partial loss of sense, it then becomes probable that the first complaints were from concussion, and that the latter are from extravasation; and the greater the distance of time between the two the greater is the probability not only that an extravasation is the cause, but that the extravasation is of the limpid kind, made gradatim, and within the brain.

Whoever seriously reflects on the nature of these two causes of evil within the cranium, and considers them as liable to frequent combination in the same subject, and at the same time considers that, in many instances, no degree of information can be obtained from the only person capable of giving it, (the patient) will immediately be sensible how very difficult a part a practitioner has to act in many of these cases, and how very unjust it must be to call that ignorance which is only a just diffidence arising from the obscurity of the subject, and the impossibility of attaining materials to form a clear judgment.

Abernethy observes, that in cases of simple concussion, the insensibility is not so great, as where compression exists, the pupils are more contracted, the muscles less relaxed, little or no stertor attends, but the pulse is very intermitting, and in slight cases there is often considerable sickness.

Very different modes of treating these accidents have been practised, and no doubt the same means should not be pursued indiscriminately. Much must depend on the state of the patient, when he received the injury, the degree of this, the time which has elapsed since, and other circumstances. Abernethy considers, that in the first stage little should be done; that the stimulants often employed may be even injurious; but more especially so in the second stage, increasing the tendency to inflammation; and where this has come on, that the antiphlogistic plan must be actively pursued. However, a moderate abstraction of blood, general or topical, will be commonly proper at first, where the habit will allow it, as congestion may be suspected, and to obviate inflammation, especially where the person was intoxicated at the time of the accident; and the effect of this measure may influence the subsequent treatment. If the pulse rose after it, and the patient became more sensible, we should be led to pursue the evacuating plan, taking perhaps more blood, exhibiting active cathartics, as the bowels will be found very torpid, applying cold lotions to the head, &c. These means, however, will be especially called for, when marks of inflammation appear. Sometimes brisk emetics have been very beneficial, as sulphate of zinc, &c.: they are particularly recommended, where the person was under the influence of anger; or the stomach full, when the accident happened; but they are liable to objection, where there are marks of congestion, or increased action in the vessels of the head. If bleeding should lower the pulse, and render the patient worse, evacuations must not be pursued; it may be better generally to wait the gradual return of sensibility, unless the torpor be alarming, like a state of syncope: in which case, or if it continue very long, stimulants appear justified, as ammonia, or others of transient operation, with a blister to the head, to restore some degree of sensibility. If, in the sequel, marks of irritation appear, as spasms or convulsions, opium joined with antimony, or in the form of Dover's powder, will probably be useful, the necessary evacuations being premised, and the warm bath. In all cases the head should be kept quiet; as the patient is convalescent, tonics, and the shower-bath may be employed with advantage; and it will be particularly necessary to avoid great bodily exertion, stimulating liquors, &c. Should paralytic symptoms remain, stimulants, general or local, may be required. Where alarming symptoms follow an injury to the head, extravasation may be suspected: and the operation of trepanning, skilfully performed, will do no harm to the patient, but may materially relieve, even by the loss of blood attending.

CONDENSA'TION. (*Condensatio; from condenso*, to make thick.) A thickening of any fluid.

CONDIME'NTUM. (From *condio*, to preserve, or season.) A condiment, preserve, or sweetmeat.

Condu'ctio. (From *conduco*, to draw along.) In Cœlius Aurelianus, it is a spasm, or convulsion, drawing the muscles out of their proper positions.

CONDU'CTOR. (From *conduco*, to lead, or guide.) A surgical instrument, the use of which is to direct the knife in certain operations. It is more commonly called a director.

CONDUPLICATUS. Folded. Applied to leaves, when the margins are clapped flatly together; as in *Roscœa purpurea*, and the bases of sword-shaped leaves. See *Leaf*.

CO'NDYLE. (*Condylus;* from κονδυ, an ancient cup, shaped like a joint.) A round eminence of a bone in any of the joints.

CONDYLO'MA. (*Condyloma, atis.* n.; from κονδυλος, a tubercle, or knot.) A soft, wart-like excrescence, that appears about the anus and pudendum of both sexes. There are several species of condylomata, which have received names from their appearances; as *ficus*, *crystæ*, *thymus*, from their resemblance to a fig, &c.

CONE. See *Strobilus*.

Conei'on. (From κωναν, to turn round.) In Hippocrates it imports hemlock. It is said to be thus named, because it produces a vertigo in those who take it inwardly. See *Conium*.

Cone'ssi cortex. See *Nerium antidysentericum*.

CONFE'CTION. (*Confectio, onis.* f.; from *conficio*, to make up.) A confection. In general, it means any thing made up with sugar. The term, in the new London Pharmacopœia, includes those articles which were formerly called electuaries and conserves, between which there do not appear to be sufficient grounds to make a distinction.

[" *Confections* are soft solids, in the composition of which sugar forms a principal article. The term includes what have been called *conserves*, made from recent vegetable substances, beaten with sugar as a preservative; and *electuaries*, which were formed of dry powders, &c. brought to a proper consistence with syrup, either to facilitate their deglutition, or to conceal their taste."—*Big. Mat. Med.*

The Pharmacopœia of the United States has the following:—*Confectio aromatica, Confectio aurantii corticis, Confectio cassiæ, Confectio rosæ, Confectio scammoniæ, Confectio sennæ.* A.]

Confectio amygdalarum. Confection of almonds. Take of sweet almonds, an ounce; Acacia gum powdered, a drachm; refined sugar, half an ounce. The almonds having been previously macerated in water and their external coat removed, beat the whole together, until they are thoroughly incorporated. It has been objected to the almond mixture, which is an article of very general use, that it requires considerable time for its extemporaneous preparation, and that it spoils, and cannot be kept when it is made. This will be obviated by the present form, which does keep for a sufficient length of time, and rubs down into the mixture immediately.

Confectio aromatica. This preparation was formerly called *Confectio cardiaca. Confectio Raleighana.* Take of cinnamon bark, nutmegs, of each two ounces; cloves, an ounce; cardamom seeds, half an ounce; saffron dried, two ounces; prepared shells, sixteen ounces; refined sugar powdered, two pounds; water, a pint. Reduce the dry substances, mixed together, to very fine powder; then add the water gradually, and mix the whole, until it is incorporated. This preparation is now much simplified by the London college. It is an excellent medicine, possessing stimulant, antispasmodic, and adstringent virtues; and is exhibited with these views to children and adults, in a vast variety of diseases, mixed with other medicines. It may be given in doses of 10 gr. to a drachm.

Confectio aurantiorum. *Conserva corticis exterioris aurantii hispalensis. Conserva flavedinus corticum aurantiorum.* Take of fresh external rind of oranges, separated by rasping, a pound; refined sugar, three pounds. Bruise the rind with a wooden pestle, in a stone mortar; then, after adding the sugar, bruise it again, until the whole is thoroughly incorporated. This is well calculated to form the basis of a tonic and stomachic confection, and may be given alone in doses of from two to five drachms, twice or three times a day.

Confectio cardiaca. See *Confectio aromatica.*

Confectio cassiæ. *Electuarium cassiæ. Electuarium e cassia.* Confection of cassia. Take of fresh cassia pulp, half a pound; manna, two ounces; tamarind pulp, an ounce; syrup of roses, half a pint. Bruise the manna; melt it in the syrup by a water-bath; then mix in the pulps, and evaporate down to a proper consistence. This is a very elegant, pleasant, and mild aperient for the feeble, and for children. Dose from two drachms to an ounce.

Confectio opii. *Confectio opiata. Philonium Londinense. Philonium Romanum.* Confection of opium. Take of hard opium powdered, six drachms; long pepper, an ounce; ginger root, two ounces; caraway-seeds, three ounces; syrup, a pint. Rub together the opium and the syrup previously heated; then add the remaining articles reduced to powder, and mix. To the credit of modern pharmacy, this is the only one that remains of all those complicated and confused preparations called mithridate, theriaca, &c.; it more nearly approximates, in its composition, the philonium than any other, and may be considered as an effectual substitute for them in practice. This very warm and stimulating confection is admirably calculated to relieve diarrhœa, or spasms of the stomach and bowels, and is frequently ordered in doses of from 10 grs. to half a drachm. About 36 grains contain one of opium.

Confectio piperis nigri. Confection of black pepper. Take of black pepper; elecampane, of each a pound; fennel seeds, three pounds; honey; refined sugar, of each two pounds. Rub the dry ingredients together, so as to reduce them to a very fine powder; then, having added the honey, rub them again so that the whole may incorporate. This confection is given internally against a relaxed condition of the extremity of the rectum, producing partial prolapse, and against that piley state which results from weakness. A similar compound has been long celebrated and sold under the name of Ward's paste.

Confectio rosæ caninæ. *Conserva cynosbati. Conserva fructus cynosbati.* Conserve of hips. Confection of dog-rose. Take of dog-rose pulp, a pound; refined sugar powdered, twenty ounces. Expose the pulp in a water bath to a gentle heat; then add the sugar gradually, and rub them together until they are thoroughly incorporated. This preparation is cooling and adstringent; it is seldom given alone, but mostly joined to some other medicine, in the form of linctus, or electuary.

Confectio rosæ gallicæ. *Conserva rosæ. Conserva rosarum rubrarum.* Conserve of red rose. Take of the petals of the red rose, before it is expanded, and without the claws, a pound; refined sugar, three pounds. Bruise the petals in a stone mortar; then, having added the sugar, beat them again together, until they are thoroughly incorporated. This is an excellent sub-astringent composition. Rubbed down with water, it forms an excellent drink, with some lemon juice, in hæmorrhagic complaints; it may also be given with vitriolated zinc, in the form of an electuary.

Confectio rutæ. *Electuarium e baccis lauri.* Confection of rue. Take of rue leaves dried, caraway seeds, bay-berries, of each an ounce and a half; sagapenum, half an ounce; black pepper, two drachms; clarified honey, sixteen ounces. Rub the dry articles together, into a very fine powder; then add the honey, and mix the whole. Its use is confined to clysters.

Confectio scammoneæ. *Electuarium scammonii. Electuarium e scammonio. Electuarium caryocostinum.* Confection of scammony. Take of scammony gum resin powdered, an ounce and a half; cloves bruised, ginger root powdered, of each, six drachms; oil of caraway, half a drachm; syrup of roses, as much as is sufficient. Rub the dry articles together, into very fine powder; next rub them again while the syrup is gradually added; then add the oil of caraway, and mix the whole well together. This is a strong stimulating cathartic, and calculated to remove worms from the primæ viæ, with which view it is mostly exhibited. Dose from ℈ss. to ℈j.

Confectio sennæ. *Electuarium sennæ. Electuarium lenitivum.* Confection of senna. Take of senna leaves, eight ounces; figs, a pound; tamarind pulp, pulp of prunes, cassia pulp, of each half a pound; coriander seeds, four ounces; liquorice root, three ounces; refined sugar, two pounds and a half. Powder the senna leaves with the coriander seeds, and separate, by sifting ten ounces of the mixed powder. Boil the remainder with the figs and the liquorice-root, in four pints of water, until it be reduced to half; then press out and strain the liquor. Evaporate the liquor, until a pint and a half only remains of the whole; then add the sugar, to make syrup. Lastly, mix the pulps gradually with the syrup, and, having added the sifted powder, mix the whole together. This is a mild and elegant aperient, well adapted for pregnant women, and those whose bowels are easily moved. Dose, ℈ss. ℥ss.

CONFERTUS. Clustered, or crowded together: applied to leaves. See *Leaf.*

CONFE'RVA. (From *conferveo*, to knit together.) 1. The name of a genus of plants in the Linnæan system. Class, *Cryptogamia;* Order, *Algæ.*

2. A kind of moss: named from its use formerly in healing broken bones

Conferva helminthocortos. See *Corallina corsicana.*

Conferva rivalis. This plant, *Conferva; filamentis simplicissimus æqualibus longissimus*, of Linnæus, has been recommended in cases of spasmodic asthma, phthisis, &c. on account of the great quantity of vital air it contains.

CONFIRMA'NTIA. (From *con*, and *firmo*, to strengthen.) 1. Restoratives.

2. Medicines which fasten the teeth in their sockets.

CONFLUENT. Running together. Applied to eruptions. See *Variola.*

CONFLU'XION. Much used by Hippocrates, and his interpreter Galen, from a notion that parts at a distance have mutual consent with one another, and that they are all perspirable by many subtle streams. Paracelsus, according to his way, expressed the former by confederation.

CONFORMA'TIO. (From *conformo*, to shape or fashion.) Conformation. The natural shape and form of any part.

Conforta'ntia. (From *conforto*, to strengthen. Cordial and strengthening medicines.

Confortati'va. The same.

Confu'sio. (From *confundo*, to mix together.) A confusion, or disorder in the eyes, proceeding from a rupture of the membranes, which include the humours, by which means they are all confounded together.

Congela'ti. (From *congelo*, to freeze.) *Congelatici.* Persons afflicted with a catalepsy are so called, by which all sensation seems to be taken away.

CONGELA'TION. (*Congelatio;* from *congelo*, to freeze.) That change of liquid bodies which takes place when they pass to a solid state, by losing the caloric which kept them in a state of fluidity.

Congelati'va. (From *congelo*, to congeal.) Medicines that inspissate humours, and stop fluxions and rheums.

CO'NGENER. (From *con*, and *genus*, kind.) Of the same kind; concurring in the same action. It is usually said of the muscles.

CONGE'STION. (From *congero*, to amass.) A collection of blood or other fluid; thus we say a congestion of blood in the vessels, when they are over distended, and the motion is slow.

CONGLOBA'TE. *Conglobatus;* from *conglobo*, to gather into a ball.) 1. A term applied to a gland, *Glandula conglobata*, which is formed of a contortion of lymphatic vessels, connected together by cellular structure, having neither a cavity nor any excretory duct: such are the mesenteric, inguinal, axillary glands, &c. See *Gland.*

2. A conglobate *flower*, is a compound one growing in the form of a sphere or globe.

CONGLOMERATE. (*Conglomeratus;* from *conglomero*, to heap upon one.) 1. Applied to a gland, *Glandula conglomerata*, which consists of a number of smaller glomerate glands, the excretory ducts of which all unite into one common duct: such are the salival, parotid glands, &c.

2. Conglomerate *flowers*, are such as are heaped together on a footstalk, to which they are irregularly, but closely connected. See *Panicula.*

CONGLOMERITE. A compound mineral mass, in which angular fragments of rocks are imbedded. The Italian term *brecchia*, has the same meaning. In pudding stone, the imbedded fragments are round, bearing the marks of having been polished by attrition.

CONGLUTINA'NTIA. (From *conglutino*, to glue together.) Healing medicines; and such as unite parts disjoined by accident.

CONICUS. Conical. Applied to leaves, nectaries, receptacles, &c.—Nectarium conicum, in the *Utricularia foliosa*, and the receptacle of the daisy, *Anthemis arvensis, cotula*, and *Matricaria chamomilla.*

CONIFERÆ. Cone-bearing plants. The name of an order in Linnæus's Fragments of a Natural Method.

CO'NIS. Κονις. Dust; fine powder; ashes; a nit in the hair; scurf from the head; and sometimes it signifies lime.

CONITE. 1. An ash or greenish-gray coloured mineral, which becomes brown on exposure to air. It is found in Saxony and Iceland.

2. Dr. Macculloch has given this name to a pulverulent mineral, as fusible as glass into a transparent bead,

which he found in the trap hills of Kilpatrick, and the Isle of Sky.

[3. The petrifaction of a conus. See *Organic relics*. A.]

CONI'UM. (From κονια, dust, according to Linnæus; or from κωναω, *circumago*, on account of its inebriating and poisonous quality.) Hemlock.

1. The name of a genus of plants in the Linnæan system. Class, *Pentandria; Order, Digynia.*

2. The pharmacopœial name of the officinal hemlock. See *Conium maculatum.*

CONIUM MACULATUM. The systematic name for the *cicuta* of the pharmacopœias. It is called by some *camaran;* by others *abiotos;* and, according to Erotian, *cambeion* is an old Sicilian word for cicuta. *Cicuta major fœtida. Conium—seminibus striatis*, of Linnæus.

Hemlock is found in every part of England, and is distinguished from those plants which bear some resemblance to it, by the spotted stem. It is generally believed to be a very active poison. In a very moderate dose it is apt to occasion sickness and vertigo: in a larger quantity it produces anxiety, cardialgia, vomiting, convulsions, coma, and death. Baron Stoerk was the first who brought hemlock into repute as a medicine of extraordinary efficacy: and although we have not in this country any direct facts, like those mentioned by Stoerk, proving that inveterate scirrhuses, cancers, ulcers, and many other diseases hitherto deemed irremediable, are to be completely cured by the cicuta; we have however the testimonies of several eminent physicians, showing that some complaints which had resisted other powerful remedies, yielded to hemlock; and that even some disorders, which if not really cancerous, were at least suspected to be of that tendency, were greatly benefited by this remedy. In chronic rheumatisms, some glandular swellings, and in various fixed and periodical pains, the cicuta is now very generally employed; and from daily experience, it appears in such cases to be a very efficacious remedy. It has also been of singular use in the hooping-cough. Nor is it less efficacious when applied externally; a poultice made of oatmeal and the expressed juice, (or a decoction of the extract, when the other cannot be obtained,) allays the most excruciating torturing pains of a cancer, and thus gives rest to the distracted patient.

The proper method of administering conium internally, is to begin with a few grains of the powder or inspissated juice, and gradually to increase the dose until a giddiness affects the head, a motion is felt in the eyes as if pressed outwards, with a slight sickness and trembling agitation of the body. One or more of these symptoms are the evidence of a full dose, which should be continued until they have ceased, and then after a few days the dose may be increased; for little advantage can be expected but by a continuance of the greatest quantity the patient can bear. In some constitutions even small doses greatly offend, occasioning spasms, heat and thirst; in such instances it will be of no service. As the powder of the dried leaves has been thought to act, and may be depended upon with more certainty than the extract, the following direction should be observed in the preparation:—Gather the plant about the end of June, when it is in flower; pick off the little leaves, and throw away the leaf-stalks: dry the small selected leaves in a hot sun, or in a tin or pewter dish before the fire. Preserve them in bags made of strong brown paper, or powder them and keep the powder in glass phials where the light is excluded; for light dissipates the beautiful green colour very soon, and thus the medicine loses its appearance, if not its efficacy: this mode is recommended by Dr. Withering. The extract should also be made of the plant gathered at this period. From 2 to 20 grains of the powder may be taken twice or thrice a day.

CONJUGATUS. Conjugate or yoked: applied to leaves, which are said to be conjugate or binate. They consist of one pair of leaflets; as in the *Mimosa.*

CONJUNCTIVA. *Membrana conjunctiva.* The conjunctive membrane of the eye; a thin, transparent, delicate membrane, that lines the internal superficies of one eyelid, and is reflected from thence over the anterior part of the bulb, then reflected again to the edge of the other eyelid. That portion which covers the transparent cornea cannot, without much difficulty, be separated from it. Inflammation of this membrane is called *ophthalmia.*

CONJUNCTUS. Conjoined. A botanical term applied to a tuber which is said to be conjoined when in immediate contact with another, as in many of the *Orchides.*

CONNA'TUS. (From *con*, and *nascor*, to grow together.) 1. Born with a person; the same with *congenitus.*

2. In botany it is applied to leaves, which are said to be connate when united at their base; as in *Chlora perfoliata.*

CONNEXION. See *Articulation.*

CONNIVENS. (From *conniveo*, to make as if he did not see.) In botany applied to petals of flowers, as in those of the *Rumex*, and to the receptacle of the fig, which the fruit really is, being a fleshy connivent receptacle, enclosing and hiding the florets.

CONNUTRI'TUS. (From *con*, and *nutrior*, to be nourished with.) It is what becomes habitual to a person from his particular nourishment, or what breaks out into a disease in process of time, which gradually had its foundation in the first aliments, as from sucking a distempered nurse, or the like.

CONQUASSA'TIO. Conquassation. In pharmacy it is a species of comminution, or an operation by which moist concrete substances, as recent vegetables, fruits, the softer parts of animals, &c. are agitated and bruised, till, partly by their proper succulence, or by the affusion of some liquor, they are reduced to a soft pulp.

CONRI'NGIUS, HERMAN, was born at Norden, in East Friesland, 1606, and graduated in medicine at Helmstat, where he soon after became professor in that science, and subsequently in physics, law, and politics. He was also made physician and aulic counsellor to the Queen of Sweden, the King of Denmark, and several of the German princes. He wrote numerous works in philosophy, medicine, and history, displaying great learning, and long highly esteemed. In one treatise he refers the degeneracy of the modern Germans to their altered mode of living, the use of stoves, tobacco, &c. He published also an "Introduction to the whole Art of Medicine, and its several Parts," containing a History of Bibliotheca Medica, with numerous Dissertations on particular Diseases. He died in 1681.

CONSENT. Consent of parts. See *Sympathy.*

CONSE'RVA. (From *conservo*, to keep.) A conserve. A composition of some recent vegetable and sugar, beat together into a uniform mass of the consistence of honey; as conserve of hips, orange peel, &c. Conserves are called confections in the last edition of the London Pharmacopœia. See *Confectio.*

CONSERVA ABSINTHII MARITIMI. See *Artemisia maritima.*

CONSERVA ARI. This is occasionally exhibited as a stimulant and diuretic. See *Arum maculatum.*

CONSERVA AURANTII HISPALENSIS. See *Confectio aurantiorum.*

CONSERVA CYNOSBATI. See *Confectio rosæ caninæ.*

CONSERVA LUJULÆ. A preparation of woodsorrel, possessing acid, cooling, and antiseptic qualities. See *Oxalis acetosella.*

CONSERVA MENTHÆ. This preparation of mint is given occasionally as a stomachic, in sickness and weakness of the stomach. See *Mentha viridis.*

CONSERVA PRUNI SYLVESTRIS. Astringent virtues are ascribed to this medicine, which is now seldom used but in private formulæ.

CONSERVA ROSÆ. This conserve, rubbed down with water, to which is added some lemon-juice, forms an excellent drink in hæmorrhagic complaints. See *Confectio rosæ gallicæ.*

CONSERVA SCILLÆ. A preparation of squills, which affords an excellent basis for an electuary, possessing expectorant and diuretic qualities.

[CONSERVATIVES. See *Organic relics.* A.]

CONSISTE'NTIA. (From *consisto*, to abide.) The state or acme of a disease. The appearance or state of the humours and excrements.

CONSO'LIDA. (So called, *quia consolidandi et conglutinandi vi pollet;* from its power in agglutinating and joining together things broken.) See *Symphytum.*

CONSOLIDA AUREA. See *Solidago virga aurea.*
CONSOLIDA MAJOR. See *Symphytum.*
CONSOLIDA MEDIA. See *Ajuga pyramidalis*
CONSOLIDA MINOR. See *Prunella.*

CONSOLIDA REGALIS. See *Delphinium consolida.*

CONSOLIDA SARACENICA. See *Solidago virga aurea.*

CONSOUND. See *Symphytum.*

Consound middle. See *Ajuga pyramidalis.*

CONSTANTI'NUS, AFRICANUS, was born at Carthage, towards the middle of the 11th century. He lived near forty years at Babylon, and was celebrated for his knowledge of the Eastern languages. Among the sciences, medicine appears to have principally occupied his attention; and two of his works were thought deserving of being printed at Bâle, about 4 1-2 centuries after his death, which occurred in 1087. They are thought however to have been chiefly translated from Arabian writers.

CONSTIPATION. (*Constipatio:* from *constipo,* to crowd together.) *Obstipatio.* Costiveness. A person is said to be costive when the alvine excrements are not expelled daily, and when the fæces are so hardened as not to receive their form from the impression of the rectum upon them.

CONSTITUTION. *Constitutio.* The general condition of the body, as evinced by the peculiarities in the performance of its functions: such are, the peculiar predisposition to certain diseases, or liability of particular organs to disease; the varieties in digestion, in muscular power and motion, in sleep, in the appetite, &c. Some marked peculiarities of constitution are observed to be accompanied with certain external characters, such as a particular colour and texture of the skin, and of the hair, and also with a peculiarity of form and disposition of mind; all of which have been observed from the earliest time, and divided into classes: and which received names during the prevalence of the humeral pathology which they still retain. See *Temperament.*

CONSTRICTI'VA. (From *constringo,* to bind together.) Styptics.

CONSTRI'CTOR. (From *constringo,* to bind together.) A name given to those muscles which contract any opening of the body.

CONSTRICTOR ALÆ NASI. See *Depressor labii superioris alæque nasi.*

CONSTRICTOR ANI. See *Sphincter ani.*

CONSTRICTOR ISTHMI FAUCIUM. *Glosso-staphilinus.* of Winslow, Douglas, and Cowper; and *Glosso staphilin* of Dumas. A muscle situated at the side of the entry of the fauces, that draws the *velum pendulum palati* towards the root of the tongue, which it raises at the same time, and with its fellow contracts the passage between the two arches, by which it shuts the opening of the fauces.

CONSTRICTOR LABIORUM. See *Orbicularis oris.*

CONSTRICTOR ORIS. See *Orbicularis oris.*

CONSTRICTOR PALPEBRARUM. See *Orbicularis palpebrarum.*

CONSTRICTORES PHARYNGÆI. The muscles of the œsophagus.

CONSTRICTOR PHARYNGIS INFERIOR. *Crico pharyngeus; Thyro-pharyngeus* of Douglas and Winslow. *Cricothyropharyngien* of Dumas. A muscle situated on the posterior part of the pharynx. It arises from the side of the thyroid cartilage, near the attachment of the sterno-hyoideus and thyro-hyoideus muscles; and from the cricoid cartilage, near the crico-thyroideus; it is inserted into the white line, where it joins with its fellow, the superior fibres running obliquely upwards, covering nearly one-half of the middle constrictor, and terminating in a point; the inferior fibres run more transversely, and cover the beginning of the œsophagus. Its use is to compress that part of the pharynx which it covers, and to raise it with the larynx a little upwards.

CONSTRICTOR PHARYNGIS MEDIUS. *Hyopharyngeus* and *cephalo-pharyngeus* of Douglas and Winslow. *Chondro-pharyngeus* of Douglas. *Syndesmopharyngeus* of Winslow. *Cephalo-pharyngeus* of Winslow and Douglas. *Hyo-glosso basi pharyngien* of Dumas. A muscle situated on the posterior part of the pharynx. It arises from the appendix of the os hyoides, from the cornu of that bone, and from the ligament which connects it to the thyroid cartilage; the fibres of the superior part running obliquely upwards, and covering a considerable part of the superior constrictor, terminate in a point; and it is inserted into the middle of the cuneiform process of the os occipitis, before the foramen magnum, and joined to its fellow at a white line in the middle part of the pharynx. This muscle compresses that part of the pharynx which it covers, and draws it and the os hyoides upwards.

CONSTRICTOR PHARYNGIS SUPERIOR. *Glosso-pharyngeus; Mylo-pharyngeus; Pterygo-pharyngeus* of Douglas and Winslow, and *Pterigo syndesmo staphili pharyngien* of Dumas. A muscle situated on the posterior part of the pharynx. It arises above, from the cuneiform process of the os occipitis, before the foramen magnum, from the pterygoid process of the sphenoid bone, from the upper and under jaw, near the roots of the last dentes molares, and between the jaws. It is inserted in the middle of the pharynx. Its use is to compress the upper part of the pharynx, and to draw it forwards and upwards.

CONSTRICTOR VESICÆ URINARIÆ. See *Detrusor urinæ.*

CONSTRICTO'RIUS. A disease attended with constriction, or spasm.

CONSTRINGEN'TIA. (From *constringo,* to bind together.) Astringent medicines. See *Astringent.*

CONSUMPTION. (From *consumo,* to waste away.) See *Phthisis.*

CONTABESCE'NTIA. (From *contabesco,* to pine or waste away.) An atrophy, or nervous consumption.

CONTAGION. (*Contagio;* from *contango,* to meet or touch each other.) This word properly imports the application of any poisonous matter to the body through the medium of touch. It is applied to those very subtile particles arising from putrid substances, or from persons labouring under certain diseases, which communicate the disease to others; as the contagion of putrid fever, the effluvia of dead animal or vegetable substances, the miasm of bogs and fens, the virus of smallpox, lues venerea, &c. &c.

The principal diseases excited by poisonous miasmata are, intermittent, remittent, and yellow fevers, dysentery, and typhus. That of the last is generated in the human body itself, and is sometimes called the typhoid fomes. The other miasmata are produced from moist vegetable matter, in some unknown state of decomposition. The contagious *virus* of the plague, smallpox, measles, chincough, cynanche maligna, and scarlet fever, as well as of typhus and the jail fever, operates to a much more limited distance through the intermedium of the atmosphere, than the marsh miasmata. Contact of a diseased person is said to be necessary for the communication of plague; and approach within 2 or 3 yards of him, for that of typhus. The Walcheren miasmata extended their pestilential influence to vessels riding at anchor, fully a quarter of a mile from the shore.

The chemical nature of all these poisonous effluvia is little understood. They undoubtedly consist, however, of hydrogen, united with sulphur, phosphorus, carbon, and azot, in unknown proportions, and unknown states of combination. The proper neutralizers or destroyers of these gasiform poisons, are nitric acid vapour, muriatic acid gas, and chlorine. The last two are the most efficacious; but require to be used in situations from which the patients can be removed at the time of the application. Nitric acid vapour may, however, be diffused in the apartments of the sick, without much inconvenience. Bed-clothes, particularly blankets, can retain the contagious fomes, in an active state, for almost any length of time. Hence, they ought to be fumigated with peculiar care. The vapour of burning sulphur or sulphurous acid is used in the East, against the plague. It is much inferior in power to the other antiloimic reagents.

There does not appear to be any distinction commonly made between contagious and infectious diseases.

[The very evident distinction has long since been made and employed in this country. *Contagion* is applied to those diseases which are propagated from one to another by contact or close approach, and which produces a like disease; as the venereal disease, itch, smallpox, measles, &c. Diseases produced by *infection,* are those contracted from a vitiated atmosphere, as intermittent, remittent, bilious, and yellow fevers. In 1819 and 1822, we had the yellow-fever in New-York, and the board of health shut up that part of the city where the disease prevailed, by running fences across the streets leading to it. This was called the *infected district,* from the local causes contaminating the atmosphere and producing the infection.

Beyond this district the city was not unhealthy, and those who were taken sick in the infected district, when removed to other parts not infected, recovered, and did not communicate the disease to others. A.]

CONTE'NSIO. (From *contineo*, to restrain.) It is sometimes used to express a tension or stricture.

CO'NTINENS FEBRIS. A continent fever, which proceeds regularly in the same tenor, without either exacerbation or remission. This rarely, if ever, happens.

CONTI'NUA FEBRIS. (From *continuo*, to persevere.) A continued fever. See *Febris continua.*

CONTINUED. *Continuus;* from *continuo*, to persevere.) A term applied in pathology to diseases which go on with a regular tenor of symptoms, but mostly to fevers, the symptoms of which continue, without intermission, until the disease terminates: hence continual fevers in distinction to intermittent fevers.

CONTINUUS. See *Continued.*

CONTO'RSIO. (From *contorqueo*, to twist about.) A contortion, or twisting. In medicine this word has various significations, and is applied to the iliac passion, to luxation of the vertebræ, head, &c.

CONTORTÆ. Twisted plants. The name of an order in Linnæus's Fragments of a Natural Method, consisting of plants which have a single petal that is twisted or bent toward the side, as *Nerium Vinca*, &c.

CONTORTUS. (From *con*, and *torqueo*, to twist.) Twisted. Applied to the seed-vessel of plants: as the *legumen contortum* of the *Medicago sativa*

CONTRA-APERTURA. (From *contra*, against, and *aperio*, to open.) A counter-opening. An opening made opposite to the one that already exists.

CONTRACTILITY. *Contractilitas.* A property in bodies, the effect of the cohesive power, by which their particles resume their former propinquity when the force ceases which was applied to separate them. It also denotes the power which muscular fibres possess of shortening themselves.

CONTRACTION. (From *contraho*, to draw together.) *Contractura; Beriberia.* A rigid contraction of the joints. It is a genus of disease in the class *Locales*, and order *Dyscinesiæ* of Cullen. The species are,

1. *Contractura primaria*, from a rigid contraction of the muscles, called also obstipitas; a word that, with any other annexed, distinguishes the variety of the contraction. Of this species he forms four varieties. 1. *Contractura ab inflammatione*, when it arises from inflammation. 2. *Contractura à spasmo*, called also tonic spasm and cramp, when it depends upon spasm. 3. *Contractura ob antagonistas paraliticos*, from the antagonist muscles losing their action. 4. *Contractura ab acrimoniâ irritante*, which is induced by some irritating cause.

2. *Contractura articularis*, originating from a disease of the joint.

CONTRAFISSU'RA. (From *contra*, against, and *findo*, to cleave.) *Contre-coup* of French writers. A fracture in a part opposite to that in which the blow is received; as when the frontal bone is broken by a fall on the occiput, where the bone remains sound.

CONTRAHE'NTIA. (From *contraho*, to contract.) Medicines which shorten and strengthen the fibres. Astringents are the only medicines of this nature.

CONTRA-INDICATION. (*Contra-indicatio;* from *contra*, against, and *indico*, to show.) A symptom attending a disease, which forbids the exhibition of a remedy which would otherwise be employed; for instance, bark and acids are usually given in putrid fevers; but if there be difficulty of breathing, or inflammation of any viscus, they are contra-indications to their use.

CONTRA-LUNA'RIS. (From *contra*, and *luna*, the moon.) An epithet given by Dietericus to a woman who conceives during the menstrual discharge.

CONTRA-SEMEN. See *Artemisia Santonica.*

CONTRAYE'RVA. (From *contra*, against, and *yerva*, poison, Span.; *i. e.* an herb good against poison.) See *Dorstenia.*

CONTRAYERVA ALBA. *Cantrayerva Germanorum.* A name for a species of asclepias.

CONTRAYERVA NOVA. Mexican contrayerva. See *Psoralea pentaphylla.*

CONTRAYERVA VIRGINIANA. See *Aristolochia serpentaria.*

Contre-coup. See *Contrafissura.*

CONTRI'TIO. The act of grinding, or reducing to powder.

CONTUSION. (*Contusio;* from *contundo*, to knock together.) A bruise, or contused wound.

CONUS. A cone. See *Strobilus*

CONVALESCENCE. (*Convalescentia;* from *con valesco*, to grow well.) The recovery of health after the cure of a disease. The period of convalescence is that space from the departure of a disease, to the recovery of the strength lost by it.

CONVALESCENT. Recovering or returning to a state of health after the cure of a disease.

CONVALLA'RIA. (From *convallis*, a valley; named from its abounding in valleys and marshes.) The name of a genus of plants in the Linnæan system. Class, *Hexandria;* Order, *Monogynia.*

CONVALLARIA MAJALIS. The systematic name of the lily of the valley. *Lillium convallium; Convallaria; Maianthemum.* May-lily. The flowers of this plant, *Convallaria—scapo nudo* of Linnæus, have a penetrating bitter taste, and are given in nervous and catarrhal disorders. When dried and powdered, they prove strongly purgative. Watery or spirituous extracts made from them, given in doses of a scruple, or drachm, act as gentle stimulating aperients and laxatives; and seem to partake of the purgative virtue, as well as the bitterness of aloes. The roots, in the form of tincture, or infusion, act as a sternutatory when snuffed up the nose, and as a laxative or purgative when taken internally.

CONVALLARIA POLYGONATUM. The systematic name of Solomon's seal. *Sigillum Salomonis; Convallaria—foliis alternis amplexicaulibus, caule ancipiti, pedunculis axillaribus subunifloris*, of Linnæus. The roots are applied externally as adstringents, and are administered internally as corroborants.

CONVEXUS. Convex. A term in very general use in anatomy, botany, &c.

CONVOLU'TA OSSA. See *Spongiosa ossa.*

CONVOLU'TUS. Rolled up or folded. Applied to bones, membranes, leaves, &c.

CONVO'LVULUS (From *convolvo*, to roll together, or entwine.)

1. A name for the iliac passion.

2. The name of a genus of plants in the Linnæan system, so called from their twisting round others, (Class, *Pentandria;* Order, *Monogynia*,) which affords the Jalapa, mechoacanna, turbith, and scammony. The whole genus consists of plants containing a milky juice strongly cathartic and caustic.

CONVOLVULUS AMERICANUS. The jalap root. See *Convolvulus jalapa.*

CONVOLVULUS BATATAS. *Batatas.* A native of the West Indies. Its root is firm and of a pale brown on the outside, and white within. When boiled it is sweet, like chesnuts, and is esteemed by some as an esculent.

[This is the sweet potato, extensively cultivated and eaten in all the southern parts of the United States, even as far north as New-Jersey. It is commonly called the *Carolina potato.* See *Batatas.* A.]

CONVOLVULUS CANTABRICA. A name for the cantabrica. *Convolvulus minimus spicæ foliis; Convolvulus linariæ folio; Convolvulus Cantabrica* of Linnæus. Lavender-leaved bind-weed. Pliny says it was discovered in the time of Augustus, in the country of the Cantabri in Spain; whence its name. It is anthelmintic and actively cathartic.

CONVOLVULUS COLUBRINUS. The pariera brava. See *Cissampelos pareira.*

CONVOLVULUS JALAPA. The systematic name of the jalap plant. *Jalapium mechoacanna nigra. Convolvulus; caule volubli; foliis ovatis, subcordatis, obtusis, obsolete repandis, subtus villosis; pedunculis unifloris* of Linnæus. It is a native of South America. In the shops, the root is found both cut into slices and whole, of an oval shape, solid, ponderous, blackish on the outside, but gray within, and marked with several dark veins, by the number of which, and by its hardness, heaviness, and dark colour, the goodness of the root is to be estimated. It has scarcely any smell, and very little taste, but to the tongue, and to the throat, manifests a slight degree of pungency. The medicinal activity of jalap resides principally, if not wholly, in the resin, which, though given in small doses, occasions violent tormina. The root powdered is a very common, efficacious, and safe purgative, as daily experience evinces; but, according as it contains more or less resin, its effects must of course vary. In large doses, or when joined with calomel, it is recommended as an anthelmintic and hydragogue. In the pharmacopœias, this root is ordered in the form of tincture and extract; and the Edinburgh College directs it also in powder with twice its weight of crystals of tartar.

CONVOLVULUS MAJOR ALBUS. See *Convolvulus sepium.*

CONVOLVULUS MARITIMUS. The brassica maritima, or sea colewort.

CONVOLVULUS MECHOACAN. *Mechoacanna; Jalapa alba;* or *Bryonia alba Peruviana; Rhabarbarum album.* Mechoacan. The root of this species of convolvulus is brought from Mexico. It possesses aperient properties, and was long used as the common purge of this country, but is now wholly superseded by jalap.

["CONVOLVULUS PANDURATUS. *Wild potato.* The affinity of this plant to jalap, in its botanical character, has caused a medicinal quality to be ascribed to it which it does not possess. It is one of the weakest of our indigenous cathartics, and requires too large a dose to be of much use in that character. It is said to mitigate strangury and gravel, and to operate as a diuretic." —*Big. Mat. Med.* A.]

CONVOLVULUS SCAMMONIA. The systematic name of the scammony plant. See *Scammonium; Convolvulus syriacus; Scammonium syriacum; Diagrydium.* This plant, *Convolvulus—foliis sagittatis postice truncatis, pedunculis teretibus subtifloris* of Linnæus, affords the concrete gummi-resinous juice termed scammony. It grows plentifully about Maraash, Antioch, Edlib, and towards Tripoli, in Syria. No part of the dried plant possesses any medicinal quality, but the root, which Dr. Russel administered in decoction, and found it to be a pleasant and mild cathartic. It is from the milky juice of the root that we obtain the officinal scammony, which is procured in the following manner by the peasants, who collect it in the beginning of June. Having cleared away the earth from about the root, they cut off the top in an oblique direction, about two inches below where the stalks spring from it. Under the most depending part of the slope, they fix a shell, or some other convenient receptacle, into which the milky juice gradually flows. It is left there about twelve hours, which time is sufficient for draining off the whole juice; this, however, is in small quantity, each root affording but a very few drachms. This juice from the several roots is put together, often into the leg of an old boot, for want of some more proper vessel, where, in a little time, it grows hard, and is the genuine scammony. The smell of scammony is rather unpleasant, and the taste bitterish and slightly acrid. The different proportions of gum and resin, of which it consists, have been variously stated; but, as proof spirit is the best menstruum for it, these substances are supposed to be nearly in equal parts. It is brought from Aleppo and Smyrna in masses, generally of a light shining gray colour, and friable texture; of rather an unpleasant smell, and bitterish and slightly acrid taste. The scammony of Aleppo is by far the purest. That of Smyrna is ponderous, black, and mixed with extraneous matters. Scammony appears to have been well known to the Greek and Arabian physicians, and was exhibited internally as a purgative, and externally for the itch, tinea, fixed pains, &c. It is seldom given alone, but enters several compounds, which are administered as purgatives.

CONVOLVULUS SEPIUM. *Convolvulus major albus.* The juice of this plant, *Convolvulus—foliis sagittatis postice truncatis pedunculis tetragonis, unifloris,* of Linnæus, is violently purgative, and given in dropsical affections. A poultice of the herb, made with oil, is recommended in white swellings of the knee joint.

CONVOLVULUS SOLDANELLA. The systematic name of the sea convolvulus. Κραμβη θαλασσια. *Brassica marina; Convolvulus maritimus; Soldanella.* Soldanella. This plant, *Convolvulus—foliis reniformibus, pedunculis unifloris,* of Linnæus, is a native of our coasts. The leaves are said to be a drastic purge. It is only used by the common people, the pharmacopœias having now substituted more safe and valuable remedies in its place.

CONVOLVULUS SYRIACUS. The scammony plant. See *Convolvulus scammonia.*

CONVOLVULUS TURPETHUM. The systematic name of the turbith plant. *Turpethum.* The cortical part of the root of a species of convolvulus, brought from the East Indies, in oblong pieces: it is of a brown or ash colour on the outside, and whitish within. The best is ponderous, not wrinkled, easy to break, and discovers to the eye a large quantity of resinous matter. When chewed, it at first imparts a sweetish taste, which is followed by a nauseous acrimony. It is considered as a purgative liable to much irregularity of action.

CONVULSION. (*Convulsio;* from *convello,* to pull together.) *Hieranosos; Distentio nervorum; Syspacia convulsio* of Good. Clonic spasm. A diseased action of muscular fibres, known by alternate relaxations, with violent and involuntary contractions of the muscular parts, without sleep. Cullen arranges convulsion in the class *Neuroses,* and order *Spasmi.* Convulsions are universal or partial, and have obtained different names, according to the parts affected, or the symptoms; as the *risus sardonicus,* when the muscles of the face are affected; St. Vitus's dance, when the muscles of the arm are thrown into involuntary motions, with lameness and rotations. The hysterical epilepsy, or other epilepsies, arising from different causes, are convulsive diseases of the universal kind: the muscles of the globe of the eye, throwing the eye into involuntary distortions in defiance of the direction of the will, are instances of partial convulsion. The muscles principally affected in all species of convulsions, are those immediately under the direction of the will; as those of the eyelids, eye, face, jaws, neck, superior and inferior extremities. The muscles of respiration, acting both voluntarily and involuntarily, are not unfrequently convulsed; as the diaphragm, intercostals, &c. The more immediate causes of convulsions are, 1. Either mental affection, or any irritating cause exciting a greater action in the arterial system of the brain and nerves. 2. An increase of nervous energy, which seems to hold pace or be equipotent with the increased arterial energy excited in the brain. 3. This increased energy, conveying its augmented effects, without the direction of the will, to any muscles destined to voluntary motion, over-irritates them. 4. The muscles, irritated by the increased nervous energy and arterial influx, contract more forcibly and involuntarily by their excited vis insita, conjointly with other causes, as long as the increased nervous energy continues. 5. This increased energy in the nervous system may be excited either by the mind, or by any acrimony in the blood, or other stimuli sufficiently irritating to increase the arterial action, nervous influence, and the vires insitæ of muscles. 6. After muscles have been once accustomed to act involuntarily, and with increased action, the same causes can readily produce the same effects on those organs. 7. All parts that have muscular fibres may be convulsed. 8. The sensations in the mind most capable of producing convulsions, are timidity, horror, anger, great sensibility of the soul, &c.

CONVULSIO CANINA. A wry mouth.

CONVULSIO CEREALIS. Cereal convulsion is a singular disorder of the spasmodic convulsive kind, not common to this country, but mentioned by Cartheuser under this title, from the peculiar tingling and formication perceived in the arms and legs. *Motus spasmodicus* of Hoffman. It is endemial in some places in Germany; but more a rural than urbanical disorder, said to arise from the use of spoiled corn.

CONVULSIO HABITUALIS. Saint Vitus's dance. See *Chorea Sancti Viti.*

CONY'ZA. (From κονις, dust; because its powder is sprinkled to kill fleas in places where they are troublesome.) The name of a genus of plants in the Linnæan system. Class *Syngenesia;* Order, *Polygamia superflua.* There is some difficulty in ascertaining the plants called conyzas by the older practitioners: they are either of the genus conyza, inula, gnaphalium, erigeron, or chrysocoma.

CONYZA ÆTHIOPICA. The plant so called is most probably the *Chrysocoma comaurea* of Willdenow, a shrub which grows wild about the Cape of Good Hope, and is cultivated in our green-houses, because it flowers the greater part of the year.

CONYZA CŒRULEA. The *Erigeron acre* of Linnæus answers to the description of this plant.

CONYZA MAJOR. Supposed to be the *Inula viscosa* of Linnæus.

CONYZA MAJOR VULGARIS. See *Inula dysenterica*.

CONYZA MEDIA. See *Inula dysenterica*.

CONYZA MINOR. The *Inula pulicaris* of Linnæus answers to the description given of this plant in most books. Its chief use is to destroy fleas and gnats.

COOPERTO RIA. (From *co-operio*, to cover over.) The thyroid cartilage.

COO'STRUM. The centre of the diaphragm.

COPA'IBA. (*Copaiba*, *æ*. fœm.; from *copal*, the American name for any odoriferous gum, and *iba*, or *iva*, a tree.) The name given by the College of Physicians of London to the balsam of copaiva. See *Copaifera officinalis*.

COPAI'FERA. (From *Copaiva*, the Indian name, and *fero*, to bear.) The name of a genus of plants in the Linnæan system. Class, *Decandria*; Order, *Monogynia*.

COPAIFERA OFFICINALIS. The systematic name of the plant from which the Copaiba balsam, *Balsamum Braziliense; Balsamum. copaibæ; Balsamum de copaibu; Balsamum capivi*; Copaiba; Capevi; is obtained.

Copaiba is a yellow resinous juice, of a moderately agreeable smell, and a bitterish biting taste, very permanent on the tongue. The tree which affords it grows in Brazil, New-Spain. It is obtained by making deep incisions near its trunk, when the balsam immediately issues, and, at the proper season, flows in such abundance, that sometimes, in three hours, twelve pounds have been procured. The older trees afford the best balsam, and yield it two or three times in the same year. The balsam supplied by the young and vigorous trees, which abound with the most juice, is crude and watery, and is, therefore, accounted less valuable. While flowing from the tree, this balsam is a colourless fluid; in time, however, it acquires a yellowish tinge, and the consistence of oil; but, though by age it has been found thick, like honey, yet it never becomes solid, like other resinous fluids. By distillation in water, the oil is separated from the resin; and, in the former, the taste and smell of the balsam are concentrated. If the operation is carefully performed, about one-half of the balsam rises into the receiver, in the form of oil. The balsam unites with fixed and volatile oils, and with spirit of wine. It is given in all diseases of the urinary organs, when no inflammation is present. In gleets, and in gonorrhœa, it was once a favourite remedy, but is now disused. In diseases of the kidneys it is still employed, though less frequently than usual; and in hæmorrhoids it is occasionally trusted. The dose is from 20 to 30 drops, twice or three times a day, mixed with water, by means of an egg, or any mucilage. The balsam of copaiva is occasionally adulterated with turpentine, but its virtues are not greatly injured by the fraud.

COPAIVA. See *Copaiba*.

COPAL. (The American name of all clear odoriferous gums.) Gum copal. This resinous substance is imported from Guinea, where it is found in the sand on the shore. It is a hard, shining, transparent, citron-coloured, odoriferous, concrete juice of an American tree, but which has neither the solubility in water common to gums, nor the solubility in alkohol common to resins, at least in any considerable degree. By these properties it resembles amber. It may be dissolved by digestion in linseed oil, rendered drying by quicklime, with a heat very little less than sufficient to boil or decompose the oil. This solution, diluted with oil of turpentine, forms a beautiful transparent varnish, which, when properly applied, and slowly dried, is very hard, and very durable. This varnish is applied to snuff-boxes, tea-boards, and other utensils. It preserves and gives lustre to paintings, and greatly restores the decayed colours of old pictures, by filling up the cracks, and rendering the surfaces capable of reflecting light more uniformly.

COPE'LLA. See *Cupel*.

CO'PHER. A name for camphor.

CO'PHOS. (Κωφος, dumb.) Deaf or dumb. Also a dulness in any of the senses.

COPHO'SIS. (From κωφος, deaf.) A difficulty of hearing. It is often symptomatic of some disease. See *Dysecœa*.

COPPER. (*Cuprum*, *i*. neut. *quasi æs Cyprium*; so named from the island of Cyprus, whence it was formerly brought.) "A metal of a peculiar reddish brown colour; hard, sonorous, very malleable and ductile; of considerable tenacity, and of a specific gravity from 8.6 to 8 9. At a degree of heat far below ignition, the surface of a piece of polished copper becomes covered with various ranges of prismatic colours, the red of each order being nearest the end which has been most heated; an effect which must doubtless be attributed to oxidation, the stratum of oxide being thickest where the heat is greatest, and growing gradually thinner and thinner towards the colder part. A greater degree of heat oxidizes it more rapidly, so that it contracts thin powdery scales on its surface, which may easily be rubbed off; the flame of the fuel becoming at the same time of a beautiful bluish-green colour. In a heat, nearly the same as is necessary to melt gold or silver, it melts, and exhibits a bluish-green flame; by a violent heat it boils and is volatilized partly in the metallic state.

Copper rusts in the air; but the corroded part is very thin, and preserves the metal beneath from farther corrosion.

There are two oxides of copper:

1st, The black, procurable by heat, or by drying the hydratic oxide precipitated by potassa from the nitrate. It consists of 8 copper+2 oxygen. It is a *deutoxide*.

2dly, The *protoxide* is obtained by digesting a solution of muriate of copper with copper turnings, in a close phial. The colour passes from green to dark brown, and gray crystalline grains are deposited. The solution of these yields, by potassa, a precipitate of an orange colour, which is the protoxide. It consists of 8 copper +1 oxygen. Protoxyde of copper has been lately found by Mushet, in a mass of copper, which had been exposed to heat for a considerable time, in one of the melting furnaces of the mint under his superintendence.

Copper, in filings, or thin laminæ, introduced into chlorine, unites with flame into the chloride, of which there are two varieties; the protochloride, a fixed yellow substance, and the deutochloride, a yellowish-brown pulverulent sublimate.

1. The crystalline grains deposited from the above muriatic solution, are *protochloride*. The protochloride is conveniently made by heating together two parts of corrosive sublimate, and one of copper filings. An amber-coloured translucent substance, first discovered by Boyle, who called it resin of copper, is obtained. It is fusible at a heat just below redness; and in a close vessel, or a vessel with a narrow orifice, is not decomposed or sublimed by a strong red heat. But if air be admitted, it is dissipated in dense white fumes. It is insoluble in water. It effervesces in nitric acid. It dissolves silently in muriatic acid, from which it may be precipitated by water. By slow cooling of the fused mass, Dr. John Davy obtained it crystallized, apparently in small plates, semi-transparent, and of a light yellow colour. It consists, by the same ingenious chemist, of

Chlorine,	36	or 1 prime	=4.45	35.8
Copper,	64	or 1 prime	8.00	64.2
	100		12.45	100.0

2. *Deutochloride* is best made by slowly evaporating to dryness, at a temperature not much above 400° Fahr. the deliquescent muriate of copper. It is a yellow powder. By absorption of moisture from the air, it passes from yellow to white, and then green, reproducing common muriate. Heat converts it into protochloride, with the disengagement of chlorine. Dr. Davy ascertained the chemical constitution of both these compounds, by separating the copper with iron, and the chlorine by nitrate of silver. The deutochloride consists of

Chlorine,	53	2 primes	8.9	52.7
Copper,	47	1 do.	8.0	47.3
	100		16.9	100.0

The *iodide* of copper is formed by dropping aqueous hydriodate of potassa into a solution of any cupreous salt. It is an insoluble dark brown powder.

Phosphuret of copper is made by projecting phosphorus into red-hot copper.

Sulphuret of copper is formed by mixing together eight parts of copper filings, and two of sulphur, and exposing the mixture to a gentle heat.

The sulphuric acid, when concentrated and boiling, dissolves copper.

Nitric acid dissolves copper with great rapidity, and disengages a large quantity of nitrous gas. Part of the metal falls down in the form of an oxide; and the filtrated or decanted solution, which is of a much deeper blue colour than the sulphuric solution; affords crystals by slow evaporation. This salt is deliquescent, very soluble in water, but most plentifully when the fluid is heated.

The saline combinations of copper were formerly called *sales veneres*, because Venus was the mythological name of copper. They have the following general characters:

1. They are mostly soluble in water, and their solutions have a green or blue colour, or acquire one of these colours on exposure to air.

2. Ammonia added to the solutions, produces a deep blue colour.

3. Ferroprussiate of potassa gives a reddish-brown precipitate, with cupreous salts.

4. Gallic acid gives a brown precipitate.

5. Hydrosulphuret of potassa gives a black precipitate.

6. A plate of iron immersed in these solutions throws down metallic copper, and very rapidly if there be a slight excess of acid. The protoxide of copper can be combined with the acids only by very particular management. All the ordinary salts of copper have the peroxide for a base.

The joint agency of air and acetic acid, is necessary to the production of the cupreous *acetates*. By exposing copper plates to the vapours of vinegar, the bluish-green *verdigris* is formed, which, by solution in vinegar, constitutes *acetate of copper*.

Arseniate of copper presents us with many subspecies which are found native. The arseniate may be formed artificially by digesting arsenic acid on copper, or by adding arseniate of potassa to a cupreous saline solution.

Carbonate of copper. Of this compound there are three native varieties, the green, the blue, and the anhydrous.

Chlorate of copper is a deflagrating deliquescent green salt.

Fluate of copper is in small blue-coloured crystals.

Hydriodate of copper is a grayish-white powder.

Protomuriate of copper has already been described in treating of the chlorides.

Deutomuriate of copper, formed by dissolving the deutoxide in muriatic acid, or by heating muriatic acid on copper filings, yields by evaporation crystals of a grass-green colour.

The *ammonio-nitrate* evaporated, yields a fulminating copper. Crystals of nitrate, mixed with phosphorus, and struck with a hammer, detonate.

Subnitrate of copper is the blue precipitate, occasioned by adding a little potassa to the neutral nitric solution.

Nitrate of copper is formed by mixing nitrate of lead with sulphate of copper.

The *sulphate*, or blue vitriol of commerce, is a bisulphate.

A mixed solution of this sulphate and salammoniac, forms an ink, whose traces are invisible in the cold, but become yellow when heated; and vanish again as the paper cools.

Protosulphite of copper is formed by passing a current of sulphurous acid gas through the deutoxide of copper diffused in water. It is deprived of a part of its oxygen, and combines with the acid. The sulphate, simultaneously produced, dissolves in the water; while the sulphite forms small red crystals, from which merely long ebullition in water expels the acid.

Sulphite of potassa and copper is made by adding the sulphite of potassa to nitrate of copper. A yellow flocculent precipitate, consisting of minute crystals, falls.

Ammonia-sulphate of copper is the salt formed by adding water of ammonia to solution of the bisulphate. It consists, according to Berzelius, of 1 prime of the cupreous, and 1 of the ammoniacal sulphate, combined together; or 20.0+7.13+14.625 of water.

Subsulphate of ammonia and copper is formed by adding alkohol to the solution of the preceding salt, which precipitates the subsulphate. It is the *cuprum ammoniacum* of the pharmacopœia.

Sulphate of potassa and copper is formed by digesting bisulphate of potassa on the deutoxide or carbonate of copper.

The following acids, antimonic, antimonious, boracic, chromic, molybdic, phosphoric, tungstic, form insoluble salts with deutoxide of copper. The first two are green, the third is brown, the fourth and fifth green, and the sixth white. The benzoate is in green crystals, sparingly soluble. The oxalate is also green The binoxalates of potassa and soda, with oxide of copper, give triple salts, in green needle-form crystals. There are also ammonia-oxalates in different varieties. Tartrate of copper forms dark bluish-green crystals Cream-tartrate of copper is a bluish-green powder, commonly called Brunswick green.

To obtain pure copper for experiments, we precipitate it in the metallic state, by immersing a plate of iron in a solution of the deutomuriate. The pulverulent copper must be washed with dilute muriatic acid.

This metal combines very readily with *gold*, *silver*, and *mercury*. It unites imperfectly with *iron* in the way of fusion. *Tin* combines with copper, at a temperature much lower than is necessary to fuse the copper alone. On this is grounded the method of tinning copper vessels. For this purpose, they are first scraped or scoured; after which they are rubbed with sal-ammoniac. They are then heated, and sprinkled with powdered resin, which defends the clean surface of the copper from acquiring the slight film of oxide that would prevent the adhesion of the tin to its surface. The melted tin is then poured in, and spread about. An extremely small quantity adheres to the copper, which may perhaps be supposed insufficient to prevent the noxious effects of the copper as perfectly as might be wished.

When tin is melted with copper, it composes the compound called *bronze*.

Copper unites with *bismuth*, and forms a reddish-white alloy. With *arsenic* it forms a white brittle compound, called tombac. With *zinc* it forms the compound called brass, and distinguished by various other names, according to the proportions of the two ingredients.

Copper unites readily with antimony, and affords a compound of a beautiful violet colour. It does not readily unite with *manganese*. With *tungsten* it forms a dark brown spongy alloy, which is somewhat ductile.

Verdigris, and other preparations of copper, act as virulent poisons, when introduced in very small quantities into the stomachs of animals. A few grains are sufficient for this effect. Death is commonly preceded by very decided nervous disorders, such as convulsive movements, tetanus, general insensibility, or a palsy of the lower extremities. This event happens frequently so soon, that it could not be occasioned by inflammation or erosion of the *primæ viæ;* and indeed, where these parts are apparently sound. It is probable that the poison is absorbed, and, through the circulation, acts on the brain and nerves. The cupreous preparations are no doubt very acrid, and if death do not follow their immediate impression on the sentient system, they will certainly inflame the intestinal canal. The symptoms produced by a dangerous dose of copper are exactly similar to those which are enumerated under arsenic, only the taste of copper is strongly felt. The only chemical antidote to cupreous solutions, whose operation is well understood, is water strongly impregnated with sulphuretted hydrogen. The alkaline hydrosulphurets are acrid, and ought not to be prescribed.

But we possess, in sugar, an antidote to this poison, of undoubted efficacy, though its mode of action be obscure. Duval introduced into the stomach of a dog, by means of a caoutchouc tube, a solution in acetic acid, of four French drachms of oxide of copper. Some minutes afterward he injected into it four ounces of strong syrup. He repeated this injection every half-hour, and employed altogether 12 ounces of syrup. The animal experienced some tremblings and convulsive movements. But the last injection was followed by a perfect calm. The animal fell asleep, and awakened free from any ailment.

Orfila relates several cases of individuals who had by accident or intention swallowed poisonous doses of acetate of copper, and who recovered by getting large doses of sugar. He uniformly found, that a dose of verdigris which would kill a dog in the course of an hour or two, might be swallowed with impunity, provided it was mixed with a considerable quantity of sugar.

As alcohol has the power of completely neutralizing, in the æthers, the strongest muriatic and hydriodic acids, so it would appear that sugar can neutralize the oxides of copper and lead. The neutral saccharite of lead, indeed, was employed by Berzelius in his experiments, to determine the prime equivalent of sugar. If we boil for half an hour, in a flask, an ounce of white sugar, an ounce of water, and 10 grains of verdigris, we obtain a green liquid, which is not affected by the nicest tests of copper, such as ferroprussiate of potassa, ammonia, and the hydrosulphurets. An insoluble green carbonate of copper remains at the bottom of the flask."—*Ure's Chem. Dict.*

Copper, ammoniated solution of. See *Cupri ammoniati liquor.*

CO'PPERAS. A name given to blue, green, and white vitriol.

COPRAGO'GA. (From κοπρος, dung, and αγω, to bring away.) Purgatives. *Copragogum* is the name of a gently-purging electuary, mentioned by Rulandus.

COPRIE'MESIS. (From κοπρος, excrement, and εμεω, to vomit.) A vomiting of fæces.

COPROCRI'TICA. (From κοπρος, excrement, and κρινω, to separate.) Mild cathartic medicines.

COPROPHO'RIA. (From κοπρος, excrement, and φορεω, to bring away.) A purging.

CO'PROS. Κοπρος. The fæces, or excrements from the bowels.

COPROSTA'SIA. (From κοπρος, fæces, and ιϛημι, to remain.) Costiveness, or a constriction of the belly.

COPTA'RIOM. (Κοπ7η, a small cake.) *Coptarium.* A lozenge.

CO'PTE. (Κοπ7η, a small cake.) 1. The form of a medicine used by the ancients.

2. A cataplasm generally made of vegetable substances, and applied externally to the stomach, and on many occasions given internally.

["COPTIS TRIFOLIA. *Gold thread.* The *coptis trifolia*, which was arranged among the *Hellebores* by Linnæus, is a beautiful native, evergreen plant, of the northern States. Its roots are creeping, thread-shaped, and of a bright yellow colour. They have an intensely bitter taste, without warmth or astringency. Alcohol is the best *solvent* of this article, forming a bright yellow tincture. Water also extracts the bitterness, but less perfectly. Gold thread is a pleasant tonic, and promotes appetite and digestion. It is a popular remedy in apthous mouths and ulcers of the throat, though it does not appear to be very powerful in these complaints. As a tonic it may be given in the *dose* of ten or twenty grains of the powder. It is, however, somewhat difficult to pulverize, owing to the tenacity of the fibres. A tincture, formed by an ounce of the root in a pint of diluted alkohol, may be given in *doses* of a drachm."—*Big. Mat. Med.* A.]

CO'PULA. (*Quasi compula*; from *compello*, to restrain.) A name for a ligament.

COQUE'NTIA. (From *coquo*, to digest.) Medicines which promote concoction.

COR. (*Cor, dis.* neut.)

1. The heart. See *Heart.*

2. Gold.

3. An intense fire.

CORACI'NE. (From κοραξ, a crow; so named from its black colour.) A name for a lozenge, quoted by Galen from Asclepiades.

CORACO. The first part of the name of some muscles which are attached to the coracoid process of the blade-bone.

CORACO-BRACHIALIS. *Coraco-humeral* of Dumas. *Coraco-brachiæus.* A muscle, so called from its origin and insertion. It is situated on the humerus, before the scapula. It arises, tendinous and fleshy, from the forepart of the coracoid process of the scapula, adhering, in its descent, to the short head of the biceps; inserted, tendinous and fleshy, about the middle of the internal part of the os humeri, near the origin of the third head of the triceps, called *brachialis externus*, where it sends down a thin tendinous expansion to the internal condyle of the os humeri. Its use is to raise the arm upwards and forwards.

CORACO HYOIDEUS. See *Omo hyoideus.*

CO'RACOID. (*Coracoideus;* from κοραξ, a crow, and ειδος, resemblance: shaped like the beak of a crow.) Some processes of the bones are so named which were supposed to resemble the beak of a crow.

CORACOID PROCESS. *Processus coracoides.* See *Scapula.*

CO'RAL. See *Corallium.*

CORALLI'NA. (Diminutive of *corallium.*) *Muscus maritimus; Corallina officinalis; Corallina alba.* Sea coralline; Sea moss; White wormseed. A marine production, or fucus, resembling a small plant without leaves, consisting of numerous brittle cretaceous substances, friable betwixt the fingers, and crackling between the teeth. Powdered, it is administered to children as an anthelminthic, in the dose of half a drachm to a drachm once or twice a day.

CORALLINA CORSICANA. *Helmintho-corton; Conferva helmintho-cortos: Corallina rubra; Corallina melito-corton; Lemitho-corton; Mouse de Corse.* Corsican wormweed. *Fucus helmintho-corton* of De la Tourrette. This plant has gained great repute in destroying all species of intestinal worms. Its virtues are extolled by many; but impartial experimentalists have frequently been disappointed of its efficacy. The Geneva Pharmacopœia directs a syrup to be made of it.

CORALLINA MELITO-CORTON. See *Corallina corsicana.*

CORALLINA RUBRA. See *Corallina corsicana.*

CORALLINE. See *Corallina.*

Coralline, Corsican. See *Corallina corsicana.*

[CORALLINITE. See *Organic relics.*]

CORA'LLIUM. (*Corallium, i.* n.; from κορη, a daughter, and αλς, the sea, because it is the production of the sea.) Coral.

CORALLIUM ALBUM. A hard, white, calcareous brittle substance; the nidus of the *Madrepora oculata.* Class, *Vermes;* Order, *Lithophyta.* It is sometimes exhibited as an absorbent earth.

CORALLIUM RUBRUM. *Acmo. Azur.* The red coral is mostly employed medicinally. It is a hard, brittle, calcareous substance, resembling the stalk of a plant, and is the habitation of the *Isis nobilis.* Class, *Vermes;* Order, *Zoophyta.* When powdered, it is exhibited as an absorbent earth to children; but does not appear to claim any preference to common chalk.

CORALLODE'NDRON. (From κοραλλιον, coral, and δενδρον, a tree, resembling in hardness and colour a piece of coral.) The coral-tree of America; antivenereal.

CORALLOI'DES. (From κοραλλιον, coral, and ειδος, likeness.) Coral-like. See *Clavaria coralloides.*

CO'RCHORON. (From κορη, the pupil of the eye, and κορεω, to purge; so called because it was thought to purge away rheum from the eyes.) The herb pimpernel, or chickweed.

CORCULUM. (*Corculum*, a little heart; diminutive of *cor*, a heart.) An essential part of a germinating seed, called also the *embryo*, or germ. It lies between the cotyledons. It is the point from which the life and organization of the future plant originate. In some seeds it is much more conspicuous than in others. The walnut, bean, pea, and lupine show it in perfection. Its internal structure, before it begins to vegetate, is observed to be very simple, consisting of a uniformly medullary substance, enclosed in its appropriate bark or skin. Vessels are formed in it as soon as the vital principle is excited to action, and parts are then developed which seemed not previously to exist. There are observed in it,

1. The *rostellum*, or little beak, which penetrates into the earth and becomes the root.

2. The *plumula*, which shoots above the ground, and becomes a tuft of young leaves, with which the young stem, if there be any, ascends. See *Cotyledon.*

CO'RDA. See *Chorda.*

CORDA TYMPANI. See *Chorda tympani.*

CORDA WILLISII. See *Dura mater.*

CORDATUS. Heart-shaped. Applied to leaves, petals, &c. which are ovate, hollowed out at the base, according to the vulgar idea of a heart: a form very frequent in leaves; as in those of *Arctium lappa*, and

Tamus communis, and the petals of the *Sium Selinum*.

A leaf is called *obcordate*, when the apex of the heart-shaped leaf is fixed to the petiole.

CO'RDIA. (So called by Plumier in honour of Euricius Cordius and his son Valerius, two eminent German botanists.) The name of a genus of plants. Class, *Pentandria;* Order, *Monogynia.*

CORDIA MYXA. The systematic name of the Sebesten plant. *Sebesten; Sebestina; Cordia—foliis ovatis, supra glabris; corymbis lateralibus; calycibus decemstriatis* of Linnæus. The dark black fruit possesses glutinous and aperient qualities, and is exhibited in form of decoction in various diseases of the chest, hoarseness, cough, difficult respiration, &c.

CORDIAL. *Cardiacus.* Medicines are generally so termed, which possess warm and stimulating properties, and that are given to raise the spirits.

CORDINE'MA. (From καρα, the head, and δινεω, to move about.) A headache attended with a vertigo.

CORDO'LIUM. (From *cor*, the heart, and *dolor*, pain.) A name formerly applied to cardialgia, or heartburn.

CORDUS, VALERIUS, was born in 1515, of a Hessian family. After studying in some of the German universities, he travelled through Italy, chiefly engaged in botanical researches. He died at the early age of 29, leaving several works; a "History of Plants," many of them never before described; "Annotations on Dioscorides;" a Nuremberg Dispensatory, &c.

CO'RE. Κορη. The pupil of the eye.

CORE'MATA. (From κορεω, to cleanse.) Medicines for cleansing the skin.

CORIACEUS. Leathery. Applied to leaves and pods that are thick and tough without being pulpy, or succulent; as in the leaves of *Magnolia grandiflora, Aucuba*, &c. and the pods of the Lupin.

CORIANDER. See *Coriandrum.*

CORIA'NDRUM. (*Coriandrum, i.* n.; from κορη, a pupil, and ανηρ, a man: because of its roundness, like the pupil of a man's eye; or probably so called from κορις, *cimex*, a bug, because the green herb, seed and all, stinks intolerably of bugs.) Coriander.

1. The name of a genus of plants in the Linnean system. Class, *Pentandria;* Order, *Dygynia.*

2. The pharmacopœial name of the officinal coriander. See *Coriandrum sativum.*

CORIANDRUM SATIVUM. The systematic name of the plant called *coriandrum* in the pharmacopœias. *Cassibor; Corianon.* The *Coriandrum—fructibus globosis*, of Linnæus. This plant is a native of the South of Europe, where, in some places, it is said to grow in such abundance as frequently to choke the growth of wheat and other grain. From being cultivated here as a medicinal plant, it has for some time become naturalized to this country, where it is usually found in corn fields, the sides of roads, and about dunghills. Every part of the plant, when fresh, has a very offensive odour, but, upon being dried, the seeds have a tolerably grateful smell, and their taste is moderately warm and slightly pungent. They give out their virtue totally to rectified spirit, but only partially to water. In distillation with water, they yield a small quantity of a yellowish essential oil, which smells strongly and pretty agreeably of the coriander.

Dioscorides asserts, that the seeds, when taken in a considerable quantity, produce deleterious effects; and, in some parts of Spain and Egypt, where the fresh herb is eaten as a cordial, instances of fatuity, lethargy, &c. are observed to occur very frequently; but these qualities seem to have been unjustly ascribed to the coriander; and Dr. Withering informs us, that he has known six drachms of the seeds taken at once, without any remarkable effect. These seeds, and indeed most of those of the umbelliferous plants, possess a stomachic and carminative power. They are directed in the infusum amarum, the infusum sennæ tartarizatum, and some other compositions of the pharmacopœias; and according to Dr. Cullen, the principal use of these seeds is, "that infused along with senna, they more powerfully correct the odour and taste of this than any other aromatic that I have employed, and are, I believe, equally powerful in obviating the griping that senna is very ready to produce."

CORIA'NON. See *Coriandrum.*

CO'RIS. (From κειρω, to cleave, or cut; so called because it was said to heal wounds.) The herb St. John's wort. See *Hypericum.*

CORIS CRETICA. See *Hypericum Saxatile.*

CORIS LUTEA. See *Hypericum coris.*

CORIS MONSPELIENSIS. *Symphetumpœtreum.* Heath pine. This plant is intensely bitter and nauseous, but apparently, an active medicine, and employed, it is said, with success in syphilis.

CORK. *Suber.* The bark of the *Quercus suber* of Linnæus, formerly employed as an astringent, but now disused. By the action of nitric acid it is acidified. See *Suberic acid.*

Cork has been recently analyzed by Chevreuil by digestion, first in water and then in alkohol. By distillation there came over an aromatic principle, and a little acetic acid. The watery extract contained a yellow and a red colouring matter, an undetermined acid, gallic acid, an astringent substance, a substance containing azot, a substance soluble in water and insoluble in alkohol, gallate of iron, lime, and traces of magnesia. 20 parts of cork treated in this way, left 17.15 of insoluble matter. The undissolved residue being treated a sufficient number of times with alkohol, *yielded* a variety of bodies, but which seem reducible to three; namely, *cerin*, resin, and an oil. The ligneous portion of the cork still weighed 14 parts, which are called *suber.*

[CORK, when burnt and reduced to a black coal, may be pulverized and given as a medicine. It produces a light and delicate carbon, which may be given by the tea-spoonful, in a little syrup or milk, to children with cholera infantum or sour stomach. It is an excellent corrector of acidity, and is a useful domestic remedy for complaints of the bowels in children during warm weather. A.]

Cork, fossil. See *Asbestos.*

CORN. *Clavus.* A hardened portion of cuticle, produced by pressure: so called because a piece can be picked out like a corn of barley.

Corn salad. See *Valeriana locusta.*

CORNACHINI PULVIS. Scammony, antimony, and cream of tartar.

CORNARIUS, JOHN, was born in Upper Saxony, in the year 1500. According to Haller his real name was Haguenbot, or Hanbut. He is said to have been led to the study of medicine from the delicacy of his own constitution. He graduated at Padua, after attending several other universities. Besides translating Hippocrates, and some other Greek writers into Latin, he was author of several works on medicine; and is said to have had an extensive practice. He died in 1558, leaving a son, DIOMEDE, who succeeded him, and was afterward professor of medicine at Vienna, and physician to Maximilian II.

CORNARO, LEWIS, of a noble Venetian family, was born in 1467. Having impaired his constitution by a debauched and voluptuous life, and brought on at last a severe illness, on recovering from this, at the age of more than 40, he adopted a strict, abstemious regimen, limiting himself to twelve ounces of solid food, and fourteen of wine, daily; which quantity he rather diminished in the latter part of his life. He carefully avoided also the extremes of heat or cold, with all violent exercise; and took care to live in a pure dry air. He thus preserved a considerable share of health and activity to the great age of 98. His wife, by whom he had an only child, a daughter, when they were both advanced in years, survived him, and attained nearly the same period. When he was 83, he published a short treatise in commendation of temperance, which has been repeatedly translated, and printed in every country of Europe. He then states himself to have been able to mount his horse, without assistance, from any rising ground. He wrote three other discourses on similar subjects at subsequent periods, the last only three years before his death. The best English translation is said to be that of 1779.

CO'RNEA. The sclerotic membrane of the eye is so called, because it is of a horny consistence. See *Sclerotic coat.*

CORNEA OPACA. See *Sclerotic coat.*

CORNEA TRANSPARENS. *Sclerotica ceratoides.* The transparent portion of the sclerotic membrane, through which the rays of light pass, is so called, to distinguish it from that which is opaque. See *Sclerotic coat.*

["CORNEA TUNICA. (From *cornu*, a horn.) The an

terior transparent convex part of the eye, which, in texture, is tough like horn. It has a structure peculiar to itself, being composed of a number of concentric cellular lamellæ, in the cells of which is deposited a particular sort of fluid. It is covered externally by a continuation of the conjunctiva, which belongs to the class of mucous membranes; and it is lined by a membrane, the tunica humoris aquei, which seems to belong to the serous class."—*Cooper's Surg. Dict.* A.]

CORNE'STA. A chemical retort.

CORNFLOWER. See *Centaurea cyanus.*

CORNI'CULA. (From *cornu*, a horn.) A cupping instrument, made of horn.

CORNICULA'RIS. (From *cornu*, a horn.) Shaped like a horn; the coracoid process of the scapula.

CORNIFORMIS. (From *cornu*, a horn, and *forma* resemblance.) Horn-shaped: applied to the nectary of plants:—*nectarium corniforme*, in the orchis tribe.

CO'RNU. A horn. This term is used both in anatomy, surgery, and materia medica. 1. A wart. See *Verruca.*

2. A corn or horny induration of the cuticle. See *Corn.*

3. The horn of the stag.

4. The cavities of the brain.

CORNU AMMONIS. *Cornu arietis.* When the pes hippocampi of the human brain is cut transversely through, the cortical substance is so disposed as to resemble a ram's horn. This is the true cornu ammonis, though the name is often applied to the *pes hippocampi.*

[This name is also applied to the chambered shells found in a petrified state, and designated among the organic relics of another world as Ammonites. They are very abundant in Yorkshire, England, and have been found in some places in this country. A.]

CORNU ARIETIS. See *Cornu ammonis.*

CORNU CERVI. Hartshorn. The horns of several species of stag, as the *Cervus alces*, *Cervus dama*, *Cervus elaphus*, and *Cervus taranda*, are used medicinally. Boiled, they impart to the water a nutritious jelly, which is frequently served at table. Hartshorn jelly is made thus:—Boil half a pound of the shavings of hartshorn, in six pints of water, to a quart; to the strained liquor add one ounce of the juice of lemon, or of Seville orange, four ounces of mountain wine and half a pound of sugar; then boil the whole to a proper consistence. The chief use of the horns is for calcination, and to afford the *liquor volatilis cornu cervi* and subcarbonate of ammonia.

CORNU CERVI CALCINATUM. See *Cornu ustum.*

CORNU USTUM. *Cornu cervi calcinatum.* Burn pieces of hartshorn in an open fire, till they become thoroughly white; then powder, and prepare them in the same manner as is directed for chalk. Burnt hartshorn shavings possess absorbent, antacid, and adstringent properties, and are given in the form of decoction, as a common drink in diarrhœas, pyrosis, &c.

CORNUA UTERI. *Plectenæ.* In comparative anatomy, the horns of the womb; the womb being in some animals triangular, and its angles resembling horns.

CORNUMU'SA. A retort.

CO'RNUS. 1. The name of a genus of plants in the Linnæan system. Class, *Tetrandria;* Order, *Monogynia.*

2. The pharmacopœial name of the cornel-tree. See *Cornus sanguinea.*

["CORNUS FLORIDA. *Dogwood.* This is a small native tree, well known for its ornamental flowers in most parts of the country, but more particularly in the middle and southern states. The bark of the trunk is rough externally, and of a brownish colour within. Its taste is a strong bitter, with some astringent and aromatic flavour. It appears to contain a bitter extractive substance, tannin, gallic acid, and a small portion of resin. This bark has been much employed as a tonic in various parts of the interior country. It is particularly used in intermittent fevers, and is applied to various other cases of debility, in which tonics are indicated. When fresh, it is sometimes liable to disorder the stomach and bowels, which tendency it is thought to lose by age. It may be given in powder in doses of one or two scruples. Although this species has been most attended to, there are several others of the same genus, which, from their bitterness, promise quite as much efficacy"—*Big. Mat. Med.* A.]

["CORNUS CIRCINATA. *Round-leafed dogwood.* This species of dogwood is a native shrub, distinguished from others of its genus by its round leaves and beautifully spotted twigs. The bark is not exceeded by any other in bitterness, and unites with this property the chemical and sensible evidences of astringency. It is highly valuable as a tonic and stomachic, and appears to be largely in use in some parts of the United States, particularly in Connecticut, where it is employed as a substitute for cinchona, and has become an officinal article. It is exhibited in the same way as *Cornus florida.*"—*Big. Mat. Med.* A.]

["CORNUS SERICEA. *Swamp dogwood.* This is another of the bitter *cornels*, native in the United States. Its properties resemble the preceding so much, that it is unnecessary to repeat them. Indeed, the genus *Cornus* in the northern hemisphere, like *Cinchona* in the southern, appears to have the same medical character pervading all its species, differing only in degree."—*Big. Mat. Med.* A.]

CORNUS SANGUINEA. The fruit is moderately cooling and astringent.

CORNU'TA. (From *cornu;* from its resemblance to a horn.) A retort.

COROLLA. (From *coronula*, a little crown.) The leaves of a flower which consist of those more delicate and dilated, generally more coloured leaves, which are always internal with respect to the calyx, between it and the internal organs of the flower, and which constitute its chief beauty. It always consists of one or more coloured leaves, which are termed *petals.*

A coloured calyx is to be distinguished from a corolla, which may be readily done in the *Allyssum alpestre*, and *Lamium orvala.*

There are four general divisions of corols.

1. *Monopetalous*, which consists of one petal, as in *Nicotiana tabacum.*

2. *Polypetalous*, having many; as in *Lillium candidum.*

3. *Compound*, consisting of many corolla, which are not calyculated, and are on a common receptacle, and calyx; as in *Helianthus annuus.*

4. *Aggregate*, consisting of many calyculated corolla placed on a common calyx; as in *Scabiosa arvensis*, and *Echinops spærocephalus.*

A. *Corolla monopetala*, formed of one petal, which, for the most part, forms a cavity, and is divided into,

a. *Limbus*, the limb, which is the margin, or horizontal spreading portion.

b. *Tubus*, the tube, which is the cylindrical and inferior part, and is enclosed in the calyx.

c. *Fauces*, or the orifice of the tube.

From the figure of a regular or uniform limb are derived the following terms:

1. *Corolla campanulata*, bell-shaped; as in *Campanula* and *Atropa.*

2. *C. globosa*, globular; as in *Hyacynthus botryoides* and *Erica ramentacea.*

3. *C. Tubulosa*, tubular, as in *Primula* and *Erica Massoni.*

4. *C. claviculata;* as in *Erica tubiflora.*

5. *C. cyathiformis*, cup-shaped; as in *Sympathum officinale.*

6. *C. infundibuliformis*, funnel-shaped; as in *Nicotiana tabacum*, and *Datura stramonium.*

7. *C. hypocrateriformis*, salver-shaped, a flat limb upon a long tube; as in *Vinca rosea.*

8. *C. rotata:* wheel-shaped, that is, salver-shaped, with scarcely any tube; as in *Borago-officinalis*, and *Physalis alkekengi.*

9. *C. urceolata*, saucer-like; as in *Evolvulus alcinoides.*

10. *C. contorta*, obliquely bent; as in *Vinca minor* and *Nerium oleander.*

11. *C. ligulata*, the tube very short, and ending suddenly in an oblong petal; as in the corolla of the radius of the *Helianthus annuus.*

From the figure of an *unequal limb:*

1. *Corolla ringens*, irregular and gaping like the mouth of an animal; as in *Lamium album*, and *Salvia sclarea.*

2. *C. personata*, irregular and closed by a kind of palate; as in *Antirrhinum majus.*

In the ringent and personate corollæ are to be noticed the following parts:

a. *Tubus*, the inferior part.

b. *Rictus*, the space between the two lips.

c. *Faux*, the orifice of the tube in the rectus.

d. *Galea*, the helmet or superior arched lip.
e. *Labellum* or *barba*, the inferior lip.
f. *Palatum*, the palate, an eminence in the inferior lip which shuts the rictus of a personate corolla.
g. *Calcar*, the spur which forms an obtuse or acute bag at the side of the receptacle.
3. *C. bilabiata*, two-lipped, the tube divided into two irregular lips opposite each other, without any visible rictus; as in *Aristolochia bilabiata.*
In the bilabiate corolla are to be noticed,
a. The *tubus*.
b. The *faux*.
c. The *superior lip*, formed of one or two lobes.
d. The *inferior lip*, mostly three-lobed.
e. *One-lipped*, the upper or lower wanting, as in *Aristolochia clematitis*, and *Teucrium*.
Corolla infera, means that it is below the germen, which is the most common place of the corolla; and *corolla supera*, above the germen, as in roses.
B. *Corolla polypetala*, formed of many petals.
In the petal of this division are noticed,
a The *unguis*, the claw, the thin inferior part.
b The *lamina* or border, the broader and superior part; example, *Dianthus caryophyllis*.
From the *number* of *uniform* petals, the corol of this division is named,
1 *Dipetalous;* as in *Euphorbia graminea.*
2. *Tripetalous:* as in *Tradescantia virginica.*
3. *Tetrapetalous;* as in *Chieranthus incanus.*
4. *Pentapetalous;* as in *Pæonia officinalis.*
5. *Hexapetalous;* as in *Lilium candidum.*
6. *Polypetalous;* as in *Rosa centifolia.*
From the *figure*,
1. *Malvaceous;* pentapetalous, with its claws united laterally, so that it appears monopetalous; as in *Malva sylvestris*, and *Alcea*.
2. *Rosaceous*, spreading like a rose, pentapetalous, almost destitute of claws; as in *Rosa canina*, and *Pæonia officinalis.*
3. *Liliaceous;* six-petalled, sometimes three without a calyx; as in *Lilium candidum.*
4. *Caryophyllaceous:* five-petalled, with a long claw, spreading border, and a monophyllous tubular calyx; as in *Dianthus caryophyllus*, and *Saponaria officinalis.*
5. *Cruciform;* three-petalled, like a cross; as in *Sinapis alba*, and *Lunaria alba.*
6. *Manifold*, many corols lying one on another; as in *Cactus flagelliformis.*
From the *figure* of *unequal petals:*
1. *Orchideal*, five petals, three of which are bent backward, and two are lateral and in the middle of these: the labellum is bent back on the nectary.
2. *Papilionaceous*, four petals, irregular and spreading, somewhat like a butterfly; as in *Lathyrus latifolius*, and *Robinii pseudacacia.*
In a *papilionaceous* corolla, observe,
a. The *vexillum*, the standard or large concave one at the bark.
b. *Alæ*, the wings or two side-petals, placed in the middle.
c. The *carina*, or keel, consisting of two petals, united or separate, embracing the internal organs.
3. *Calcarate* or spurred, pentapetalous, one petal formed into a spur-like tube.
C. *Compound corolla;* consisting of numerous florets, not calyculate, and within a common perianthium.
It affords,
a. The *discus*, disk, or middle.
b. The *radius*, which forms the circumference. The marginal white florets of the daisy exemplify the rays, and the central yellow ones the disk.
From the difference in the florets of a compound flower it is said to be,
a. *Tubulate*, when all the florets are cylindrical.
b. *Ligulate* or *semiflosculose*, shaped like a strap or riband; as in *Leontodon taraxacum.*
c. *Radiate*, if the florets in the radius are ligulate, and those in the disk tubular.
d. *Semiradiate*, the radius consisting of only a few ligulate florets on one side; as in *Bidens*. See also *Petala.*

COROLLULA (A diminutive of *corolla*, a little wreath or crown.) The partial petal, or floret of a compound flower.

CORO'NA A crown. This term is used in anatomy to designate the basis of some parts; and in botany, to parts of plants, from their resemblance. In the writings of some botanists, it is synonymous with *radius.*

CORONA CILIARIS. The ciliar ligament.

CORONA GLANDIS. The margin of the glans penis.

CORONA IMPERIALIS. A name for crown-imperial The Turks use it as an emetic. The whole plant is poisonous.

CORONA REGIA. The melilotus.

CORONA SOLIS. See *Helianthus annuus.*

CORONA VENERIS. Venereal blotches on the forehead are so termed.

CORONAL. (*Coronalis;* from *corona*, a crown or garland.) Belonging to a crown or garland: so named because the ancients wore their garlands in its direction.

CORONAL SUTURE. *Sutura coronalis; Sutura arcualis.* The suture of the head, that extends from one temple across to the other, uniting the two parietal bones with the frontal.

CORONA'RIUS. See *Coronary.*

CORONARIÆ. The name of an order of plants in Linnæus's Fragments of a Natural Method, consisting of such as have beautiful flowers, thus forming a floral crown.

CORONARY. (*Coronarius;* from *corona*, a crown.) This term is applied to vessels and nerves, which supply the corona or basis of parts, or because they spread round the part like a garland or crown.

CORONARY LIGAMENTS. (From *corona*, a crown.) Ligaments uniting the radius and ulna. The term ligamentum coronarium is also applied to a ligament of the liver.

CORONARY VESSELS. *Vasa coronaria.* The arteries and veins of the heart and stomach.

CORONATUS. Little crown-like eminences on the surface of the petal; or in *Nerium oleander.*

CORONATI. *Coronaticus.* The name of a class of plants in Linnæus's Fragments of a Natural Method, consisting of plants which have the seed-bud placed under the flower-cup which serves it for a crown.

CORO'NE. (Κορωνη, a crow: so named from its supposed likeness to a crow's bill.) The acute process of the lower jaw-bone.

CORONOID. (*Coronoideus;* from κορωνη, a crow, and ειδος, likeness. Processes of bones are so called, that have any resemblance to a crow's beak; as coronoid process of the ulna, jaw, &c.

CORONO'PUS. (From κορωνη, a carrion crow, and πoυ, a foot; the plant being said to resemble a crow's foot.) See *Plantago.*

CORONULA. The hem or border which surrounds the seeds of some flowers in the form of a crown.

CO'RPUS. 1. The body. See *Body.*
2. Many parts and substances are also distinguished by this name: as *corpus callosum*, *corpus luteum*, &c.

CORPUS ALBICANS. Two white eminences in the basis of the brain, discovered by Willis, and called *corpora albicanta Willisii.*

CORPUS ANNULARE. A synonyme of the pons Varolii. See *Pons Varolii.*

CORPUS CALLOSUM. *Commissura magna cerebri.* The white medullary part joining the two hemispheres of the brain, and coming into view under the falx of the dura mater when the hemispheres are drawn from each other. On the surface of the *corpus callosum* two lines are conspicuous, called the *raphe.*

CORPUS CAVERNOSUS CLITORIDIS. See *Clitoris.*

CORPUS CAVERNOSUS PENIS. See *Penis.*

CORPUS FIMBRIATUM. The flattened terminations of the posterior crura of the fornix of the brain, which turn round into the inferior cavity of the lateral ventricle, and end in the *pedes hippocampi.*

CORPUS GLANDULOSUM. The prostate gland.

CORPUS LOBOSUM. Part of the cortical part of the kidney.

CORPUS LUTEUM. A yellow spot found in that part of the ovarium of females, from whence an ovum has proceeded; hence their presence determines that the female has been impregnated. The number of the *corpora lutea* corresponds with the number of impregnations. It is, however, asserted by a modern writer, that *corpora lutea* have been detected in young virgins, where no impregnations could possibly have taken place.

CORPUS MUCOSUM. See *Rete mucosum.*

Corpus nerveo-spongiosum. The cavernous substance of the penis.

Corpus nervosum. The cavernous substance of the clitoris.

Corpus olivare. Two external prominences of the medulla oblongata, shaped somewhat like an olive, are called corpora olivaria.

Corpus pampiniforme. Applied to the spermatic chord and thoracic duct; also to the plexus of veins surrounding the spermatic artery in the cavity of the adbomen.

Corpus pyramidale. Two internal prominences of the medulla oblongata, which are of a pyramidal shape, are called corpora pyramidalia.

Corpus quadrigeminum. See *Tubercula quadrigemina.*

Corpus reticulare. See *Rete mucosum.*

Corpus sesamoideum. A little prominence at the entry of the pulmonary artery.

Corpus spongiosum urethræ. *Substantia spongiosa urethræ. Corpus spongiosum penis.* This substance originates before the prostate gland, surrounds the urethra, and forms the *bulb;* then proceeds to the end of the corpora cavernosa, and terminates in the *glans penis*, which it forms.

Corpus striatum. So named from its appearance. See *Cerebrum.*

Corpus varicosum. The spermatic chord.

Corra'go. (From *cor*, the heart; it being supposed to have a good effect in comforting the heart.) See *Borago officinalis.*

Co'rre. (From κειρω, to shave.) The temples. That part of the jaws where the beard grows, and which it is usual to shave.

CORROBORANT. (*Corroborans.*) Whatever gives strength to the body; as bark, wine, beef, cold-bath, &c. See *Tonic.*

CORROSIVE. (*Corrosivus; from corrodo*, to eat away.) See *Escharotic.*

Corrosive sublimate. The oxymuriate of mercury. See *Hydrargyri oxymurias.*

CORRUGA'TOR. (From *corrugo*, to wrinkle.) The name of muscles, the office of which is to wrinkle or corrugate the parts they act on.

Corrugator supercilii. A small muscle situated on the forehead. *Musculus supercilii* of Winslow; *Musculus frontalis verus, seu corrugator coiterii* of Douglas; and *Cutanio sourcillier* of Dumas. When one muscle acts, it is drawn towards the other, and projects over the inner canthus of the eye. When both muscles act, they pull down the skin of the forehead, and make it wrinkle, particularly between the eyebrows.

CO'RTEX. (*Cortex, icis.* m. or f.) This term is generally, though improperly, given to the Peruvian bark. It applies to any rind, or bark.

Cortex angelinæ. The bark of a tree growing in Grenada. A decoction of it is recommended as a vermifuge. It excites tormina, similar to jalap, and operates by purging.

Cortex angusturæ. See *Cusparia.*

Cortex antiscorbuticus. The canella alba. See *Winteria aromatica.*

Cortex aromaticus. See *Winteria aromatica.*

Cortex bela-aye. See *Nerium antidysentericum.*

Cortex canellæ malabaricæ. See *Laurus cassia.*

Cortex cardinalis de lugo. The Peruvian bark: so called, because the Cardinal Lugo had testimonials of above a thousand cures performed by it in the year 1653.

Cortex cerebri. The cortical substance of the brain. See *Cerebrum.*

Cortex chinæ regius. See *Cinchona.*

Cortex chinæ surinamensis. This bark is remarkably bitter, and preferable to the other species in intermittent fevers.

Cortex chinchinæ. See *Cinchona.*

Cortex elutheriæ. See *Croton cascarilla.*

Cortex geoffroyæ jamaicensis. See *Geoffroya jamaicensis.*

Cortex jamaicensis. See *Acras sapota.*

Cortex lavola. The bark bearing this name is supposed to be the produce of the tree which affords the *Anisum stellatum* Its virtues are similar.

Cortex magellanicus. See *Winteria aromatica.*

Cortex massoy. The produce of New Guinea, where it is beaten into a pultaceous mass with water, and rubbed upon the abdomen to allay pain of the bowels. It has the smell and flavour of cinnamon.

Cortex patrum. See *Cinchona.*

Cortex peruvianus. See *Cinchona.*

Cortex peruvianus flavus. See *Cinchona.*

Cortex peruvianus ruber. See *Cinchona.*

Cortex pocgerebæ. A bark sent from America; said to be serviceable in diarrhœas, and dysenteries.

Cortex quassiæ. See *Quassia amara.*

Cortex winterianus. See *Winteria aromatica*

CO'RTICAL. *Corticalis.* 1. Belonging to the bark of a plant or tree.

2. Embracing or surrounding any part like the bark of a tree; as the cortical substance of the brain, kidney, &c.

CORTICO'SUS. Like bark or rind. Applied to the hard pod of the *Cassia fistularis.*

Cortu'sa. See *Sanicula europæa.*

Co'ru canarica. A quince-like tree of Malabar; it is antidysenteric.

CORUNDUM. A genus of minerals, which, according to Jameson, contains three species; the octohedral, rhomboidal, and prismatic.

CORYDALES. (From κορυς, a helmet.) The name of an order of plants in Linnæus's Fragments of a Natural Method, consisting of plants which have flowers somewhat resembling a helmet or hood.

CO'RYLUS. (Derivation uncertain: according to some, from καρυα, a walnut.) 1. The name of a genus of plants in the Linnæan system. Class, *Monœcia;* Order, *Polyandria.*

2. The pharmacopœial name of the hazel-tree. See *Corylus avellana.*

Corylus avellana. The hazel-nut tree. The nuts of this tree are much eaten in this country; they are hard of digestion, and often pass the bowels very little altered; if, however, they are well chewed, they give out a nutritious oil. An oil is also obtained from the wood of this tree, *Corylus avellana stipulis ovatis, obtusis*, of Linnæus; which is efficacious against the toothache, and is said to kill worms.

CORYMBIFERÆ. (From *corymbus;* a species of florescence, and *fero*, to bear.) Plants which bear corymbal flowers.

CORYMBUS. (Κορυμβον, or κορυμβος, a branch or cluster crowning the summit of a plant; from κορυς, a helmet.) A corymb. That species of inflorescence formed by many flowers, the partial flower-stalks of which are gradually longer, as they stand lower on the common stalk, so that all the flowers are nearly on a level; as in the *Crysanthemum corymbosum.* It is said to be *simple*, when not divided into branches; as in *Thlaspi arvense*, and *Gnaphalium dentatum:* and *compound*, when it has branches; as in *Gnaphalium stæchas.*

Co'ryphe. Κορυφη. The vertex of the head.—*Galen.*

CORY'ZA. (Κορυζα; from καρα, the head, and ζεω, to boil.) An increased discharge of mucus from the nose. See *Catarrh.* Dr. Good makes this a genus of disease; running at the nose. It has two species, *Coryza entonica*, and *atonica.*

Coscu'lia. The grains of kermes.

COSME'TIC. *Cosmeticus.* A term applied to remedies against blotches and freckles.

Co'smos. A regular series. In Hippocrates it is the order and series of critical days.

Co'ssis. A little tubercle in the face, like the head of a worm.

Co'ssum. A malignant ulcer of the nose, mentioned by Paracelsus.

COSTA. A rib. 1. The rib of an animal. See *Ribs.*

2. The thick middle nerve-like cord of a leaf, which proceeds from its base to the apex. See *Leaf.*

Costa herba. The *Hypochœris radicata.*

COSTALIS. (From *costa*, a rib.) Belonging to a rib: applied to muscles, arteries, nerves, &c.

Costa pulmonaria. Very probably the *Hypochæris radicata*, or long-rooted hawk-weed, which was used in pulmonary affections, and pains of the side.

COSTA'TUS. Ribbed. Applied to leaves, and is synonymous with *nervous:* the leaf having simple lines extended from the base to the point. See *Leaf.*

Costo-hyoideus. A muscle, so named from its origin and insertion. See *Omohyoideus.*

COSTUS. (From *kasta*, Arabian.) The name of a genus of plants in the Linnæan system. Class, *Monandria;* Order, *Monogynia.*

Costus amarus. See *Costus arabicus.*

Costus arabicus. The systematic name of the *Costus indicus; amarus; dulcis; orientalis.* Sweet and bitter costus. The root of this tree possesses bitter and aromatic virtues, and is considered as a good stomachic. Formerly there were two other species, the *bitter* and *sweet*, distinguished for use. At present, the Arabic only is known, and that is seldom employed. It is, however, said to be stomachic, diaphoretic, and diuretic

Costus corticosus. The canella alba.

Costus hortorum minor. The *Achillæa ageratum.*

Costus nigra. The artichoke.

Cotaro'nium. A word coined by Paracelsus, implying a liquor into which all bodies, and even their elements, may be dissolved.

Co'tis. (From κοτ]η, the head.) The back part of the head; sometimes the hollow of the neck.

CO'TULA. (*Cotula*, diminutive of *cos*, a whetstone, from the resemblance of its leaves to a whetstone; or from κο]υλη, a hollow.) Stinking chamomile.

["Cotula. *Mayweed.* The *anthemis cotula* is an annual weed imported from Europe, and now very common by road sides throughout the United States. Its taste is strong, disagreeable, and bitter. In small quantities it is tonic, stimulating, and diaphoretic; in large ones emetic and sudorific. It is commonly given in infusion."—*Big. Mat. Med.* A.]

CO'TULE. (Κοτυλη, the name of an old measure.) The socket of the hipbone. See *Acetabulum.*

Cottula fœtida. See *Anthemis cotula.*

COTYLEDON. (*Cotyledon, onis.* f.; from κοτυλη, a cavity.) Seed-lobe, or cotyledon. The *cotyledones* are the two halves of a seed, which, when germinating, become two pulpy leaves, called the *seminal leaves.* These leaves are often of a different *form* from those which are about to appear; as in the *Raphanus sativus;* and sometimes they are of another *colour;* as in *Cannabis sativa*, the seminal leaves of which are white.

Almost all the cotyledons wither and fall off, as the plant grows up.

These bodies are spoken of in the plural, because it it is much doubted whether any plant can be said to have a solitary cotyledon, so that most plants are *dicotyledonous.* Plants without any, are called *acotyledones.* Those with more than two, *polycotyledonous.*

Between the two cotyledons of the germinating seed, is seated the *embryo*, or germ of the plant, called by Linnæus, *corculum*, or little heart, in allusion to the heart of the walnut. Mr. Knight denominates it the germen: but that term is appropriated to a very different part, the rudiment of the fruit. The expanding embryo, resembling a little feather, has, for that reason, been called by Linnæus, *plumula:* it soon becomes a tuft of young leaves, with which the young stem ascends. See *Corculum.*

COTYLOID. (*Cotyloides;* from κοτυλη, the name of an old measure, and ειδος, resemblance.) Resembling the old measure, or *cotule.*

Cotyloid cavity. The acetabulum. See *Innominatum os.*

COTYLOI'DES.—See *Cotyloid.*

COUCHING. A surgical operation that consists in removing the opaque lens out of the axis of vision, by means of a needle constructed for the purpose.

Couch-grass. See *Triticum repens.*

COUGH. *Tussis.* A sonorous concussion of the thorax, produced by the sudden expulsion of the air from the chest through the fauces. See *Catarrh.*

Co'um. The meadow-saffron.

COUNTER-OPENING. *Contra-apertura.* An opening made in any part of an abscess opposite to one already in it. This is often done in order to afford a readier egress to the collected pus.

Coup de soleil. The French for an erysipelas or apoplexy, or any affection produced instantaneously from a scorching sun.

Cou'rap. (Indian.) The provincial name of a disease of the skin common in Java, and other parts of the East Indies, accompanied by a perpetual itching and discharge of matter.

Cou'rbaril. The tree which produces the gum anime See *Anime.*

Couro'ndi. An evergreen tree of India, said to be antidysenteric.

Couroy moelli. A shrub of India, said to be antivenomous.

Cou'scous. An African food, much used about the river Senegal. It is a composition of the flour of millet, with some flesh, and what is there called lalo.

Covola'm. See *Cratæva marmelos.*

COWHAGE. See *Dolichos pruriens.*

COW-ITCH. See *Dolichos pruriens.*

COWPER, William, was born about the middle of the 17th century, and became distinguished as a surgeon and anatomist in this metropolis. His first work, entitled "Myotomia Reformata," in 1694, far excelled any which preceded it on that subject in correctness, though since surpassed by Albinus. Three years after, he published at Oxford "the Anatomy of Human Bodies," with splendid plates, chiefly from Bidloo; but forty of the figures were from drawings made by himself; he added also some ingenious and useful anatomical and surgical observations. Having been accused of plagiarism by Bidloo, he wrote an apology, called "Eucharistia;" preceded by a description of some glands, near the neck of the bladder, which have been called by his name. He was also author of several communications to the Royal Society, and some observations inserted in the anthropologia of Drake. He died in 1710.

Cowper's glands. (*Cowperi glandulæ;* named from Cowper, who first described them.) Three large muciparous glands of the male, two of which are situated before the prostate gland under the accelerator muscles of the urine, and the third more forward, before the bulb of the urethra. They excrete a fluid, similar to that of the prostate gland, during the venereal orgasm.

Cowpe'ri glandulæ. See *Cowper's glands.*

CO'XA. The ischium is sometimes so called, and sometimes the os coccygis.

COXE'NDIX. (From *coxa*, the hip.) The ischium; the hip-joint.

Crablouse. A species of pediculus which infests the axillæ and pudenda.

[The crab-louse is not a pediculus, but belongs to the genus of *acarus.* If the parts infested by them be washed with an infusion of tobacco, it will soon kill these vermin. A.]

Crab-yaws. A name in Jamaica for a kind of ulcer on the soles of the feet, with callous lips, so hard that it is difficult to cut them.

["CRAIK, James, M.D. Dr. Craik was born in Scotland, where he received his education for the medical service of the British army. He came to the colony of Virginia in early life, and had the honour to accompany the youthful Washington in his expedition against the French and Indians in 1754, and returned in safety after the battle of the Meadows, and surrender of Fort Necessity. In 1755, he attended Braddock in his march through the wilderness, and on the 9th of July, assisted in dressing the wounds of that brave, but unfortunate commander. At the close of the French war, the subject of this article resumed and continued his professional labours till the commencement of the Revolution in 1775. By the aid of his early and fast friend, General Washington, he was transferred to the Medical Department in the Continental army, and rose to the first rank and distinction. In 1777, he had an opportunity, which he gladly embraced, to show his fidelity to his General, and to his adopted country, by taking an active part in the developement of a nefarious conspiracy, the object of which was the removal of the commander in chief. In 1780, he was deputed to visit Count de Rochambeau, then recently arrived at Rhode-Island, and to make arrangements for the establishment of Hospitals to accommodate the French army. Having performed this difficult duty, he continued in the army to the end of the war, and was present at the surrender of Cornwallis, on the memorable 19th October, 1781.

After the cessation of hostilities, the Doctor settled as a physician in Charles County, in Maryland, but soon removed to the neighbourhood of his illustrious friend and companion, the farmer of Mount Vernon, at his particular, repeated, and urgent request. In 1798, when, like a guardian angel, the never to be for gotten Washington again stepped forth to redress the wrongs of his country; the venerable Craik was once more appointed to his former station in the medical staff. With the disbandment of the army, then called into service, ceased the public professional labours of the subject of this memoir, whose life, for nearly half a century, has been devoted with zeal and high reputation to the cause of his country.

One trying duty yet remained to be performed; it was to witness the closing scene, and to receive the last sigh of his revered commander, the most distinguished man of his age. Their youthful commissions had been signed on the same day; they had served together in the ranks of war; their friendship was cemented by a social intercourse of fifty years' continuance, and they were greatly endeared to each other by common toils, privations, and honours. At length the moment of parting arrived; it was tender, affectionate, solemn, and impressive. In reference to that painful event, the Doctor is said to have expressed himself in this manner: "I, who was bred amid scenes of human calamity, who had so often witnessed death in its direst and most awful forms, believed that its terrors were too familiar to my eye to shake my fortitude; but when I saw this great man die, it seemed as if the bonds of my nature were rent asunder, and that the pillar of my country's happiness had fallen to the ground."

As a physician, Dr. Craik was greatly distinguished by his skill and success, and his professional merits were highly and justly appreciated. In the various relations of private life, his character was truly estimable, and his memory is precious to all who had the happiness and the honour of his acquaintance. He was one, and what a proud eulogy it is, of whom the immortal Washington was pleased to write, "my compatriot in arms, my old and intimate friend." He departed this life at the place of his residence in Fairfax county, on the 6th February, 1814, in the 84th year of his age."—*Thach. Med. Biog.* A.]

CRA'MBE. (Κραμβη, the name given by Dioscorides, Galen, and others, to the cabbage; the derivation is uncertain.) The name of a genus of plants in the Linnæan system. Class, *Tetradynamia;* Order, *Siliculosa.* Cabbage.

Crambe maritima. The systematic name for the sea-cole, or sea-kale. A delicious vegetable when forced and blanched. It is brought to table about Christmas, has a delicate flavour, and is much esteemed. Like to all oleraceous plants, it is flatulent and watery.

CRAMP. (From *krempen*, to contract. Germ.) See *Spasm.*

CRANESBILL. See *Geranium.*

Cranesbill, bloody. See *Geranium sanguineum.*

CRA'NIUM. (Κρανιον, *quasi* καρανιον; from καρα, the head.) The skull or superior part of the head. See *Caput.*

Crante'res. (From κραινω, to perform.) A name given to the dentes sapientiæ and other molares, from their office of masticating the food.

CRA'PULA. (Κραιπυλα.) A surfeit; drunkenness.

CRA'SIS. (From κεραννυμι, to mix.) Mixture. A term applied to the humours of the body, when there is such an admixture of their principles as to constitute a healthy state: hence, in dropsies, scurvy, &c. the crasis, or healthy mixture of the principles of the blood, is said to be destroyed.

Cra'spedon. (Κρασπεδον, the hem of a garment; from κρεμαω, to hang down, and πεδον, the ground.) A relaxation of the uvula, when it hangs down in a thin, long membrane, like the hem of a garment.

CRASSAME'NTUM. (From *crassus*, thick.) See *Blood.*

CRA'SSULA. (From *crassus*, thick: so named from the thickness of its leaves.) See *Sedum telephium.*

CRATÆ'GUS. (From κρατος, strength: so called from the strength and hardness of its wood.) The wild service-tree, of which there are many, are all species of the genus *Prunus.* The fruits are most of them astringent.

CRATEVA. (So called from Cratevas, a Greek physician, celebrated by Hippocrates for his knowledge of plants.) The name of a genus of plants. Class, *Polyandria;* Order, *Monogynia.*

Crateva marmelos. The fruit is astringent while unripe; but when ripe, of a delicious taste. The bark of the tree strengthens the stomach, and relieves hypochondriac languors.

Crati'cula. (From *crates*, a hurdle.) The bars or grate which covers the ash-hole in a chemical furnace.

CRATON, John, called also Craftheim, was born at Breslaw in 1519. He was intended for the church, but preferring the study of medicine, went to graduate at Padua, and then settled at Breslaw. But after a few years he was called to Vienna, and made physician and aulic counsellor to the Emperor Ferdinand I.: which offices also he held under the two succeeding emperors, and died in 1585. His works were numerous: the principal are, "A Commentary on Syphilis;" "A Treatise on Contagious Fever;" another on "Therapeutics;" and seven volumes of Epistles and Consultations.

Cream of tartar. See *Potassæ supertartras.*

CREMA'STER. (From κρεμαω, to suspend.) A muscle of the testicle, by which it is suspended, and drawn up and compressed, in the act of coition. It arises from Poupart's ligament, passes over the spermatic chord, and is lost in the cellular membrane of the scrotum, covering the testicles.

Cre'mnus. (From κρημνος, a precipice, or shelving place.) 1. The lip of an ulcer.

2. The labium pudendi.

CRE'MOR. 1. Cream. The oily part of milk which rises to the surface of that liquid, mixed with a little curd and serum. When churned, butter is obtained. See *Milk.*

2. Any substance floating on the top, and skimmed off.

CRENATUS. Crenate or notched, applied to a leaf or petal, when the indentations are blunted or rounded, and not directed toward either end of the leaf; as in *Glecoma hederacea.* The two British species of *Salvia* are examples of doubly crenate leaves The petals of the *Linum usitatissimum* are crenate.

CRE'PITUS. (From *crepo*, to make a noise.) A puff or little noise. The word is generally employed to express the pothognamonic symptoms of air being collected in the cellular membrane of the body; for when air is in these cavities, and the part is pressed, a little cracking noise, or crepitus, is heard.

Crepitus lupi. See *Lycoperdon bovista.*

Crescent-shaped. See *Leaf.*

CRESS. There are several kinds of cresses eaten at the table, and used medicinally, as antiscorbutics.

Cress, water. See *Sisymbrium nasturtium aquaticum.*

CRE'TA. Chalk. An impure carbonate of lime. See *Creta præparata.*

Creta præparate. Take of chalk a pound; add a little water, and rub it to a fine powder. Throw this into a large vessel full of water; then shake them, and after a little while pour the still turbid liquor into another vessel, and set it by that the powder may subside; lastly, pouring off the water, dry this powder Prepared chalk is absorbent, and possesses antacid qualities: it is exhibited in form of electuary, mixture, or bolus, in pyrosis, cardialgia, diarrhœa, acidities of the primæ viæ, rachitis, crusta lactea, &c. and is said by some to be an antidote against white arsenic.

Cretaceous acid. See *Carbonic acid.*

Crete, dittany of. See *Origanum dictamnus.*

CRETINISMUS. Cretinism. A species of *Cyrtosis* in Dr. Good's Nosology: a disease affecting chiefly the head and neck; countenance vacant and stupid; mental faculties feeble, or idiotic; sensibility obtuse, mostly with enlargement of the thyroid gland.

CRIBRIFO'RM. (*Cribriformis;* from *cribrum*, a sieve, and *forma*, likeness; because it is perforated like a sieve.) Perforated like a sieve. See *Ethmoid bone.*

CRICHTONITE. A mineral named after Dr. Crichton, which Jameson thinks is a new species of titanium ore. It is of a splendent velvet black colour.

CRI'CO. Names compounded of this word belong to muscles which are attached to the cricoid cartilage.

Crico-arytænoideus lateralis. *Crico-lateri arithenoidien* of Dumas. A muscle of the glottis, that opens the *rima* by pulling the ligaments from each other.

Crico-arytænoideus posticus. *Crico-creti ari thenoidien* of Dumas. A muscle of the glottis, that opens the *rima glottidis* a little, and by pulling back the arytænoid cartilage, stretches the ligament so as to make it tense.

CRICO-PHARYNGEUS. See *Constrictor pharyngis inferior*.

CRICO-THYROIDEUS. *Crico-thyroidien* of Dumas. The last of the second layer of muscles between the os hyoides and trunk, that pulls forward and depresses the thyroid cartilage, or elevates and draws backwards the cricoid cartilage.

CRICOI'D. (*Cricoides;* from κρικος, a ring, and ειδος, resemblance.) A round ring-like cartilage of the larynx is called the cricoid. See *Larynx*.

CRIMNO'DES. (From κριμνον, bran.) A term applied to urine, which deposites a sediment like bran.

CRINA'TUS. (From κρινον, the lily.) A term given to a suffumigation mentioned by P. Ægineta, composed chiefly of the roots of lilies.

CRI'NIS. The hair. See *Capillus*.

CRINOMY'RON. (From κρινον, a lily, and μυρον, ointment.) An ointment composed chiefly of lilies.

CRINONES. (From *crinis*, the hair.) *Malis gordii* of Good. *Morbus pilaris* of Horst. *Malis à crinonibus* of Elmuller and Sauvages. Collections of a sebaceous fluid in the cutaneous follicles upon the face and breast, which appear like black spots, and when pressed out, look like small worms, or, as they are commonly called, maggots.

CRIO'GENES. An epithet for certain troches, mentioned by P. Ægineta, and which he commends for cleansing ulcers.

CRIPSO'RCHIS. (From κρυπτω, to conceal, and ορχις, a testicle.) Having the testicle concealed, or not yet descended from the abdomen into the scrotum.

CRI'SIS. (From κρινω, to judge.) The judgment. The change of symptoms in acute diseases, from which the recovery or death is prognosticated or judged of.

CRISPATU'RA. (From *crispo*, to curl.) A spasmodic contraction or curling of the membranes and fibres.

CRISPUS. Curled. Applied to a leaf, when the border is so much more dilated than the disk, that it necessarily becomes curled and twisted; as in *Malva crispa*, &c.

CRI'STA. (*Quasi cerista;* from κερας, a horn, or *carista;* from καρα, the head, as being on the top of the head.) Any thing which has the appearance of a crest, or the comb upon the head of a cock. 1. In anatomy it is thus applied to a process of the ethmoid bone, *christa galli*, and to a part of the *nymphæ;*—*crista clitoridis*.

2. In surgery, to excrescences, like the comb of a cock, about the anus.

3. In botany, to several accessary parts or appendages, chiefly belonging to the antheræ of plants; as the pod of the *Hedysarum crista galli*, &c.

CRISTA GALLI. An eminence of the ethmoid bone, so called from its resemblance to a cock's comb. See *Ethmoid bone*.

CRISTATUS. Crested. Applied to several parts of plants.

CRI'THAMUM. See *Crithmum*.

CRI'THE. (Κριθη, barley.) A stye or tumour on the eyelid, in the shape and of the size of a barley-corn.

CRITHE'RION. (From κρινω, to judge.) The same as crisis.

CRI'THMUM. (From κρινω, to secrete; so named from its supposed virtues in promoting a discharge of the urine and menses.) Samphire or sea-fennel.

CRITHMUM MARITIMUM. The Linnæan name of the samphire or sea-fennel. *Crithmum* of the pharmacopœias. It is a low perennial plant, and grows about the sea-coast in several parts of the island. It has a spicy aromatic flavour, which induces the common people to use it as a pot-herb. Pickled with vinegar and spice, it makes a wholesome and elegant condiment, which is in much esteem.

CRITHO'DES. (From κριθη, barley, and ειδος, resemblance.) Resembling a barley-corn. It is applied to small protuberances.

CRI'TICAL. (*Criticus;* from *crisis;* from κεινω, to judge.) Determining the event of a disease. Many physicians have been of opinion, that there is something in the nature of fevers which generally determines them to be of a certain duration; and, therefore, that their terminations, whether salutary or fatal, happen at certain periods of the disease, rather than at others. These periods, which were carefully marked by Hippocrates, are called *critical days*. The critical days, or those on which we suppose the termination of continued fevers especially to happen, are the third, fifth, seventh, ninth, eleventh, fourteenth, seventeenth, and twentieth.

CROCIDI'XIS. (From κροκιδιζω, to gather wool.) Floccilation. A fatal symptom in some diseases, where the patient gathers up the bed-clothes, and seems to pick up substances from them.

CRO'CINUM. (From κροκος, saffron.) A mixture of oil, myrrh, and saffron.

CROCO'DES. (From κροκος, saffron; so called from the quantity of saffron they contain.) A name of some old troches.

CROCOMA'GMA. (From κροκος, saffron, and μαγμα, the thick oil or dregs.) A troch made of oil of saffron and spices.

CRO'CUS. (Κροκος of Theophrastus. The story of the young Crocus, turned into this flower, may be seen in the fourth book of Ovid's Metamorphoses Some derive this name from κροκη or κροκις, a thread; whence the stamens of flowers are called κροκιδες Others, again, derive it from *Coriscus*, a city and mountain of Cilicia, and others from *crokin*, Chald.) Saffron.

1. The name of a genus of plants in the Linnæan system. Class, *Triandria:* Order, *Monogynia*. Saffron.

2. The pharmacopœial name of the prepared stigmata of the saffron plant. See *Crocus sativus*.

3. A term given by the older chemists to several preparations of metallic substances, from their resemblance: thus, *Crocus martis*, *Crocus veneris*.

CROCUS ANTIMONII. A sulphuretted oxide of antimony.

CROCUS GERMANICUS. See *Carthamus*.

CROCUS INDICUS. See *Curcuma*.

CROCUS MARTIS. Burnt green vitriol.

CROCUS METALLORUM. A sulphuretted oxide of antimony.

CROCUS OFFICINALIS. See *Crocus sativus*.

CROCUS SARACENICUS. See *Carthamus*.

CROCUS SATIVUS. The systematic name of the saffron plant. *Crocus:—spatha univalvi radicali, corollæ tubo longissimo*, of Linnæus. Saffron has a powerful, penetrating, diffusive smell, and a warm, pungent, bitterish taste. Many virtues were formerly attributed to this medicine, but little confidence is now placed in it. The Edinburgh College directs a tincture, and that of London a syrup of this drug.

CROCUS VENERIS. Copper calcined to a red powder.

CRO'MMYON. (Παρα το τας κορας μυειν, because it makes the eyes wink.) An onion.

CROMMYOXYRE'GMA. (From κρομμυον, an onion, οξυς, acid, and ρηγνυμι, to break out.) An acid eructation accompanied with a taste resembling onions.

CROONE, WILLIAM, was born in London, where he settled as a physician, after studying at Cambridge. In 1659, he was chosen rhetoric professor of Gresham College, and soon after register of the Royal Society, which then assembled there. In 1662, he was created doctor in medicine by mandate of the king, and the same year elected fellow of the Royal Society, and of the College of Physicians. In 1670, he was appointed lecturer on anatomy to the Company of Surgeons. On his death, in 1684, he bequeathed them 100*l.*; his books on Medicine to the College of Physicians, as also the profits of a house, for Lectures, to be read annually, on Muscular Motion; and donations to seven of the colleges at Cambridge, to found Mathematical Lectures. He left several papers on philosophical subjects, but his only publication was a small tract, "De Ratione Motus Musculorum."

CROSS-STONE. Harmotome; Pyramidal zeolite. A crystallized grayish-white mineral, harder than fluor-spar, but not so hard as apatite, found only in mineral veins and agate balls in the Hartz, Norway, and Scotland.

CROTALUS. The name of a genus of reptiles.

CROTALUS HORRIDUS. The rattle-snake; the stone out of the head of which is erroneously said to be an antidote to the poison of venomous animals. A name also of the Cobra de capella, the *Coluber naja* of Linnæus.

Crotaphica arteria. The tendon of the temporal muscle.

CROTAPHI'TES. (From κροταφος, the temple.) See *Temporalis.*

Crota'phium. (From κροτεω, to pulsate; so named from the pulsation which in the temples is eminently discernible.) *Crotaphos. Crotaphus.* A pain in the temples.

Cro'taphos. See *Crotaphium.*

Cro'taphus. See *Crotaphium.*

CROTCHET. A curved instrument with a sharp hook to extract the fœtus.

CRO'TON. (From κροτεω, to beat.)

1. An insect called a tick, from the noise it makes by beating its head against wood.

2. A name of the ricinus or castor-oil berry, from its likeness to a tick.

3. The name of a genus of plants in the Linnæan system. Class, *Monœcia;* Order, *Monadelphia.*

Croton benzoe. See *Styrax benzoe.*

Croton cascarilla. The systematic name of the plant which affords the Cascarilla bark. *Cascarilla; Chocarilla; Elutheria; Eluteria.* The bark comes to us in quills, covered upon the outside with a rough, whitish matter, and brownish on the inner side, exhibiting, when broken, a smooth, close, blackish-brown surface. It has a light agreeable smell, and a moderately bitter taste, accompanied with a considerable aromatic warmth. It is a very excellent tonic, adstringent, and stomachic, and is deserving of a more general use than it has hitherto met with.

Croton lacciferum. The systematic name of the plant upon which gum-lac is deposited. See *Lacca.*

Croton tiglium. The systematic name of the tree which affords the pavana wood, and tiglia seeds. *Croton—foliis ovatis glabris acuminatis serratis, caule arboreo* of Linnæus.

1. Pavana wood. *Lignum pavanæ; Lignum pavanum; Lignum moluccense.* The wood is of a light spongy texture, white within, but covered with a grayish bark: and possesses a pungent, caustic taste, and a disagreeable smell. It is said to be useful as a purgative in hydropical complaints.

2. *Grana tiglia. Grana tilli. Grana tiglii.* The grana tiglia are seeds of a dark gray colour, in shape very like the seed of the *ricinus communis.* They abound with an oil which is far more purgative than castor-oil, which has been lately imported from the East Indies, where it has been long used, and is now admitted into the London pharmacopœia. One drop proves a drastic purge, but it may be so managed as to become a valuable addition to the materia medica.

[The oil of Croton is the produce of a shrub or arborescent plant well known to botanists, and the oil when taken into the stomach acts as a powerful cathartic. The shrub belongs to the Class *Monœcia,* and Order, *Monadelphia,* of Linnæus's sexual system.

Persoon enumerates 82 species of this genus of plants. The specific character of the Tilgium is, that "The leaves are ovate, smooth, acuminated, serrated, and the stem arborescent." It is a native of the East Indies, China, and other Australasian islands. Ceylon, and the Moluccas are particularly quoted as affording this species of Croton. It is also well known in Amboyna and Batavia, and, indeed, generally through the distant east. Several parts of the plant possess medicinal virtue.

1. *Radix,* the root, or pulvis radicis croti. The powdered root of Croton is a drastic cathartic, when exhibited in the small quantity of even a few grains, on which account it has been considered by the Asiatics as a grand remedy for dropsy, upon the same principle by which the operation of scammony and gamboge is explained.

2. *The Wood* of the Croton. Lignum croti tiglii. This is also efficacious, for in small doses it acts as a sudorific, by relaxing the pores of the skin; while in large ones it purges severely.

3. *The Leaves.* Folia croti tiglii. Pulvis foliorum tiglii siccatorum. The dried leaves when powdered are reputed an antidote against the bite of that formidable and venomous serpent the Copra de Capello.

4. *The Seeds.* Semina vel grana croti tiglii. They are the part of the plant most known and employed in medicine. They are of a date at least as old as the age of Serapion, one of the earliest physicians of Arabia who wrote on the Materia Medica, and he flourished about 1000 years ago, or probably in the 8th century. When they were introduced into Europe long since, they were known by the name of "*Molucca grains or seeds,* and as the grains or seeds of Tilium or Tiglium.

It appears that they were freely administered, not merely for the purpose as a cathartic, but for the accomplishment of mischievous and deleterious ends. It is even stated by the accomplished Rumphius, the Dutch physician and botanist, that a dose of *four grains* had been administered for the working of destruction by women who wished to kill their husbands. Though the seeds were freely administered at that age and after, the extreme violence of their operation seems to have induced a very unfavourable opinion of them. This no doubt arose from injudicious doses; as, under similar circumstances, the digitalis purpurea, or purple fox-glove, had undergone a similar fate. It had been frequently administered, and was even popular, but from the bad consequences of injudicious prescription, was condemned as noxious, and was neglected as unfit for use. So, cubebs (amomum cubeba) were once in use, then discontinued from a supposed want of power, and latterly revived and rendered fashionable. It nevertheless appears, that molucca grains are still used in the East Indies as an effectual cathartic.

5. *The baked Seeds.* Semina tosta vel furno cocta. The baked or roasted seeds of the Croton Tiglium. By these operations the shell or hull was removed, the seed rendered capable of being powdered, and, according to Ainslie's Materia Medica of Hindostan, the acrimonious and vehement qualities very much moderated.

The medicinal history of this plant seems to have rested a long time. At length, however, as the seeds were replete with oil, it occurred to somebody to express it, and this oil was known to the celebrated pharmacians, Lemery and Geoffroy. Yet it lay dormant, until a revival was made by Mr. E. Conwell, of the English East India Company's service on the Madras Establishment. Having prescribed the Croton oil for many years with advantage, he sent a parcel of it to London for experiment.

6. *The Oil of Tiglium,* or oil of Croton. Oleum, croti tiglii expressum. The oil has a yellowish hue, but a faint smell, and an acrimonious taste. Though these qualities have some variation, caused probably by the degree of heat, or torrefaction, employed in the process for obtaining it.

7. *Gustus olei tiglii.* Touching the tongue with the oil. It is reported, that in some constitutions the mere application of a particle to the tongue, is sufficient to produce a cathartic effect, thereby evincing an extraordinary power of sympathy between the organ of taste and the alimentary canal. There are, however, very striking analogies to illustrate its action. Tobacco, for example, in the form of a segar, applied to the mouth of some persons, moves the intestines to evacuation. A drop of the Prussic acid applied to the mouth of a rat causes instant death. The poison of a rattlesnake, as witnessed by Dr. Mitchill, infused in a wound, destroys the life of a rat, or other small animal in an exceedingly short time. It is reported, that a man who had been in the habit of using enemas, had been brought to a stool by the sight of a clysterpipe.

8. *Pills of the Oil of Tiglium.* Pillulæ olei tiglii. A single drop, or at most two, is a sufficient dose. A safe method is to take the pills, to contain each one drop, with a crumb of bread; or, for more expeditious practice, the prescriber may prepare them containing two drops. He can thus administer with an assurance that the laxative effect will be produced without the fear of exciting any alarming commotion. In cases where there is an aversion to taking medicines, and where the bulk and repetition of the doses are objectionable, this remedy therefore possesses advantages which highly recommend it. The quantity of even half a drop, or in other words half a grain, will frequently move the intestines to discharge; and the effect, which is generally speedy, more resembles that of the saline cathartics than the other drastics, such as elaterium, gamboge, and scammony.

9. *Tincture of the Oil of Tiglium.* Solutio olei

tiglii in alcohol. Chemistry has proved that this oil is composed of two principal constituent parts: 1. *A fixed oil*, resembling that of the olive, destitute of cathartic qualities; and, 2. *An acrid purgative principle*, in which its virtue resides. The proportions are stated by Dr. Nimmo thus,

Fixed oil,............ 55 parts.
Acrid principle,...... 45 do.
———
100

The latter has been denominated *Tiglin*, in the modern nomenclature. Alkohol is capable of decomposing this native oil; the tiglin being dissolved with a minute quantity only of the fixed oil, and the rest of it left uncombined. This discovery enables us to form a tincture upon a well-ascertained principle. It is accordingly proposed to form the tincture, by adding *two drops of the oil* (as it comes to us) *to a fluid drachm of rectified spirit*. After digesting long enough to secure the union between the spirit and the tiglin, the tincture must be filtered. Yet, as a fluid so volatile as the spirit will suffer some loss by evaporation, it is calculated that half a fluid drachm of the tincture is equal to a drop and an half of the oil. It is found that the alkohol does not impair the cathartic power of the *tiglin*. This solution may therefore be exactly apportioned to the nature of the disorder, and the wish of the physician, and thus be regulated with the greatest exactness. If taken in quantity corresponding to the number of drops decomposed, experience has decided that the same effects were produced as by the same quantity of undecompounded and entire oil.

An article so expensive as this in comparison with other fixed oils, holds out a strong temptation for fraud by adulteration. This has been practised to a considerable extent by mixing it with the cheaper kinds. A method, however, has been proposed for detecting such vitiation by Dr. Nimmo, by means of alkonol, a phial, a balance, and an evaporating process, of which an abstract will be found in the Pharmacologia of Dr. Paris, vol. 2, p. 338. New-York edit. by Dr. Ives. This writer's opinion is, on the whole matter, "that this oil does not appear to produce any effects which cannot be commanded by other drastic purgatives. Its value depends upon the facility with which it may be administered.—*Notes from Dr. Mitchill's Lectures on Mat. Med.* A.]

Croton tinctorium. The systematic name of the lacmus plant. *Croton—foliis rhombeis repandis, capsulis pendulis, caule herbaceo*, of Linnæus. *Bezetta cærulea.* This plant yields the *Succus heliotropii; Lacmus seu tornæ; Lacca cærulea; Litmus.* It is much used by chemists as a test.

Crotu'ne. (From κροτον, the tick.) A fungus on trees produced by an insect like a tick; and by metaphor applied to tumours and small fungous excrescences on the periosteum.

Crotopus. (From κροτος, *pulsus*.) Painful pulsation.

Crotophium. (From κροτος, the pulse.) Painful pulsation.

CROUP. See *Synanche.*

Crousis. (From κρουω, to beat, or pulsate.) Pulsation.

Crou'smata. (From κρουω, to pulsate.) Rheums or defluxions from the head.

CROWFOOT. See *Ranunculus.*

Crowfoot-cranesbill. See *Geranium pratense.*

CRUCIAL. (*Crucialis; from crus*, the leg.) 1. Cross-like. Some parts of the body are so called when they cross one another, as the crucial ligaments of the thigh.

2. A name of the mugweed or crosswort.

CRUCIA'LIS. See *Crucial.*

CRUCIBLE. (*Crucibulum;* from *crucio*, to torment: so named, because, in the language of old chemists, metals are tormented in it, and tortured, to yield up their powers and virtues.) A chemical vessel made mostly of earth to bear the greatest heat. They are of various shapes and composition.

CRUCIFORMIS. Cross-like. Applied to leaves, flowers, &c. which have that shape.

CRU'DITAS. (From *crudus*, raw.) It is applied to undigested substances in the stomach, and formerly to humours in the body unprepared for concoction.

CRUICKSHANK, William, was born at Edinburgh, in 1746. He was intended for the church, and made great proficiency in classical learning; but showing a partiality to medicine, he was placed with a surgeon at Glasgow. In 1771, he came to London, and was soon after made librarian to Dr. William Hunter; and, on the secession of Mr. Hewson, became assistant, and then joint lecturer in anatomy, with the Doctor. He contributed largely to enrich the Museum, particularly by his curious injections of the lymphatic vessels. He published, in 1786, a work on this subject, which is highly valued for its correctness. In 1795, he communicated to the Royal Society an Account of the Regeneration of the Nerves; and the same year published a pamphlet on Insensible Perspiration; and in 1797, an Account of Appearances in the Ovaria of Rabbits in different Stages of Pregnancy. He died in 1800.

Cru'nion. (From κρουνος, a torrent.) A medicine mentioned by Aëtius, and named from the violence of its operations as a diuretic.

CRU'OR. (From κρυος, *frigus*, it being that which appears like a coagulum as the blood cools.) The red part of the blood. See *Blood.*

CRU'RA. The plural of *crus.*

Crura clitoridis. See *Clitoris.*

Crura medullæ oblongatæ. The roots of the medulla oblongata.

CRURÆ'US. (From *crus*, a leg; so named, because it covers almost the whole foreside of the upper part of the leg or thigh.) *Cruralis.* A muscle of the leg, situated on the forepart of the thigh. It arises, fleshy, from between the two trochanters of the os femoris, but nearer the lesser, firmly adhering to most of the forepart of the os femoris; and is inserted, tendinous, into the upper part of the patella, behind the rectus. Its use is to assist the vasti and rectus muscles in the extension of the leg.

CRURAL. (*Cruralis;* from crus, the leg.) Belonging to the crus, leg, or lower extremity.

Crural hernia. See *Hernia cruralis.*

CRURA'LIS. See *Cruræus.*

CRUS. 1. The leg.

2. The root or origin of some parts of the body, from their resemblance to a leg or root; as *Crura cerebri, Crura cerebelli; Crura* of the diaphragm, &c.

CRU'STA. 1. A shell.

2. A scab.

3. The scum or surface of a fluid.

Crusta lactea. A disease that mostly attacks some part of the face of infants at the breast. It is known by an eruption of broad pustules, full of a glutinous liquor, which form white scabs when they are ruptured. It is cured by mineral alteratives.

Crusta villosa. The inner coat of the stomach and intestines has been so called.

Crustula. (Dim. of *crusta*, a shell.) A discoloration of the flesh from a bruise, where the skin is entire, and covers it over like a shell.

Crustumina'tum. (From *Crustuminum*, a town where they grew.) 1. A kind of Catherine pear.

2. A rob or electuary made of this pear and apples boiled up with honey.

Crymo'des. (From κρυος, cold.) An epithet for a fever, wherein the external parts are cold.

CRYOLITE. A white or yellowish brown mineral, composed of alumina, soda, and fluoric acid. It is curious and rare, and found hitherto only at West Greenland.

CRYOPHORUS. (From κρυος, cold, and φερω, to bear.) The frost-bearer, or carrier of cold; an elegant instrument invented by Dr. Wollaston, to demonstrate the relation between evaporation at low temperatures, and the production of cold.

CRYPSO'RCHIS. (From κρυπτω, to conceal, and ορχις, a testicle.) A term applied to a man whose testicles are hid in the belly, or have not descended into the scrotum.

CRY'PTA. (From κρυπτω, to hide.) The little rounded appearances at the end of the small arteries of the cortical substance of the kidneys, that appear as if formed by the artery being convoluted upon itself.

CRYPTOGAMIA. (From κρυπτω, to conceal, and γαμος, a marriage.) The twenty-fourth and last class of the sexual or Linnæan system of plants, containing several numerous genera, in which the parts essential to their fructification have not been sufficiently ascertained to admit of their being referred to the other class. It is divided by Linnæus into four orders, *Filices*, *Musci*, *Algæ*, and *Fungi*.

Cryso'rchis. Κρυσορχις. 1. A retraction or retrocession of one of the testicles.

2. See *Crypsorchis*.

CRYSTAL. See *Crystallus*.

CRYSTALLINE. (*Crystallinus*; from its crystal-like appearance.) Crystal-like.

Crystalline lens. A lentiform pellucid part of the eye, enclosed in a membranous capsule, called the capsule of the crystalline lens, and situated in a peculiar depression in the anterior part of the vitreous humour. Its use is to transmit and refract the rays of light. See *Eye*.

Crystalli'num (From κρυςαλλος, a crystal: so called from its transparency.) White arsenic.

CRYSTALLIZATION. (*Crystallizatio*; from *crystallus*, a crystal.) A property by which crystallizable bodies tend to assume a regular form, when placed in circumstances favourable to that particular disposition of their particles. Almost all minerals possess this property, but it is most eminent in saline substances. The circumstances which are favourable to the crystallization of salts, and without which it cannot take place, are two: 1. Their particles must be divided and separated by a fluid, in order that the corresponding faces of those particles may meet and unite. 2. In order that this union may take place, the fluid which separates the integrant parts of the salt must be gradually carried off. so that it may no longer divide them.

["*Crystallization*, in the most limited extent of the term, is that process by which the particles of bodies unite in such a manner as to produce determinate and regular solids. But it is equally true, that those minerals, which possess a foliated or fibrous structure, are the products of crystallization, under circumstances which have rendered the process more or less imperfect, and prevented the appearance of distinct and regular forms.

The ancients believed crystallized quartz (rock crystal) to be water, congealed by exposure to intense cold; and accordingly applied to it the term κρυςαλλος, which signified ice. Hence the etymology of the word crystal. Now, as a beautiful regularity of form is one of the most striking properties of crystallized quartz, the name crystal has been extended to all mineral and other inorganic substances, which exhibit themselves under the form of regular geometrical solids.

A crystal may therefore be defined an inorganic body, which, by the operation of affinity, has assumed the form of a regular solid, terminated by a number of plane and polished faces. The corresponding faces of all crystals, which possess the same variety of form, and belong to the same substance, are inclined to each other in angles of a constant quantity. This constancy of angles remains, even in those cases where the faces themselves, from some accidental causes, have changed their dimensions or number of sides. Transparency, though many crystals possess it in a greater or less degree, is not a necessary property. But plane surfaces, bounded by right lines, are so essential to the crystalline form, that their absence decidedly indicates imperfection in the process of crystallization. The lustre and smoothness of the faces may also be diminished by accidental causes."—*Cleav. Min.* A.]

CRYSTA'LLUS. (*Crystallus*, *i.* m.; from κρυος, cold, and ςελλω, to contract: *i. e.* contracted by cold into ice.) A crystal. "When fluid substances are suffered to pass with adequate slowness to the solid state, the attractive forces frequently arrange their ultimate particles, so as to form regular polyhedral figures or geometrical solids, to which the name of crystals has been given. Most of the solids which compose the mineral crust of the earth are found in the crystallized state. Thus granite consists of crystals of quartz, felspar, and mica. Even mountain masses like clay-slate, have a regular tabulated form. Perfect mobility among the corpuscles is essential to crystallization. The chemist produces it either by igneous fusion, or by solution in a liquid. When the temperature is slowly lowered in the former case, or the liquid slowly abstracted by evaporation in the latter, the attractive forces resume the ascendency, and arrange the particles in symmetrical forms. Mere approximation of the particles, however, is not alone sufficient for crystallization. A hot saturated saline solution, when screened from all agitation, will contract by cooling into a volume much smaller than what it occupies in the solid state, without crystallizing. Hence the molecules must not only be brought within a certain limit of each other, for their concreting into crystals; but they must also change the direction of their poles, from the fluid collocation to their position in the solid state.

This reversion of the poles may be effected, 1st, By contact of any part of the fluid with a point of a solid, of similar composition, previously formed. 2d, Vibratory motions communicated, either from the atmosphere or any other moving body, by deranging, however slightly, the fluid polar direction, will instantly determine the solid polar arrangement, when the balance had been rendered nearly even by previous removal of the interstitial fluid. On this principle we explain the regular figures which particles of dust or iron assume, when they are placed on a vibrating plane, in the neighbourhood of electrized or magnetized bodies. 3d, Negative or resinous voltaic electricity instantly determines the crystalline arrangement, while positive voltaic electricity counteracts it. Light also favours crystallization, as is exemplified with camphor dissolved in spirits, which crystallizes in bright and re-dissolves in gloomy weather

It might be imagined, that the same body would always concrete in the same, or at least in a similar crystalline form. This position is true, in general, for the salts crystallized in the laboratory; and on this uniformity of figure, one of the principal criteria between different salts depends. But even these forms are liable to many modifications, from causes apparently slight; and in nature we find frequently the same chemical substance crystallized in forms apparently very dissimilar. Thus, carbonate of lime assumes the form of a rhomboid, of a regular hexaëdral prism, of a solid terminated by 12 scalene angles, or of a dodecahedron with pentagonal faces, &c. Bisulphuret of iron or martial pyrites produces sometimes cubes and sometimes regular octohedrons, at one time dodecahedrons with pentagonal faces, at another icosahedrons with triangular faces, &c.

While one and the same substance lends itself to so many transformations, we meet with very different substances, which present absolutely the same form Thus fluate of lime, muriate of soda, sulphuret of iron, sulphuret of lead, &c. crystallize in cubes, under certain circumstances; and in other cases, the same minerals, as well as sulphate of alumina and the diamond, assume the form of a regular octohedron.

Romé de l'Isle first referred the study of crystallization to principles conformable to observation. He arranged together, as far as possible, crystals of the same nature. Among the different forms relative to each species, he chose one as the most proper, from its simplicity, to be regarded as the primitive form; and by supposing it truncated in different ways, he deduced the other forms from it, and determined a gradation, a series of transitions between this same form and that of polyhedrons, which seem to be still further removed from it. To the descriptions and figures which he gave of the crystalline forms, he added the results of the mechanical measurement of their principal angles, and showed that these angles were constant in each variety.

The illustrious Bergmann, by endeavouring to penetrate to the mechanism of the structure of crystals, considered the different forms relative to one and the same substance, as produced by a superposition of planes, sometimes constant and sometimes variable, and decreasing around one and the same primitive form. He applied this primary idea to a small number of crystalline forms, and verified it with respect to a variety of calcareous spar by fractures, which enabled him to ascertain the position of the nucleus, or of the primitive form, and the successive order of the laminæ covering this nucleus. Bergmann, however, stopped here, and did not trouble himself either with determining the laws of structure, or applying calculation to it. It was a simple sketch of the most prominent point of view in mineralogy, but in which we see the hand of the same master who so successfully filled up the outlines of chemistry.

In the researches which Haüy undertook, about the same period, on the structure of crystals, he proposed combining the form and dimensions of integrant molecules with simple and regular laws of arrangement, and submitting these laws to calculation. This work produced a mathematical theory, which he reduced to analytical formulæ, representing every possible case, and the application of which to known forms leads to valuations of angles, constantly agreeing with observation."—*Ure's Chem. Dict.*

2. An eruption over the body of white transparent pustules.

["CRYSTALLOGRAPHY. Of the physical properties of minerals, no one is so important in itself, and extensive in its influence and application, as that by which crystals or regular solids are produced. To investigate and describe these solids is the object of crystallography, and constitutes, without doubt, the most interesting branch of mineralogical research."—*Cleav. Mineralogy.* A.]

CTE'DONES. (From κτηδων, a rake.) The fibres are so called from their pectinated course.

CTEIS. Κτεις. A comb or rake. *Ctenes*, in the plural number, implies those teeth which are called incisores, from their likeness to a rake.

CUBE ORE. Hexaëdral olivenite. *Wurfelerz* of Werner. A mineral arseniate of iron, of a pistachio-green colour.

CUBE SPAR. See *Anhydrite.*

CUBEB. See *Piper cubeba.*

CUBE'BA. (From *cubabah*, Arab.) See *Piper cubeba.*

CUBITÆUS EXTERNUS. An extensor muscle of the fingers. See *Extensor digitorum communis.*

CUBITÆUS INTERNUS. A flexor muscle of the fingers. See *Flexor sublimis*, and *profundus.*

CUBITAL. (*Cubitalis;* from *cubitus*, the fore-arm.) Belonging to the forearm.

CUBITAL ARTERY. *Arteria cubitalis; Arteria ulnaris.* A branch of the brachial that proceeds in the forearm, and gives off the recurrent and interosseals, and forms the palmary arch, from which arise branches going to the fingers, called digitals.

CUBITAL NERVE. *Nervus cubitalis; Nervus ulnaris.* It arises from the brachial plexus, and proceeds along the ulna.

CUBITALIS MUSCULUS. An extensor muscle of the fingers. See *Extensor.*

CU'BITUS. (From *cubo*, to lie down, because the ancients used to lie down on that part at their meals.) 1. The forearm, or that part between the elbow and wrist.

2. The larger bone of the forearm is called *os cubiti.* See *Ulna.*

CUBOI'DES OS. (From κυβος, a cube or die, and ειδος, likeness.) A tarsal bone of the foot, so called from its resemblance.

CUCKOW FLOWER. See *Cardamine.*

CUCU'BALUS. The name of an herb mentioned by Pliny. The name of a genus or family of plants in the Linnæan system. Class, *Decandria;* Order *Trygynia.*

CUCUBALUS BACCIFERUS. The systematic name of the berry-bearing chick-weed, which is sometimes used as an emollient poultice.

CUCUBALUS BEHEN. The systematic name of the *Behen officinarum*, or spatling poppy, formerly used as a cordial and alexipharmic.

CUCULLA'RIS. (From *cucullis*, a hood: so named, because it is shaped like a hood.) See *Trapezius.*

CUCULLATUS. Hooded. Applied to a leaf, when the edges meet in the lower part, and expand in the upper, forming a sheath or hood, of which the genus *Sarcacenia* are an example; to the nectary of the aconite tribe, &c.

CUCU'LLUS. 1. A hood.

2. An odoriferous cap for the head.

CUCUMBER. See *Cucumis.*

Cucumber, bitter. See *Cucumis colocynthis.*

Cucumber, squirting. See *Momordica elaterium.*

Cucumber, wild. See *Momordica elaterium.*

CU'CUMIS. (*Cucumis, mis.* m.; also *cucumer, ris.; quasi curvimeres*, from their curvature.) The cucumber. 1. The name of a genus of plants in the Linnæan system. Class, *Monœcia;* Order, *Syngenesia.* The cucumber.

2. The pharmacopœial name of the garden cucumber. See *Cucumis sativus.*

CUCUMIS AGRESTIS. See *Momordica elaterium.*

CUCUMIS ASININUS. See *Momordica elaterium.*

CUCUMIS COLOCYNTHIS. The systematic name for the officinal bitter apple. *Colocynthis; Alhandula* of the Arabians. *Coloquintida.* Bitter apple; bitter gourd; bitter cucumber. The fruit, which is the medicinal part of this plant, *Cucumis—foliis multifidis, pomis globosis glabris*, of Linnæus, is imported from Turkey. Its spongy membranous medulla or pith, is directed for use; it has a nauseous, acrid, and intensely bitter taste; and is a powerful irritating cathartic. In doses of ten or twelve grains, it operates with great vehemence, frequently producing violent gripes, bloody stools, and disordering the whole system. It is recommended in various complaints, as worms, mania, dropsy, epilepsy, &c.; but is seldom resorted to, except where other more mild remedies have been used without success, and then only in the form of the *extractum colocynthidis compositum*, and the *pilulæ ex colocynthide cum aloë* of the pharmacopœias.

CUCUMIS MELO. The systematic name of the melon plant. *Melo.* Musk-melon. This fruit, when ripe, has a delicious refrigerating taste, but must be eaten moderately, with pepper, or some aromatic, as all this class of fruits are obnoxious to the stomach, producing spasms and colic. The seeds possess mucilaginous qualities.

CUCUMIS SATIVUS. The systematic name of the cucumber plant. *Cucumis. Cucumis—foliorum angulis rectis; pomis oblongis scabris* of Linnæus. It is cooling and aperient, but very apt to disagree with bilious stomachs. It should always be eaten with pepper and oil. The seeds were formerly used medicinally.

CUCUMIS SYLVESTRIS. See *Momordica elaterium.*

CU'CUPHA. A hood. An odoriferous cap for the head, composed of aromatic drugs.

CUCU'RBITA. (*A curvitate*, according to Scaliger, the first syllable being doubled; as in *Cacula, Populus*, &c.) 1. The name of a genus of plants in the Linnæan system. Class, *Monœcia;* Order, *Syngenesia.* The pumpion.

2. The pharmacopœial name of the common gourd. See *Cucurbita pepo.*

3. A chemical distilling vessel, shaped like a gourd.

CUCURBITA CITRULLUS. The systematic name of the water-melon plant. *Citrullus; Angura; Jace brasilientibus; Tetranguria.* Sicilian citrul, or water-melon. The seeds of this plant, *Cucurbita—foliis multipartitis* of Linnæus, were formerly used medicinally, but now only to reproduce the plant. Water-melon is cooling and somewhat nutritious; but so soon begins to ferment, as to prove highly noxious to some stomachs, and bring on spasms, diarrhœas, cholera, colics, &c.

CUCURBITA LAGENARIA. The systematic name of the bottle-gourd plant. See *Cucurbita pepo.*

CUCURBITA PEPO. The systematic name of the common pumpion or gourd. *Cucurbita.* The seeds of this plant, *Cucurbita—foliis lobatis, pomis lævibus*, are used indifferently with those of the *Cucurbita lagenaria—foliis subangulatis, tomentosis, basi subtus biglandulosus; pomis lignosis.* They contain a large proportion of oil, which may be made into emulsions; but is superseded by that of sweet almonds.

CUCURBITACEÆ. (From *cucurbita*, a gourd.) The name of an order of Linnæus's Fragments of a Natural Method, consisting of plants which resemble the gourd.

CUCURBI'TINUS. A species of worm, so called from its resemblance to the seed of the gourd. See *Tænia.*

CUCURBI'TULA. (A diminutive of *cucurbita*, a gourd; so called from its shape.) A cupping-glass.

CUCURBITULA CRUENTA. A cupping-glass, with scarification to procure blood.

CUCURBITULA CUM FERRO. A cupping-glass, with scarification to draw out blood.

CUCURBITULA SICCA. A cupping-glass without scarification.

CUE'MA. (From κυω, to carry in the womb.) The conception, or rather, as Hippocrates signifies by this word, the complete rudiments of the fœtus.

CULBI'CIO. A sort of stranguary, or rather heat of urine.

CULILA'WAN. See *Laurus culilawan.*

CULI'NARY. (*Culinarius*, from *culina*, a kitchen.) Any thing belonging to the kitchen, as salt, pot-herbs, &c.

CULLEN, William, was born at Lanark, Scotland, in 1712, of respectable, but not wealthy parents. After the usual school education, he was apprenticed to a surgeon and apothecary at Glasgow, and then, made several voyages, as surgeon, to the West Indies. He afterward settled in practice at Hamilton, and formed a connexion with the celebrated William Hunter; but their business being scanty, they agreed to pass a winter alternately at some university. Cullen went first to Edinburgh, and attended the classes so diligently, that he was soon after able to commence teacher. Hunter came the next winter to London, and engaged as assistant in the dissecting-room of Dr. William Douglas, who was so pleased with his assiduity and talent, as to offer him a share in his lectures: but though the partnership with Cullen was thus dissolved, they continued ever after a friendly correspondence. Cullen had the good fortune, while at Hamilton, to assist the Duke of Argyle in some chemical pursuits: and still more of being sent for to the Duke of Hamilton, in a sudden alarming illness, which he speedily relieved by his judicious treatment, and gained the entire approbation of Dr. Clarke, who afterward arrived. About the same time he married the daughter of a neighbouring clergyman, who bore him several children. In 1746 he took the degree of doctor in medicine, and was appointed teacher of chemistry at Glasgow. His talents were peculiarly fitted for this office; his systematic genius, distinct enunciation, lively manner, and extensive knowledge of the subject, rendered his lectures highly interesting. In the mean time his reputation as a physician increased, so that he was consulted in most difficult cases. In 1751, he was chosen professor in medicine to the university; and, five years after, the chemical chair at Edinburgh was offered him, on the death of Dr. Plummer, which was too advantageous to be refused. He soon became equally popular there, and his class increased, so as to exceed that of any other professor, except the anatomical. This success was owing not only to his assiduity, and his being so well qualified for the office, but also in a great measure to the kindness which he showed to his pupils, and partly to the new Views on the Theory of Medicine, which he occasionally introduced into his lectures. He appears also, about this time, to have given Clinical Lectures at the Infirmary. On the death of Dr. Alston, Lecturer on the Materia Medica, he was appointed to succeed him: and six years afterward, jointly with Dr. Gregory, to lecture on the Theory and Practice of Medicine, when he resigned the Chemical Chair to his pupil, Dr. Black. Dr. Gregory having died the following year, he continued the Medical Lectures alone, till within a few months of his death, which happened in February 1790, in his seventy-seventh year; and he is said, even at the last, to have shown no deficiency in his delivery, nor in his memory, being accustomed to lecture from short notes. His Lectures on the Materia Medica being surreptitiously printed, he obtained an injunction against their being issued until he had corrected them, which was accomplished in 1772: but they were afterward much improved, and appeared in 1789, in two quarto volumes. Fearing a similar fate to his Lectures on Medicine, he published an outline of them in 1784, in four volumes, octavo, entitled "First Lines of the Practice of Physic." He wrote also the "Institutions of Medicine," in one volume, octavo: and a "Letter to Lord Cathcart, on the Recovery of drowned Persons" But his most celebrated work is his "Synopsis Nosologiæ Methodicæ," successively improved in different editions; the fourth, published in 1785, in two octavo volumes, contains the Systems of other Nosologists till that period, followed by his own, which certainly, as a practical arrangement of diseases, greatly surpasses them.

CULMUS. Culm. Straw. The stem of grasses, rushes, and plants nearly allied to them. It bears both leaves and flowers, and its nature is more easily understood than defined. Its varieties are,

1. *Culmus teres*, round; as in *Carex uliginosa.*
2. *C. tetragonus;* as in *Festuca ovina.*
3. *C. triangularis;* as in *Eriocaulon triangulare.*
4. *C. capillaris;* as in *Scirpus capillaris.*
5. *C. prostratus;* as in *Agrostis canina.*
6. *C. repens;* as in *Agrostis stolonifera.*
7. *C. nudus*, as in *Carex montana.*
8. *C. enodis*, without joints; as in *Juncus conglomeratus.*
9. *C. articulatus*, jointed; as in *Agrostis alba.*
10. *C. geniculatus*, bent like the knee; as in *Alopecurus geniculatus.*

It is also either solid or hollow, rough or smooth, sometimes hairy or downy, scarcely woolly.

Culmiferæ. Plants which have smooth soft stems.

CULPEPER, Nicholas, was the son of a clergyman, who put him apprentice to an apothecary; after serving his time, he settled in Spitalfields, London, about the year 1642. In the troubles prevailing at that period, he appears to have favoured the Puritans; but his decided warfare was with the College of Physicians, whom he accuses of keeping the people in ignorance, like the Popish clergy. He therefore published a translation of their Dispensary, with practical remarks; also an Herbal, pointing out, among other matters, under what planet the plants should be gathered; and a directory to midwives, showing the method of ensuring a healthy progeny, &c. These works were for some time popular. He died in 1654.

CU'LTER. (From *colo*, to cultivate.)

1. A knife or shear.
2. The third lobe of the liver is so called from its supposed resemblance.

CU'LUS. (From κουλος.) The anus or fundament.

Cu'mamus. See *Piper cubeba.*

CUMIN. See *Cuminum.*

CU'MINUM. (From κυω, to bring forth; because it was said to cure sterility.)

1. The name of a genus of plants in the Linnæan system. Class, *Heptandria;* Order, *Digynia.* The cumin plant.
2. The pharmacopœial name of the cumin plant. See *Cuminum cyminum.*

Cuminum æthiopicum. A name for the ammi verum. See *Sison ammi.*

Cuminum cyminum. The systematic name of the cumin plant. *Cuminum; Fœniculum orientale.* A native of Egypt and Ethiopia, but cultivated in Sicily and Malta, from whence it is brought to us. The seeds of cumin, which are the only part of the plant in use, have a bitterish taste, accompanied with an aromatic flavour, but not agreeable. They are generally preferred to other seeds for external use in discussing indolent tumours, as the encysted scrofulous, &c. and give name both to a plaster and cataplasm in the pharmacopœias.

Cunea'dis sutura. The suture by which the os sphenoides is joined to the os frontis.

CUNEIFORMIS. (From *cuneus*, a wedge, and *forma*, likeness.) Cuneiform, wedge-like. Applied to bones, leaves, &c. which are broad and abrupt at the extremity. See *Sphenoid bone; Tarsus*, and *Carpus; Leaf; Petalum.*

Cune'olus. (From *cuneo*, to wedge.) A crooked tent to put into a fistula.

["Cunila. Pennyroyal. The plant called *pennyroyal*, in England, is a species of mint, *Mentha pulegium;* while the American plant, which bears the same common appellation, belongs to the genus *Cunila*, of Linnæus, and *Hedeoma*, of Persoon. American pennyroyal is a warm aromatic, possessing a pungent flavour, which is common to many of the labiate plants of other genera. Like them, it is heating, carminative, and diaphoretic. It is in popular repute as an emmenagogue."—*Big. Mat. Med.* A.]

Cup of the flower. See *Calyx.*

CUPEL. (*Kuppel*, a cup, German.) *Copella; Catellus cinereus; Cineritium; Patella docimastica; Testa probatrix, exploratrix*, or *docimastica.* A shallow earthen vessel like a cup, made of phosphate of lime, which suffers the baser metals to pass through it, when exposed to heat, and retains the pure metal. This process is termed cupellation.

CUPELLATION. *Cupellatio.* The purifying of perfect metals by means of an addition of lead, which, at a due heat, becomes vitrified, and promotes the vitrification and calcination of such imperfect metals as may be in the mixture, so that these last are carried off in the fusible glass that is formed, and the perfect metals are left nearly pure. The name of this operation is taken from the vessels made use of, which are called cupels.

Cu'phos. Κουφος. Light. When applied to aliments, it imports their being easily digested; when to distempers, that they are mild.

[Cupping. Topical bleeding. "This is done by means of a scarificator, and a glass, shaped somewhat like a bell. The scarificator is an instrument containing a number of lancets, sometimes as many as twenty, which are so contrived, that when the instrument is applied to any part of the surface of the body, and a spring is pressed, they suddenly start out, and make the necessary punctures. The instrument is so constructed, that the depth, to which the lancets penetrate, may be made greater or less, at the option of the practitioner. As only small vessels can be thus opened, a very inconsiderable quantity of blood would be discharged, were not some method taken to promote the evacuation. This is commonly done with a cupping-glass, the air within the cavity of which is rarefied by the flame of a little lamp, containing spirit of wine, and furnished with a thick wick. This plan is preferable to that of setting on fire a piece of tow, dipped in this fluid, and put in the cavity of the glass. The larger the glass, if properly exhausted, the less pain does the patient suffer, and the more freely does the blood flow. When the mouth of the glass is placed over the scarifications, and the rarefied air in it becomes condensed as it cools, the glass is forced down on the skin, and a considerable suction takes place."—*Cooper's Surg. Dict.* A.]

CUPRE'SSUS. (So called, *απο του κυειν παρισους τους ακρεμονας*, because it produces equal branches.) Cypress.

1. The name of a genus of plants in the Linnæan system. Class, *Monœcia*; Order, *Monadelphia*. The cypress-tree.

2. The pharmacopœial name of the cypress-tree. See *Cupressus sempervirens*.

Cupressus sempervirens. The systematic name of the cupressus of the shops. *Cupressus—foliis imbricatis squamis quadrangulis*, of Linnæus; called also *cyparissus*. Every part of the plant abounds with a bitter, aromatic, terebinthinate fluid; and is said to be a remedy against intermittents. Its wood is extremely durable, and constitutes the cases of Egyptian mummies.

Cupri ammoniati liquor. Solution of ammoniated copper. *Aqua cupri ammoniati* of Pharm. Lond. 1787, and formerly called *Aqua sapphirina*. Take of ammoniated copper, a drachm; distilled water, a pint. Dissolve the ammoniated copper in the water, and filter the solution through paper. This preparation is employed by surgeons for cleansing foul ulcers, and disposing them to heal.

Cupri rubigo. Verdigris.

Cupri sulphas. *Vitriolum cupri; Vitriolum cæruleum; Vitriolum Romanum; Cuprum vitriolatum.* Sulphate of copper. It possesses acrid and styptic qualities; is esteemed as a tonic, emetic, adstringent, and escharotic, and is exhibited internally in the cure of dropsies, hæmorrhages, and as a speedy emetic. Externally it is applied to stop hæmorrhages, to hæmorrhoids, leucorrhœa, phagedænic ulcers, proud flesh, and condylomata.

CU'PRUM. (*Quasi æs Cyprium;* so called from the island of Cyprus, whence it was formerly brought.) See *Copper*.

Cuprum ammoniacale. See *Cuprum ammoniatum*.

Cuprum ammoniatum. *Cuprum ammoniacale.* Ammoniated copper. Ammoniacal sulphate of copper Take of sulphate of copper, half an ounce; subcarbonate of ammonia, six drachms; rub them together in a glass mortar, till the effervescence ceases; then dry the ammoniated copper, wrapped up in bibulous paper, by a gentle heat. In this process the carbonic acid is expelled from the ammonia, which forms a triple compound with the sulphuric acid and oxide of copper. This preparation is much milder than the sulphate of copper. It is found to produce tonic and astringent effects on the human body. Its principal internal use has been in epilepsy, and other obstinate spasmodic diseases, given in doses of half a grain, gradually increased to five grains or more, two or three times a day. For its external application, see *Cupri ammoniati liquor*.

Cuprum vitriolatum. See *Cupri sulphas*.

CUPULA. An accidental part of a seed, being a rough calyculus, surrounding the lower part of a gland, as that of the oak, of which it is the cup.

Cura avanacea. A decoction of oats and succory roots, in which a little nitre and sugar were dissolved, was formerly used in fevers, and was thus named.

Cu'rcas. See *Jatropha curcas*.

Cu'rculio. (From *karkarah*, Hebrew.) The throat and the aspera arteria.

[Also the name of a genus of coleopterous insects, according to Linnæus's system. A.]

Cu'rcum. See *Cheledonium majus*.

CURCU'MA. (From the Arabic *curcum* or *hercum*.) Turmeric. 1. The name of a genus of plants in the Linnæan system. Class, *Monandria;* Order, *Monogynia*.

2. The pharmacopœial name of the turmeric-tree. See *Curcuma longa*.

Curcuma longa. The systematic name of the turmeric plant. *Crocus Indicus; Terra marita; Cannacorus radice croceo; Curcuma rotunda; Mayella; Kua kaha* of the Indians. *Curcuma—foliis lanceolatis; nervis lateralibus numerossimis* of Linnæus. The Arabians call every root of a saffron colour by the name of *curcum*. The root of this plant is imported here in its dried state from the East Indies, in various forms. Externally it is of a pale yellow colour, wrinkled, solid, ponderous, and the inner substance of a deep saffron or gold colour: its odour is somewhat fragrant; to the taste it is bitterish, slightly acrid, exciting a moderate degree of warmth in the mouth, and on being chewed, it tinges the saliva yellow. It is an ingredient in the composition of *Curry powder*, is valuable as a dying dru and furnishes a chemical test of the presence of uncombined alkalies. It is now very seldom used medicinally, but retains a place in our pharmacopœias.

Curcuma rotunda. See *Curcuma longa*.

CURD. The coagulum, which separates from milk, upon the addition of acid or other substances.

["Curette. (French.) An instrument shaped like a minute spoon, or scoop, invented by Daviel, and used in the extraction of the cataract, for taking away any opaque matter, which may remain behind the pupil, immediately after the crystalline has been taken out."—*Cooper's Surg. Dict.* A.]

Curled leaf. See *Leaf*.

CU'RMI. (From *κεραω*, to mix.) Ale. A drink made of barley, according to Dioscorides.

CURRANT. See *Ribes*.

Cu'rsuma. *Curtuma.* The *Ranunculus ficaria* of Linnæus.

Cursu'ta. (Corrupted from *cassuta*, *kasuth*, Arabian.) The root of the *Gentiana purpurea* of Linnæus.

Curva'tor coccygis. A muscle bending the coccyx. See *Coccygeus*.

CURVATUS. (From *curvus*, a curve.) Curvate, bent. Applied to the form of a pepo or gourd seed-vessel; as in *Cucumi flexuosus*.

CUSCU'TA. (According to Linnæus, a corruption from the Greek *Κασυτας*, or *Καδυτας*, which is from the Arabic *Chessuth*, or *Chasuth*.) Dodder. 1. The name of a genus of plants in the Linnæan system. Class, *Tetrandria;* Order, *Digynia*.

2. The pharmacopœial name of dodder of thyme. See *Cuscuta epithymum*.

Cuscuta epithymum. The systematic name of dodder of thyme. *Epythymum. Cuscuta—foliis sessilibus, quinquifidis, bracteis obvallaiis.* A parasitical plant, possessing a strong disagreeable smell, and a pungent taste, very durable in the mouth. Recommended in melancholia, as cathartics.

Cuscuta europæa. The systematic name of a species of dodder of thyme. *Cuscuta—floribus sessilibus*, of Linnæus.

CUSPA'RIA. The name given by Messrs. Humboldt and Bonpland to a genus of plants in which is the tree we obtain the Angustura bark from.

Cusparia febrifuga. This is the tree said to yield the bark called Angustura.—*Cortex cuspariæ*, and imported from Angustura in South America. Its external appearances vary considerably. The best is not fibrous, but hard, compact, and of a yellowish-brown colour, and externally of a whitish hue. When reduced into powder, it resembles that of Indian rhubarb. It is very generally employed as a febrifuge, tonic, and adstringent. While some deny its virtue in curing intermittents, by many it is preferred to the Peruvian bark; and it has been found useful in diarrhœa, dyspepsia, and scrofula. It was thought to be the bark of the *Brucea antidysenterica*, or *ferruginea*. Wildenow suspected it to be the *Magnalia plumieri;* but Humboldt and Bonpland, the celebrated travellers in South America, have ascertained it to belong to a tree not before known, and which they promise to describe by the name of *Cusparia febrifuga.*

CUSPIDA'TUS. (From *cuspis*, a point.) 1. Four of the teeth are called *cuspidati*, from their form. See *Teeth.*

2. Sharp-pointed. Applied to leaves which are tipped with a spine, as in thistles. See *Leaf.*

CU'SPIS. (From *cuspa*, Chaldean, a shell, or bone, with which spears were formerly pointed.) 1. The glans penis was so called, from its likeness to the point of a spear.

2. The name of a bandage.

CU'STOS OCULI. An instrument to fix the eye during an operation.

CUTA'MBULUS. (From *cutis*, the skin, and *ambulo*, to walk.) 1. A cutaneous worm.

2. Scorbutic itching.

CUTANEOUS. (*Cutaneus;* from *cutis*, the skin.) Belonging to the skin.

CUTA'NEUS MUSCULUS. See *Platysma myoides.*

CUTICLE. *Cuticula.* (A diminutive of *cutis*, the skin.) *Epidermis.* Scarf-skin. A thin, pellucid, insensible membrane, of a white colour, that covers and defends the true skin, with which it is connected by the hairs, exhaling and inhaling vessels, and the rete mucosum.

CUTICULA. See *Cuticle.*

CU'TIS. (*Cutis, tis.* fœm.) See *Skin.*

CUTIS ANSERINA. The rough state the skin is sometimes thrown into from the action of cold, or other cause, in which it looks like the skin of the goose.

CUTIS VERA. The true skin under the cuticle.

CYANIA. The trivial name in Good's arrangement of diseases of a species called *Exangia cyania*, or blue skin. Class, *Hœmatica;* Order, *Struma.*

CYANIC ACID. *Acidum cyanicum.* See *Prussic acid.*

CYANITE. Kyanite. Disthene of Haüy. A mineral of a Berlin blue colour, found in India and Europe.

CYANOGEN. (From κυανος, blue, and γινομαι, to form.) Production of blue. See *Prussine.*

CY'ANUS. (Κυανος, cærulean, or sky-blue; so called from its colour.) Blue-bottle. See *Centauria cyanus.*

CY'AR. (From κεω, to pour out.) 1. The lip of a vessel.

2. The eye of a needle.

3. The orifice of the internal ear, from its likeness to the eye of a needle.

CYA'SMA. Spots on the skin of pregnant women.

CYATHI'SCUS. (From κυαθος, a cup.) The hollow part of a probe, formed in the shape of a small spoon, as an ear-picker.

CY'BITOS. See *Cubitus.*

CY'BITUM. See *Cubitus.*

CY'BITUS. See *Cubitus.*

CYBOI'DES. See *Cuboides.*

CYCAS. (Κυκας, of Theophrastus. The name of a palm, said to grow in Ethiopia.) The name of a genus of plants, one of the *Palmæ pinnatifoliæ*, of Linnæus; but afterward removed by him to the *felices.*

CYCAS CIRCINALIS. The systematic name of a palm-tree which affords a sago, called also *Sagus; Sagu:*—a dry fecula, obtained from the pith of this palm, in the islands of Java, Molucca, and the Philippines. The same substance is also brought from the West Indies, but it is inferior to that brought from the East. Sago becomes soft and transparent by boiling in water, and forms a light and agreeable liquid, much recommended in febrile, phthisical and calculous disorders, &c. To make it palatable, it is customary to add to it, when boiled or softened with water, some lemon juice, sugar, and wine.

CY'CEUM. (From κυκαω, to mix.) *Cyceon.* A mixture of the consistence of pap.

CY'CIMA. (From κυκαω, to mix.) So called from the mixture of the ore with lead, by which litharge is made.

CY'CLAMEN. (From κυκλος, circular; either on account of the round form of the leaves, or of the roots.) Cyclamen.

1. The name of a genus of plants in the Linnæan system. Class, *Pentandria;* Order, *Monogynia.*

2. The pharmacopœial name of the sow-bread. See *Cyclamen Europæum.*

CYCLAMEN EUROPÆUM. The systematic name of the sow-bread. *Arthanita* of the pharmacopœias. The root is a drastic purge and errhine; and by the common people it has been used to procure abortion.

CYCLI'SCUS. (From κυκλος, a circle.) An instrument in the form of a half-moon, formerly used for scraping the rotten bones.

CYCLI'SMUS. (From κυκλος, a circle.) A lozenge.

CYCLOPHO'RIA. (From κυκλος, a circle, and φερω, to bear.) The circulation of the blood, or other fluids.

CYCLO'PION. (From κυκλοω, to surround, and ωψ, the eye.) The white of the eye.

CY'CLOS. *Cyclus.* A circle. Hippocrates uses this word to signify the cheeks, and the orbits of the eyes.

CYCLUS METASYNCRITICUS. A long protracted course of remedies, persisted in with a view of restoring the particles of the body to such a state as is necessary to health.

CYDO'NIA. (From *Cydon*, a town in Crete, where the tree grows wild.) The quince-tree. See *Pyrus cydonia.*

CYDONIUM MALUM. The quince. See *Pyrus cydonia.*

CYE'MA. (From κυω, to bring forth.) Parturition

CYLI'CHNIS. (From κυλιξ, a cup.) A gallipot or vessel to hold medicines.

Cylindrical Leaf. See *Leaf.*

CYLI'NDRUS. (From κυλιω, to roll round.) A cylinder. A tent for a wound, equal at the top and bottom.

CYLLO'SIS. (From κυλλοω, to make lame.) A tibia or leg bending outwards.

CY'LUS. (From κυλλοω, to make lame.) In Hippocrates, it is one affected with a kind of luxation, which bends outwards, and is hollowed inward. Such a defect in the tibia is called *Cyllosis*, and the person to whom it belongs, is called by the Latins *Varus*, which term is opposed to *Valgus.*

CYMA. A cyme. A species of inflorescence of plants, consisting of several flower-stalks, all springing from one centre or point, but each stalk is variously subdivided; and in this last respect, a cyme differs essentially from an umbel, the subdivisions of the latter being formed like its primary divisions, of several stalks springing from one point. This difference is of great importance in nature. The mode of inflorescence agrees also with a corymbus in general aspect; but in the latter the primary stalks have no common centre, though the partial ones may sometimes be umbellate, which last case is precisely the reverse of a cyme.

From its division into primary stalks or branches, it is distinguished into,

1. *Trifid;* as in *Sedum acre.*
2. *Quadrifid;* as in *Crassula rubens.*
3. *Tripartite*, having three less cymes; as in *Sambucus ebulus.*
4. *Quinquipartite;* as in *Sambucus nigra.*
5. *Sessile*, or without stalk; as in *Gnaphalium frutescens.*

Comus sanguinea and *sericea* afford examples of the *Cyma nuda.*

CYMATO'DES. Is applied by Galen and others to an unequal fluctuating pulse.

CY'MBA. (From κυμβος, hollow.) A boat, pinnace, or skiff. A bone of the wrist is so called, from its supposed likeness to a skiff. See *Naviculare os.*

CYMBIFORMIS. (From *cymba*, a boat or skiff, and *forma*, likeness.) Skiff or boat-like. Applied to the seeds of the *Calendula officinalis.*

CY'MINUM. See *Cuminum.*

CYMOPHANE. See *Chrysoberyl.*

CYMOSUS. Having the character of a cyme. Applied to aggregate flowers.

CYNA'NCHE. (From κυων, a dog, and αγχω, to suffocate, or strangle; so called from dogs being said to be subject to it.) Sore throat. A genus of disease in the class *Pyrexiæ*, and order *Phlegmasiæ* of Cullen. It is known by pain and redness of the throat, attended with a difficulty of swallowing and breathing.

The species of this disease are:—

1. *Cynanche trachealis; Cynanche laryngea; Suffocatio stridula; Angina perniciosa; Asthma infantum; Cynanche stridula; Morbus strangulatorius; Catarrhus suffocatius; Barbadensis; Angina polyposa sive membranacea.* The croup. A disease that mostly attacks infants, who are suddenly seized with a difficulty of breathing and a crouping noise: it is an inflammation of the mucous membrane of the trachea that induces the secretion of a very tenacious coagulable lymph, which lines the trachea and bronchia, and impedes respiration. The croup does not appear to be contagious, whatever some physicians may think to the contrary; but it sometimes prevails epidemically. It seems, however, peculiar to some families; and a child having once been attacked, is very liable to its returns. It is likewise peculiar to young children, and has never been known to attack a person arrived at the age of puberty.

The application of cold seems to be the general cause which produces this disorder, and therefore it occurs more frequently in the winter and spring, than in the other seasons. It has been said, that it is most prevalent near the sea-coast; but it is frequently met with in inland situations, and particularly those which are marshy.

Some days previous to an attack of the disease, the child appears drowsy, inactive, and fretful; the eyes are somewhat suffused and heavy; and there is a cough, which, from the first, has a peculiar shrill sound; this, in the course of two days, becomes more violent and troublesome, and likewise more shrill. Every fit of coughing agitates the patient very much; the face is flushed and swelled, the eyes are protuberant, a general tremor takes place, and there is a kind of convulsive endeavour to renew respiration at the close of each fit. As the disease advances, a constant difficulty of breathing prevails, accompanied sometimes with a swelling and inflammation in the tonsils, uvula, and velum pendulum palati; and the head is thrown back, in the agony of attempting to escape suffocation. There is not only an unusual sound produced by the cough, (something between the yelping and barking of a dog,) but respiration is performed with a hissing noise, as if the trachea was closed up by some slight spongy substance. The cough is generally dry; but if any thing is spit up, it has either a purulent appearance, or seems to consist of films resembling portions of a membrane. Where great nausea and frequent retchings prevail, coagulated matter of the same nature is brought up. With these symptoms, there is much thirst, an uneasy sense of heat over the whole body, a continual inclination to change from place to place, great restlessness, and frequency of the pulse.

In an advanced stage of the disease, respiration becomes more stridulous, and is performed with still greater difficulty, being repeated at longer periods, and with greater exertions, until at last it ceases entirely.

The croup generally proves fatal by suffocation, induced either by spasm affecting the glottis, or by a quantity of matter blocking up by the trachea or bronchia; but when it terminates in health, it is by a resolution of the inflammation, by a ceasing of the spasms, and by a free expectoration of the matter exuding from the trachea, or of the crusts formed there.

The disease has, in a few instances, terminated fatally within twenty-four hours after its attack; but it more usually happens, that where it proves fatal, it runs on to the fourth or fifth day. Where considerable portions of the membranous films, formed on the surface of the trachea, are thrown up, life is sometimes protracted for a day or two longer than would otherwise have happened.

Dissections of children who have died of the croup, have mostly shown a preternatural membrane, lining the whole internal surface of the upper part of the trachea, which may always be easily separated from the proper membrane. There is likewise usually found a good deal of mucus, with a mixture of pus, in the trachea and its ramifications.

The treatment of this disease must be conducted on the strictly antiphlogistic plan. It will commonly be proper, where the patient is not very young, to begin by taking blood from the arm, or the jugular vein; several leeches should be applied along the forepart of the neck. It will then be right to give a nauseating emetic, ipecacuanha with tartarized antimony, or with squill in divided doses; this may be followed up by cathartics, diaphoretics, digitalis, &c. Large blisters ought to be applied near the affected part, and a discharge kept up by savine cerate, or other stimulant dressing. Mercury, carried speedily to salivation, has in several instances arrested the progress of the disease, when it appeared proceeding to a fatal termination. As the inflammation is declining, it is very important that free expectoration should take place; this may be promoted by nauseating medicines, by inhaling steam, and by stimulating gargles; for which the decoction of senna is particularly recommended. Where there is much wheezing, an occasional emetic may relieve the patient considerably, and under symptoms of threatening suffocation, the operation of bronchotomy has sometimes saved life.—Should fits of spasmodic difficulty of breathing occur in the latter periods of the disease, opium joined with diaphoretics would be most likely to do good.

2. *Cynanche tonsillaris.* The inflammatory quinsy, called also *angina inflammatoria.* In this complaint, the inflammation principally occupies the tonsils; but often extends through the whole mucous membrane of the fauces, so as essentially to interrupt the speech, respiration, and deglutition of the patient.

The causes which usually give rise to it are, exposure to cold, either from sudden vicissitudes of weather, from being placed in a partial current of air, wearing damp linen, sitting in wet rooms, or getting wet in the feet; all of which may give a sudden check to perspiration. It principally attacks those of a full and plethoric habit, and is chiefly confined to cold climates, occurring usually in the spring and autumn; whereas the ulcerated sore throat chiefly attacks those of a weak irritable habit, and is most prevalent in warm climates. The former differs from the latter likewise in not being contagious. In many people there seems to be a particular tendency to this disease; as from every considerable application of cold it is readily induced.

An inflammatory sore throat discovers itself by a difficulty of swallowing and breathing, accompanied by a redness and tumour in one or both tonsils, dryness of the throat, foulness of the tongue, lancinating pains in the parts affected, a frequent but difficult excretion of mucus, and some small degree of fever. As the disease advances, the difficulty of swallowing and breathing becomes greater, the speech is very indistinct, the dryness of the throat and thirst increases, the tongue swells and is incrusted with a dark fur, and the pulse is full and frequent. In some cases, a few white, sloughy spots are to be observed on the tonsils. If the inflammation proceeds to such a height as to put a total stop to respiration, the face will become livid, the pulse will sink, and the patient will quickly be destroyed.

The chief danger arising from this species of quinsy is, the inflammation occupying both tonsils, and proceeding to such a degree as to prevent a sufficient quantity of nourishment for the support of nature from being taken, or to occasion suffocation; but this seldom happens, and its usual termination is either in resolution or suppuration. When proper steps are adopted, it will in general readily go off by the former.

Where the disease has proved fatal by suffocation, little more than a highly inflamed state of the parts affected, with some morbid phenomena in the head, have been observed on dissection.

This is usually a complaint not requiring very active treatment. If, however, the inflammation run high, in a tolerably strong and plethoric adult, a moderate quantity of blood should be drawn from the arm, or the jugular vein: but still more frequently leeches will be required; or scarifying the tonsils may afford more effectual relief. An emetic will often be very beneficial, sometimes apparently check the progress of the complaint: likewise cathartics must be employed, diaphoretics, and the general antiphlogistic regimen. A blister to the throat, or behind the neck, sometimes has a very excellent effect: but in milder cases, the linimentum ammoniæ, or other rubefacient application, applied every six or eight hours, and wearing flannel round the throat, may produce a sufficient determination from the part affected. The use of proper gargles generally contributes materially to the cure. If there be much tension and pain in the fauces, a solution of nitrate of potassa will be best; otherwise dilute acids, a weak solution of alum, &c. Should the disease proceed to suppuration, warm emollient gargles ought to be employed, and perhaps similar external applications may be of some service: but it is particularly important to make an early opening into the abscess for the discharge of the pus. When deglutition is prevented by the tumefaction of the tonsils, it is recommended to exhibit nutritious clysters; and when suffocation is threatened, an emetic or inhaling æther may cause a rupture of the abscess, or this may be opened; but if relief be not thereby obtained, bronchotomy will become necessary.

3. *Cynanche pharyngea.* This species is so called when the pharynx is chiefly affected. Dr. Wilson, in his Treatise on Febrile Diseases, includes in his definition of cynanche tonsillaris, that of cynanche pharyngea. These varieties of cynanche differ considerably when they are exquisitely formed. But the one is seldom present in any considerable degree, without being attended with more or less of the other. Dr. Cullen declares, indeed, that he never saw a case of true cynanche pharyngea; that is, a case in which the inflammation was confined to the pharynx; it constantly spread in a greater or less degree to the tonsils and neighbouring parts. Besides, the mode of treatment is, in almost every instance, the same in both cases. And if we admit the cynanche pharyngea to be a distinct variety, we must admit another, the cynanche œsophagea; for inflammation frequently attacks the œsophagus, and is sometimes even confined to it.

4. *Cynanche parotidea.* The mumps. A swelling on the cheek and under the jaw, extending over the neck, from inflammation of the parotid and other salivary glands, rendering deglutition, or even respiration, sometimes difficult, declining the fourth day. Epidemic and contagious.

The disease is subject to a metastasis occasionally, in females to the mammæ, in males to the testes; and in a few instances, repelled from these parts, it has affected the brain, and even proved fatal. In general, however, the disease is without danger, and scarcely calls for medical aid. Keeping a flannel over the part, and the antiphlogistic regimen, with mild laxatives, will be sufficient. Should the mammæ, or the testes, be affected, more active evacuations may be necessary to prevent the destruction of those organs, bleeding general and topical, &c. but avoiding cold applications, lest it should be driven to the brain. And where this part is unfortunately attacked, besides the means explained under *Phrenitis*, it may be useful to endeavour to recall the inflammation to its former seat by warm fomentations, stimulant liniments, &c.

5. *Cynanche maligna.* The malignant, putrid, or ulcerous sore throat. Called also *Cynanche gangrænosa; Angina ulcerosa; Febris epidemica cum angina ulcusculosa; Angina epidemica; Angina gangrænosa; Angina suffocativa; Angina maligna.* This disease is readily to be distinguished from the inflammatory quincy, by the soreness and specks which appear in the fauces, together with the great debility of the system, and small fluttering pulse, which are not to be observed in the former. In the inflammatory sore throat there is always great difficulty of swallowing, a considerable degree of tumour, with a tendency in the parts affected to suppurate, and a hard, full pulse. Moreover in the former affection the disease is seated principally in the mucous membrane of the mouth and throat; whereas in the latter the inflammation chiefly occupies the glandular parts.

The putrid sore throat often arises from a peculiar state of the atmosphere, and so becomes epidemical; making its attacks chiefly on children, and those of a weak relaxed habit. It is produced likewise by contagion, as it is found to run through a whole family, when it has once seized any person in it; and it proves often fatal, particularly to those in an infantile state.

It appears, however, that under this head two different complaints have been included; the one, especially fatal to children, is an aggravated form of scarlatina; the other, a combination of inflammation of the fauces with typhus fever; the former is perhaps always, the latter certainly often, contagious. See *Scarlatina* and *Typhus*.

CYNA'NCHICA. (*Cinanchicus;* from κυναγχη, the quincy.) Medicines which relieve a quincy.

CYNANTHRO'PIA. (From κυων, a dog, and ανθρωπος, a man.) It is used by Bellini, De Morbis Capitas, to express a particular kind of melancholy, when men fancy themselves changed into dogs, and imitate their actions.

CY'NARA. See *Cinara*.

CYNAROCEPHALUS. (From κιναρα, the artichoke, and κεφαλη, a head.) Having a head like the *Cinara*, or artichoke; as the thistle, globe thistle, burdock, blue bottle.

CY'NCHNIS. Κυγχνις. A vessel of any kind to hold medicines in.

CYNOCRA'MBE. (From κυων, a dog, and κραμβη, cabbage; an herb of the cabbage tribe, with which dogs are said to physic themselves.) See *Mercurialis perennis*.

CYNO'CTANUM. (From κυων, a dog, and κτεινω, to kill.) A species of aconitum, said to destroy dogs. See *Aconitum napellus*.

CYNOCY'TISIS. (From κυων, a dog, and κυτισος, the cytisis: so named because it was said to cure the distemper of dogs.) The dog-rose. See *Rosa canina*

CYNODE'CTOS. (From κυων, a dog, and δακνω, to bite.) So Dioscorides calls a person bit by a mad dog.

CYNODE'SMION. (From κυων, a dog, and δεω, to bind; so named because in dogs it is very discernible and strong.) A ligature by which the prepuce is bound to the glands. See *Frænum*.

CYNODO'NTES. (Κυνοδοντες: from κυων, a dog, and οδους, a tooth.) The canine teeth. See *Teeth*.

CYNOGLO'SSUM. (From κυων, a dog, and γλωσσα, a tongue; so named from its supposed resemblance.) Hound's tongue.

1. The name of a genus of plants in the Linnæan system. Class, *Pentandria;* Order, *Monogynia*.

2. The pharmacopœial name of the hound's tongue See *Cynoglossum officinale*.

CYNOGLOSSUM OFFICINALE. The systematic name for hound's tongue. *Cynoglossum; Lingua canina; Cynoglossum—staminibus corolla brevioribus; foliis lato lanceolatis tomentosis, sessilibus*, of Linnæus It possesses narcotic powers, but is seldom employed medicinally. Acids are said to counteract the ill effects of an over-dose more speedily than any thing else, after clearing the stomach.

CYNO'LOPHUS. (From κυων, a dog, and λοφος, a protuberance: so called because in dogs they are peculiarly eminent.) The asperities and prominences of the vertebræ.

CYNOLY'SSA. (From κυων, a dog, and λυσση, madness.) Canine madness.

CYNOMO'RIUM. The name of a genus of plants in the Linnæan system. Class, *Monœcia;* Order *Monandria*.

CYNOMORIUM COCCINEUM. The systematic name of the *Fungus melitensis;* improperly called a fungus It is a small plant which grows only on a little rock adjoining Malta. A drachm of the powder is given for a dose in dysenteries and hæmorrhages, and with remarkable success.

CYNORE'XIA. (From κυων, a dog, and ορεξις, appetite.) A voracious or canine appetite. See *Bulimia*.

CYNO'SBATOS. See *Cynosbatus*.

CYNO'SBATUS. (From κυων, a dog, and βατος, a thorn: so called because dogs are said to be attracted by its smell.) The dog-rose. See *Rosa canina*.

CYNOSPA'STUM. (From κυων, a dog, and σπαω, to attract.) See *Rosa canina*.

CYOPHO'RIA. (From κυος, a fœtus, and φερω, to bear.) Pregnancy.

CYPARI'SSUS. See *Cupressus*.

CY'PERUS. (From κυπαρος, a little round vessel, which its roots are said to resemble.) Cyperus. The name of a genus of plants in the Linnæan system. Class, *Triandria;* Order, *Monogynia*.

CYPERUS ESCULENTUS. The rush-nut. This plant is a native of Italy, where the fruit is collected and eaten, and said to be a greater delicacy than the chesnut.

CYPERUS LONGUS. The systematic and pharmacopœial name of the English galangale. *Cyperus—culmo triquetro folioso, umbella foliosa supra-decomposita: pedunculis nudis, spicis alternis*, of Linnæus. The smell of the root of this plant is aromatic, and its taste warm, and sometimes bitter. It is now totally fallen into disuse.

Cyperus rotundus. This species, the round cyperus, *Cyperus—culmo triquetro subnudo, umbella decomposita; spicis alternis linearibus*, of Linnæus, is generally preferred to the former, being a more gratefully aromatic bitter. It is chiefly used as a stomachic.

CYPHELLA. A peculiar sort of pit or pore on the under side of the frond, in that section of lichens called *stricta*.

CYPHO'MA. (From κυπ7ω, to bend.) A gibbosity, or curvature of the spine.

CYPHO'SIS. An incurvation of the spine.

CYPRESS. See *Cyprus*.

Cypress spurge. See *Esula minor*.

Cy'prinum oleum. Flowers of cypress, calamus, cardamoms, &c. boiled in olive oil, now fallen into disuse.

Cy'prium. (From κυπρος, Cyprus, an island where it is said formerly to have abounded.) Copper.

CY'PRUS. (So called from the island of Cyprus, where it grew abundantly.) The cypress-tree, or Eastern privet.

[CYPRŒITE. Petrifaction of a Cyprœa or Cowrey. See *Organic relics*. A.]

CY'PSELIS. (From κυψελη, a beehive.) The aperture of the ear, also the wax of the ear.

Cyrcne'sis. (From κυρκναω, to mix.) A mixture, or composition.

Cyrto'ma. (From κυρ7ος, curved.) 1. An unnatural convex tumour.

2. Tympanites.

Cyrtono'sus. (From κυρ7ος, curved, and νοσος, a disease.) 1. The rickets.

2. Curved spine.

CYRTOSIS. (*Cyrtosis, is.* f.; from κυρτος, *curvus, incurvus, gibbosus*, and among the ancients particularly imputed recurvation of the spine, or posterior crookedness, as λορδασις, imputed procurvation of the head and shoulders, or anterior crookedness.) The name of a genus of diseases in Good's Nosology. Class, *Eccritioa*; Order, *Mesotica*. Contortion of the bones; defined, head bulky, especially anteriorly; stature short and incurvated; flesh flabby, pale, and wrinkled. It has two species, *Cyrtosis rhachia*, and *C. cretenismus*, cretenism.

Cy'ssarus. (From κυσος, the anus.) The intestinum rectum is so called, because it reaches to the anus.

Cysso'tis. (From κυσος, the anus.) An inflammation of the anus.

CYSTEOLI'THUS. (Prom κυςις, the bladder, and λιθος, a stone.) A stone in the bladder, either urinary or gall-bladder.

Cy'sthus. Κυσθος. The anus.

CYSTIC. (*Cysticus*; from κυςις, a bag.) Belonging to the urinary or gall-bladder.

Cystic duct. See *Ductus cysticus*.

Cystic oxide. A peculiar animal product discovered by Dr. Wollaston. See *Calculus, urinary*.

Cy'stica. (*Cysticus*; from κυςις, the bladder.) Remedies for diseases of the bladder.

CY'STIDES. (*Cystis, idis.* f.; from κυςις, a bag.) Encysted tumours.

CYSTIPHLO'GIA. (From κυςις, the bladder, and φλεγω, to burn.) An inflammation in the bladder See *Cystitis*.

CYSTIRRHA'GIA. (From κυςις, the bladder, and ρηγνυμι, to burst forth.) A discharge from the bladder.

CY'STIS. (Κυςις, a bag.) 1. Cyst or bladder.

2. The urinary bladder.

3. The membranous or cyst surrounding or containing any morbid substance.

Cystis choledocha. See *Gall-bladder*

Cystis fellea. See *Gall-bladder*.

Cystis urinaria. See *Urinary bladder*.

CYSTI'TIS. (From κυςις, the bladder.) Inflammation of the bladder. A genus of disease arranged by Cullen in the class *Pyrexiæ*, and order *Phlegmasiæ*. It is known by great pain in the region of the bladder, attended with fever and hard pulse, a frequent and painful discharge of urine, or a suppression, and generally tenesmus. This is rarely a primary disease, and when it occurs, the above character of it will readily point it out. There also is frequently nausea and vomiting, and, in some cases, delirium. It most generally arises in consequence of inflammation of the adjacent parts, or from calculi in the bladder. The treatment is very similar to that of *Nephritis*; which see. When suppression of urine attends, the catheter must be occasionally introduced.

CYSTOCE'LE. (From κυςις, the bladder, and κηλη, a tumour.) A hernia formed by the protusion of the urinary bladder.

CYSTOLI'THICUS. (From κυςις, the bladder, and λιθος, a stone.) Having a stone in the bladder.

CYSTOPHLE'GICUS. (From κυςις, the bladder, and φλεγω, to burn.) An inflammation of the bladder.

CYSTOPHLEGMA'TICUS. (From κυςις, the bladder, and φλεγμα, phlegm.) Having matter or mucus in the bladder.

CYSTOPRO'CTICUS. (From κυςις, the bladder, and πρωκ7ος, the anus, or rectum.) A disease of the bladder and rectum.

CYSTOPTO'SIS. (From κυςις, the bladder, and πιπ7ω, to fall.) A protrusion of the inner membrane of the bladder, through the urethra.

CYSTOSPA'STICUS. (From κυςις, the bladder, and σπασμα, a spasm.) A spasm in the sphincter of the bladder.

CYSTOSPY'ICUS. (From κυςις, the bladder, and πυον, pus.) Purulent matter in the bladder.

CYSTOTHROMBOI'DES. (From κυςις, the bladder, and θρομβος, a coagulation of blood.) A concretion of grumous blood in the bladder.

CYSTOTO'MIA. (From κυςις, the bladder, and 7εμνω, to cut.) The operation of cutting or piercing the bladder.

Cy'thion. An eye-wash.

CY'TINUS. (Perhaps, as Martyn suggests, from κυ7ινοι, a name given by Theophrastus to the blossoms of the pomegranate, the calyx of which the flower in question resembles in shape.) The name of a genus of plants. Class, *Gynandria*; Order, *Octandria* of Linnæus.

Cytinus hypocistis. Rape of Cystus. A fleshy pale-yellowish plant, parasitical on the roots of several species of cystus in the south of Europe, from which the *succus hypocistidus* is obtained.

Cytiso-genista. Common broom. See *Spartium scoparium*.

Cyzemer. A swelling of the wrists.

Cyzice'nus. A plaster for wounds of the nerves.

D

DACNE'RUS. (From δακνω, to bite.) Biting. Pungent. An epithet for a sharp eye-wash, composed of burnt copper, pepper, cadmia, myrrh, and opium.

Dacry'dium. (From δακρυ, a tear.) The inspissated juice of scammony, in small drops, and therefore called a tear.

DACRYGELO'SIS. (From δακρυω, to weep, and γελαω, to laugh.) A species of insanity, in which the patient weeps and laughs at the same time.

Dacryo'des. (From δακρυω, to weep.) A sanious, or weeping ulcer.

DACRYO'MA. (From δακρυω, to weep.) A closing of one or more of the puncta lachrymalia, causing an effusion of tears.

Dactyle'thra (From δακ7υλος, a finger.) A species of bougies shaped like a finger, to excite vomiting.

Dactyle'tus. (From δακ7υλος, the date.) The hermodactyl. See *Hermodactylus*.

Da'ctylius. (From δακ7υλος, a finger.) A round pastil, troche, or lozenge, shaped like a finger.

DA'CTYLUS. (From δακ7υλος, a finger; so called

from the likeness of its fruit to a finger.) 1. A finger. See *Digitus*.

2. The date. See *Phœnix dactylifera*.

DÆ'DIUM. (From δαις, a torch. A small torch or candle. A bougie.

DÆMONOMA'NIA. (From δαιμων, a dæmon, and μανια, madness.) That species of melancholy where the patient supposes himself to be possessed by devils.

DAISY. See *Bellis perennis*.

Daisy, ox-eye. See *Chrysanthemum leucanthemum*.

DALE, SAMUEL, was born in 1659. After practising as an apothecary, he became a licentiate of the college of physicians, and settled at Bocking, where he continued till his death in 1739. He was also chosen a fellow of the Royal Society. In 1693, he published his "Pharmacologia," an Introduction to the Materia Medica, which he afterward much enlarged and improved; the work was well received, and passed through many editions. He also gave a good account of the natural productions about Harwich and Dover Court.

Damask rose. See *Rosa centifolia*.

DAMNA'TUS. (From *damno*, to condemn.) The dry useless fæces, left in a vessel after the moisture has been distilled from it, is called terra damnata, or *caput mortuum*.

DAMSON. The fruit of a variety of the *Prunus domestica*.

[DANA, JAMES FREEMAN, M. D., was the oldest son of Luther Dana, Esq., and was born in Amherst, in the state of New-Hampshire, in September 1793. After his graduation, he commenced the study of medicine under Dr. John Gorham, at that time Professor of Chemistry in Harvard University. In the year 1815, before he had completed his professional studies, he had become so well known as a practical chemist, that he was selected by the University to go to London, as an agent, for the purpose of procuring a new apparatus for the chemical department. While in England, where he remained several months, he prosecuted the study of chemistry in the Laboratory of Accum, a celebrated operative chemist.

With Dartmouth College he remained connected, in the capacity of Lecturer on Chemistry, until the year 1820, when he received the appointment of Professor of Chemistry and Mineralogy in the same institution. This office he held until the year 1826; and those who enjoyed the privilege of hearing his admirable lectures, will long remember with what ability and success he discharged its duties. In 1826 he was appointed one of the Board of Visiters of the Military Academy at West Point; and, immediately after his return from the discharge of this duty, he was appointed Professor of Chemistry in the University of New-York. This appointment, which opened a wide field for the exertion of his talents, he readily accepted, and removed with his family to the city, in the autumn of the same year. About six months after his removal to New-York, he sunk under an attack of erysipelas, at the early age of 33, and when just entering upon an extended sphere of usefulness and honour.

His principal publications were the following, viz. "Outlines of the Mineralogy and Geology of Boston and its Vicinity:" "Epitome of Chemical Philosophy:" "Report on a singular Disease of horned Cattle, in the Town of Burton, New-Hampshire." Besides these publications, he contributed several papers to the American Journal of Science, the New-England Journal of Medicine, and the Annals of the Lyceum of Natural History of New-York, some of them of very considerable merit, and some of which have been reprinted in Europe."—*Thatch. Med. Biog*. A.]

DANDELION. See *Leontodon Taraxacum*.

DANDRIF. See *Pityriasis*.

DANEWORT. See *Sambucus Ebulus*.

DAOURITE. A variety of red schorl from Siberia.

DA'PHNE. (*Daphne*, δαφνη; from δαω, to burn, and φωνη, a noise: because of the noise it makes when burnt.) The name of a genus of plants in the Linnæan system. Class, *Octandria*; Order, *Monogynia*. The laurel, or bay-tree.

DAPHNE ALPINA. *Chamælea*; *Chamelæa*. This species of dwarf olive-tree is said to be purgative in the dose of ℈ij, and is sometimes given by country people. The French chemists have lately examined it chemically. See *Daphnin*.

2. The mezereon is also so called, because it has leaves like the olive-tree. See *Daphne mezereum*.

Daphne, flax-leaved. See *Daphne gnidium*.

DAPHNE GNIDIUM. The systematic name of the tree which affords the Garou bark. *Daphne:—panicula terminali foliis lineari-lanceolatis acuminatis* of Linnæus. *Thymelæa; Oneoron*. Spurge-flax; Flax-leaved Daphne. Garou bark, which very much resembles that of our mezereum, is to be immersed in vinegar for about an hour before it is wanted; a small piece, the size of a sixpence, thus steeped, is applied to the arm or any other part, and renewed once a day in winter and twice in summer. It produces a serous exudation from the skin without irritating or blistering. It is recommended, and is in frequent use in France and Russia, against some diseases of the eyes.

DAPHNE LAUREOLA. The systematic name of the spurge-laurel. *Laureola daphnoides*. The bark of this plant is recommended to excite a discharge from the skin, in the same way as that of the *Daphne gnidium*.

DAPHNE MEZEREUM. The systematic name of the mezereon. Spurge-olive; Widow-wail. *Mezereum*. *Daphne—floribus sessilibus ternis caulinis, foliis lanceolatis deciduis*, of Linnæus. This plant is extremely acrid, especially when fresh, and, if retained in the mouth, excites great and long-continued heat and inflammation, particularly of the mouth and fauces; the berries, *grana cnidii* of old writers, also have the same effects, and, when swallowed, prove a powerful corrosive poison, not only to man, but to dogs, wolves, and foxes. The bark of the root is the part employed medicinally in the *decoctum sarsaparillæ compositum*, intended to assist mercury in resolving nodes and other obstinate symptoms of syphilis. The antisyphilitic virtues of mezereum, however, have been by many writers very justly doubted. "The result of my own experience (says Mr. Pearson, of the Lock Hospital) by no means accords with the representation given of this root by former writers. From all that I have been able to collect, in the course of many years' observation, I feel myself authorized to assert, unequivocally, that the mezereum has not the power of curing the venereal disease in any one stage, or under any one form. If a decoction of this root should ever reduce a venereal node, where no mercury has been previously given, yet the patient will by no means be exempted from the necessity of employing mercury for as long a space of time, and in as large a quantity, as if no mezereum had been taken. With respect to the power it is said to possess, of alleviating the pain, and diminishing the bulk of membraneous nodes, nothing peculiar and appropriate can be ascribed to the mezereum on these accounts, since we obtain the same good effects from sarsaparilla, guaiacum, volatile alkali, blistering plasters, &c. Nevertheless, venereal nodes, which have subsided under the use of any of these articles of the materia medica, will appear again, and often with additional symptoms, if a full and efficacious course of mercury be not submitted to. It has, indeed, been alleged, that mezereum always alleviates the pain occasioned by a venereal node, and generally reduces it, where the periosteum only is affected; and that it seldom fails of removing those enlargements of the periosteum which have not yielded during the administration of mercury.

That some instances of success, in cases like these, may have fallen to the share of those who made the assertion, it would not become me to deny; but I have met with few such agreeable evidences of the efficacy of this medicine. I have given the mezereum in the form of a simple decoction, and also as an ingredient in compound decoctions of the woods, in many cases, where no mercury had been previously employed, but never with advantage to a single patient. I have also tried it, in numerous instances, after the completion of a course of mercury; yet, with the exception of two cases, where the thickened state of the periosteum was removed during the exhibition of it, I never saw the least benefit derived from taking this medicine In a few cases of anomalous pains, which I supposed were derived from irregularities during a mercurial course, the mezereum was of service, after I had tried the common decoction of the woods without success; but even in this description of cases, I have always found it a very uncertain remedy. I have made trial of this vegetable in a great number of scrofulous cases, where the membranes covering the bones were in a diseased state, and I am not sure that one single patient obtained any evident and material benefit from it.

The late Dr. Cullen, whose reports may justly claim attention from all medical men, when treating of the mezereum, in his Materia Medica, says, "I have frequently employed it in several cutaneous affections, and sometimes with success." It were to have been wished, that the professor of medicine had specified what those diseases of the skin were, in which the mezereum was sometimes employed with success; for, if I except an instance or two of lepra, in which the decoction of this plant conferred a temporary benefit, I have very seldom found it possessed of medicinal virtue, either in syphilis, or in the sequelæ of that disease, in scrofula or in cutaneous affections. Indeed the mezereum is of so acrimonious a nature, often producing heat and other disagreeable sensations in the fauces, and, on many occasions, disordering the primæ viæ, that I do not often subject my patients, to the certain inconveniences which are connected with the primary effects of this medicine, as they are rarely compensated by any other important and useful qualities."

DAPHNELÆ'ON. (From δαφνη, the laurel, and ελαιον, oil.) The oil of bay-berries.

DAPHNIN. The bitter principle of the *Daphne alpina*, discovered by Vauquelin. From the alkoholic infusion of this bark, the resin was separated by its concentration. On diluting the tincture with water, filtering and adding acetate of lead, a yellow *daphnate* of lead fell, from which sulphuretted hydrogen separated the lead, and left the daphnin in small transparent crystals. They are hard, of a grayish colour, a bitter taste when heated, evaporate in acrid acid vapours, sparingly soluble in cold, but moderately in boiling water. It is stated, that its solution is not precipitated by acetate of lead; yet acetate of lead is employed in the first process to throw it down.

DAPHNI'TIS. (From δαφνη, the laurel.) A sort of cassia resembling the laurel.

DAPHNOI'DES. (From δαφνη, the laurel, and ειδος, a likeness.) The herb spurge laurel. See *Daphne laureola*.

DA'RSIN. (From *darzin*, Arabian.) The grosser sort of cinnamon.

DA'RSIS. (From δερω, to excoriate.) An excoriation.

DA'RTOS. (From δερω, to excoriate: so called from its raw and excoriated appearance.) The part so called, under the skin of the scrotum, is by some anatomists considered as a muscle, although it appears to be no more than a condensation of the cellular membrane lining the scrotum. It is by means of the dartos that the skin of the scrotum is corrugated and relaxed.

DARWIN, ERASMUS, was born at Elton, in Nottinghamshire, in 1731. After studying at Cambridge and Edinburgh, and becoming doctor of medicine, he went to settle at Litchfield. He had soon after the good fortune to succeed in the cure of a gentleman in the neighbourhood, who was so ill of a fever, as to have been given over by the physician previously in attendance: this speedily procured him very extensive practice. He soon after married, and by his first wife had three sons, of whom only one survived him. At the age of 50, he married again, and removed to Derby, where he continued till his death in 1802, leaving six children by his second wife. The active life he led, and his very temperate habits, preserved his health and faculties in a great degree unimpaired. He distinguished himself more as a poet, than by professional improvements: though he certainly suggested some ingenious methods of practice; but, warned by preceding examples, he avoided publishing any material poem, till his medical fame was thoroughly established. His "Botanic Garden," and "Zoonomia," are well known, but they have long ceased to be popular: and the philosophy of the latter work, which advocates materialism, is justly censured. He communicated to the College of Physicians an account of his successful use of digitalis in dropsy, and some other diseases, which was published in their Transactions. His son *Charles*, who died while studying at Edinburgh, obtained a gold medal by an Essay on the distinction of Pus and Mucus; and left another unfinished on the Retrograde Action of the Absorbents: which were published after his death by his father.

DASY'MNA. (From δασυς, rough.) A scabby roughness of the eyelids.

DA'SYS. (Δασυς, rough.) 1. A dry, parched tongue, 2. Difficult respiration.

DATE. See *Dactylus*.

Date plum, Indian. See *Dyospyrus lotus*.

DATOLYTE. Datholit of Werner. A species of silicious ore divided into common datolyte and botroidal datolyte.

[This is the silicious borate of lime, called *Datholit*, by Werner and Brogniart. It was discovered by Esmark. "It is sometimes in prismatic crystals, with ten sides, having two opposite solid angles on each base truncated. The primitive form is a right prism, whose bases are rhombs, with angles of 109° 28′ and 70° 32′. It also appears in large granular concretions, which frequently discover indications of a prismatic form; also in grains or amorphous. The surface of the concretions is rough and glimmering.

Its hardness enables it to scratch fluate of lime, and its specific gravity is 2.98. Its fracture is imperfectly conchoidal, shining, and nearly vitreous. Its colour is white, shaded with gray or green, often very delicately.

When exposed to the flame of a candle, it assumes a dull white colour, and becomes very brittle, even between the fingers. Before the blowpipe it swells into a milk-white mass, and then melts into a pale rose-coloured glass. It is composed of

Lime	35.5
Silex	36.5
Boracic acid	24.0
Water	4.0
	——100

Cleav. Min. A.]

DATU'RA. (Blanchard says, it is derived from the Indian word *datiro*, of which he knows not the meaning.) The name of a genus of plants in the Linnæan system. Class, *Pentandria*; Order, *Monogynia*.

DATURA STRAMONIUM. The systematic name of the thorn-apple. *Stramonium; Dutray; Barryo coccalon; Solanum maniacum* of Dioscorides. *Stramonium spinosum* of Gerard. *Solanum fœtidum* of Bauhin. *Stramonium majus album.* Common thorn-apple *Datura—pericarpiis spinosis erectis ovatis, foliis ovatis glabris*, of Linnæus. This plant has been long known as a powerful narcotic poison. In its recent state it has a bitterish taste, and a smell somewhat resembling that of poppies, especially if the leaves be rubbed between the fingers. Instances of the deleterious effects of the plant are numerous, more particularly of the seed. An extract prepared from the seeds is recommended by Baron Stoerck in maniacal, epileptic, and convulsive affections; and is said by some to succeed, while, in the hands of others, it has failed. In this country, says Dr. Woodville, we are unacquainted with any practitioners whose experience tends to throw light on the medical character of this plant. It appears to us, continues Dr. Woodville, that its effects as a medicine are to be referred to no other power than that of a narcotic. And Dr. Cullen, speaking on this subject, says, "I have no doubt that narcotics may be a remedy in certain cases of mania and epilepsy; but I have not, and I doubt if any other person has, learned to distinguish the cases to which such remedies are properly adapted. It is therefore that we find the other narcotics, as well as the stramonium, to fail in the same hands in which they had in other cases seemed to succeed. It is this consideration that has occasioned my neglecting the use of stramonium, and therefore prevented me from speaking more precisely from my own experience on this subject."

The extract of this plant has been the preparation usually employed from one to ten grains and upwards a day; but the powdered leaves, prepared after the manner of those of hemlock, would seem to be more certain and convenient. Greding found the strength of the extract to vary exceedingly; that which he obtaintained from Ludwig was much more powerful than that which he had of Stoerck. Externally, the leaves of stramonium have been applied to inflammatory tumours and burns, and it is said with success, and of late, the dried leaves have been smoked as a remedy in asthma; but it does not appear that they have been more efficacious in this way than tobacco.

[The *Stramonium* is known in different parts of the United States, by the name of *Thorn-apple, Jamestown-*

weed, *Stink-weed*, &c. All parts of the plant appear to be poisonous. Some soldiers died, during the revolutionary war, by eating the young plants, for greens, early in the spring. I have seen children labouring under the effects of the poison from having swallowed the seeds, and from drinking a decoction of herbs in which some of the young seed-vessels, and small leaves, of the stramonium had been accidentally mixed.

The poison of the stramonium produces, in children, a peculiar spasmodic delirium, attended with dilatation of the pupils of the eyes, heat of the skin, and a flush of the face. The ripe or unripe seeds, or the leaves, produce the same effect, and the only remedy is to discharge them from the stomach by emetics, as soon as possible. A.]

DAUBENTON, Lewis Mary, was born in Burgundy, 1716. Having become doctor in medicine at the age of 24, he went to Paris, and being very zealous in the study of comparative anatomy, the office of keeper of the royal cabinet of natural history was procured for him by the celebrated Buffon. He contributed materially to enrich the splendid work of that eminent naturalist, by furnishing the anatomy both of man and animals. He was a member of several distinguished societies, among others of the Royal Academy of Sciences at Paris, to which he made some useful communications. Having escaped the revolutionary horrors in France, he was chosen, in 1799, a member of the Conservative Senate: but he died towards the end of the same year.

Dauc'ites vinum. Wild-carrot seeds, steeped in must.

DAU'CUS. Απου του δαυειν, from its relieving the colic, and discussing flatulencies.) The carrot. 1. The name of a genus of plants in the Linnæan system. Class, *Pentandria;* Order, *Digynia.*

2. The pharmacopœial name of the garden carrot. See *Daucus carota.*

Daucus alsaticus. The *Oreoselinum pratense*, of Linnæus.

Daucus annuus minor. The *Caucalis anthriscus*, of Linnæus.

Daucus carota. The systematic name of the carrot plant. *Daucus; Daucus sylvestris; Pastinaca sylvestris tenuifolia officinarum; Daucus—seminibus hispidis, petiolis subtus nervosis*, of Linnæus. The cultivated root, scraped, and applied in the form of a poultice, is a useful application to phagedænic ulcers, and to cancers and putrid sores. The seeds, which obtain a place in the materia medica, have a light aromatic smell, and a warm acrid taste, and are esteemed for their diuretic qualities, and for their utility in calculous and nephritic complaints, in which an infusion of three spoonfuls of the seeds, in a pint of boiling water, has been recommended; or the seeds may be fermented in malt liquor, which receives from them an agreeable flavour, resembling that of lemon-peel. The boiled root is said by many to be difficult of digestion; but this is the case only when the stomach is weak. It contains a considerable quantity of the saccharine principle, and is very nutritious.

Daucus creticus. See *Athamanta cretensis.*

Daucus sativus. A variety of the *Daucus carota*, the seeds of which are preferred by some practitioners,

Daucus seprinius. Common chervil.

Daucus sylvestris. Wild carrot, or bird's nest. The seeds of the wild plant are said to be more efficacious than those of the garden carrot; they possess demulcent and aromatic qualities, and are given, in infusion, or decoction, in calculous complaints.

DAY-MARE. See *Ephialtes.*

DAY-SIGHT. See *Paropsis noctifuga.*

Dead nettle. See *Lamium album.*

Deadly nightshade. See *Atropa belladonna.*

DEAFNESS. *Surditas.* See *Paracusis.*

Deaf-dumbness. Speechlessness, from deafness.

Dearticula'tio. (From *de*, and *articulus*, a joint.) Articulation admitting evident motion.

Deascia'tio. (From *de*, and *ascio*, to chip, as with a hatchet.) A bone splintered on its side.

DECAGY'NIA. (From δεκα, ten, and γυνη, a woman.) The name of an order of the class *Decandria*, of the sexual system of plants. See *Plants.*

Decamy'ron. (From δεκα, ten, and 'μυρον, an ointment.) An aromatic ointment, mentioned by Oribasius, containing ten ingredients.

DECA'NDRIA. (From δεκα, ten, and ανηρ, a man.) The name of a class, and also of an order of plants in the sexual system. See *Plants.*

Decide'ntia. (From *decido*, to fall down.) Any change prolonging acute diseases.

DECI'DUA. (*Deciduus;* from *decido*, to fall off.) *Membrana decidua.* A very thin and delicate membrane or tunic, which adheres to the gravid uterus, and is said to be a reflection of the chorion, and, on that account, is called *decidua reflexa.* The tunica decidua comes away after delivery, in small pieces, mixed with the *lochia.*

DECI'DUUS. (From *decido*, to fall off, or down: to die.) Deciduous; falling off. Applied to trees and shrubs, which, in most European countries, lose their leaves as winter approaches, and to the *perianthium* of *Tilia europæa*, which does not fall off until after the flower is expanded.

This term is expressive of the second stage of duration, and, like *caducous*, has a different application according to the particular part to which it refers: thus leaves are deciduous which drop off in the autumn, petals which fall off with the stamina and pistils; and calyces are *deciduous* which fall off after the the expansion, and before the dropping of the flower.

DECIMA'NUS. (From *decem*, ten, and *mane*, the morning.) Returning every tenth day, applied to some erratic fevers.

DECLI'VIS. (From *de*, and *clivis*, a hill.) Declining, descending. A name of an abdominal muscle, because of its posture.

DECO'CTUM. (From *decoquo*, to boil.) A decoction. Any medicine made by boiling in a watery fluid. In a chemical point of view, it is a continued ebullition with water, to separate such parts of bodies as are only soluble at that degree of heat. The following are among the most approved decoctions.

Decoctum album. See *Mistura cornu usti.*

Decoctum aloes compositum. Compound decoction of aloes. Take of extract of liquorice, half an ounce; subcarbonate of potassa, two scruples; extract of spiked aloe powdered, myrrh powdered, saffron stigmata, of each a drachm; water, a pint. Boil down to twelve fluid ounces, and strain; then add compound tincture of cardamoms, four fluid ounces. This decoction, now first introduced into the London Pharmacopœia, is analogous to an article in very frequent use, invented by the late Dr. Devalingin, and sold under the name of *Beaume de vie.* By the proportion of tincture which is added, it will keep unchanged for any length of time.

Decoctum althææ. Decoction of marsh mallows. Take of dried marsh-mallow roots, ℥ iv; raisins of the sun, stoned, ℥ ij; water ℔vij. Boil to five pounds; place apart the strained liquor, till the fæces have subsided, then pour off the clear part. This preparation, directed in the Edinburgh Pharmacopœia, may be exhibited as a common drink in nephralgia, and many diseases of the urinary passages, with advantage.

Decoctum anthemidis. See *Decoctum chamæmeli.*

Decoctum astragali. Take of the root of the astragalus escapus, ℥ j; distilled water, ℔iij. These are to be boiled, till only a quart of fluid remain. The whole is to be taken, a little warmed, in the course of 24 hours. This remedy was tried very extensively in Germany, and said to evince very powerful effects, as an antisyphilitic.

Decoctum bardanæ. Take of bardana root, ℥ vj; of distilled water, ℔vj. These are to be boiled till only two quarts remain. From a pint to a quart in a day is given, in those cases where sarsaparilla and other remedies, that are called alterative, are supposed to be requisite.

Decoctum chamæmeli. Chamomile decoction. Take of chamomile flowers, ℥ j; caraway seeds, ℥ ss; water, ℔v. Boil fifteen minutes, and strain. A very common and excellent vehicle for tonic powders, pills, &c. It is also in very frequent use for fomentation, and clysters.

Decoctum cinchonæ. Decoction of cinchona, commonly called decoction of Peruvian bark. Take of lance-leaved cinchona bark bruised, an ounce; water, a pint. Boil for ten minutes, in a vessel slightly covered, and strain the decoction while hot. According to the option of the practitioner, the bark of either of the other species of cinchona, the cordifolia, or *yellow*, or the oblongifolia, or *red*, may be substituted for the lancifolia, or *quilled;* which is here directed. This way of administering the bark is very general, as all the other preparations may be mixed with it, as necessity requires. It is a very proper fomentation for prolapsus of the uterus and rectum.

Decoctum cornu. See *Mistura cornu usti.*

Decoctum cydoniæ. *Mucilago seminis cydonii malii. Mucilago seminum cydoniorum.* Decoction of quince seeds. Take of quince seeds, two drachms; water, a pint. Boil over a gentle fire for ten minutes, then strain. This decoction, in the new London Pharmacopœia, has been removed from among the mucilages, as being less dense than either of the others, and as being employed in larger doses, like other mucilaginous decoctions. In addition to gum, it contains other constituent parts of the seeds, and is, therefore, more apt to spoil than common mucilage, over which it possesses no other advantages, than that it is more grateful, and sufficiently thin, without further dilution, to form the bulk of any liquid medicine. Its virtues are demulcent. Joined with syrup of mulberry and a little borax, it is useful against aphthæ of the mouth and fauces.

Decoctum daphnes mezerei. Decoction of mezereon. Take of the bark of mezereon root, ℥ij; liquorice root, bruised, ℥ss; water, ℔iij. Boil it, with a gentle heat, down to two pounds, and strain it. From four to eight ounces of this decoction may be given four times a day, in some obstinate venereal and rheumatic affections. It operates chiefly by perspiration.

Decoctum dulcamaræ. Decoction of woody nightshade. Take of woody nightshade stalks, newly gathered, ℥j; distilled water, ℔iss. These are to be boiled away to a pint, and strained. The dose is half an ounce to two ounces, mixed with an equal quantity of milk. This remedy is employed in inveterate cases of scrofula; in cancer and phagedæna; in lepra, and other cutaneous affections; and in anomalous local diseases, originating in venereal lues.

Decoctum geoffrææ inermis. Decoction of cabbage-tree plant. Take of bark of the cabbage-tree, powdered, ℥j; water, ℔ij. Boil it, with a gentle fire, down to one pound, and strain. This is a powerful anthelmintic. It may be given in doses of one tablespoonful to children, and four to adults. If disagreeable symptoms should arise from an over-dose, or from drinking cold water during its action, we must immediately purge with castor oil, and dilute with acidulated drinks.

Decoctum guaiaci officinalis compositum. *Decoctum lignorum.* Compound decoction of guaiacum, commonly called decoction of the woods. Take of guaiacum raspings, ℥iij; raisins, stoned, ℥ij; sassafras root, liquorice, each, ℥j; water, ℔x. Boil the guaiacum and raisins with the water, over a gentle fire, to the consumption of one half; adding, towards the end, the sassafras and liquorice. Strain the liquor without expression. This decoction possesses stimulant and diaphoretic qualities, and is generally exhibited in rheumatic and cutaneous diseases, which are dependent on a vitiated state of the humours. It may be taken by itself, to the quantity of a quarter of a pint, twice or thrice a day, or used as an assistant in a course of mercurial or antimonial alteratives; the patient, in either case, keeping warm, in order to promote the operation of the medicine.

Decoctum hellebori albi. Decoction of white hellebore. Take of the root of white hellebore, powdered, by weight, ℥j; water, two pints; rectified spirits of wine, ℥ij, by measure. Boil the water, with the root, to one pint; and the liquor being cold and strained, add to it the spirit. This decoction, in the last London Pharmacopœia, is called decoctum veratri. It is a very efficacious application, externally, as a wash, in tinea capitis, lepra, psora, &c. When the skin is very tender and irritable, it should be diluted with an equal quantity of water.

Decoctum hordei. *Decoctum hordei distichi. Aqua hordeata.* Take of pearl barley, ℥ij; water, four pints and a half. First wash away any adhering extraneous substances with cold water; next, having poured upon the barley half a pint of water, boil for a few minutes. Let this water be thrown away, and add the remainder of the water boiling; then boil down to two pints, and strain. Barley-water is a nutritive and softening drink, and the most proper of all liquors in inflammatory diseases. It is an excellent gargle in inflammatory sore throats, mixed with a little nitre.

Decoctum hordei compositum. *Decoctum pectorale.* Compound decoction of barley. Take of decoction of barley, two pints; figs, sliced, ℥ij; liquorice root, sliced and bruised, ℥ss; raisins, stoned, ℥ij; water, a pint. Boil down to two pints and strain. From the pectoral and demulcent qualities of this decoction, it may be administered as a common drink in fevers and other acute disorders, in catarrh, and several affections of the chest.

Decoctum hordei cum gummi. Barley-water, ℔ij; gum arab., ℥j. The gum is to be dissolved in the barley decoction, while warm. It then forms a suitable diluent in strangury, dysury, &c. for the gum, finding a passage into the bladder, in an unaltered state, mixes with the urine, and prevents the action of its neutral salts on the urinary canal.

Decoctum lichenis. Decoction of Iceland moss or liverwort. Take of liverwort, one ounce; water, a pint and a half. Boil down to a pint, and strain. The dose is from ℥j to ℥iv.

[The Iceland moss was once in great repute as a remedy in consumption, the decoction being made with milk, but it is no longer in repute, being considered a weak mucilagious bitter of little or no efficacy. A.]

Decoctum lobeliæ. Take a handful of the roots of the *Lobelia syphilitica;* distilled water, ℔xij. These are to be boiled in the usual way, till only four quarts remain. The very desirable property of curing the venereal disease has been attributed to this medicine, but it is not more to be depended on than guaiacum, or other vegetable substances, of which the same thing has been alleged. The effects of this decoction are purgative, and the manner of taking it, as described by Swediaur, is as follows:—The patient is to begin with half a pint, twice a day. The same quantity is then to be taken, four times a day, and continued so long as its purgative effect is not too considerable. When the case is otherwise, it is to be discontinued for three or four days, and then had recourse to again till the cure is completed. As this is a remedy on the old system, and not admitted into our pharmacopœias, little confidence ought to be placed in it.

Decoctum lusitanicum. Take of sliced sarsaparilla, lignum sassafras, lignum santalum rubrum, officinal lignum guaiacum, of each one ounce and a half; of the root of mezereon, coriander seed, of each half an ounce; distilled water, ten pounds. These are to be boiled till only half the fluid remains. The dose is a quart or more in a day.

Take of sliced sarsaparilla, lignum santalum rubrum, lignum santalum citrinum, of each, ℥iss; of the root of glycirrhiza and mezereon, of each, ʒij; of lignum rhodii, officinal lignum guaiacum, and lignum sassafras, of each, ℥ss; of antimony, ℥j; distilled water, ℔v. These ingredients are to be macerated for twenty-four hours, and afterward boiled, till the fluid is reduced to half its original quantity. From one to four pints are given daily.

The late Mr. Hunter notices this, and also the following formula, in his Treatise on the Venereal Disease.

Take of sliced sarsaparilla, of the root of China, of each ℥j; walnut peels dried, xx; antimony, ℥ij, pumice-stone, powdered, ℥j; distilled water, ℔x. The powdered antimony and pumice-stone are to be tied in separate pieces of rag, and boiled, along with the other ingredients. This last decoction is reckoned to be the genuine Lisbon diet drink, the qualities of which have been the subject of so much encomium.

Decoctum malvæ compositum. *Decoctum pro enemate. Decoctum commune pro clystere.* Compound decoction of mallows. Take of mallows dried, an ounce; chamomile flowers dried, half an ounce; water, a pint. Boil for a quarter of an hour, and strain. A very excellent form for an emollient clyster. A variety of medicines may be added to answer particular indications.

Decoctum mezerei. See *Decoctum daphnes mezerei.*

Decoctum papaveris. *Decoctum pro fomento. Fotus communis.* Decoction of poppy. Take of white poppy capsules bruised, ℥iv; water, four pints Boil for a quarter of an hour, and strain. This pre paration possesses sedative and antiseptic properties, and may be directed with advantage in sphacelus, &c.

DECOCTUM PRO ENEMATE. See *Decoctum malvæ compositum.*

DECOCTUM PRO FOMENTO. See *Decoctum papaveris.*

DECOCTUM QUERCUS. Decoction of oak bark. Take of oak bark, ℥j; water, two pints. Boil down to a pint, and strain. This astringent decoction has lately been added to the Lond. Pharm., and is chiefly used for external purposes. It is a good remedy in prolapsus ani, and may be used also in some cases as an injection.

DECOCTUM SARSAPARILLÆ. Decoction of sarsaparilla. Take of sarsaparilla root, sliced, ℥iv; boiling water, four pints. Macerate for four hours, in a vessel lightly covered, near the fire; then take out the sarsaparilla and bruise it. After it is bruised, put it again into the liquor, and macerate it in a similar manner for two hours more; then boil it down to two pints, and strain.

This decoction is much extolled by some practitioners, in phthisis, and to restore the strength after a long course of mercury.

DECOCTUM SARSAPARILLÆ COMPOSITUM. Compound decoction of sarsaparilla. Take of decoction of sarsaparilla boiling, four pints; sassafras root sliced, guaiacum wood shavings, liquorice root bruised, of each an ounce; mezereon root bark, ʒiij. Boil for a quarter of an hour, and strain. The alterative property of the compound is very great; it is generally given after a course of mercury, where there have been nodes and indolent ulcerations, and with great benefit. The dose is from half a pint to a pint in twenty-four hours.

DECOCTUM SENEGÆ. Decoction of senega. Take of senega root, ℥j; water, two pints. Boil down to a pint, and strain. This is now first introduced into the Lond. Pharm. as being a useful medicine, especially in affections of the lungs, attended with debility and inordinate secretion.

DECOCTUM ULMI. Decoction of elm bark. Take of fresh elm bark bruised, four ounces; water, four pints. Boil down to two pints, and strain. This may be employed with great advantage as a collyrium in chronic ophthalmia. It is given internally in some cutaneous eruptions.

DECOCTUM VERATRI. See *Decoctum hellebori albi.*

[The Pharmacopœia of the United States contains the following decoctions.

DECOCTUM ARALIÆ NUDICAULIS. *Decoction of false sarsaparilla.*

DECOCTUM CINCHONÆ. *Decoction of Peruvian bark.*

DECOCTUM COLOMBÆ COMPOSITUM. *Compound decoction of Columbo.*

DECOCTUM DULCAMARÆ. *Decoction of bitter-sweet.*

DECOCTUM GUAIACI. *Decoction of guaiacum.*

DECOCTUM HORDEI. *Decoction of barley.*

DECOCTUM HORDEI COMPOSITUM. *Compound decoction of barley.*

DECOCTUM LICHENIS. *Decoction of Iceland moss.*

DECOCTUM MEZEREI. *Decoction of mezereon.*

DECOCTUM SARSAPARILLÆ. *Decoction of sarsaparilla.*

DECOCTUM SARSAPARILLÆ COMPOSITUM. *Compound decoction of sarsaparilla.*

DECOCTUM SCILLÆ. *Decoction of squill.*

DECOCTUM SENEGÆ. *Decoction of seneca snake root.*

DECOCTUM VERATRI. *Decoction of white hellebore.* A.]

DECOLLA'TIO. (From *decollo*, to behead.) The loss of a part of the skull.

DECOMPOSITÆ. The name of a class in Sauvage's Methodus Foliorum, consisting of such as have twice compounded leaves; that is, have a common footstalk supporting a number of less leaves, each of which is compounded; as in *Fumaria*, and many umbelliferous plants.

DECOMPOSITION. *Decompositio.* The separation of the component parts or principles of bodies from each other. The decomposition of bodies forms a very large part of chemical science. It seems probable, from the operations we are acquainted with, that it seldom takes place but in consequence of some combinations or composition having been effected. It would be difficult to point out an instance of the separation of any of the principles of bodies which has been effected, unless in consequence of some new combination. The only exceptions seem to consist in those separations which are made by heat, and voltaic electricity.

DECOMPOSITUS. A term applied to leaves, and means doubly compound. Sir James Smith observes, that Linnæus, in his Philosophia Botanica, gives an erroneous definition of this term which does not agree with his own use of it. The *Ægopodium podagraria* and *Fulmaria claviculata*, afford examples of the decomposite leaves. *Supra decompositum*, means thrice compound, or more; as in *Caucalis anthriscus*. The decomposite flowers are such as contain within a common calyx a number of less or partial flower-cups, each of which is composed of many florets.

DECORTICATION. (*Decorticatio;* from *de*, from, and *cortex*, bark.) The stripping of any thing of its bark, husk, or shell; thus almonds, and the like, are decorticated, that is, deprived of their pellicle, when ordered for medicinal purposes.

[There is a natural and artificial decortication performed on certain trees. The shag-bark hickory-tree (juglans alba) throws off its bark by a natural and spontaneous decortication. So does the button-wood (platanus occidentalis) or plane-tree. The cork-tree is deprived of its bark artificially every few years, and lives longer than those trees which are suffered to grow without molestation. Those not decorticated become shaggy and hide-bound, while the others form a new bark and improve in appearance and vigour. These facts suggested the idea of improving fruit-trees that had become hide-bound and shaggy, and appeared to be in a state of decay. Dr. Mitchill first tried the experiment on an old apple-tree, and by removing the old bark, in the warm season, from the body of the tree, and protecting it from external injury for a time, he succeeded in producing a new bark and in regenerating a tree which was considered as past bearing. The tree became vigorous, again put forth blossoms and bore fruit. Since that experiment, it has become common in apple orchards to improve old trees by a similar process. A.]

DECREPITATION. (*Decrepitatio;* from *decrepo*, to crackle.) A kind of crackling noise, which takes place in some bodies, when heated: it is peculiar to some kinds of salts, as muriate of soda, sulphate of barytes, &c.

DECUMBENS. (From *decumbo*, to lie down.) Drooping: a term applied to flowers which incline to one side and downwards.

DECURRENS. Decurrent. A term applied by botanists to leaves which run down the stem or leafy border or wing; as in *Onopordium acanthium*, and many thistles, great mullein, and comfrey: and to leafstalks; as in *Pisum ochrus.*

DECURSIVE. Decurrently. Applied to leaflets that run down the stem; as in *Eryngium campestre.*

DECUSSATION. (*Decussatio;* from *decutio*, to divide.) When nerves, or muscular fibres cross one another, they are said to decussate each other.

DECUSSATUS. Decussated. Applied to leaves and spines which are in pairs, alternately crossing each other; as in *Veronica decussata*, and *Genista lucitanica.*

DECUSSO'RIUM. (From *decusso*, to divide.) An instrument to depress the dura mater, after trepanning.

DEFENSI'VA. (From *defendo*, to preserve.) Cordial medicines, or such as resist infection.

DE'FERENS. (From *defero*, to convey; because it conveys the semen to the vesiculæ seminales.) See *Vas deferens.*

DEFLAGRATION. (*Deflagratio;* From *deflagro*, to burn.) A chemical term, chiefly employed to express the burning or setting fire to any substance; as nitre, sulphur, &c.

DEFLUXION. (*Defluxio;* from *defluo*, to run off.) A falling down of humours from a superior to an inferior part. Many writers mean nothing more by it than inflammation.

DEFOLIATIO. (From *de*, and *folium*, a leaf.) The fall of the leaf. A term opposed to *frondescentia*, or the renovation of the leaf.

DEGLUTITION. (*Deglutitio;* from *degluto*, to swallow down.) A natural action. "It is understood to be the passage of a substance, either solid, liquid, or gaseous, from the mouth to the stomach

Though deglutition is very simple in appearance, it is nevertheless the most complicated of all the muscular actions that serve for digestion. It is produced by the contraction of a great number of muscles, and requires the concurrence of many important organs.

All the muscles of the tongue, those of the *velum* of the palate, of the pharynx, of the larynx, and the muscular layer of the œsophagus, are employed in deglutition.

The *velum* is a sort of valve attached to the posterior edge of the roof of the palate; its form is nearly quadrilateral; its free or inferior edge is pointed, and forms the *uvula*. Like the other valves of the intestinal canal, the *velum* is essentially formed by a duplicature of the digestive mucous membrane; there are many mucous follicles that enter into its composition, particularly in the uvula. Eight muscles move it; it is raised by the two internal *pterygoid:* the external *pterygoid* hold it transversely; the two *palato-pharyngei*, and the two *constrictores isthmi faucium* carry it downwards. These four are seen at the bottom of the throat, where they raise the mucous membrane, and form the pillars os of the *velum* of the palate, between which are situated the *amygdalæ*, a mass of mucous follicles. The opening between the base of the tongue below, the *velum* of the palate above, and the pillars laterally, is called the isthmus of the throat. By means of its muscular apparatus, the *velum* of the palate may have many changes of position. In the most common state it is placed vertically, one of its faces is anterior, the other posterior; in certain cases it becomes horizontal: it has then a superior and inferior aspect, and its free edge corresponds to the concavity of the pharynx. This last position is determined by the contraction of the elevating muscles.

The *pharynx* is a vestibule into which open the nostrils, the Eustachian tubes, the mouth, the larynx, and the œsophagus, and which performs very important functions in the production of voice, in respiration, hearing, and digestion.

The pharynx extends from top to bottom, from the basilar process of the occipital bone, to which it is attached, to the level of the middle part of the neck.

Its transverse dimensions are determined by the os hyoides, the larynx, and the pterygo-maxillary aponeurosis, to which it is fixed. The mucous membrane which covers it interiorly is remarkable for the developement of its veins, which form a very apparent plexus. Round this membrane is the muscular layer, the circular fibres of which form the three constrictor muscles of the pharynx, the longitudinal fibres of which are represented by the stylo-pharyngeus and constrictores isthmi faucium. The contractions of these different muscles are not generally subject to the will.

The *œsophagus* is the immediate continuation of the pharynx, and is prolonged as far as the stomach, where it terminates. Its form is cylindrical; it is united to the surrounding parts by a slack and extending cellular tissue, which gives way to its dilatation and its motions. To penetrate into the abdomen the œsophagus passes between the pillars of the diaphragm, with which it is closely united. The mucous membrane of the œsophagus is white, thin, and smooth; it forms longitudinal folds very proper for favouring the dilatation of the canal. Above it is confounded with that of the pharynx.

There are found in it a great number of mucous follicles, and at its surface there are perceived the orifices of many excretive canals of the mucous glands.

The muscular layer of the œsophagus is thick, its tissue is denser than that of the pharynx; the longitudinal fibres are the most external and the least numerous; the circular are placed in the interior and are very numerous.

Round the pectoral and inferior portion of the œsophagus, the two nerves of the eighth pair form a plexus which embraces the canal, and sends many filaments into it.

The contraction of the œsophagus takes place without the participation of the will.

Mechanism of Deglutition. Deglutition is divided into three periods. In the first, the food passes from the mouth to the pharynx; in the second, it passes the opening of the glottis, that of the nasal canals, and arrives at the œsophagus; in the the third it passes through this tube and enters the stomach.

Let us suppose the most common case, that in which we swallow at several times the food which is in the mouth, and according as mastication takes place.

As soon as a certain quantity of food is sufficiently chewed, it is placed, by the effects of the motions of mastication, in part upon the superior face of the tongue, without the necessity, as some think, of its being collected by the point of the tongue from the different parts of the mouth. Mastication then stops, the tongue is raised and applied to the roof of the palate, in succession, from the point towards the base. The portion of food, or the alimentary bolus placed upon its superior surface, having no other way to escape from the force that presses, is directed towards the pharynx; it soon meets the velum of the palate applied to the base of the tongue and raises it; the velum becomes horizontal, so as to make a continuation of the palate. The tongue, continuing to press the food, would carry it towards the nasal canals, if the velum did not prevent this by the tension that it receives from the external peristaphyline muscles, and particularly by the contraction of its pillars; it thus becomes capable of resisting the action of the tongue, and of contributing to the direction of the food towards the pharynx.

The muscles which determine more particularly the application of the tongue to the top of the palate, and to the velum of the palate, are the proper muscles of the organ, aided by the mylo-hyoideus. Here the first time of deglutition terminates. Its motions are voluntary, except those of the velum of the palate. The phenomena happen slowly and in succession; they are few and easily noticed.

The second period is not the same; in it the phenomena are simultaneous, multiplied, and are produced with such promptitude, that Boerhaave considered them as a sort of convulsion.

The space that the alimentary bolus passes through in this time is very short, for it passes only from the middle to the inferior part of the pharynx; but it was necessary to avoid the opening of the glottis and that of the nasal canals, where its presence would be injurious. Besides, its passage ought to be sufficiently rapid, in order that the communication between the larynx and the external air may not be interrupted, except for an instant.

Let us see how nature has arrived at this important result. The alimentary bole no sooner touches the pharynx than every thing is in motion. First, the pharynx contracts, embraces and retains the bole; the velum of the palate, drawn down by its pillars, acts in the same way. On the other hand, and in the same instant, the base of the tongue, the os hyoides, the larynx, are raised and carried forward to meet the bole, in order to render its passage more rapid over the opening of the glottis. While the os hyoides, and the larynx are raised, they approach each other, that is, the superior edge of the thyroid cartilage engages itself behind the body of the os hyoides: the epiglottic gland is pushed back; the epiglottis descends, inclines downwards and backwards, so as to cover the entrance of the larynx. The cricoid cartilage makes a motion of rotation upon the inferior horns of the thyroid, whence it results that the entrance of the larynx becomes oblique downwards and backwards. The bole slides along its surface, and being always pressed by the contraction of the pharynx and of the velum of the palate, it arrives at the œsophagus.

It is not long since the position that the epiglottis takes in this place was considered as the only obstacle opposed to the entrance of the food into the larynx, at the instant of deglutition; but Dr. Magendie has shown, by a series of experiments, that this cause ought to be considered as only accessary. In fact, the epiglottis may be entirely taken away from an animal without deglutition suffering any injury from it. What is the reason, then, that no part of the food is introduced into the larynx the instant that we swallow? The reason is this. In the instant that the larynx is raised and engaged behind the os hyoides, the glottis shuts with the greatest closeness. This motion is produced by the same muscles that press the glottis in the production of the voice; so that if an animal has the recurrents and nerves of the larynx divided, while the epiglottis is untouched, its deglutition is rendered very difficult, because the principal cause is removed which opposes the introduction of food into the glottis.

Immediately after the alimentary bole has passed the glottis, the larynx descends, the epiglottis is raised, and the glottis is opened to give passage to the air.

After what has been said, it is easy to conceive why the food reaches the œsophagus without entering any of the openings which end in the pharynx. The velum of the palate, which, in contracting, embraces the pharynx, protects the posterior nostrils, and the orifices of the Eustachian tubes; the epiglottis, and particularly the motion by which the glottis shuts, preserves the larynx.

Thus, the second period of deglutition is accomplished; by the effects of which the alimentary bole passes the pharynx, and is engaged in the superior part of the œsophagus. All the phenomena which concur in it take place simultaneously, and with great promptitude: they are not subject to the will; they are then different in many respects from the phenomena that belong to the first period.

The third period of deglutition is that which has been studied with the least care, probably on account of the situation of the œsophagus, which is difficult to be observed except in its cervical portion.

The phenomena which are connected with it are not complicated. The pharynx, by its contraction, presses the alimentary bole into the œsophagus with sufficient force to give a suitable dilatation to the superior part of this organ. Excited by the presence of the bolus, its superior circular fibres very soon contract, and press the food towards the stomach, thereby producing the distension of those more inferior. These contract in their turn, and the same thing continues in succession until the bolus arrives at the stomach. In the upper two-thirds of the œsophagus, the relaxation of the circular fibres follows immediately the contraction by which they displaced the alimentary bolus. It is not the same with the inferior third; this remains some moments contracted after the introduction of food into the stomach.

All the extent of the mucous surface that the alimentary bolus passes in the three periods of deglutition is lubricated by an abundant mucosity. In the way that the bolus passes, it presses more or less the follicles that it meets in its passage, it empties them of the fluid that they contain, and slides more easily upon the mucous membrane. We remark that in those places where the bolus passes more rapidly, and is pressed with greater force, the organs for secreting mucus are much more abundant. For example, in the narrow space where the second period of deglutition takes place, there are found the tonsils, the fungous papillæ of the base of the tongue, the follicles of the velum of the palate, and the uvula, those of the epiglottis, and the arytenoid glands. In this case the saliva and the mucosity fulfil uses analogous to those of the synovia.

The mechanism by which we swallow the succeeding mouthfuls of food does not differ from that which we have explained.

Nothing is more easy than the performance of deglutition, and, nevertheless, all the acts of which it is composed are beyond the influence of the will and of instinct. We cannot make an empty motion of deglutition. If the substance contained in the mouth is not sufficiently chewed, if it has not the form, the consistence, and the dimensions of the alimentary bolus, if the motions of mastication which immediately precede deglutition have not been made, we will frequently find it impossible to swallow it, whatever efforts we make. How many people do we not find who cannot swallow a pill, or medicinal bolus, and who are obliged to fall upon other methods to introduce it into the œsophagus?—*Magendie.*

DE'GMUS. (From δακνω, to bite.) A biting pain in the orifice of the stomach.

DEHISCENTIA. (From *dehisco*, to gape wide.) A spitting, or bursting open. Applied to capsules, anthers, &c. of plants.

DEIDIER, ANTHONY, was son of a surgeon of Montpelier. Having graduated in medicine in 1691, he was six years after made professor of chemistry. In 1732, being appointed physician to the galleys, he went to Marseilles, where he died in 1746. He published, among many other works on different branches of medicine, "Experiments on the Bile, and the Bodies of those who died of the Plague," which occurred while he was at Marseilles. He states that he tried mercurial inunctions, but they had no effect on the disease. There are three volumes of consultations and observations by him deserving of perusal. The rest of his works are scarcely now referred to.

DEINO'SIS. (From δεινοω, to exaggerate.) An enlargement of the supercilia.

DEJE'CTIO. A discharge of any excrementitious matter; generally applied to the fæces: hence *dejectio alvina.*

DEJECTO'RIA. (From *dejicio*, to cast out.) Purging medicines.

DELACHRYMATI'VA. (From *de*, and *lachryma*, a tear.) Medicines which dry the eyes, first purging them of tears.

DELA'PSIO. (From *delabor*, to slip down.) A falling down of any part, as the anus, uterus, or intestines.

DELETERIOUS. (*Deleterius;* from δηλεω, to hurt or injure.) Of a poisonous nature; as opium, hemlock, henbane, &c.

[DELIQUESCE. To deliquesce is that action by which certain bodies become liquid by absorbing moisture from the atmosphere. Potash for instance by exposure to the air will absorb so much water as to change from a solid to a fluid state. This is common to many saline bodies. A.]

DELIQUESCENCE. Deliquation, or the spontaneous assumption of the fluid state of certain saline bodies, when left exposed to the air, in consequence of their attracting water from it.

DELI'QUIUM. (*Deliquium;* from *delinquo*, to leave.) A fainting. See *Syncope.*

DELI'RIUM. (From *deliro*, to rave.) A febrile symptom, consisting in the person's acting or talking unreasonably. It is to be carefully distinguished from an alienation of the mind, without fever.

DELIVERY. See *Parturition.*

DELOCA'TIO. (From *de*, from, and *locus*, a place.) A dislocation.

DELPHIA. See *Delphinia.*

DELPHINE. See *Delphinia.*

DELPHINIA. *Delphia.* Delphine. A new vegetable alkali, recently discovered by Lasseigne and Feneulle, in Stavesacre. See *Delphinium staphysagria.*

DELPHINIC ACID *Acidum delphinicum.* The name of an acid, extracted from the oil of the dolphin. It resembles a volatile oil; has a light lemon colour, and a strong aromatic odour, analogous to that of rancid butter. Its taste is pungent, and its vapour has a sweetened taste of æther. It is slightly soluble in water, and very soluble in alkohol. The latter solution strongly reddens litmus. 100 parts of delphinic acid neutralize a quantity of base, which contains 9 of oxygen, whence its prime equivalent appears to be 11.11.

DELPHINITE. See *Epidote.*

DELPHI'NIUM (From δελφινος, the dolphin.) Larkspur; so called from the likeness of its flower to the dolphin's head. The name of a genus of plants in the Linnæan system. Class, *Polyandria;* Order, *Trigynia.*

["DELPHINIUM OR LARKSPUR. The botanical alliance of the larkspur of our gardens with aconite and some other poisonous plants, would justify, *a priori*, a belief, that it possesses active properties. This is found on experiment to be the case. A tincture formed by infusing an ounce of the bruised seeds in a pound of spirit has been found an antispasmodic in asthma, and an active diuretic in dropsy. The *dose* is from ten to twenty drops. Larger doses are liable to nauseate, and would, not improbably, produce narcotic symptoms."—*Big. Mat. Med.* A.]

DELPHINIUM CONSOLIDA. The systematic name of the *Consolida regalis. Calcatrippa. Delphinium—nectariis monophyllis, caule subdiviso,* of Linnæus. Many virtues have been attributed to this plant. The flowers are bitter, and a water distilled from them is recommended in ophthalmia. The herb has been administered in calculous cases, obstructed menses, and visceral diseases.

DELPHINIUM STAPHISAGRIA. The systematic name of stavesacre. *Staphisagria; Staphis; Pedicularia; Delphinium—nectariis tetraphyllis petalo brevioribus, foliis palmatis, lobis obtusis*, of Linnæus. The seeds, which are the only parts directed for medicinal use, are usually imported here from Italy; they are large, rough, of an irregular triangular figure, and of a blackish colour on the outside, but yellowish within; their smell is disagreeable, and somewhat fœtid; to the taste they are very bitter, acrid, and nauseous. It was formerly employed as a masticatory, but is now confined to external use, in some kinds of cutaneous eruptions, but more especially for destroying lice and other insects: hence, by the vulgar, it is called louse-wort.

A new vegetable alkali has lately been discovered in this plant by Lasseigne and Feneulle. It is thus obtained:

The seeds, deprived of their husks, and ground, are to be boiled in a small quantity of distilled water, and then pressed in a cloth. The decoction is to be filtered, and boiled for a few minutes with pure magnesia. It must then be refiltered, and the residuum left on the filter is to be well washed, and then boiled with highly rectified alkohol, which dissolves out the alkali. By evaporation, a white pulverulent substance, presenting a few crystalline points, is obtained.

It may also be procured by the action of dilute sulphuric acid, on the bruised but unshelled seeds. The solution of sulphate thus formed, is precipitated by subcarbonate of potassa. Alkohol separates from this precipitate the vegetable alkali in an impure state.

Pure delphinia obtained by the first process, is crystalline while wet, but becomes opake on exposure to air. Its taste is bitter and acrid. When heated it melts; and on cooling becomes hard and brittle like resin. If more highly heated, it blackens and is decomposed. Water dissolves a very small portion of it. Alkohol and æther dissolve it very readily. The alkoholic solution renders syrup of violets green, and restores the blue tint of litmus reddened by an acid. It forms soluble neutral salts with acids. Alkalies precipitate the delphinia in a white gelatinous state, like alumina.

Sulphate of delphinia evaporates in the air, does not crystallize, but becomes a transparent mass like gum. It dissolves in alkohol and water, and its solution has a bitter acrid taste. In the voltaic circuit it is decomposed, giving up its alkali at the negative pole.

Nitrate of delphinia, when evaporated to dryness, is a yellow crystalline mass. If treated with excess of nitric acid, it becomes converted into a yellow matter, little soluble in water, but soluble in boiling alkohol, This solution is bitter, is not precipitated by potassa, ammonia, or lime-water, and appears to contain no nitric acid, though itself is not alkaline. It is not destroyed by further quantities of acid, nor does it form oxalic acid. Strychnia and morphia take a red colour from nitric acid, but delphinia never does. The muriate is very soluble in water.

The acetate of delphinia does not crystallize, but forms a hard transparent mass, bitter and acrid, and readily decomposed by cold sulphuric acid. The oxalate forms small white plates, resembling in taste the preceding salts.

Delphinia, calcined with oxide of copper, gave no other gas than carbonic acid. It exists in the seeds of the stavesacre, in combination with malic acid, and associated with the following principles: 1. A brown bitter principle, precipitable by acetate of lead. 2. Volatile oil. 3. Fixed oil. 4. Albumen. 5. Animalized matter. 6. Mucus. 7. Saccharine mucus. 8. Yellow bitter principle, not precipitable by acetate of ead. 9. Mineral salts.—*Annales de Chimie et de Physique*, vol. xii. p. 358.

DE'LPHYS. Δελφυς. The uterus, or pudendum muliebre.

DE'LTA. (The Greek letter, Δ.) The external pudendum muliebre is so called, from the triangular shape of its hair.

DELTOI'DES. (From δελτα, the Greek letter Δ, and ειδος, a likeness; shaped like the Greek delta.) 1. A muscle of the superior extremity, situated on the shoulder. *Sous-acromio-clavi-humeral* of Dumas. It arises exactly opposite to the trapezius, from one-third part of the clavicle, from the acromion and spine of the scapula, and is inserted, tendinous, into the middle of the os humeri, which bone it lifts up directly; and it assists with the supraspinatus and coracobrachialis n all the actions of the humerus, except the depression; it being convenient that the arm should be raised and sustained, in order to its moving on any side.

2. A leaf is so called, *folium deltoides*, which is trowel shaped, or like the letter delta, having three angles, of which the terminal one is much further from the base than the lateral ones; as in *Chenopodium bonus-henricus*.

DEME'NTIA. (From *de*, and *mens*, without mind.) Absence of intellect; madness; fatuity.

DEMERSUS. A leaf which is naturally under water, and different from those above, is so called; *folia immersa*, and *submersa*, are the same as *demersa*. See *Natans*.

DEMULCENT. (*Demulcens;* from *demulceo*, to soften.) Medicines suited to obviate and prevent the action of acrid and stimulant matters; and that not by correcting or changing their acrimony, but by involving it in a mild and viscid matter, which prevents it from acting upon the sensible parts of our bodies, or by covering the surface exposed to their action.

Where these substances are directly applied to the parts affected, it is easy to perceive how benefit may be derived from their application. But where they are received by the medium of the stomach, into the circulating system, it has been supposed that they can be of no utility, as they must lose that viscidity on which their lubricating quality depends. Hence it has been concluded that they can be of no service in gonorrhœa, and some similar affections. It is certain, however, says J. Murray, in his Elements of Materia Medica and Pharmacy, that many substances which undergo the process of digestion are afterward separated, in their entire state, from the blood, by particular secreting organs, especially by the kidneys; and it is possible, that mucilaginous substances, which are the principal demulcents, may be separated in this manner. There can be no doubt, however, but that a great share of the relief demulcents afford, in irritation or inflammation of the urinary passages, is owing to the large quantities of water in which they are diffused, by which the urine is rendered less stimulating from dilution. In general, demulcents may be considered merely as substances less stimulating than the fluids usually applied.

Catarrh, diarrhœa, dysentery, calculus, and gonorrhœa, are the diseases in which demulcents are employed. As they are medicines of no great power, they may be taken in as large quantities as the stomach can bear.

The particular demulcents may be reduced to the two divisions of mucilages and expressed oils. The principal demulcents are, the acacia vera, astragalus, tragacanthe, linum usitatissimum, althœa officinalis, malva, sylvestris, glycyrrhiza glabra, cycas circinalis, orchis mascula, maranta arundinacea, triticum hybernum, ichthyocolla, olea Europæa, amygdalus communis, cetaceum, and cera.

[DENDRITIC. (From δενδρον, a tree.) A term used in mineralogy to designate those appearances frequently found in minerals resembling trees or clusters of trees. A.]

DENDROLI'BANUS. (From δενδρον, a tree, and ολιβανος, frankincense.) Frankincense-tree. See *Rosmarinus officinalis*.

DENS. (*Dens, tis.* m.; *quasi edens;* from *edo*, to eat, or from οδους, οδοντος.)

1. A tooth. See *Teeth*.

2. Many herbs have this specific name, from their fancied resemblance to the tooth of some animal, as *Dens leonis*, the dandelion; *Dens canis*, dog's tooth, &c.

Dens caninus. See *Teeth*.

Dens cuspidatus. See *Teeth*.

Dens incisor. See *Teeth*.

Dens lacteus. See *Teeth*, and *Dentition*

Dens leonis. See *Leontodon Taraxacum*.

Dens molaris. See *Teeth*.

DENTA'GRA. (*Dentagra*, οδονταγρα; from οδους, a tooth, and αγρα, a seizure.) 1. The toothache.

2. An instrument for drawing the teeth.

DENTA'RIA. (*Dentaria;* from *dens*, a tooth. so called because its root is denticulated.) See *Plumbago europæa*.

DENTARPA'GA. (From οδους, a tooth, and αρπαζω, to fasten upon.) An instrument for drawing of teeth.

Dentata. See *Dentatus*.

DENTA'TUS (From *dens*, a tooth; from its tooth-like process.) 1. The second vertebra of the neck. *Dentata; Epistrophæus.* It differs from the other cervical vetebræ, by having a tooth-like process at the upper part of the body. See *Vertebræ.*

2. Toothed: applied to roots, leaves, petals, &c. which are beset with projecting, horizontal, rather distant teeth of its own substance; as in the leaf of *Atriplex lacinata*, and the perianthium of *Marrubium vulgare*, and *Ereca denticulata*, and the petals of the *Silene lucitanica.* The *Ophris corallorhiza* has a toothed root.

DENTELLA'RIA. (From *dentella*, a little tooth; so called because its root is denticulated.) The herb tooth-wort. See *Plumbago europæa.*

DENTIDU'CUM. (From *dens*, a tooth, and *duco*, to draw.) An instrument for drawing of teeth.

DENTIFRICE. (*Dentifricus;* from *dens*, a tooth, and *frigo*, to rub.) A medicine to clean the teeth.

DENTISCA'LPIUM. (From *dens*, a tooth, and *scalpo*, to scrape.) An instrument for scaling teeth.

DENTITION. (*Dentitio;* from *dentio*, to breed teeth.) *Odontiasis; Odontophica.* The breeding or cutting of the teeth. The first dentition begins about the sixth or seventh month, and the teeth are termed the *primary* or *milk* teeth. About the seventh year, these fall out, and are succeeded by others, which remain during life, and are called the *secondary* or *perennial* teeth. The last dentition takes place between the ages of twenty and five-and-twenty, when the four last grinders appear; they are called *dentes sapientiæ.* See also *Teeth.*

DENTODU'CUM. See *Dentiducum.*

DENUDATÆ PLANTÆ. The name of an order of Linnæus's Fragments of a Natural Method, embracing those plants, the flowers of which are naked, or without a flower-cup.

DENUDA'TIO. (From *denudo*, to make bare.) The laying bare any part; usually applied to a bone.

DENUDATUS. (From *denudo*, to strip naked.) Denude; naked.

DEOBSTRUENT. (*Deobstruens;* from *de*, and *obstruo*, to obstruct.) A medicine that is exhibited with a view of removing any obstruction.

DEOPPILA'NTIA. (From *de*, and *oppilo*, to stop.) *Deoppilativa.* Medicines which remove obstructions.

DEPARTI'TIO. (From *de*, and *partior*, to divide.) Separating metals.

DEPERDI'TIO. (From *deperdo*, to lose.) Abortion, or the undue loss of the fœtus.

DEPETI'GO. (From *de*, and *petigo*, a running scab.) A ringworm, tetter, scurf, or itch, where the skin is rough.

DEPHLEGMA'TION. (*Dephlegmatio;* from *de*, and *phlegma*, phlegm.) The operation of rectifying or freeing spirits from their watery parts, or any method by which bodies are deprived of their water.

DEPHLOGISTICATED. A term of the old chemistry, implying deprived of phlogiston or the inflammable principle.

Dephlogisticated air. See *Oxygen gas.*

Dephlogisticated muriatic acid. See *Chlorine.*

DEPILATORY. (*Depilatorius;* from *de*, of, and *pilus*, the hair.) Any application which removes the hairs from any part of the body; thus, a pitch cap pulls the hairs of the head out by the roots.

[A depilatory ointment is sometimes used to remove hairs from inconvenient places. The French call it *Pate depilatoire*, a depilatory paste. It is made with quick lime, lapis calaminaris, and arsenic, intimately united and made into a thin paste with a little water, and a thin coat spread upon the surface. The hairs are removed by the action of the arsenic as a caustic, but its action is modified by the other ingredients. A.]

DEPLU'MATIO. (From *de*, and *pluma*, a feather.) A disease of the eyelids, which causes the hair to fall off.

DEPREHE'NSIO. (From *deprehendo*, to catch unawares.) The epilepsy is so called, from the suddenness with which persons are seized with it.

DEPRESSION. (*Depressio;* from *deprimo*, to press down.) When the bones of the skull are forced inwards by fracture, they are said to be depressed.

DEPRE'SSOR. (From *deprimo*, to press down.) A muscle is so termed, which depresses the part on which it acts.

DEPRESSOR ALÆ NASI. See *Depressor labii superioris alæque nasi.*

DEPRESSOR ANGULI ORIS. A muscle of the mouth and lip, situated below the under lip. *Triangularis*, of Winslow. *Depressor labiorum communis*, of Douglas. *Depressor labiorum*, of Cowper. *Sous-maxillo-labial* of Dumas. It arises broad and fleshy, from the lower edge of the lower jaw, near the chin; and is inserted into the angle of the mouth, which it pulls downwards.

DEPRESSOR LABII INFERIORIS. A muscle of the mouth and lip. *Quadratus*, of Winslow. *Depressor labii inferioris proprius*, of Douglas and Cowper. *Mentonier labial*, of Dumas. It pulls the under lip and skin of the side of the chin downwards, and a little outwards.

DEPRESSOR LABII SUPERIORIS ALÆQUE NASI. A muscle of the mouth and lip. *Depressor alæ nasi*, of Albinus. *Incisivus medius*, of Winslow. *Depressor labii superioris proprius*, of Douglas. *Constrictores alarum nasi, ac depressores labii superiores*, of Cowper. *Maxillo-alveoli nasal*, of Dumas. It is situated above the mouth, draws the upper lip and ala nasi downwards and backwards. It arises, thin and fleshy, from the superior maxillary bone, immediately above the joining of the gums, with the two incisor teeth and cuspidatus; from thence it runs upwards, and is inserted into the upper lip and root of the ala of the nose.

DEPRESSOR LABII SUPERIORIS PROPRIUS. See *Depressor labii superioris alæque nasi.*

DEPRESSOR LABIORUM COMMUNIS. See *Depressor anguli oris.*

DEPRESSOR OCULI. See *Rectus inferior oculi.*

DEPRESSUS. Depressed; flattened vertically, as the leaves of the *Mesembryanthemum linguiforme.* *Folia depressa* is applied also to radical leaves which are pressed close to the ground, as is seen in *Plantago media;* but when applied to stem leaves, it regards their shape only, as being vertically flattened in opposition to *compressa.*

DE'PRIMENS. See *Rectus inferior oculi.*

DEPURA'NTIA. (*Depurans;* from *depuro*, to make clean.) Medicines which evacuate impurities.

DEPURA'TION. *Depuratio.* The freeing a liquor or solid from its foulness.

DEPURATO'RIUS. (From *de*, and *purus*, pure.) Depuritory: applied to fevers, which terminate in perspiration.

DERBYSHIRE SPAR. A mineral formed of calcareous earth with fluoric acid.

DE'RIS. (Δερις; from δερω, to excoriate.) The skin.

DERIVATION. (*Derivatio;* from *derivo*, to drain off.) The doctrines of derivation and revulsion talked of by the ancients, are now, in their sense of the terms, wholly exploded. Derivation means the drawing away any disease from its original seat to another part.

DE'RMA. Δερμα. The skin. See *Skin.*

DERMATO'DES. (From δερμα, skin, and ειδος, a likeness.) Resembling skin, or leather; applied to the dura mater.

DERMATOLO'GIA. (From δερμα, the skin, and λογος, a discourse.) A discourse or treatise on the skin.

DE'RTRON. (From δερις, skin.) The omentum, and peritonæum, are so named, from their skin-like consistence.

DESAULT, PETER, was a native of Bordeaux, where he graduated, and became distinguished as a practitioner in medicine about the beginning of the last century. He was author of some popular and useful dissertations on medical subjects. In syphilis he maintained that a cure could be effected without salivation; and in calculous complaints, by the patient drinking the Bareges water, this being also injected into the bladder; but it probably merely palliated the symptoms. He exposed also some of the prevailing errors concerning hydrophobia; as that the patient barked like a dog, and had a propensity to bite his attendants. The precise period of his death is not mentioned.

DESAULT, PETER JOSEPH, was chief surgeon to the Hôtel-Dieu at Paris. He published several numbers of a surgical journal, in 1791, &c.; also, jointly with Chopart, in 1794, "A Treatise on Chirurgical

Diseases, and the Operations required in their Cure;" which is allowed to have considerable merit. He attended the young King of France, Lewis XVII., in the temple; and died under suspicious circumstances, shortly before his royal patient, in 1795.

DESCENSO'RIUM. (From *descendo*, to move downwards.) A vessel in which the distillation by descent is performed.

DESCE'NSUS. (From *descendo*, to move downwards.) The same chemists call it a distillation *per descensum*, by descent, when the fire is applied at the top and round the vessel, the orifice of which is at the bottom.

DESICCATI'VE. (*Desicativus; from desicco*, to dry up.) An application to dry up the humours and moisture running from a wound or ulcer.

DESIPIE'NTIA. (From *desipio*, to dote.) A defect of reason.

DESIRE. Will. We give the name of will to that modification of the faculty of perception by which we form desires. It is generally the effect of our judgment; but what is remarkable, our happiness or our misery are necessarily connected with it. When we satisfy our desires we are happy; but we are miserable if our desires be not fulfilled; it is then necessary to give such a direction to our desires that we may be enabled to obtain happiness. We ought not to desire things which cannot be obtained; we ought to avoid, even with greater care, those things which are hurtful; for in such cases we must be unhappy, whether our desires are satisfied or not. Morality is a science which tends to give the best possible direction to our desires.

DE'SME. (From δεω, to bind up.) A bandage, or ligature.

DESMI'DION. (From δεσμη, a handful.) A small bundle, or little bandage.

DE'SMOS (From δεω, to bind up.) 1. A bandage.

2. An inflammatory stricture of a joint, after luxation.

DE'SPUMATION. (*Despumatio;* from *despumo*, to clarify.) The clarifying a fluid, or separating its foul parts from it.

DESQUAMATION. (*Desquamatio;* from *desquamo*, to scale off.) The separating of laminæ, or scales, from a bone. Exfoliation.

DESQUAMATO'RIUM. (From *desquamo*, to scale off.) A trepan, or instrument to take a piece out of the skull.

DESTILLA'TION. See *Distillation.*

DESUDA'TIO. (From *desudo*, to sweat much.) An unnatural and morbid sweating.

DETE'NTIO. (From *detineo*, to stop, or hinder.) Epilepsy is so called, from the suddenness with which the patient is seized.

DETERGENT. (From *detergo*, to wipe away.) 1. A medicine which cleanses and removes such viscid humours as adhere to and obstruct the vessels.

2. An application that clears away foulness from ulcers.

DETERMINATE`. Applied by botanists to branches and stems: *determinatè ramosus* is abruptly branched, when each branch, after terminating in flowers, produces a number of fresh shoots, in a circular order, from just below the origin of those flowers. The term occurs frequently in the latter publication of Linnæus, particularly the second *Mantissa;* but he does not appear to have any where explained its meaning.—*Smith.*

DETONATION. (*Detonatio;* from *detono*, to make a noise.) A sudden combustion and explosion.

DETRA'CTOR. (From *detraho*, to draw.) Applied to a muscle, the office of which is to draw the part to which it is attached.

DE'TRAHENS. (From *detraho*, to draw.) The name of a muscle, the office of which is to draw the part it is attached to.

DETRAHENS QUADRATUS. See *Platysma myoides.*

DETRU'SOR URINÆ. (From *detrudo*, to thrust out.) 1. The name of a muscle, the office of which is to squeeze out the urine.

2. The muscular coat of the urinary bladder was formerly so called.

DEU'TERI. (From δευτερος, second: because it is discharged next after the fœtus.) The secundines, or after-birth.

DEUTEROPA'THIA. (From δευτερος, second, and παθος, a suffering.) An affection or suffering by consent, where a second part suffers, from consent, with the part originally affected, as where the stomach is disturbed through a wound in the head.

DEUTOXIDE. See *Oxide.*

Deutoxide of azot. See *Nitrogen.*

DEVENTER, HENRY, was born in Holland, toward the end of the 17th century. He took a degree in medicine, but his practice was principally in surgery, and at last almost confined to midwifery. He distinguished himself much by his improvements in this art, as well as by his mechanical inventions for obviating deformities in children. He published some obstetrical works several years prior to his death, which occurred in 1739; after which appeared a Treatise on the Rickets in his native language, of which Haller makes favourable mention.

Devil's dung. See *Ferula assafœtida.*

Dewberry. See *Blackberry.*

DIA. Δια. Many terms in medicine, surgery, and pharmacy, commence with this word, when they signify composition and mixture; as *Diacassia, Diacastoreum,* &c.

[DIABASE. The Diabase of some French mineralogists is the greenstone of Werner and Jameson. Greenstone abounds in the United States. There is a long ridge of this kind of rock in Connecticut running northward from New-Haven. There are several ridges of this formation of superincumbent rocks in New-Jersey. The most remarkable is the ridge bordering the Hudson river on the west side, running north from New-York city to the extent of thirty or forty miles, and known by the common appellation of the Palisado Rocks. There is a sublime show of this kind of rock on the south side of Lake Superior.

Diabase or "Greenstone is essentially composed of *hornblende* and *felspar*, in the state of grains, or sometimes of small crystals. The proportions are somewhat various; but the hornblende predominates, and very frequently gives to this aggregate more or less of a greenish tinge, especially when it is moistened. Hence the name of this rock (Greenstone). Sometimes the tinge of green is considerably lively, and may arise either from the hornblende, or from Epidote disseminated through the mass. Sometimes also its colour is dark gray, or grayish black. In fine, its colour, especially at the surface, is often modified by the presence of oxide of iron.

"This rock presents a considerable variety of aspect, depending on the general structure, or on the size, proportion, disposition, and more or less intimate mixture of its constituent parts.

"In some of the more common varieties, the two ingredients are in distinct grains of considerable size, like those of granite; and the foliated structure both of the hornblende and felspar is often distinctly visible. The proportion of felspar is sometimes very small.

"From Greenstone with a coarse granular structure. to those varieties whose texture is so finely granular that the two ingredients can scarcely be perceived, there is a gradual passage, exhibiting every intermediate step. Indeed the grains are sometimes so minute, and so uniformly and intimately mingled, that the mass is altogether homogeneous, and the different ingredients are hardly perceptible, even with a glass. Hence the texture of this rock is sometimes distinctly crystalline, and sometimes almost compact and earthy.

"Greenstone, like basalt, sometimes presents itself in *prisms*, or *columns* of various sizes. These prisms may have from three to seven sides, and are sometimes as regular as those of basalt.

"The general aspect of Greenstone is sometimes much diversified by the foreign ingredients, which it admits into its composition. Among these are quartz, epidote, mica, talc, carbonate of lime, and almost always sulphuret of iron, which is sometimes magnetic.—The quartz is, in some cases, abundant, and seems almost to take the place of felspar. Iron frequently enters into the composition of this rock. Hence by exposure to the weather, its exterior becomes brownish or reddish brown; and sometimes Green stones are gradually decomposed.

"Many Greenstones are susceptible of a polish;—and that variety which admits *epidote* into its composition, often forms a very beautiful mineral, when polished, especially if it be porphyritic. Its colour is often a fine dark green, resembling serpentine. The epidote, either crystallized or compact, is sometimes in very narrow veins; and sometimes it is uniformly disseminated in very minute grains. In other cases, the epidote and felspar form a kind of base, containing acicular crystals of hornblende; or the three ingredients are distinct, as in granite."—*Cleaveland's Mineral.* A.]

DIABE'CUS. (From διαβεβαιοω, to strengthen; so called, as affording the chief support to the foot.) The ankle-bone.

DIABETES. (From δια, through, and βαινω, to pass.) An immoderate flow of urine. A genus of disease in the class *Neuroses*, and order *Spasmi* of Cullen.

There are two species in this complaint:

1. *Diabetes insipidus*, in which there is a superabundant discharge of limpid urine, of its usual urinary taste.

2. *Diabetes mellitus*, in which the urine is very sweet, and contains a great quantity of sugar.

Great thirst, with a voracious appetite, gradual emaciation of the whole body, and a frequent discharge of urine, containing a large proportion of saccharine and other matter, which is voided in a quantity even exceeding that of the aliment or fluid introduced, are the characteristics of this disease. Those of a shattered constitution, and those who are in the decline of life, are most subject to its attacks. It not unfrequently attends on hysteria, hypochondriasis, dyspepsia, and asthma: but it is always much milder when symptomatic, than when it appears as a primary affection.

Diabetes may be occasioned by the use of strong diuretic medicines, intemperance of life, and hard drinking; excess in venery, severe evacuations, or by any thing that tends to produce an impoverished state of the blood, or general debility. It has, however, taken place, in many instances, without any obvious cause.

That which immediately gives rise to the disease, has ever been considered as obscure, and various theories have been advanced on the occasion. It has been usual to consider diabetes as the effect of relaxation of the kidneys, or as depending on a general colliquation of the fluids. Dr. Richter, professor of medicine in the university of Gottingen, supposes the disease to be generally of a spasmodic nature, occasioned by a stimulus acting on the kidneys; hence a *secretio aucta urinæ*, and sometimes *perversa*, is the consequence. Dr. Darwin thinks that it is owing to an *inverted* action of the urinary branch of the lymphatics; which doctrine, although it did not escape the censure of the best anatomists and experienced physiologists, met, nevertheless, with a very favourable reception on its being first announced. The late Dr. Cullen offered it as his opinion, that the proximate cause of this disease might be some fault in the assimilatory powers, or in those employed in converting alimentary matters into the proper animal fluids, which theory has since been adopted by Dr. Dobson, and still later by Dr. Rolla, surgeon-general to the royal artillery. The liver has been thought, by some, to be the chief source of the disease; but diabetes is hardly ever attended with any affection of this organ, as has been proved by frequent dissections; and when observed, it is to be considered as accidental.

The primary seat of the disease is, however, far from being absolutely determined in favour of any hypothesis yet advanced; and, from the most attentive consideration of all the circumstances, the weight of evidence appears to induce the majority of practitioners to consider diabetes as depending on a primary affection of the kidneys.

Diabetes sometimes comes on slowly and imperceptibly, without any previous disorder; and it now and then arises to a considerable degree, and subsists long without being accompanied with evident disorder in any particular part of the system; the great thirst which always, and the voracious appetite which frequently occur in it, being often the only remarkable symptoms; but it more generally happens, that a considerable affection of the stomach precedes the coming on of the disease; and that, in its progress, besides the symptoms already mentioned, there is a great dryness in the skin, with a sense of weight in the kidneys, and a pain in the ureters, and the other urinary passages.

Under a long continuance of the disease, the body becomes much emaciated, the feet œdematous, great debility arises, the pulse is frequent and small, and an obscure fever, with all the appearance of hectic, prevails.

The urine in diabetes mellitus, from being at first insipid, clear, and colourless, soon acquires a sweetish or saccharine taste, its leading characteristic; and, when subjected to experiment, a considerable quantity of saccharine matter is to be extracted from it. Sometimes it is so loaded with sugar, as to be capable of being fermented into a vinous liquor Upwards of one-twelfth of its weight of sugar was extracted from some diabetic urine, by Cruickshank, which was at the rate of twenty-nine ounces troy a day, from one patient.

In some instances, the quantity of urine in diabetes is much greater than can be accounted for from all the sources united. Cases are recorded, in which 25 to 30 pints were discharged in the space of a natural day, for many successive weeks, and even months; and in which the whole ingesta, as was said, did not amount to half the weight of the urine. To account for this overplus, it has been alleged that water is absorbed from the air by the surface of the body; as also that a quantity of water is compounded in the lungs themselves.

Dissections of diabetes have usually shown the kidneys to be much affected. In some instances, they have been found in a loose flabby state, much enlarged in size, and of a pale ash colour; in others, they have been discovered much more vascular than in a healthy state, approaching a good deal to what takes place in inflammation, and containing, in their infundibula, a quantity of whitish fluid, somewhat resembling pus, but without any sign of ulceration whatever. At the same time that these appearances have been observed in their interior, the veins on their surface were found to be much fuller of blood than usual, forming a most beautiful net-work of vessels, the larger branches of which exhibited an absorbent appearance. In many cases of dissection, the whole of the mesentery has been discovered to be much diseased, and its glands remarkably enlarged; some of them being very hard, and of an irregular texture; others softer, and of a uniform spherical shape. Many of the lacteals have likewise been seen considerably enlarged. The liver, pancreas, spleen, and stomach, are in general perceived to be in a natural state; when they are not so, the occurrence is to be considered as accidental. The bladder, in many cases, is found to contain a considerable quantity of muddy urine.

A great variety of remedies has been proposed for this disease; but their success is generally precarious, or only temporary, at least in the mellitic form of the complaint. The treatment has been generally conducted on the principles of determining the fluids to other outlets, particularly the skin, and of increasing the tone of the kidneys. Diaphoretics are certainly very proper remedies, especially the combination of opium with ipecacuanha, or antimonials, assisted by the warm bath, suitable clothing, and perhaps removal to a milder climate: in the insipid form of diabetes, this plan has sometimes effected a cure; and it appears that the large use of opium has even the power of correcting, for the time, the saccharine quality of the urine. Cathartics are hardly of service, farther than to keep the bowels regular. Tonics are generally indicated by obvious marks of debility; and if the patient be troubled with acidity in the primæ viæ, alkaline medicines will be properly joined with them, preferring those which have no diuretic power. Astringents have been highly extolled by some practitioners, but do not appear likely to prevail, except those which pass off by the urine, as uva ursi; or the milder stimulants, which can be directed to the kidneys, as copaiba, &c. may correct the laxity of those organs, if the disease depend on this cause. The tinctura lyttæ must be used with great caution, and its efficacy is not well established: and blisters to the loins can only be useful as counter-irritants, though not the most suitable. Frequent friction, especially over the kidneys, wearing a tight belt, and gentle exercise, may assist the recovery of the patient; and when the function of the skin is restored, using the bath gradually of a lower temperature, will tend greatly to obviate its suppression afterward. It is likewise highly important to regulate the diet, especially in the mellitic diabetes. Dr Rolla first pointed out the advantage derived from restricting the patient to a diet principally of animal food, avoiding especially those vegetables which might afford saccharine matter, the urine becoming thereby of a more healthy quality, and diminishing in quantity: but unfortunately the benefit appears but temporary, and the plan is not persevered in without distress to the patient. The same gentleman recommended also the sulphuret of potassa, and still more the hydrosulphuret of ammonia; but they are very nauseous medicines, and of doubtful efficacy. Another plan of treating the disease has been more recently proposed, namely, by bleeding, and other antiphlogistic measures; and some cases of its success have been recorded: but farther experience is certainly required, before we should be justified in relying much upon it.

DIA'BOLUS METALLORUM. Tin.

DIABO'TANUM. (From δια, and βοτανη, an herb.) A plaster made of herbs.

DIACA'DMIAS. (From δια, and καδμια, cadmia.) The name of a plaster, the basis of which is cadmia.

DIACALAMI'NTHES. (From δια, and καλαμινθη, calamint.) The name of an antidote, the chief ingredient in which is calamint.

DIACA'RCINUM. (From δια, and καρκινος, a crab.) The name of an antidote prepared from the flesh of crabs and cray-fish.

DIACA'RYON. (From δια, and καρυον, a nut.) Rob of nuts, or walnuts.

DIACA'SSIA. (From δια, and κασσια, cassia.) Electuary of cassia.

DIACASTO'RIUM. (From δια, and καςωρ, castor.) An antidote, the basis of which is castor.

DIACATHO'LICON. (From δια, and καθολικος, universal.) The name of a purge, so called from its general usefulness.

DIACENTAU'RIUM. (From δια, and κενταυριον, centaury.) The Duke of Portland's powder is so called, because its chief ingredient is centaury.

DIACENTRO'TUM. (From δια, and κεντροω, to prick.) A collyrium, so called from its pungency and stimulating qualities.

DIACHALCI'TIS. (From δια, and χαλκιτις, chalcitis.) A plaster, the chief ingredient in which is chalcitis.

DIACHA'LSIS. (From διαχαλω, to be relaxed.) 1. A relaxation.

2. The opening of the sutures of the head.

DIACHEIRI'SMUS. (From δια, and χειρ, the hand.) Any operation performed by the hand.

DIACHELIDO'NIUM. (From δια, and χελιδωνιον, celandine.) A plaster, the chief ingredient in which was the herb celandine.

DIACHORE'MA. (From διαχωρεω, to separate from.) *Diachoresis.* Any excretion, or excrement, but chiefly that by stool.

DIACHORE'SIS. See *Diachorema.*

DIACHRI'STA. (From δια, and χριω, to anoint.) Medicines to anoint parts.

DIACHRY'SUM. (From δια, and χρυσος, gold.) A plaster for fractured limbs; so named from its yellow colour.

DIA'CHYLUM. (From δια, and χυλος, juice.) A plaster formerly made of certain juices, but it now means an emollient digestive plaster.

DIA'CHYSIS. (From δια, and χυω, to pour out.) Fusion or melting.

DIACHY'TICA. (From διαχυω, to dissolve.) Medicines which discuss tumours.

DIACINE'MA. (From δια, and κινεω, to move.) A slight dislocation.

DIACI'SSUM. (From δια, and κισσος, ivy.) An application composed of ivy leaves.

DIA'CLASIS. (From δια, and χλαω, to break.) A small fracture.

DIACLY'SMA. (From διακλυζω, to wash out.) A gargle or wash for the mouth.

DIACOCCYME'LON. (From δια, and κοκκυμηλον, a plum.) An electuary made of prunes.

DIACO'DIUM. (From δια, and κωδια, a poppy head.) A composition made of the heads of poppies.

DIACOLOCY'NTHIS. (From δια, and κολοκυνθις, the colocynth.) A preparation, the chief ingredient of which is colocynth.

DIACO'MMA. (From διακοπτω, to cut through.) *Diacope.* A deep cut or wound.

DIA'COPE. See *Diacomma.*

DIACOPRÆ'GIA. (From δια, κοπρος, dung, and αιξ, a goat.) A preparation with goat's dung.

DIACORA'LLUM. (From δια, and κοραλλιον, coral.) A preparation in which coral is a chief ingredient.

DIA'CRISIS. (From διακρινω, to distinguish.) The distinguishing diseases one from another by their symptoms.

DIACRO'CIUM. (From δια, and κροκος, saffron.) A collyrium in which is saffron.

DIACURCU'MA. (From δια, and κυρκουμα, turmeric.) An antidote in which is turmeric or saffron.

DIACYDO'NIUM. (From δια, and κυδωνια, a quince.) Marmalade of quinces.

DIADAPHNI'DION. (From δια, and δαφνις, the laurel-tree.) A drawing plaster in which were bay-berries.

DIADE'LPHIA. (From δις, twice, and αδελφις, a brotherhood; two brotherhoods.) The name of a class in the sexual system of plants, embracing those the flowers of which are hermaphrodites, and have the male organs united below in two sets of cylindrical filaments.

DIADE'MA. (From διαδεω, to surround.) 1. A diadem or crown.

2. A bandage to put round the head.

DIADE'XIS. (From διαδεχομαι, to transfer.) *Diadoche.* A transposition of humours from one place to another.

DIA'DOCHE. See *Diadexis.*

DIA'DOSIS. (From διαδιδωμι, to distribute.) The remission of a disorder.

DIÆ'RESIS. (From διαιρεω, to divide or separate.) A solution of continuity of the soft parts of the human body.

DIÆRE'TICA. (From διαιρεω, to divide.) Corrosive medicines.

DIÆ'TA. (From διαιταω, to nourish.) Diet; food. It means also the whole of the non-naturals. See *Diet.*

DIAGLAU'CIUM. (From δια, and γλαυκιον, the blue juice of an herb.) An eye-water made of the purging thistle.

DIAGNO'SIS. (From διαγινωσκω, to discern or distinguish.) The science which delivers the signs by which a disease may be distinguished from another disease: hence those symptoms which distinguish such affections are termed *diagnostic.*

DIAGRY'DIUM. Corrupted from dacrydium or scammony.

DIAHERMODA'CTYLUN. (From δια, and ερμοδακτυλος, the hermodactyl.) A purging medicine, the basis of which is the hermodactyl.

DIAI'REON. (From δια, and ιρις, the lily.) An antidote in which is the root of the lily.

DIAI'UM. (From δια, and ιον, a violet.) A pastil, the chief ingredient of which is violets.

DIALA'CCA. (From δια, and λακκα.) An antidote in which is the lacca.

DIALAGO'UM. (From δια, and λαγως, a hare.) A medicine in which is the dung of a hare.

DIALE'MMA. (From διαλαμβανω, to interrupt.) The remission of a disease.

DIALE'PSIS. (From διαλαμβανω, to interrupt.) 1. An intermission.

2. A space left between a bandage.

DIALI'BANUM. (From δια, and λιβανον, frankincense.) A medicine in which frankincense is a chief ingredient.

DIALLAGE. Smaragdite of Saussure. *Verde di Corsica duro* of artists. A species of the genus Schiller spar. It is a mineral of a greenish colour, composed of silica, alumina, magnesia, lime, oxide of iron, oxide of copper, and oxide of chrome. It is found principally in Corsica.

DIA'LOES. (From δια, and αλοη, the aloe.) A medicine chiefly composed of aloes.

DIALTHÆ'A. (From δια, and αλθαια, the mallow.) An ointment composed chiefly of marsh-mallows.

DIA'LYSIS. (From διαλυω, to dissolve.) A solution of continuity, or a destruction of parts.

DIA'LYSES. The plural of dialysis. The name of an order in the class *Locales* of Cullen's Nosology.

DIALY'TICA. (From διαλυω, to dissolve.) Medicines which heal wounds and fractures.

DIAMARGARI'TON. (From δια, and μαργαριτις, pearl.) An antidote in which pearls are the chief ingredient.

DIAMASSE'MA. (From δια, and μασσομαι, to chew.) A masticatory, or substance put into the mouth, and chewed to excite a discharge of the saliva.

Dia'mbra. (From $\delta\iota\alpha$, and $\alpha\mu\beta\rho\alpha$, amber.) An aromatic composition in which was ambergris.

Diame'lon. (From $\delta\iota\alpha$, and $\mu\eta\lambda o\nu$, a quince.) A composition of quinces.

DIAMOND. The diamond, which was well known to the ancients, is principally found in the western peninsula of India, on the coast of Coromandel, in the kingdoms of Golconda and Visapour, in the island of Borneo, and in the Brazils. It is the most valued of all minerals.

Diamonds are generally found bedded in yellow ochre or in rocks of freestone, or quartz, and sometimes in the beds of running waters. When taken out of the earth, they are incrusted with an exterior earthly covering, under which is another, consisting of carbonate of lime.

In the Brazils, it is supposed that diamonds might be obtained in greater quantities than at present, if the sufficient working of the diamond-mines was not prohibited, in order to prevent that diminution of their commercial value, which a greater abundance of them might occasion.

Brazilian diamonds are, in commercial estimation, inferior to the oriental ones.

In the rough, diamonds are worth two pounds sterling the carat, or four grains, provided they are without blemish. The expense of cutting and polishing amounts to about four pounds more. The value however is far above what is now stated when they become considerable in size. The greatest sum that has been given for a single diamond is one hundred and fifty thousand pounds.

The usual method of calculating the value of diamonds is by squaring the number of carats, and then multiplying the amount by the price of a single carat: thus supposing one carat to be 2*l.* a diamond of 8 carats is worth 128*l.* being $8 \times 8 \times 2$.

The famous Pigot diamond weighs 188 1-8th grains.

Physical Properties of Diamond.

Diamond is always crystallized, but sometimes so imperfectly, that, at first sight, it might appear amorphous. The figure of diamond, when perfect, is an eight-sided prism. There are also cubical, flat, and round diamonds. It is the oriental diamond which crystallizes into octohedra, and exhibits all the varieties of this primitive figure. The diamond of Brazil crystallizes into dodecahedra.

The texture of the diamond is lamellated, for it may be split or cleft with an instrument of well-tempered steel, by a swift blow in a particular direction. There are however some diamonds which do not appear to be formed of *laminæ*, but of twisted and interwoven fibres, like those of knots in wood. These exceed the others greatly in hardness, they cannot be cut or polished, and are therefore called by the lapidaries *diamonds of nature.*

The diamond is one of the hardest bodies known. It resists the most highly-tempered steel file, which circumstance renders it necessary to attack it with diamond powder. It takes an exquisite and lasting polish. It has a great refractive power, and hence its lustre, when cut into the form of a regular solid, is uncommonly great. The usual colour of diamonds is a light gray, often inclining to yellow, at times lemon colour, violet, or black, seldomer rose-red, and still more rarely green or blue, but more frequently pale brown. The purest diamonds are perfectly transparent. The colourless diamond has a specific gravity which is in proportion to that of water as 3.512 to 1.000, according to Brisson. This varies however considerably. When rubbed it becomes *positively* electric, even before it has been cut by the lapidary.

Diamond is not acted upon by acids, or by any chemical agent, oxygen excepted; and this requires a very great increase of temperature to produce any effect.

The diamond burns by a strong heat, with a sensible flame, like other combustible bodies, attracting oxygen, and becoming wholly converted into carbonic acid gas during that process.

It combines with iron by fusion, and converts it, like common charcoal, into steel; but diamond requires a much higher temperature for its combustion than common charcoal does, and even then it consumes but slowly, and ceases to burn the instant its temperature is lowered.

"From the high refractive power of the diamond, Bigot and Arago supposed that it might contain hydrogen. Sir H. Davy, from the action of potassium on it, and its non-conduction of electricity, suggested in his third Bakerian lecture, that a minute portion of oxygen might exist in it; and in his new experiments on the fluoric compounds, he threw out the idea, that it might be the carbonaceous principle, combined with some new, light, and subtle element of the oxygenous and chlorine class

This unrivalled chemist, during his residence at Florence in March 1814, made several experiments on the combustion of the diamond and of plumbago, by means of the great lens in the cabinet of natural history; the same instrument as that employed in the first trials on the action of the solar heat on the diamond, instituted in 1694 by Cosmo III. Grand Duke of Tuscany. He subsequently made a series of researches on the combustion of different kinds of charcoal at Rome. His mode of investigation was peculiarly elegant, and led to the most decisive results.

He found that diamond, when strongly ignited by the lens, in a thin capsule of platinum, perforated with many orifices, so as to admit a free circulation of air, continued to burn with a steady brilliant red light, visible in the brightest sunshine, after it was withdrawn from the focus. Some time after the diamonds were removed out of the focus, indeed, a wire of platina that attached them to the tray was fused, though their weight was only 1.84 grains. His apparatus consisted of clear glass globes of the capacity of from 14 to 40 cubic inches, having single apertures to which stop-cocks were attached. A small hollow cylinder of platinum was attached to one end of the stop-cock, and was mounted with the little perforated capsule for containing the diamond. When the experiment was to be made, the globe containing the capsule and the substance to be burned was exhausted by an excellent air-pump, and pure oxygen, from chlorate of potassa, was then introduced. The change of volume in the gas after combustion was estimated by means of a fine tube connected with a stop-cock, adapted by a proper screw to the stop-cock of the globe, and the absorption was judged of by the quantity of mercury that entered the tube which afforded a measure so exact, that no alteration however minute could be overlooked. He had previously satisfied himself that a quantity of moisture, less than 1-100th of a grain, is rendered evident by deposition on a polished surface of glass; for a piece of paper weighing one grain was introduced into a tube of about four cubic inches' capacity, whose exterior was slightly heated by a candle. A dew was immediately perceptible on the inside of the glass, though the paper, when weighed in a balance turning with 1-100th of a grain, indicated no appreciable diminution.

The diamonds were also heated to redness before they were introduced into the capsule. During their combustion, the glass globe was kept cool by the application of water to that part of it immediately above the capsule, and where the heat was greatest.

From the results of his different experiments, conducted with the most unexceptionable precision, it is demonstrated, that diamond affords no other substance by its combustion than pure carbonic acid gas; and that the process is merely a solution of diamond in oxygen, without any change in the volume of the gas. It likewise appears, that in the combustion of the different kinds of charcoal, water is produced; and that from the diminution of the volume of the oxygen, there is every reason to believe that the water is formed by the combustion of hydrogen existing in strongly ignited charcoal. As the charcoal from oil of turpentine left no residuum, no other cause but the presence of hydrogen can be assigned for the diminution occasioned in the volume of the gas during its combustion.

The only chemical difference perceptible between diamond and the purest charcoal is, that the last contains a minute portion of hydrogen; but can a quantity of an element, less in some cases than 1-50,000th part of the weight of the substance, occasion so great a difference in physical and chemical characters? The opinions of Tennant, that the difference depends on crystallization, seems to be correct. Transparent solid bodies are in general non-conductors of electricity; and it is probable that the same corpuscular arrangements which give to matter the power of transmitting and polurizing light, are likewise connected with its relations to electricity. Thus water, the hydrates of the alkalies, and a number of other bodies which are conductors of electricity when fluid, become non-conductors in their crystallized form.

That charcoal is more inflammable than the diamond, may be explained from the looseness of its texture, and from the hydrogen it contains. But the diamond appears to burn in oxygen with as much facility as plumbago, so that at least one distinction supposed to exist between the diamond and common carbonaceous substances is done away by these researches. The power possessed by certain carbonaceous substances of absorbing gases, and separating colouring matters from fluids, is probably mechanical and dependent on their porous organic structure; for it belongs in the highest degree to vegetable and animal charcoal, and it does not exist in plumbago, coke, or anthracite.

The nature of the chemical difference between the diamond and other carbonaceous substances, may be demonstrated by igniting them in chlorine, when muriatic acid is produced from the latter, but not from the former. The visible acid vapour is owing to the moisture present in the chlorine uniting to the dry muriatic gas. But charcoal, after being intensely ignited in chlorine, is not altered in its conducting power of colour. This circumstance is in favour of the opinion, that the minute quantity of hydrogen is not the cause of the great difference between the physical properties of the diamond and charcoal." See *Carbon.*

Diamond-shaped. See *Leaf.*

DIAMO'RON. (From δια, and μωρον, a mulberry.) A preparation of mulberries.

DIAMO'SCHUM. (From δια, and μοσχος, musk.) An antidote in which musk is a chief ingredient.

DIAMOTO'SIS. (From δια, and μοτος, lint.) The introduction of lint into an ulcer or wound.

DIA'NA. 1. The moon.

2. The chemical name for silver from its white shining appearance.

DIANANCA'SMUS. (From δια, and αναγκαζω, to force.) 1. The forcible restoration of a luxated part into its proper place.

2. An instrument to reduce a distorted spine.

DIA'NDRIA. (From δις twice, and ανηρ, a man.) The name of a class in the sexual system, consisting of hermaphrodite plants which have flowers with two staminæ.

DIA'NTHUS. (From Δις, διος, Jove, and ανθος, a flower: so called from the elegance and fragrance of its flower.) The name of a genus of plants in the Linnæan system. Class, *Decandria*; Order, *Digynia.*

DIANTHUS CARYOPHYLLUS. The systematic name of the clove-pink. *Caryophyllum rubrum; Tunica; Vetonica; Betonica; Coronaria; Caryophyllus hortensis.* Clove gilliflower. Clove July flower. This fragrant plant, *Dianthus—floribus solitariis, squamis calycinus subovatis, brevissimus, corollis crenatis*, of Linnæus, grows wild in several parts of England; but the flowers, which are pharmaceutically employed, are usually produced in gardens: they have a pleasant aromatic smell, somewhat allied to that of clove-spice; their taste is bitterish and sub-adstringent. These flowers were formerly in extensive use, but are now merely employed in form of syrup, as a useful and pleasant vehicle for other medicines.

DIAPA'SMA. (From διαπασσω, to sprinkle.) A medicine reduced to powder and sprinkled over the body, or any part.

DIAPEDE'SIS. (From διαπηδαω, to leap through.) The transudation or escape of blood through the coats of an artery.

DIAPE'GMA. (From διαπηγνυω, to close together.) A surgical instrument for closing together broken bones.

DIAPE'NTE. (From δια, and πεντε, five.) A medicine composed of five ingredients.

DIAPHANOUS. (*Diaphanosus*; from δια, through, and φαινω, to shine.) A term applied to any substance which is transparent; as the hyaloid membrane covering the vitreous humour of the eye, which is as transparent as glass.

DIAPHŒ'NICUM. From δια, and φοινιξ, a date.) A medicine made of dates.

DIA'PHORA. (From διαφερω, to distinguish.) The distinction of diseases by their characteristic marks and symptoms.

DIAPHORE'SIS (From διαφορεω, to carry through.) Perspiration.

DIAPHORETIC. (*Diaphoreticus*; from διαφορεω, to carry through.) That which, from being taken internally, increases the discharge by the skin. When this is carried so far as to be condensed on the surface, it forms sweat: and the medicine producing it is named sudorific. Between diaphoretic and sudorific, there is no distinction; the operation is in both cases the same, and differs only in degree from augmentation of dose, or employment of assistant means. This class of medicines comprehends five orders.

1. *Pungent diaphoretics*, as the *volatile salts*, and *essential oils*, which are well adapted for the aged; those in whose system there is little sensibility; those who are difficultly affected by other diaphoretics; and those whose stomachs will not bear large doses of medicines.

2. *Calefacient diaphoretics*, such as *serpentaria contrayerva*, and *guaiacum*: these are given in cases where the circulation is low and languid.

3. *Stimulant diaphoretics*, as antimonial and mercurial preparations, which are best fitted for the vigorous and plethoric.

4. *Antispasmodic diaphoretics*, as *opium*, *musk*, and *camphire*, which are given to produce a diaphoresis, when the momentum of the blood is increased.

5. *Diluent diaphoretics*, as water, whey, &c. which are best calculated for that habit in which a predisposition to sweating is wanted, and in which no diaphoresis takes place, although there be evident causes to produce it.

DIAPHRA'GMA. (*Diaphragma, matis.* n.; from δια, and φραττω, to divide.) *Septum transversum.* The midriff, or diaphragm. A muscle that divides the thorax from the abdomen. It is composed of two muscles; the first and superior of these arises from the sternum, and the ends of the last ribs on each side. Its fibres, from this semicircular origination, tend towards their centre, and terminate in a tendon, or aponeurosis, which is termed the *centrum tendinosum.* The second and inferior muscle comes from the vertebræ of the loins by two productions, of which that on the right side comes from the first, second, and third vertebræ of the loins; that on the left side is somewhat shorter, and both these portions join and make the lower part of the diaphragm, which joins its tendons with the tendon of the other, so that they make but one muscular partition. It is covered by the pleura on its upper side, and by the peritonæum on the lower side. It is pierced in the middle for the passage of the vena cava; in its lower part for the œsophagus, and the nerves, which go to the upper orifice of the stomach, and between the productions of the inferior muscle, passes the aorta, the thoracic duct, and the vena azygos. It receives arteries and veins called phrenic or diaphragmatic, from the cava and aorta: and sometimes on its lower part two branches from the vena adiposa, and two arteries from the lumbares. It has two nerves which come from the third vertebra of the neck, which pass through the cavity of the thorax, and are lost in its substance. In its natural situation, the diaphragm is convex on the upper side towards the breast, and concave on its lower side towards the belly; therefore, when its fibres swell and contract, it must become plain on each side, and consequently the cavity of the breast is enlarged to give liberty to the lungs to receive air in inspiration; and the stomach and intestines are pressed for the distribution of their contents; hence the use of this muscle is very considerable; it is the principal agent in respiration, particularly in inspiration; for when it is in action the cavity of the thorax is enlarged, particularly at the sides, where the lungs are chiefly situated; and as the lungs must always be contiguous to the inside of the thorax and upper side of the diaphragm, the air rushes into them, in order to fill up the increased space. In expiration it is relaxed and pushed up by the pressure of the abdominal muscles upon the viscera of the abdomen; and at the same time that they press it upwards, they pull down the ribs, by which the cavity of the thorax is diminished, and the air suddenly pushed out of the lungs.

DIAPHRAGMATI'TIS. (From διαφραγμα, the diaphragm.) Inflammation of the diaphragm. See *Paraphrenitis.*

DIA'PHTHORA. (From διαφθειρω to corrupt.) An abortion where the fœtus is corrupted in the womb.

DIAPHYLA'CTICA. (From διαφυλασσω, to preserve.) Medicines which resist putrefaction or prevent infection.

DIA'PHYSIS. (From διαφυω, to divide.) An interstice or partition between the joints.

DIAPISSELÆ'UM. (From δια, and πισσελαιον, the oil of pitch, or liquid pitch.) A composition in which is liquid pitch.

DIA'PLASIS. (From διαπλασσω, to put together.) The replacing a luxated or fractured bone in its proper situation.

DIAPLA'SMA. (From διαπλασσω, to anoint.) An unction or fomentation applied to the whole body or any part.

DIA'PNE. (From διαπνεω, to blow through, or pass gently as the breath does.) An insensible discharge of the urine.

DIA'PNOE. (From διαπνεω, to breathe through.) The transpiration of vapour through the pores of the skin.

DIAPNO'ICA. (From διαπνεω, to transpire.) Diaphoretics or medicines which promote perspiration.

DIAPORE'MA. (From διαπορεω, to be in doubt.) Nervous anxiety.

DIAPORON. (From δια, and οπωρα, autumnal fruits.) A composition in which are several autumnal fruits, as quinces, medlars, and services.

DIAPRA'SSIUM. (From δια, and πρασσιον, hoarhound.) A composition in which hoarhound is the principal ingredient.

DIAPRU'NUM. (From δια, and προυνη, a prune.) An electuary of prunes.

DIAPSO'RICUM. (From δια, and ψωρα, the itch or scurvy.) A medicine for the itch or scurvy.

DIAPTE'RNES. (From δια, and πτερνα, the heel.) A composition of cow heel and cheese.

DIAPTERO'SIS. (From δια, and πτερον, a feather.) The cleaning the ears with a feather.

DIAPYE'MA. (From δια, and πυον, pus.) A suppuration or abscess.

DIAPYE'MATA. (From διαπυημα, a suppuration.) Suppurating medicines.

DIAPYE'TICA. (From διαπυημα, a suppuration.) Suppurating applications.

DIARHO'CHA. (From δια, and ρηχος, a space.) The space between the foldings of a bandage.

DIA'RIUS. (From *dies*, a day.) A term applied to fevers which last but one day.

DIAROMA'TICUM. (From δια, and αρωματικον, an aromatic.) A composition of spices.

DIA'RRHAGE. (From διαρρηγνυμι, to break asunder.) A fracture.

DIARRHODO'MELI. (From δια, ροδον, a rose, and μελι, honey.) Scammony, agaric, pepper, and honey.

DIA'RRHODON. (From δια, and ροδον, a rose.) A composition of roses.

DIARRHŒ'A. (From διαρρεω, to flow through.) A purging. It is distinguished by frequent stools with the natural excrement, not contagious, and seldom attended with pyrexia. It is a genus of disease in the class *Neuroses*, and order *Spasmi* of Cullen, containing the following species:

1. *Diarrhœa crapulosa.* The feculent diarrhœa, from *crapulus*, one who overloads his stomach.

2. *Diarrhœa biliosa.* The bilious, from an increased secretion of bile.

3. *Diarrhœa mucosa.* The mucous, from a quantity of slime being voided.

4. *Diarrhœa hepatirrhœa.* The hepatic, in which there is a quantity of serous matter, somewhat resembling the washings of flesh, voided; the liver being primarily affected.

5. *Diarrhœa lienterica.* The lientery; when the food passes unchanged.

6. *Diarrhœa cœliaca.* The cœliac passion: the food passes off in this affection in a white liquid state like chyle.

7. *Diarrhœa verminosa.* Arising from worms.

Diarrhœa seems evidently to depend on an increase of the peristaltic motion, or of the secretion of the intestines; and besides the causes already noticed, it may arise from many others, influencing the system generally, or the particular seat of the disease. Of the former kind are cold, checking perspiration, certain passions of the mind, and other disorders as dentition, gout, fever, &c. To the latter belong various acrid ingesta, drastic cathartics, spontaneous acidity, &c. In this complaint each discharge is usually preceded by a murmuring noise, with a sense of weight and uneasiness in the hypogastrium. When it is protracted, the stomach usually becomes affected with sickness, or sometimes vomiting, the countenance grows pale or sallow, and the skin generally dry and rigid. Ultimately great debility and emaciation, with dropsy of the lower extremities, often supervene. Dissections of diarrhœa, where it terminated fatally, have shown ulcerations of the internal surface of the intestines, sometimes to a considerable extent, especially about the follicular glands; in which occasionally a cancerous character has been observable. The treatment of this complaint must vary greatly according to circumstances: sometimes we can only hope to palliate, as when it occurs in the advanced period of phthisis pulmonalis; sometimes it is rather to be encouraged, relieving more serious symptoms, as a bilious diarrhœa coming on in fever, though still some limits must be put to the discharge. Where, however, we are warranted in using the most speedy means of stopping it, the objects are, 1. To obviate the several causes. 2. To lessen the inordinate action, and give tone to the intestine.

I. Emetics may sometimes be useful, clearing out the stomach, and liver, as well as determining to the skin. Cathartics also, expelling worms, or indurated fæces; but any acrimony in the intestine would probably cause its own discharge, and where there is much irritability, they might aggravate the disease: however, in protracted cases, the alvine contents speedily become vitiated, and renew the irritation; which may be best obviated by an occasional mild aperient, particularly rhubarb. If, however, the liver do not perform its office, the intestine will hardly recover its healthy condition: and that may most probably be effected by the cautious use of mercury. Likewise articles which determine the fluids to other outlets, diuretics, and particularly diaphoretics, in many cases contribute materially to recovery; the latter perhaps assisted by bathing, warm clothing, gentle exercise, &c. Diluent, demulcent, antacid, and other chemical remedies, may be employed to correct acrimony, according to its particular nature. In children teething, the gums should be lanced; and if the bowels have been attacked on the repulsion of some other disease, it may often be proper to endeavour to restore this. But a matter of the greatest importance is the due regulation of the diet, carefully avoiding those articles, which are likely to disagree, or irritate the bowels, and preferring such as have a mild astringent effect. Fish, milk, and vegetables, little acescent, as rice, bread, &c. are best; and for the drink, madeira or brandy, sufficiently diluted, rather than malt liquors.

II. Some of the means already noticed will help to fulfil the second indication also, as a wholesome diet, exercise, diaphoretics, &c.: but there are others of more power, which must be resorted to in urgent cases. At the head of these is opium, a full dose of which frequently at once effects a cure; but where there is some more fixed cause, and the complaint of any standing, moderate quantities repeated at proper intervals will answer better, and other subsidiary means ought not to be neglected; aromatics may prevent its disordering the stomach, rhubarb obviate its causing permanent constipation, &c. Tonics are generally proper, the discharge itself inducing debility, and where there is a deficiency of bile particularly, the lighter forms of the aromatic bitters, as the infusum calumbæ, &c. will materially assist; and mild chalybeates are sometimes serviceable. In protracted cases astringents come in aid of the general plan, and where opium disagrees, they may be more necessary: but the milder ones should be employed at first, the more powerful only where the patient appears sinking. Chalk and lime-water answer best where there is acidity; otherwise the pomegranate rind, logwood extract, catechu, kino, tormentil, &c. may be given: where these fail, alum, sulphate of zinc, galls, or superacetate of lead.

DIARTHRO'SIS. (From διαρθροω, to articulate.) A moveable connexion of bones. This genus has five species, viz. enarthrosis, arthrodia, ginglymus, trochoides, and amphiarthrosis.

DIASAPO'NIUM. (From δια, and σαπων, soap.) An ointment of soap.

DIASATY'RIUM. (From $\delta\iota\alpha$, and $\sigma\alpha\tau\upsilon\rho\iota o\nu$, the orchis.) An ointment of the orchis-root.

DIASCI'LLIUM. (From $\delta\iota\alpha$, and $\sigma\kappa\iota\lambda\lambda\alpha$, the squill.) Oxymel and vinegar of squills.

DIASCI'NCUS. (From $\delta\iota\alpha$, and $\sigma\kappa\iota\gamma\kappa o\varsigma$, the crocodile.) A name for the mithridate, in the composition of which there was a part of the crocodile.

DIASCO'RDIUM. (From $\delta\iota\alpha$, and $\sigma\kappa o\rho\delta\iota o\nu$, the water germander.) Electuary of scordium.

DIASE'NA. (From $\delta\iota\alpha$, and *sena.*) A medicine in which is senna.

DIASMY'RNUM. (From $\delta\iota\alpha$, and $\sigma\mu\upsilon\rho\nu\eta$, myrrh.) *Diasmyrnes.* A wash for the eyes, composed of myrrh.

DIASO'STICUS. (From $\delta\iota\alpha\sigma\omega\zeta\omega$, to preserve.) That which preserves health.

DIASPE'RMATUM. (From $\delta\iota\alpha$, and $\sigma\pi\epsilon\rho\mu\alpha$, seed.) A medicine composed chiefly of seeds.

DIA'SPHAGE. (From $\delta\iota\alpha\sigma\phi\alpha\zeta\omega$, to separate.) *Diasphaxis.* The interstice between two veins.

DIASPHY'XIS. (From $\delta\iota\alpha$, and $\sigma\phi\upsilon\zeta\omega$, to strike.) The pulsation of an artery.

[*Diaspore*, of Haüy, Brogniart, Cleaveland, &c. "This mineral is but little known. It is composed of laminæ, somewhat curved, easily separable from each other, and possessing a pearly gray colour, with considerable lustre. These laminæ according to the natural joints, which they present, when examined by a light, seem to have separated in the direction of the smaller diagonals of the bases of a rhomboidal prism. The edges or angles of its fragments are capable of scratching glass. Its specific gravity is 3.43.

"A small fragment, placed in the flame of a candle, almost instantly decrepitates, and is *dispersed* in numerous little spangles. Hence its name from the Greek $\Delta\iota\alpha\delta\pi\epsilon\iota\rho\omega$. It is composed of alumine 80, water 17, iron 3. Nothing is known of its geological situation. Its gangue, is a rock, both argillaceous and ferruginous."—*Cleav. Min.* A.]

DIA'STASIS. (From $\delta\iota\iota\sigma\tau\eta\mu\iota$, to separate.) *Diastema.* A separation. A separation of the ends of the bones; as that which occasionally happens to the bones of the cranium, in some cases of hydrocephalus.

DIASTE'ATON. (From $\delta\iota\alpha$, and $\varsigma\epsilon\alpha\rho$, fat.) An ointment of the fat of animals.

DIASTE'MA. See *Diastasis.*

DIASTOLE. (From $\delta\iota\alpha$, and $\sigma\tau\epsilon\lambda\lambda\omega$, to stretch.) The dilatation of the heart and arteries. See *Circulation.*

DIASTOMO'SIS. (From $\delta\iota\alpha\varsigma o\mu o\omega$, to dilate.) Any dilatation, or dilating instrument.

DIASTRE'MMA. (From $\delta\iota\alpha\varsigma\rho\epsilon\phi\omega$, to turn aside.) *Diastrophe.* A distortion of any limb or part.

DIA'STROPHE. See *Diastremma.*

DIA'TASIS. (From $\delta\iota\alpha\tau\epsilon\iota\nu\omega$, to distend.) The extension of a fractured limb, in order to reduce it.

DIATECOLI'THUM. (From $\delta\iota\alpha$, and $\tau\eta\kappa o\lambda\iota\theta o\varsigma$, the Jew's stone.) An antidote containing lapis judaicus.

DIATERE'SIS. (From $\delta\iota\alpha$, and $\tau\epsilon\rho\epsilon\omega$, to perforate.) A perforation or aperture.

DIATERE'TICA. (From $\delta\iota\alpha$ and $\tau\epsilon\rho\epsilon\omega$, to preserve.) Medicines which preserve health and prevent disease.

DIATE'SSARON. (From $\delta\iota\alpha$, and $\tau\epsilon\sigma\sigma\alpha\rho\epsilon\varsigma$, four.) A medicine compounded of four simple ingredients.

DIATE'TTIGUM. (From $\delta\iota\alpha$, and $\tau\epsilon\tau\tau\iota\gamma\omega\nu$, a grasshopper.) A medicine in the composition of which were grasshoppers, given as an antidote to some nephritic complaints, by Ægineta.

DIA'THESIS. (From $\delta\iota\alpha\tau\iota\theta\eta\mu\iota$, to dispose.) Any particular state of the body: thus, in inflammatory fever, there is an inflammatory diathesis, and, during putrid fever, a putrid diathesis.

DIATHE'SMUS. (From $\delta\iota\alpha\theta\epsilon\omega$, to run through.) A rupture through which some fluid escapes.

DIATRAGACA'NTHUM. From $\delta\iota\alpha$, and $\tau\rho\alpha\gamma\alpha\kappa\alpha\nu\theta\alpha$, tragacanth.) A medicine composed of gum-tragacanth.

DIA'TRIUM. (From $\delta\iota\alpha$, and $\tau\rho\epsilon\iota\varsigma$, three.) A medicine composed of three simple ingredients.

DIAXYLA'LOES. (From $\delta\iota\alpha$, and $\xi\upsilon\lambda\alpha\lambda o\eta$, the lignum aloes.) A medicine in which is lignum aloes.

DIAZO'MA. (From $\delta\iota\alpha\zeta\omega\nu\nu\upsilon\mu\iota$, to surround; because it surrounds the cavity of the thorax.) The diaphragm

DIAZO'STER. (From $\delta\iota\alpha\zeta\omega\nu\nu\upsilon\mu\iota$, to surround; because, when the body is girded, the belt usually lies upon it.) A name of the twelfth vertebra of the back.

DICENTE'TUM. (From $\delta\iota\alpha$, and $\kappa\epsilon\nu\tau\epsilon\omega$, to stimulate.) A pungent or stimulating wash for the eyes.

DICHASTE'RES. (From $\delta\iota\chi\alpha\zeta\omega$, to divide, because they divide the food.) A name of the foreteeth.

DICHOPHY'IA. (From $\delta\iota\chi\alpha$, double, and $\phi\upsilon\omega$, to grow.) A distemper of the hairs, in which they split and grow forked.

DICHOTOMUS. (From $\delta\iota\varsigma$, twice, and $\tau\epsilon\mu\nu\omega$, to cut; that is, cut into two.) Dichotomous or bifurcated. Applied to stems, styles, &c. which are forked or divided into two.

DICHROITE. A species of iolite.

DICOTYLEDONES. Two cotyledons. See *Cotyledon.*

DICROTIC. (*Dicroticus;* from $\delta\iota\varsigma$, twice, and $\kappa\rho o\upsilon\omega$, to strike.) A term given to a pulse in which the artery rebounds after striking, so as to convey the sensation of a double pulsation.

DICTAMNI'TES. (From $\delta\iota\kappa\tau\alpha\mu\nu o\varsigma$, dittany.) A wine medicated with dittany.

DICTA'MNUS. (From *Dictamnus*, a city in Crete, on whose mountains it grows.) The name of a genus of plants in the Linnæan system. Class, *Decandria;* Order, *Monogynia.* Dittany.

DICTAMNUS ALBUS. White fraxinella, or bastard dittany. *Fraxinella. Dictamnus albus—foliis pinnatis, caule simplici*, of Linnæus. The root of this plant is the part directed for medicinal use; when fresh, it has a moderately strong, not disagreeable smell. Formerly it was much used as a stomachic, tonic, and alexipharmic, and was supposed to be a medicine of much efficacy in removing uterine obstructions, and destroying worms; but its medicinal powers became so little regarded by modern physicians, that it had fallen almost entirely into disuse, till Baron Stoerck brought it into notice, by publishing several cases of its success, viz. in tertian intermittents, worms, (lumbrici) and menstrual suppressions. In all these cases, he employed the powdered root to the extent of a scruple twice a day. He also made use of a tincture, prepared of two ounces of the fresh root digested in 14 ounces of spirit of wine; of this 20 to 50 drops, two or three times a day, were successfully employed in epilepsies, and, when joined with steel, this root, we are told, was of great service to chlorotic patients. The dictamnus undoubtedly, says Dr. Woodville, is a medicine of considerable power; but notwithstanding the account of it given by Stoerck, who seems to have paid little attention to its modus operandi, we may still say with Haller, "*nondum autem vires pro dignitate exploratus est,*" and it is now fallen into disuse.

DICTAMNUS CRETICUS. See *Origanum dictamnus.*

DIDYMÆ'A. (From $\delta\iota\delta\upsilon\mu o\varsigma$, double.) A cataplasm; so called by Galen, from the double use to which he puts it.

DI'DYMI. (From $\delta\iota\delta\upsilon\mu o\varsigma$, double.) Twins. An old name of the testicles, and two eminences of the brain, from their double protuberance.

DIDYNAMIA. (From $\delta\iota\varsigma$, twice, and $\delta\upsilon\nu\alpha\mu\iota\varsigma$, power, two powers.) The name of a class in the sexual system of plants, consisting of those with hermaphrodite flowers, which have four stamina, two of which are long, and two short.

DIECBO'LIUM. (From $\delta\iota\alpha$, and $\epsilon\kappa\beta\alpha\lambda\lambda\omega$, to cast out.) A medicine causing an abortion.

DIELE'CTRON. (From $\delta\iota\alpha$, and $\epsilon\lambda\epsilon\kappa\tau\rho o\nu$, amber.) A name of a troche, in which amber is an ingredient.

DIEMERBROECK, ISBRAND, was born near Utrecht, in 1609. After graduating at Angers, he went to Nimeguen in 1636, and for some years continued freely attending those who were ill of the plague, which raged with great violence, and of which he subsequently published an account. This obtained him much credit: and, in 1642, he was made professor extraordinary in medicine at Utrecht; when he gave lectures on that subject, as well as on anatomy, which rendered him very popular. He received also other distinctions at that university, and continued in high esteem till his death, in 1674. He was author, besides, of a system of anatomy, and several other works in medicine and surgery; part of which were published after his death by his son, especially his treatise on the measles and smallpox.

DIERVI'LLA. (Named in honour of Mr. Dierville, who first brought it from Arcadia.) See *Lonicera diervilla.*

DIET. *Diæta.* The dietetic part of medicine is no inconsiderable branch, and seems to require a much greater share of regard than it commonly meets with. A great variety of diseases might be removed by the observance of a proper diet and regimen, without the assistance of medicine, were it not for the impatience of the sufferers. However, it may on all occasions come in as a proper assistant to the cure, which sometimes cannot be performed without a due observance of the non-naturals. That food is, in general, thought the best and most conducive to long life, which is most simple, pure, and free from irritating qualities, and such as approaches nearest to the nature of our own bodies in a healthy state, or is capable of being easiest converted into their substance by the vis vitæ, after it has been duly prepared by the art of cookery; but the nature, composition, virtues, and uses of particular aliments, can never be learnt to satisfaction, without the assistance of practical chemistry.

Diet drink. An alterative decoction employed daily in considerable quantities, at least from a pint to a quart. The decoction of sarsaparilla and mezereon, the Lisbon diet drink, is the most common and most useful.

DIETE'TIC. *Dieteticus.* That part of medicine which considers the way of living with relation to food, or diet, suitable to any particular case.

Die'xodos. (From δια, and εξοδος, a way to pass out.) *Diodos.* In Hippocrates it means evacuation by stool.

Diffla'tio. (From *difflo*, to blow away.) Perspiration.

DIFFUSUS. Diffused; spreading. Applied to panicles and stems. *Panicula diffusa*, that is, lax and spreading; as in *Saxifraga umbrosa;* the London pride, so common in our gardens; and many grasses, especially the common cultivated oat. The *Bunias kakile*, or sea rocket, has the *caulis diffusus.*

DIGA'STRICUS. (From δις, twice, and γαστηρ, a belly: so called from its having two bellies.) *Biventer maxillæ* of Albinus. *Mastoido-hygenien* of Dumas. A muscle situated externally between the lower jaw and *os hyoides.* It arises, by a fleshy belly, from the upper part of the processus mastoideus, and descending, it contracts into a round tendon, which passes through the stylohyoideus, and an annular ligament which is fastened to the os hyoides: then it grows fleshy again, and ascends towards the middle of the edge of the lower jaw, where it is inserted. Its use is to open the mouth by pulling the lower jaw downwards and backwards; and when the jaws are shut, to raise the larynx, and consequently the pharynx, upwards, as in deglutition.

Digere'ntia. (From *digero*, to digest.) Medicines which promote the secretion of proper pus in wounds and ulcers.

DIGESTER. A strong and tight iron kettle or copper, furnished with a valve of safety, in which bodies may be subjected to the vapour of water, alcohol, or æther, at a pressure above that of the atmosphere.

DIGESTION. (*Digestio;* from *digero*, to dissolve.)

1. An operation in chemistry and pharmacy, in which such matters as are intended to act slowly on each other, are exposed to a heat, continued for some time.

2. In physiology, the change that the food undergoes in the stomach, by which it is converted into chyme.

"The immediate object of digestion is the formation of chyle, a matter destined for the reparation of the continual waste of the animal economy. The digestive organs contribute also in many other ways to nutrition.

If we judge of the importance of a function by the number and variety of its organs, digestion ought to be placed in the first rank; no other function of the animal economy presents such a complicated apparatus.

There always exists an evident relation between the sort of aliment proper for an animal and the disposition of its digestive organs. If, by their nature, the aliments are very different from the elements which compose the animal: if, for example, it is graminivorous, the dimensions of the apparatus will be more complicated, and more considerable; if, on the contrary, the animal feeds on flesh, the digestive organs will be fewer and more simple, as is seen in the carnivorous animals. Man, called to use equally animal and vegetable aliments, keeps a mean between the graminivorous and carnivorous animals, as to the disposition and complication of his digestive apparatus, without deserving, on that account, to be called omnivorous.

We may represent the digestive apparatus as a long canal differently twisted upon itself, wide in certain points, narrow in others, susceptible of contracting or enlarging its dimensions, and into which a great quantity of fluids are poured by means of different ducts. The canal is divided into many parts by anatomists;

1. The mouth.
2. The pharynx.
3. The œsophagus.
4. The stomach.
5. The small intestines.
6. The great intestines.
7. The anus.

Two membranous layers form the sides of the digestive canal in its whole length. The inner layer, which is intended to be in contact with the aliments, consists of a mucous membrane, the appearance and structure of which vary in every one of the portions of the canal, so that it is not the same in the pharynx as in the mouth, nor is it in the stomach like what it is in the œsophagus, &c. In the lips and the anus this membrane becomes confounded with the skin. The second layer of the sides of the digestive canal is muscular; it is composed of two layers of fibres, one longitudinal, the other circular. The arrangement, the thickness, the nature of the fibres which enter into the composition of these strata are different, according as they are observed in the mouth, in the œsophagus, or in the large intestine, &c. A great number of blood-vessels go to, or come from the digestive canal; but the abdominal portion of this canal receives a quantity incomparably greater than the superior parts. This presents only what are necessary for its nutrition, and the inconsiderable secretion, of which it is the seat; while the number and the volume of the vessels that belong to the abdominal portion show that it must be the agent of a considerable secretion. The chyliferous vessels arise exclusively from the small intestine.

As to the nerves, they are distributed to the digestive canal in an order inverse to that of the vessels; that is, the cephalic parts, *cervical* and *pectoral*, receive a great deal more than the abdominal portion, the stomach excepted, where the two nerves of the eighth pair terminate. The other parts of the canal scarcely receive any branch of the cerebral nerves. The only nerves that are observed, proceed from the *subdiaphragmatic* ganglions of the great sympathetic. We will see, farther on, the relation that exists between the mode of distribution of the nerves, and the functions of the superior and inferior portions of the digestive canal.

The bodies that pour fluids into the digestive canal, are,

1. The *digestive mucous membrane.*
2. *Isolated follicles* that are spread in great numbers in the whole length of this membrane.
3. The *agglomerated follicles* which are found at the isthmus of the throat, between the *pillars* of the *velum* of the palate, and sometimes at the junction of the œsophagus and the stomach.
4. The *mucous glands* which exist in a greater or less number in the sides of the cheeks, in the roof of the palate, around the œsophagus.
5. The *parotid*, the *submaxillary*, and *sublingual glands*, which secrete the saliva of the mouth, the liver, and the pancreas; the first of which pours the bile, the second the pancreatic juice, by distinct canals, into the superior part of the small intestine, called duodenum.

All the digestive organs contained in the abdominal cavity are immediately covered, more or less completely, by the serous membrane called the peritonæum. This membrane, by the manner in which it is disposed, and by its physical and vital properties, is very useful in the act of digestion, by preserving to the organs their respective relations, by favouring their changes of volume, by rendering easy the sliding motions which they perform upon each other, and upon the adjoining parts.

The surface of the mucous digestive membrane is

always lubrified by a glutinous adhesive matter, more or less abundant, than is seen in greatest quantity where there exist no follicles,—a circumstance which seems to indicate that these are not the only secreting organs. A part of this matter, to which is given generally the name of *mucus*, continually evaporates, so that there exists habitually a certain quantity of vapours in all the points of the digestive canal. The chemical nature of this substance, as taken at the intestinal surface, is still very little known. It is transparent, with a light gray tint; it adheres to the membrane which forms it; its taste is salt, and its acidity is shown by the re-agents: its formation still continues some time after death. That which is formed in the mouth, in the pharynx, and in the œsophagus, goes into the stomach mixed with the saliva, and the fluids of the mucous glands, by movements of deglutition, which succeed each other at near intervals. According to this detail, it would appear that the stomach ought to contain, after it has been some time empty of aliments, a considerable quantity of a mixture of mucus, of saliva, and follicular fluid. This observation is not proved, at least in the greatest number of individuals. However, in a number of persons, who are evidently in a particular state, there exist, in the morning, in the stomach, many ounces of this mixture. In certain cases it is foamy, slightly troubled, very little viscous, holding suspended some flakes of mucus; its taste is quite acid, not disagreeable, very sensible in the throat, acting upon the teeth, so as to diminish the polish of their surface, and rendering their motion upon each other more difficult. This liquid reddens paper stained with turnsol.

In the same individual, in other circumstances, and with the same appearances as to colour, transparency, and consistency, the liquid of the stomach had no savour, nor any acid property; it is a little salt: the solution of potassa, as well as the nitric and sulphuric acids, produced in it no apparent change.

When we examine the dead bodies of persons killed by accident, the stomach not having received any aliments nor drink for some time, this organ contains only a very few acid mucosities adhering to the coats of the stomach, part of which, in the pyloric portion of that viscus, appears reduced to chyme. It is, then, very probable, that the liquid which ought to be in the stomach is digested by this viscus as an alimentary substance, and that this is the reason why it does not accumulate there.

In animals the organization of which approaches to that of man, such as dogs and cats, there is no liquid found in the stomach after one, or many days of complete abstinence; there is seen only a small quantity of viscous mucosity adhering to the sides of the organ, towards its *splenic* extremity. This matter has the greatest analogy, both chemical and physical, with that which is found in the stomach of man. But, if we make these animals swallow a body which is not susceptible of being digested, as a pebble for example, there forms, after some time, in the cavity of the stomach, a certain quantity of an acid liquid mucus of a grayish colour, sensibly salt, which, in its composition, is nearly the same as that found sometimes in man.

This liquid, resulting from the mixture of the mucosities of the mouth, of the pharynx, of the œsophagus and the stomach, with the liquid secreted by the follicles of the same parts and with the saliva, has been called by physiologists the *gastric juice*, and to which they have attributed particular properties.

In the small intestine there is also formed a great quantity of mucous matter, which rests habitually attached to the sides of the intestine; it differs little from that of which we have spoken above; it is viscid, tough, and has a salt and acid savour; it is renewed with great rapidity. If the mucous membrane of this intestine is laid bare, in a dog, and the layer of mucus absorbed by a sponge, it will appear again in a minute. This observation may be repeated as often as we please, until the intestine becomes inflamed by the contact of the air, and foreign bodies.

The mucus of the stomach penetrates into the cavity of the small intestine only under the form of a pulpous matter, grayish and opaque, which has all the appearance of a particular chyme.

It is at the surface of this same portion of the digestive canal that the bile is delivered as well as the liquid secreted by the pancreas. In animals, such as dogs, the flowing of these liquids takes place at intervals; that is, about twice in a minute, there is seen to spring from the orifice of the ductus choledochus, or biliary canal, a drop of bile, which immediately spreads itself uniformly in a sheet upon the surrounding parts, which are already impregnated with it; there is, also, constantly found a certain quantity of bile in the small intestine.

The flowing of the liquid formed by the pancreas takes place much in the same manner, but it is much slower; sometimes a quarter of an hour passes before a drop of this fluid springs from the orifice of the canal which pours it into the intestine

The different fluids deposited in the small intestine, which are, the chymous matter that comes from the stomach, the mucus, the follicular fluid, the bile, and the pancreatic liquid, all mix together; but, on account of its properties, and perhaps of its proportions, the bile predominates, and gives to the mixture its proper taste and colour. A great part of this mixture descends towards the large intestine, and passes into it; in this passage, it becomes more consistent, and the clear yellow colour which it had before becomes dark, and afterward greenish. There are, however, in this respect, strong individual differences.

In the large intestine, the mucous and follicular secretion appears less active than in the small intestine; the mixture of fluids which comes from the small intestine acquires in it more consistence; it contracts a fœtid odour, analogous to that of ordinary excrements: it has, besides, the appearance of it, by its colour, odour, &c.

The knowledge of these facts enables us to understand how a person who uses no aliments can continue to produce excrements, and how, in certain diseases, their quantity is very considerable, though the sick person has been long deprived of every alimentary substance, even of a liquid kind. Round the anus exist follicles, which secrete a fatty matter of a singularly powerful odour.

We find gas almost always in the intestinal canal; the stomach contains only very little. The chemical nature of these gases has not yet been examined with care; but as the saliva that we swallow is always more or less impregnated with atmospheric air, it is probably the atmospheric air, more or less changed, which is found in the stomach. At least, it contains carbonic acid. The small intestine contains only a small quantity of gas; it is a mixture of carbonic acid, of azote and hydrogen. The large intestine contains carbonic acid, azote, and hydrogen, sometimes carburetted, sometimes sulphuretted. Twenty-three per cent. of this gas was found in the rectum of an individual, whose large intestine contained no excrement.

The muscular layer of the digestive canal deserves to be remarked, in respect to the different modes o contraction it presents. The lips, the jaws, in mos cases the tongue, the cheeks, are moved by a contrac tion, entirely like that of the muscles of locomotion. The roof of the palate, the pharynx, the œsophagus, and the tongue in certain particular circumstances, offer many motions, which have a manifest analogy with muscular contraction, but which are very different from it, because they take place without the participation of the will.

This does not imply that the motions of the parts just named are beyond the influence of the nerves; experience proves directly the contrary. If, for example, the nerves that come to the œsophagus are cut, this tube is deprived of its contractile faculty.

The muscles of the velum of the palate, those of the pharynx, the superior two-thirds of the œsophagus, scarcely contract like digestive organs, but when they act in permitting substances to pass from the mouth into the stomach. The inferior third of the œsophagus presents a phenomenon which is important to be known: this is an alternate motion of contraction and relaxation which exists in a constant manner. The contraction commences at the union of the *superior two-thirds* of the canal with the *inferior third;* it is continued, with a certain rapidity, to the insertion of the œsophagus into the stomach: when it is once produced, it continues for a time, which is variable; its mean duration is, at least, thirty seconds. Being so contracted in its inferior third, the œsophagus is hard and elastic, like a cord strongly stretched. The relaxation which succeeds the contraction happens all at once, and simultaneously in all the contracted fibres; in certain cases, however, it seems to take place from the superior to the inferior fibres. In the state of relaxation, the œsophagus presents a remarkable flaccidity, which makes a singular contrast with its state of contraction.

This motion of the œsophagus depends on the nerves of the eighth pair. When these nerves of an animal are cut, the œsophagus no longer contracts, but neither is it in the relaxed state that we have described; its fibres being separated from nervous influence, shorten themselves with a certain force, and the canal is found in an intermediate state between contraction and relaxation. The vacuity, or distention of the stomach, has an influence upon the duration and intensity of the contraction of the œsophagus.

From the inferior extremity of the stomach to the end of the intestine rectum, the intestinal canal presents a mode of contraction which differs, in almost every respect, from the contraction of the sub-diaphragmatic portion of the canal. This contraction always takes place slowly, and in an irregular manner; sometimes an hour passes before any trace of it can be perceived; at other times many intestinal portions contract at once. It appears to be very little influenced by the nervous system: for example,—it continues in the stomach after the section of the nerves of the eighth pair; it becomes more active by the weakness of animals, and even by their death; in some, by this cause it becomes considerably accelerated; it continues though the intestinal canal is entirely separated from the body. The pyloric portion of the stomach, the small intestine, are the points of the intestinal canal where it is presented oftenest, and most constantly. This motion, which arises from the successive or simultaneous contraction of the longitudinal or circular fibres of the intestinal canal, has been differently denominated by authors: some have named it *vermicular*, others *peristaltic*, others again, *sensible organic contractility*, &c. Whatever it is, the will appears to exert no sensible influence upon it.

The muscles of the anus contract voluntarily.

The supra-diaphragmatic portion of the digestive canal is not susceptible of undergoing any considerable dilatation; we may easily see, by its structure, and the mode of contraction of its muscular coat, that it is not intended to allow the aliments to remain in its cavity, but that it is rather formed to carry these substances from the mouth into the stomach: this last organ, and the large intestine, are evidently prepared to undergo a very great distention; substances, also, which are introduced into the alimentary canal, accumulate, and remain for a time, more or less, in their interior.

The diaphragm, and the abdominal muscles, produce a sort of perpetual agitation of the digestive organs contained in the abdominal cavity; they exert, upon them, a continual pressure, which becomes sometimes very considerable.

The digestive actions which by their union constitute digestion, are—

1. The apprehension of aliments.
2. Mastication.
3. Insalivation.
4. Deglutition.
5. The action of the stomach.
6. The action of the small intestines.
7. The action of the large intestines.
8. The expulsion of the fœcal matter.

All the digestive actions do not equally contribute to the production of chyle; the action of the stomach and that of the small intestines, are alone absolutely necessary.

The digestion of solid food requires generally the eight digestive actions; that of drinks is much more simple; it comprehends only apprehension, deglutition, the action of the stomach, and that of the small intestine.

The mastication and deglutition of the food being effected, we have now to notice the action of the stomach on the aliment: chemical alterations will now present themselves to our examination. In the stomach the food is transformed into a matter proper to animals, which is named *chyme*.

Before showing the changes that the food undergoes in the stomach, it is necessary to know the phenomena of their accumulation in this viscus, as well as the local and general effects that result from it.

The first mouthfuls of food swallowed are easily lodged in the stomach. This organ is not much compressed by the surrounding viscera; its sides separate easily, and give way to the force which presses the alimentary bole; but its distention becomes more difficult in proportion as new food arrives, for this is accompanied by the pressing together of the abdominal viscera, and the extension of the sides of the abdomen. This accumulation takes place particularly towards the right extremity and the middle part: the pyloric half gives way with more difficulty.

While the stomach is distended, its form, its relations, and even its positions, undergo alterations: in place of being flattened on its aspects, of occupying only the epigastrium and a part of the left *hypochondrium*, it assumes a round form; its great *cul de sac* is thrust into this *hypochondrium*, and fills it almost completely; the greater *curvature* descends towards the umbilicus, particularly on the left side; the pylorus, alone, fixed by a fold of the *peritonæum*, preserves its motion and its relations with the surrounding parts. On account of the resistance that the vertebral column presents behind, the posterior surface of the stomach cannot distend itself on that side: for that reason this viscus is wholly carried forward; and as the pylorus and the œsophagus cannot be displaced in this direction, it makes a motion of rotation, by which its great curve is directed a little forward; its posterior aspect inclines downwards, and its superior upwards.

Though it undergoes these changes of position and relation, it, nevertheless, preserves the recurved conoid form which is proper to it. This effect depends on the manner in which the three tunics contribute to its dilatation. The two plates of the serous membrane separate and give place to the stomach. The muscular layer suffers a real distention; its fibres are prolonged, but so as to preserve the particular form of the stomach. Lastly, the mucous membrane gives way, particularly in the points where the folds are multiplied. It will be noticed that these are found particularly along the larger curve, as well as at the splenic extremity.

The dilatation of the stomach alone produces very important changes in the abdomen. The total volume of this cavity augments; the belly juts out; the abdominal viscera are compressed with greater force; often the necessity of passing urine, or fæces, is felt. The diaphragm is pressed towards the breast, it descends with some difficulty; thence the motions of respiration, and the phenomena which depend on it, are more incommoded, such as speech, singing, &c.

In certain cases, the dilatation of the stomach may be carried so far that the sides of the abdomen are painfully distended, and respiration becomes difficult.

To produce such effects, the contraction of the œsophagus, which presses the food in the stomach, must be very energetic. We have remarked above the considerable thickness of the muscular layer of this canal, and the great number of nerves which go to it; nothing less than this disposition is necessary to account for the force with which the food distends the stomach. For more certainty, the finger has only to be introduced into the œsophagus of an animal by the cardiac orifice, and the force of the contraction will be found striking.

But if the food exerts so marked an influence upon the sides of the stomach and the abdomen, they ought themselves to suffer a proportionate reaction, and tend to escape by the two openings of the stomach. Why does this effect not take place? It is generally said that the cardia and pylorus shut; but this phenomenon has not been submitted to any particular researches. Here is what Dr. Magendie's experiments have produced in this respect.

The alternate motion of the œsophagus prevents the return of the food into this cavity. The more the stomach is distended, contraction becomes the more intense and prolonged, and the relaxation of shorter duration. Its contraction generally coincides with the instant of inspiration, when the stomach is most forcibly compressed. Its relaxation ordinarily happens at the instant of expiration.

We may have an idea of this mechanism by laying bare the stomach of a dog, and endeavouring to make the food pass into the œsophagus by compressing the stomach with both hands It will be nearly impossible to succeed, whatever force is used, if it is done at the instant when the œsophagus is contracted: but the passage will take place, in a certain degree, of itself; if the stomach is compressed at the instant of relaxation.

The resistance that the pylorus presents to the passage of the aliments is of another kind. In living animals, whether the stomach is empty or full, this opening is habitually shut, by the constriction of its fibrous ring, and the contraction of its circular fibres. There is frequently seen another constriction in the stomach, at the distance of one or two inches, which appears intended to prevent the food from reaching the pylorus; we perceive, also, irregular and peristaltic contractions, which commence at the duodenum, and are continued into the pyloric portion of the stomach, the effect of which is to press the food towards the splenic part. Besides, should the pylorus not be naturally shut, the food would have little tendency to enter it, for it only endeavours to escape into a place where the pressure is less; and this would be equally great in the small intestine as in the stomach, since it is nearly equally distributed over all the abdominal cavity.

Among the number of phenomena produced by the food in the stomach, there are several, the existence of which, though generally admitted, do not appear sufficiently demonstrated; such is the diminution of the volume of the spleen, and that of the blood-vessels of the liver, or the *omenta*, &c.; such is also a motion of the stomach, which should preside over the reception of the food, distribute it equally by exerting upon it a gentle pressure, so that its dilatation, far from being a passive phenomenon, must be essentially active. Dr. Magendie has frequently opened animals the stomachs of which were filled with food; he has examined the bodies of executed persons, a short time after death, and has seen nothing favourable to these assertions.

The accumulation of food in the stomach is accompanied by many sensations, of which it is necessary to take account:—at first, it is an agreeable feeling, or the pleasure of a want satisfied. Hunger is appeased by degrees; the general weakness that accompanied it is replaced by an active state, and a feeling of new force. If the introduction of food is continued, we experience a sensation of fulness and satiety which indicates that the stomach is sufficiently replenished; and if, contrary to this instinctive information, we still persist to make use of food, disgust and nausea soon arrive, and they are very soon followed by vomiting. These different impressions must not be attributed to the volume of the aliments alone. Every thing being equal in other respects, food very nutritive occasions, more promptly, the feeling of satiety. A substance which is not very nourishing does not easily calm hunger, though it is taken in great quantity.

The mucous membrane of the stomach, then, is endowed with considerable sensibility, since it distinguishes the nature of substances which come in contact with it. This property is very strongly marked if an irritating poisonous substance is swallowed: intolerable pain is then felt. We also know that the stomach is sensible to the temperature of food.

We cannot doubt that the presence of the aliments of the stomach causes a great excitement, from the redness of the mucous membrane, from the quantity of fluid it secretes, and the volume of vessels directed there; but this is favourable to chymification. This excitement of the stomach influences the general state of the functions.

The time that the aliments remain in the stomach is considerable, generally several hours; it is during this stay that they are transformed into chyme.

Changes of the aliments in the stomach:—

It is more than an hour before the food suffers any apparent change in the stomach, more than what results from the perspiratory and mucous fluids with which they are mixed, and which are continually renewed.

The stomach is uniformly distended during this time; but the whole extent of the pyloric portion afterward contracts, particularly that nearest the splenic portion, into which the food is pressed. Afterward, there is nothing found in the pyloric portion but chyme, mixed with a small quantity of unchanged food.

The best authors have agreed to consider the chyme as a homogeneous substance, pultaceous, grayish, of a sweetish taste, insipid, slightly acid, and preserving some of the properties of the food. This description leaves much to be explained.

The result of Dr. Magendie's experiments are as follows:

A. There are as many sorts of chyme as there are different sorts of food, if we judge by the colour, consistence, appearance, &c.; as we may easily ascertain, by giving different simple alimentary substances to dogs to eat, and killing them during the operation of digestion. He frequently found the same result in man, in the dead bodies of criminals, or persons dead by accident.

B. Animal substances are generally more easily and completely changed than vegetable substances. It frequently happens that these last traverse the whole intestinal canal without changing their apparent properties. He has frequently seen in the rectum, and in the small intestine, the vegetables which are used in soup, spinage, sorrel, &c., which had preserved the most part of their properties: their colour alone appeared sensibly changed by the contact of the bile.

Chyme is formed particularly in the pyloric portion. The food appears to be introduced slowly into it, and during the time they remain they undergo transformation. The Doctor believes, however, that he has observed frequently chymous matter at the surface of the mass of aliments which fill the splenic portion; but the aliments in general preserve their properties in this part of the stomach.

It would be difficult to tell why the pyloric portion is better adapted to the formation of chyme than the rest of the stomach; perhaps the great number of follicles that are seen in it modify the quantity or the nature of the fluid that is there secreted. The transformation of alimentary substances into chyme takes place generally from the superficies to the centre. On the surface of portions of food swallowed, there is formed a soft layer easy to be detached. The substances seem to be attacked and corroded by a reagent capable of dissolving them. The white of a hard egg, for instance, becomes in a little time as if plunged in vinegar, or in a solution of potassa.

C. Whatever is the alimentary substance employed, the chyme has always a sharp odour and taste, and reddens paper coloured with turnsol.

D. There is only a small quantity of gas found in the stomach during the formation of chyme; sometimes there exists none. Generally, it forms a small bubble at the superior part of the splenic portion Once only in the body of a criminal a short time after death he gathered with proper precautions a quantity sufficient to be analyzed. Chevreuil found it composed of:

Oxygen,	11.00
Carbonic acid,	14.00
Pure hydrogen,	3.55
Azote,	71.45
Total,	100.00

There is rarely any gas found in the stomach of a dog. We cannot then believe, with Professor Chaussier, that we swallow a bubble of air at every motion of deglutition, which is pressed into the stomach by the alimentary bole. Were it so, there ought to be found a considerable quantity of air in this organ after a meal: now the contrary is to be seen.

E. There is never a great quantity of chyme accumulated in the pyloric portion: the most that the Doctor ever saw in it was scarcely equal in volume to two or three ounces of water. The contraction of the stomach appears to have an influence upon the production of chyme. The following is what he observed in this respect. After having been some time immoveable, the extremity of the duodenum contracts, the pylorus and the pyloric portion contract also; this motion presses the chyme towards the splenic portion but it afterward presses it in a contrary direction, that is, after being distended, and having permitted the chyme to enter again into its cavity, the pyloric portion contracts from left to right, and directs the chyme towards the duodenum, which immediately passes the pylorus and enters the intestine.

The same phenomenon is repeated a certain number of times, but it stops to begin again, after a certain time. When the stomach contains much food, this motion is limited to the parts of the organ nearest the pylorus; but in proportion as it becomes empty, the motion extends farther, and is seen even in the splenic portion when the stomach is almost entirely empty. It becomes generally more strong about the end of chymification. Some persons have a distinct feeling of it at this moment.

The pylorus has been made to play a very important part in the passage of the chyme from the stomach to the intestine. It judges, they say, of the chymification of the food; it opens to those that have the required qualities, and shuts against those that have not. However, as we daily observe substances not digestible traverse it easily, such as stones of cherries, it is added, that becoming accustomed to a substance not chymified, which presents itself repeatedly, it at last opens a passage. These considerations, consecrated in a certain degree by the word *pylorus, a porter*, may please the fancy, but they are purely hypothetical.

F. All the alimentary substances are not transformed into chyme with the same promptitude.

Generally the fat substances, the tendons, the cartilages, the concrete albumen, the mucilaginous and sweet vegetables, resist more the action of the stomach than the caseous, fibrinous, and glutinous substances. Even some substances appear refractory: such as the bones, the epidermis of fruits, their stones, and whole seeds, &c.

In determining the digestibility of food, the volume of the portions swallowed ought to be taken into account. The largest pieces, of whatever nature, remain longest in the stomach; on the contrary, a substance which is not digestible, if it is very small, such as grape stones, does not rest in the stomach, but passes quickly with the chyme into the intestine.

In respect of the facility and quickness of the formation of chyme, it is different in every different individual. It is evident, after what has been said, that to fix the necessary time for the chymification of all the food contained in the stomach, we ought to take into account their quantity, their chemical nature, the manner in which the mastication acts upon them, and the individual disposition. However, in four or five hours after an ordinary meal, the transformation of the whole of the food into chyme is generally effected.

The nature of the chemical changes that the food undergoes in the stomach is unknown. It is not because there have been no attempts at different periods to give explanations of them more or less plausible. The ancient philosophers said that the food became putrified in the stomach; Hippocrates attributed the digestive process to coction; Galen assigned the stomach attractive, retentive, concoctive, expulsive faculties, and by their help he attempted to explain digestion. The doctrine of Galen reigned in the schools until the middle of the seventeenth century, when it was attacked and overturned by the *fermenting chemists*, who established in the stomach an *effervescence*, a particular fermentation, by means of which the food was *macerated*, *dissolved*, *precipitated*, &c.

This system was not long in repute; it was replaced by ideas much less reasonable. Digestion was supposed to be only a trituration, a bruising performed by the stomach; an innumerable quantity of little worms was supposed to attack and divide the food. Boerhaave thought he had found the truth, by combining the different opinions that had reigned before him. Haller did not follow the ideas of his master; he considered digestion a simple *maceration*. He knew that vegetable and animal matters, plunged into water, are soon covered with a soft homogeneous layer; he believed that the food underwent a like change, by macerating in the saliva and fluids secreted by the stomach.

Reaumur and Spallanzani made experiments on animals, and demonstrated the falsity of the ancient systems; they showed that food, contained in hollow metallic balls pierced with small holes, was digested the same as if it was free in the cavity of the stomach. They proved that the stomach contains a particular fluid, which they call *gastric juice*, and that this fluid was the principal agent of digestion; but they much exaggerated its properties, and they were mistaken when they thought to have explained digestion in considering it as a *solution:* because, in not explaining this solution, they did not explain the changes of food in the stomach.

In the formation of chyme, it is necessary to consider, 1st, The circumstances in which the food is found in the stomach. 2dly, The chemical nature of it.

The circumstances affecting the food in the stomach, during its stay there, are not numerous: 1st, it suffers a pressure more or less strong, either from the sides of the abdomen, or from those of the stomach; 2dly, the whole is entirely moved by the motions of respiration; 3dly, it is exposed to a temperature of thirty to thirty-two degrees of Reaumur; 4thly, it is exposed to the action of the saliva, of the mucosities proceeding from the mouth and the œsophagus, as well as the fluid secreted by the mucous membrane of the stomach.

It will be remembered that this fluid is slightly viscous, that it contains much water, mucus, salts, with a base of soda and ammonia, and lactic acid of Berzelius.

With regard to the nature of the food, we have already seen how variable it is, since all the immediate principles, animal or vegetable, may be carried into the stomach, in different forms and proportions, and serve usefully in the formation of chyme. Now, making allowance for the nature of the food, and the circumstances in which it is placed in the stomach, shall we be able to account for the known phenomena of the formation of chyme? The temperature of thirty to thirty-two degrees, R. = 100 to 104 F.; the pressure, and the tossing that the food sustains, cannot be considered as the principal cause of its transformation into chyme; it is probable that they only co-operate in this; the action of the saliva and that of the fluid secreted in the stomach remain; but after the known composition of the saliva, it is hardly possible that it can attack and change the nature of the food; at most, it can only serve to divide, to imbibe it in such a manner as to separate its particles: i must then be the action of the fluid formed by the internal membrane of the stomach. It appears certain that this fluid, in acting chemically upon the alimentary substances, dissolves them from the surface towards the centre.

To produce a palpable proof of it, with this fluid of which we speak, there have been attempts made to produce what is called in physiology, *artificial digestions*, that is, after having macerated food, it is mixed with gastric juice, and then exposed in a tube, or any other vase, to a temperature equal to that of the stomach. Spallanzani advanced, that these digestions succeeded, and that the food was reduced to chyme; but, according to the researches of de Montegre, it appears that they are not; and that, on the contrary, the substances employed undergo no alteration analogous to chymification; this is agreeable to experiments made by Reaumur. But because the gastric juice does not dissolve the food when put with it into a tube, we ought not to conclude that the same fluid cannot dissolve the food when it is introduced into the stomach; the circumstances are indeed far from being the same: in the stomach, the temperature is constant, the food is pressed and agitated, and the saliva and gastric juice are constantly renewed; as soon as the chyme is formed, it is carried away and pressed in the duodenum. Nothing of this takes place in the tube or vase which contains the food mixed with gastric juice; therefore, the want of success in artificial digestions, proves nothing which tends to explain the formation of chyme.

But how does it happen that the same fluid can act in a manner similar upon the great variety of alimentary substances, animal and vegetable? The acidity which characterizes it, though fit to dissolve certain matters, as albumen, for example, would not be suitable for dissolving fat.

To this it may be answered, that nothing proves the gastric juice to continue always the same; the small number of analyses that have been made of it demonstrate, on the contrary, that it presents considerable varieties in its properties. The contact of different sorts of food upon the mucous membrane of the stomach, may possibly influence its composition, it is at least certain, that this varies in the different animals For example, that of man is incapable of acting on bones; it is well known that the dog digests these substances perfectly.

Generally speaking, the action by which the chyme is formed prevents the reaction of the constituent elements of the food upon each other: but this effort takes place only in good digestions; in bad digestion, fermentation, and even putrefaction may take place: this may be suspected by the great quantity of inodorous gases that are developed in certain cases, and the sulphuretted hydrogen which is disengaged in others.

The nerves of the eighth pair have long been considered to direct the act of chymification: in fact, if these nerves are cut, or tied in the neck, the matters introduced into the stomach undergo no alteration. But the consequence, (says Dr. Magendie) that is deduced from this fact, does not appear to me to be rigorous. Is not the effect produced upon the stomach by the injury done to respiration, confounded here with the direct influence of the section of the nerves of the eighth pair upon this organ? I am inclined to believe it: for, as I have many times done, if the two eighth pairs be cut in the breast *below* the branches which go to the lungs, the food which is introduced afterward into the stomach is transformed into chyme, and ultimately furnishes an abundant chyle.

Some persons imagine that electricity may have an influence in the production of chyme, and that the nerves we mention may be the conductors: there is no established fact to justify this conjecture. The most probable use of the nerves of the eighth pair is, to establish intimate relations between the stomach and the brain, to give notice whether any noxious substances have entered along with the food, and whether they are capable of being digested.

In a strong person, the operation of the formation of chyme takes place without his knowledge; it is merely perceived that the sensation of fulness, and the difficulty of respiration produced by the distention of the stomach, disappear by degrees; but frequently, with people of a delicate temperament, digestion is accompanied with feebleness in the action of the senses, with a general coldness, and slight shiverings; the activity of the mind diminishes, and seems to become drowsy, and there is a disposition to sleep. The vital powers are then said to be concentrated in the organ that acts, and to abandon for an instant the others. To those general effects are joined the production of the gas that escapes by the mouth, a feeling of weight, of heat, of giddiness, and sometimes of burning, followed by an analogous sensation along the œsophagus, &c. These effects are felt particularly towards the end of the chymification. It does not appear, however, that these laborious digestions are much less beneficial than the others.

From the stomach, the food is received into the *small intestine*, which is the longest portion of the digestive canal; it establishes a communication between the stomach and the large intestine. Not being susceptible of much distention, it is twisted a great many times upon itself, being much longer than the place in which it is contained. It is fixed to the vertebral column by a fold of the peritonæum, which limits, yet aids its motions; its longitudinal and circular fibres are not separated as in the stomach; its mucous membrane, which presents many villi, and a great number of mucous follicles, forms irregular circular folds, the number of which are greater in proportion as the intestine is examined nearer the pyloric orifice: these folds are called *valvulæ conniventes*.

The small intestine receives many blood-vessels; its nerves come from the *ganglions* of the *great sympathetic*. At its internal surface, the numerous orifices of the chyliferous vessels open.

This intestine is divided into three parts, called the *duodenum*, *jejunum*, and *ileum*. The mucous membrane of the small intestine, like that of the stomach, secretes abundance of mucus; viscous, thready, of a salt taste, and reddens strongly turnsol paper; all which properties are also in the liquid secreted by the stomach. Haller gave this fluid the name of *intestinal juice;* the quantity that is formed in twenty-four hours he estimated at eight pounds.

Not far from the gastric extremity of this intestine is the common orifice of the biliary and pancreatic canals, by which the fluid secreted by the liver and the pancreas flow into the intestinal cavity. If the formation of the chyme is still a mystery, the nature of the phenomena that take place in the small intestine are little better known.

In the experiments which have been made on dogs and rabbits, the chyme is seen to pass from the stomach into the duodenum. The phenomena are these. At intervals, more or less distant, a contractile motion commences towards the middle of the duodenum; it is propagated rapidly to the site of the pylorus: this ring contracts itself, as also the pyloric part of the stomach; by this motion, the matters contained in the duodenum are pressed back towards the pylorus, where they are stopped by the valve, and those that are found in the *pyloric* part, are partly pressed towards the *splenic* part; but this motion, directed from the intestine towards the stomach, is very soon replaced by another in a contrary direction, that is, which propagates itself from the stomach towards the duodenum, the result of which is to make a considerable quantity of chyme pass the pylorus.

This fact seems to indicate that the valve of the pylorus serves as much to prevent the matters contained in the small intestine from flowing back into the stomach, as to retain the chyme and the food in the cavity of this organ.

The motion that we have described, is generally repeated many times following, and modified as to the rapidity, the intensity of the contraction, &c.; it then ceases to begin again after some time. It is not very marked in the first moments of the formation of the chyme; the extremity only of the pyloric part participates in it. It augments in proportion as the stomach becomes empty; and, towards the end of chymification, it often takes place over the whole stomach. It is not suspended by the section of the nerves of the eighth pair.

Thus the entrance of chyme into the small intestine is not perpetual. According as it is repeated, the chyme accumulates in the first portion of the intestine, it distends its sides a little, and presses into the intervals of the valves; its presence very soon excites the organ to contract, and by this means one part advances into the intestine; the other remains attached to the surface of its membrane, and afterward takes the same direction. The same phenomenon continues down to the large intestine; but, as the duodenum receives new portions of the chyme, it happens at last that the small intestine is filled in its whole length with this matter. It is observed only to be much less abundant near the *cæcum* than at the pyloric extremity.

The motion that determines the progress of the chyme through the small intestine, has a great analogy with that of the pylorus: it is irregular, returns at periods which are variable, is sometimes in one direction, sometimes in another, takes place sometimes in many parts at once; it is always slow, more or less; it causes relative changes among the intestinal circumvolutions. It is beyond the influence of the will.

We should form a false idea of it were we merely to examine the intestine of an animal recently dead; it has then a much greater activity than during life. Nevertheless, in weak digestions it appears to acquire more than ordinary energy and velocity.

In whatever manner this motion takes place, the chyme appears to move very slowly in the small intestine: the numerous valves that it contains, the multitude of asperities that cover the mucous membrane, the many bendings of the canal, are so many circumstances that ought to contribute to retard its progress, but which ought to favour its mixture with the fluids contained in the intestine, and the production of the chyle which results from it.

Changes that the chyme undergoes in the small intestine.—It is only about the height of the orifice of the choledochus and pancreatic canal that the chyme begins to change its properties. Before this, it preserves its colour, its semi-fluid consistence, its sharp odour, its slightly acid savour; but, in mixing with the bile and the pancreatic juice, it assumes new qualities: its colour becomes yellowish, its taste bitter, and its sharp odour diminishes much. If it proceeds from animal or vegetable matters, which contained grease or oil, irregular filaments are seen to form here and there upon its surface; they are sometimes flat, at other times rounded, attach themselves quickly to the surface of the valve, and appear to consist of crude chyle. This matter is not seen when the chyme proceeds from matter that contained no fat: it is a grayish layer, more or less thick, which adheres to the mucous membrane, and appears to contain the elements of chyle. The same phenomena are observed in the *two superior thirds* of the small intestine: but in the *inferior third*, the chymous matter is more consistent; its yellow colour becomes more deep; it ends sometimes by becoming of a greenish brown, which pierces through the intestinal parietes, and gives an appearance to the *ileum*, distinct from that of the *duodenum* and *jejunum*. When it is examined near the *cæcum*, there are few or no whitish chylous striæ seen; it seems, in this place, to be only the remainder of the matter which has served in the formation of the chyle.

After what has been said above, upon the varieties that the chyme presents, we may understand that the changes it undergoes in the small intestine are variable according to its properties; in fact, the phenomena of digestion in the small intestine, vary according to the nature of the food. The chyme, however, preserves its acid property; and if it contains small quantities of food or other bodies that have resisted the action of the stomach, they traverse the small intestine without undergoing any alteration. The same phenomena appear when the same substances have been used. Dr. Magendie has ascertained this fact upon the bodies of two criminals, who, two hours before death, had taken an ordinary meal, in which they had eaten the same food nearly in equal quantity; the matters contained in the stomach, the chyme in the pyloric portion and in the small intestine, appeared to him exactly the same as to consistence, colour, taste, odour, &c.

There is generally gas found in the small intestine during the formation of chyle. Drs. Magendie and Chevreuil have made experiments upon the bodies of criminals opened shortly after death, and who, being young and vigorous, presented the most favourable conditions for such researches. In a subject of twenty-four years, who had eaten, two hours before his death, bread, and some Swiss cheese, and drank water reddened with wine, they found in the small intestine:

Oxygen	0.00
Carbonic acid	24.39
Pure hydrogen	55.53
Azote	20.08
Total	100.00

In a second subject, aged twenty-three years, who had eaten of the same food at the same hour, and whose punishment took place at the same time:

Oxygen	0.00
Carbonic acid	40.00
Pure hydrogen	51.15
Azote	8.85
Total	100.00

In a third experiment, made upon a young man of twenty-eight years, who, four hours before death had eaten bread, beef, lentiles, and drank red wine, they found in the same intestine:

Oxygen	0.00
Carbonic acid	25.00
Pure hydrogen	8 40
Azote	66.60
Total	100.00

They never observed any other gases in the small intestine. These gases might have different origins. They might possibly come from the stomach with the chyme; or they were, perhaps, secreted by the intestinal mucous membrane; they might arise from the reciprocal action of the matters contained in the intestine; or perhaps they might come from all these sources at once.

However, the stomach contains oxygen, and very little hydrogen, while they have almost always found much hydrogen in the small intestine, and never any oxygen. Besides, it is a daily observation, that the little gas that the stomach contains is generally passed by the mouth towards the end of chymification, probably, because at this instant it can more easily advance into the œsophagus.

The probability of the formation of gases by the secretion of the mucous membrane could not be at all admissible, except for carbonic acid, which seems to be formed in this manner in respiration. With regard to the action of matters contained in the intestine, Dr. Magendie says he has many times seen the chymous matter let bubbles of gas escape very rapidly. This took place from the orifice of the ductus choledochus to the commencement of the *ileum* · there was no trace of it perceived in this last intestine, nor in the superior part of the duodenum, nor the stomach. He made this observation again upon the body of a criminal four hours after death; it presented no traces of putrefaction.

The alteration which chyme undergoes in the small intestine is unknown; it is easily seen to be the result of the action of the bile, of the pancreatic juice, and of the fluid secreted by the mucous membrane, upon the chyme. But what is the play of the affinities in this real chemical operation, and why is the chyle precipitated against the surface of the *valvulæ conniventes*, while the rest remains in the intestine to be afterward expelled? This is completely unknown.

We have learned something more of the time that is necessary for this alteration of the chyme. The phenomenon does not take place quickly: in animals, it often happens that we do not find any chyle formed three or four hours after the meal.

After what has been said, we see that in the small intestine, the chyme is divided into two parts: the one which attaches itself to the sides, and which is the chyle still impure; the other the true refuse, which is destined to be thrown into the large intestine, and afterward entirely carried out of the body.

The manner in which drinks accumulate in the stomach differs little from that of the aliments; it is generally quicker, more equal, and more easy; probably because the liquids spread, and distend the stomach more uniformly. In the same manner as the food, they occupy more particularly its left and middle portion; the pyloric, or right extremity, contains always much less.

The distention of the stomach must not, however, be carried to a great degree, for the liquid would be expelled by vomiting. This frequently happens to persons that swallow a great quantity of drink quickly. When we wish to excite vomiting in persons who have taken an emetic, one of the best means is to make them drink a number of glasses of liquid quickly.

The presence of drinks in the stomach produces local phenomena like those which take place from the *accumulation of the aliments;* the same changes in the form and position of the organ, the same distention of the abdomen, the same contraction of the pylorus and the œsophagus, &c.

The general phenomena are different from those produced by the aliments: this depends on the action of the liquids upon the sides of the stomach, and the quickness with which they are carried into the blood.

Potations, in passing rapidly through the mouth and the œsophagus, preserve more than the food their proper temperature until they arrive in the stomach. We therefore prefer them to those, when we wish to experience in this organ a feeling of heat or of cold · hence arises the preference that we give to hot drinks in winter, and cold drinks in summer.

Every one knows that the drinks remain a much shorter time in the stomach than the aliments; but the manner of their passage out of this viscus is still very little known. It is generally supposed that they traverse the pylorus and pass into the small intestine, where they are absorbed with the chyle; nevertheless a ligature applied round the pylorus in such a manner as to hinder it from penetrating into the duodenum, does not much retard its disappearance from the cavity of the stomach.

Alteration of drinks in the stomach.—Fluids, in respect of the alterations that they prove in the stomach, may be divided into two classes: the one sort do not form any chyme, and the other are chymified wholly or in part.

To the first class belong pure water, alcohol, sufficiently weak to be considered as a drink, the vegetable acids, &c. During its stay in the stomach, water assumes an equilibrium of temperature with the sides of this viscus: it mixes at the same time with mucus, the gastric juice, and the saliva which are found in it; it becomes muddy, and afterward disappears slowly without suffering any other transformation. One part passes into the small intestine; the other appears to be directly absorbed. There remains after its disappearance a certain quantity of mucus, which is very soon reduced to chyme like the aliments. By observation we know that water deprived of atmospheric air, as distilled water, or water charged with a great quantity of salts, as well-water, remain long in the stomach and produce a feeling of weight.

Alkohol acts quite in a different manner. We know the impression of burning heat that it causes at first in its passage through the mouth, the pharynx, the œsophagus; and that which it excites when it enters the stomach: the effects of this action determine the contraction of this organ, irritate the mucous membrane, and augment the secretion of which it is the seat; it coagulates at the same time all the albuminous parts with which it is in contact; and as the different liquids in the stomach contain a considerable proportion of this matter, it happens that a short time after alkohol has been swallowed, there is in this viscus a certain quantity of concrete albumen. The mucus undergoes a modification analogous to that of the albumen; it becomes hard, forms irregular elastic filaments, which preserve a certain transparency.

In producing these phenomena, the alkohol mixes with the water that the saliva and the gastric juice contain; probably it dissolves a part of the elements that enter into their composition, so that it ought to be much weakened by its stay in the stomach. It disappears very quickly; its general effects are also very rapid, and drunkenness or death follow almost immediately the introduction of too great a quantity of alkohol into the stomach.

The matters coagulated by the action of the alkohol are, after its disappearance, digested like solid aliments.

Among the drinks that are reduced to chyme, some are reduced in part and some wholly.

Oil is in this last case; it is transformed, in the pyloric part, into a matter analogous in appearance with that which is drawn from the purification of oils by sulphuric acid; this matter is evidently the chyme of oil. On account of this transformation, oil is perhaps the liquid that remains longest in the stomach.

Every one knows that milk curdles soon after it is swallowed; this curd then becomes a solid aliment, which is digested in the ordinary manner. Whey only can be considered as drink

The greatest number of drinks that we use are formed of water, or of alkohol, in which are in suspension or dissolution, immediate animal or vegetable principles, such as gelatine, albumen, osmazome, sugar, gum, fecula, colouring or astringent matters, &c. These drinks contain salts of lime, of soda, of potassa, &c.

The result of several experiments that have been made upon animals, and some observations that have been made on man, is, that there is a separation of the water and the alkohol in the stomach from the matters that these liquids hold in suspension or solution. These matters remain in the stomach, where they are transformed into chyme, like the aliments; while the liquids with which they were united are absorbed, or pass into the small intestine; lastly, they are conducted, as we have just now seen, in treating of water and alkohol.

Salts that are in solution in water do not abandon this liquid, and are absorbed with it. Red wine, for example, becomes muddy at first by its mixture with juices that are formed in, or carried into the stomach; it very soon coagulates the albumen of these fluids, and becomes flaky; afterward, its colouring matter, carried perhaps by the mucus and the albumen, is deposited upon the mucous membrane: there is a certain quantity of it seen at least in the pyloric portion; the watery and alkoholic parts disappear with rapidity.

The broth of meat undergoes the same changes. The water that it contains is absorbed; the gelatine, the albumen, the fat, and probably the osmazome, remain in the stomach, where they are reduced into chyme.

Action of the small intestine upon drinks.—After what has been read, it is clear that fluids penetrate, under two forms, into the small intestine: 1st, under that of liquid; 2dly, under that of chyme.

The liquids that pass from the stomach into the intestine remain but a short time, except under particular circumstances; they do not appear to undergo any other alteration than their mixture with the intestinal juice, the chyme, the pancreatic liquid, and the bile; they do not form any sort of chyle; they are generally absorbed in the duodenum, and the commencement of the jejunum; they are rarely seen in the ilium, and still more rarely in the large intestine. It appears that this last case does not happen except in the state of sickness; for example, during the action of a purgative.

The chyme that proceeds from drinks follows the same rule, and appears to undergo the same changes as that of the food; it therefore produces chyle.

Such are the principal phenomena of the digestion of drinks: we see how necessary it was to distinguish them from those that belong to the digestion of the aliments.

But we do not always digest the aliments and the drinks separately, as we have supposed; very frequently the two digestions take place at the same time.

Drink favours the digestion of the aliments; this effect is probably produced in various manners. Those that are watery, soften, divide, dissolve even certain foods; they aid in this manner their chymification and their passage through the pylorus.

Wine fulfils analogous uses, but only for the substances that it is capable of dissolving; besides, it excites by its contact the mucous membrane of the stomach, and causes a greater secretion of the gastric juice. Alkohol acts much in the same manner as wine, only it is more intense. It is thus that those liquors which are used after meals, are useful in exciting the action of the stomach."—*Magendie's Physiology.*

DIGESTIVE. *Digestivus;* from *digero*, to dissolve.) A term applied by surgeons to those substances which, when applied to an ulcer or wound, promote suppuration: such are the *ceratum resinæ*, *unguentum elemi*, warm poultices, fomentations, &c

Digestive salt. The muriate of potassa.

Digestive salt of Sylvius. The muriate of potassa.

DIGESTI'VUM SAL. See *Potassæ murias.*

DIGITA'LIS. (From *digitus*, a finger; because its flower represents a finger.)

1. The name of a genus of plants in the Linnæan system. Class, *Didynamia;* Order, *Angiospermia.* Fox-glove.

2. The pharmacopœial name of the common fox-glove. See *Digitalis purpurea.*

DIGITALIS PURPUREA. The systematic name of the fox-glove. *Digitalis—calycinis foliolis ovatis acutis, corollis obtusis, labio superiore integro,* of Linnæus. The leaves of this plant have a bitter nauseous taste, but no remarkable smell; they have been long used externally to ulcers and scrofulous tumours with considerable advantage. When properly dried, their colour is a lively green. They ought to be collected when the plant begins to blossom, to be dried quickly before the fire, and preserved unpowdered.

Of all the narcotics, digitalis is that which diminishes most powerfully the actions of the system; and it does so without occasioning any previous excitement. Even in the most moderate dose, it diminishes the force and frequency of the pulse, and, in a large dose, reduces it to a great extent, as from 70 beats to 40 or 35 in a minute, occasioning, at the same time, vertigo, indistinct vision, violent and durable sickness, with vomiting. In a still larger quantity, it induces convulsions, coldness of the body, and insensibility; symptoms which have sometimes terminated fatally As a narcotic, fox-glove has been recommended in epilepsy, insanity, and in some acute inflammatory diseases. Lately it has been very extensively employed in phthisis, and the beneficial effects which it produces in that disease, are probably owing to its narcotic power, by which it reduces the force of the circulation through the lungs and general system. It is administered so as to produce this effect. One grain of the powdered leaves, or ten drops of the saturated tincture, may be given night and morning. This dose is increased one half every second day, till its action on the system becomes apparent As soon as the pulse begins to be diminished, the increase of dose must be made with more caution: and, whenever nausea is induced, it ought rather to be reduced, or, if necessary, intermitted for a short time. If the sickness become urgent, it is best relieved by stimulants, particularly large doses of brandy, with aromatics. The tincture has been supposed to be the best form of administering digitalis, when the remedy is designed to act as a nar cotic: it is also more manageable in its dose, and more uniform in its strength, than the dried leaves.

Besides its narcotic effects, digitalis acts as one of the most certain diuretics in dropsy, apparently from its power of promoting absorption. It has frequently succeeded where the other diuretics have failed. Dr. Withering has an undoubted claim to this discovery; and the numerous cases of dropsy related by him, and other practitioners of established reputation, afford incontestable evidence of its diuretic powers, and of its practical importance in the cure of those disorders. From Dr. Withering's extensive experience of the use of the digitalis in dropsies, he has been able to judge of its success by the following circumstances;—"It seldom succeeds in men of great natural strength, of tense fibre, of warm skin, of florid complexion, or in those with a tight and cordy pulse. If the belly in ascites be tense, hard, and circumscribed, or the limbs in anasarca solid and resisting, we have but little hope. On the contrary, if the pulse be feeble, or intermitting, the countenance pale, the lips livid, the skin cold, the swollen belly soft and fluctuating, the anasarcous limbs readily pitting under the pressure of the finger, we may expect the diuretic effects to follow in a kindly manner." Of the inferences which he deduces, the fourth is, "that if it (digitalis) fails, there is but little chance of any other medicine succeeding." Although the digitalis is now generally admitted to be a very powerful diuretic, yet it is but justice to acknowledge that this medicine has more frequently failed than could have been reasonably expected, from a comparison of the facts stated by Dr. Withering. The dose of the dried leaves in powder is from one to three grains, twice a day. But if a liquid medicine be preferred, a drachm of the dried leaves is to be infused for four hours, in half a pint of boiling water, adding to the strained liquor an ounce of any spirituous water. One ounce of this infusion, given twice a day, is a medium dose. It is to be continued in these doses till it either acts upon the kidneys, the stomach, the pulse (which, as has been said, it has a remarkable power of lowering,) or the bowels.

The administration of this remedy requires to be conducted with much caution. Its effects do not immediately appear; and when the doses are too frequent, or too quickly augmented, its action is concentrated so as to produce frequently the most violent symptoms. The general rules are, to begin with a small dose, to increase it gradually, till the action is apparent on the kidneys, stomach, intestines, or vascular system; and immediately suspending its exhibition, when its effects on any of these parts take place.

The symptoms arising from too large a dose of digitalis are, extreme sickness, vertigo, indistinct vision, incessant vomiting, and a great reduction of the force of the circulation, terminating sometimes in syncope, or convulsions. They are relieved by frequent and small doses of opium, brandy, aromatics, and strong bitters, and by a blister applied to the region of the stomach.

DIGITATUS. Digitate or fingered. A leaf is called *folium digitatum*, when several leaflets proceed from the summit of a common footstalk, as in *Potentilla verna;* and *reptans*.

DIGITIFORMIS. Finger-like. Applied to the receptacle of the *Arum maculatum*, and *Calla æthiopica*.

DIGI'TIUM. (From *digitus*, a finger.)

1. A contraction of the finger-joint.
2. A whitlow, or other sore upon the finger.

DI'GITUS. (From *digero*, to direct.) A finger. *Digitus manus*, is the finger, properly so called; and *digitus pedis*, the toe.

DIGITUS MANUS. A finger. The *fingers* and thumb in each hand consist of fourteen bones, there being three to each *finger*, and two to the thumb; they are a little convex and round towards the back of the hand, but hollow and plain towards the palm, except the last, where the nails are. The order of their disposition is called first, second, and third *phalanx*. The first is longer than the second, and the second longer than the third. What has been said of the fingers, applies to the toes also.

DIGITUS PEDIS. A toe. See *Digitus Manus*.

DIGLO'SSUM. (From δις, double, and γλωσσα, a tongue: so called because above its leaf there grows a less leaf, like two tongues.) 1. The *Laurus alexandrina*.

2. Galen makes mention of a man born with two tongues.

DIGNO'TIO. (From *dignosco*, to distinguish.) See *Diagnosis*.

DIGY'NIA. (From δις, twice, and γυνη, a woman.) The name of an order of several classes of the sexual system of plants, embracing those plants which to the character of the class, whatever it may be, add the circumstance of having two styles.

DIHÆ'MATON. (From δια and αιμα, blood.) An antidote in which is the blood of many animals.

DIHA'LON. (From δια and αλς, salt.) A plaster prepared with salt and nitre, adapted to foul ulcers.

DII'PETES. (From Ζευς, διος heaven, and πιπτω, to fall: *i. e.* falling as rain.) An epithet applied by Hippocrates to semen, when it is discharged like a shower of rain.

DILATA'TIO. (From *dilato*, to enlarge.)

1. Dilatation, or enlargement.
2. The diastole of the heart.

DILA'TOR. (From *dilato*, to enlarge.) The name of some muscles, the office of which is to open and enlarge parts.

DILATOR ALÆ NASI. See *Levator labii superioris*.

DILATO'RIUM. (From *dilato*, to enlarge.) A surgical instrument for enlarging any part.

DILL. See *Anethum*.

DILUENT. (*Diluens;* from *diluo*, to wash away.) Those substances which increase the proportion of fluid in the blood. It is evident that this must be done by watery liquors. Water is, indeed, properly speaking, the only diluent. Various additions are made to it, to render it pleasant, and frequently to give it a slightly demulcent quality. But these are not sufficiently important to require to be noticed, or to be classed as medicines.

Diluents are merely secondary remedies. They are given in acute inflammatory diseases, to lessen the stimulant quality of the blood. They are used to promote the action of diuretics in dropsy, and to favour the operation of sweating.

DI'NICA. (From δινος, giddiness.) Medicines which relieve a giddiness.

DI'NOS. See *Dinus*.

DI'NUS. (From δινεω, to turn round.) *Dinos*. Dizziness. The name of a genus of disease in Good's Nosology. Class, *Neurotica;* Order, *Systatica*. It has only one species. *Dinus vertigo*. Vertigo, or giddiness.

DIO'CRES. The name of a lozenge.

DI'ODOS. (From δια, and οδος, the way through.) Evacuation by stool.

DIŒ'CIA. (From δις, double, and οικια, a house.) The name of a class of plants in the sexual system of Linnæus, containing such as have barren, or male, flowers on one individual, and fertile, or female, ones on another of the same species.

DIŒNA'NTHES. (From δια, and οιvανθη, the flower of the vine.) A remedy said to be good for cholera, in which was the flower of the vine-tree.

DIO'GMUS. (From διωκω, to persecute.) A distressing palpitation of the heart.

DIOI'CUS. (From δις, double, and οικια, a house.) Dioecious. Plants and flowers are so called when the barren and fertile flowers grow from two separate roots.

DIONIS, PETER, was born about the middle of the 17th century, and educated to the practice of surgery. He was appointed to read the lectures in anatomy, &c. in the royal gardens at Paris, instituted by Lewis XIV., and after this, surgeon to the queen, and other branches of the royal family, which offices he held, with great credit, till his death, in 1718. His first publication gave an account of a woman who died in the sixth month of pregnancy, of what he considered to be a ruptured uterus; but as he states that there were two uteri, it is suspected that the ruptured part was one of the Fallopian tubes much enlarged. He afterward gave a useful epitome of anatomy, which was very favourably received, passed through several editions, and was even translated into the Tartar language, by order of the emperor of China. His next work, a course of surgical operations, obtained still more celebrity, which it even now in some degree retains, especially as commented upon by Heister. Besides these a dissertation on sudden death, and a treatise on midwifery, were published by this author.

DIONYSI'SCUS. (From Διονυσος, Bacchus, who was of old represented as having horns.) Certain bony excrescences, near the temples, were called dionysisci.

DIONYSONY'MPHAS. (From Διονυσος, Bacchus, and νυμφα, a nymph.) An herb which, if bruised, smells of wine, and yet resists drunkenness.

DIOPO'RUM. (From δια, and οπωρα, autumnal fruits.) A medicine composed of ripe fruits for quinsy.

DIOPSIDE. A subspecies of oblique-edged augite, found near Piedmont.

DIOPTASE. Emerald, copper ore.

DIO'PTRA. (From διοπ7ομαι, to see through.) *Dioptron.* 1. Speculum ani, oris, or uteri.

2. The lapis specularis.

DIO'PTRICS. (*Dioptricus;* from διοπ7ομαι, to see through.) The doctrine of the refraction of light.

DIOPTRI'SMUS. (From διοπ7ομαι, to see through.) Dilatation of any natural passage.

DIO'ROBUM. (From δια, and οροβος, a vetch.) A medicine, in the composition of which there are vetches.

DIORRHO'SIS. (From δια, and ορρος, the serum.) *Diorosis.* 1. A dissolved state of the blood.

2. A conversion of the humours into serum and water.

DIORTHRO'SIS. (From διορθροω, to direct.) The reduction of a fracture.

DIOSCO'REA. (Named in honour of Dioscorides.) The name of a genus of plants in the Linnæan system. Class, *Diœcia;* Order, *Hexandria.*

DIOSCOREA ALATA. The name of the plant which affords the esculent root, called the yam. It is obtained, however, from three species; the *alata*, *bulbifera*, and *sativa.* They grow spontaneously in both Indies, and their roots are promiscuously eaten, as the potato is with us. There is great variety in the colour, size, and shape of yams; some are generally blue or brown, round or oblong, and weigh from one pound to two. They are esteemed, when dressed, as being nutritious and easy of digestion, and are preferred to wheaten bread. Their taste is somewhat like the potato, but more luscious. The negroes, whose common food is yams, boil and mash them. They are also ground and made into bread and puddings.

When they are to be kept for some time, they are exposed upon the ground to the sun, as we do onions, and when sufficiently withered, they are put into dry sand in casks, and placed in a dry garret, where they remain often for many seasons without losing any of their primitive goodness.

DIOSCOREA BULBIFERA. See *Dioscorea alata.*

DIOSCOREA SATIVA. See *Dioscorea alata.*

DIOSCORI'DES, PEDACIUS, or PEDANIUS, a celebrated Greek physician and botanist of Anazarba, in Cilicia, now Caramania, who is supposed to have lived in the time of Nero. He is said to have been originally a soldier, but soon became eminent as a physician, and travelled much to improve his knowledge. He paid particular attention to the materia medica, and especially to botany, as subservient to medicine. He profited much by the writings of Theophrastus, who appears to have been a more philosophical botanist. Dioscorides has left a treatise on the materia medica, in five books, chiefly considering plants; also two books on the composition and application of medicines, an essay on antidotes, and another on venomous animals. His works have been often printed in modern times, and commented upon, especially by Matthiolus. He notices about 600 plants, but his descriptions are often so slight and superficial, as to leave their identity a matter of conjecture; which is perhaps of no very great medical importance; though their virtues being generally handed down from the Greeks, it might be useful to ascertain which particular plants they meant.

DIOSCU'RI. (*i. e.* Διος, Κουροι, the sons of Jupiter, or Castor and Pollux.) The parotid glands were so named from their twin-like equality in shape and position.

["DIOSPYROS. *Persimmon.* The persimmon-tree is very common in the middle and western states, and grows also in the southern parts of our country. The bark is bitter, and has been added to our numerous list of native tonics. It is recommended in intermittents and ulcerated sore throats, and may be exhibited in the same manner as cinchona."—*Bigelow's Mat. Med.* A.]

DIOSPY'ROS LOTUS. The Indian date plum. The fruit, when ripe, has an agreeable taste, and is very nutritious.

DIOXELÆ'UM. (From δια, οξυς, acid, and ελαιον, oil.) A medicine composed of oil and vinegar

DIO'XOS. (From δια, and οξυς, acid.) A collyrium composed chiefly of vinegar.

DIPHYLLUS. (From δις, double, and φυλλον, a leaf.) Diphyllous, or two-leaved. Applied to the perianthium of flowers, when there are two calyces; as in *Papaver rhœas.*

DIPLASIA'SMUS. (From διπλοω, to double.) The re-exacerbation of a disease.

DI'PLOE. (From διπλοω, to double.) The spongy substance between the two tables of the skull.

DIPLO'PIA. (From διπλοος, double, and οπτομαι, to see.) *Visus duplicatus.* A disease of the eye, in which the person sees an object double or triple. Dr. Cullen makes it a variety of the second species of pseudoblepsis, which he calls mutans, in which objects appear changed from what they really are; and the disease varies according to the variety of the remote causes.

DI'PNOOS. (From δις, twice, and πνεω, to breathe.) A wound which is perforated quite through, and admits the air at both ends.

Dipple's animal oil. See *Animal oil.*

DI'PSACUS. (From διψα, thirst; so called from the concave situation of its leaves, which hold water, by which the thirst of the traveller may be relieved.) *Dipsacum.*

1. The name of a genus of plants in the Linnæan system. Class, *Syngenesia;* Order, *Polygamia.* The teasel.

2. A diabetes, from the continual thirst attending it.

DIPSOSIS. (From διψα, thirst.) The name of a genus of diseases in Good's Nosology, known by the desire for drinking being excessive or impaired. It has two species, *Dipsosis avens*, and *Dipsosis expers.*

DIPYRE. Schmelstein. A mineral found in white or reddish steatite in the Western Pyrenees, composed of silica, alumina, and lime.

DIPYRE'NUM. (From δις, twice, and πυρην, a berry.) 1. A berry, or kernel.

2. A probe with two buttons.

DIPYRI'TES. (From δις, twice, and πυρ, fire.) *Dipyros.* An epithet given by Hippocrates to bread twice baked, and which he recommended in dropsies

DIRE'CTOR. (From *dirigo*, to direct.)

1. A hollow instrument for guiding an incisor-knife.

2. The name of a muscle.

DIRECTOR PENIS. (From *dirigo*, to direct.) The same as erector penis.

DIRI'NGA. A name, in the isle of Java, for the *Calamus aromaticus.* See *Acorus calamus.*

DISCE'SSUS. (From *discedo*, to depart.) The separation of any two bodies, before united, by chemical operation.

DISCIFO'RMIS. (From *discus*, a quoit, and *forma*, likeness.) Resembling a disk, or quoit, in shape. It is applied to the knee-pan.

DISCOI'DES. (From δισκος, a quoit, and ειδος, resemblance.) Resembling a disk, or quoit, in shape It is applied to the crystalline humour of the eye

DISCRI'MEN. 1. A small roller.

2. The diaphragm.

DISCUS. (From δισκος, a quoit and disk, and from its flat and round appearance like the circumference of the sun.) The disk, or central part of a leaf, and of a compound flower. In the common daisy, the white leaflets of the flower surround the disk.

The disk of a leaf is the whole flat surface within the margin.

DISCU'TIENT. (*Discutiens;* from *discutio*, to shake in pieces.) *Discusorius; Diachyticus.* A term in surgery, applied to those substances which possess a power of repelling or resolving tumours.

DISEASE. *Morbus.* Any alteration from a perfect state of health. A disease is variously termed: when it pervades the whole system, as fever does, it is called a *general disease*, to distinguish it from inflammation of the eye, or any other viscus, which is a *partial*, or *local* one. When it does not depend on another disease, it is termed *idiopathic*, which may be either general or partial, to distinguish it from a *symptomatic* one, which depends upon another disease. See also *Endemic*, *Epidemic*, *Sporadic*, &c.

[DISINTEGRATION. This is a geological term, and means the crumbling down of rock by their decomposition, and the consequent formation of alluvial soil. A.]

DISK. See *Discus*.

DISLOCA'TION. (*Dislocatio*; from *disloco*, to put out of place.) Luxation. The secession of a bone of a moveable articulation from its natural cavity.

DISPE'NSARY. (*Dispensarium*; from *dispendo*, to distribute.) 1. The shop or place in which medicines are prepared.

2. The name of an institution, in which the poor are supplied with medicines and advice.

DISPE'NSATORY. (*Dispensatorium*; from *dispendo*, to distribute.) *Antidotarium*. A book which treats of the composition of medicines.

DISSE'CTION (*Dissectio*; from *disseco*, to cut asunder.) The cutting to pieces of any part of an animal, or vegetable, for the purpose of examining its structure. See *Anatomy*.

DISSECTUS. Cut. A term used by botanists synonymously with *incised* and *laciniated*, to leaves which are cut, as it were, into numerous irregular portions. See *Leaf*.

DISSEPIMENTUM. (From *dissepio*, to separate.) A partition. Applied by botanists to partitions which separate the cells of a capsule. See *Capsula*.

DISSE'PTUM. (From *dissepio*, to enclose round.) The diaphragm, or membrane, which divides the cavity of the thorax from the abdomen.

DISSOLVE'NTIA. (From *dissolvo*, to loosen.)

1. Medicines which loosen and dissolve morbid concretions in the body.

2. In chemistry, it means menstrua.

DISSOLU'TUS. (From *dissolvo*, to loosen.) Loose, morbus dissolutus. An epithet applied to dysentery.

DISTANS. Distant. Applied to petals from their direction; as in *Cucubalus bacciferus*.

DISTE'NTIO. (From *distendo*, to stretch out.) 1. Distention, or dilatation.

2. A convulsion.

DISTHENE. See *Cyanite*.

DISTI'CHIA. See *Distichiasis*.

DISTICHI'ASIS. (From διστιχια: from δις, double, and ϛιχος, a row.) *Districhiasis*; *Distichia*. A disease of the eyelash, in which there is a double row of hairs, the one row growing outwards, the other inwards towards the eye.

DISTICHUS. Two-ranked. Applied to stems, leaves, &c. when they spread in two horizontal directions; as the branches of the *Pinus picea*, or silver fur, and the leaves of the *Taxus baccata*, or yew.

DISTILLA'TION. (*Distillatio*; from *distillo*, to drop little by little.) *Alsacta*; *Catastagmos*. A chemical process, very similar to evaporation, instituted to separate the volatile from the fixed principles, by means of heat. Distillatory vessels are either alembics or retorts; the former consist of an inferior vessel called a cucurbit designed to contain the matter to be examined, and having an upper part fixed to it, called the capital, or head. In this last, the vapours are condensed by the contact of the surrounding air, or, in other cases, by the assistance of cold water surrounding the head, and contained in a vessel called the refrigeratory. From the lower part of the capital proceeds a tube called the nose, beak, or spout, through which the vapours, after condensation, are, by a proper figure of the capital, made to flow into a vessel called the receiver, which is usually spherical. These receivers have different names, according to their figure, being called mattresses, balloons, &c. Retorts are a kind of bottle of glass, pottery, or metal, the bottom being spherical, and the upper part gradually diminishing into a neck, which is turned on one side.

Distilled vinegar. See *Acetum*.

DISTO'RTION. (*Distortio*; from *distorqueo*, to wrest aside.) A term applied to the eyes, when a person seems to turn them from the object he would look at, and is then called squinting, or strabismus. It also signifies the bending of a bone preternaturally to one side; as distortion of the spine, or vertebræ.

DISTO'RTOR. (From *distorqueo*, to wrest aside.) A muscle, the office of which is to draw the mouth awry.

DISTORTOR ORIS. See *Zygomaticus minor*.

DISTRICHI'ASIS. See *Distichiasis*.

DI'STRIX. (From δις, double, and θριξ, the hair.) A disease of the hair, when it splits and divides at the end.

DITTANDER. See *Lepidium sativum*.

DITTANY. See *Dictamnus*.

Dittany, bastard. See *Dictamnus albus*.

Dittany of Crete. See *Origanum dictamnus*.

Dittany, white. See *Dictamnus albus*.

DIURE'SIS. (From δια, through, and ουρεω, to make water.) An increased secretion of urine. It is also applied to a diabetes.

DIURETIC. (*Diureticus*. Διουρητικος; from διουρησις, a discharge of urine.) That which, when taken internally, augments the flow of urine from the kidneys It is obvious that such an effect will be produced by any substance capable of stimulating the secreting vessels of the kidneys. All the saline diuretics seem to act in this manner. They are received into the circulation; and passing off with the urine, stimulate the vessels, and increase the quantity secreted.

There are other diuretics, the effect of which appears not to arise from direct application, but from an action excited in the stomach, and propagated by nervous communication to the secreting urinary vessels.

The diuretic operation of squill, and other vegetables, appears to be of this kind.

There is still, perhaps, another mode in which certain substances produce a diuretic effect; that is, by promoting absorption. When a large quantity of watery fluid is introduced into the circulating mass, it stimulates the secreting vessels of the kidneys, and is carried off by urine. If, therefore, absorption be promoted, and if a portion of serous fluid, perhaps previously effused, be taken up, the quantity of fluid secreted by the kidneys will be increased. In this way digitalis seems to act: its diuretic effect, it has been said, is greater when exhibited in dropsy than it is in health.

On the same principle (the effect arising from stimulating the absorbent system) may probably be explained the utility of mercury in promoting the action of several diuretics.

The action of these remedies is promoted by drinking freely of mild diluents. It is also influenced by the state of the surface of the body. If external heat be applied, diuresis is frequently prevented, and diaphoresis produced. Hence the doses of them should be given in the course of the day, and the patient, if possible, be kept out of bed.

The direct effects of diuretics are sufficiently evident. They discharge the watery part of the blood; and, by that discharge, they indirectly promote absorption over the whole system.

Dropsy is the disease in which they are principally employed; and when they can be brought to act, the disease is removed with less injury to the patient than it can be by exciting any other evacuation. Their success is very precarious, the most powerful often failing; and, as the disease is so frequently connected with organic affection, even the removal of the effused fluid, when it takes place, only palliates without effecting a cure.

Diuretics have been likewise occasionally used in calculous affections, in gonorrhœa, and with a view of diminishing plethora, or checking profuse perspiration.

Murray, in his Elements of Materia Medica, classes the supertartrate of potassa, or cream of tartar, and nitrate of potassa, or nitre, the muriate of ammonia, or crude sal-ammoniac, potassa, and the acetate of potassa, or kali acetatum, among the *saline* diuretics; and selects the following from the *vegetable* kingdom: —scilla maritima, digitalis purpurea, nicotiana tabacum, solanum dulcamara, lactuca virosa, colchicum autumnale, gratiola officinalis, spartium scoparium juniperis communis, copaifera officinalis, pinus balsamea, and pinus larix; and the lytta vesicatoria from the *animal* kingdom.

In speaking of particular diuretics, Dr. Cullen says, the diuretic vegetables, mentioned by writers, are of very little power, and are employed with very little success. Of the umbellatæ, the medicinal power resides especially in their seeds; but he never found any of them very efficacious. The semen dauci sylvestris has been commended as a diuretic; but its powers as such are not very remarkable. In like manner, some of the *plantæ stellatæ* have been commended as diuretics; but none of them deserve our notice, except the *rubia tinctorium*, the root of which passes so much by the kidneys as to give its colour to the urine. Hence it may fairly be supposed to stimulate the secretories; but Dr. Cullen found its diuretic powers did not always appear, and never to any considerable degree; and as, in brute animals, it has always appeared hurtful to the system, he does not think it fit to be employed to any extent in human diseases. The bardana, lithospermum, ononis, asparagus, enula campana, are all substances which seem to pass, in some measure, by the kidneys; but their diuretic powers are hardly worth notice.

The principal articles included by Dr. Cullen, in his catalogue of diuretics, are dulcamara, digitalis, scilla; some of the alliaceæ and siliquosæ; the balsams and resins; cantharides, and the diuretic salts.

DIVAPORA'TIO. Evaporation.

DIVARICATION. The crossing of any two things: thus when the muscular or tendinous fibres intersect each other at different angles, they are said to divaricate.

Divellent affinity. See *Affinity quiescent.*

DIVERSO'RIUM. (From *diversor*, to resort to.) The receptaculum chyli.

DIVERTI'CULUM. A mal-formation or diseased appearance of a part, in which a portion goes out of the regular course; and thereby forms a diverticulum, or deviation from the usual course. It is generally applied to the alimentary canal.

DIVERTICULUM NUCKII. The opening through which the round ligaments of the uterus pass. Nuck asserted that it remained open a long time after birth; to these openings he gave the name of *diverticula.*

DIVI'NUS. A pompous epithet of many compositions, from their supposed excellence.

DIVU'LSIO. (From *divello*, to pull asunder.) Urine with uneven sediment.

DOCIMASTIC. *Ars docimastica.* The art of examining fossils, in order to discover what metals, &c. they contain.

DOCK. See *Rumex.*

Dock-cresses. See *Lapsana.*

Dock, sour. See *Rumex acetosa.*

Dock, water. See *Rumex hydrolapathum.*

DODDER. See *Cuscuta epithymum.*

DODECADA'CTYLUS. (From δωδεκα, twelve, and δακ7υλος, a finger; so named because its length is about the breadth of twelve fingers.) The duodenum, an intestine so called. It must be observed, that at the time this name was given, anatomy consisted in the dissection of brutes; and the length was therefore probably adjudged from the gut of some animal, and not of man.

DODECA'NDRIA. (From δωδεκα, twelve, and ανηρ, a man.) The name of a class of plants in the sexual system, embracing those with hermaphrodite flowers, and twelve stamina.

DODECAPHA'RMACUM. (From δωδεκα, twelve, and φαρμακον, a medicine.) An ointment consisting of twelve ingredients, for which reason it was called the ointment of the twelve apostles.

DODECA'THEON. (From δωδεκα, twelve, and 7ιθημι, to put.) An antidote consisting of twelve simples.

DODONÆUS, REMBERTUS, (or DODOENS,) was born at Mechlin, in 1517. He became physician to two succeeding emperors, and, in 1582, was appointed professor of physic in the newly-founded University of Leyden, the duties of which he performed with credit, till his death, three years after. His fame at present chiefly rests on his botanical publications, particularly his "Pemptades," or 30 books of the history of plants. The "Frugum Historia," "Herbarium Belgicum," &c. are of much inferior merit.

DOG. See *Canis.*

Dog's-bane, Syrian. See *Asclepias syriaca.*

Dog's-grass. See *Triticum repens.*

Dog's-mercury. See *Mercurialis perennis.*

Dog-rose. See *Rosa canina.*

Dog-stones. See *Orchis mascula.*

[*Dogwood.* See *Cornus Florida.* A.]

DO'GMA. (From δοκεω, to be of opinion.) A dogma, or opinion, founded on reason and experience.

DOLERITE. When volcanic masses are composed of grains distinct from each other, and contain besides felspar, much pyroxene, black oxide of iron, amphibole, &c., they are called, by the French geologist, *dolerite.*

DO'LICHOS. (From δολιχος, long: so called from its long shape.) 1. The name of a genus of plants in the Linnæan system. Class, *Diadelphia;* Order, *Decandria.*

2. The pharmacopœial name of the cowhage. See *Dolichos pruriens.*

DOLICHOS PRURIENS. The systematic name of the cowhage. *Dolichos; Dolichos—volubilis, leguminibus racemosis, valvulis subcarinatis hirtis, pedunculis ternis*, of Linnæus. The pods of this plant are covered with sharp hairs, which are the parts employed medicinally in form of electuary, as anthelmintics. The manner in which these hairy spicula act, seems to be purely mechanical: for neither the tincture, nor the docoction, possess the least anthelmintic power.

DOLICHOS SOJA. The plant which affords the soy. It is much cultivated in Japan, where it is called *daidsu:* and where the pods supply their kitchens with various productions; but the two principal are, a sort of butter, termed *miso*, and a pickle called *sooju.*

DOLABRIFORMIS. (From *dolabella*, a hatchet, and *forma*, resemblance.) Hatchet-shaped. A term applied to a leaf, which is compressed with a very prominent dilated keel, and a cylindrical base; as in *Mesembryanthemum dolabriforme.*

DOLOMITE. A calcareo-magnesian carbonate

DO'LOR. (*Dolor, oris.* f.) Pain.

DOLOR FACIEI. See *Tic douloureux.*

DORO'NICUM. (From *dorongi*, Arab.) Leopard's bane. See *Arnica montana.*

DORONICUM GERMANICUM. See *Arnica montana.*

DORONICUM ROMANUM. The pharmacopœial name of the Roman leopard's bane. See *Doronicum pardalianches.*

DORONICUM PARDALIANCHES. The systematic name of the Roman leopard's bane. *Doronicum romanum; Doronicum—foliis cordatis, obtucis, denticulatis; radicalibus petiolatis; caulinis amplexicaulibus*, of Linnæus. The root of this plant, if given in a full dose, possesses poisonous properties; but instances are related of its efficacy in epileptical and other nervous diseases.

DO'RSAL. (*Dorsalis;* from *dorsum*, the back.) Belonging to the back.

DORSALIS NERVUS. The nerve which passes out from the vertebræ of the back.

[DORSEY, JOHN SYNG, M.D., Professor of anatomy in the university of Pennsylvania, was born in the city of Philadelphia, in December, 1783. In early life he received an excellent elementary and classical education at a school in Philadelphia, of the society of Friends, then in high repute, and here manifested the same vivacity of genius and quickness in learning, with the mild and gracious dispositions, for which he was subsequently so conspicuous. At the age of 15 years, he entered the office of his relation, the celebrated Dr. Physick.

Not long after receiving his degree, the yellow fever reappeared in the city, and prevailed so widely that an hospital was opened for the accommodation exclusively of the sick with this disease, to which he was appointed resident physician. So great was the value attached to his services, that it is difficult to speak too highly of the manner in which he discharged the duties of his office of hazardous benevolence. At the close of the same season, he proceeded to Europe, for the purpose of improving his medical knowledge. In December, 1804, he returned home, and immediately entered on the practice of his profession. The reputation he brought with him, his amiable temper, and popular manners, his fidelity and attention, speedily introduced him into a large share of business. From this period professional honours were heaped on him with profusion. He was appointed surgeon to the dispensary, the alms-house, and hospitals, and in all our medical associations he held some elevated office. But there was reserved for him a still higher and more dignified station. In 1807 he was elected adjunct professor of surgery, in which office he continued till he was raised to the chair of anatomy, by the lamented death of the venerable Dr. Wistar

"Considering himself now placed for the first time

in the proper sphere for the exercise of his talents and the gratification of a generous ambition, the appointment gave him much delight; and with ample preparation, he opened the session by one of the finest exhibitions of eloquence ever heard within the walls of the college. But here his bright and prosperous career ended, and the expectations of success thus created were not permitted to be realized. Elevated to a position above which he could hardly ascend, and surrounded by all that we most value, Providence seems to have selected him as an instance to teach a salutary lesson of the shortness of life, the insignificance of things transitory, and the importance of that eternity which absorbs all being and all time. On the evening of the same day that he pronounced his introductory lecture, and while the praises of it still resounded, he was attacked with a fever of such vehemence, that in one short week it closed his existance, leaving to us only his enviable name and inestimable example. He died in November, 1818, aged 35 years."—*Thach. Med. Biog.* A.]

DORSTE'NIA. (Named in honour of Dr. Dorsten.) The name of a genus of plants in the Linnæan system. Class, *Tetrandria;* Order, *Monogynia.*

DORSTENIA BRAZILIENSIS. The root of this plant is used by the natives of Brazil, internally and externally. They call it *Caa apia.* When chewed, it has the same effects as ipecacuanha. The wounds from poisoned darts are said to be cured with the juice of the root, which they pour into the wound.

DORSTENIA CONTRAYERVA. The systematic name of the plant which affords the contrayerva root; *Contrayerva; Drakena: Cyperus longus, odorus, peruanus; Bezoardica radix.* The contrayerva root was first brought into Europe about the year 1581, by Sir Francis Drake, whence its name Drakena. It is the root of a small plant found in Peru, and other parts of the Spanish West Indies. Dr. Houston observes, that the roots of different species of dorstenia are promiscuously gathered and exported for those of the contrayerva, and, as all the species bear a great resemblance to each other, they are generally used for medical purposes in this country. The tuberous parts of these roots are the strongest, and should be chosen for use. They have an agreeable aromatic smell; a rough, bitter, penetrating taste; and, when chewed, they give out a sweetish kind of acrimony.

It is diaphoretic and antiseptic; and was formerly used in low nervous fevers, and those of the malignant kind; but its use is superseded by the cinchona.

Dr. Cullen observes, that this and serpentaria are powerful stimulants; and both have been employed in fevers in which debility prevailed. However, he thinks, wine may always supersede the stimulant powers of these medicines; and that debility is better remedied by the tonic and antiseptic powers of cold and Peruvian bark, than by any stimulants.

By the assistance of heat, both spirit and water extract all its virtues; but they carry little or nothing in distillation; extracts made by inspissating the decoction, retain all the virtues of the root.

The London College forms the compound powder of contrayerva, by combining five ounces of contrayerva root with a pound and a half of prepared shells. This powder was formerly made up in balls, and called *lapis contrayervæ*, employed in the decline of ardent fevers, and through the whole course of low and nervous ones. The radix serpentariæ virginiensis, in all cases, may be substituted for the contrayerva.

DORSTENIA DRAKENA. The systematic name for one sort of the contrayerva.

DORSTENIA HOUSTONII. See *Dorstenia contrayerva.*

DO'THIEN. A name for the furunculus.

DOUGLAS, JAMES, M. D. was born in Scotland in 1675. After completing his education, he came to London, and applied himself diligently to the study of anatomy and surgery, which he both taught and practised several years with success. Haller has spoken very highly of his preparations, to show the motion of the joints, and the structure of the bones. He patronised the celebrated William Hunter; who assisted him shortly before his death in 1742. He was reader of Anatomy to the Company of Surgeons, and a Fellow of the Royal Society, to which he made several communications. He published, in 1707, a more correct description of the muscles than had before appeared; eight years after, a tolerable account of preceding anatomical writers; in 1726, a History of the lateral Operation for the Stone; and in 1730, a very accurate Description of the Peritonæum, &c.

DOUGLAS, JOHN, brother of the preceding, was surgeon to the Westminster Infirmary, and author of several controversial pieces. In one of them, called "Remarks on a late pompous Work," he censures, with no small degree of severity, Cheselden's Anatomy of the Bones; in another, he criticises, with equal asperity, the works of Chamberlen and Chapman; and in a third, he decries the new forceps of Dr. Smellie. He also wrote a work on the high operation for the stone, which he practised; a Dissertation on the Venereal Disease; and an Account of the Efficacy of Bark in stopping Gangrene.

DOVE'S FOOT. See *Geranium rotundifolium.*

Dover's powder. See *Pulvis ipecacuanhæ compositus.*

Down of seed. See *Pappus.*

DRA'BA. (From δρασσω, to seize; so called from its sudden effect upon the nose of those who eat it.) The name of a genus of plants in the Linnæan system. Class, *Tetradynamia;* Order, *Siliculosa.*

DRABA VERNA. A common plant on most walls. The seed is hot and stimulating, and might be used for pepper.

DRA'CO. (*Draco, onis.* m. Δρακων, the dragon.) The dragon.

DRACO MITIGATUS. The submuriate of mercury.

DRACO SYLVESTRIS. See *Achillea Ptarmica.*

DRACOCE'PHALUM. (From δρακων, a dragon, and κεφαλη, a head.) The name of a genus of plants in the Linnæan system. Class, *Didynamia;* Order, *Gymnospermia.*

DRACOCEPHALUM CANARIENSE. The systematic name of the balm of Gilead. Turkey-balsam; Canary balsam; Balsam of Gilead. *Moldavica; Melissa Turcica. Dracocephalum moldavica—floribus verticellatis, bracteis lanceolatis, serraturis capillaceis* of Linnæus. This plant affords a fragrant essential oil, by distillation, known in Germany by the name of *oleum syriæ.* The whole herb abounds with an aromatic smell, and an agreeable taste, joined with an aromatic flavour; it is recommended to give tone to the stomach and nervous system.

DRACONIS SANGUIS. Dragon's blood. See *Calamus rotang.*

DRACONTIA. The dracontia of the Greeks, according to Pliny, was the Guinea-worm, or *dracunculus.* See *Medinensis vena.*

DRACO'NTIUM. (From δρακων, a dragon; so called because its roots resemble a dragon's tail.) See *Arum dracunculus.*

["DRACONTIUM. *Skunk Cabbage.* The skunk cabbage is an indigenous plant, very common in wet meadows throughout the United States, and well known for its offensive odour, perfectly resembling that of the animal whose name it bears. Its odour resides in a volatile substance not easily obtained in a separate state, and soon dissipated by heat or by drying. It contains likewise an acrid principle like that of the genus *arum;* also a portion of resin and mucilage.

"This plant in small doses is a stimulant and antispasmodic, and in large doses a narcotic. Thirty grains of the powdered root, if freshly prepared, will bring on vertigo, nausea, and frequently vomiting. Age and exposure, however, diminish its activity. In medicine this vegetable has been found of important use in certain forms of asthma, and in chronic catarrh, in which diseases it has succeeded, even when the cases had previously been of great obstinacy. It has also been recommended in rheumatism, in hysteria, and in dropsy.

"A popular form of using this medicine is that of a syrup. This is an uncertain preparation, owing to the volatility of the active ingredients. It is better given in powder made from the dried root a short time before it is wanted. Ten grains may be taken at a *dose,* in honey or treacle, and the quantity gradually increased as long as the stomach and head remain unaffected."—*Big. Mat. Med.* A.]

DRACU'NCULUS. (From δρακων, a serpent.) *Gordius medinensis; Vermis medinensis; Vena medinensis; Vermiculus capillaris.* The Guinea worm. This animalcule is common in both Indies, in most parts of Africa, occasionally at Genoa, and other hot countries. It resembles the common worm, but is much larger; is commonly found in the legs, but sometimes in the muscular part of the arms. It principally affects children, and its generation is not unlike that of the broad worms of the belly. While it moves under the skin, it creates no trouble; but, in length of time, the place near the dracunculus suppurates, and the animal puts forth its head. If it be drawn, it excites considerable uneasiness, especially if drawn so forcibly as to break it; for the part left within creates intolerable pain. These worms are of different lengths. In the Edin. Med. Essays, mention is made of one that was three yards and a half in length.

DRACUNCULUS PRATENSIS. See *Achillea ptarmica.*

DRAGACA'NTHA. See *Astragalus.*

Dragant gum. See *Astragalus.*

DRAGON. See *Draco.*

Dragon's blood. See *Calamus rotang.*

Dragon's wort. See *Arum dracunculus.*

DRAKE, JAMES, M. D. Fellow of the College of Physicians, and of the Royal Society, published, in 1707, "A New System of Anatomy," which, though taken principally from Cowper, being on a reduced plan, and more within the reach of students, was pretty favourably received. In the third edition, it was styled "Anthropologia Nova." In abscesses of the antrum maxillare, he advised drawing one of the molar teeth, to let out the matter. The description of the internal nostrils, and of the cavities entering them, is new; as are also the plates of the abominal viscera.

DRAKE'NA. See *Dorstenia contrayerva.*

DRA'STIC. (*Drasticus.* Δραστικος, active, brisk; from δραω, to effect.) A term generally applied to those medicines which are very violent in their action; thus, drastic purges, emetics, &c.

Drawing slate. See *Chalk, black.*

DRELINGCOURT, CHARLES, was born at Paris in 1633; and after studying some years at Saumur, he went to graduate at Montpelier. He soon after attended the celebrated Turenne in his campaigns, and was by him made physician to the army. He was also appointed one of the physicians to Lewis XIV. But in 1688 he was chosen to succeed Vander Linden, as professor of medicine at Leyden; and two years after he was advanced to the chair of anatomy. He was also made physician to William, then Prince of Orange, and his consort; and on their accession to the throne of England, he spoke the congratulatory oration to them, as rector of the university. He continued in his professorship, giving general satisfaction, to the period of his death in 1697. He was a voluminous and learned, but hardly an original writer; yet his works were very much read at the time. In one of his orations, he exculpates medical men from the charge of impiety, observing that the contemplation of the works of God tends to blind them more to religion. In his "Apologia Medica," he refutes the notion, that physicians were excluded from Rome for six hundred years. He strenuously opposed the introduction of chemical preparations into medicine, which was then very prevalent. His son, *Charles*, succeeded him in practice, but has left no publication, except his thesis "De Lienosis."

DRO'MA. The name of a plaster described by Myrepsus.

DROPACI'SMUS. (From δρεπω, to remove.) *Dropax.* A stimulant plaster of pitch, wax, &c. to take off hair.

DRO'PAX. See *Dropacismus.*

DRO'PSY. *Hydrops.* A collection of a serous fluid in the cellular membrane; in the viscera and the circumscribed cavities of the body. See *Hydrops, Ascites, Anasarca, Hydrocephalus, Hydrothorax, Hydrocele.*

Dropsy of the belly. See *Ascites.*

Dropsy of the brain. See *Hydrocephalus.*

Dropsy of the chest. See *Hydrothorax.*

Dropsy of the ovary. See *Ascites.*

Dropsy of the skin. See *Anasarca.*

Dropsy of the testicle. See *Hydrocele.*

DROPWORT. See *Œnanthe*, and *Spiræa.*

Dropwort, hemlock. See *Œnanthe.*

Dropwort, water. See *Œnanthe.*

DRO'SERA. (From δροσερα, dewy; which is from δροσος, dew; drops hanging on the leaves like dew.) The name of a genus of plants. Class, *Pentandria*, Order, *Hexagynia.* Sun-dew.

DROSERA ROTUNDIFOLIA. The sytematic name of the sun-dew. *Ros solis; Rosella.* Sun-dew. *Drosera rotundifolia—scapis radicatis; foliis orbiculatis* of Linnæus. This elegant little plant is said to be so acrid as to ulcerate the skin, and remove warts and corns; and to excite a fatal coughing and delirium in sheep who eat it. It is seldom given medicinally in this country but by the lower orders, who esteem a decoction of it as serviceable in asthmas and coughs.

DROSOBO'TANUM. (From δροσος, dew, and βοτανη, an herb: so called from its being covered with an aromatic dew.) The herb betony. See *Betonica.*

DROSSO'MELI. (From δροσος, dew, and μελι, honey.) Honey-dew. Manna.

DRUPA. (*Drupæ*, unripe olives.) A stone fruit formed of a fleshy or coriaceous seed-vessel, enclosing a nut.

It is distinguished into,

1. *Drupa succosa*, when of a succulent fleshy consistence; as the cherry, plum, peach, and nectarine.

2. *D. fibrosa*, the nut being fibrose; as in *Cocus nucifera.*

3. *D. exsicca*, dry and subcoriaceous; as the almond and horse-chesnut.

4. *D. dehiscens*, opening; as in *Juglans regia*, and *Myristica moschata.*

From the number of nuts it contains, the *drupa* is said to be *monosperma*, when there is but one, as in the olive and pistachia; and *disperma* when there are two, as in *Styrax.*

DRUPACEUS. Drupaceous; resembling a drupe, or stone fruit. Applied to the pod of *Erugago* and *Bunias.*

DUCT. See *Ductus.*

Duct, biliary. See *Biliary duct.*

DUCTI'LITY. *Ductilitas.* A property by which bodies are elongated by repeated or continued pressure. It is peculiar to metals. Most authors confound the words malleability, laminability, and ductility, together, and use them in a loose indiscriminate way; but they are very different. Malleability is the property of a body which enlarges one or two of its three dimensions, by a blow or pressure very suddenly applied. Laminability belongs to bodies extensible in dimension by a gradually applied pressure; and ductility is properly to be attributed to such bodies as can be rendered longer and thinner by drawing them through a hole of less area than the transverse section of the body so drawn.

DU'CTUS. A canal or duct.

DUCTUS ARTERIOSUS. A great artery-like canal found only in the fœtus, and very young children, between the pulmonary artery and the aorta. In adults it is closed up.

DUCTUS AURIS PALATINUS. The Eustachian tube.

DUCTUS BILIARIS. See *Choledochus ductus.*

DUCTUS COMMUNIS CHOLEDOCHUS. See *Choledochus ductus.*

DUCTUS CYSTICUS. The trunk of the biliary ducts in the liver which carries the bile from them into the gall-bladder.

DUCTUS HEPATICUS. See *Hepatic duct.*

DUCTUS LACHRYMALIS. See *Lachrymal ducts.*

DUCTUS LACTIFERUS. *Ductus galactophorus.* The excretory ducts of the glandular substance composing the female breast. The milk passes along these ducts to the nipple.

DUCTUS AD NASUM. See *Canalis nasalis.*

DUCTUS PANCREATICUS. The pancreatic duct. It is white and small, and arises from the sharp extremity of the pancreas, runs through the middle of the gland towards the duodenum, into which it pours its contents by an opening common to it and the *ductus communis choledochus.*

DUCTUS SALIVALES. The excretory ducts of the salivary glands, which convey the saliva into the mouth.

DUCTUS STENONIS. The Stenonian duct, which was so called after its discoverer, *Steno.* It arises from all the small excretory ducts of the parotid gland, and passes transversely over the masseter muscle, penetrates the buccinator, and opens into the mouth.

DUCTUS THORACICUS. See *Thoracic duct.*

DUCTUS VENOSUS. When the vena cava passes th.

liver in the fœtus, it sends off the ductus venosus, which communicates with the sinus of the vena portæ; but, in adults, it becomes a flat ligament.

Ductus warthonianus. The excretory duct of the maxillary glands; so named after its discoverer.

Dulcacidum. (From *dulcis*, sweet, and *acidus*, sour.) A medicine composed of a sweet and sour ingredient.

DULCAMA'RA. (From *dulcis*, sweet, and *amarus*, bitter.) Bitter-sweet. See *Solanum dulcamara*.

Dumbness. See *Aphonia* and *Paracusis*.

DUMOSUS. (From *dumus* a bush.) Bushy.

Dumosæ. The name of an order of plants in Linnæus's Fragments of a Natural Method, consisting of shrubby plants, which are thick set with irregular branches, and bushy.

DUNCAN, Daniel, was born at Montaubon, in Languedoc, in 1649, son of a professor of physic in that city, but of a family originally Scotch. Having lost both his parents in early infancy, he was taken under the protection of his maternal uncle, and at a proper age sent to study medicine at Montpelier, where he took his degree. He afterward resided seven years at Paris, where he published his first work, upon the principle of motion in animal bodies. He then visited London, partly to arrange some family affairs, partly to obtain information concerning the plague, and intended to have settled there; but after two years he was summoned to attend his patron, the great Colbert. He soon after made public two works, in which he attempted to explain the Annual Functions on Chemical and Mechanical Principles. On the death of Colbert, he resided for some years in his native city; but the persecution of the Protestants in 1690 drove him to Switzerland, and he was appointed Professor of Anatomy and Chemistry at Berne, where he got into considerable practice. In 1699 he was sent for to attend the Princess of Hesse-Cassel, who had symptoms of threatening consumption, induced by the excessive use of tea, and other hot liquors; which led him to write a Treatise against that practice, published subsequently by the persuasion of his friend, Boerhaave. He remained there three years, affording meanwhile much relief to the French refugees; and the fame of his liberality procured his invitation to the court of Berlin: but a regard to his health and to economy soon obliged him to remove to the Hague. In 1714 he accomplished his favourite object of settling in London, and when he reached his 70th year, put in practice his previous resolution of giving his professional services only gratuitously: in which he steadily persevered during the remaining sixteen years of his life, though, in 1721, he lost the third part of his property by the South-sea scheme.

DUNG. See *Fæx*.

Dung, devil's. See *Ferula assafœtida*.

DUO. (Δυω, two.) Some compositions consisting of two ingredients, are distinguished by this term; as pilulæ ex duobus.

DUODE'NUM. (From *duodenus*, consisting of twelve; so called because it was supposed not to exceed the breadth of twelve fingers: but as the ancients dissected only animals, this does not hold good in the human subject.) The first portion of the small intestines. See *Intestines*.

DUPLEX. (From *duo*, two, and *plico*, to fold.) Double or two-fold. In botany applied to leaves, petals, perianths, &c. The *perianthum duplex* is seen in *Malva althæa* and *Hibiscus*.

Duplica'na. (From *duplex*, double.) A name of the double tertian fever.

DUPLICATUS. (From *duplex*, double.) This term is applied to a flower which has two series or rows of petals.

DU'RA MATER. (From *durus*, hard, and *mater*, a mother: called *dura*, from its comparative hardness with the *pia mater;* and *mater*, from its being supposed to be the source of all the other membranes. Other parts have received the trivial name of dura, from their comparative hardness; as portio dura, a branch of the seventh pair of nerves.) *Dura meninx; Dermatodes.* A thick and somewhat opaque and insensible membrane, formed of two layers, that surrounds and defends the brain, and adheres strongly to the internal surface of the cranium. It has three considerable processes, the falciform, the tentorium, and the septum cerebelli; and several sinuses, of which the longitudinal, lateral, and inferior longitudinal, are the principal. Upon the external surface of the dura mater, there are little holes, from which emerge fleshy-coloured papillæ, and which, upon examining the skull-cap, will be found to have corresponding foveæ. These are the external glandulæ Pacchioni. They are in number from ten to fifteen on each side, and are chiefly lateral to the course of the longitudinal sinus. The arteries which supply this membrane with vessels for its own nourishment, for that of the contiguous bone, and for the perpetual exudation of the fluid, or halitus rather, which moistens or bedews its internal surface, may be divided into anterior, middle, and posterior. The first proceeds from the ophthalmic and ethmoidal branches; the second from the internal maxillary and superior pharyngeal; the posterior from the occipital and vertebral arteries.

The principal artery of the dura mater, named, by way of distinction, the great artery of the dura mater, is derived from the internal maxillary artery, a branch of the external carotid. It is called the spinalis, or spheno-spinalis, from its passing into the head through the spinous hole of the sphenoid bone, or meninga media, from its relative situation, as it rises in the great middle fossa of the skull. This artery, though it sometimes enters the skull in two branches, usually enters in one considerable branch, and divides, soon after it reaches the dura mater, into three or four branches, of which the anterior is the largest; and these spread their ramifications beautifully upon the dura mater, over all that part which is opposite to the anterior, middle, and posterior lobes of the brain. Its larger trunks run upon the internal surface of the parietal bone, and are sometimes for a considerable space buried in its substance. The extreme branches of this artery extend so as to inosculate with the anterior and posterior arteries of the dura mater; and through the bones (chiefly parietal and temporal bones), they inosculate with the temporal and occipital arteries. The meningeal artery has been known to become aneurismal, and distended at intervals; it has formed an aneurism, destroying the bones and causing epilepsy.

Dura meninx. See *dura mater*.

DWALE. See *Atropa belladonna*.

Dwarf elder. See *Sambucus ebulus*.

Dyo'ta. (From δυω, two, and ους, ωτος, an ear.) A chemical instrument with two ears, or handles.

DYSÆSTHE'SIA. (From δυς, difficulty, and αισθανομαι, to feel or perceive.) Impaired feeling.

Dysæsthesiæ. (The plural of *Dysæsthesia.*) The name of an order in the class *Locales* of Dr. Cullen's Nosology, containing those diseases, in which the senses are depraved, or destroyed, from a defect of the external organs.

Dysanago'gus. (From δυς, with difficulty, and αναγω, to subdue.) Viscid expectoration.

DYSCATAPO'TIA. (From δυς, and καταπινω, to drink.) A difficulty of swallowing liquids, which Dr. Mead thinks a more proper term than that generally used for canine madness, viz. hydrophobia; as it is more particularly descriptive of the affection under which the unhappy patients labour; for, in reality, they dread water from the difficulty of swallowing it.

DYSCINE'SIA. (From δυς, bad, and κινεω, to move.) Bad or imperfect motion.

Dyscinesiæ. (The plural of *dyscinesia.*) Applied to an order in the class *Locales* of Cullen's Nosology; embracing diseases in which the motion is impeded, or depraved, from an imperfection of the organ.

DYSCOPHO'SIS. (From δυς, with difficulty, and κωφοω, to be deaf) A defect in the sense of hearing.

DYSCRA'SIA. (From δυς, with difficulty, and κεραννυμι, to mix.) A bad habit of body.

DYSECŒ'A. (From δυς, difficulty, and ακοη, hearing). *Cophosis.* Deafness. Hearing diminished, or destroyed. A genus of disease in the class *Locales* and order *Dysæsthesiæ* of Cullen, containing two species: *Dysecœa organica*, which arises from wax in the meatus, injuries of the membrane, or inflammation and obstruction of the tube: *Dysecœa atonica*, when without any discernible injury of the organ.

Dyse'lcia. (From δυς, with difficulty, and ελκος an ulcer.) An inveterate ulcer, or one difficult to heal.

Dyse'metus. (From δυς, with difficulty, and εμεω, to vomit.) A person not easily made to vomit.

DYSENTE'RIA. See *Dysentery*.

DYSENTERY. (*Dysenteria;* from δυς, difficulty

and εν7ερα, the bowels.) *Dissolutus morbus. Diarrhœa carnosa.* The flux. A genus of disease in the class *Pyrexiæ*, and order *Profluvia* of Cullen's Nosology. It is known by contagious pyrexia; frequent griping stools; tenesmus; stools, chiefly mucous, sometimes mixed with blood, the natural fæces being retained or voided in small, compact, hard substances, known by the name of scybala, loss of appetite, and nausea. It occurs chiefly in summer and autumn, and is often occasioned by much moisture succeeding quickly intense heat, or great drought; whereby the perspiration is suddenly checked, and a determination made to the intestines. It is likewise occasioned by the use of unwholesome and putrid food, and by noxious exhalations and vapours; hence it appears often in armies encamped in the neighbourhood of low marshy ground, and proves highly destructive; but the cause which most usually gives rise to it, is a specific contagion; and when it once makes its appearance, where numbers of people are collected together, it not unfrequently spreads with great rapidity. A peculiar disposition in the atmosphere seems often to predispose, or give rise to the dysentery, in which case it prevails epidemically.

It frequently occurs about the same time with autumnal intermittent and remittent fevers, and with these, it is often complicated.

The disease, however, is much more prevalent in warm climates than in cold ones; and in the months of August, September, and October, which is the rainy season of the year in the West Indies, it is very apt to break out and to become very general among the negroes on the different plantations in the colonies. The body having been rendered irritable by the great heat of the summer, and being exposed suddenly to much moisture with open pores, the blood is thereby thrown from the exterior vessels upon the interior, so as to give rise to dysenteries.

An attack of dysentery is sometimes preceded by loss of appetite, costiveness, flatulency, sickness at the stomach, and a slight vomiting, and comes on with chills, succeeded by heat in the skin, and frequency of the pulse. These symptoms are in general the forerunners of the griping and increased evacuations which afterward occur.

When the inflammation begins to occupy the lower part of the intestinal tube, the stools become more frequent, and less abundant; and, in passing through the inflamed parts, they occasion great pain, so that every evacuation is preceded by a severe griping, as also a rumbling noise.

The motions vary both in colour and consistence, being sometimes composed of frothy mucus, streaked with blood, and at other times of an acrid watery humour, like the washings of meat, and with a very fœtid smell. Sometimes pure blood is voided; now and then lumps of coagulated mucus, resembling bits of cheese, are to be observed in the evacuations, and in some instances a quantity of purulent matter is passed.

Sometimes what is voided consists merely of a mucous matter, without any appearance of blood, exhibiting that disease which is known by the name of dysenteria alba, or morbus mucosus.

While the stools consist of these various matters, and are voided frequently, it is seldom that we can perceive any natural fæces among them, and when we do, they appear in small hard balls, called scybala, which being passed, the patient is sure to experience some temporary relief from the griping and tenesmus.

It frequently happens, from the violent efforts which are made to discharge the irritating matters, that a portion of the gut is forced beyond the verge of the anus, which, in the progress of the disease, proves a troublesome and distressing symptom; as does likewise the tenesmus, there being a constant inclination to go to stool, without the ability of voiding any thing, except perhaps a little mucus.

More or less pyrexia usually attends with the symptoms which have been described, throughout the whole of the disease, where it is inclined to terminate fatally; and is either of an inflammatory or putrid tendency. In other cases, the febrile state wholly disappears after a time, while the proper dysenteric symptoms probably will be of long continuance. Hence the distinction into acute and chronic dysentery.

When the symptoms run high, produce great loss of strength and are accompanied with a putrid tendency and a fœtid and involuntary discharge, the disease often terminates fatally in the course of a few days; but when they are more moderate, it is often protracted to a considerable length of time, and so goes off at last by a gentle perspiration, diffused equally over the whole body; the fever, thirst, and griping then ceasing, and the stools becoming of a natural colour and consistence. When the disease is of long standing, and has become habitual, it seldom admits of any cure; and when it attacks a person labouring under an advanced stage of scurvy, or pulmonary consumption, or whose constitution has been much impaired by any other disorder, it is sure to prove fatal. It sometimes appears at the same time with autumnal intermittent and remittent fevers, as has been observed, and is then more complicated and difficult to remove.

Upon opening the bodies of those who die of dysentery, the internal coat of the intestines (but more particularly of the colon and rectum) appears to be affected with inflammation and its consequences, such as ulceration, gangrene, and contractions. The peritonæum, and other coverings of the abdomen, seem likewise, in many instances, to be affected by inflammation.

In the treatment of the acute dysentery, when not arising from contagion, but attended by considerable pyrexia and pain, in persons of a strong and full habit, it will be right to commence by a moderate venæsection; but in general, leeches to the abdomen will abstract a sufficient quantity of blood followed by fomentations, or the warm bath, which may produce a powerful determination to the surface as well as counteract spasm; also blisters or rubefacients should not be neglected. With regard to internal remedies, a brisk emetic will often be advisable, particularly where the tongue is very foul, the stomach loaded, or marks of congestion in the liver appear: it may also, by inducing diaphoresis, materially check the violence of the symptoms, nay sometimes cut short the disease at once. The next object is effectually to clear out the bowels: for which purpose calomel, joined with opium in quantity sufficient to relieve the pain may be given, and followed up by castor oil, neutral salts, &c. till they operate. In the mean time, mucilaginous demulcents may help to moderate the irritation. When the bowels have been thoroughly evacuated, it will be important to procure a steady determination to the surface, and the compound powder of ipecacuanha is perhaps the best medicine; assisted by warm clothing, friction, exercise, &c. Should the liver not perform its office properly, the continued use of mercury may be necessary; to restore the strength, and relieve dyspeptic symptoms, tonics and antacids will be useful, with a mild nutritious diet; and great care must be taken to obviate accumulation of fæces. In the chronic form of the disease, demulcents and sedatives may be freely employed by the mouth, or in the form of clyster; the bowels may be occasionally relieved by rhubarb, or other mild aperients; mercury should be cautiously employed, where the discharge of bile is indicated, or if that cannot be borne, nitric acid may be tried; and besides great attention to regimen, as in the decline of acute dysentery, mild astringents, with tonics, &c. may contribute materially to the recovery of the patient.

DYSEPULO'TICUS. (From δυς, with difficulty, and επυλοω, to cicatrize.) *Dysepulotus.* An inveterate ulcer difficult to be healed.

DYSHÆMORRHO'IS. (From δυς, with difficulty, and αιμορροις, the piles.) Suppression of the bleeding from piles.

DYSLO'CHIA. (From δυς, difficulty, and λοχια, the lochia.) A suppression of the lochia.

DYSMENORRHÆ'A. (From δυς, with difficulty, and μηνορροια, the menses.) A difficult or painful menstruation, accompanied with severe pains in the back, loins, and bottom of the belly.

DYSO'DES. (From δυς, bad, and οζω, to smell.) 1. A bad smell. Fœtid.

2. Hippocrates applies it to a fœtid disorder of the small intestines.

3. The name of a malagma and acopon in Galen and Paulus Ægineta.

DYSO'PIA. (From δυς, bad, and ωψ, an eye.) *Parorasis.* Difficult sight. Sight depraved, requiring one certain quantity of light one particular distance, or one position. A genus of disease in the class *Locales*, and order *Dysæsthesiæ* of Cullen, containing the five following species:

1 *Dysopia tenebrarum*, called also *Amblyopia crepuscularis*, requiring objects to be placed in a strong light.

2. *Dysopia luminis*, likewise termed *Amblyopia meridiana*, objects only discernible in a weak light.

3. *Dysopia dissitorum*, in which distant objects are not perceived.

4. *Dysopia proximorum*, or *Dysopia amblyopia*, in which objects too near are not perceived.

5. *Dysopia lateralis*, called also *Amblyopia luscorum*, in which objects are not seen, unless placed in an oblique position.

DYSORE'XIA. (From δυς, bad, and ορεξις, appetite.) A depraved appetite.

Dysorexiæ. (The plural of *Dysorexia*.) The name of an order in the class *Locales* of Cullen's Nosology, which he divides into two sections, appetitus erronei and deficientes.

DYSPE'PSIA. (From δυς, bad, and πεπτω, to concoct.) *Apepsia*. Indigestion. Dr. Cullen arranges this genus of disease in the class *Neuroses*, and order *Adynamiæ*. It chiefly arises in persons between thirty and forty years of age, and is principally to be met with in those who devote much time to study, or who lead either a very sedentary or irregular life. A great singularity attendant on it is, that it may and often does continue a great length of time, without any aggravation or emission of the symptoms.

Great grief and uneasiness of mind, intense study, profuse evacuations, excess in venery, hard drinking, particularly of spirituous liquors, and of tea, tobacco, opium, and other narcotics, immoderate repletion, and over distention of the stomach, a deficiency in the secretion of the bile, or gastric juice, and the being much exposed to moist and cold air, when without exercise, are the causes which usually occasion dyspepsia.

A long train of nervous symptoms generally attend on this disease, such as a loss of appetite, nausea, heart-burn, flatulency, acid, fœtid, or indorous eructations, a gnawing in the stomach when empty, a sense of constriction and uneasiness in the throat, with pain in the side, or sternum, so that the patient at times can only lie on his right side; great costiveness, habitual chilliness, paleness of the countenance, languor, unwillingness to move about, lowness of spirits, palpitations, and disturbed sleep.

The number of these symptoms varies in different cases, with some, being felt only in part; in others, being accompanied even with additional ones, equally unpleasant, such as severe transient pains in the head and breast, and various affections of the sight, as blindness, double vision, &c.

Dyspepsia never proves fatal, unless when, by a very long continuance, it produces great general debility and weakness; and so passes into some other disease, such as dropsy; but it is at all times very difficult to remove, but more particularly so in warm climates.

The morbid appearances to be observed on dissections of this disease, are principally confined to that part of the stomach which is called the pylorus; which is often found either in a contracted, scirrhous, or ulcerated state. In every instance, the stomach is perceived to be considerably distended with air.

The treatment of dyspepsia consists, 1. In obviating the several exciting causes. 2. In relieving urgent symptoms, some of which may tend to prolong the disease. 3. In restoring the tone of the stomach, or of the general system, and thus getting rid of the liability to relapse.

I. In fulfilling the first indication, we are often much circumscribed by the circumstances or habits of the patient; and particularly when they have been accustomed to drink spirits, which they can hardly relinquish, or only in a very gradual manner. The diet must be regulated by the particular form of the disease; in those who are liable to acidity, it should be chiefly of an animal nature, with the least acescent vegetable substances, and for drink, toast and water, or soda water, adding a little brandy, if really necessary; where the opposite, or septic tendency appears, which happens especially in persons of a florid complexion, it should consist principally of vegetable matter, particularly the ripe subacid fruits, with the meat of young animals occasionally, and if plain water be not agreeable, table-beer, cider, &c. may be allowed for drink; and in those of the phlegmatic temperament the most nutritious and digestible articles must be selected, mostly of an animal nature, assisted by the warmer condiments, and the more generous fermented liquors in moderation. It will be generally better to take food oftener, rather than to load the stomach too much at once; but more than four meals a day can hardly be requisite; if at any other time a craving should occur, a crust of bread or a piece of biscuit may be eaten.

II. Among the symptoms requiring palliation, heart-burn is frequent, resulting from acrimony in the stomach, and to be relieved by antacid, or antiseptic remedies, according to circumstances, or diluents and demulcents may answer the purpose. A sense of weight at the stomach, with nausea, may occasionally indicate a gentle emetic; but will be less likely to occur if the bowels are kept regular. Flatulence may be relieved by aromatics, æther, &c.; and these will be proper for spasmodic, or nervous pains; but if ineffectual, opium should be had recourse to. Vomiting is generally best checked by carbonic acid. When diarrhœa occurs, the aromatic confection is mostly proper, sometimes with a little opium. But the bowels are much more commonly confined, and mild cathartics should be frequently exhibited, as castor oil, rhubarb, aloes, &c.; sometimes the more active, where these do not answer. In those of a florid complexion a laxative diet, with the supertartrate of potassa, or other saline cathartic occasionally, may agree better: and where the liver is torpid, mercurials should be resorted to.

III. The third object is to be attempted by tonics, particularly the aromatic bitters, the mineral acids, or the preparations of iron; by the cold bath prudently regulated; by gentle exercise steadily persevered in, particularly walking or riding on horseback; by a careful attention to the diet; by seeking a pure mild air, keeping regular hours, with relaxation and amusement of the mind, &c.

DYSPERMATI'SMUS. (From δυς, bad, and σπερμα, seed.) *Agenesia*. Slow, or impeded emission of semen, during coition, insufficient for the purpose of generation. A genus of disease in the class *Locales*, and order *Epischeses* of Cullen. The species are:

1. *Dyspermatismus urethralis*, when the obstruction is in the urethra.

2. *Dyspermatismus nodosus*, when a tumour is formed in either corpus cavernosum penis.

3. *Dyspermatismus præputialis*, when the impediment is from a straightness of the orifice of the præpuce.

4. *Dyspermatismus mucosus*, when the urethra is obstructed by a viscid mucus.

4. *Dyspermatismus hypertonicus*, when there is an excess of erection of the penis.

6. *Dyspermatismus epilepticus*, from epileptic fits coming on during coition.

7. *Dyspermatismus apractodes*, from a want of vigour in the genitals.

8. *Dyspermatismus refluus*, in which the semen is thrown back into the urinary bladder.

DYSPHA'GIA. (From δυς, with difficulty, and φαγω, to eat.) A difficulty of deglutition. A genus of disease in Good's Nosology, embracing five species *Dysphagia constricta; atonica; globosa; uvulosa; linguosa*.

DYSPHO'NIA. (From δυς, bad, and φωνη, the voice.) A difficulty of speaking. Dissonant voice The sound of the voice imperfect or depraved. A genus of disease in Good's Nosology, embracing three species *Dysphonia susurrans*, *puberans*, and *immodulata*.

DYSPHORIA. (From δυς, and φορεω, *gesto*.) Restlessness. A genus of disease in Good's Nosology, it has two species, *Dysphorea simplex* and *anxietas*.

DYSPNŒ'A. (From δυς, difficult, and πνεω, to breathe.) *Dyspnoon*. Difficult respiration, without sense of stricture, and accompanied with cough through the whole course of the disease. A genus of disease in the class *Neuroses*, and order *Spasmi* of Cullen. He distinguishes eight species.

1. *Dyspnœa catarrhalis*, when with a cough there are copious discharges of viscid mucus, called also *asthma catarrhale*, *pneumodes*, *pneumonicum*, and *pituitosum*.

2. *Dyspnœa sicca*, when there is a cough without any considerable discharge.

3. *Dyspnœa aërea*, when the disease is much increased by slight changes of the weather

4. *Dyspnœa terrea*, when earthy or calculous matters are spit up.

5. *Dyspnœa aquosa*, when there is a scarcity of urine and œdematous feet, without the other symptoms of a dropsy in the chest.

6. *Dyspnœa pinguedinosa*, from corpulency.

7. *Dyspnœa thoracica*, when parts surrounding the chest are injured, or deformed.

8. *Dyspnœa extrinseca*, from manifest external causes.

DY'SPNOON. See *Dyspnœa*.

DYSTHETICA. (Δυσθετικα, an ill-conditioned state of the body.) The name of the fourth order of the class *Hæmatica* in Good's Nosology. Cachexies. Its genera are *Plethora; Hæmorrhagia; Marasmus; Struma; Carcinus; Lues; Elephantius; Bucnemia; Catacausis; Porphyra; Exangia; Gangrena; Ulcus.*

DYSTHY'MIA. (From δυς, bad, and θυμος, mind.) Insanity.

DYSTO'CHIA. (From δυς, with difficulty, and τικτω, to bring forth.) Difficult labour.

DYSTŒCHI'ASIS. (From δυς, bad, and ϛοιχος, order.) An irregular disposition of the hairs in the eyelids.

DYSU'RIA. (From δυς, difficulty, and ουρον, urine.) *Stillicidium; Ardor urinæ; Culbicio.* A suppression or difficulty in discharging the urine. A total suppression is called ischuria; a partial suppression, dysuria: and this may be with or without heat. When there are frequent, painful, or uneasy urgings to discharge the urine, and it passes off only by drops, or in very small quantities, the disease is called strangury. When a sense of pain, or heat, attends the discharge, it passes with difficulty, and is styled ardor urinæ, heat of the urine. The dysuria is acute, or chronic. Dr. Cullen places this disease in the class *Locales*, and order *Epischeses*, containing six species:

1. *Dysuria ardens*, with a sense of heat, without any manifest disorder of the bladder.

2. *Dysuria spasmodica*, from spasm.

3. *Dysuria compressionis*, from a compression of the neighbouring parts.

4. *Dysuria phlogistica*, from violent inflammation.

5. *Dysuria calculosa*, from stone in the bladder.

6. *Dysuria mucosa*, from an abundant secretion of mucus.

The causes which give rise to these diseases are, an inflammation of the urethra, occasioned either by venereal sores, or by the use of acrid injections, tumour, ulcer of the prostate gland, inflammation of the kidneys, or bladder, considerable enlargements of the hæmorrhoidal veins, a lodgment of indurated fæces in the rectum, spasm at the neck of the bladder, the absorption of cantharides, applied externally or taken internally, and excess in drinking either spirituous or vinous liquors; but particles of gravel, sticking at the neck of the bladder, or lodging in the urethra, and thereby producing irritation, prove the most frequent cause. Gouty matter falling on the neck of the bladder, will sometimes occasion these complaints.

In dysury, there is a frequent inclination to make water, with a smarting pain, heat, and difficulty in voiding it, together with a sense of fulness in the region of the bladder. The symptoms often vary, however, according to the cause which has given rise to it. If it proceeds from a calculus in the kidney or ureter, besides the affections mentioned, it will be accompanied with nausea, vomiting, and acute pains in the loins and region of the ureter and kidney of the side affected. When a stone in the bladder, or gravel in the urethra, is the cause, an acute pain will be felt at the end of the penis, particularly on voiding the last drops of urine, and the stream of water will either be divided into two, or be discharged in a twisted manner, not unlike a corkscrew. If a scirrhus of the prostate gland has occasioned the suppression or difficulty of urine, a hard indolent tumour, unattended with any acute pain, may readily be felt in the perinæum, or by introducing the finger into the rectum

E

EAGLE STONE. An argillaceous iron stone.

EAR. *Auris.* The ear is the organ of hearing. It is situated at the side of the head, and is divided into external and internal ear. The *auricula*, or *pinna*, commonly called the ear, constitutes the external part. It is of a greater or less size, according to the individual. Its external face, which, in a well-formed ear, is a little anterior, presents five eminences, the *helix*, *anti-helix*, *tragus*, *anti-tragus*, *lobula*; and three cavities, those of the *helix*, *fossa navicularis*, *concha*.

The pinna is formed of a *fibrous cartilage*, elastic and pliant; the skin which covers it is thin and dry; adheres to the fibro-cartilage by a cellular tissue, which is compact, and contains very little adipose substance: the lobule alone contains it in considerable quantity. There are seen under the skin a number of sebaceous follicles, which furnish a micaceous white matter, that produces the polish and suppleness of the skin.

There are also seen, upon the different projections of the cartilaginous ear, certain muscular fibres, to which the name of *muscles* have been given, but which are only *vestigia*. The pinna, receiving many vessels and nerves, is very sensible, and easily becomes red. It is fixed to the head by the cellular tissue, and by muscles, which are called according to their position, *anterior*, *superior*, and *posterior*. These muscles are much developed in many animals: in man they may be considered as simple vestiges.

The *meatus auditorius* extends from the *concha* to the membrane of the *tympanum*; its length, variable according to age, is from ten to twelve lines in the adult; it is narrower in the middle than at the ends; it presents a slight curve above, and in front. Its external orifice is commonly covered with hairs, like the entrance to the other cavities. It is composed of an osseous part, of a fibro-cartilaginous substance, which is confounded with that of the pinna, of a fibrous part, which completes it above. The skin sinks into it, becoming thinner, and terminates in covering the external surface of the membrane of the *tympanum*. Below this skin exist a great number of sebaceous follicles, which furnish the *cerumen*, a yellow, bitter matter.

The middle ear comprehends the cavity of the tympanum, the little bones which are contained in this cavity, the mastoid cells, the Eustachian tube, &c.

The *tympanum* is a cavity which separates the external from the internal ear. Its form is that of a portion of a cylinder, but a little irregular. Its external partition presents, on the upper part, the *fenestra ovalis*, which communicates with the vestibule, and which is formed by a membrane; immediately below, a projection which is called *promontory*; below this projection, a little groove, which lodges a small nerve; still lower, an opening called the *fenestra rotunda*, which corresponds to the external winding of the cochlea: and which is also shut by a membrane. The external side presents the *membrana tympani.* This membrane is directed obliquely downward and inward; it is bent, very slender and transparent, covered on the outside by a continuation of the skin, on the inside by the narrow membrane which covers the tympanum; it is also covered on this side by the nerve called *chorda tympani*: its centre serves as a point of fixation for the extremity of the handle of the malleus; its circumference is fixed to the bony extremity of the meatus auditorius: it adheres equally in every point, and presents no opening that might admit a communication between the external and middle ear. Its tissue is dry, brittle, and has nothing analogous in the animal economy; there are neither fibres, vessels, nor nerves, found in it. The circumference of the tympanum presents, in the forepart, 1st, The opening of the Eustachian tube, by which the cavity communicates with the superior part of the pharynx; 2dly, The opening by which the tendon of the internal muscle of the malleus enters. Behind are seen, 1st, The opening of the mastoid cells,—irregular winding cavities, which are formed in the mastoid process, and which are always filled with air; 2dly, The pyramid, a little hollow projection, which lodges the muscle of the *stapes;* 3dly, The opening by which the *chorda tympani* enters into the hollow of the tympanum. Below, the tympanum presents a slit, called *glenoid*, by which the tendon of the anterior muscle of the *malleus* enters, and the *chorda tympani* passes out, and goes to unite itself with the lingual nerve of the fifth pair.

Above, the circumference presents only a few small openings, by which blood-vessels pass. The cavity of the tympanum, and all the canals which end there, are covered with a very slender mucous membrane: this cavity, which is always full of air, contains besides four small bones, (the *malleus*, *incus*, *os orbiculare*, and *stapes*,) which form a chain from the membrana tympani to the fenestra ovalis, where the base of the stapes is fixed. There are some little muscles for the purpose of moving this osseous chain, of stretching and slackening the membranes to which they are attached: thus, the internal muscle of the malleus draws it forward, bends the chain in this direction, and stretches the membranes; the anterior muscle produces the contrary effect: it is also supposed that the small muscle which is placed in the pyramid, and which is attached to the neck of the *stapes*, may give a slight tension to the chain, in drawing it towards itself.

The *internal ear*, or *labyrinth*, is composed of the *cochlea*, of the *semicircular canals*, and of the *vestibule.*

The cochlea is a bony cavity, in form of a spiral, from which it has taken its name. This cavity is divided into two others, called the *gyri* of the cochlea, and which are distinguished into external and internal. The partition which separates them is a plate set edgeways, and which in its whole length is partly bony, and partly membranous. The external gyration communicates by the fenestra rotunda with the cavity of the tympanum; the internal gyration ends in the vestibule.

The *semicircular canals* are, three cylindrical cavities, bent in a semicircular form, two of which are disposed horizontally, and the others vertically. These canals terminate by their extremities in the vestibule. They contain bodies of a gray colour, the extremities of which are terminated by swellings.

The *vestibule* is the central cavity, the point of union of all the others. It communicates with the tympanum by the fenestra ovalis, with the internal gyration of the cochlea, with the semicircular canals, and with the internal meatus auditorius, by a great number of little openings.

The whole of the cavities of the internal ear are hollowed out of the hardest part of the petrous portion of the temporal bone: they are covered with an extremely thin membrane, and are full of a very thin and limpid fluid, called *Liquor of Cotunnius*, which can flow out by two narrow apertures, known by the name of the *aquæducts of the cochlea*, and *of the vestibule:* they contain, besides, the acoustic nerve.

The *acoustic nerve* proceeds from the fourth ventricle; it enters into the labyrinth by the holes that the internal auditory meatus presents in its bottom. Having entered into the vestibule, it separates itself into a number of branches, one of which remains in the vestibule, another enters into the cochlea, and two go to the semicircular canals. Scarpa has very minutely described the distribution of these different branches in the cavities of the internal ear.

In terminating this short description, we remark that the internal and middle ear are traversed by several nervous threads, the presence of which is, perhaps, useful to hearing. It is known that the facial nerve proceeds a considerable space in a canal of the petrous portion. In this canal it receives a small thread of the vidian nerve; it furnishes the chorda tympani, which attaches itself to this membrane. There are two other nervous inosculations in the ear; to one of which Ribes called the attention of anatomists not long since; the other was recently discovered by Jacobson.

Ear-wax. See *Cerumen aurium.*

EARI'TES. Hæmatites, or blood-stone.

EARTH. *Terra.* Although there seems to be an almost infinite variety of earthy substances scattered on the surface of this globe, yet when we examine them with a chemical eye, we find, not without surprise, that all the earth and stones which we tread under our feet, and which compose the largest rocks, as well as the numerous different specimens which adorn the cabinets of the curious, are composed of a very few simple or elementary earths. "Analysis has shown, that the various stony or pulverulent masses, which form our mountains, valleys, and plains, might be considered as resulting from the combination or intermixture, in various numbers and proportions, of nine primitive earths, to which the following names were given:

1. Barytes. 2. Strontites. 3. Lime. 4. Magnesia. 5. Alumina, or clay. 6. Silica. 7. Glucina. 8. Zirconia. 9. Yttria.

Alkalies, acids, metallic ores, and native metals, were supposed to be of an entirely dissimilar constitution.

The brilliant discovery by Sir H. Davy, in 1808, of the metallic bases of potassa, soda, barytes, strontites, and lime, subverted the ancient ideas regarding the earths, and taught us to regard them as all belonging, by most probable analogies, to the metallic class.

To the above nine earthy substances, Berzelius has lately added a tenth, which he calls *thorina.* Whatever may be the revolutions of chemical nomenclature, mankind will never cease to consider as *earths*, those solid bodies composing the mineral strata, which are incombustible, colourless, not convertible into metals by all the ordinary methods of reduction, or when reduced by scientific refinements, possessing but an evanescent metallic existence, and which either alone, or at least when combined with carbonic acid, are insipid and insoluble in water.

Earth, absorbent. See *Absorbent.*

Earth, aluminous. See *Alumina.*

Earth, animal calcareous. This term is applied to crab's-claws, &c. which contain calcareous earth, and are obtained from the animal kingdom.

Earth, argillaceous. See *Alumina.*

Earth-bath. A remedy recommended by some writers on the continent, as a specific in consumption.

Earth, bolar. See *Bole.*

Earth, fullers'. *Cimolia purpurescens.* A compact bolar earth, commonly of a grayish colour. It is sometimes applied by the common people to inflamed breasts, legs, &c. with a view of cooling them.

Earth, heavy. See *Barytes.*

Earth, Japan. See *Acacia catechu.*

Earth, mineral calcareous. Those calcareous earths which are obtained from the mineral kingdom. The term is applied in opposition to those obtained from animals.

Earth-nut. See *Bunium bulbocastanum.*

Earth, sealed. *Terra sigillata.* Little cakes of earths, which are stamped with impressions. They were formerly in high estimation as absorbents, but now fallen into disuse.

Earth-worm. See *Lumbricus terrestris.*

Eaton's styptic. French brandy highly impregnated with calcined green vitriol. A remedy for checking hæmorrhages.

[EATON, AMOS, professor in the Rensselaer school, at Troy, in the state of New-York. Although Professor Eaton is still living, we deem it but justice to say, that he is one of the most industrious and indefatigable votaries of natural science in the state. He has lectured a number of years at Albany and Troy, on botany, mineralogy, and geology. He has published a valuable Manual of Botany for the Northern States, a Geological Section of the Country from Boston to Lake Erie, and a pamphlet, containing a "Geological Nomenclature for North America." He has been employed for seven years past, under the direction of the Hon. Stephen Van Rensselaer, in travelling over different parts of the state of New-York, and those adjoining, and in making geological surveys and examinations of strata. He has probably done more in this way than any geologist in the country. He promises to publish a System of American Geology, in which will be displayed some peculiarities of the formations in this country, and show how they differ from those of the Eastern continent. A.]

Eau-de-luce. See *Spiritus ammoniæ succinatus.*

Eau-de-rabel. This is composed of one part of sulphurous acid to three of rectified spirit of wine. It s much used in France, when diluted, in the cure of gonorrhœas, leucorrhœa, &c.

Ebi'scus. See *Hibiscus abelmoschus.*

EBULLI'TION. (*Ebullitio.* From *ebullio,* to bubble up.) Boiling. This consists in the change which a fluid undergoes from a state of liquidity to that of an elastic fluid, in consequence of the application of heat, which dilates and converts it into vapour.

E'BULUS. (From *ebullio,* to make boil: so called because of its supposed use in purifying the humours of the body.) See *Sambucus ebulus.*

Ecbo'lica. (From εκβαλλω, to cast out.) Medicines which cause abortion.

Ecbo'lios. (From εκβαλλω, to cast out.) Miscarriage.

Ecbra'smata. (From εκβραζω, to be very hot.) *Ecchymata.* Painful fiery pimples in the face, or surface of the body.

Ecbra'smus. (From εκβραζω, to become hot.) Fermentation.

Ecbyrso'mata. (Prom εκ, and βυρσα, the skin.) Protuberances of the bones at the joints, which appear through the skin.

Ecchylo'ma. (From εκ, and χυλος, juice.) An extract.

Ecchy'mata. (From εκχυω, to pour out.) See *Ecbrasmata.*

ECCHYMO'MA. (Εκχυμωμα; from εκχυω, to pour out.) *Ecchymosis; Crustula; Sugillatio.* Extravasation. A black and blue swelling, either from a bruise or spontaneous extravasation of blood. A genus of disease in the class *Locales,* and order *Tumores* of Cullen.

Ecchymoma arteriosum. The false aneurism.

ECCHYMO'SIS. See *Ecchymoma.*

E'CCLISIS. (From εκκλινω, to turn aside.) A luxation or dislocation.

E'CCOPE. (From εκκοπ7ω, to cut off.) The cutting off any part.

Ecco'peus. (From εκκοπ7ω, to cut off.) An ancient instrument, the raspatory, used in trepanning.

ECCOPRO'TIC. (*Eccoproticus;* from εκ, and κοπρος, dung.) An opening medicine, the operation of which is very gentle; such as manna, senna, &c.

ECCRINOCRI'TICA. (From εκκρινω, to secrete, and κρινω, to judge.) Judgments formed from the secretions.

ECCRINOLO'GIA. (From εκκρινω, to secrete, and λογος, a discourse.) *Eccrinologica.* The doctrine of secretions.

E'CCRISIS. (From εκκρινω, to secrete.) A secretion of any kind.

ECCRITICA. (From εκκρινω, to secern, or strain off.) Dr. Good applies this name to a class of diseases of the excernent system. It has three orders, viz. *Mesotica, Catotica, Acrotica.*

ECCYESIS. (From εκ, and κυησις, *gravidity.*) Extra-uterine fœtation. The name of a genus of diseases in Good's Nosology. It has three species: *Eccyesis ovariæ, tubalis, abdominalis.*

ECCYMO'SIS. See *Ecchymoma.*

E'CDORA. (From εκδερω, to excoriate.) An excoriation: and particularly used for an excoriation of the urethra.

Ecdo'ria. (From εκδερω, to excoriate.) Medicines which excoriate and burn through the skin.

Echeco'llon. (From εχω, to have, and κολλα, glue.) *Echecollum.* Any topical glutinous remedy.

Echetro'sis. So Hippocrates calls the white briony.

ECHINATUS. Bristly. Applied in botany to any thing beset with bristles, as the pod of *Glycyrrhiza echinata,* and to the gourd seed-vessel, or *pepo.*

Echini'des. In Hippocrates it is mentioned as what be used for purging the womb with.

ECHINOPHTHA'LMIA. (From εχινος, a hedgehog, and οφθαλμια, an inflammation of the eye.) An inflammation of that part of the eyelids, where the hairs bristle out like the quills of an echinus, or hedgehog.

ECHINOPO'DIUM. (From εχινος, a hedge-hog, and πους, a foot; so named because its flowers resemble the foot of an urchin.) A species of broom or genista.

ECHI'NOPS. (From εχινος, as beset with prickles.) The name of a genus of plants. Class, *Syngenesia;* Order, *Polygamia segregata.*

Echinops sphærocephalus. The systematic name of the globe thistle. *Crocodilion; Acanthaleuca; Scabiosa carduifolia; Sphærocephala elatis; Echinopus.* It is raised in our gardens. The root and seeds are moderately diuretic, but not used.

Echi'nopus. See *Echinops.*

ECHINUS. 1. The hedge-hog, or *Erinaceus Europæus* of Linnæus.

2. A genus in the Linnæan system, included in the molusca order of vermes.

3. The calcareous petrifaction of the sea hedge-hog.

4. The prominent points on the surface of the *pileus,* or upper part of the mushroom tribe, are called *echini.* See *Fungus.*

ECHIOIDES. (From εχις, a viper, and ειδος, resemblance.) The trivial name of some plants, from their supposed resemblance to the *Echium.*

E'CHIUM. (From εχις, a viper; so called because it was said to heal the stings of vipers.) The name of a genus of plants in the Linnæan system. Class, *Pentandria;* Order, *Monogynia.* Viper's bugloss.

Echium ægyptiacum. Wall bugloss. The *Asperugo ægyptiaca,* the root of which is sudorific, and is used with oil as a dressing for wounds.

E'CHOS. Ηχος. Sound. In Hippocrates, it signifies the same as the tinnitus aurium, or noise in the ears.

E'CHYSIS. (From εχυω, to pour out.) A fainting or swooning.

ECLA'MPSIA. (From εκλαμπω, to shine. See *Eclampsis.*

ECLA'MPSIS. (From εκλαμπω, to shine. *Eclampsia.* It signifies a splendour, brightness, effulgence flashing of light, scintillation. It is a flashing light, or those sparklings which strike the eyes of epileptic patients. Cœlius Aurelianus calls them *circuli ignei,* scintillations, or fiery circles. Though only a symptom of the epilepsy, Hippocrates puts it for epilepsy itself.

ECLE'CTIC. (*Eclecticus;* from εκλεγω, to select.) Archigenes and some others selected from all other sects what appeared to them to be the best and most rational; hence they were called *Eclectics,* and their medicine *Eclectic medicine.*

ECLE'CTOS. (From εκλειχω, to lick up. A linctus, or soft medicine, like an electuary, to be licked up.

ECLE'GMA. (From εκλειχω, to lick.) A linctus, or form of medicine made by the incorporation of oils with syrups, and which is to be taken upon a liquorice stick.

E'CLYSIS. (From εκλυω, to dissolve.) A universal faintness.

ECMA'GMA. (From εκμασσω, to form together.) A mass of substances kneaded together.

ECPEPIE'MENOS. (From εκπιεζω, to press out.) An ulcer with protuberating lips.

ECPHLYSIS. (Εκφλυσις; from εκφλυζω, to boil, or bubble up, or over.) A blain, or vesicular eruption. The name of a genus of disease in Good's Nosology. It has four species, viz. *Ecphlysis pompholex, herpes, rhypia,* and *eczema.*

ECPHRA'CTIC. (From εκφρασσω, to remove obstructions. That which attenuates tough humours, so as to promote their discharge.

ECPHRA'XIS. (From εκφρασσω, to remove obstruction.) A perspiration, an opening of obstructed pores.

ECPHRONIA. (Εκφρωνε, or εκφροσυνη, from εκφρων, *extra mentem,* out of one's mind.) The name of a genus in Good's Nosology. Insanity and craziness. It has two species: *Ecphronia melancholia,* and *Ecphronia mania.*

E'CPHYAS. (From εκ, and φυο, to produce.) 1. An appendix, or excrescence.

2. The appendicula cæci vermiformis.

ECPHYMA. (From εκφυω, *educo, egero.*) A cutaneous excrescence. The name of a genus of diseases in Good's Nosology. Class, *Eccritica;* Order, *Acrotia.* It has four species, viz. *Ecphyma caruncula, verruca, clavus,* and *callus.*

E'cphyse. (From εκφυσαω, to blow out.) Flatus from the bladder through the urethra, and from the wound through the vagina.

Ecphyse'sis. (From εκφυσαω, to breathe through.) A quick expulsion of the air from the lungs.

E'CPHYSIS. (From εκφυω, to produce.)

1. An apophysis, or appendix.

2. A process.

ECPIE'SMA. (From εκπιεζω, to press out.) A fracture of the skull, in which the bones press inwardly.

ECPIE'SMOS. (From εκπιεζω, to press out.) A disorder of the eye, in which the globe is almost pressed out of the socket by an afflux of humours.

ECPLERO'MA. (From εκπληροω, to fill.) In Hippocrates they are hard balls of leather, or other substances, adapted to fill the arm-pits, while by the help of the heels, placed against the balls, and repressing the same, the luxated os humeri is reduced into its place.

ECPLE'XIS. (From εκπλησσω, to terrify or astonish.) A stupor, or astonishment, from sudden external accidents.

E'CPNOE. (From εκπνεω, to breathe.) Expiration; that part of respiration in which the air is expelled from the lungs.

ECPTO'MA. (From εκπιπτω, to fall out.) 1. A luxation of a bone.

2. The expulsion of the secundines.

3. The falling off of gangrenous parts.

4. A hernia in the scrotum.

5. A falling down of the womb.

ECPY'CTICA. (From εκπυκαζω, to condense.) Medicines that render the fluids more solid.

ECPYE'MA. (From εκ, and πυον, pus.) A collection of pus, from the suppuration of a tumour.

ECPYESIS. (From εκπυω, to suppurate.) The name of a genus of diseases in Good's Nosology. Class, *Eccritica;* Order, *Acrotica.* Humid scalp. It has four species, *Ecpyesis impetigo, porrigo, ecthyma, scabies.*

ECRE'GMA. (From εκρηγνυμι, to break.) A rupture.

ECRE'XIS. (From εκρηγνυμι, to break.) A rupture. Hippocrates expresses by it a rupture or laceration of the womb.

ECHRY'THMOS. (From εκ, and ρυθμος, harmony.) A term applied to the pulse, and signifies that it is irregular.

E'CROE. (From εκρεω, to flow out.) An efflux, or the course by which any humour which requires purging is evacuated.

Ecrueles. The French for scrofula.

E'CRYSIS. (From εκρεω, to flow out.) In Hippocrates it is an efflux of the semen before it receives the conformation of a fœtus, and therefore is called an efflux, to distinguish it from abortion.

ECSARCO'MA. (From εκ, and σαρξ, flesh.) A fleshy excrescence.

E'CSTASIS. (*Ecstasis, eos.* f. Εκςασις; from εξιςαμαι, to be out of one's senses.) An ecstasy, or trance. In Hippocrates it signifies a delirium.

ECSTRO'PHIUS. (From εκςρεφω, to invert.) An epithet for any medicine, that makes the blind piles appear outwardly.

ECTHELY'NSIS. (From εκθελυνω, to re nder effeminate.) Softness. It is applied to the skin and flesh, when lax and soft, and to bandages, when not sufficiently tight.

ECTHLI'MMA. (From εκθλιβω, to press out against.) An ulceration caused by pressure of the skin.

ECTHLI'PSIS. (From εκθλιβω, to press out against.) Elision, or expression. It is spoken of swelled eyes, when they dart forth sparks of light.

E'CTHYMA. (*Ecthyma, atis.* n. εκθυειν, to rage, or break forth with fury.) A pustule or cutaneous eruption.

ECTILLO'TICA. (From εκτιλλω, to pull out.) Medicines which eradicate tubercles or corns, or destroy superfluous hair.

ECTO'PIA. (From εκτοπος, out of place.) Displaced.

ECTOPIÆ. (The plural of *ectopia.*) Parts displaced. An order in the class *locales* of Cullen's Nosology. See *Nosology.*

ECTRAPELOGA'STROS. (From εκτρεπομαι, to degenerate, and γαςηρ, a belly.) One who has a monstrous belly, or whose appetite is voraciously large.

ECTRI'MMA. (From εκτριβω, to rub off.) An excoriation. In Hippocrates it is an exulceration of the skin about the os sacrum.

E'CTROPE. (From εκτρεπω, to divert, pervert, or invert.) It is any duct by which the humours are diverted and drawn off. In P. Ægineta it is the same as *Ectropium.*

ECTRO'PIUM. (From εκτρεπω, to evert.) An eversion of the eyelids, so that their internal surface is outermost.

There are two species of this disease: one produced by an unnatural swelling of the lining of the eyelids, which not only pushes their edges from the eyeball, but also presses them so forcibly, that they become everted; the other arising from a contraction of the skin covering the eyelid, or of that in the vicinity, by which means the edge of the eyelid is first removed for some distance from the eye, and afterward turned completely outward, together with the whole of the affect ed eyelid.

The morbid swelling of the lining of the eyelids, which causes the first species of ectropium, arises mostly from a congenital laxity of this membrane, afterward increased by chronic ophthalmies, particularly of a scrofulous nature, in relaxed, unhealthy subjects; or else the disease originates from the small-pox affecting the eyes.

While the disease is confined to the lower eyelid, as it most commonly is, the lining of this part may be observed rising in the form of a semilunar fold, of a pale red colour like the fungous granulations of wounds, and intervening between the eye and eyelid, which latter it in some measure everts. When the swelling is afterward occasioned by the lining of both the eyelids, the disease assumes an annular shape, in the centre of which the eyeball seems sunk, while the circumference of the ring presses and everts the edges of the two eyelids, so as to cause both great uneasiness and deformity. In each of the above cases, on pressing the skin of the eyelids with the point of the finger, it becomes manifest that they are very capable of being elongated, and would readily yield, so as entirely to cover the eyeball, were they not prevented by the intervening swelling of their membranous lining.

Besides the very considerable deformity which the disease produces, it occasions a continual discharge of tears over the cheek, and, what is worse, a dryness of the eyeball, frequent exasperated attacks of chronic ophthalmy, incapacity to bear the light, and, lastly opacity and ulceration of the cornea.

The second species of ectropium, or that arising from a contraction of the integuments of the eyelids, or neighbouring parts, is not unfrequently a consequence of puckered scars, produced by a confluent small-pox, deep burns, or the excision of cancerous or encysted tumours, without saving a sufficient quantity of skin; or, lastly, the disorder is the effect of malignant carbuncles, or any kind of wound attended with much loss of substance. Each of these causes is quite enough to bring on such a contraction of the skin of the eyelids as to draw the parts towards the arches of the orbits, so as to remove them from the eyeball, and turn their edges outward. No sooner has this circumstance happened, than it is often followed by another one equally unpleasant, namely, a swelling of the internal membrane of the affected eyelids, which afterward has a great share in completing the eversion. The lining of the eyelids, though trivially everted, being continually exposed to the air, and irritation of extraneous substances, soon swells, and rises up like fungus. One side of this fungous-like tumour covers a part of the eyeball; the other pushes the eyelid so considerably outwards, that its edge is not unfrequently in contact with the margin of the orbit. The complaints induced by this second species of ectropium are the same as those brought on by the first; it being noticed, however, that in both cases, whenever the disease is very inveterate, the fungous swelling of the inside of the eyelids becomes hard, and as it were callous.

Although, in both species of ectropium, the lining of the eyelids seems equally swollen, yet the surgeon can easily distinguish to which of the two species the disease belongs. For, in the first, the skin of the eyelids, and adjoining parts, is not deformed with scars; and by pressing the everted eyelid with the point of the finger, the part would with ease cover the eye, were it not for the intervening fungous swelling. But in the second species of ectropium, besides the obvious cicatrix and contraction of the skin of the eyelids, or adjacent parts, when an effort is made to cover the eye with the everted eyelid, by pressing upon the latter part with the point of the finger, it does not give way so as completely to cover the globe, as it ought to do, only yielding for a certain extent: or it does not move in the least from its unnnatural position, by reason of the integuments of the eyelids having been so extensively destroyed, that their margin has become adherent to the arch of the orbit.

ECTRO'SIS. (Εκτρωσις; from εκτιτρωσκω, to miscarry.) A miscarriage.

Ectro'tica. (From εκτιτρωσκω, to miscarry.) *Ectyrotica; Ectylotica.* Medicines which cause abortion.

Ectylo'tica. See *Ectillotica.*

Ectyro'tica. See *Ectrotica.*

ECZE'MA. (From εκζεω, to boil out.) *Eczesma.* A hot, painful eruption, or pustule.

Ede'lphus. The prognosis of a disease from the nature of elements.

EDULCORA'NTIA. (From *edulco*, to make sweet.) Edulcorants. Medicines which purify the fluids, by depriving them of their acrimony.

EFFERVESCENCE. (*Effervescentia; from effervesco*, to grow hot.) 1. That agitation which is produced by mixing substances together, which cause the evolution of a gas.

2. A small degree of ebullition.

E'ffila. Freckles.

EFFLORESCENCE. (*Efflorescentia; from efflo- resco*, to blow as a flower.) 1. In *pathology*, it is used to express a morbid redness of the skin, and is generally synonymous with exanthema.

2. In *chemistry*, it means that effect which takes place when bodies spontaneously become converted into a dry powder. It is almost always occasioned by the loss of the water of crystallization in saline bodies.

3. In *botany*, it is applied to express the blooming of flowers, and the time of flowering.

EFFLU'VIUM. (From *effluo*, to spread abroad.) See *Contagion.*

Effractu'ra. (From *effringo*, to break down.) A fracture, in which the bone is much depressed by the blow.

EFFUSION. (*Effusio*; from *effundo*, to pour out.) In pathology it means the escape of any fluid out of the vessel, or viscus, naturally containing it, and its lodgment in another cavity, in the cellular substance, or in the substance of parts. Effusion also sometimes signifies the morbid secretion of fluids from the vessels; thus physicians frequently speak of coagulable lymph being effused on different surfaces.

EGERAN. A sub-species of pyramidal garnet of a reddish-brown colour.

Ege'ries. (From *egero*, to carry out.) *Egestio.* An excretion, or evacuation.

EGG. *Ovum.* The eggs of hens, and of birds in general, are composed of several distinct substances. 1. The shell or external coating, which is composed of carbonate of lime .72, phosphate of lime .2, gelatine .3. The remaining .23 are perhaps water. 2. A thin white and strong membrane, possessing the usual characters of animal substances. 3. The white of the egg, for which, see Albumen. 4. The yelk, which appears to consist of an oil of the nature of fat oils, united with a portion of serous matter, sufficient to render it diffusible in cold water, in the form of an emulsion, and concrecible by heat. Yelk of egg is used as the medium for rendering resins and oils diffusible in water. The eggs of poultry are chiefly used as food, the different parts are likewise employed in pharmacy and in medicine. The calcined shell is esteemed as an absorbent. The oil is softening, and is used externally to burns and chaps. The yelk renders oil miscible with water, and is triturated with the same view with resinous and other substances. Raw eggs have been much recommended as a popular remedy for jaundice.

Egrego'rsis. (From εγρηγορεω, to watch.) A watchfulness, or want of sleep.

Ei'lamis. (From ειλεω, to involve.) A membrane involving the brain.

Eile'ma. (From ειλεω, to form convolutions.) In Hippocrates, it signifies painful convolutions of the intestines from flatulence. Sometimes it signifies a covering. Vogel says, it is a fixed pain in the bowels, as if a nail was driven in.

Ei'leon. (From ειλεω, to wind.) Gorræus says it is a name of the intestinum ileum.

Ei'leos. (From ειλεω, to form convolutions.) The iliac passion.

Ei'sbole. (From εις, into, and βαλλω, to cast.) It signifies strictly an injection, but is used to express the access of a distemper, or of a particular paroxysm.

Ei'spnoe. (From εις, into, and πνεω, to breathe.) Inspiration of air.

EJACULA'NTIA. (From *ejaculo*, to cast out.) *Ejaculatoria.* The vessels which convey the seminal matter secreted in the testicles to the penis. These are the epididymis, and the vasa deferentia; the vesiculæ seminales are the receptacles of the semen.

EJE'CTIO. (From *ejicio*, to cast out.) Ejection, or the discharging of any thing from the body.

Elaca'lli. The Indian name of a cathartic shrub, the *Euphorbia nervifolia*, of Linnæus.

Elæa'gnon. (From ελαιον, oil, and αγνος, chaste.) See *Vitex agnus castus.*

Elæo'meli. (From ελαιον, oil, and μελι, honey.) A sweet purging oil, like honey.

ELÆOSA'CCHARUM. (From ελαιον, oil, and σακχαρον, sugar.) A mixture of an essential oil with sugar.

Elæoseli'num. See *Eleoselinum.*

ELAIN. The oily principle of solid fats, so named by its discoverer, Chevreuil, who dissolves tallow in very pure hot alkohol, separates the *stearin* by crystallization, and then procures the *elain* by evaporation of the spirit. Braconnot has adopted a simpler, and probably a more exact method. By squeezing tallow between the folds of porous paper, the *elain* soaks into it, while the *stearin* remains. The paper being then soaked in water, and pressed, yields up its oily impregnation. Elain has very much the appearance and properties of vegetable oil. It is liquid at the temperature of 60°. Its smell and colour are derived from the solid fats from which it is extracted.

["Mr. Pictet's method of procuring elaine, consists in pouring upon oil a concentrated solution of caustic soda, stirring the mixture, heating it slightly to separate the elaine from the soap of the stearine, pouring it on a cloth, and then separating by decantation the elaine from the excess of alkaline solution.—*Webster's Man. of Chemistry.* A.]

Elais guinee'nsis. A species of palm which grows spontaneously on the coast of Guinea, but is much cultivated in the West Indies. It is from this tree that the oil, called in the West Indies *Mackaw fat*, is obtained: and, according to some, the palm-oil, which is considered as an emollient and strengthener of all kinds of weakness of the limbs. It also is recommended against bruises, strains, cramps, pains, swellings, &c.

Elambica'tio. A method of analyzing mineral waters.

ELAOLITE. A subspecies of pyramidal felspar.

ELAPHOBO'SCUM. (From ελαφος, a stag, and βοσκω, to eat: so called, because deer eat them greedily.) See *Pastinaca.*

ELAPHOSCO'RODON. (From ελαφος, the stag, and σκοροδον, garlic.) Stag's or viper's garlic.

Ela'sma. (From ελαυνω, to drive.) A lamina of any kind. A clyster-pipe.

ELASTIC. (*Elasticus*; from ελαςης, *impulsor*, or of ελαυνειν, to impel, to push.) Springy; having the power of returning to the form from which it has been forced to deviate, or from which it is withheld; thus, a blade of steel is said to be elastic, because if it is bent to a certain degree, and then let go, it will of itself return to its former situation; the same will happen to the branch of a tree, a piece of Indian rubber, &c. See *Elasticity.*

Elastic fluid. See *Gas.*

Elastic gum. See *Caoutchouc.*

ELASTICITY. *Elasticitas.* A force in bodies, by which they endeavour to restore themselves to the posture from whence they were displaced by any external force. To solve this property, many have recourse to the universal law of nature, attraction, by which the parts of solid and firm bodies are caused to cohere together: whereby, when hard bodies are struck or bent, so that the component parts are a little moved from one another, but not quite disjoined or broken off, nor separated so far as to be out of the power of the attracting force, by which they cohere together; they certainly must, on the cessation of the external violence, spring back with a very great velocity to their former state. But in this circumstance, the atmospherical pressure will account for it as well; because such a violence, if it be not great enough to separate the constituent particles of a body far enough to let in any foreign matter, must occasion many vacuola between the separated surfaces, so that upon the removal of the external force, they will close again by the pressure of the aërial fluid upon the external parts, *i. e.* the body will come again into its natural posture. The included air, likewise, in most bodies, gives that power of resilition upon their percussion.

If two bodies perfectly *elastic* strike, one against another, there will be or remain in each the same relative velocity as before, *i. e.* they will recede with the same velocity as they met together. For the compressive force, or the magnitude of the stroke in any given bodies, arises from the relative velocity of those bodies, and is proportional to it, and bodies perfectly *elastic* will restore themselves completely to the figure they had before the shock; or, in other words, the restitutive force is equal to the compressive, and therefore must be equal to the force with which they came together, and consequently they must, by elasticity, recede again from each other with the same velocity. Hence, taking equal times before and after the shock, the distances between the bodies will be equal: and therefore the distances of them from the common centre of gravity will, in the same times, be equal. And hence the laws of percussion of bodies perfectly elastic are easily deduced.

ELATE'RIUM. (From ελαυνω, to stimulate or agitate: so named from its great purgative qualities.) See *Momordica elaterium.*

["The *Momordica elaterium* is a perennial plant, growing spontaneously in the south of Europe. The fruit, which is botanically allied to the cucumber and melon, has the curious property of separating itself, when ripe, from its stalk, and ejecting its seeds with great force through an opening in the base, where the stalk was attached. The medicinal property resides chiefly in the juice at the centre of the fruit, and about the seeds. The drug called *Elaterium* in our Pharmacopœia, and which the London College have, with some latitude of application, called an extract, is the sediment which subsides from the juice of the fruit after it has been drawn out. The quantity of genuine elaterium contained in a single fruit is extremely small, as it appears that only six grains were obtained by Dr. Clutterbuck from forty of the cucumbers. The plant might be raised in this country.

"Elaterium is sold in small, thin cakes, or fragments, of a greenish colour, and a bitter and somewhat acrid taste. It is liable to vary in strength, according to the mode of its preparation. If the juice has been extracted with much pressure, the sediment contains portions of the fruit which are comparatively inactive, and which, of course, tend to lessen its activity. In selecting *elaterium*, those specimens which have a very dark colour, are compact and heavy, and break with a shining resinous fracture, are to be rejected as bad.

"This drug is one of the most violent cathartics. It was employed by the ancients as a hydragogue in dropsy, in a form not dissimilar to that used at the present day. It was also used by the Arabians, and in more modern times by Boerhaave, Sydenham, and Lister. Quite recently it has been highly recommended in dropsy by some distinguished English physicians, and their practice has been successfully imitated in this country; although the great uncertainty of its operation has repeatedly caused it to be abandoned. It has the peculiar property of not only purging, but at the same time exciting a febrile action, which Lister describes as attended with a throbbing that is felt to the fingers' ends. Orfila found that a large dose, given to a dog, brought on inflammation of the stomach, but when injected in two cases into the cellular texture of the thigh, the rectum was the only part of the canal which became inflamed. Hence he concludes, that the medicine has some peculiar action on that organ.

"The uncertainty arising from the different preparations of this medicine may be inferred from the circumstance, that Fallopius gave it in doses of a drachm, while Dr. Clutterbuck found one-eighth of a grain to purge violently. The strength of any particular parcel ought always to be tested by small doses, before it is ventured on in any considerable quantity. Of the article imported into this country, I have given from one to two grains in a pill three times a day, without any excessive operation resulting from it."—*Big. Mat Med.* A.]

ELATHE'RIA. A name for the cascarilla bark.

ELATIN. The active principle of elaterium. See *Momordica elaterium.*

ELATI'NE. (From ελα7των, smaller, being the smaller species.) See *Antirrhinum elatine.*

ELATIO. Elevated, exalted. This term is applied in Good's Nosology, to a species of the genus *Alusio*, to designate mental extravagance.

ELATI'TES. Bloodstone.

ELCO'SIS. (From ελκος, an ulcer.) A disease attended with fœtid, carious, and chronic ulcers. The term is seldom used.

ELDER. See *Sambucus.*

Elder, dwarf. See *Sambucus Ebulus.*

ELECAMPANE. See *Inula helenium.*

ELECTIVE. That which is done, or passes, by election.

Elective affinity, double. See *Affinity double.*

Elective attraction. See *Affinity.*

Elective attraction, double. See *Affinity double*

ELECTRICITY. (*Electricitas;* from *electrum*, ηλεκτρον, from ηλεκ7ωρ, the sun, because of its bright shining colour; or from ελκω, to draw, because of its magnetic power.) A property which certain bodies possess when rubbed, heated, or otherwise excited, whereby they attract remote bodies, and frequently emit sparks or streams of light. The ancients first observed this property in amber, which they called *Electrum*, and hence arose the word electricity.

"If a piece of sealing-wax and of dry warm flannel be rubbed against each other, they both become capable of attracting and repelling light bodies. A dry and warm sheet of writing-paper, rubbed with India rubber, or a tube of glass rubbed upon silk, exhibit the same phenomena. In these cases, the bodies are said to be *electrically excited;* and when in a dark room, they always appear luminous. If two pith-balls be electrified by touching them with the sealing-wax, or with the flannel, they repel each other; but if one pith-ball be electrified by the wax, and the other by the flannel, they attract each other. The same applies to the glass and silk: it shows a difference in the electricities of the different bodies, and the experiment leads to the conclusion, that *bodies similarly electrified repel each other; but that when dissimilarly electrified, they attract each other.*

The term *electrical repulsion* is here used merely to denote the appearance of the phenomenon, the separation being probably referrible to the new attractive power which they acquire, when electrified, for the air and other surrounding bodies.

If one ball be electrified by sealing-wax rubbed by flannel, and another by silk rubbed with glass, those balls will repel each other; which proves that the electricity of the silk is the same as that of the sealing-wax. But if one ball be electrified by the sealing-wax and the other by the glass, they then attract each other, showing that they are oppositely electrified.

These experiments are most conveniently performed with a large downy feather, suspended by a silken thread. If an excited glass tube be brought near it, it will receive and retain its electricity; it will be first attracted and then repelled; and upon re-exciting the tube, and again approaching it, it will not again be attracted, but retain its state of repulsion; but upon approaching it with excited sealing-wax, it will instantly be attracted, and remain in contact with the wax till it has acquired its electricity, when it will be repelled, and in that state of repulsion it will be attracted by the glass. In these experiments, care must be taken that the feather remains freely suspended in the air, and touches nothing capable of carrying off its electricity.

The terms *vitreous* and *resinous* electricity were applied to these two phenomena; but Franklin, observing that the same electricity was not inherent in the same body, but that glass sometimes exhibited the same phenomena as wax, and *vice versâ*, adopted another term, and instead of regarding the phenomena as dependent upon two electric fluids, referred them to the presence of one fluid, in excess in some cases, and in deficiency in others. To represent these states, he used the terms *plus* and *minus*, *positive* and *negative.* When glass is rubbed with silk, a portion of electricity leaves the silk, and enters the glass; it becomes po *sitive*, therefore, and the silk *negative:* but when sealing-wax is rubbed with flannel, the wax loses, and the flannel gains; the former, therefore, is negative, and the latter positive. All bodies in nature are thus regarded as containing the electric fluid, and when its equilibrium is disturbed, they exhibit the phenomena just described. The substances enumerated in the following table become positively electrified when rubbed with those which follow them in the list; but with those which precede them they become negatively electrical.—*Biot*, *Traité de Physique*, tom ii. p. 220.

Cat's-skin.	Paper.
Polished glass.	Silk.
Woolen cloth.	Gum lac.
Feathers.	Rough glass.

Very delicate pith-balls, or strips of gold leaf, are usually employed in ascertaining the presence of electricity; and by the way in which their divergence is effected by glass or sealing-wax, the kind or state of electricity is judged of. When properly suspended or mounted for delicate experiments, they form an *electrometer* or *electroscope.* For this purpose, the slips of gold leaf are suspended by a brass cap and wire in a glass cylinder: they hang in contact when unelectrified, but when electrified they diverge.

When this instrument, as usually constructed, becomes in a small degree damp, its delicacy is much diminished, and it is rendered nearly useless.

The kind of electricity by which the gold leaves are diverged may be judged of by approaching the cap of the instrument with a stick of excited sealing-wax; if it be *negative*, the divergence will increase; if *positive*, the leaves will collapse, upon the principle of the mutual annihilation of the opposite electricities, or that bodies similarly electrified repel each other, but that when dissimilarly electrified, they become mutually attractive.

Some bodies suffer electricity to pass through their substance, and are called *conductors.* Others only receive it upon the spot touched, and are called *non-conductors.* The former do not, in general, become electrified by friction, and are called *non-electrics:* the latter, on the contrary, are *electrics*, or acquire electricity by friction. They are also called *insulators.* The metals are all conductors; dry air, glass, sulphur, and resins, are non-conductors. Water, damp wood, spirit of wine, damp air, and some oils, are imperfect conductors.

Rarified air admits of the passage of electricity; so does the Jarricellian vacuum; hence, if an electrified body be placed under the receiver of the air-pump, it loses its electricity during exhaustion. So that the air, independent of its non-conducting power, appears to influence the retentive properties of bodies, in respect to electricity, by its pressure.

There appears to be no constant relation between the state of bodies and their conducting powers: among solids, metals are conductors; but gums and resins are non-conductors: among liquids, strong alkaline acid, and saline solutions, are good conductors; pure water is an imperfect conductor, and oils are non-conductors; solid wax is almost a non-conductor; but when melted a good one.

Conducting powers belong to bodies in the most opposite states; thus, the flame of alkohol and ice are equally good conductors. Glass is a non-conductor when cold, but conducts when red-hot: the diamond is a non-conductor; but pure and well-burned charcoal is among the best conductors.

There are many mineral substances which show signs of electricity when heated, as the tourmalin, topaz, diamond, boracite, &c., and in these bodies the different surfaces exhibit different electrical states.

Whenever one part of a body, or system of bodies, is positive, another part is invariably negative; and these opposite electrical states are always such as exactly to neutralize each other. Thus, in the common electrical machine, one conductor receives the electricity of the glass-cylinder, and the other that of the silk-rubber, and the former conductor is positive, and the latter negative; but, if they be connected, all electrical phenomena cease.

Electricians generally employ the term *quantity* to indicate the absolute quantity of electric power in any body, and the term *intensity*, to signify its power of passing through a certain stratum of air, or other ill-conducting medium.

If we suppose a charged Leyden phial to furnish a spark, when discharged, of one inch in length, we should find that another uncharged Leyden phial, the inner and outer coating of which were communicated with those of the former, would, upon the same quantity of electricity being thrown in, reduce the length of the spark to half an inch; here the *quantity* of electricity remaining the same, its *intensity* is diminished by one-half, by its distribution over the larger surface.

It is obvious that the extension of surface alluded to in the last paragraph will be attended with a greater superficial exposure to the unelectrified air; and hence it might be expected that a similar diminution of intensity would result from the vicinity of the electrified surface to the ground, or to any other body of sufficient magnitude in its ordinary state. That this is the case, may be shown by diverging the leaves of the gold leaf electrometer, and in that state approaching the instrument with an uninsulated plate, which, when within half an inch of the electrometer plate, will cause the leaves to collapse; but, on removing the uninsulated plate, they will again diverge, in consequence of the electricity regaining its former intensity. The same fact is shown by the condensing electrometer.

The power of the Leyden jar is proportioned to its surface; but a very large jar is inconvenient and difficult to procure; the same end is attained by arranging several jars, so that by a communication existing between all their interior coatings, their exterior being also united, they may be charged and discharged as one jar. Such a combination is called an electrical *battery*, and is useful for exhibiting the effect of accumulated electricity.

The discharge of the battery is attended by a considerable report, and if it be passed through small animals, it instantly kills them; if through fine metallic wires, they are ignited, melted, and burned; and gunpowder, cotton sprinkled with powdered resin, and a variety of other combustibles, may be inflamed by the same means.

There are many other sources of electricity than those just noticed. When glass is rubbed by mercury, it becomes electrified; and this is the cause of the luminous appearance observed when a barometer is agitated in a dark room, in which case flashes of light are seen to traverse the empty part of the tube. Even the friction of air upon glass is attended by electrical excitation: for Wilson found, that by blowing upon a dry plate of glass with a pair of bellows, it acquired a positive electricity. Whenever bodies change their forms, their electrical states are also altered. Thus, the conversion of water into vapour, and the congelation of melted resins and sulphur are processes in which electricity is also rendered sensible.

When an insulated plate of zinc is brought into contact with one of copper or silver, it is found, after removal, to be positively electrical, and the silver or copper is left in the opposite state.

The most oxidisable metal is always positive, in relation to the least oxidisable metal, which is negative, and the more opposite the metals in these respects the greater the electrical excitation; and if the metals be placed in the following order, each will become positive by the contact of that which precedes it, and negative by the contact of that which follows it; and the greatest effect will result from the contact of the most distant metals.

Platinum.	Mercury.	Tin.
Gold.	Copper.	Lead.
Silver.	Iron.	Zinc.

If the nerve of a recently killed frog be attached to a silver probe, and a piece of zinc be brought into the contact of the muscular parts of the animal, violent convulsions are produced every time the metals thus connected are made to touch each other. Exactly the same effect is produced by an electric spark, or the discharge of a very small Leyden-phial.

If a piece of zinc be placed upon the tongue, and a piece of silver under it, a peculiar sensation will be perceived every time the two metals are made to touch.

In these cases the chemical properties of the metals are observed to be effected. If a silver and zinc wire be put into a wine glass full of dilute sulphuric acid, the zinc wire will only evolve gas; but upon bringing the two wires in contact with each other, the silver will also copiously produce air bubbles.

If a number of alterations be made of copper or sil

ver leaf, zinc leaf, and thin paper, the electricity excited by the contact of the metals will be rendered evident to the common electrometer.

If the same arrangement be made with the paper moistened with brine, or a weak acid, it will be found, on bringing a wire communicating with the last copper plate into contact with the first zinc plate, that a spark is perceptible, and also a slight shock, provided the number of alternations be sufficiently numerous. This is the voltaic apparatus.

Several modes of constructing this apparatus have been adopted with a view to render it more convenient or active. Sometimes double plates of copper and zinc soldered together, are cemented into wooden troughs in regular order, the intervening cells being filled with water, or saline, or acid solutions.

Another form consists in arranging a row of glasses, containing dilute sulphuric acid, in each of which is placed a wire, or plate of silver, or copper, and one of zinc, not touching each other, but so connected by metallic wires, that the zinc of the first cup may communicate with the copper of the second; the zinc of the second with the copper of the third; and so on throughout the series.

When the poles of the Voltaic apparatus are connected by a steel wire, it requires magnetic properties, and if by a platinum, or other metallic wire, that wire exhibits numerous magnetic poles, which attract and repel the common magnetic needle. This very curious fact was first observed by Professor Oersted, of Copenhagen.

On immersing the wires from the extremes of this apparatus into water, it is found that the fluid suffers decomposition, and that oxygen gas is liberated at the positive wire or pole, and hydrogen gas at the negative pole.

All other substances are decomposed with similar phenomena, the inflammable element being disengaged at the negatively electrical surface; hence it would appear, upon the principle of similarly electrified bodies repelling each other, and dissimilarly electrified bodies attracting each other, that the inherent or natural electrical state of the inflammable substances is positive, for they are attracted by the negative or oppositely electrified pole; while the bodies, called supporters of combustion, or acidifying principles, are attracted by the positive pole, and, therefore, may be considered as possessed of the negative power.

When bodies are thus under the influence of electrical decomposition, their usual chemical energies are suspended, and some very curious phenomena are observed.

The most difficult decomposable compounds may be thus resolved into their component parts by the electrical agency; by a weak power the proximate elements are separated, and by a stronger power these are resolved into their ultimate constituents.

All bodies which exert powerful chemical agencies upon each other when freedom of motion is given to their particles, render each other oppositely electrical when acting as masses. Hence Sir H. Davy, the great and successful investigator of this branch of chemical philosophy, has supposed that electrical and chemical phenomena, though in themselves quite distinct, may be dependent on one and the same power, acting in the former case upon masses of matter, in the other upon its particles.

The power of the Voltaic apparatus to communicate divergence to the electrometer, is most observed when it is well insulated, and filled with pure water; but its power of producing ignition and of giving shocks, and of producing the other effects observed when its poles are connected; are much augmented by the interposition of dilute acids, which act chemically upon one of the plates: here the insulation is interfered with by the production of vapour, but the quantity of electricity is much increased, a circumstance which may, perhaps, be referred to the increase of the positive energy of the most oxidisable metal by the contact of the acid. In experiments made with the great battery of the Royal Institution, it has been found that 120 plates rendered active by a mixture of one part of nitric acid, and three of water, produces effects equal to 480 plates rendered active by one part of nitric acid, and fifteen of water.

In the Voltaic pile, the *intensity* of the electricity increases with the number of alternations, but the *quantity* is increased by extending the surface of the plates. Thus, if a battery, composed of thirty pairs of plates, two inches square, be compared with another battery of thirty pairs of twelve inches square charged in the same way, no difference will be perceived in their effects upon bad or imperfect conductors; their powers of decomposing water, and of giving shocks, will be similar; but upon good conductors the effects of the large plates will be considerably greater than those of the small: they will ignite and fuse large quantities of platinum wire, and produce a very brilliant spark between charcoal points. The following experiment well illustrates the different effects of quantity and intensity in the Voltaic apparatus.

Immerse the platinum wires connected with the extremity of a charged battery composed of twelve-inch plates into water, and it will be found that the evolution of gas is nearly the same as that occasioned by a similar number of two-inch plates. Apply the moistened fingers to the wires, and the shock will be the same as if there were no connexion by the water. While the circuit exists through the human body and the water, let a wire attached to a thin slip of charcoal be made to connect the poles of the battery, and the charcoal will become vividly ignited. The water and the animal substance discharge the electricity of a surface, probably, not superior to their own surface of contact with the metals; the wires discharge all the residual electricity of the plates; and if a similar experiment be made on plates of an inch square, there will scarcely be any sensation when the hands are made to connect the ends of the battery, a circuit being previously made through water; and no spark, when charcoal is made the medium of connexion, imperfect conductors having been previously applied. These relative effects of quantity and intensity were admirably illustrated by the experiments instituted by Children, who constructed a battery, the plates of which were two feet eight inches wide, and six feet high. They were fastened to a beam, suspended by counterpoises, from the ceiling of his laboratory, so as to be easily immersed into, or withdrawn from the cells of acid. The effects upon metallic wires, and perfect conductors, were extremely intense; but upon imperfect conductors, such as the human body, and water, they were feeble.—*Phil. Trans.* 1815, p. 363.

When the extremes of a battery composed of large plates are united by wires of different metals, it is found that some are more easily ignited than others, a circumstance which has been referred to their conducting powers: thus platinum is more easily ignited than silver, and silver than zinc. If the ignition be supposed to result from the resistance to the passage of electricity, we should say that the zinc conducted better than silver, and the silver than platinum.

An important improvement has been suggested in the construction of the Voltaic apparatus, by Dr. Wollaston, (Annals of Philosophy, Sept. 1815,) by which great increase of *quantity* is obtained, without inconvenient augmentation of the size of the plates; it consists in extending the copper plate, so as to oppose it to every surface of the zinc.

With the single pair of plates, of very small dimensions, constructed upon this principle, Dr. Wollaston succeeded in fusing and igniting a fine platinum wire. This is the most economical and useful form of the Voltaic apparatus; certainly, at least, it is so for all those researches in which there is an occasional demand for quantity as well as intensity of electricity.

The theory of the Voltaic pile is involved in many difficulties. The original source of electricity appears to depend upon the contact of the metals, for we know that a plate of silver and a plate of zinc, or of any other difficultly and easily oxidisable metals, become negative and positive on contact. The accumulation must be referred to *induction*, which takes place in the electrical column, through the very thin stratum of air, or paper, and through water, when that fluid is interposed between the plates. Accordingly, we observe, that the apparatus is in the condition of the series of conductors, with interposed air, and of the Leyden phials. When the electric column is insulated, the extremities exhibit feeble negative and positive powers, but if either extremity be connected with the ground, the electricity of its poles or extremities is greatly increased, as may be shown by the increased divergence of the leaves of the electrometer which then ensues.

As general changes in the form and constitution of matter are connected with its electrical states, it is obvious that electricity must be continually active in nature. Its effects are exhibited on a magnificent scale in the thunder-storm, which results from the accumulation of electricity in the clouds, as was first experimentally demonstrated by Dr. Franklin, who also first showed the advantage of pointed conductors as safeguards to buildings. In these cases, the conducting rod, or rods, should be of copper, or iron, and from half to three-fourths of an inch diameter. Its upper end should be elevated three or four feet above the highest part of the building, and all the metallic parts of the roof should be connected with the rod, which should be perfectly continuous throughout, and passing down the side of the building, penetrate several feet below its foundation, so as always to be immersed in a moist stratum of soil, or if possible, into water. The leaden water pipes attached to houses, often might be made to answer the purpose of conductors, especially when thick enough to resist fusion.

During a thunder-storm the safest situation is in the middle of a room, at a distance from the chimney, and standing upon a woollen rug, which is a nonconductor. Blankets and feathers being nonconductors, bed is a place of comparative safety, provided the bell-wires are not too near, which are almost always melted in houses struck by lightning. When out of doors, it is dangerous to take shelter under trees: the safest situation is within some yards of them, and upon the dryest spot that can be selected.

The discharge of electricity in a thunder-storm is sometimes only from cloud to cloud; sometimes from the earth to the clouds; and sometimes from the clouds to the earth; as one or the other may be positive or negative. When aqueous vapour is condensed, the clouds formed are usually more or less electrical; and the earth below them being brought into an opposite state, by induction, a discharge takes place when the clouds approach within a certain distance, constituting lightning; and the indulation of the air, produced by the discharge, is the cause of thunder, which is more or less intense, and of longer or shorter duration, according to the quantity of air acted upon, and the distance of the place, where the report is heard from the point of the discharge. It may not be uninteresting to give a further illustration of this idea. Electrical effects take place in no sensible time. It has been found that a discharge through a circuit of four miles is instantaneous; but sound moves at the rate of about twelve miles a minute. Now, suppose the lightning to pass through a space of some miles, the explosion will be first heard from the point of the air agitated nearest to the spectator: it will gradually come from the more distant parts of the course of electricity, and last of all, will be heard from the remote extremity, and the different degrees of the agitation of the air, and likewise the difference of the distance, will account for the different intensities of the sound, and its apparent reverberations and changes.

In a violent thunder-storm, when the sound instantly succeeds the flash, the persons who witness the circumstance are in some danger; when the interval is a quarter of a minute, they are secure.

A variety of electrical apparatus has been devised to illustrate the operation of conductors for lightning, and the advantage of points over balls; the simplest consists of a model of a house having a conductor with a break in it, in which some inflammable matter should be placed; the lower end of the conductor should be communicated with the exterior of a charged Leyden phial, the knob of which, brought over its upper end, will then represent a thunder cloud. If the conductor be pointed, it will be slowly discharged, if surrounded by a ball, there will be an explosion, and the combustibles probably inflamed.

The coruscations of the *Aurora borealis* are also probably electrical, and much resemble flashes of electric light traversing rarefied air. The water-spout may be referred to the same source, and is probably the result of the operation of a weakly electrical cloud, at an inconsiderable elevation above the sea, brought into an opposite electrical state: and the attraction of the lower part of the cloud, for the surface of the water, may be the immediate cause of this extraordinary phenomenon.

In the *gymnotus*, or *electric* eel, and in the *torpedo*, or *electric ray*, are arrangements given to those remarkable animals for the purpose of defence, which certain forms of the Voltaic apparatus must resemble; for they consist of many alternations of different substances. These electrical organs are much more abundantly supplied with nerves than any other part of the animal, and the too frequent use of them is succeeded by debility and death.

That arrangements of different organic substances are capable of producing electrical effects, has been shown by various experimentalists. If the hind-legs of a frog be placed upon a glass plate, and the crural nerve dissected out of one made to communicate with another, it will be found on making occasional contacts with the remaining crural nerve, that the limbs of the animal will be agitated at each contact. These circumstances have induced some physiologists to suppose, that electricity may be concerned in some of the most recondite phenomena of vitality, and Dr. Wollaston, Sir E. Home, and myself, have made some experiments tending to confer probability on this idea.

We have as yet no plausible hypothesis concerning the *cause* of electrical phenomena, though the subject has engaged the attention of the most eminent philosophers of Europe. They have been, by some, referred to the presence of a peculiar fluid existing in all matter, and exhibiting itself by the appearances which have been described wherever its equilibrium is disturbed, presenting negative and positive electricity, when deficient, and when redundant. Others have plausibly argued for the presence of two fluids, distinct from each other. Others have considered the effects as referrible to peculiar exertions of the attractive powers of matter, and have regarded the existence of any distinct fluid, or form of matter, to be as unnecessary to the explanation of the phenomena, as it is in the question concerning the cause of gravitation.

When the flame of a candle is placed between a positive and negative surface, it is urged towards the latter; a circumstance which has been explained upon the supposition of a current of electrical matter passing from the positive to the negative pole; indeed, it has been considered as demonstrating the existence of such a current of matter. But if the flame of phosphorus be substituted for that of a candle, it takes an opposite direction; and instead of being attracted towards the negative, it bends to the positive surface. It has been shown that inflammable bodies are always attracted by negative surfaces; and acid bodies, and those in which the supporters of combustion prevail, are attracted by positive surfaces. Hence the flame of the candle throwing off carbon, is directed to the negative pole, while that of phosphorus forming acid matter goes to the positive, consistently with the ordinary laws of electro-chemical attraction.

There are other experiments opposed to the idea that electricity is a material substance. If we discharge a Leyden phial through a quire of paper, the perforation is equally burred upon both sides, and not upon the negative side only, as would have been the case if any material body had gone through in that direction. The power seems to have come from the centre of the paper, as if one half of the quire had been attracted by the positive, and the other by the negative surface.

When a pointed metallic wire is presented towards the conductor of the electrical machine, in a darkened room, a star of light is observed when the conductor is positive, but a brush of light when it is negative; a circumstance which has been referred to the reception of the electric fluid in the one case, and its escape in the other. In the Voltaic discharge the same appearances are evident upon the charcoal point; rays appearing to diverge from the negative conductor, while from the positive a spot of bright light is perceptible. But these affections of light can scarcely be considered as indicating the omission, or reception of any specific form of matter.

The efficacy of electricity in the cure of several diseases has been supported by many very respectable authorities, especially in paralytic diseases. It considerably augments the circulation of the blood, and excites the action of the absorbents."—*Brande's Chemistry.*

ELECTRO-MAGNETISM. The name given to a class of very interesting phenomena, first observed by Oersted, of Copenhagen, in the winter of 1819–20, and which have since received great illustration from the labours of Ampère, Arago, Sir H. Davy, Wollaston, Faraday, de la Rive, and several other philosophers. The following is a short outline of the fundamental facts.

Let the opposite poles of a voltaic battery be connected by a metallic wire, which may be left of such length as to suffer its being bent or turned in various directions. This is the conjunctive wire of Oersted. Let us suppose that the rectilinear portion of this wire is extended horizontally in the line of the magnetic meridian. If a freely suspended compass-needle be now introduced, with its centre *under* the conjunctive wire, the needle will instantly deviate from the magnetic meridian; and it will decline towards the *west*, under that part of the conjunctive wire which is nearest the negative electric pole, or the copper end of the voltaic apparatus. The amount of this declination depends on the strength of the electricity, and the sensibility of the needle. Its *maximum* is 90°.

We may change the direction of the conjunctive wire, out of the magnetic meridian, towards the east or the west, provided it remains above the needle, and parallel to its plane, without any change in the above result, except that of its amount. Wires of platinum, gold, silver, brass, and iron, may be equally employed; nor does the effect cease, though the electric circuit be partially formed by water. The effect of the conjunctive wire takes place across plates of glass, metal, wood, water, resin, pottery, and stone.

If the conjunctive wire be disposed horizontally *beneath* the needle, the effects are of the same nature as those which occur when it is *above* it; but they operate in an inverse direction; that is to say, the pole of the needle under which is placed the portion of the conjunctive wire which receives the negative electricity of the apparatus, declines in that case towards the *east*.

To remember these results more readily, we may employ the following proposition: *The pole,* ABOVE *which the negative electricity enters, declines towards the* WEST; *but if it enters* BENEATH *it, the needle declines towards the* EAST.

If the conjunctive wire (always supposed horizontal) is slowly turned about, so as to form a gradually increasing angle with the magnetic meridian, the declination of the needle increases, if the movement of the wire be towards the line of position of the disturbed needle; it diminishes, on the contrary, if it recede from its position.

When the conjunctive wire is stretched alongside of the needle in the same horizontal plane, it occasions no declination either to the east or west; but it causes it merely to incline in a vertical line, so that the pole adjoining the negative influence of the pile on the wire dips when the wire is on its west side, and rises when it is on the east.

If we stretch the conjunctive wire, either above or beneath the needle, in a plane perpendicular to the magnetic meridian, it remains at rest, unless the wire be very near the pole of the needle; for, in this case, it rises when the entrance takes place by the west part of the wire, and sinks when it takes place by the east part.

When we dispose the conjunctive wire in a vertical line opposite the pole of the needle, and make the upper extremity of the wire receive the electricity of the negative end of the battery, the pole of the needle moves towards the *east;* but if we place the wire opposite a point between the pole and the middle of the needle, it moves to the *west.* The phenomena are presented in an inverse order, when the upper extremity of the conjunctive wire receives the electricity of the positive side of the apparatus.

It appears from the preceding facts, says Oersted, that the electric conflict (action) is not enclosed within the conducting wire, but that it has a pretty extensive sphere of activity round it. We may also conclude from the observations, that this conflict acts by revolution; for without this supposition we could not comprehend how the same portion of the conjunctive wire, which, placed *beneath* the magnetic pole, carries the needle towards the east, when it is placed *above* this pole, should carry it towards the west. But such is the nature of the circular action, that the movements which it produces take place in directions precisely contrary to the two extremities of the same diameter. It appears also, that the circular movement, combined with a progressive movement in the direction of the length of the conjunctive wire, ought to form a kind of action, which operates *spirally* around this wire as an axis. For further information, Faraday's able and original paper, in the Journal of Science, may be consulted; as also Ampère's several ingenious memoirs in the Annales de Chimie et de Physique.

ELECTRO'DES. (From ηλεκτρον, amber.) An epithet for intestinal fæces which shine like amber.

ELECTROMETER. (From ηλεκτρον, and μετρον, a measure.) See *Electricity.*

ELECTROSCOPE. (From ελεκτρον, and σκοπεω to see.) See *Electricity.*

ELE'CTRUM. Ελεκτρον. Amber.

ELECTRUM MINERALE. The tincture of metals. It is made of tin and copper, to which some add gold, and double its quantity of martial regulus of antimony melted together; from these there results a metallic mass, to which some chemists have given the name of *electrum minerale.* This mass is powdered and detonated with nitre and charcoal to a kind of scoria; it is powdered again while hot, and then digested in spirit of wine, whence a tincture is obtained of a fine red colour.

ELECTUA'RIUM. An electuary. The London Pharmacopœia refers those articles which were formerly called electuaries to confections. See *Confectio.*

ELECTUARIUM ANTIMONII. ℞. Electuarii sennæ, ℥j; guaiaci gummi, hydrargyri cum sulphure, antimonii ppti. sing. ℥ss; syrupi simplicis q. s. misce. Of this electuary, from a drachm to about two drachms is given twice a day, in those cutaneous diseases which go under the general name of scorbutic. It is usually accompanied with the decoctions of elm bark or sarsaparilla.

ELECTUARIUM CASSIÆ. See *Confectio cassiæ.*

ELECTUARIUM CATECHU. *Confectio Japonica.* Electuary of catechu, commonly called Japonic confection. Take of mimosa catechu, four ounces; kino, three ounces; cinnamon, nutmeg, each one ounce; opium diffused in a sufficient quantity of Spanish white wine one drachm and a half; syrup of red roses boiled to the consistence of honey, two pounds and a quarter. Reduce the solids to powder, and, having mixed them with the opium and syrup, make them into an electuary. A very useful astringent, and perhaps the most efficacious way of giving the catechu to advantage. Ten scruples of this electuary contain one grain of opium.

ELECTUARIUM CINCHONÆ CUM NATRO. ℞. natri ppti. ʒij.; pulveris cinchonæ unc.: mucilaginis gummi arabici q. s. misce. In this composition, mucilage is preferred to syrup on account of its covering the taste of the bark much more advantageously. It should, for this purpose, however, be made thin, otherwise it will increase the bulk of the electuary too much.

This remedy will be found an excellent substitute for the burnt sponge, the powers of which, as a remedy in scrofula, are known solely to depend on the proportion of natron contained in it. The dose is two drachms, twice or thrice a day.

ELECTUARIUM OPIATUM. See *Confectio opii.*

ELELI'SPHACOS. (From ελελιζω, to distort, and σφακος, sage: so named from the spiral coiling of its leaves and branches.) A species of sage.

ELEMENT. Radical. First principles. A substance which can no further be divided or decomposed by chemical analysis.

E'LEMI. (It is said this is the Ethiopian name.) Gum elemi. The parent plant of this resin is supposed to be an amyris. See *Amyris elemifera.*

ELEN'GI. A tree of Malabar, which is said to possess cordial and carminative properties.

ELEOCHRY'SUM. (From ηλιος, the sun, and χρυσος, gold: so called from its gold-like, or shining yellow appearance.) Goldilocks. See *Gnaphalium stœchas.*

ELEOSELI'NUM (From ελος, a lake, and σελινον, parsley.) See *Apium.*

ELEPHA'NTIA. (From ελεφας, an elephant: so called from the great enlargement of the body in this disorder.) See *Elephantiasis.*

ELEPHANTIA ARABUM. In Dr. Cullen's Nosology it is synonymous with elephantiasis. The term is, however, occasionally confined to this disease when it affects the feet.

ELEPHANTI'ASIS. (From ελεφας, an elephant: so named from the legs of people affected with this disorder growing scaly, rough, and wonderfully large, at an advanced period, like the legs of an elephant.) *Elephas; Elephantia; Lazari morbus vel malum; Phœniceus morbus.* A disease that attacks the whole body, but mostly affects the feet, which appear somewhat like those of the elephant. It is known by the skin being thick, rough, wrinkly, unctuous, and void of hair, and mostly without the sense of feeling. It is said to be contagious. Cullen makes it a genus of disease in the class *Cachexiæ*, and order *Impetigines*.

Elephantiasis has generally been supposed to arise in consequence of some slight attack of fever, on the cessation of which the morbid matter falls on the leg, and occasions a distention and tumefaction of the limb, which is afterward overspread with uneven lumps, and deep fissures. By some authors it has been considered as a species of leprosy; but it often subsists for many years without being accompanied with any of the symptoms which characterize that disease.

It sometimes comes on gradually, without much previous indisposition; but more generally, the person is seized with a coldness and shivering, pains in the head, back, and loins, and some degree of nausea. A slight fever then ensues, and a severe pain is felt in one of the inguinal glands, which, after a short time, becomes hard, swelled, and inflamed. No suppuration, however, ensues; but a red streak may be observed running down the thigh from the swelled gland to the leg. As the inflammation increases in all the parts, the fever gradually abates; and, perhaps, after two or three days' continuance, goes off. It, however, returns again at uncertain periods, leaving the leg greatly swelled with varicose turgid veins, the skin rough and rugged, and a thickened membrana cellulosa. Scales appear also on the surface, which do not fall off, but are enlarged by the increasing thickness of the membranes; uneven lumps, with deep fissures, are formed, and the leg and foot become at last of an enormous size.

A person may labour under this disease many years without finding much alteration in the general health, except during the continuance of the attacks; and perhaps the chief inconvenience he will experience is the enormous bulky leg which he drags about with him. The incumbrance has, indeed, induced many who have laboured under this disease to submit to an amputation; but the operation seldom proves a radical cure, as the other leg frequently becomes affected.

Hilary observes, that he never saw both legs swelled at the same time. Instances where they have alike acquired a frightful and prodigious size, have, however, frequently fallen under the observation of other physicians.

ELEPHANTI'NUM EMPLASTRUM. A plaster described by Oribasius. Celsus describes one of the same name, but very different in qualities.

E'LEPHAS. (Ελεφας, the elephant.)

1. The name of an animal.

2. The name of a disease of the skin. See *Elephantiasis*.

3. Aqua fortis was so called in some old chemical books.

ELE'TTARI PRIMUM. The true amomum. See *Elettaria cardamomum*.

ELETTA'RIA. (From *elettari*.) The name of a new genus of plants formed by Dr. Maton, to which the less cardamom is referred. Class, *Monandria*; Order, *Monogynia*.

ELETTARIA CARDAMOMUM. *Cardamomum minus.* Less or officinal cardamom. *Amomum repens;* or *le cardamome de la côte de Malabar*, of Sonnerat. *Elettaria cardamomum*, of Maton, in Act. Soc. Lin. The seeds of this plant are imported in their capsules or husks, by which they are preserved, for they soon lose a part of their flavour when freed from this covering. On being chewed, they impart a glowing aromatic warmth, and grateful pungency; they are supposed gently to stimulate the stomach, and prove cordial, carminative, and antispasmodic, but without that irritation and heat which many of the other spicy aromatics are apt to produce. Simple and compound spirituous tinctures are prepared from them, and they are ordered as a spicy ingredient in many of the officinal compositions.

ELEUTHE'RIA. See *Croton cascarilla*.

ELEVA'TIO. (From *elevo*, to lift up.) Elevation. Sublimation.

ELEVA'TOR. (From *elevo*, to lift up.)

1. A muscle is so called, the office of which is to lift up the part to which it is attached.

2. A chirurgical instrument, *elevatorium*, with which surgeons raise any depressed portion of bone, but chiefly those of the cranium.

ELEVATOR LABII INFERIORIS PROPRIUS. See *Levator labii inferioris*.

ELEVATOR LABII SUPERIORIS PROPRIUS. See *Levator labii superioris alæque nasi*.

ELEVATOR LABIORUM. See *Levator anguli oris*.

ELEVATOR NASI ALARUM. See *Levator labii superioris alæque nasi*.

ELEVATOR OCULI. See *Rectus superior oculi*.

ELEVATOR PALPEBRÆ SUPERIORIS. See *Levator palpebræ superioris*.

ELEVATOR SCAPULÆ. See *Levator scapulæ*.

ELEVATO'RIUM. (From *elevo*, to lift up.) An instrument to raise a depression in the skull.

ELI'BANUM. See *Juniperus lycia*.

ELICHRY'SUM. (From ηλιος, the sun, and χρυσος, gold; so called from its gold-like, or shining yellow appearance.) See *Gnaphalium stœchas*.

ELI'DRION. Mastich. A mixture of brass.

ELI'GMA. A linctus.

ELIOSELI'NUM. See *Eleoselinum*.

ELIPTICUS. Eliptic. Applied to leaves and receptacles, which are of a somewhat oval form, but broader at each end; as in the leaf of the *Convallaria majalis*, and the receptacle of the *Dorstenia drakenia*.

ELIQUATION. An operation, by means of which a more fusible substance is separated from another, which is less fusible. It consists in the application of a degree of heat, sufficient to fuse the former, but not the latter.

["If lead be heated so as to boil and smoke, it soon dissolves pieces of copper thrown into it; the mixture when cold is brittle. The union of these two metals is remarkably slight; for upon exposing the mass to a heat no greater than that in which lead melts, the lead almost entirely runs off by itself. This process is called *eliquation*. The coarser sorts of lead, which owe their brittleness and granulated texture to an admixture of copper, throw it up to the surface on being melted by a small heat."—*Web. Man. of Chem.* A.]

ELITHROI'DES. The vaginal coat of the testicle See *Elythroides* and *Testis*.

ELIXA'TIO. (From *elixo*, to boil.) The act of seething or boiling.

ELI'XIR. (From *elekser*, an Arabic word, signifying quintessence.) A term formerly applied to many preparations similar to compound tinctures. It is now very little employed.

Elixir of health. Elixir salutis. A term formerly applied to tincture of senna.

ELIXIR PAREGORICUM. See *Tinctura camphoræ composita*.

ELIXIR PROPRIETATIS. A preparation like the compound tincture of aloes.

ELIXIR SACRUM. A tincture of rhubarb and aloes.

ELIXIR SALUTIS. See *Tinctura sennæ*.

ELIXIR STOMACHICUM. See *Tinctura gentianæ composita*.

ELIXIVA'TIO. (From *elixo*, to boil, or from *lixivium*, lye.) The extraction of a fixed salt from vegetables, by an affusion of water. See *Lixiviation*

ELLAGIC ACID. (*Acidum ellagicum;* so named by Braconnot, by reversing the word *galle*.) The deposite which forms in infusion of nut-galls, left to itself, is not composed solely of gallic acid and a matter which colours it. It contains, besides, a little gallate and sulphate of lime, and a new acid, which was pointed out for the first time by Chevreuil, in 1815, an acid on which Braconnot made observations, in 1818, and which he proposed to call acid *ellagic*, from the word *galle* reversed. Probably this acid does not exist ready formed in nut-galls. It is insoluble; and, carrying down with it the greater part of the gallic acid, forms the yellowish crystalline deposite. But boiling water removes the gallic acid from the ellagic: whence the means of separating them from one another. *Ann. de Chim. et de Phys.* ix. 181

ELLEBORUM. See *Helleborus* and *Veratrum*.

ELM. See *Ulmus*.

Elm-leaved sumach. See *Rhus coriaria.*

ELMI'NTHES. (From ειλεω, to involve, from its contortions.) A worm.

ELO'DES. (From ελος, a swamp.) A term given to a sweating fever, from its great moisture.

Elonga'tio. (From *elongo*, to lengthen out.) An imperfect luxation, where the ligament is only lengthened, and the bone not put out of its socket.

ELOY, Nicholas Francis Joseph, was born at Mons, in 1714, and died in 1788, having practised as a physician with great ability and humanity. He had the honour of attending Prince Charles of Lorraine. He was a man of extensive learning, and, notwithstanding his professional avocations, was author of several publications. The principal of these, an Historical Medical Dictionary, was originally in two octavo volumes; but in 1788, it appeared greatly improved and enlarged in four volumes quarto. An Introduction to Midwifery; a Memoir on Dysentery; Reflections on the Use of Tea; and a Medico-Political Tract on Coffee; were likewise written by this author. The latter work procured him the reward of a superb snuff-box from the estates of Hainault, inscribed "Ex dono Patriæ."

ELUTRIATION. (*Elutriatio;* from *elutrio*, to cleanse.) Washing. It is the pouring a liquor out of one vessel into another, in order to separate the lighter earthy parts, which are carried away while the heavier metallic parts subside to the bottom.

ELU'VIES. (From *eluo*, to wash out.) The effluvium from a swampy place. Also the humour discharged in fluor albus.

Eluxa'tio. (From *eluxo*, to put out of joint.) A luxation, or dislocation.

ELYMAGRO'STIS. (From ελυμος, the herb panic, and αγρωςις, wild.) Wild panic.

ELY'MUS. Ελυμος. The herb panic, or panicum of Dioscorides, but now the name of a new genus of grasses, in the Linnæan system.

ELYOT, Sir Thomas, was born of a good family in Suffolk, about the beginning of the sixteenth century. After studying at Oxford, and improving himself by travelling, he was introduced at court; and Henry VIII. conferred upon him the honour of knighthood, and employed him in several embassies. He distinguished himself in various branches of learning, as well as by patronising learned men; and was generally beloved by his contemporaries for his virtues and accomplishments. He died in 1546, and was buried in Cambridgeshire, of which he had been sheriff. Among other studies, he was partial to medicine, and made himself master of the ancient authors on that subject, though he never exercised the profession. He published a work about the year 1541, called "The Castell of Health," which was much admired, even by some of the faculty: in this he is a strong advocate for temperance, especially in sexual pleasures. He also notices, that catarrhs were much more common than they had been forty years before; which he ascribes chiefly to free living, and keeping the head too much covered. He also wrote and translated several other works, but not on medical subjects.

ELYTROCE'LE. (From ελυτρον, the vagina, and κηλη, a tumour.) A hernia in the vagina. See *Hernia vaginalis.*

ELYTROI'DES. (*Elytroides;* from ελυτρον, a sheath, and ειδος, form.) Like a sheath. The tunica vaginalis is so called by some writers, because it includes the testis like a sheath

ELY'TRON. (From ελυω, to involve.) The vagina. A sheath. The membranes which involve the spinal marrow are called ελυτρα.

EMACIATION. See *Atrophia* and *Marasmus.*

Emargina'tio. (From *emargino*, to cleanse the edges.) The cleansing of the edges of wounds from scurf and filth.

EMARGINATUS. Emarginate, nicked, that is, having a small acute notch at the summit; as the leaf of the bladder senna, *Colutea arborescens*, the petals of the *Allium roseum*, and *Agrostema flos jovis.*

EMASCULA'TUS. (From *emasculo*, to render impotent.) Having the testicles in the belly, and not fallen into the scrotum.

Emba'mma. (From εμβαπτω, to emerge in.) A medicated pickle to dip the food in.

E'mbole. (From εμβαλλω, to put in.) The setting of a dislocated bone

E'MBOLUM. (From εμβαλλω, to cast out: so named because it ejects the semen.) The penis.

Embre'gma. (From εμβρεχω, to make wet.) A fluid application to any part of the body.

EMBROCA'TIO. (From εμβρεχω, to moisten or soak in.) *Embroche.* An embrocation. A fluid application to rub any part of the body with. Many use the term, however, as synonymous with liniment. The following embrocations are in general use.

Embrocatio aluminis. ℞. Aluminis ʒ ij. Aceti, spiritus vinosi tenuioris, sing. ℔ss. For chilblains and diseased joints.

Embrocatio ammoniæ. ℞. Embrocationis ammoniæ acetatis ℥ ij. Aquæ ammoniæ puræ ʒ ij. For sprains and bruises.

Embrocatio ammoniæ acetatis. ℞. Aquæ ammoniæ acetatæ. Solutionis saponis sing. ℥ j M. For bruises with inflammation.

Embrocatio ammoniæ acetatis camphorata. ℞. Solutionis saponis cum camphora, aquæ ammoniæ acetatæ sing. ℥ j. Aquæ ammoniæ puræ ℥ ss. For sprains and bruises. It is also frequently applied to disperse chilblains which have not suppurated. It is said to be the same as Steer's opodeldoc.

Embrocatio cantharidis cum camphora ℞. Tinct. cantharidis. Spiritus camphoræ sing. ℥ j M. This may be used in any case in which the object is to stimulate the skin. The absorption of cantharides, however, may bring on a stranguary.

E'mbroche. See *Embrocatio.*

E'MBRYO. (From εμβρυω, to bud forth.) 1. The germ of a plant; called by Linnæus the *corculum.* See *Corculum* and *Cotyledon.*

2. The *fœtis in utero* is so called before the fifth month of pregnancy, because its growth resembles that of the budding of a plant.

Embryothla'stes. (From εμβρυον, the fœtus, and θλαω, to break.) *Embryorectes.* A crotchet or instrument for breaking the bones of a dead fœtus to promote its delivery.

EMBRYO'TOMY. (*Embryotomia;* from εμβρυον, a fœtus, and τεμνω, to cut.) The separating of any part of the fœtus while *in utero*, to extract it.

Embryu'lcus. (From εμβρυον, a fœtus, and ελκω, to draw.) A blunt hook or forceps, for drawing the child from the womb.

EMERALD. A beautiful genus of minerals, which contains two species.

1. *The prismatic emerald*, Euclase of Haüy. This is of a green and sky-blue colour, and is found in Peru and Brazil.

2. *Rhomboidal emerald*, of which there are two subspecies, the precious emerald and the beryl. The first is well known by its emerald green colour. The most beautiful emeralds come from Peru. As a gem, it is valued next to ruby.

["This mineral is by no means uncommon in the United States. It occurs in the primitive range, and particularly in granite, in which it is imbedded. In the State of Maine, it has been found remarkably clear and transparent, and in every respect resembling the *Siberian Beryl*, particularly that discovered at Topsham by Professor Cleveland, of Brunswick College The crystals are well defined hexaædral prisms, and are often imbedded in the smoky quartz which abound in the large-grained granite. In some instances, in point of colour, it equals the finest Peruvian emerald.

"At Chesterfield, in Massachusetts, it occurs in great abundance. Dr. J. F. Waterhouse, who has carefully examined this locality, informs us that crystals, in hexangular prisms, from an ounce and under to 6℔. in weight, are found singly disseminated through the granite. They are of various dimensions, from a small size to that of a foot in diameter; their colour light green. The Chesterfield emerald greatly resembles that lately discovered in France. If the new earth *glucine* should be required for the arts or manufactures, this emerald would furnish it in abundance; as such is the quantity occurring at this place, that Dr. Waterhouse obtained upwards of 70℔. within a very small space. The emerald occurs in other parts of Massachusetts. To the politeness of Dr. David Hunt, we are indebted for several specimens found by that indefatigable mineralogist, in the vicinity of Northampton and Goshen.

"At Haddam, in Connecticut, this mineral occurs in abundance; the crystals are from a very small size to several inches in length; they are generally of a light yellowish-green, and sometimes of an amber colour, resembling topaz. Col. Gibbs has in his possession a crystal of a deep green an inch in diameter, and several in length, it bears a strong resemblance to the Peruvian emerald. Mr. Mather, a young mineralogist of great promise, discovered one seven inches in length, by nine inches in the diagonal diameter: it is in the cabinet of Professor Silliman.

"New-York affords but few instances of the production of emerald. It now and then, though rarely, occurs in the granite veins which traverse the gneiss on the island, about four miles from the city.

"The emerald is found in the vicinity of Philadelphia, and at Chester. These are the principal localities of this mineral in the United States, which have as yet come to our knowledge. As others occur, we shall with pleasure notice them."—*Bruce's Min. Journal.* A.]

EMERSUS. (From *emergo*, to rise up or appear out of the water.) Raised above the water, as the upper leaves accompanying the flowers of the *Meriophyllum verticillatum*, while its lower ones are *demersa.*

E'MERUS. Scorpion senna. A laxative.

EMERY. A sub-species of rhomboidal corundum, found in quantities in the isle of Naxor, and at Smyrna. Its fine powder, which is used for polishing hard minerals and metals, is made by trituration and elutriation.

EMESIA. (From εμεω, to vomit.) *Emesma; Emesis.* The act of vomiting. Medicines which cause vomiting.

EME'TIC. (*Emeticus;* from εμεω, to vomit.) That which is capable of exciting vomiting, independently of any effect arising from the mere quantity of matter introduced into the stomach, or of any nauseous taste or flavour.

The susceptibility of vomiting is very different in different individuals, and is often considerably varied by disease.

Emetics are employed in many diseases.

When any morbid affection depends upon, or is connected with, over-distention of the stomach, or the presence of acrid, indigestible matters, vomiting gives speedy relief. Hence its utility in impaired appetite, acidity in the stomach, in intoxication, and where poisons have been swallowed.

From the pressure of the abdominal viscera in vomiting, emetics have been considered as serviceable in jaundice, arising from biliary calculi obstructing the ducts.

The expectorant power of emetics, and their utility in catarrh and phthisis, have been ascribed to a similar pressure extended to the thoracic viscera.

In the different varieties of febrile affections, much advantage is derived from exciting vomiting, especially in the very commencement of the disease. In high inflammatory fever it is considered as dangerous, and in the advanced stage of typhus it is prejudicial.

Emetics given in such doses, as only to excite nausea, have been found useful in restraining hæmorrhage.

Different species of dropsy have been cured by vomiting, from its having excited absorption. To the same effect, perhaps, is owing the dispersion of swelled testicle, bubo, and other swellings, which has occasionally resulted from this operation.

The operation of vomiting is dangerous, or hurtful, in the following cases: where there is determination of the blood to the head, especially in plethoric habits: in visceral inflammation; in the advanced stage of pregnancy; in hernia and prolapsus uteri; and wherever there exists extreme general debility. The frequent use of emetics weakens the tone of the stomach. An emetic should always be administered in the fluid form. Its operation may be promoted by drinking any tepid diluent, or bitter infusion.

The individual emetics may be arranged under two heads, those derived from the vegetable, and those from the mineral kingdom. From the vegetable kingdom are numbered ipecacuanha, scilla maritima, anthemis nobilis, sinapis alba, asarum Europæum, nicotiana tabacum. From the mineral kingdom, antimony, the sulphates of zinc and copper, and the subacetate of copper. To these may be added ammonia and its hydro-sulphuret.

EMETIN. *Emetine.* Digest ipecacuan root, first in æther and then in alkohol. Evaporate the alkoholic infusion to dryness, redissolve in water, and drop in acetate of lead. Wash the precipitate, and then diffusing it in water, decompose by a current of sulphuretted hydrogen gas. Sulphuret of lead falls to the bottom, and the emetin remains in solution. By evaporating the water, this substance is obtained pure.

Emetin forms transparent brownish-red scales. It has no smell, but a bitter acrid taste. At a heat somewhat above that of boiling water, it is resolved into carbonic acid, oil, and vinegar. It affords no ammonia. It is soluble both in water and alkohol, but not in æther; and uncrystallizable. It is precipitated by protonitrate of mercury and corrosive sublimate, but not by tartar emetic. Half a grain of emetin acts as a powerful emetic, followed by sleep; six grains vomit violently, and produce stupor and death. The lungs and intestines are inflamed."—*Pelletier* and *Magendie.*

Emetine. See *Emetin.*

EMETOCATHA'RTICUS. (From εμεω, to vomit, and καθαιρω, to purge.) Purging both by vomit and stool.

EMINE'NTIÆ QUADRIGEMINÆ. See *Tubercula quadrigemina.*

ENMENAGOGUE. (*Emmenagogus;* from εμμηνια, the menses, and αγω, to move.) Whatever possesses the power of promoting that monthly discharge by the uterus, which, from a law of the animal economy, should take place in certain conditions of the female system. The articles belonging to this class may be referred to four ordres:—

1. *Stimulating emmenagogues,* as *hydrargyrine* and *antimonial preparations,* which are principally adapted for the young, and those with peculiar insensibility of the uterus.

2. *Irritating emmenagogues,* as *aloes, savine,* and *Spanish flies:* these are to be preferred in torpid and chlorotic habits.

3. *Tonic emmenagogues,* as *ferruginous preparations, cold bath,* and *exercise,* which are advantageously selected for the lax and phlegmatic.

4. *Antispasmodic emmenagogues,* as *asafœtida, castor,* and *pediluvia:* the constitutions to which these are more especially suited are the delicate, the weak, and the irritable.

EMME'NIA. (From εν, in, and μην, a month.) The menstrual flux.

EMO'LLIENT. (*Emolliens;* from *emollio,* to soften.) Possessing the power of relaxing the living and animal fibre, without producing that effect from any mechanical action. The different articles belonging to this class of medicines may be comprehended under the following orders:—

1. *Humectant emollients,* as *warm water,* and *tepid vapours,* which are fitted for the robust and those in the prime of life.

2. *Relaxing emollients,* as *althæa, malva,* &c. These may be employed in all constitutions, while at the same time they do not claim a preference to others from any particular habit of body.

3. *Lubricating emollients,* as *bland oils, fat,* and *lard.* The same observation will hold of this order as was made of the last mentioned.

4. *Atonic emollients,* as *opium* and *pediluvia.* These are applicable to any constitution, but are to be preferred in habits where the effects of this class are required over the system in general.

EMPATHEMA. (Ἐμπαθης; from παθημα, *passio, affectio.*) Ungovernable passion. A genus of disease in Good's Nosology. Class, *Neurotica;* Order, *Phrenica.*

It has three species, *Empathema entonicum, atonicum, insane,* and innumerable varieties.

EMPEI'RIA. (From εν, and πειρω, to endeavour.) Professional experience.

EMPHERO'MENUS. (From εμφερω, to bear.) Urine, or other substances which have a sediment.

EMPHLYSIS. (From εμ, in, and φλυσις, a vesicular tumour or eruption.) The name of a genus, *ichorous exanthem,* of Good's Nosology, which includes six species: *Emphlysis miliaria; Aphtha; Vaccinia; Varicella; Pemphigus; Erysipelas.*

EMPHRA'CTICA. (From εμφραττω, to obstruct.) Medicines which, applied to the skin, shut up the pores.

EMPHYMA. This term, applied by Good to a genus of disease, Class, *Eccritica;* Order, *Mesotica,* of his arrangement, imports (in contradiction to *Phyma*, which, in his system, is limited to cutaneous tumours, accompanied with inflammation,) a tumour originating below the integuments, and unaccompanied with inflammation, at least in its commencement. It embraces three species, viz. *Emphyma sarcoma; Encystis; Exostosis.*

EMPHYSE'MA. (*Emphysema, atis,* n.; from εμφυσαω, to inflate.) See *Pneumatosis.*

EMPIRIC. (*Empiricus.* Εμπειρικος; from εν, in, and πειρα, experience.) One who practises the healing art upon experience, and not theory. This is the true meaning of the word empiric; but it is now applied, in a very opposite sense, to those who deviate from the line of conduct pursued by scientific and regular practitioners, and vend nostrums, or sound their own praise in the public papers.

Empla'stica. (From εμπλασσω, to obstruct.) Medicines which, spread upon the skin, stop the pores.

EMPLA'STRUM. (*Emplastrum, i.* n.; from εμπλασσω, to spread upon.) A plaster. Plasters are composed of unctuous substances, united either to powders or metallic oxides, &c. They ought to be of such a consistence as not to stick to the fingers when cold, but to become soft, so as to be spread out in a moderate degree of heat, and in that of the human body, to continue tenacious enough to adhere to the skin. They owe their consistence either to metallic oxides, especially those of lead, or to wax, resin, &c. They are usually kept in rolls wrapped in paper, and spread, when wanted for use, upon thin leather; if the plaster be not of itself sufficiently adhesive, it is to be surrounded at its margin by a boundary of resin plaster.

Emplastrum ammoniaci. Take of purified ammoniacum, five ounces; acetic acid, half a pint. Dissolve the ammoniacum in the acid, then evaporate the liquor in an iron vessel, by means of a water-bath, constantly stirring it, until it acquires a proper consistence. This plaster is now first introduced into the London Pharmacopœia; it adheres well to the skin, without irritating it, and without producing inconvenience by its smell.

Emplastrum ammoniaci cum hydrargyro. Take of purified ammoniacum, a pound; purified mercury, three ounces; sulphuretted oil, a fluid drachm. Rub the mercury with the sulphurated oil until the globules disappear; then add by degrees the ammoniacum, previously melted, and mix the whole together. This composition is said to possess resolvent virtues; and the plaster is recommended with this view to be applied to nodes, tophs, indurated glands, and tumours.

Emplastrum asafœtidæ. *Emplastrum antihystericum.* Plaster of asafœtida. Take of plaster of semi-vitrified oxide of lead, asafœtida, each two parts: galbanum, yellow wax, each one part. This plaster is said to possess anodyne and antispasmodic virtues. It is, therefore, occasionally directed to be applied to the umbilical region in hysterical cases.

Emplastrum cantharidis. Blistering-fly plaster. *Emplastrum vesicatorium.* Take of blistering flies, in very fine powder, a pound; wax plaster, a pound and a half; prepared fat, a pound. Having melted the plaster and fat together, and removed them from the fire, a little before they become solid sprinkle in the blistering flies, and mix the whole together. See *Blister* and *Cantharis.*

Emplastrum ceræ. Wax plaster. *Emplastrum attrahens.* Take of yellow wax, prepared suet, of each three pounds; yellow resin, a pound. Melt them together and strain. This is a gently-drawing preparation, calculated to promote a moderate discharge from the blistered surface, with which intention it is mostly used. Where the stronger preparations irritate, this will be found in general to agree.

Emplastrum cumini. Cumin plaster. Take of cumin-seeds, caraway-seeds, bay-berries, of each three ounces; dried pitch, three pounds; yellow wax, three ounces. Having melted the dry pitch and wax together, add the remaining articles previously powdered, and mix. A warm stomachic plaster, which, when applied to the stomach, expels flatulency. To indolent scrofulous tumours, where the object is to promote suppuration, this is an efficacious plaster.

Emplastrum galbani compositum. Compound Galbanum plaster, formerly called *emplastrum lithargyri compositum* and *diachylon magnum cum gummi.* Take of galbanum gum resin purified, eight ounces, lead plaster, three pounds; common turpentine, ten drachms; resin of the spruce fir, three ounces. Having melted the galbanum gum resin with the turpentine, mix in first the powdered resin of the spruce fir, and then the lead plaster, previously melted by a slow fire, and mix the whole. This plaster is used as a warm digestive and suppurative, calculated to promote maturation of indolent or scirrhous tumours, and to allay the pains of sciatica, arthrodynia, &c.

Emplastrum hydrargyri. Mercurial plaster. *Emplastrum lithargyri cum hydrargyro.* Take of purified mercury, three ounces; sulphurated oil, a fluid drachm; lead plaster, a pound. Rub the mercury with the sulphurated oil, until the globules disappear; then add by degrees the lead plaster, melted, and mix the whole.

Emplastrum ladani compositum. Take of soft labdanum, three ounces; of frankincense, one ounce; cinnamon and expressed oil of mace, each half an ounce; essential oil of mint, one drachm: add to the frankincense, melted first, the labdanum a little heated, till it becomes soft, and then the oil of mace; afterward mix in the cinnamon with the oil of mint, and beat them together into a mass, in a warm mortar, and keep it in a vessel well closed. This may be used with the same intentions as the cumin-plaster, to which it is in no way superior, though composed of more expensive materials. Formerly, it was considered as a very elegant stomach plaster, but is now disused.

Emplastrum lithargyri. See *Emplastrum plumbi.*

Emplastrum lithargyri compositum. See *Emplastrum Galbani compositum.*

Emplastrum lithargyri cum resina. See *Emplastrum resinæ.*

Emplastrum lyttæ. See *Emplastrum cantharidis.*

Emplastrum opii. Plaster of opium. Take of hard opium, powdered, half an ounce; resin of the spruce fir, powdered, three ounces; lead plaster, a pound. Having melted the plaster, mix in the resin of the spruce fir, and opium, and mix the whole. Opium is said to produce somewhat, though in a smaller degree, its specific effect when applied externally.

Emplastrum picis compositum. Compound pitch plaster. *Emplastrum picis Burgundicæ.* Take of dried pitch, two pounds; resin of spruce fir, a pound; yellow resin, yellow wax, of each four ounces; expressed oil of nutmegs, an ounce. Having melted together the pitch, resin, and wax, add first the resin of the spruce fir, then the oil of nutmegs, and mix the whole together. From the slight degree of redness this stimulating application produces, it is adapted to gently irritate the skin, and thus relieve rheumatic pains. Applied to the temples, it is sometimes of use in pains of the head.

Emplastrum plumbi. Lead plaster. *Emplastrum lithargyri; Emplastrum commune; Diachylon simplex.* Take of semi-vitreous oxide of lead, in very fine powder, five pounds; olive oil, a gallon; water, two pints. Boil them with a slow fire, constantly stirring until the oil and litharge unite, so as to form a plaster. Excoriations of the skin, slight burns, and the like, may be covered with this plaster: but is in more general use, as a defensive, where the skin becomes red from lying a long time on the part. This plaster is also of great importance, as forming the basis, by addition to which many other plasters are prepared.

Emplastrum resinæ. Resin plaster. *Emplastrum adhæsivum; Emplastrum lithargyri cum resina.* Take of yellow resin, half a pound; lead plaster, three pounds. Having melted the lead plaster over a slow fire, add the resin in powder, and mix. The adhesive, or sticking plaster, is chiefly used for keeping on other dressings, and for retaining the edges of recent wounds together.

Emplastrum saponis. Soap plaster. Take of hard soap sliced, half a pound; lead plaster, three pounds. Having melted the plaster, mix in the soap; then boil it down to a proper consistence. Discutient properties are attributed to this elegant plaster, with which view, it is applied to lymphatic and other indoent tumours. It forms an admirable defensive and soft application, spread on linen, to surround a fractured limb.

Emplastrum thuris compositum. Compound frankincense plaster. Take of frankincense, half a pound; dragon's blood, three ounces; litharge plaster, two pounds. To the melted lead plaster, add the rest powdered. This plaster is said to possess strengthening, as well as adhesive powers. By keeping the skin firm, it may give tone to the relaxed muscles it surrounds, but cannot, in any way, impart more strength than the common adhesive plaster.

[The pharmacopœia of the United States admits the following plasters:

Emplastrum ammoniaci.
Do. asafœtidæ.
Do. ferri.
Do. hydrargyri.
Do. plumbi.
Do. plumbi subcarbonatis compositum.
Do. resinosum.
Do. resinosum cantharidum. A.]

Empneumato'sis. From εν, in, and πνεω, to blow.) An inflation of the stomach, or any other viscus.

EMPO'RIUM. (From εμπορεω, to negotiate.) A mart. The brain is so called, as being the place where all rational and sensitive transactions are collected.

EMPRESMA. Good revives this term (used in its simple form both by Hippocrates and Galen, to express internal inflammation) to designate a genus of disease in his Class, *Hæmatica*; Order, *Phlogotica*. Visceral inflammation. It embraces inflammation of all the viscera: hence *Empresma cephalitis*; *otitis*; *parotitis*; *paristhmitis*; *laryngitis*; *bronchitis*; *pneumonitis*; *pleuritis*; *carditis*; *peritonitis*; *gastritis*; *enteritis*; *hepatitis*; *splenitis*; *nephritis*; *cystitis*; *hysteritis*; *orchitis*.

E'mprion. (From εν, and πριων, a saw.) Serrated. Formerly applied to a pulse, in which the artery at different times is unequally distended.

EMPROSTHO'TONOS. (From εμπροσθεν, before, or forwards, and τεινω, to draw.) A clonic spasm of several muscles, so as to keep the body in a fixed position and bent forward. Cullen considers it as a species of tetanus. See *Tetanus*.

E'MPTYSIS. (From εμπτυω, to spit out.) A discharge of blood from the mouth.

EMPYE'MA. (From εν, within, and πυον, pus.) A collection of pus in the cavity of the thorax. It is one of the terminations of pleuritis. There is reason for believing that matter is contained in the cavity of the chest, when, after a pleurisy, or inflammation in the thorax, the patient has a difficulty of breathing, particularly on lying on the side opposite the affected one; and when an œdematous swelling is externally perceptible.

EMPYE'MATA. (From εν, and πυον, pus.) Suppurating medicines.

EMPYESIS. (From εμπυοω, or εμπυεω, *suppuro*.) Good has given this term (found in the fifth book of Hippocrates's aphorisms) to a genus of disease, class, *Hæmatica*; order, *Exanthematica*, characterized by phlegmonous pimples, which gradually fill with a purulent fluid. It has only one species, small-pox—*Empyesis variola*.

Empyreal air. Scheele gave this name to oxygen gas.

EMPYREU'MA. (From εμπυρευω, to kindle, from πυρ, fire.) A peculiar and offensive smell that distilled waters and other substances receive from being exposed to heat in closed vessels, or when burned under circumstances which prevent the accession of air to a considerable part of the mass.

EMPYREUMA'TIC. *Empyreumaticus*; from εμπυρευω, to kindle.) Smelling as it were burnt; thus empyreumatic oils are those distilled with a great heat, and impregnated with a smell of the fire.

EMU'LGENT. (*Emulgens*; from *emulgeo*, to melt out; applied to the artery and vein which go from the aorta and vena cava to the kidneys, because the ancients supposed they strained, and, as it were, milked the serum through the kidneys.) The vessels of the kidneys are so termed. The emulgent artery is a branch of the aorta. The emulgent vein evacuates its blood into the ascending cava.

EMU'LSIO. (*Emulsio*, *onis*. f.; from *emulgeo*, to milk) An emulsion. A soft and somewhat oily medicine resembling milk. An imperfect combination of oil and water, by the intervention of some other substance capable of combining with both these substances.

Emulsio acaciæ. This is made in the same manner as the almond emulsion, only adding while beating the almonds, two ounces of gum arabic. This cooling and demulcent emulsion, ordered in the Edinburgh Pharmacopœia, may be drank ad libitum to mitigate ardor urinæ, whether from the venereal virus or any other cause. In difficult and painful micturition, and strangury, it is of infinite service.

Emulsio amygdalæ. Almond emulsion. Take of almonds, one ounce; water, two pounds and a half. Beat the blanched almonds in a stone mortar, gradually pouring on them the water; then strain off the liquor. It possesses cooling and demulcent properties.

Emulsio camphorata. Take of camphor, one scruple; sweet almonds, blanched, two drachms; double refined sugar, one drachm; water, six ounces. This is to be made in the same manner as the common emulsion. It is calculated for the stomachs of those who can only bear small quantities of camphire.

EMULSION. See *Emulsio*.

Emulsion, almond. See *Emulsio amygdalæ*.

Emulsion, Arabic. See *Emulsio acaciæ*.

Emulsion of asafœtida. See *Mistura asafœtidæ*

Emulsion, camphorated. See *Emulsio camphorata*.

Emulsion of gum-ammoniac. See *Mistura ammoniaci*.

EMU'NCTORY. (*Emunctorium*; from *emungo*, to drain off.) The excretory ducts of the body are so termed; thus the exhaling arteries of the skin constitute the great emunctory of the body.

Enæ'ma. (From εν, and αιμα, blood.) *Enæmos*. So Hippocrates and Galen call such topical medicines as are appropriated to bleeding wounds.

Enæore'ma. (From εν, and αιωρεω, to lift up.) The pendulous substance which floats in the middle of the urine.

ENA'MEL. See *Teeth*.

ENANTHE'SIS. 1. (From εν, *in*, *intra*, and ανθεω, *floreo*; efflorescence from within, or from internal affection.) A genus of disease, Class, *Hæmatica*; Order, *Exanthematica*, in Good's Nosology. Rash exanthem. It comprehends three species: viz. *Enanthesis rosalia*; *rubeola*; *urticaria*.

2. (From εν, and αντaω, to meet.) The near approach of ascending and descending vessels.

ENARTHRO'SIS. (From εν, in, and αρθρον, a joint.) The ball and socket-joint. A species of diarthrosis, or moveable connexion of bones, in which the round head of one is received into the deeper cavity of another, so as to admit of motion in every direction; as the head of the os femoris with the acetabulum of the os innominatum. See *Articulation*.

ENCA'NTHIS. (From εν, and κανθος, the angle of the eye.) A disease of the caruncula lachrymalis, of which there are two species. *Encanthis benigna*, and *Encanthis maligna seu inveterata*. The encanthis, at its commencement, is nothing more than a small, soft, red, and sometimes rather livid excrescence which grows from the caruncula lachrymalis, and at the same time from the neighbouring semilunar fold of the conjunctiva. This excrescence on its first appearance is commonly granulated, like a mulberry, or is of a ragged and fringed structure. Afterward, when it has acquired a certain size, one part of it represents a granulated tumour, while the rest appears like a smooth, whitish, or ash-coloured substance, streaked with varicose vessels, sometimes advancing as far over the conjunctiva, covering the side of the eye next to the nose, as where the cornea and sclerotica unite.

The encanthis keeps up a chronic ophthalmy, impedes the action of the eyelids, and prevents, in particular, the complete closure of the eye. Besides, partly by compressing and partly by displacing the orifices of the puncta lachrymalia, it obstructs the free passage of the tears into the nose. The inveterate encanthis is ordinarily of a very considerable magnitude; its roots extend beyond the caruncula lachrymalis and semilunar fold to the membraneous lining of one or both eyelids. The patient experiences very serious inconvenience from its origin and interposition between the commissure of the eyelids, which it necessarily keeps asunder on the side towards the nose. Sometimes the disease assumes a cancerous malignancy. This character is evinced by the dull red, and, as it were, leaden colour of the excrescence; by its exceeding hardness, and the lancinating pains which occur in it, and extend to the forehead, the whole eyeball and the temple, especially when the tumour has been, though slightly, touched. It is also shown, by the propensity of the excrescence to bleed, by the partial ulcerations on its surface, which emit a fungous substance, and a thin and exceedingly acrid discharge.

ENCATALE'PSIS. (From εν, and καταλαμβανω, to seize.) A catalepsy.

ENCATHI'SMA. (From εν, and καθιζω, to sit in.) A semicupium, or bath for half the body.

ENCAU'MA. (From εν, in, and καιω, to burn.) A burn. See *Burn.*

ENCAU'SIS. (From εν, and καιω, to burn.) A burn. See *Burn.*

ENCEPHALOCE'LE. (From εγκεφαλον, the brain, and κηλη, a tumour.) A rupture of the brain.

ENCE'PHALON. (From εν, in, and κεφαλη, the head.) *Encephalum.* By some writers the cerebrum only is so called; and others express by this term the contents of the cranium.

ENCE'RIS. (From εν, and κηρος, wax.) A roll of wax for making plasters.

ENCERO'SIS. (From εν, and κεροω, to wax.) The covering of a plaster with wax.

ENCHARA'XIS. (From εν, and χαρασσω, to scarify.) A scarification.

ENCHEIRE'SIS. (From εν, and χειρ, the hand.) *Encheira.* Galen uses this word as a part of the title to one of his works, which treats of dissection. The word imports the manual treatment of any subject.

ENCHEI'RIA. See *Encheiresis.*

ENCHILO'MA. See *Enchyloma.*

ENCHO'NDRUS. (From εν, and χονδρος, a cartilage.) A cartilage.

ENCHRIS'TA. (From εγχριω, to anoint.) Ointments.

ENCHYLO'MA. (From εν, and χυλος, juice.) An inspissated juice. An elixir, according to Lemery.

E'NCHYMA. (From εν, and χεω, to infuse.) *Enchysis.* 1. An infusion.

2. A sanguineous plethora.

ENCHY'MATA. (From εγχυω, to infuse.) Injections for the eyes and ears.

ENCHYMO'MA. (From εν, and χυω, to pour in.) In the writings of the ancient physicians, it is a word by which they express that sudden effusion of blood into the cutaneous vessels, which arises from joy, anger, or shame; and, in the last instance, is what we usually call blushing.

ENCHYMO'SIS. Εγχυμωσις. 1. Blushing.

2. An extravasation of blood, which makes the part appear livid.

E'NCHYSIS. See *Enchyma.*

ENCLY'SMA. (From εν, and κλυζω, to cleanse out.) A clyster.

ENCŒ'LIA. (From εν, within, and κοιλια, the belly.) The abdominal viscera.

ENCOLPI'SMUS. (From εγκολπεω, to insinuate.) A uterine injection.

ENCRA'NIUM. (From εν, within, and κρανιον, the skull.) The cerebrum and the whole contents of the skull.

ENCRASI'CHOLUS. (From εν, in, κερας, the head, and χολη, bile; because it is said to have the gall in its head.) The anchovy. See *Clupea.*

E'NCRIS. Εγκρις. A cake of meal, oil, and honey.

E'NCYMON. (From εν, and κυω, to conceive.) Pregnancy.

E'NCYSIS. (From εν, and κυω, to bring forth.) Parturition.

ENCY'STED. *Saccatus.* A term applied to those tumours which consist of a fluid or other matter, enclosed in a sac or cyst.

ENCY'STIS. (From εν, in, and κυστις, a bag.) An encysted tumour.

ENDE'MIC. (*Endemicus*, sc. *morbus;* from εν, in, and δημος, people.) A disease is so termed that is peculiar to a certain class of persons, or country: thus struma is endemial to the inhabitants of Derbyshire and the Alps; scurvy to seafaring people; and the plica polonica is met with in Poland.

E'NDESIS. (From εν, and δεω, to tie up.) A ligature. A bandage.

ENDIVE. See *Cichorium.*

ENDI'VIA. (*Quasi eundo via, quia passim nascitur;* named from the quickness of its growth.) See *Cichorium.*

E'NDOSIS. (From εν, and διδωμι, to give.) A remission, disorder.

ENECIA. (From Ηνεκης, continued.) A genus of disease in Good's Nosology. Class, *Hæmatica;* Order, *Pyretica:* continued fever. It comprehends three species, *Enecia cauma; typhus; synochus.*

ENELLA'GMENUS. (From εναλλαττω, to interchange.) An epithet applied to the union of the joints of the vertebræ.

E'NEMA. (*Enema, matis.* neut.; from ενιημι, to inject.) A clyster. A well-known form of conveying both nourishment and medicine to the system, under certain morbid circumstances. The former takes place where obstruction of the passage to the stomach is so great as to render access to that organ impossible, such as occurs in lockjaw, diseased œsophagus, &c. By these means the body can be supported for a few weeks, while an attempt is made at effecting a cure. It is composed, in such cases, of animal broths, gruels made of farinaceous seeds, mucilages, &c. As a form of medicine, clysters are no less useful; and, according to the intention with which they are prescribed, they are either of an emollient, anodyne, or purgative nature. The following forms are in general use.

ENEMA ANODYNUM. Take of starch jelly, half a pint; tincture of opium, forty to sixty drops. Mix. The whole to be injected by means of a clyster-syringe, in cases of dysentery or violent purging, and pain in the bowels.

ENEMA ANTISPASMODICUM. Take of tincture of asafœtida, half an ounce; tincture of opium, forty drops; gruel, half a pint. Mix. For spasmodic affections of the bowels.

ENEMA LAXATIVUM. Take of sulphate of magnesia, two ounces; dissolve in three quarters of a pint of warm gruel, or broth, with an ounce of fresh butter, or sweet oil.

ENEMA NICOTIANÆ. Take of the infusion of tobacco from a half to a whole pint. Employed in cases of strangulated hernia.

ENEMA NUTRIENS. Take of strong beef tea, twelve ounces; thicken with hartshorn shavings, or arrow-root.

ENEMA TEREBINTHINÆ. Take of common turpentine, half an ounce; the yelk of one egg, and half a pint of gruel. The turpentine being first incorporated with the egg, add to them the gruel. This clyster is generally used, and with great good effect, in violent fits of the stone.

ENEREI'SIS. (From ενερειδω, to adhere to a compression.) A tight ligature.

E'NERGY. (*Energia;* from ενεργεω, to act.) The degree of force exercised by any power: thus, nervous energy, muscular energy, &c.

ENERVATING. The act of destroying the force, use, or office of the nerves, either by cutting them, or breaking them by violence or abuse of the non-naturals.

ENEURE'SIS. See *Enuresis.*

ENERVIS. Ribless: applied to leaves which are without lines or ribs.

ENGALA'CTUM. (From εν, and γαλα, milk; so called, because it is eaten by nurses to increase their milk.) The herb saltwort. See *Salsola.*

ENGASTRIMY'THUS. (From εν, in, γαστηρ, the belly, and μυθεομαι, to discourse.) A ventriloquist; one who appears to speak from his belly.

ENGISO'MA. (From εγγιζω, to approach.)

1. An instrument for making the parts of a broken clavicle meet.

2. A fracture of the cranium.

English Mercury. See *Mercurialis.*

ENGLOTTO-GASTOR. (From εν, γλωττη, the tongue, and γαστηρ, the belly.) A ventriloquist.

ENGOMPHO'SIS. (From εν, and γομφος, a nail.) That species of articulation which resembles a nail driven into wood, as a tooth in its socket.

ENGO'NIOS. (From εν, and γωνια, an angle.) The flexure, or angle made by the bending of a joint.

ENI'XUM PARACELSI. The caput mortuum of the distillation of nitric acid, which is a super-sulphate of potassa.

ENNEANDRIA. (From εννεα, nine, and ανηρ, a man.) The name of a class of plants in the sexual system, containing such as have hermaphrodite flowers with nine stamina.

Ennbapha'rmacum. (From εννεα, nine, and φαρμακον, a medicine.) A medicine composed of nine simple ingredients.

ENNEAPHY'LLUM. (From εννεα, nine, and φυλλον, a leaf; because its flower consists of nine leaves.) A name for helleboraster, or bear's-foot.

ENODIS. Without knots: applied to stems of plants, as *Culmus enodis;* that is, a smooth culm, as in our common rushes.

Enry'thmus. (From εν, and ρυθμος, number.) A pulse in some respect regular.

ENS. This word denoted in ancient chemistry the most efficacious part of any natural mixed body, whether animal, vegetable, or fossil, wherein all the qualities or virtues of the ingredients of the mixed are comprehended in a small compass.

ENSATÆ. (From *ensis*, a sword.) The name of a natural order of plants, consisting of such as have sword-shaped leaves.

E'NSIFORM. (*Ensiformis;* from *ensis*, a sword, and *forma*, resemblance.) Sword-like. 1. A term applied to some parts from their resemblance; as the ensiform cartilage.

2. In botany, a leaf is called *folium ensiforme*, which has two edges, and tapers to a point, like a sword. See *Leaf.*

Ensta'ctum. (From εν, and ςαζω, to instil.) A liquid medicine, which is applied *instillatim*, or drop by drop.

ENTASIA. (From εντασις, *intentio vehementia.*) A name of a genus of diseases in Good's Nosology. Class, *Neurotica;* Order, *Cinetica.* Constrictive spasm. It has eight species, viz. *Entasia priapismus; loxia; articularis; systremma; trismus; tetanus; lyssa; acrotismus.*

Enta'tica. (From εντεινω, to strain.) Provocatives, or whatever excites venereal inclination.

E'NTERA. (From εντος, within.)

1. The bowels.

2. Hippocrates calls by this name the bags in which medicines for fomentations were formerly enclosed.

ENTERADE'NES. (From εντερον, an intestine, and αδην, a gland.) The intestinal glands.

Entere'nchyta. (From εντερα, the bowels, and εγχυω, to infuse into.) An instrument for administering clysters. A clyster-pipe.

ENTERICA. (From εντερον, *intestinum*, *alvus.*) The name of the first order, class *Cœliaca*, of Good's Nosology. Diseases affecting the alimentary canal. Its genera are, *Odontia; Ptyalismus; Dysphagia; Dipsosis; Limosis; Colica; Coprostasis; Diarrhœa; Cholera; Enterolithus; Helminthia; Proctica.*

ENTERI'TIS. (From εντερον, an intestine.) Inflammation of the intestines. It is a genus of disease in the class *Pyrexiæ*, and order *Phlegmasiæ* of Cullen, and is known by the presence of pyrexia, fixed pain in the abdomen, costiveness, and vomiting. The causes of enteritis are much the same as those of gastritis, being occasioned by acrid substances, indurated fæces, long-continued and obstinate costiveness, spasmodic colic, and a strangulation of any part of the intestinal canal; but another very general cause is the application of cold to the lower extremities, or to the belly itself. It is a disease which is most apt to occur at an advanced period of life, and is very liable to a relapse.

It comes on with an acute pain, extending in general over the whole of the abdomen; but more especially round the navel, accompanied with eructations, sickness at the stomach, a vomiting of bilious matter, obstinate costiveness, thirst, heat, great anxiety, and a quick and hard small pulse. After a short time the pain becomes more severe, the bowels seem drawn together by a kind of spasm, the whole region of the abdomen is highly painful to the touch, and seems drawn together in lumpy contractions; invincible costiveness prevails, and the urine is voided with great difficulty and pain.

The inflammation continuing to proceed with violence, terminates at last in gangrene; or abating gradually, it goes off by resolution.

Enteritis is always attended with considerable danger, as it often terminates in gangrene in the space of a few hours from its commencement; which event is marked by the sudden remission of pain, sinking of the pulse, shrinking of the features, and distention of the belly, and it frequently proves fatal likewise, during the inflammatory stage. If the pains abate gradually, if natural stools be passed, if a universal sweat, attended with a firm equal pulse, comes on, or if a copious discharge of loaded urine, with the same kind of pulse, takes place, a resolution and favourable termination may be expected.

Dissections of this disease show, that the inflammation pervades the intestinal tube to a very considerable extent; that adhesions of the diseased portion to contiguous parts are formed; and that, in some cases, the intestines are in a gangrenous state, or that ulcerations have formed. They likewise show, that, besides obstinate obstructions, introsusception, constrictions, and twistings, are often to be met with; and that, in most cases, the peritonæum is more or less affected, and is perceived, at times, to be covered with a layer of coagulable lymph. The treatment must be begun by taking blood freely from the arm, as far as the strength of the patient will allow; but the disease occurring more frequently in persons rather advanced in years, and of a constitution somewhat impaired, it becomes more important to limit this evacuation and rely in a great measure on the effects of a number of leeches, applied to the abdomen. Another very useful step is to put the patient into a hot bath, which may presently induce faintness; or where this cannot be procured, fomenting the abdomen assiduously. When the symptoms are thus materially relieved, an ample blister should be applied. It becomes also of the first importance to clear out the bowels: a copious laxative clyster will evacuate the inferior part of the canal, and solicit the peristaltic motion downwards; and the milder cathartics, as castor oil, neutral salts, &c. in divided doses, may gradually procure a passage. But where the disease has been preceded by costiveness, more active articles will probably be necessary, as calomel, compound extract of colocynth, infusion of senna, with salts, &c. If the stomach be irritable, the effervescing saline draught may enable it to retain the requisite cathartics. Another plan, often very successful, is giving opium in a full dose, particularly in conjunction with calomel, taking care to follow it up by some of the remedies above mentioned, till the bowels are relieved; which effect it appears to promote by its soothing artispasmodic power. Afterward we may endeavour to keep up diaphoresis, and recruit the strength of the patient by a mild nourishing diet; taking care to guard against accumulation of fæces, exposure to cold, or any thing else likely to occasion a relapse.

ENTERO'. (From εντερον, an intestine.) Names compounded of this word belong to things which resemble an intestine; or to parts connected with, or diseases of some part of the intestine.

ENTEROCE'LE. (From εντερον, an intestine, and κηλη, a tumour.) An intestinal rupture or hernia. Every hernia may be so called that is produced by the protrusion of a portion of intestine, whether it is in the groin, navel, or elsewhere.

Entero-epiplocele. (From εντερον, an intestine, επιπλοον, the epiploon, and κηλη, a tumour.) A rupture formed by the protrusion of part of an intestine, with a portion of the epiploon.

Entero-hydrocele. (From εντερον, an intestine, υδωρ, water, and κηλη, a tumour.) This must mean a common scrotal hernia, with a good deal of water in the hernial sac; or else a hernia congenita, (in which the bowels descend into the tunica vaginalis testis,) attended with a collection of fluid in the cavity of this membrane.

ENTEROLITHUS. (From εντερον, an intestine, and λιθος, a stone.) The name of a genus of disease, Class, *Cœliaca;* Order, *Enterica*, in Good's Nosology Intestinal concretion. It embraces three species, viz *Enterolithus bezoar; calculus; scybalum*

ENTERO'MPHALUS. (From εντερον, an intestine, and ομφαλος, the navel.) An umbilical hernia, produced by the protrusion of a portion of intestine.

ENTERO'PHYTUM. (From εντερον, an intestine, and φυτον, a plant.) A plant which grows in the form of a gut, the sea-chitterling.

ENTERORA'PHIA. (From εντερον, an intestine, and ραφη, a suture.) A suture of the intestines, or the sewing together the divided edges of an intestine.

ENTEROSCHEOCE'LE. (From εντερον, an intestine, οσχεον, the scrotum, and κηλη, a rupture.) A scrotal hernia, or rupture of the intestines into the scrotum.

ENTHE'MATA. (From ενϳιθημι, to put in.) Anti-inflammatory styptics.

E'NTHLASIS. A contusion with the impression of the instrument by which it happened.

Entire Leaf. See *Integerrimus*.

ENTROCHI. A genus of extraneous fossils, made up of round joints, which, when separate and loose, are called *trochitæ*.

ENTRO'PIUM (*Entropium, i.* n.; from εν, and τρεπω, to turn.) A disease of the eyelids, occasioned by the eyelashes and eyelid being inverted towards the bulb of the eye.

ENTYPO'SIS. (From ενϳυποω, to make an impression.) 1. The acetabulum.

2. The scapula, or concave bone of the shoulder.

E'NULA. (A corruption of *henula*, or *Helenium*, from *Helene*, the island where it grew.) See *Inula helenium*.

ENULA CAMPANA. See *Inula helenium*.

ENU'LON. (From εν, and ουλον, the gums.) The internal flesh of the gums, or that part of them which is within the mouth.

ENURE'SIS. (*Eneuresis, is.* f.; from ενουρεω, to make water.) An incontinency, or involuntary flow of urine. This disease usually proceeds either from relaxation or a paralytic affection of the sphincter of the bladder, induced by various debilitating causes, as too free a use of spirituous liquors, manustupration, and excess in venery; or it arises from compression on the bladder, from the diseased state of the organ, or from some irritating substance contained in its cavity. It is arranged in the class *Locales*, and order *Apocenoses* of Cullen, and contains two species: 1. *Enuresis atonica*, the sphincter of the bladder having lost its tone from some previous disease. 2. *Enuresis ab irritatione, vel compressione vesicæ*, from an irritation or compression of the bladder.

EPACMA'STICUS. (From επι, and ακμαζω, to increase.) A fever which is increasing in malignity.

EPA'CME. (From επακμαζω, to increase.) The increase, or exacerbation of a disease.

EPAGO'GIUM. (From επαγω, to draw over.) The præpuce, or that part of the penis which is drawn over the glans, according to Dioscorides.

EPANADIDO'NTES. (From επαναδιδωμι, to increase.) A term applied to fevers which continue to increase in their degree of heat.

EPANADIPLO'SIS. (From επαναδιπλοω, to reduplicate.) The reduplication of a fit of a semitertian fever; that is, the return of the cold fit before the hot fit is ended.

EPANA'STASIS. (From επι, and ανιςημι, to excite.) A tubercle, or small pustule upon the skin.

EPANCYLO'TUS. (From επι, and αγκυλος, crooked.) A sort of crooked bandage in Oribasius.

EPANETUS. (From Ἐπανειμι, to return.) The name of a genus, Class *Hæmatica*; Order, *Pyretica*, in Good's Nosology. Remittent fever. It has three species, viz. *Epanetus nutis*; *malignus*; *hectica*.

EPA'RMA. (From επαιρω, to elevate.) *Eparsis*. Any kind of tumour, but frequently applied to one of the parotid gland.

EPA'RSIS. See *Eparma*.

EPASMA'STIGA FEBRIS. A fever is so called by Bellini, and others, while it is in its increase. See *Epacmasticus*.

EPE'NCRANIS. (From επι, εν, in, and κρανιον, the skull.) The name of the cerebellum.

EPHEBÆ'UM. (From επι, and ηβη, the groin.) The hair upon the pubes.

E'PHEDRA. (From εφεζομαι, to sit upon.) *Ephedrana*. 1. The buttocks.

2. A species of horse-tail.

EPHE'DRANA. See *Ephedra*.

EPHE'LCIS. (From επι, upon, and ελκος, an ulcer.) 1. The crust of an ulcer.

2. Hardened purulent expectoration.

EPHE'LIS. (*Ephelis*; from επι, and ηλιος, the sun.) A sun spot. A solitary, or aggregated spot, attacking most commonly the face, back of the hand, and breast, from exposure to the sun.

EPHE'MERA. (From επι, upon, and ημερα, a day.) A disease of a day's duration.

2. A fever which begins, is perfectly formed, and runs through its course in the space of twelve hours.

EPHEME'RIDES. (*Ephemeris, idis. f.*; from εφημερις, an almanac: so called because, like the moon's age, they may be foretold by the almanac. Diseases which return at particular times of the moon.

EPHIA'LTES. (From εφαλλομαι, to leap upon: so called because it was thought a dæmon leaped upon the breast.) Incubus, or nightmare. See *Oneirodynia*.

EPHIA'LTIA. (From *ephialtes*, the nightmare; so called because it was said to cure the nightmare.) The herb peony.

EPHIDRO'SIS. (From εφιδροω, to perspire.) *Sudatio*. *Mador*. A violent and morbid perspiration. A genus of disease in the class *Locales*, and order *Apocenoses* of Cullen.

EPHI'PPIUM. A saddle, which it is thought to resemble. See *Sella turcica*.

E'PHODOS. (From επι and οδος, a way.) In Hippocrates it hath three significations:

1. The ducts or passages, by which the excrements of the body are evacuated.

2. The periodical attack of a fever, from the common use of it to express the attack of thieves.

3. The access of similar or dissimilar things, which may be useful or hurtful to the body.

EPIA'LTES. See *Ephialtes*.

EPI'ALUS. (From ηπιον, gently, and αλκαζω, to heat.) *Epialos*. An ardent fever, in which both heat and cold are felt in the same part at the same time. Galen defines it to be a fever in which the patient labours under a preternatural heat and a coldness at the same time. The ancient Latins call it *Quercera*.

EPI'BOLE. (From επιβαλλω, to press upon.) The nightmare, or ephialtes.

EPICA'NTHIS. (From επι, and κανθος, the angle of the eye.) The angle of the eye.

EPICA'RPIUM. (From επι, upon, and καρπος, the wrist.) A medicine applied to the wrist.

EPICA'UMA. (From επι, and καιω, to burn.) A burn.

EPICAU'SIS. A burn.

EPI'CERAS. (From επι, and κερας, a horn: so called because its pods are shaped like a horn.) See *Trigonella fœnum græcum*.

EPICERA'STICA. (From επι, and κεραννυμι, to mix.) Medicines which, by mixing with acrimonious juices, temper them and render them less troublesome; as emollients.

EPICHEIRE'SIS. (From επι, and χειρ, the hand.) A manual operation.

EPI'CHOLUS. (From επι, and χολη, the bile.) Bilious.

EPICHO'RDIS. (From επι, upon, and χορδη, a gut.) The mesentery.

EPICHO'RIOS. (From επι, upon, and χορα, a region.) The same as epidermis.

EPICHROSIS. (From επιχρωσις, a coloured or spotted surface.) The name of a genus of disease, Class, *Eccritica*; Order, *Acrotica*, in Good's Nosology. Macular skin, or simple discoloration of the surface It embraces seven species, viz. *Epichrosis leucasmus*, *spilus*; *lenticula*; *ephelis*; *aurigo*; *pœcilia*; *alphosis*.

EPICŒLIS. (From επι, upon, and κοιλις, the eyelid.) The upper eyelid.

EPICO'LIC. (*Epicolicus*; from επι, upon, and κωλον, the colon.) That part of the abdomen which lies over the head of the cœcum and the sigmoid flexure of the colon, is called the epicolic region.

EPICOPHO'SIS. (From επι, and κωφος, deaf.) A total deafness.

EPICRA'NIUM. (From επι, and κρανιον, the cranium.) The common integuments, aponeurosis, and muscular expansion which lie upon the cranium.

EPICRA'NIUS. See *Occipito frontalis*.

EPI'CRASIS. (From επι, and κεραννυμι, to temper.) A critical evacuation of bad humours, an attemperation of bad ones. When a cure is performed in the alterative way, it is called *per Epicrasin*.

EPICRISIS. (From επι, and κρινω, to judge from.) A judgment of the termination of a disease from present symptoms.

EPICTE'NIUM. (From επι, about, and κϳεις, the pubes.) The parts above and about the pubes.

EPICYE'MA. (From επι, upon, and κυω, to conceive.) *Epicyesis*. Superfœtation.

EPICYE'SIS. See *Epicyema*.

EPIDE'MIC. (*Epidemicus*; from επι, upon, and δημος, the people.) A contagious disease is so termed, that attacks many people at the same season, and in the same place; thus, putrid fever, plague, dysentery, &c. are often epidemic.

EPIDE'NDRUM. (From επι, upon, and δενδρον, a tree; because all this genus of plants grow parasitically on the trunks or branches of trees.) The name of a genus of plants in the Linnæan system. Class, *Gynandria;* Order, *Monandria.*

Epidendrum vanilla. The systematic name of the vanelloe plant. *Vanilla; Banlia; Banilas; Aracus aromaticus; Epidendrum—scandens, foliis ovato oblongis nervosis sessilibus caulinis, cirrhis spiralibus* of Linnæus. The vanelloe is a long, flattish pod, containing, under a wrinkled brittle shell, a reddish brown pulp, with small shining black seeds, which have an unctuous aromatic taste, and a fragrant smell like that of some of the finer balsams heightened with musk. Although chiefly used as perfumes, they are said to possess aphrodisiac virtues.

Epi'deris. (From επι, and δερας, the skin.) The clitoris.

EPIDE'RMIS, (From επι, upon, and δερμα, the true skin.) The scarf-skin. See *Cuticle.*

Epi'desis. (From επι, upon, and δεω, to bind.) A bandage to stop a discharge of blood.

Epide'smus. (From επι, upon, and δεω, to bind.) A bandage by which splints, bolsters, &c. are secured.

EPIDI'DYMIS. (From επι, upon, and διδυμος, a testicle.) A hard, vascular, oblong substance, that lies upon the testicle, formed of a convolution of the *vas deferens.* It has a thick end, which is convex, and situated posteriorly; and a thin end, which is rather flat, and situated inferiorly. The epididymis adheres to the testicle by its two extremities only, for its middle part is free, forming a bag, to which the tunica vaginalis of the testicle is attached.

Epi'dosis. (From επιδιδωμι, to grow upon.) A preternatural enlargement of any part.

EPIDOTE. Pistacite of Werner. Acanticone from Norway. A sub-species of prismatoidal augite. A compounded ore, containing silica, alumina, lime, oxide of iron, oxide of manganese, found in primitive beds and veins, along with augite, hornblende, calcareous spar, &c.

Epi'drome. (From επιδρεμω, to run upon.) An afflux of humours.

EPIGA'STRIC. (*Epigastricus;* from επι, upon, or above, and γαςηρ, the stomach.) That part of the abdomen that lies over the stomach, is called the epigastric region; it reaches from the pit of the stomach to an imaginary line above the navel, supposed to be drawn from one extremity of the last of the false ribs to the other. Its sides are called hypochondria, and are covered by the false ribs, between which lies the epigastrium.

EPIGA'STRIUM. (From επι, upon, or above, and γαςηρ, the belly.) The part immediately over the stomach.

EPIGENESIS. A name given by the ancients, to that theory of generation which consists in regarding the fœtus as the joint production of matter afforded by both sexes.

EPIGENNE'MA. (From επιγινομαι, to generate upon.) 1. The fur on the tongue.

2. An accessory symptom.

EPIGENNE'SIS. See *Epigennema.*

EPIGINO'MENA. (From επιγινομαι, to succeed or supervene.) Galen says, they are those symptoms which naturally succeed, or may be expected in the progress of a disease; but Foesius says, they are accessions of some other affection to diseases, which never happen but in stubborn and malignant diseases.

EPIGLO'SSUM. (From επι, upon, and γλωσσα, the tongue: so called because a less leaf grows above the larger in the shape of a tongue.) The Alexandrian laurel, a species of *Ruscus.*

EPIGLO'TTIS. (From επι, upon, and γλωττις, the tongue.) The cartilage at the root of the tongue that falls upon the glottis or superior opening of the larynx. Its figure is nearly oval; it is concave posteriorly, and convex anteriorly. Its apex or superior extremity is loose, and is always elevated upwards by its own elasticity. While the back of the tongue is drawn backwards in swallowing, the epiglottis is put over the aperture of the larynx, hence it shuts up the passage from the mouth into the larynx. The base of the epiglottis is fixed to the thyroid cartilage, the os hyoides, and the base of the tongue, by a strong ligament.

Epiglo'ttum. (From επιγλωττις, the epiglottis, which it resembles in shape.) An instrument mentioned by Paracelsus for elevating the eyelids.

EPIGLOU'TIS. (From επι, upon, and γλουτος, the buttocks.) The superior parts of the buttocks.

Epigo'natis. (From επι, upon, and γονυ, the knee.) The patella or knee-pan.

Epigo'nides. (From επι, and γονυ, the knee.) The muscles inserted into the knees.

Epi'gonum. (From επιγινομαι, to proceed upon.) A superfœtation.

Epile'mpsis. See *Epilepsy.*

Epile'ntia. Corrupted from epilepsia.

EPILEPSY. (*Epilepsia, æ,* f.; from επιλαμβανω, to seize upon: so called, from the suddenness of its attack.) It is also called falling sickness, from the patient suddenly falling to the ground on an attack of this disease. By the ancients it was termed, from its affecting the mind, the most noble part of the rational creature, the sacred disease. It consists of convulsions with sleep, and usually froth issuing from the mouth. It is a genus of disease in the class *Neuroses,* and order *Spasmi,* of Cullen, and contains three species:

1. *Epilepsia cerebralis;* attacking suddenly without manifest cause, and not preceded by any unpleasant sensation, unless perhaps some giddiness or dimness of sight.

2. *Epilepsia sympathica;* without manifest cause, but preceded by a sensation of an aura ascending from some part of the body to the head.

3. *Epilepsio occasionalis;* arising from manifest irritation, and ceasing on the removal of this. It comprehends several varieties:—a. *Epilepsia traumatica,* arising from an injury of the head: b. *Epilepsia à dolore,* from pain: c. *Epilepsia verminosa,* from the irritation of worms: d. *Epilepsia à veneno,* from poisons: e. *Epilepsia exanthematica,* from the repulsion of cutaneous eruptions: f. *Epilepsia à cruditate ventriculi,* from crudities of the stomach: g. *Epilepsia ab inanitione,* from debility: h. *Epilepsia uterina,* from hysterical affections: i. *Epilepsia ex onanismo,* from onanism, &c.

Epilepsy attacks by fits, and after a certain duration goes off, leaving the person most commonly in his usual state; but sometimes a considerable degree of stupor and weakness remain behind, particularly where the disease has frequent recurrences. It is oftener met with among children than grown persons, and boys seem more subject to its attacks than girls. Its returns are periodical, and its paroxysms commence more frequently in the night than in the day, being somewhat connected with sleep. It is sometimes counterfeited, in order to extort charity or excite compassion.

Epilepsy is properly distinguished into sympathetic and idiopathic, being considered as sympathetic, when produced by an affection in some other part of the body, such as acidities in the stomach, worms, teething, &c. as idiopathic when it is a primary disease, neither dependent on nor proceeding from any other.

The causes which give rise to epilepsy are blows, wounds, fractures, and other injuries, done to the head by external violence, together with lodgments of water in the brain, tumours, concretions, and polypi. Violent affections of the nervous system, sudden frights, fits of passion, great emotions of the mind, acute pains in any part, worms in the stomach or intestines, teething, the suppression of long-accustomed evacuations, too great emptiness or repletion, and poisons received into the body, are causes which likewise produce epilepsy. Sometimes it is hereditary, and at others it depends on a predisposition arising from mobility of the sensorium, which is occasioned either by plethora, or a state of debility.

An attack of epilepsy is now and then preceded by a heavy pain in the head, dimness of sight, noise in the ears, palpitations, flatulency in the stomach and intestines, weariness, and a small degree of stupor, and in some cases, there prevails a sense of something like a cold vapour or aura arising up to the head; but it more generally happens that the patient falls down suddenly without much previous notice; his eyes are distorted, or turns so that only the whites of them can be seen; his fingers are closely clenched, and the trunk of his body, particularly on one side, is much agitated; he foams at the mouth, and thrusts out his tongue, which often suffers great injury from the muscles of the lower jaw being affected; he loses all sense of feeling, and not unfrequently voids both urine and fæces involuntarily.

The spasms abating, he recovers gradually; but on coming to himself feels languid and exhausted, and retains not the smallest recollection of what has passed during the fit.

When the disease arises from an hereditary disposition, or comes on after the age of puberty, or where the fits recur frequently, and are of long duration, it will be very difficult to effect a cure: but when its attacks are at an early age, and occasioned by worms, or any accidental cause, it may in general be removed with ease. In some cases, it has been entirely carried off by the occurrence of a fever, or by the appearance of a cutaneous eruption. It has been known to terminate in apoplexy, and in some instances to produce a loss of the powers of the mind, and to bring on idiotism.

The appearances usually to be observed on dissection, are serous and sanguineous effusion, a turgid tense state of the vessels of the brain without any effusion, a dilatation of some particular part of the brain, excrescences, polypi, and hydatids, adhering to it, and obstructing its functions, and likewise ulcerations.

During the epileptic paroxysm in general, little or nothing is to be done, except using precautions, that the patient may not injure himself; and it will be prudent to remove any thing which may compress the veins of the neck, to obviate congestion in the head. Should there be a considerable determination of blood to this part, or the patient very plethoric, it may be proper, if you can keep him steady, to open a vein, or the temporal artery; and in weakly constitutions the most powerful antispasmodics may be tried in the form of clyster, as they could hardly be swallowed: but there is very seldom time for such measures. In the intervals, the treatment consists: 1. In obviating the several exciting causes. 2. In correcting any observable predisposition. 3. In the use of those means, which are most likely to break through the habit of recurrence.

I. The manner of fulfilling the first indication requires little explanation; after an injury to the head, or where there is disease of the bone, an operation may be necessary, to remove irritation from the brain; in children teething, the gums ought to be lanced: where the bowels are foul, or worms suspected, active purgatives should be exhibited, &c. In those instances in which the aura epileptica is perceived, it has been recommended to destroy the part, where it originates, or divide the nerve going to it, or correct the morbid action by a blister, &c.; such means would certainly be proper when there is any disease discoverable in it. Making a tight ligature on the limb above has sometimes prevented a fit; but, perhaps, only through the medium of the imagination.

II. Where a plethoric state appears to lay the foundation of the disease, which is often the case, the patient must be restricted to a low diet, frequent purges exhibited, and the other excretions kept up, and he should take regular moderate exercise, avoiding whatever may determine the blood to the head; and to counteract such a tendency, occasional cupping, blisters, issues, &c. may be useful, as well as the shower-bath; but in urgent circumstances, the lancet ought to be freely used. If, on the contrary, there are marks of inanition and debility, a generous diet, with tonic medicines, and other means of strengthening the system, will be proper. The vegetable tonics have not been so successful in this disease as the metallic preparations, particularly the sulphate of zinc, the nitrate of silver, and the ammoniated copper, but this cannot perhaps be so safely persevered in: where the patient is remarkably exsanguineous, chalybeates may answer better; and, in obstinate cases, the arsenical solution might have a cautious trial. In irritable constitutions, sedatives are indicated, as digitalis, opium, &c.: but the free use of opium is restricted by a tendency to congestion in the head. Where syphilis appears to be concerned, a course of mercury is proper; in scrofulous habits, bark, or steel, with iodine, soda, and sea-bathing; and so on.

III. The third division of remedies comes especially in use, where the fits are frequent, or where their recurrence can be anticipated; emetics will often prevent them, or a full dose of opium; also other powerful antispasmodics, as æther, musk, valerian, &c.: or strong odours, and in short any thing producing a considerable impression on the system. Bark, taken largely, might perhaps be more successful on this principle. The disease has sometimes been cured, especially when originating from sympathy, by inspiring fear or horror; and many frivolous charms may, no doubt have taken effect through the medium of the imagination. Also long voyages have removed it, which might especially be hoped for at the age of puberty, particularly if a considerable change in the mode of life were made in other respects; those who had lived indolently being obliged to exert themselves, the diet properly adapted to the state of the system, &c.

EPILO'BIUM. (From επι λοβου ιον, a violet or beautiful flower, growing on a pod.) The name of a genus of plants in the Linnæan system. Class, *Octandria*; Order, *Monogynia*.

Epilobium angustifolium. Rose-bay-willow herb. The young tender shoots cut in the spring, and dressed as asparagus, are little inferior to it.

Epime'dium. The plant barren-wort.

Epimo'rius. (Fro επι, and μειρω, to divide.) An obsolete term, formerly applied to an unequal pulse.

Epimy'lis. (From επι, and μυλη, the knee.) The patella or knee-bone.

Epineneu'cus. (From επινευω, to nod or incline.) An unequal pulse.

Epino'tium. (From επι, upon, and νωτος, the back.) The shoulder-blade.

EPINY'CTIS. (From επι, and νυξ, night.) A pustule, which rises in the night, forming an angry tumour on the skin of the arms, hands, and thighs, of the size of a lupine, of a dusky red, and sometimes of a livid and pale colour, with great inflammation and pain. In a few days it breaks, and sloughs away.

Epipa'ctis. (From επιπακτοω, to coagulate.) A plant mentioned by Dioscorides; and so named because its juice was said to coagulate milk.

Epiparoxy'smus. (From επι, upon, and παροξυσμος, a paroxysm.) An unusual frequency of febrile exacerbation.

Epipa'stum. (From επι, upon, and πασσω, to sprinkle.) Any powdered drug sprinkled on the body.

Epipe'chys. (From επι, above, and πηχυς, the cubit.) That part of the arm above the cubit.

Epiphlogi'sma. (From επι, upon, and φλογιζω, to inflame.) 1. Violent inflammation, or burning heat in any part, attended with pain, tumour, and redness.

2. A name given by Hippocrates to the shingles.

EPI'PHORA. (From επιφερω, to carry forcibly.) The watery eye. An involuntary flow of tears. A superabundant flowing of a serous or aqueous humour from the eyes. A genus of disease in the class *Locales*, and order *Apocenoses*, of Cullen. The humour which flows very copiously from the eye in epiphora, appears to be furnished, not only by the lachrymal gland, but from the whole surface of the conjunctive membrane, Meibomius's glands, and the caruncula lachrymalis; which increased and morbid secretion may be induced from any stimulus seated between the globe of the eye and lids, as sand, acrid fumes, and the like; or it may arise from the stimulus of active inflammation; or from the acrimony of scrofula, measles, small-pox, &c., or from general relaxation. The disease may also arise from a more copious secretion of tears, than the puncta lachrymalia can absorb, or, as is most common, from an obstruction in the lachrymal canal, in consequence of which the tears are prevented from passing freely from the eye into the nose.

EPIPHRAGMA. The slender membrane which sometimes shuts the peristoma of mosses, as is seen in *Polytricum*.

EPI'PHYSIS. (From επι, upon, and φυω, to grow.) Any portion of bone growing upon another, but separated from it by a cartilage.

Epipla'sma. (From επι, upon, and πλασσω, to spread.) 1. A poultice.

2. A name for an application of wheat meal, boiled in hydrelæum, to wounds.

EPIPLO. (From επιπλοον, the omentum.) Names compounded of this word belong to parts connected with, or disease of, the epiploon.

EPIPLOCE'LE. (From επιπλοον, the omentum,

and κηλη, a tumour.) An omental hernia. A rupture produced by the protrusion of a portion of the omentum See *Hernia omentalis*.

EPIPLOCOMI'STIS. (From επιπλοον, the omentum, and κομιζω, to carry.) One who has the omentum morbidly large.

Epiploic appendages. See *Appendiculæ epiploicæ.*

EPIPLOI'TIS. (From επιπλοον, the omentum.) An inflammation of the process of the peritonæum, that forms the epiploon or omentum. See *Peritonitis.*

EPIPLOO'MPHALON. (From επιπλοον, the omentum, and ομφαλος, the navel.) An omental hernia protruding at the navel.

EPI'PLOON. (From επιπλοω, to sail over, because it is mostly found floating, as it were, upon the intestines.) See *Omentum.*

EPIPLOSCHEOCE'LE. (From επιπλοον, the omentum, οσχεον, the scrotum, and κηλη, a tumour or hernia.) A rupture of the omentum into the scrotum, or a scrotal hernia containing omentum.

EPIPO'LASIS. (From επιπολαζω, to swim on the top.) 1. A fluctuation of humours.

2. A species of chemical sublimation.

EPIPO'MA. (From επι, upon, and πωμα, a lid.) An instrument to cover the shoulder in a luxation.

EPIPORO'MA. (From επιπωρεω, to harden.) A hard tumour about the joints.

EPIPTY'XIS. (From επιπτυσσω, to close up.) A spasmodic closing of the lips.

EPIPYRE'XIS. (From επι, and πυρεττω, to be feverish.) A rapid exacerbation in a fever.

EPIRIGE'SIS. (From επι, and ριγεω, to become cold.) An unusual degree of cold, or repetition of rigors.

EPI'RRHOE. (From επι, upon, and ρεω, to flow.) An influx or afflux of humours to any part.

EPISARCI'DIUM. (From επι, upon, and σαρξ, the flesh.) An anasarca, or dropsy, spread between the skin and flesh.

EPISCHE'SES. (From επισχεω, to restrain.) A suppression of excretions. It is an order in the class *Locales* of Cullen's Nosology.

EPI'SCHIUM. (From επι, upon, and ισχιον, the hip-bone.) The os pubis.

EPISCOPA'L. (From *episcopus*, a bishop, or mitred dignitary.) Of, or belonging to a bishop: applied to a valve at the orifice between the left auricle and ventricle of the heart. See *Mitral valve.*

EPISPA'SMUS. (From επισπαω, to draw together.) A quick inspiration.

EPISPA'STIC. (*Epispasticus;* from επισπαω, to draw together.) Those substances which are capable, when applied to the surface of the body, of producing a serous or puriform discharge, by exciting a previous state of inflammation. The term, though comprehending likewise issues and setons, is more commonly restricted to blisters—those applications which, exciting inflammation on the skin, occasion a thin serous fluid to be poured from the exhalants, raise the cuticle, and form the appearance of a vesicle. This effect arises from their strong stimulating power, and to this stimulant operation and the pain they excite, are to be ascribed the advantages derived from them in the treatment of disease. The evacuation they occasion is too inconsiderable to have any material effect. See *Blister.*

EPISPHÆ'RIA. (From επι, and σφαιρα, a sphere: so called from the spherical shape of the brain.) The windings of the exterior surface of the brain; or the winding vessels upon it.

EPISTA'GMUS. (From επι, and ςαζω, to trickle down.) A catarrh.

EPISTAPHYLI'NUS. (From επι, and ςαφυλη, the uvula.) See *Uvula.*

EPISTA'XIS. (From επιςαζω, to distil from.) Bleeding at the nose, with pain or fulness of the head. A genus of disease arranged by Cullen in the class *Pyrexiæ*, and order *Hæmorrhagiæ.*

Persons of a sanguine and plethoric habit, and not yet advanced to manhood, are very liable to be attacked with this complaint: females being much less subject to it than males, particularly after menstruation.

Epistaxis comes on at times without any previous warning; but at others, it is preceded by a pain and heaviness in the head, flushing in the face, heat and itching in the nostrils, a throbbing of the temporal arteries, and a quickness of the pulse. In some instances a coldness of the feet, and shivering over the whole body, together with a costive belly, are observed to precede an attack of this hæmorrhage.

This complaint is to be considered as of little consequence, when occurring in young persons, being never attended with any danger; but when it arises in those who are advanced in life, flows profusely, and returns frequently, it indicates too great fulness of the vessels of the head, and not unfrequently precedes apoplexy, palsy, &c. and, therefore, in such cases, is to be regarded as a dangerous disease. When this hæmorrhage arises in any putrid disorder, it is to be considered as a fatal symptom.

In general, we need not be very anxious to stop a discharge of blood from the nose, particularly where there are marks of fulness of the vessels of the head: but if it occurs under a debilitated state of the system, or becomes very profuse, means must be employed to suppress it. These are chiefly of a local nature; applying pressure to the bleeding vessels, introducing astringents into the nostrils, as solutions of alum, sulphate of zinc, sulphate of copper, &c. applying cold to the head, or to some very sensible part of the skin, as in the course of the spine, &c. At the same time the patient should be kept in the erect position. If the hæmorrhage be of an active character, the antiphlogistic regimen should be carefully observed: the patient kept cool and quiet; the saline cathartics, refrigerants, as nitrate of potassa and the acids, digitalis, diaphoretics, &c. administered internally; and blood may be taken from the temples by leeches, or even from the arm, if the patient be very plethoric. Sometimes, after the failure of other means, closing the posterior as well as anterior outlets from the nose, and preventing the escape of the blood for some time mechanically, has been successful; and this might be particularly proper, where it was discharged copiously into the fauces, so as to endanger suffocation, on the patient falling asleep.

EPISTHO'TONOS. (From επισθεν, forwards, and τεινω, to extend.) A spasmodic affection of muscles drawing the body forwards. See *Tetanus.*

EPISTO'MION. (From επι, upon, and ςομα, a mouth.) 1. A stopper for a bottle.

2. A venthole of a furnace, called the register.

EPISTRO'PHALUS. (From επι, upon, and ςρεφω, to turn about.) *Epistrophia*, and *Epistrophis.* Applied to the first vertebra of the neck, because it turns about upon the second as upon an axis.

EPI'STROPHE. (From επιςρεφω, to invert.) 1. An inversion of any part, as when the neck is turned round.

2. A return of a disorder which has ceased.

EPI'STROPHEUS. (From επιςροφαω, to turn round, because the head is turned upon it.) The second cervical vertebra. See *Dentatus.*

EPI'STROPHIS. See *Epistrophalus.*

EPI'TASIS. (From επι, and τεινω, to extend.) The beginning and increase of a paroxysm or disease.

EPITHE'LIUM. The cuticle on the red part of the lips.

EPITHE'MA. (From επι, upon, and τιθημι, to apply.) A term formerly applied to a lotion, fomentation, or any external application.

EPITHEMA'TIUM. The same.

EPI'THESIS. (From επι, and τιθημι, to cover, or lay upon.) The rectification of crooked limbs by means of instruments.

EPITHY'MUM. (From επι, upon, and θυμος, the herb thyme.) See *Cuscuta epithymum.*

EPO'DE. (From επι, over, and ωδη, a song.) *Epodos.* The method of curing distempers by incantation.

EPOM'IS. (From επι, upon, and ωμος, the shoulder.) The acromion, or upper part of the shoulder.

EPOMPHA'LIUM. (From επι, upon, and ομφαλος, the navel.) An application to the navel.

EPSOM. The name of a village in Surrey, about eighteen miles from London, in the neighbourhood of which is a considerable mineral spring, called Epsom water. *Aqua Epsomensis.* This water evaporated to dryness leaves a residuum, the quantity of which has been estimated from an ounce and a half in the gallon, to five drachms and one scruple. Of the total residuum, by far the greater part, about four or five-sixths, is sulphate of magnesia mixed with a very few muriates, such as that of lime, and probably magnesia, which render it very deliquescent, and increase the bitterness of taste, till purified by repeated crystalliza tions. There is nothing sulphurous or metallic ever found in this spring. The diseases in which it is employed are similar to those in which we use Seidlitz water. There are many other of the simple saline springs that might be enumerated, all of which agree with that of Epsom, in containing a notable proportion of some purging salt, which, for the most part, is either sulphate of magnesia, or sulphate of soda, or often a mixture of both, such as Acton, Kilburne, Bagnigge Wells, Dog and Duck, St. George's Fields, &c.

Epsom salt. A purging salt formerly obtained by boiling down the mineral water found in the vicinity of Epsom in Surrey. It is at present prepared from sea water, which, after being boiled down, and the muriate of soda separated, deposites numerous crystals, that consist chiefly of sulphate of magnesia, and sold in the shops under the name of sal catharticus amarus, or bitter purging salt. See *Magnesiæ sulphas.*

EPU'LIS. (From επι, and ουλα, the gums.) A small tubercle on the gums. It is said sometimes to become cancerous.

EPULO'TIC. (*Epuloticus; from* επουλοω, to cicatrize.) A term given by surgeons to those applications which promote the formation of skin.

EQUISE'TUM. (From *equus*, a horse, and *seta*, a bristle: so named from its resemblance to a horse's tail.) 1. The name of a genus of plants in the Linnæan system. Class, *Cryptogamia;* Order, *Filices.*

2. The pharmacopœial name of the *Cauda equina.* See *Hippuris vulgaris.*

Equisetum arvense. See *Hippuris ulgaris.*

EQUITANS. Equitant. This term is applied to leaves, which are disposed in two opposite rows, and clasp each other by their compressed base; as in *Narthecium ossifragum.*

EQUIVALENTS. A term introduced into chemistry by Dr. Wollaston, to express the system of definite ratios, in which the corpuscular objects of this science reciprocally combine, referred to a common standard, reckoned unity. See *Atomic system.*

E'QUUS. 1. The horse.

2. The name of a genus of animals of the order *Belluæ.*

Equus asinus. The systematic name of the animal called an ass; the female affords a light and nutritious milk. See *Milk, asses'.*

Era'nthemus. (From ηρ, the spring, and ανθεμος, a flower: so called because it flowers in the spring.) A sort of chamomile.

ERASIS'TRATUS. A celebrated Greek physician, said to have been born in the island of Ceos, and to have been the most distinguished pupil of Chrysippus, of the Cnidian school. He was the first, in conjunction with Herophilus, to dissect human bodies, anatomy having been before studied only in brutes; but the Ptolemies having allowed them to examine malefactors, they were enabled to make many important discoveries. Celsus notices a very improbable report, that they opened the bodies of those persons alive, to observe the internal motions; they could hardly then have maintained, that the arteries and left ventricle, do not naturally contain blood, but air only. The works of Erasistratus, which were numerous, are lost; but, from the account of Galen, he appears to have very accurately described the brain, which he considered as the common sensorium; also the heart and large vessels; and pointed out the office of the liver and kidneys; but he supposed digestion performed by trituration. He imagined inflammation and fever to arise from the blood being forced through the minute veins into the corresponding arteries. He was averse to blood-letting, or the use of active medicines, but sometimes employed mild clysters; trusting, however, principally to abstinence, and proper exercise. Being tormented with an ulcer in the foot, at an extreme old age, he is said to have terminated his existence by poison.

Erate'va marmelos. This plant, a native of several parts of India, affords a fruit about the size of an orange, and covered with a hard bony shell, containing a yellow viscus pulp, of a most agreeable flavour; which, when scooped out, and mixed with sugar and orange, is brought to the tables of the grandees in India, who eat it as a great delicacy. It is also esteemed as a sovereign remedy against dysentery.

Erebi'nthus. Ερεβινθος. The vetch.

ERE'CTOR. The name of several muscles, the office of which is to raise up the part to which they are inserted.

Erector clitoridis. First muscle of the clitoris of Douglas. *Ischio-cavernosus* of Winslow, and *Ischio-clitoridien* of Dumas. A muscle of the clitoris that draws it downwards and backwards, and serves to make the body of the clitoris more tense, by squeezing the blood into it from its crus. It arises from the tuberosity of the ischium, and is inserted into the clitoris.

Erector penis. *Ischio-cavernosus* of Winslow, and *Ischio-caverneux* of Dumas. A muscle of the penis that drives the urine or semen forwards, and, by grasping the bulb of the urethra, pushes the blood towards the corpus cavernosum and the glans, and thus distends them. It arises from the tuberosity of the ischium, and is inserted into the sides of the cavernous substance of the penis.

ERECTUS. Upright. Botanists use this to express the direction of the stem, branches, leaves, petals, stamens, pistils, &c.; as *Caulis erectus*, an upright stem, as in *Lysimachia vulgaris; folium erectum*, forming an acute angle with the stem, as in *Juncus articulatus*, &c. The petals of the *Brassica erecta.*

ERETHI'SMUS. (From ερεθιζω, to excite or irritate.) Increased sensibility and irritability. It is variously applied by modern writers. Mr. Pearson has described a state of the constitution produced by mercury acting on it as a poison. He calls it the mercurial erithismus, and mentions that it is characterized by great depression of strength, anxiety about the præcordia, irregular action of the heart, frequent sighing, trembling, a small, quick, sometimes intermitting pulse, occasional vomiting, a pale, contracted countenance, a sense of coldness; but the tongue is seldom furred, nor are the vital and natural functions much disturbed. In this state, any sudden exertion will sometimes prove fatal.

Ergaste'rium. (From εργον, work.) A laboratory: that part of the furnace in which is contained the matter to be acted upon.

ERI'CA. (From ερεικω, to break; so named from its fragility, or because it is broken into rods to make besoms of.) The name of a genus of plants in the Linnæan system. Class, *Octandria;* Order, *Monogynia.* Heath.

Erice'rum. (From ερεικη, heath.) A medicine in which heath is an ingredient.

ERI'GERON. (Ηριγερων, of the ancient Greeks; from ηρ the spring, and γερων, an old man, because, in the spring, it has a white, hoary blossom, like the hair of an old man.) 1. The name of a genus of plants. Class, *Syngenesia;* Order, *Polygamia superflua.*

2. The common chick-weed is so called in old books. See *Senecio vulgaris.*

Erigerum. See *Senecio vulgaris.*

ERO'SION. (*Erosio;* from *erodo*, to gnaw off.) This word is very often used in the same sense as ulceration, viz. the formation of a breach or chasm in the substance of parts, by the action of the absorbents.

EROSUS. Jagged. A leaf is called *folium erosum*, the margin of which is irregularly cut or notched, especially when otherwise divided besides; as in *Senecio squalidus.*

EROTIA'NUS, the author of a Glossary, containing an explanation of the terms in Hippocrates, lived in the reign of Nero. The work was printed at Venice, in 1566; and also annexed to Foesius's Edition of Hippocrates.

EROTOMA'NIA. (From ερως, love, and μανια, madness.) That melancholy, or madness, which is the effect of love.

E'rpes. (From ερπω, to creep: so named from their gradually increasing in size. See *Herpes.*

ERRA'TIC. (*Erraticus;* from *erro*, to wander.) Wandering; irregular. A term occasionally applied to pains, or any disease which is not fixed, but moves from one part to another, as gout, rheumatism, &c.

E'RRHINE. (*Errhinus;* ερρινα, from εν, in, and ριν, the nose.) By errhines are to be understood those medicines which, when topically applied to the internal membrane of the nose, excite sneezing, and increase the secretion, independent of any mechanical irritation. The articles belonging to this class may be referred to two orders.

1. *Sternutatory errhines;* as *nicotiana, helleborus, euphorbium*, which are selected for the torpid, the vigorous, but not plethoric, and those to whom any degree of evacuation would not be hurtful.

2. *Evacuating errhines;* as *asarum*, &c. which are calculated for the phlegmatic and infirm.

E'RROR LOCI. Boerhaave is said to have introduced this term, from the opinion that the vessels were of different sizes, for the circulation of blood, lymph, and serum, and that when the larger sized globules were forced into the less vessels, they became obstructed, by an *error of place.* But this opinion does not appear to be well-grounded.

ERU'CA. (From *erugo*, to make smooth; so named from the smoothness of its leaves, or from *uro*, to burn, because of its biting quality.) See *Brassica eruca.*

ERUCA SYL'VESTRIS. The wild rocket. See *Brassica eruca.*

ERUCTATION. Belching.

ERUPTION. *Eruptio.* A discoloration, or spots on the skin; as the eruption of small-pox, measles, nettle-rash, &c.

ERUTHEMA. (From ερυθω, to make red.) A fiery red tumour, or pustules on the skin.

E'RVUM. (*Quasi arvum*, a field, because it grows wild in the fields; or from *eruo*, to pluck out, because it is diligently plucked from corn.) The tare. 1. The name of a genus of plants in the Linnæan system. Class, *Diadelphia;* Order, *Decandria.*

2. The pharmacopœial name of tare. See *Ervum ervilia.*

ERVUM ERVILIA. *Orobus.* The seeds of this plant, *Ervum ervilia—germinibus undatoplicatis, foliis imparipinnatis* of Linnæus, have been made into bread in times of scarcity, which is not the most salubrious. The meal was formerly among the resolvent remedies by way of poultice.

ERVUM LENS. The systematic name of the lentil. *Lens.* Φακος of the Greeks. *Ervum—pedunculis subbifloris; seminibus compressis, convexis*, of Linnæus. There are two varieties; the one with large, the other with small seeds. They are eaten in many places as we eat pease, than which they are more flatulent, and more difficult to digest. A decoction of these seeds is used as a lotion to the ulcerations after small-pox and, it is said, with success.

ERY'NGIUM. (From ερυγγανω, to eructate.) Eryngo, or sea-holly. 1. The name of a genus of plants in the Linnæan system. Class *Pentandria;* Order, *Digynia.*

2. The pharmacopœial name of the sea-holly. See *Eryngium maritimum.*

["ERYNGIUM AQUATICUM. *Button snake-root.* The Eryngium aquaticum is a native of the southern states. We are told in Mr. Elliott's botany, that the root is of a pungent, bitter, and aromatic taste. When chewed, it very sensibly excites a flow of saliva. A decoction of it is diaphoretic and expectorant, and sometimes proves emetic. It is preferred by some physicians to the Seneca snake-root, which it much resembles in its effects." A.]

ERYNGIUM CAMPESTRE. The root of this plant, *Eryngium—foliis radicalibus, amplexicaulibus, pinnato-lanceolatis*, of Linnæus, is used in many places for that of the sea-eryngo. See *Eryngium.*

ERYNGIUM MARITIMUM. The systematic name of the sea-holly or eryngo. *Eryngium—foliis radicalibus subrotundis, plicatis spinosis, capitulis pedunculatis, paleis tricuspidatis*, of Linnæus. The root of this plant is directed for medical use. It has no particular smell, but to the taste it manifests a grateful sweetness; and, on being chewed for some time, it discovers a light aromatic warmth or pungency. It was formerly celebrated for its supposed aphrodisiac powers, but it is now very rarely employed.

ERYNGO. See *Eryngium.*

Eryngo, sea. See *Eryngium.*

Eryngo-leaved lichen. See *Lichen islandicus.*

ERY'SIMUM. (From ερυω, to draw, so called from its power of drawing and producing blisters. Others derive it from απο του ερεικειν, because the leaves are much cut; others from εριτιμον, precious.) 1. The name of a genus of plants in the Linnæan system. Class, *Tetradynamia;* Order, *Siliquosa.*

2. The pharmacopœial name of the hedge-mustard See *Erysimum officinale.*

ERYSIMUM ALLIARIA. The systematic name of Jack-in-the-hedge. *Alliaria; Chamæplion* of Oribasius. Sauce alone, or stinking hedge-mustard. The plant to which this name is given, is the *Erysimum foliis cordatis*, of Linnæus; it is sometimes exhibited in humid asthma and dyspnœa, with success. Its virtues are powerfully diaphoretic, diuretic, and antiscorbutic.

ERYSIMUM BARBAREA. The systematic name of the *barbarea* of the shops. The leaves of this plant, *Erysimum—foliis lyratis, extimo subrotundo* of Linnæus, may be ranked among the antiscorbutics. They are seldom used in practice.

ERYSIMUM OFFICINALE. The systematic name of the hedge-mustard. *Erysimum—siliquis spicæ adpressis, foliis runcinatis*, of Linnæus. It was formerly much used for its expectorant and diuretic qualities, which are now forgotten. The seeds are warm and pungent, and very similar to those of mustard in their sensible effects.

ERYSI'PELAS. (From ερυω, to draw, and πελας, adjoining: named from the neighbouring parts being affected by the eruption.) *Ignis sacer.* The rose, or St. Anthony's fire. A genus of disease in the class *Pyrexiæ*, and order *Exanthemata* of Cullen. It is known by synocha of two or three days' continuance, with drowsiness, and sometimes with delirium; pulse commonly full and hard; then erythema of the face, or some other part, with continuance of synocha, tending either to abscess or gangrene. There are two species of this disease, according to Cullen: 1. *Erysipelas vesiculosum*, with large blisters: 2. *Erysipelas phlyctænodes*, the shingles or an erysipelas with phlyctænæ, or small blisters.

This disease is an inflammatory affection, principally of the skin, when it makes its appearance externally, and of the mucous membrane when it is seated internally; and is more liable to attack women and children, and those of an irritable habit, than those of a plethoric and robust constitution.

It is remarkable that erysipelas sometimes returns periodically, attacking the patient once or twice a year, or even once every month, and then by its repeated attacks it often gradually exhausts the strength, especially if he be old and of a bad habit.

When the inflammation is principally confined to the skin, and is unattended by any affection of the system, it is then called erythema; but when the system is affected, it is named erysipelas.

Every part of the body is equally liable to it, but it more frequently appears on the face, legs, and feet, than any where else, when seated externally; and it occurs oftener in warm climates than phlegmonous inflammation

It is brought on by all the causes that are apt to excite inflammation, such as injuries of all kinds, the external application of stimulants, exposure to cold, and obstructed perspiration; and it may likewise be occasioned by a certain matter generated within the body, and thrown out on its surface. A particular state of the atmosphere seems sometimes to render it epidemical.

In slight cases, where it attacks the extremities, it makes its appearance with a roughness, heat, pain, and redness of the skin, which becomes pale when the finger is pressed upon it, and again returns to its former colour, when it is removed. There prevails likewise a small febrile disposition, and the patient is rather hot and thirsty. If the attack is mild, these symptoms will continue only for a few days, the surface of the part affected will become yellow, the cuticle or scarf-skin will fall off in scales, and no further inconvenience will perhaps be experienced; but if the attack has been severe, and the inflammatory symptoms have run high, then there will ensue pains in the head and back, great heat, thirst, and restlessness; the part affected will slightly swell: the pulse will become small and frequent; and about the fourth day, a number of little vesicles, containing a limpid, and, in some cases, a yellowish fluid, will arise. In some instances, the fluid is viscid, and instead of running out, as generally happens when the blister is broken, it adheres to and dries upon the skin.

In unfavourable cases, these blisters sometimes degenerate into obstinate ulcers, which now and then become gangrenous. This, however, does not happen frequently; for although it is not uncommon for the surface of the skin and the blistered places to appear livid, or even blackish, yet this usually disappears with the other symptoms.

The period at which the vesicles show themselves is very uncertain. The same may be said of the duration of the eruption. In mild cases, it often disappears gradually, or is carried off by spontaneous sweating. In some cases it continues, without showing any disposition to decline, for twelve or fourteen days, or longer.

The trunk of the body is sometimes attacked with erysipelatous inflammation, but less frequently so than the extremities. It is not uncommon, however, for infants to be attacked in this manner a few days after birth; and in these it makes its appearance about the genitals. The inflamed skin is hard, and apparently very painful to the touch. The belly often becomes uniformly tense, and sphacelated spots sometimes are to be observed. From dissections made by Dr. Underwood, it appears, that in this form of the disease the inflammation frequently spreads to the abdominal viscera.

Another species of erysipelatous inflammation, which most usually attacks the trunk of the body, is that vulgarly known by the name of *shingles*, being a corruption of the French word *ceingle*, which implies a belt. Instead of appearing a uniform inflamed surface, it consists of a number of little pimples extending round the body a little above the umbilicus, which have vesicles formed on them in a short time. Little or no danger ever attends this species of erysipelas.

When erysipelas attacks the face, it comes on with chilliness, succeeded by heat, restlessness, thirst, and other febrile symptoms, with a drowsiness or tendency to coma or delirium, and the pulse is very frequent and full. At the end of two or three days, a fiery redness appears on some part of the face, and this extends at length to the scalp, and then gradually down the neck, leaving a tumefaction in every part the redness has occupied. The whole face at length becomes turgid, and the eyelids are so much swelled as to deprive the patient of sight. When the redness and swelling have continued for some time, blisters of different sizes, containing a thin colourless acrid liquor, arise on different parts of the face, and the skin puts on a livid appearance in the blistered places; but in those not affected with blisters, the cuticle, towards the close of the disease, falls off in scales.

No remission of the fever takes place on the appearance of the inflammation on the face; but, on the contrary, it is increased as the latter extends, and both will continue probably for the space of eight or ten days. In the course of the inflammation, the disposition to coma and delirium are sometimes so increased as to destroy the patient between the seventh and eleventh days of the disease. When the complaint is mild, and not leading to a fatal event, the inflammation and fever generally cease gradually without any evident crisis.

If the disease arises in a bad habit of body, occupies a part possessed of great sensibility, is accompanied with much inflammation, fever, and delirium, and these take place at an early period, we may suppose the patient exposed to imminent danger. Where translations of the morbid matter take place, and the inflammation falls on either the brain, lungs, or abdominal viscera, we may entertain the same unfavourable opinion. Erysipelas never terminates in suppuration, unless combined with a considerable degree of phlegmonous inflammation, which is, however, sometimes the case; but in a bad habit, it is apt to terminate in gangrene, in which case there will be also great danger. When the febrile symptoms are mild, and unaccompanied by delirium or coma, and the inflammation does not run high, we need not be apprehensive of danger.

Where the disease has occupied the face, and proves fatal, inflammation of the brain, and its consequences, are in some cases met with on dissection.

The treatment of erysipelas must proceed on the antiphlogistic plan, varied however in its activity according to the type of the disease. When it occurs in robust plethoric constitutions, partaking of the phlegmonous character, with severe synochal fever, it will be proper to begin by taking a moderate quantity of blood, then direct cooling saline purgatives, antimonial diaphoretics, a light vegetable diet, &c. When the disorder attacks the face, it may be better to use cupping behind the neck, and keep the head somewhat raised. But if the disease exhibits rather the typhoid type, and particularly where there is a tendency to gangrene, the patient's strength must be supported: after clearing out the primæ viæ, and endeavouring to promote the other secretions by mild evacuants, when the pulse begins to fail, a more nutritious diet, with a moderate quantity of wine, and the decoction of bark with sulphuric acid, or other tonic medicine, may be resorted to; nay, even the bark in substance, and the more powerful stimulants, as ammonia, &c. ought to be tried, if the preceding fail. Should the inflammation, quitting the skin, attack an internal part, a blister, or some rubefacient, may help to relieve the patient; and stimulants to the lower extremities will likewise be proper, where the head is severely affected. To the inflamed part of the skin, applications must not be too freely made: where there is much pain and heat, cooling it occasionally, with plain water, is perhaps best; and where an acrid discharge occurs, washing it away from time to time with warm milk and water. Should suppuration happen, it is important to make an early opening for the escape of the matter, to obviate the extensive sloughings otherwise apt to follow, and where gangrene occurs, the fermenting cataplasm may be applied.

ERYTHE'MA. (From ερυθρος, red.) Inflammatory blush. A morbid redness of the skin, as is observed upon the cheeks of hectic patients after eating, and the skin covering bubo, phlegmon, &c.

ERYTHRO'DANUM. (From ερυθρος, red: so called from the colour of its juice.) See *Rubia tinctorum*.

ERYTHROEI'DES. (From ερυθρος, red, and ειδος, a likeness: so called from its colour.) A name given to the tunica vaginalis testis.

ERYTHRO'NIUM. (From ερυθρος, red: so called from the red colour of its juice.) A species of satyrion.

["ERYTHRONIUM AMERICANUM. The Erythronium Americanum is an emetic in its recent state, producing vomiting in the *dose* of thirty or forty grains. This property is impaired by drying. The affinity of the plant to *Colchicum*, and some others of known activity, renders it deserving of further investigation. The bulbs should be dug when the leaves first appear, before flowering. A pure fecula may be obtained from them."—*Big. Mat. Med.* A.]

ERYTHRO'XYLUM. (From ερυθρος, red, and ξυλον, wood: so named from its colour.) Logwood. See *Hæmatoxylum*.

E'RYTHRUS. (From ερυθρος, red: so named from the red colour of its juice.) The sumach. See *Rhus coriaria*.

E'SAPHE. (From εσαφαω, to feel.) The touch; or feeling the mouth of the womb, to ascertain its condition.

E'SCHAR. (Εσχαρα; from εσχαροω, to scab over.) *Eschara*. The portion of flesh that is destroyed by the application of a caustic, and which sloughs away.

ESCHARO'TIC. (*Escharoticus;* from εσχαροω, to scab over.) Caustic; corrosive. A term given by surgeons to those substances which possess a power of destroying the texture of the various solid parts of the animal body to which they are directly applied. The articles of this class of substances may be arranged under two orders:

1. *Eroding escharotics;* as blue vitriol, *alumen ustum*, &c.

2. *Caustic escharotics;* as *lapis infernalis, argenti nitras, acidum sulphuricum, nitricum*, &c.

ESCULENT. *Esculentus*. An appellation given to such animals, fishes, and plants, or any part of them, that may be eaten for food.

E'SOX. The name of a genus of fishes. Class, *Pisces;* Order, *Abdominales*.

ESOX LUCIUS. The systematic name of the pike fish, from the liver of which an oil is separated spontaneously, which is termed, in some pharmacopœias, *oleum lucii piscis*. It is used in some countries, by surgeons, to destroy spots of the transparent cornea.

E'SSENCE. Several of the volatile or essential oils are called by this name.

ESSENTIAL. *Essentialis*. Something that is necessary to constitute a thing, or that has such a connexion with the nature of a thing, that is found wherever the thing itself is; thus the heart, brain, spinal marrow, lungs, stomach, &c. are parts essential to life.

In natural history, it is applied to those circumstances which mark or distinguish an animal or plant from all others in the same order or genus.

Esse'ntial oil. See *Oil*.

E'SSERA. (*Essera*, from *Eshera*, an Arabian word literally meaning *papulæ*.) A species of cutaneous eruption, distinguished by broad, shining, smooth, red spots, mostly without fever, and differing from the nettle-rash in not being elevated. It generally attacks the face and hands.

Esthiomenos. (From εσθιω, to eat.) A term formerly applied to any disease which rapidly destroyed, or, as it were, ate away the flesh, as some forms of herpes, lupus, cancer.

E'SULA. (From esus, eaten, because it is eaten by some as a medicine.) Spurge.

Esula major. See *Euphorbia palustris*.

Esula minor. See *Euphorbia cyparissias*.

E'THER. See *Æther*.

Ether, acetic. Acetic naphtha. An ethereal fluid, drawn over from an equal admixture of alkohol and acetic acid, distilled with a gentle heat from a glass retort in a sand-bath It has a grateful smell, is extremely light, volatile, and inflammable.

Ether muriatic. Marine æther. Muriatic æther is obtained by fixing and distilling alkohol with extremely concentrated muriate of tin. It is stimulant, antiseptic, and diuretic.

Ether, nitrous. Nitric naphtha. This is only a stronger preparation than the spiritus ætheris nitrici of the London Pharmacopœia; it is produced by the distillation of two parts of alkohol to one part and a half of fuming nitric acid.

Ether, sulphuric. See *Æther sulphuricus*.

Ether, vitriolic. See *Æther sulphuricus*.

ETHEREAL. A term applied to any highly rectified essential oil, or spirit. See *Oleum æthereum*.

Ethiops, antimonia. See *Æthiops antimonialis*.

Ethiops, martial. The black oxide of iron.

Ethiops mineral. See *Hydrargyri sulphuretum nigrum*.

Ethiops per se. See *Hydrargyri oxydum cinereum*.

ETHMOID. (*Ethmoides*; from εφμος, a sieve, and ειδος, form: because it is perforated like a sieve.) Sieve-like.

Ethmoid bone. *Os ethmoideum; os æthmoides*. Cribriform bone. A bone of the head. This is, perhaps, one of the most curious bones of the human body. It appears almost a cube, not of solid bone, but exceedingly light, spongy, and consisting of many convoluted plates, which form a net-work, like honey-comb. It is curiously enclosed in the os frontis, between the orbitary processes of that bone. One horizontal plate receives the olfactory nerves, which perforate that plate with such a number of small holes, that it resembles a sieve; whence the bone is named cribriform, or ethmoid bone. Other plates dropping perpendicularly from this one, receive the divided nerves, and gave them an opportunity of expanding into the organ of smelling; and these bones, upon which the olfactory nerves are spread out, are so much convoluted as to extend the surface of this sense very greatly, and are named spongy bones. Another flat plate lies in the orbit of the eye; and being very smooth, by the rolling of the eye, it is named the os planum, or smooth bone. So that the ethmoid bone supports the forepart of the brain, receives the olfactory nerves, forms the organ of smelling, and makes the chief part of the orbit of the eye; and the spongy bones, and the os planum, are neither of them distinct bones, but parts of this ethmoid bone.

The *cribriform plate* is exceedingly delicate and thin; lies horizontally over the root of the nose; and fills up neatly the space between the two orbitary plates of the frontal-bone. The olfactory nerves, like two small flat lobes, lie out upon this plate, and, adhering to it, shoot down like many roots through this bone, so as to perforate it with numerous small holes, as if it had been dotted with the point of a pin, or like a nutmeg-grater. This plate is horizontal; but its processes are perpendicular, one above, and three below.

1. The first perpendicular process is what is called *crista galli*; a small perpendicular projection, somewhat like a cock's comb, but exceedingly small, standing directly upwards from the middle of the cribriform plate, and dividing that plate into two; so that one olfactory nerve lies upon each side of the crista galli; and the root of the falx, or septum, between the two hemispheres of the brain, begins from this process. The foramen cæcum, or blind hole of the frontal bone, is formed partly by the root of the crista galli, which is very smooth, and sometimes, it is said, hollow, or cellular.

3. Exactly opposite this, and in the same direction with it, *i. e.* perpendicular to the ethmoid plate, stands out the *nasal plate* of the ethmoid bone. It is sometimes called azygous, or single process of the ethmoid, and forms the beginning of that septum, or partition, which divides the two nostrils. This process is thin but firm, and composed of solid bone; it is commonly inclined a little to one side, so as to make the nostrils of unequal size. The azygous process is united with the vomer, which forms the chief part of the partition; so that the septum, or partition of the nose, consists of the azygous process of the ethmoid bone above, of the vomer below, and of the cartilage in the fore or projecting part of the nose; but the cartilage rots away, so that whatever is seen of the septum in the skull must be part either of the ethmoid bone or vomer.

2. Upon either side of the septum, there hangs down a *spongy bone*, one hanging in each nostril. They are each rolled up like a scroll of parchment; they are very spongy; are covered with a delicate and sensible membrane; and when the olfactory nerves depart from the clibriform plate of the ethmoid bone, they attach themselves to the septum, and to these upper spongy bones, and expand upon them so that the convolutions of these bones are of material use in expanding the organ of swelling, and detaining the odorous effluvia till the impression be perfect. Their convolutions are more numerous in the lower animals, in proportion as they need a more acute sense. They are named spongy or turbinated bones, from their convolutions resembling the many folds of a turban.

The spongy bones have a great many honey-comb-like cells connected with them, which belong also to the organ of smell, and which are useful perhaps by detaining the effluvia of odorous bodies, and also by reverberating the voice. Thus, in a common cold, while the voice is hurt by an affection of these cells, the sense of smelling is almost lost.

4. The *orbitary plate*, of the ethmoid bone, is a large surface; consisting of a very firm plate of bone, of a regular square form: exceedingly smooth and polished; it forms a great part of the socket for the eye, lying on its inner side. When we see it in the detached bone, we know it to be just the flat side of the ethmoid bone; but while it is incased in the socket of the eye, we should believe it to be a small square bone: and from this, and from its smoothness, it has got the distinct name of os planum.

The cells of the ethmoid bone, which form so important a share of the organ of smell, are arranged in great numbers along the spongy bone. They are small neat cells, much like a honey-comb, and regularly arranged in two rows, parted from each other by a thin partition; so that the os planum seems to have one set of cells attached to it, while another regular set of cells belongs in like manner to the spongy bones. There are thus twelve in number opening into each other, and into the nose.

These cells are frequently the seat of venereal ulcers; and the spongy bones are the surface where polypi often sprout up. And from the general connexions and forms of the bone, we can easily understand how the venereal ulcer, when deep in the nose, having got to these cells, cannot be cured, but undermines all the face; how the venereal disease, having affected the nose, soon spreads to the eye: and how even the brain itself is not safe. We see the danger of a blow upon the nose, which, by a force upon the septum, or middle partition, may depress the delicate cribriform plate, so as to oppress the brain with all the effects of a fractured skull, and without any operation which can give relief. And we also see the danger of pulling away polypi, which are firmly attached to the upper spongy bone.

ETHMOI'DES. See *Ethmoid bone*.

ETMULLER, Michael, was born at Leipsic, in 1644. He graduated there at the age of twenty-four, after going through the requisite studies, and much improving himself by travelling through different parts of Europe. Eight years after he was appointed professor of botany in that University, as well as extraordinary professor of surgery and anatomy. He fulfilled those offices with great applause, and his death, which happened in 1683, was generally regretted by the faculty of Leipsic. He was a very voluminous writer, and his works were considered to have sufficient merit to be translated into most European languages.

E'TRON. (From εδω, to eat, as containing the receptacles of the food.) The hypogastrium.

EUA'NTHEMUM. (From ευ, well, and ανθεμος, a flower: so named from the beauty of its flowers.) The chamomile.

EUA'PHIUM. (From ευ, well, and αφη, the touch, so called because its touch was supposed to give ease.) A medicine for the piles.

EUCHLORINE. See *Chlorous oxide.*

EUCLASE. The prismatic emerald.

EUDIALITE. A brownish red-coloured mineral, belonging to the tessular system of Mohs.

EUDIO'METER. An instrument by which the quantity of oxygen and nitrogen in atmospherical air can be ascertained. Several methods have been employed, all founded upon the principle of decomposing common air by means of a body which has a greater affinity for the oxygen. See *Eudiometry.*

EUDIOMETRY. The method of ascertaining the purity of atmospheric air.

No sooner was the composition of the atmosphere known, than it became an inquiry of importance to find out a method of ascertaining, with facility and precision, the relative quantity of oxygen gas contained in a given bulk of atmospheric air.

The instruments in which the oxygen gas of a determined quantity of air was ascertained, received the name of *Eudiometers*, because they were considered as measures of the purity of air. They are, however, more properly called *Oximeters.*

The eudiometers proposed by different chemists, are the following.

1. *Priestley's Eudiometer.*—The first eudiometer was made in consequence of Dr. Priestley's discovery, that when nitrous gas is mixed with atmospheric air over water, the bulk of the mixture diminishes rapidly, in consequence of the combination of the gas with the oxygen of the air, and the absorption of the nitric acid thus formed by the water.

When nitrous gas is mixed with nitrogen gas, no diminution takes place; but when it is mixed with oxygen gas, in proper proportions, the absorption is complete. Hence it is evident, that in all cases of a mixture of these two gases, the diminution will be proportional to the quantity of the oxygen. Of course it will indicate the proportion of oxygen in air; and, by mixing it with different portions of air, it will indicate the different quantities of oxygen which they contain, provided the component parts of air be susceptible of variation.

Dr. Priestley's method was to mix together equal bulks of air and nitrous gas in a low jar, and then transfer the mixture into a narrow graduated glass tube about three feet long, in order to measure the diminution of bulk. He expressed this diminution by the number of hundredth parts remaining. Thus, suppose he had mixed together equal parts of nitrous gas and air, and that the sum total was 200 (or 2.00): suppose the residuum, when measured in the graduated tube, to amount to 104 (or 1.04), and of course that 96 parts of the whole had disappeared, he denoted the purity of the air thus tried by 104.

This method of analyzing air by means of nitrous gas is liable to many errors. For the water over which the experiment is made may contain more or less carbonic acid, atmospheric air, or other heterogeneous substance. The nitrous gas is not always of the same purity, and is partly absorbed by the nitrous acid which is formed; the figure of the vessel, and many other circumstances are capable of occasioning considerable differences in the results.

Fontana, Cavendish, Ladriani, Magellan, Von Humboldt, and Dr. Falconer, have made series of laborious experiments to bring the test of nitrous gas to a state of complete accuracy; but, notwithstanding the exertions of these philosophers, the methods of analyzing air by means of nitrous gas are liable to so many anomalies, that it is unnecessary to give a particular description of the different instruments invented by them.

2. *Scheele's Eudiometer.*—This is merely a graduated glass cylinder, containing a given quantity of air, exposed to a mixture of iron filings and sulphur, formed into a paste with water. The substances may be made use of in the following manner:

Make a quantity of sulphur in powder, and iron filings, into a paste with water, and place the mixture in a saucer, or plate, over water, on a stand raised above the fluid; then invert over it a graduated bell-glass, and allow this to stand for a few days. The air contained in the bell-glass will gradually diminish, as will appear from the ascent of the water.

When no further diminution takes place, the vessel containing the sulphuret must be removed, and the remaining air will be found to be nitrogen gas, which was contained in that quantity of atmospheric air.

In this process, the moistened sulphuret of iron has a great affinity to oxygen; it attracts and separates it from the atmospheric air, and the nitrogen gas is left behind; the sulphur, during the experiment, is converted into sulphuric acid, and the iron oxidized, and sulphate of iron results.

The air which is exposed to moistened iron and sulphur, gradually becomes diminished, on account of its oxygen combining with a portion of the sulphur and iron, while its nitrogen remains behind. The quantity of oxygen contained in the air examined becomes thus obvious, by the diminution of bulk, which the volume of air submitted to examination has undergone.

A material error to which this method is liable, is that the sulphuric acid which is formed, acts partly on the iron, and produces hydrogen gas, which joins to some of the nitrogen forming ammonia; and hence it is that the absorption amounts in general to 0.27 parts, although the true quantity of oxygen is no more than from 0.21 to 0.22.

3. *De Marti's Eudiometer.*—De Marti obviated the errors to which the method of Scheele was liable. He availed himself, for that purpose, of an hydroguretted sulphuret, formed by boiling sulphur and liquid potassa, or lime water, together. These substances, when newly prepared, have the property of absorbing a minute portion of nitrogen gas; but they lose this property when saturated with that gas, which is easily effected by agitating them for a few minutes in contact with a small portion of atmospheric air.

The apparatus is merely a glass tube, ten inches long, and rather less than half an inch in diameter, open at one end, and hermetically sealed at the other. The close end is divided into one hundred equal parts, having an interval of one line between each division. The use of this tube is to measure the portion of air to be employed in the experiment. The tube is filled with water; and by allowing the water to run out gradually, while the tube is inverted, and the open end kept shut with the finger, the graduated part is exactly filled with air. These hundredth parts of air are introduced into a glass bottle, filled with liquid sulphuret of lime previously saturated with nitrogen gas, and capable of holding from two to four times the bulk of the air introduced. The bottle is then to be closed with a ground glass stopper, and agitated for five minutes. After this, the stopper is to be withdrawn, while the mouth of the phial is under water; and, for the greater accuracy, it may be closed and agitated again. Lastly, the air is to be again transferred to the graduated glass tube, in order to ascertain the diminution of its bulk.

4. *Humboldt's Eudiometer* consists in decomposing a definite quantity of atmospheric air, by means of the combustion of phosphorus, after which, the portion of gas which remains must be measured.

Take a glass cylinder, closed at the top, and whose capacity must be measured into sufficiently small portions by a graduated scale fixed on it. If the instrument be destined solely for examining atmospheric air, it will be sufficient to apply the scale from the orifice of the cylinder down to about half its length, or to sketch that scale on a slip of paper pasted on the outside of the tube, and to varnish it over with a transparent varnish.

This half of the eudiometrical tube is divided into fifty equidistant parts, which in this case indicate hundredth parts of the whole capacity of the instrument.

Into this vessel, full of atmospheric air, put a piece of dry phosphorus (one grain to every twelve cubic inches), close it air-tight, and heat it gradually, first the sides near the bottom, and afterward the bottom itself. The phosphorus will take fire and burn rapidly. After every thing is cold, invert the mouth of the eudiometer-tube into a basin of water, and withdraw the cork. The water will ascend in proportion to the loss of oxygen gas the air has sustained, and thus its quantity may be ascertained.

Analogous to this is,

5. *Seguin's Eudiometer*, which consists of a glass tube, of about one inch in diameter, and eight or ten inches high, closed at the upper extremity. It is filled with mercury, and kept inverted in this fluid in the mercurial trough. A small bit of phosphorus is introduced into it, which, on account of its specific gravity being less than that of mercury, will rise up in it to the top. The phosphorus is then melted by means of a red-hot poker, or burning coal applied to the outside of the tube. When the phosphorus is liquefied, small portions of air destined to be examined, and which have been previously measured in a vessel graduated to the cubic inch, or into grains, are introduced into the tube. As soon as the air which is sent up reaches the phosphorus, a combustion will take place, and the mercury will rise again. The combustion continues till the end of the operation; but, for the greater exactness, Seguin directs the residuum to be heated strongly. When cold, it is introduced into the graduated vessel to ascertain its volume. The difference of the two volumes gives the quantity of the oxygen gas contained in the air subjected to examination.

6. *Berthollet's Eudiometer.*—Instead of the rapid combustion of phosphorus, Berthollet has substituted its spontaneous combustion, which absorbs the oxygen of atmospheric air completely; and, when the quantity of air operated on is small, the process is accomplished in a short time.

Berthollet's apparatus consists of a narrow graduated glass tube, containing the air to be examined, into which is introduced a cylinder, or stick of phosphorus, supported upon a glass rod, while the tube stands inverted in water. The phosphorus should be nearly as long as the tube. Immediately after the introduction of the phosphorus, white vapours are formed which fill the tube; these vapours gradually descend, and become absorbed by the water. When no more white vapours appear, the process is at an end, for all the oxygen gas which was present in the confined quantity of air, has united with the phosphorus: the residuum is the quantity of nitrogen of the air submitted to examination.

This eudiometer, though excellent of the kind, is nevertheless not absolutely to be depended upon; for, as soon as the absorption of oxygen is completed, the nitrogen gas exercises an action upon the phosphorus, and thus its bulk becomes increased. It has been ascertained, that the volume of nitrogen gas is increased by 1-40th part; consequently the bulk of the residuum, diminished by 1-40th, gives us the bulk of the nitrogen gas of the air examined; which bulk, subtracted from the original mass of air, gives us the proportion of oxygen gas contained in it. The same allowance must be made in the eudiometer of Seguin.

7. *Davy's Eudiometer.*—Until very lately, the preceding processes were the methods of determining the relative proportions of the two gases which compose our atmosphere.

Some of these methods, though very ingenious, are so extremely slow in their action, that it is difficult to ascertain the precise time at which the operation ceases. Others have frequently involved inaccuracies, not easily removed.

The eudiometer of Davy is not only free from these objections, but the result it offers is always constant; it requires little address, and is very expeditious; the apparatus is portable, simple, and convenient.

Take a small glass tube, graduated into one hundred equidistant parts; fill this tube with the air to be examined, and plunge it into a bottle, or any other convenient vessel, containing a concentrated solution of green muriate or sulphate of iron, strongly impregnated with nitrous gas. All that is necessary to be done, is to move the tube in the solution a little backwards and forwards; under these circumstances, the oxygen gas contained in the air will be rapidly absorbed, and condensed by the nitrous gas in the solution, in the form of nitrous acid.

N. B. The state of the greatest absorption should be marked, as the mixture afterward emits a little gas which would alter the result.

This circumstance depends upon the slow decomposition of the nitrous acid (formed during the experiment,) by the oxide of iron, and the consequent production of a small quantity of aëriform fluid (chiefly nitrous gas); which, having no affinity with the red muriate, or sulphate of iron, produced by the combination of oxygen, is gradually evolved and mingled with the residual nitrogen gas. However, the nitrous gas evolved might be abstracted by exposing the residuum to a fresh solution of green sulphate or muriate of iron.

The impregnated solution with green muriate, is more rapid in its operation than the solution with green sulphate. In cases when these salts cannot be obtained in a state of absolute purity, the common sulphate of iron of commerce may be employed. One cubic inch of moderately impregnated solution, is capable of absorbing five or six cubic inches of oxygen, in common processes; but the same quantity must never be employed for more than one experiment.

In all these different methods of analyzing air, it is necessary to operate on air of a determinate density, and to take care that the residuum be neither more condensed nor dilated than the air was when first operated on. If these things are not attended to, no dependence whatever can be placed upon the result of the experiments, how carefully soever they may have been performed. It is, therefore, necessary to place the air, before and after the examination, into water of the same temperature. If this, and several other little circumstances, have been attended to, for instance, a change in the height of the barometer, &c. we find that air is composed of about 0.21 of oxygen gas, and 0.79 of nitrogen gas by bulk. But as the weight of these two gases is not exactly the same, the proportion of the component parts by weight will differ a little; for as the specific gravity of oxygen gas is to that of nitrogen gas as 8 to 7 nearly, it follows that 100 parts of air are composed *by weight* of about 76 nitrogen gas, and 24 oxygen gas.

The air of this metropolis, examined by means of Davy's eudiometer, was found, in all the different seasons of the year, to contain 0.21 of oxygen: and the same was the case with air taken at Islington and Highgate; in the solitary cells in Cold-Bath-Fields prison, and on the river Thames. But the quantity of water contained in a given bulk of air from these places, differed considerably.

EUGALENUS, Severinus, a physician of Doccum, in Friesland, known chiefly as the author of a Treatise on the Scurvy, in 1604, which once maintained a considerable character: but the publication of Dr. Lind, pointing out his numerous errors, has entirely superseded it.

EUGE'NIA. (So named by Micheli, in compliment to Prince Eugene of Savoy, who sent him from Germany almost all the plants described by Clusius.) The name of a genus of plants in the Linnæan system. Class, *Icosandria;* Order, *Monogynia.*

Eugenia caryophyllata. The systematic name of the tree which affords the clove. *Caryophyllus aromaticus.* It grows in the East Indies, the Moluccas, &c. The clove is the unexpanded flower, or rather the calyx; it has a strong agreeable smell, and a bitterish, hot, not very pungent, taste. The oil of cloves, commonly met with in the shops, and received from the Dutch, is highly acrimonious and sophisticated. Clove is accounted the hottest and most acrid of the aromatics; and, by acting as a powerful stimulant to the muscular fibres, may, in some cases of atonic gout, paralysis, &c. supersede most others of the aromatic class; and the foreign oil, by its great acrimony, is also well adapted for several external purposes; it is directed by several pharmacopœias, and the clove itself enters many officinal preparations.

Eugenia jambos. The systematic name of the Malabar plum-tree. The fruit smells, when ripe, like roses. On the coast of Malabar, where the trees grow plentifully, these plums are in great esteem. They are not only eaten fresh off the trees, but are preserved in sugar, in order to have them eatable all the year.

Of the flowers, a conserve is prepared, which is used medicinally as a mild adstringent.

Euge'us. (From ευ, well, and γη, the earth: so called because of its fertility.) The uterus.

EUKAIRITE. A new mineral, composed of silver, selenium, copper, and alumina, found in the copper mine of Shrickerum, in Switzerland.

Eu'le. (From ευλαζω, to putrefy.) A worm bred in foul and putrid ulcers.

Eunu'chium. (From ευνουχος, a eunuch: so called because it was formerly said to render those who eat it impotent, like a eunuch.) The lettuce. See *Lactuca.*

Eupatoriopha'lacron (From ευπατωριον, agrimony, and φαλακρος, bald.) A species of agrimony with naked heads.

EUPATO'RIUM. (From *Eupator*, its discoverer: or *quasi hepatorium*, from ηπαρ, the liver; because it was said to be useful in diseases of the liver.) 1. The name of a genus of plants in the Linnæan system. Class, *Syngenesia;* Order, *Polygamia æqualis.*

2. The pharmacopœial name of the *Eupatorium.* See *Eupatorium cannabinum.*

Eupatorium arabicum. See *Eupatorium cannabinum.*

Eupatorium cannabinum. The systematic name of the hemp agrimony. *Eupatorium; Eupatorium arabicum.* The juice of this very bitter and strong-smelling plant, *Eupatorium—foliis digitatis* of Linnæus, proves violently emetic and purgative, if taken in sufficient quantity, and promotes the secretions generally. It is recommended in dropsies, jaundices, agues, &c. and is in common use in Holland among the lower orders, as a purifier of the blood in old ulcers, scurvy, and anasarca.

Eupatorium mesues. See *Achillea ageratum.*

["Eupatorium perfoliatum. *Thoroughwort.* The *Eupatorium perfoliatum* is an indigenous vegetable, growing in wet meadows throughout the United States. The whole plant is medicinal, but the leaves and flowers are most active. The taste is intensely bitter, accompanied by a flavour peculiar to the plant, but without astringency or acrimony. A kind of extractive matter appears to contain its sensible and medicinal properties, and of this water is an adequate solvent.

"The medicinal powers of this plant are, such as its sensible qualities would seem to indicate, those of a tonic stimulant. Given in moderate quantities, either in substance, in cold infusion or decoction, it promotes digestion, strengthens the viscera, and restores tone to the system. Like other vegetable bitters, if given in large quantities, especially in warm infusion or decoction, it proves emetic, cathartic, and sudorific. Even in cold infusion, it brings on diaphoresis more readily than most tonics. It is an efficacious article in the cure of intermittents, and is much employed for this use in districts where fever and ague prevail. Cures effected by it appear to have been as speedy as those from any of the medicines in common use. Thoroughwort has been employed in small doses with benefit in other febrile complaints attended with prostration of strength in their advanced stages. Its action upon the skin has acquired for it some confidence in the treatment of cutaneous diseases.

"As a tonic, twenty or thirty grains of the powder may be given in milk or wine, or two fluid ounces of the infusion. When intended to act as an emetic, a strong decoction may be made from an ounce of the plant in a quart of water boiled to a pint. The decoction is a disagreeable, but popular and effectual medicine in catarrhs, rheumatism, and febrile attacks. It is powerfully emetic, cathartic, and sudorific."—*Big. Mat. Med.* A.]

["Eupatorium purpureum. *Gravel root.* This is a taller plant than the species already cited. Its taste is bitter, astringent, and aromatic. I am informed that it operates as a diuretic, and is employed by different country physicians as a palliative in dysury and calculous diseases."—*Big. Mat. Med.* A.]

["Eupatorium teucrium. *Wild hoarhound.* Many of the species of *Eupatorium*, which nearly resemble Eupatorium perfoliatum, in botanical habit, are likewise similar to it in medicinal properties. The present species is one of this kind. It is tonic, diaphoretic, and cathartic, and in small doses sits well on the stomach. It is extensively used in the southern states in the cure of fever and ague."—*Bigelow's Materia Medica.* A.]

["Euphorbia ipecacuanha. *Ipecacuanha spurge.* This is a low tufted plant, growing native in sandy soils in the middle and southern parts of the United States. It was at one time supposed to be the plant from which the officinal ipecacuanha is derived.

"The root is very large in proportion to the plant, fleshy, irregular, and branched. When dried, it is of a grayish colour outside, and white within. It is light and brittle, without a ligneous centre, and has about the hardness of cork. To the taste it is sweetish, and not particularly unpleasant. It contains a substance of the nature of caoutchouc, which is soluble in ether, and precipitated by alkohol; likewise resin, mucus, and probably fæcula.

"Most of the species of the extensive genus Euphorbia, are violent emetics and cathartics. The lactescent juice, which they exude when wounded, is acrid and virulent, so as to blister and ulcerate the skin when externally applied. Taken internally in large doses, they produce the violent symptoms which are common to other acrid narcotics. The Euphorbia ipecacuanha is milder in its operation than many of the other species, and has lately been revived in practice as an effectual emetic. With a view of becoming acquainted with the mode of operation of this plant, I performed a series of experiments on its action, assisted by some medical gentlemen of the Boston Dispensary and Alms-house. These trials have led to the conclusion, that this root, in doses of from ten to twenty grains, is both an emetic and cathartic; that it is more active than ipecacuanha, in proportion to the number of grains administered; that in small doses it operates with as much ease as most emetics in a majority of instances. If it fails, however, at first, it is not so safely repeated as many of the emetics in common use. If accumulated in the stomach to the amount of two or three scruples, it finally excites active and long continued vomiting, attended with a sense of heat, vertigo, indistinct vision, and great prostration of strength. Its operation seems exactly proportionate to the quantity taken, and vomiting is not checked by the powder being thrown off in the first efforts of the stomach.

"From ten to twenty grains constitute an emetic, to be given at once. If this quantity fails to vomit, it generally purges. It may be quickened by a little tartarized antimony, but ought not to be repeated to the amount of more than twenty-five or thirty grains."—*Big. Mat. Med.* A.]

EUPE'PSIA. (From ευ, well, and πεπτω, to concoct.) A good digestion.

EUPE'PTIC. (*Eupepticus;* from ευ, good, and πεπτω, to digest.) That which is of easy digestion.

EUPHODITE. A species of rock, composed of felspar and diallage.

EUPHO'RBIA. The name of a genus of plants in the Linnæan system. Class, *Dodecandria;* Order, *Trigynia.*

Euphorbia antiquorum. The systematic name of a plant supposed to produce the *Euphorbium.*

Euphorbia canariensis. In the Canary islands this species of spurge affords the gum euphorbium.

Euphorbia cyparissias. The systematic name of the cypress spurge. *Esula minor; Tithymalus cyparissius.* This, like most of the spurges, is very acrimonious, inflaming the eyes and œsophagus after touching them. It is now fallen into disuse, whatever were its virtues formerly, which, no doubt, among some others, was that of opening the bowels, for among rustics, it was called poor man's rhubarb.

["Euphorbia corollata. Large flowering spurge. The *Euphorbia corollata* is a tall species, with a five-rayed umbel, and white flowers. It grows spontaneously in dry fields from Pennsylvania to Carolina.

"The soft brittle texture of the root, and its sweetish taste, are similar to those of *Euphorbia ipecacuanha* Its chemical constitution is nearly the same, except that the quantity of resin is apparently somewhat greater.

"This is a very active medicine, of the evacuating class, operating in small doses as a cathartic, and in large ones as an emetic. It has been thought to possess about twice the strength of jalap. It exerts its cathartic efficacy in doses of less than ten grains, and if given to the amount of fifteen or twenty, it is as sure to vomit as other common emetics in their proper quantities. The only inconveniences attending these doses, which have come to my knowledge, are, that when given in small quantities, for a cathartic, it is liable to produce nausea; and in large ones, suitable for an emetic, it has sometimes induced a degree of hypercatharsis. But similar inconveniences may occur from jalap and tartarized antimony. The effects which large doses of this root may produce on the nervous system, I have not had occasion to witness. The *Euphorbia corollata*, like many others of its genus, if applied in a contused state to the skin, excites inflammation and vesication. Its volatile particles possess a certain degree of virulence, so that inflammation of the face has been brought on by handling the root. It remains to be ascertained whether the vesicating powers of this and the other species are equally definite and manageable, with those of the more common epispastic substances."—*Big. Mat. Med.* A.]

Euphorbia lathyris. The systematic name of the plant which affords the less cataputia seeds. *Cataputia minor; Euphorbia—umbella quadrifida, dichotoma, foliis oppositis integerrimis* of Linnæus. The seeds possess purgative properties; but if exhibited in an over-dose, prove drastic and poisonous: a quality peculiar to all the *Euphorbiæ*.

Euphorbia officinarum. The systematic name of the plant which affords the euphorbium in the greatest abundance. Euphorbium is an inodorous gum-resin, in yellow tears, which have the appearance of being worm-eaten; said to be obtained from several species of euphorbiæ, but principally from the *Euphorbia officinarum; aculatea nuda multangularis, aculeis germinatis* of Linnæus: it is imported from Ethiopia, Libya, and Mauritania. It contains an active resin, and is very seldom employed internally, but, as an ingredient, it enters into many resolvent and discutient plasters.

Euphorbia palustris. The systematic name of the greater spurge. The officinal plant ordered by the name, *Esula major*, in some pharmacopœias, is the *Euphorbia palustris; umbella multifida, bifida, involucellis ovatis, foliis lanceolatis, ramis sterilibus* of Linnæus. The juice is exhibited in Russia as a common purge; and the plant is given, in some places, in the cure of intermittents.

Euphorbia paralias. *Tithymalus paralios.* Sea-purge. Every part of this plant is violently cathartic and irritating, inflaming the mouth and fauces. It is seldom employed in the practice of this country; but where it is used, vinegar is recommended to correct its irritating power.

EUPHO'RBIUM. (From *Euphorbus*, the physician of king Juba, in honour of whom it was named.) See *Euphorbia officinarum.*

EUPHRA'SIA. (Corrupted from *Euphrosyne*, ευφροσυνη, from ευφρων, joyful: so called because it exhilarates the spirits.)

1. The name of a genus of plants in the Linnæan system. Class, *Didynamia;* Order, *Angiospermia.*

2. The pharmacopœial name of eye-bright. See *Euphrasia officinalis.*

Euphrasia officinalis. The systematic name of the eye-bright. This beautiful little plant, *Euphrasia—foliis ovatis, lineatis, argute dentatis* of Linnæus, has been greatly esteemed by the common people, as a remedy for all diseases of the eyes; yet, notwithstanding this, and the encomiums of some medical writers, it is now wholly fallen into disuse. It is an ingredient in the British herb-tobacco.

Eustachian tube. *Tuba eustachiana.* The tube so called was discovered by the great Eustachius. It begins, one in each ear, from the anterior extremity of the tympanum, and runs forwards and inwards in a bony canal, which terminates with the petrous portion of the temporal bone. It then goes on, partly cartilaginous, and partly membranous, gradually becoming larger, and at length ends behind the soft palate. Through this tube the air passes to the tympanum.

Eustachian valve. See *Valvula Eustachii.*

EUSTACHIUS, Bartholomew, one of the most celebrated anatomists of the 16th century, was born at San Severino, in Italy. He studied at Rome, and made himself such a proficient in anatomy, that he was chosen professor of that branch of medicine there, where he died in 1574. He was author of several works, many of which are lost, especially his treatise "De Controversiis Anatomicorum," which is much regretted. He made several discoveries in anatomy; having first described the renal capsules, and the thoracic duct; also the passage from the throat to the internal ear, named after him the Eustachian tube. A series of copperplates, to which he alludes in his "Opuscula," were recovered by Lancisi, and published in the beginning of the 18th century. He edited the Lexicon of Erotian with a commentary.

Euthypo'ria. (From Ευθυς, straight, and πορος, a passage.) *Euthiporos.* An extension made in a straight line, to put in place a fracture, or dislocation.

EVAPORA'TION. A chemical operation usually performed by applying heat to any compound substance, in order to dispel the volatile parts. "It differs from distillation in its object, which chiefly consists in preserving the more fixed matters, while the volatile substances are dissipated and lost. And the vessels are accordingly different; evaporation being commonly made in open shallow vessels, and distillation in an apparatus nearly closed from the external air.

The degree of heat must be duly regulated in evaporation. When the fixed and more volatile matters do not greatly differ in their tendency to fly off, the heat must be very carefully adjusted; but in other cases this is less necessary.

As evaporation consists in the assumption of the elastic form, its rapidity will be in proportion to the degree of heat, and the diminution of the pressure of the atmosphere. A current of air is likewise of service in this process.

Barry has lately obtained a patent for an apparatus, by which vegetable extracts for the apothecary may be made at a very gentle heat, and *in vacuo*. From these two circumstances, extracts thus prepared differ from those in common use, not only in their physical, but medicinal properties. The taste and smell of the extract of hemlock made in this way are remarkably different, as is the colour both of the soluble and feculent parts. The form of apparatus is as follows:—

The evaporating-pan, or still, is a hemispherical dish of cast-iron, polished on its inner surface, and furnished with an air-tight flat lid. From the centre of this a pipe rises, and bending like the neck of a retort, it forms a declining tube, which terminates in a copper sphere of a capacity three (four ?), times greater than that of the still. There is a stop-cock on that pipe, midway between the still and the globe, and another at the under side of the latter.

The manner of setting it to work is this:—The juice, or infusion, is introduced through a large opening into the polished iron still, which is then closed, made air-tight, and covered with water. The stop-cock which leads to the sphere is also shut. In order to produce the vacuum, steam from a separate apparatus is made to rush by a pipe through the sphere, till it has expelled all the air, for which five minutes are commonly sufficient. This is known to be effected, by the steam issuing uncondensed. At that instant, the copper sphere is closed, the steam shut off, and cold water admitted on its external surface. The vacuum thus produced in the copper sphere, which contains four-fifths of the air of the whole apparatus, is now partially transferred to the still, by opening the intermediate stop-cock. Thus, four-fifths of the air in the still rush into the sphere, and the stop-cock being shut again, a second exhaustion is effected by steam in the same manner as the first was; after which a momentary communication is again allowed between the iron still and the receiver; by this means, four-fifths of the air remaining after the former exhaustion, are expelled. These exhaustions, repeated five or six times, are usually found sufficient to raise the mercurial column to the height of 28 inches. The water-bath, in which the iron still is immersed, is now to be heated, until the fluid that is to be inspissated begins to boil which is known by inspection through a window in the apparatus, made by fastening on, air-tight, a piece of very strong glass; and the temperature at which the boiling point is kept up, is determined by a thermometer. *Ebullition* is continued until the fluid is inspissated to the proper degree of consistence, which also is tolerably judged of by its appearance through the glass window. The temperature of the boiling fluid is usually about 100° F., but it might be reduced to nearly 90°.

In the Medico-chirurgical Transactions for 1819,

(vol. x.) there is a paper by J. T. Barry on a new method of preparing Pharmaceutical Extracts. It consists in performing the evaporation *in vacuo*. For this purpose he employed apparatus which was found to answer so well, that, contemplating its application to other manufacturers, he was induced to take out a patent for it, that is to say, *for the apparatus*. As it has been erroneously supposed that the patent is for preparing extracts *in vacuo*, it may not be improper to correct the statement by a short quotation from the above paper. 'On that account, I have been induced to take out a patent for it (the apparatus). It is, however, to be recollected by this society, that I have declined having a patent for its pharmaceutical products Chemists, desirous of inspissating extracts *in vacuo*, are therefore at liberty to do it in any apparatus differing from that which has been made the subject of my patent; and thus these substances may continue the object of fair competition as to quality and price.'

The apparatus combines two striking improvements. The first consists in producing a vacuum by the agency of *steam only*, so that the use of air-pumps and the machinery requisite for working them, is superseded.

The other improvement is a contrivance for superseding the injection of water during the process of evaporation *in vacuo*."

Evergreen leaf. See *Sempervirens*.

EVERRICULUM. (From *everro*, to sweep away.) A sort of spoon, used to clear the bladder from gravel.

EXACERBATION. (*Exacerbatio*; from *exacerbo*, to become violent.) An increase of the force or violence of the symptoms of a disease. The term is generally applied to an increase of febrile symptoms.

EXÆ'RESIS. (From εξαιρεω, to remove.) One of the divisions of surgery adopted by the old surgeons; the term implies the removal of parts.

EXA'LMA. (From εξαλλομαι, to leap out.) Hippocrates applies it to the starting of the vertebræ out of their places.

EXAMBLO'MA. (From εξαμβλοω, to miscarry.) An abortion.

EXAMBLO'SIS. An abortion.

EXANASTOMO'SIS. (From εξαναστομοω, to relax, or open.) The opening of the mouths of vessels, to discharge their contents.

EXANGIA. (*Exangia*; from εξ, and αγγειον, a vessel.) The name of a genus; class, *Hæmatica*; order, *Dysthetica*, in Good's Nosology. It embraces three species, *Exangia aneurisma, varix, cyania*.

EXANTHE'MA. (*Exanthema, atis*. n.; from εξανθεω, *effloresco*, to effloresce, or break forth on a surface.) *Exanthisma*. An eruption of the skin, called a rash. It consists of red patches on the skin, variously figured; in general confluent, and diffused irregularly over the body, leaving interstices of a natural colour. Portions of the cuticle are often elevated in a rash, but the elevations are not acuminated. The eruption is usually accompanied with a general disorder of the constitution, and terminates in a few days by cuticular exfoliations.

EXANTHE'MATA. (The plural of *exanthema*.) The name of an order of diseases of the class *Pyrexiæ* in Cullen's Nosology. It includes diseases, beginning with fever, and followed by an eruption on the skin.

EXAN'THEMATICA. The name of an order of diseases, class, *Hæmatica*, in Good's Nosology. Eruptive fevers. It comprehends four genera, viz. *Exanthesis, Emphlyis, Empyesis, Anthracia*.

EXANTHESIS. (From εξ, *extra*, and ανθεω, *floreo*.) The name of a genus of disease, class, *Eccritica*; order, *Acrotica*, in Good's Nosology. Cutaneous blush. It affords only one species, *Exanthesis roseola*.

EXANTHI'SMA. See *Exanthema*.

EXANTHRO'PIA. (From εξ, without, and ανθρωπος, a man, *i. e.* having lost the faculties of a man.) A species of melancholy, in which the patient fancies himself some kind of brute.

EXARA'GMA. (From εξαραττω, to break.) A fracture.

EXA'RMA. (From εξαιρω, to lift up.) A tumour or swelling.

EXARTE'MA. (From εξαρταω, to suspend.) A charm, hung round the neck.

EXARTHRE'MA. (From εξαρθροω, to put out of joint.) *Exarthroma; Exarthrosis*. A dislocation, or luxation.

EXARTHRO'MA. See *Exarthrema*.

EXARTHRO'SIS. See *Exarthrema*.

EXARTICULA'TIO. (From *ex*, out of, and *articulus*, a joint.) A luxation, or dislocation of a bone from its socket.

EXCI'PULUM. (From *excipio*, to receive.) A chemical receiver.

EXCITABI'LITY. That condition of living bodies wherein they can be made to exhibit the functions and phenomena which distinguish them from inanimate matter, or the capacity of organized beings to be affected by various agents called *exciting powers*.

Much confusion seems to have arisen in medical controversies from the application of the word *stimuli*, to denote the means necessary to the support of life: and particularly by Brown, in his celebrated attempt to reduce the varied and complicated states of the system to the reciprocal action of the exciting powers upon the excitability. By this hypothesis, instead of regarding life as a continued series of actions, which cannot go on without certain agents constantly ministering to them, we are to suppose a substance or quality, called *excitability*, which is superadded or assigned to every being upon the commencement of its living state. The founder of the Brunonian school considers that this substance or quality is expanded by the incessant action of the exciting powers. These are—air, food, and drink, the blood and the secretions, as well as muscular exertion, sensation, thought, and passions, or emotion, or other functions of the system itself; and these powers, which exhaust the excitability or produce *excitement* (according to the language of the school), are strangely enough called *stimuli*. We are told, that it is in the due balance between the exciting powers and the excitability that health consists: for if the exciting powers be in excess, *indirect debility* is produced; and where, on the other hand the stimuli are deficient and the excitability accumulated, there ensues a state of *direct debility*.

EXCITATION. (*Excitatio*; from *excito*, to excite.) The act of awakening, rousing, or producing some power or action: thus we say, the excitation of motion, excitation of heat, excitation of the passions, &c. In natural philosophy, it is principally used in the subjects of action of living parts, and in electricity and heat.

EXCI'TEMENT. According to the opinion of Brown, excitement is the continual exhaustion of the *matter of life*, or excitability by certain agents, which have received the name of *stimuli* or exciting powers The due degree of this expension or excitement is the condition necessary to health: the excessive action of stimuli causing indirect debility and generating *sthenic* diseases, while the opposite state of deficient excitement produces direct debility, and gives birth to *asthenic* diseases: and death is said to result equally from complete exhaustion of the excitability, and from total absence of the exciting powers. Excitement is in this view equivalent to that *forced* state which is supposed by the Brunonian school to constitute life.

It has been objected to this hypothesis, that by simplifying too much the varied phenomena of healthy functions and of diseases, it necessarily classed together conditions of the system which have been considered as widely different, and of opposite tendencies, by the more patient observer. And though gladly caught at by many, as pointing out in a few general rules the mode of cure in all diseases, namely, by restoring the proper equilibrium between excitability and the action of stimuli, the Brunonian theories seem now to be considered, by those who are suspicious of bold classifications, as an example of the observation, "that the most ingenious way of becoming foolish is by a system; and the surest way to prevent truth, is to set up something in the room of it."

EXCITING. That which has the power of impressing the solids, so as to alter their action, and thus produce disease.

EXCITING CAUSE. That which, when applied to the body, excites a disease.

EXCORIA'TION. (*Excoriatio*; from *excorio*, to take off the skin.) An abrasion of the skin.

E'XCREMENT. (*Excrementum*; from *excerno*, to separate from.) The alvine fæces.

EXCRE'SCENCE. (*Excrescentia*; from *excresco*, to grow from.) Any preternatural formation of flesh, or any part of the body, as wens, warts, &c.

EXCRE'TION. (*Excretio*; from *excerno*, to separate from.) This term is applied to the separation of those fluids from the blood of an animal, that are supposed to be useless, as the urine, perspiration, and alvine fæces. The process is the same with that of secretion, except with the alvine fæces; but the term excretion is applied to those substances which, when separated from the blood, are not applied to any useful purposes in the animal economy.

EXCRETORY. (*Excretorius;* from *excerno*, to purge, sift, &c.) This name is applied to certain little ducts or vessels in the fabric of glands; thus the tubes which convey the secretion out of the testicle into the vesiculæ seminales are called the excretory ducts.

EXERCISE. See *Æora*

EXFOLIA'TION. (*Exfoliatio;* from *exfolio*, to cast the leaf.) The separation of a dead piece of bone from the living.

EXFOLIATI'VUM. (From *exfolio*, to shed the leaf.) A raspatory, or instrument for scraping exfoliating portions of bone.

EXI'SCHIOS. (From εξ, out of, and ισχιον, the ischium.) A luxation of the thigh-bone.

EXITU'RA. (From *exeo*, to come from.) A running abscess.

E'XITUS. (From *exeo*, to come out.) A prolapsus, or falling down of a part of the womb or bowel.

E'XOCHAS. (From εξω, without, and εχω, to have.) *Exoche.* A tubercle on the outside of the anus.

E'XOCHE See *Exochas.*

EXOCY'STE. See *Exocystis.*

EXOCY'STIS. (From εξω, without, and κυςις, the bladder.) *Exocyste.* A prolapsus of the inner membrane of the bladder.

EXO'MPHALUS. (From εξ, out, and ομφαλος, the navel.) *Exomphalos.* An umbilical hernia. See *Hernia umbilicalis.*

EXONCHO'MA. (From εξ, and ογχος, a tumour.) A large prominent tumour.

EXOPHTHA'LMIA. (From εξ, out, and οφθαλμος, the eye.) A swelling or protrusion of the bulb of the eye, to such a degree that the eyelids cannot cover it. It may be caused by inflammation, when it is termed *exophthalmia inflammatoria;* or from a collection of pus in the globe of the eye, when it is termed the *exophthalmia purulenta;* or from a congestion of blood within the globe of the eye, *exophthalmia sanguinea.*

EXORMIA. (Εξορμια; from εξορμαω, to break out.) The name of a genus of disease, class, *Eccritica;* order, *Acrotica*, in Good's Nosology. Papulous skin. It has four species, viz. *Exormia strophalus, lichen, prurigo, milium.*

EXOSTO'SIS. (From εξ, and οστεον, a bone.) *Hyperostosis.* A morbid enlargement, or hard tumour of a bone. A genus of disease arranged by Cullen in the class *Locales*, and order *Tumores.* The bones most frequently affected with exostosis, are those of the cranium, the lower jaw, sternum, humerus, radius, ulna, bones of the carpus, the femur, and tibia. There is, however, no bone of the body which may not become the seat of this disease. It is not uncommon to find the bones of the cranium affected with exostosis, in their whole extent. The ossa parietalia sometimes become an inch thick.

The exostosis, however, mostly rises from the surface of the bone, in the form of a hard round tumour; and venereal exostoses, or nodes, are observed to arise chiefly on compact bones, and such of these as are only superficially covered with soft parts; as, for instance, the bones of the cranium, and the front surface of the tibia.

EXPANSION. The increase of surface, or of bulk, to which natural bodies are susceptible.

EXPE'CTORANT. (*Expectorans;* from *expectoro*, to discharge from the breast.) Those medicines which increase the discharge of mucus from the lungs. The different articles referred to this class may be divided into the following orders:

1. *Nauseating expectorants;* as squill, ammoniacum, and garlic, which are to be preferred for the aged and phlegmatic.

2. *Stimulating expectorants;* as marrubium, which is adapted to the young and irritable, and those easily affected by expectorants.

3. *Antispasmodic expectorants;* as vesicatories, pediluvium, and watery vapours: these are best calculated for the plethoric and irritable, and those liable to spasmodic affections.

4. *Irritating expectorants;* as fumes of tobacco and acid vapours. The constitutions to which these are chiefly adapted, are those past the period of youth, and those in whom there are evident marks of torpor, either in the system generally, or in the lungs in particular.

[These are remedies which promote, or are administered to facilitate the discharge from the lungs both by secretion or expectoration.

This secretion is of two kinds, first the Halitus or watery vapour, and secondly the Muscus or slime. In cases of disease there are other secretions, or rather fluids to be excreted; such as,

1. Blood or sanguineous mixtures.
2. Pus or purulent mixtures.
3. Lymphatic or coagulated films, as in croup
4. Stony or calculous concretions.
5. Hydatids.

There may be too little vascular or grandular action in consequence of which the organ of respiration may be too dry, or secrete less than it ought; and also there may be too little power to throw out the secreted matters. Under the title therefore of Expectorants, are comprehended all the remedies which promote *secretion* or *excretion* in the lungs.

Respiration may be considered as a perspiratory function, and acting in conjunction with, or vicarious to, the skin, and as having also a somewhat to perform analogous to the alimentary canal. For which purpose the lungs and intestines may be strictly and properly considered as external surfaces.

When the pulmonary and bronchial vessels are considered as to the amount of blood they convey, the importance of the function, the proximity of the heart, the frequency and seriousness of the diseases to which the lungs are subjected, it will be evident that this class of remedies is worthy of being well understood.

The function of respiration in my view has an analogy to respiration.

Remedies therefore which determine the fluids to the skin, or excite the cuticular surface to secretory action, may be considered as almost *pari passu* encouraging pulmonary exhalation. This argument derives force from the common remark of the suppressed perspiration falling upon the lungs. There is no doubt that the pulmonic surface and the cuticular surface (both of which are to be considered as external) are frequently both disordered at once. But the true interpretation probably is, that the lungs do not suffer in consequence of the fluids repelled from the skin, but from the same cause which disturbs the skin: the cold, for example, which acts injuriously upon the former, produces a like mischief in the latter. They are cutaneous disorders, and are to be removed as far as the restoration of their respective secretions are concerned by corresponding means.

I therefore class *Sudorifics* among the expectorants.

Emetics are to be placed in the same class, and for a very good reason. Their action in inverting the motion of the stomach is favourable to the excretion of fluids from the trachea and bronchiæ, as well as from the stomach and fauces. This may be explained from the action of the belly, the diaphragm, and intercostals, and the compression they make upon the chest, and forcing out its contents. The same solution seems to apply, at least as far as secretion goes, to the operation of nauseating doses. Upon the same principle that they relax the skin, they relax the pulmonary surfaces.

Some expectorants are directly applied to the lungs; among which are,

1. Warm air, of a thermometric temperature to suit the patient's case.

2. Respirable air, medicated by carbonic acid to diminish its too stimulant quality.

3. Respirable air, quickened by a mixture of oxygenous gas to excite the bronchiæ and rouse them from torpor. The same may be done by ether.

4. Air qualified and tempered by the vapour of water and infused herbs, as in Mudges inhaler.

5. Teas and medicated drinks, sipped slowly, and swallowed gradually, so that a portion of their vapour may enter the trachea with the breath.

6. Dry fumes, as those of tobacco, stramonium, &c., a part of which undoubtedly enters the trachea, and cannot be excluded, as of cinnabar, frankincense, &c.

7. A medicated atmosphere, into which the odours

of plants and flowers, as of geraniums and oranges, or of gums and drugs, such as camphor and musk, may be set loose and mingled.

Other expectorants act upon the mouth and fauces by virtue of the sympathy between those parts and the lungs; such as,

1 Saccharine substances, as honey, syrups, dry sugars and their lozenges, liquorice, &c.

2. Mucilaginous substances, as gum arabic, gum tragacanth, &c.

Others again act through the medium of the stomach, as any of the before-mentioned substances when they are swallowed, and others bringing the lungs by consent into a relaxed and expectorating state.

The rules recommended in the administration of expectorants may be reduced to two.

1. To keep the patient in a warm and comfortable temperature.

2. To avoid the administration of such cathartics as seem to act contrariwise to expectorants. Can they not however be so employed as to supersede expectorants to a certain degree?

Excessive expectoration will frequently require your interposition, as,

1. In catarrhal affections of the chronic kind, where the secreted mucus must be evacuated by hawking or coughing; and the quantity of slime in chronic cases is very considerable. The disease is troublesome, and sometimes ends in hemoptysis or phthisis.

2. In phthisis pulmonalis; in which the excretion of mucus, pus, &c. is one of the most distressing symptoms, and thus often without vomica or ulceration.

3. In occasional rushes or determination of fluids to the trachea and bronchia, where prodigious quantities of slime are effused and excreted, with great exertion and straining.

The course of proceeding in each case will depend upon the particular state of the constitution, the idiosyncrasy of the patient, the acquired habits of living and physicking; and the connexion of this particular symptom, with the other symptoms of the dominant malady.

The following are the principal of the expectorants: 1. Lichen islandicus, Iceland moss. 2. Glycyrrhiza glabra, Liquorice. 3. Mimosa nilotica, Gum arabic. 4. Ulmus aspera, Slippery elm. 5. Heracleum gummosiferum, Gum ammoniac. 6. Scilla maritima, the Squill. 7. Allium sativum, Garlic. 8. Ferula, Assafœtida. 9. Arum tryphillum, March turnip. 10. Polygala Senega, Seneca snakeroot. 11. Carbonate of ammonia. 12. Carbonate of potash. 13. Carbonate of soda. 14. Colchicum-autumnale or meadow saffron. 15. Balsams of Tolu, Capivi, &c. 16. Inhalations of water, vinegar, medicated infusions. 17. Syrups and saccharine compositions, as honey and vinegar, molasses and vinegar, &c.—*Notes from Dr. Mitchill's Lect. on Mat. Med.* A]

EXPERIENCE. A kind of knowledge acquired by long use, without any teacher. Experience consists in the ideas of things we have seen or read, which the judgment has reflected on, to form for itself a rule or method.

EXPERS. Wanting; destitute. The trivial name of some diseases; as dipsosis expers, in which the thirst is wanting.

EXPIRA'TION. (*Expiratio;* from *expiro*, to breathe.) That part of respiration in which the air is thrust out from the lungs. See *Respiration.*

Expressed oil. Such oils as are obtained by pressing the substance containing them; as olives, which give out olive oil, almonds, &c.

EXSUCCA'TIO. (From *ex*, out of, and *succus*, humour.) An ecchymosis, or extravasation of humours, under the integuments.

EXTE'NSOR. (From *extendo*, to stretch out.) A term given to those muscles, the office of which is to extend any part; the term is in opposition to flexor.

EXTENSOR BREVIS DIGITORUM PEDIS. A muscle of the toes, situated on the foot. *Extensor brevis*, of Douglas. *Calcanò phalanginien commune*, of Dumas. It arises fleshy and tendinous from the fore and upper part of the os calcis, and soon forms a fleshy belly, divisible into four portions, which send off an equal number of tendons that pass over the upper part of the foot, under the tendons of the extensor longus digitorum pedis, to be inserted into its tendinous expansion. Its office is to extend the toes.

EXTENSOR CARPI RADIALIS BREVIOR. An extensor muscle of the wrist, situated on the forearm. *Radialis externus brevior*, of Albinus. *Radialis secundus*, of Winslow. It arises tendinous from the external condyle of the humerus, and from the ligament that connects the radius to it, and runs along the outside of the radius. It is inserted by a long tendon into the upper and back part of the metacarpal bone of the middle finger. It assists in extending and bringing the hand backward.

EXTENSOR CARPI RADIALIS LONGIOR. An extensor muscle of the carpus, situated on the forearm, that acts in conjunction with the former. *Radialis externus longior*, of Albinus. *Radialis externus primus*, of Winslow. It arises thin, broad, and fleshy, from the lower part of the external ridge of the os humeri, above its external condyle, and is inserted by a round tendon into the posterior and upper part of the metacarpal bone that sustains the forefingers.

EXTENSOR CARPI ULNARIS. *Ulnaris externus*, of Albinus and Winslow. It arises from the outer condyle of the os humeri, and then receives an origin from the edge of the ulna: its tendon passes in a groove behind the styloid process of the ulna, to be inserted into the inside of the basis of the metacarpal bone of the little finger.

EXTENSOR DIGITORUM COMMUNIS. A muscle situated on the forearm, that extends all the joints of the fingers. *Extensor digitorum communis manus*, of Douglas and Winslow. *Extensor digitorum communis, seu digitorum tensor*, of Cowper, and *Epichondylo-suspha-langettien commune*, of Dumas. *Cum extensore proprio auricularis*, of Albinus. It arises from the external protuberance of the humerus: and at the wrist it divides into three flat tendons, which pass under the annular ligament, to be inserted into all the bones of the fore, middle, and ring fingers.

EXTENSOR DIGITORUM LONGUS. See *Extensor longus digitorum pedis.*

EXTENSOR INDICIS. See *Indicator.*

EXTENSOR LONGUS DIGITORUM PEDIS. A muscle situated on the leg, that extends all the joints of the four small toes. *Extensor digitorum longus. Peroneo-tibisus-phalangittien commune*, of Dumas. It arises from the upper part of the tibia and fibula, and the interosseous ligament; its tendon passes under the annular ligament, and then divides into five, four of which are inserted into the second and third phalanges of the toes, and the fifth goes to the basis of the metatarsal bone. This last, Winslow reckons a distinct muscle, and calls it *Peroneus brevis.*

EXTENSOR LONGUS POLLICIS PEDIS. See *Extensor proprius pollicis pedis.*

EXTENSOR MAGNUS. See *Gastrocnemius internus.*

EXTENSOR MAJOR POLLICIS MANUS. See *Extensor secundi internodii.*

EXTENSOR MINOR POLLICIS MANUS. See *Extensor primi internodii.*

EXTENSOR OSSIS METACARPI POLLICIS MANUS. An extensor muscle of the wrist, situated on the forearm. *Abductor longus pollicis manus*, of Albinus. *Extensor primi internodii*, of Douglas. *Extensor primus pollicis*, of Winslow. *Extensor primi internodii pollicis*, of Cowper. *Cubito-radisus metacarpien du pouce*, of Dumas. It arises fleshy from the middle and posterior part of the ulna, from the posterior part of the middle of the radius, and from the interosseous ligament, and is inserted into the os trapezium, and upper part of the metacarpal bone of the thumb.

EXTENSOR POLLICIS PRIMUS. See *Extensor primi internodii.*

EXTENSOR POLLICIS SECUNDUS. See *Extensor secundi internodii.*

EXTENSOR PRIMI INTERNODII. A muscle of the thumb situated on the hand, that extends the first bone of the thumb obliquely outwards. *Extensor minor pollicis manus* of Albinus. This muscle, and the *Extensor ossis metacarpi pollicis manus*, are called *Extensor pollicis primus* by Winslow; *Extensor secundi internodii* by Douglas; *Extensor secundi internodii ossis pollicis* of Cowper. *Cubito-susphalangien du pouce* of Dumas. It arises fleshy from the posterior part of the ulna, and from the interosseous ligament, and is inserted tendinous into the posterior part of the first bone of the thumb.

Extensor proprius pollicis pedis. An exterior muscle of the great toe, situated on the foot. *Extensor longus* of Douglas. *Extensor pollicis longus* of Winslow and Cowper. *Peroneo susphalangien du pouce* of Dumas. It arises by an acute, tendinous, and fleshy beginning, some way below the head, and anterior part of the fibula, along which it runs to near its lower extremity, connected to it by a number of fleshy fibres, which descend obliquely, and form a tendon, which is inserted into the posterior part of the first and last joint of the great toe.

Extensor secundi internodii. A muscle of the thumb, situated on the hand, that extends the last joint of the thumb obliquely backwards. *Extensor major pollicis manus* of Albinus. *Extensor pollicis secundus* of Winslow. *Extensor tertii internodii* of Douglas. *Extensor internodii ossis pollicis* of Cowper. *Cubito susphalangettien du pouce* of Dumas. It arises tendinous and fleshy from the middle part of the ulna, and interosseous ligament; it then forms a tendon, which runs through a small groove at the inner and back part of the radius, to be inserted into the last bone of the thumb. Its use is to extend the last phalanx of the thumb obliquely backwards.

Extensor secundi internodii indicis proprius. See *Indicator.*

Extensor tarsi minor. See *Plantaris.*

Extensor tarsi suralis. See *Gastrocnemius internus.*

Extensor tertii internodii indicis. See *Prior indicis.*

Extensor tertii internodii minimi digiti. See *Abductor minimi digiti manus.*

Externus mallei. See *Laxator tympani.*

EXTIPULATUS. Without stipulæ. A botanical term. Applied to stems.

EXTIRPA'TION. (*Extirpatio;* from *extirpo,* to eradicate.) The complete removal or destruction of any part, either by cutting instruments, or the action of caustics.

E'XTRACT. *Extractum.* 1. When chemists use this term, they generally mean the product of an aqueous decoction.

2. In pharmacy it includes all those preparations from vegetables which are separated by the agency of various liquids, and afterward obtained from such solutions, in a solid state, by evaporation of the menstruum. It also includes those substances which are held in solution by the natural juices of fresh plants, as well as those to which some menstruum is added at the time of preparation. Now, such soluble matters are various, and mostly complicated; so that chemical accuracy is not to be looked for in the application of the term. Some chemists, however, have affixed this name to one peculiar modification of vegetable matter, which has been called *extractive,* or extract, or extractive principle; and, as this forms one constituent part of common extracts, and possesses certain characters, it will be proper to mention such of them as may influence its pharmaceutical relations. The extractive principle has a strong taste, differing in different plants: it is soluble in water, and its solution speedily runs into a state of putrefaction, by which it is destroyed. Repeated evaporations and solutions render it at last insoluble, in consequence of its combination with oxygen from the atmosphere. It is soluble in alkohol, but insoluble in æther. It unites with alumine, and if boiled with neutral salts thereof, precipitates them. It precipitates with strong acids, and with the oxides from solutions of most metallic salts, especially muriate of tin. It readily unites with alkalies, and forms compounds with them, which are soluble in water. No part, however, of this subject has been hitherto sufficiently examined.

In the preparation of all the extracts, the London Pharmacopœia requires that the water be evaporated as speedily as possible, in a broad, shallow dish, by means of a water-bath, until they have acquired a consistence proper for making pills; and, towards the end of the inspissation, that they should be constantly stirred with a wooden rod. These general rules require minute and accurate attention, more particularly in the immediate evaporation of the solution, whether prepared by expression or decoction, in the manner as well as the degree of heat by which it is performed, and the promotion of it by changing the surface by constant stirring, when the liquor begins to thicken, and even by directing a strong current of air over its surface, if it can conveniently be done. It is impossible to regulate the temperature over a naked fire, or, if it be used, to prevent the extract from burning; the use of a water-bath is, therefore, absolutely necessary, and not to be dispensed with, and the beauty and precision of extracts so prepared, will demonstrate their superiority.

EXTRAC'TION. (*Extractio;* from *extraho,* to draw out.) The taking extraneous substances out of the body. Thus bullets and splinters are said to be *extracted* from wounds; stones from the urethra, or bladder. Surgeons also sometimes apply the term *extraction* to the removal of tumours out of cavities, as, for instance, to the taking of cartilaginous tumours out of the joints. They seldom speak of extracting any diseased original part of the body; though they do so in one example, viz. the cataract.

EXTRA'CTIVE. See *Extract.*

EXTRA'CTUM. (From *extraho,* to draw out.) An extract. See *Extract.*

Extractum aconiti. Extract of aconite. Take of aconite leaves, fresh, a pound; bruise them in a stone mortar, sprinkling on a little water; then press out the juice, and, without any separation of the sediment, evaporate it to a proper consistence. The dose is from one grain to five grains. For its virtues, see *Aconitum.*

Extractum aloes purificatum. Purified extract of aloes. Take of extract of spike aloe, powdered, half a pound; boiling water, four pints. Macerate for three days in a gentle heat, then strain the solution, and set it by, that the dregs may subside. Pour off the clear solution, and evaporate it to a proper consistence. The dose, from five to fifteen grains. *See Aloës.*

Extractum anthemidis. Extract of chamomile, formerly called extractum chamæmeli. Take of chamomile flowers, dried, a pound; water, a gallon; boil down to four pints, and strain the solution while it is hot, then evaporate it to a proper consistence. The dose is ten grains to a scruple. For its virtues, see *Anthemis nobilis.*

Extractum belladonnæ. Extract of belladonna. Take of deadly night-shade leaves, fresh, a pound. Bruise them in a stone mortar, sprinkling on a little water; then press out the juice, and without any previous separation of the sediment, evaporate it to a proper consistence. The dose is from one to five grains. For its virtues, see *Atropa belladonna.*

Extractum cinchonæ. Extract of bark. Take of lance-leaved cinchona bark, bruised, a pound; water a gallon; boil down to six pints, and strain the liquor, while hot. In the same manner, with an equal quantity of water, four times boil down, and strain. Lastly, consume all the liquors, mixed together, to a proper consistence. This extract should be kept soft, for making pills, and hard to be reduced to powder.

Extractum cinchonæ resinosum. Resinous extract of bark. Take of lance-leaved cinchona bark, bruised, a pound; rectified spirit, four pints; macerate for four days and strain. Distil the tincture in the heat of a water-bath, until the extract has acquired a proper consistence. This is considered by many as much more grateful to the stomach, and, at the same time, producing all the effects of bark in substance, and by the distillation of it, it is intended that the spirit which passes over shall be collected and preserved. The dose is from ten grains to half a drachm. See *Cinchona.*

Extractum colocynthidis. Extract of colocynth. Take of colocynth pulp, a pound; water, a gallon; boil down to four pints, and strain the solution while it is hot, and evaporate it to a proper consistence. The dose is from five to thirty grains. For its virtues, see *Cucumis colocynthis.*

Extractum colocynthidis compositum. Compound extract of colocynth. Take of colocynth pulp, sliced, six drachms; extract of spike aloe, powdered, an ounce and half; scammony gum-resin, powdered, half an ounce; cardamom seeds, powdered, a drachm; proof spirit, a pint. Macerate the colocynth pulp in the spirit, for four days, in a gentle heat: strain the solution, and add it to the aloes and scammony; then, by means of a water-bath, evaporate it to a proper consistence, constantly stirring, and about the end of the inspissation, mix in the cardamom-seeds. The dose from five to thirty grains.

Extractum conii. Extract of hemlock, formerly called succus cicutæ spissatus. Take of fresh hemlock, a pound. Bruise it in a stone mortar, sprinkling on a little water; then press out the juice, and, without any separation to the sediment, evaporate it to a proper consistence. The dose, from five grains to a scruple.

EXTRACTUM ELATERII. Extract of elaterium. Cut the ripe, wild cucumbers into slices, and pass the juice, very gently expressed, through a very fine hair sieve, into a glass vessel; then set it by for some hours, until the thicker part has subsided. Pour off, and throw away the thinner part, which swims at the top. Dry the thicker part which remains in a gentle heat. The dose, from half a grain to three grains. For its virtues, see *Momordica elaterium*.

EXTRACTUM GENTIANÆ. Extract of gentian. Take of gentian root, sliced, a pound; boiling water, a gallon; macerate for twenty-four hours, then boil down to four pints; strain the hot liquor, and evaporate it to a proper consistence. Dose, from ten to thirty grains. See *Gentiana*.

EXTRACTUM GLYCYRRHIZÆ. Extract of liquorice. Take of liquorice root, sliced, a pound; boiling water, a gallon; macerate for twenty-four hours, then boil down to four pints; strain the hot liquor, and evaporate it to a proper consistence. Dose, from one drachm to half an ounce. See *Glycyrrhiza*.

EXTRACTUM HÆMATOXYLI. Extract of logwood, formerly called extractum ligni campechensis. Take of logwood, powdered, a pound; boiling water, a gallon; macerate for twenty-four hours; then boil down to four pints; strain the hot liquor, and evaporate it to a proper consistence. Dose, from ten grains to half a drachm. For its virtues, see *Hæmatoxylon campechianum*.

EXTRACTUM HUMULI. Extract of hops. Take of hops, four ounces; boiling water, a gallon; boil down to four pints; strain the hot liquor, and evaporate it to a proper consistence. This extract is said to produce a tonic and sedative power combined; the dose is from five grains to one scruple. See *Humulus lupulus*.

EXTRACTUM HYOSCYAMI. Extract of henbane. Take of fresh henbane leaves, a pound; bruise them in a stone mortar, sprinkling on a little water; then press out the juice, and, without separating the fæculencies, evaporate it to a proper consistence. Dose, from five to thirty grains. For its virtues, see *Hyoscyamus*.

EXTRACTUM JALAPÆ. Extract of jalap. Take of jalap-root powdered, a pound; rectified spirit, four pints; water, ten pints; macerate the jalap-root in the spirits for four days, and pour off the tincture; boil the remaining powder in the water, until it be reduced to two pints; then strain the tincture and decoction separately, and let the former be distilled and the latter evaporated; until each begins to grow thick. Lastly, mix the extract with the resin, and reduce it to a proper consistence. Let this extract be kept in a soft state, fit for forming pills, and in a hard one, so that it it may be reduced to powder. The dose, from ten to twenty grains. For its virtues, see *Convolvulus jalapa*.

EXTRACTUM OPII. Extract of opium, formerly called extractum thebaicum. Opium colatum. Take of opium, sliced, half a pound; water, three pints; pour a small quantity of the water upon the opium, and macerate it for twelve hours, that it may become soft; then, adding the remaining water gradually, rub them together until the mixture be complete. Set it by, that the fæculencies may subside; then strain the liquor, and evaporate it to a proper consistence. Dose, from half a grain to five grains.

EXTRACTUM PAPAVERIS. Extract of white poppy. Take of white poppy capsules bruised, and freed from the seeds, a pound; boiling water a gallon. Macerate for twenty-four hours, then boil down to four pints; strain the hot liquor, and evaporate it to a proper consistence. Six grains are about equivalent to one of opium. For its virtues, see *Papaver album*.

EXTRACTUM RHEI. Extract of rhubarb. Take of rhubarb root, powdered, a pound; proof spirit, a pint; water, seven pints. Macerate for four days in a gentle heat; then strain and set it by, that the fæculencies may subside. Pour off the clear liquor, and evaporate to a proper consistence. This extract possesses the purgative properties of the root, and the fibrous and earthy parts are separated; it is therefore, a useful basis for pills, as well as given separately. Dose, from ten to thirty grains. See *Rheum*.

EXTRACTUM SARSAPARILLÆ. Extract of sarsaparilla. Take of sarsaparilla root, sliced, a pound; boiling water, a gallon; macerate for twenty-four hours, then boil down to four pints; strain the hot liquor, and evaporate it to a proper consistence. In practice this is much used, to render the common decoction of the same root stronger and more efficacious. Dose, from ten grains to a drachm. For its virtues, see *Smilax sarsaparilla*.

EXTRACTUM SATURNI. See *Plumbi acetatis liquor*

EXTRACTUM TARAXACI. Take of dandelion root, fresh and bruised, a pound; boiling water, a gallon; macerate for twenty-four hours; boil down to four pints, and strain the hot liquor; then evaporate it to a proper consistence. Dose, from ten grains to a drachm. For its virtues, see *Leontodon taraxacum*.

[The Pharmacopœia of the United States admits the following extracts.

Extractum aconiti.
.. belladonnæ.
.. conii.
.. hyoscyami.
.. stramonii.
.. anthemidis.
.. gentianæ.
.. hæmatoxyli.
.. hellebori nigri.
.. juglandis.
.. quassiæ.
.. cinchonæ.
.. colocynthidis compositum.
.. jalapæ.
.. podophylli.
.. sambuci. A.]

EXTRAFOLIACEUS. Applied to stipulæ, which are below the footstalk, and external with respect to the leaf; as in *Astragalus onobrichis*.

EXTRAVASA'TION. (*Extravasatio;* from *extra*, without, and *vas*, a vessel.) A term applied by surgeons to fluids, which are out of their proper vessels, or receptacles. Thus, when blood is effused on the surface, or in the ventricles of the brain, it is said that there is an extravasation. When blood is poured from the vessels into the cavity of the peritonæum, in wounds of the abdomen, surgeons call this accident *extravasation*. The urine is also said to be *extravasated*, when, in consequence of a wound, or of slough ing, or ulceration, it makes its way into the cellular substance or among the abdominal viscera. When the bile spreads among the convolutions of the bowels, in wounds of the gall-bladder, it is also a species of extravasation.

EXTREMITIES. This term is applied to the limbs, as distinguishing them from the other divisions of the animal, the head and trunk. The extremities are four in number, divided in man into upper and lower; in other animals into anterior and posterior. Each extremity is divided into four parts; the upper into the shoulder, the arm, the forearm and the hand: the lower into the hip, the thigh, the leg, and the foot.

EYE. *Oculus*. The parts which constitute the eye are divided into external and internal. The external parts are:

1. The *eyebrows*, or *supercilia*, which form arches of hair above the orbit, at the lower part of the forehead. Their use is to prevent the sweat falling into the eyes, and for moderating the light above.

2. The eyelashes, or *cilia*, are the short hairs that grow on the margin of the eyelids; they keep external bodies out of the eyes and moderate the influx of light.

3. The eyelids, or *palpebræ*, of which, one is superior or upper, and the other inferior, or under; where they join outwardly, it is called the *external canthus;* inwardly, towards the nose, the *internal canthus;* they cover and defend the eyes.

The margin of the eyelids, which is cartilaginous, is called *tarsus*.

In the *tarsus*, and internal surface of the eyelids, small glands are situated, called *glandulæ Meibomianæ*, because Meibomius discovered them; they secrete an oily or mucilaginous fluid, which prevents the attrition of the eyes and eyelids, and facilitates their motions.

4. The lachrymal glands, or *glandulæ lachrymales* which are placed near the external canthus, or corner of the eyes, in a little depression of the os frontis.

From these glands six or more canals issue, which are called lachrymal ducts, or *ductus lachrymales*, and they open on the internal surface of the upper eyelid.

5. The lachrymal caruncle, or *caruncula lachrymalis*, which is situated in the internal angle, or canthus of the eyelids.

6. *Puncta lachrymalia*, are two callous orifices or openings, which appear at the internal angle of the tarsus of the eyelids; the one in the superior, the other in the inferior eyelid.

7. The *canales lachrymales*, or lachrymal ducts, are two small canals, which proceed from the lachrymal points into the lachrymal sac.

8. The *saccus lachrymalis*, or lachrymal sac, is a membraneous sac, which is situated in the internal canthus of the eye.

9. The *ductus nasalis*, or nasal duct, is a membraneous canal, which goes from the inferior part of the lachrymal sac through the bony canal below, and a little behind, into the cavity of the nose, and opens under the inferior spongy bone into the nostril.

10. The *membrana conjunctiva*, or conjunctive membrane, which, from its white colour is called also *albuginea*, or white of the eye, is a membrane which lines the internal superficies of the eyelids, and covers the whole forepart of the globe of the eye: it is very vascular, as may be seen in inflammations.

The bulb, or globe of the eye, is composed of eight membranes, or coverings, two chambers, or *cameræ*, and three humours, improperly so called.

The membranes of the globe of the eye, are, *four* in the hinder or posterior part of the bulb, or globe, viz. *sclerotica*, *choroidea*, *retina*, and *hyaloidea*, or *arachnoidea*; *four* in the fore or anterior part of the bulb, viz. *cornea transparens*, *iris*, *uvea*, and *capsule of the crystalline lens*.

The *membrana sclerotica*, or the sclerotic or horny membrane, is the outermost. It begins from the optic nerve, forms the spherical or globular cavity, and terminates in the circular margin of the transparent cornea.

The *membrana choroidea*, or *choroides*, is the middle tonic of the bulb, of a black colour, beginning from the optic nerve, and covering the internal superficies of the sclerotica, to the margin of the transparent cornea. In this place it secedes from the cornea, and deflects transversely and inwardly, and in the middle forms a round foramen. This circular continuation of the choroidea in the anterior surface is called *iris*, in the posterior superficies, *uvea*.

The round opening in the centre is called the *pupil*, or *pupilla*. This foramen, or round opening, can be dilated, or contracted by the moving powers of almost invisible muscular fibres.

The *membrana retina*, is the innermost tunic of a white colour, and similar to mucus, being an expansion of the optic nerve, chiefly composed of its medullary part. It covers the inward surface of the choroides, to the margin of the crystalline lens, and there terminates.

The *chambers*, or *cameræ* of the eyes are:

1. *Camera anterior*, or fore-chamber; an open space, which is formed anteriorly, by the hollow surface of the *cornea transparens*, and posteriorly, by the surface of the *iris*.

2. *Camera posterior*, that small space which is bounded anteriorly by the *tunica uvea*, and *pupilla*, or pupil; posteriorly by the anterior surface of the crystalline lens.

Both these chambers are filled with an aqueous humour. The humours of the eye, as they are called, are in number three:

1. The *aqueous humour*, which fills both chambers.

2. The *crystalline lens*, or humour, is a pellucid body, about the size of a lentil, which is included in an exceedingly fine membrane, or *capsula*, and lodged in a concave depression of the vitreous humour.

3. The *vitreous humour*, is a pellucid, beautifully transparent substance, which fills the whole bulb of the eye behind the crystalline lens. Its external surface is surrounded with a most pellucid membrane, which is called *membrana hyaloidea*, or *arachnoidea*. In the anterior part is a fovea, or bed, for the crystalline lens.

The connexion of the bulb is made anteriorly, by means of the conjunctive membrane, with the inner surface of the eyelids, or *palpebræ*; posteriorly, by the adhesion of six muscles of the bulb and the optic nerve with the orbit.

The optic nerve, or *nervus opticus*, perforates the sclerotica and choroides, and then constitutes the retina, by spreading itself on the whole posterior part of the internal globe of the eye.

The muscles by which the eye is moved in the orbit, are six; much fat surrounds them, and fills up the cavities in which the eyes are seated. The arteries are the internal orbital, the central, and the ciliary arteries. The veins empty themselves into the external jugulars. The nerves are the optic, and branches from the third, fourth, fifth, and six pair.

The use of the eye is to form the organ of vision See *Vision*.

Externally, the globe of the eye and the transparent cornea are moistened with a most limpid fluid, called *lachrymæ*, or tears; the same pellucid subtile fluid exactly fills all the pores of the transparent cornea; for, deprived of this fluid, and being exposed to the air, that coat of the eye becomes dry, shrivelled, and cloudy, impeding the rays of light.

EYE-BRIGHT. See *Euphrasia*.

EYE-BROW. *Supercilium*. See *Eye*.

EYE-LID. *Palpebra*. See *Eye*.

Eye-tooth. The fangs of the two upper cuspidati are very much larger than those on each side, and extend up near to the orbit, on which account they have have been called eye-teeth. See *Teeth*.

F

F. or ft. In a prescription these letters are abbreviations of *fiat*, or *fiant*, let it, or them, be made; thus *f. bolus*, let the substance or substances prescribed be made into a bolus.

FA'BA. A bean. See *Bean*.

Faba crassa. See *Sedum telephium*.

Faba ægyptiaca. See *Nymphæa nelumbo*.

Faba febrifuga. See *Ignatia amara*.

Faba indica. See *Ignatia amara*.

Faba major. The garden-bean. See *Bean*.

Faba minor. The horse-bean. It differs no otherwise from the garden-bean than in being less.

Faba pechurim. *Faba pichurim; Faba pechuris*. Brazilian bean. An oblong oval, brown, and ponderous seed, supposed to be the produce of a *Laurus*, brought from the Brazils. Their smell is like that of musk, between it and the scent of sassafras. They are exhibited as carminatives in flatulent colics, diarrhœas, and dysenteries.

Faba purgatrix. See *Ricinus*.

Faba sancti ignatii. See *Ignatia amara*.

Faba suilla. See *Hyoscyamus*.

Faba'ria. (From *faba*, a bean, which it resembles.) See *Sedum telephium*.

FABRICIUS, Hieronymus, born at *Aquapendente* in Italy, 1537. He studied at Padua under Fallopius, whom he succeeded as professor of anatomy and surgery there; which office he held for nearly half a century with great credit, and died at the advanced age of eighty-two, universally regretted. The republic of Venice also conferred many honours upon him. He is thought to have been the first to notice the valves of the veins, which he demonstrated in 1574. But his surgical works obtained him most reputation; indeed he has been called the father of modern surgery. His first publication in 1592 contained five Dissertations on Tumours, Wounds, Ulcers, Fractures, and Dislocations. He afterward added another part, treating of all the diseases which are curable by manual operation. This work passed through seventeen editions in different languages.

FABRICIUS, James, was born at Rostock, in 1577. After travelling through different parts of Europe, he graduated at Jena, and soon gained extensive practice. He was professor of medicine and the mathematics at Rostock during forty years, and first physician to the Duke of Mecklenburgh; afterward went to Copenhagen, and was made physician to the kings of Norway and Denmark, and died there, in 1652. He has left several tracts on medical subjects.

FABRICIUS, Philip Conrad, professor of medicine at Helmstadt, was author of several useful works in anatomy and surgery. His first treatise, "Idea Anatomes Practicæ," 1741, contained some new directions in the Art of Injection, and described several branches of the Portio Dura, &c. In another work he has some good observations on the Abuse of Trepanning.

FABRICIUS, William, better known by the name of *Hildanus*, from Hilden, in Switzerland, where he was born in 1560. He repaired to Lausanne, to complete his knowledge of surgery, at the age of twenty-six; and distinguished himself there by his assiduity, and the successful treatment of many difficult cases. He studied medicine also, and went to practise both arts at Payenne, in 1605; but ten years after was invited to Berne by the senate, who granted him a pension. In the latter part of his life, severe illness prevented his professional exertions, which had procured him general esteem and high reputation. His death occurred in 1634. His works were written in German, but have been mostly translated into Latin. He published five "Centuries of Observations," which present many curious facts, as also several instruments invented by him.

FACE. *Facies*. The lower and anterior part of the cranium, or skull.

FA'CIAL. *Facialis*. Belonging to the face; as facial nerve, &c.

Facial nerve. *Nervus facialis. Portio dura* of the auditory nerve. These nerves are two in number, and are properly the eighth pair: but are commonly called the seventh, being reckoned with the auditory, which is the portio mollis of the seventh pair. They arise from the fourth ventricle of the brain, pass through the petrous portion of the temporal bone to the face, where they form the pes anserinus, which supplies the integuments of the face and forehead.

FA'CIES. The face. See *Face*.

Facies hippocratica. That particular disposition of the features which immediately precedes the stroke of death is so called, because it has been so admirably described by Hippocrates.

Facies rubra. See *Gutta rosacea*.

FACTI'TIOUS. A term applied to any thing which is made by art, in opposition to that which is native, or found already made in nature.

FA'CULTY. *Facultas*. The power or ability by which any action is performed.

Fæ'ces. (The plural of *fæx*.) The alvine excretions.

FÆ'CULA. (Diminutive of *fæx*.) A substance obtained by bruising or grinding certain vegetables in water. It is that part which, after a little, falls to the bottom. The fæcula of plants differs principally from gum or mucus in being insoluble in cold water, in which it falls with wonderful quickness. There are few plants which do not contain fæcula; but the seeds of gramineous and leguminous vegetables, and all tuberose roots contain it most plentifully.

FÆX. (*Fæx, æcis*, f. an excretion.) The alvine excretions are called *fæces*.

FAGA'RA. (From *fagus*, the breech, which it resembles.) The name of a genus of plants in the Linnæan system. Class, *Tetrandria*; Order, *Monogynia*.

Fagara major. See *Fagara plerota*.

Fagara octandra. The systematic name of the plant which affords *Tacamahaca*, which is a resinous substance that exudes both spontaneously, and when incisions are made into the stem of this tree: *Fagara foliolis tomentosis*, of Linnæus, and not, as was formerly supposed, from the *Populus balsamifera*. Two kinds of a tacamahaca are met with in the shops. The best, called, from its being collected in a kind of gourd-shell, tacamahaca in shells, is somewhat unctuous and soft, of a pale yellowish or greenish colour, a bitterish aromatic taste, and a fragrant delightful smell, approaching to that of lavender and ambergris. The more common sort is in semi-transparent grains, of a whitish, yellowish, brownish, or greenish colour, and of a less grateful smell than the former. Tacamahaca was formerly in high estimation as an ingredient in warm stimulating plasters; and although seldom used internally, it may be given with advantage as a corroborant and astringent balsamic.

Fagara plerota. *Fagara major; Castana Luzonis; Cubebis*. This plant is found in the Philippine islands. The berries are aromatic, and, according to Avicenna, heating, drying, good for cold, weak stomachs, and astringent to the bowels.

FAGOPY'RUM. (From φαγος, the beech, and πυρος, wheat; because its seeds were supposed to resemble the mast, *i. e.* fruit of beech.) See *Polygonum fagopyrum*.

Fagotri'ticum. See *Polygonum fagopyrum*.

FA'GUS. (From φαγω, to eat; its nut being one of the first fruits used by man.)

1. The name of a genus of plants in the Linnæan system. Class, *Monœcia*; Order, *Polyandria*.

2. The pharmacopœial name of the beech See *Fagus sylvatica*.

Fagus castanea. The systematic name of the chesnut-tree. *Castanea; Lopima; Mota; Glans Jovis Theophrasti*. Jupiter's acorn; Sardinian acorn; the common chesnut. The fruit of this plant, *Fagus —foliis lanceolatis, acuminato-serratis, subtus nudis*, of Linnæus, are much esteemed as an article of luxury after dinner. Toasting renders them more easy of digestion; but, notwithstanding, they must be considered as improper for weak stomachs. They are moderately nourishing, as containing sugar, and much farinaceous substance.

Fagus sylvatica. The systematic name of the beech-tree. *Fagus; Oxya; Balanda; Valanida*. The fruit and interior bark of this tree, *Fagus—foliis ovatis, obsolete serratis*, of Linnæus, are occasionally used medicinally, the former in obstinate headache, and the latter in the cure of hectic fever. The oil expressed from beech-nuts is supposed to destroy worms; a child may take two drachms of it night and morning; an adult an ounce. The poor people of Silesia use this oil instead of butter.

FAHLUMITE. A sub-species of octohedral corundum.

FAINTING. See *Syncope*.

FAIRBURN. The name of a village in the county of Ross, in the north of Britain, where there is a sulphureous spring.

FA'LCIFORM. (*Falciformis*; from *falx*, a scythe, and *forma*, resemblance.) Resembling a scythe.

Falciform process. The falx. A process of the dura mater, that arises from the crista galli, separates the hemispheres of the brain, and terminates in the tentorium.

Falde'lla. Lint, used as a compress.

Falling-sickness. See *Epilepsia*.

Fallopian tube. See *Tuba Fallopiana*.

Fallopian ligament. See *Poupart's ligament*.

FALLOPIUS, Gabriel, a physician of Modena, was born about the year 1523. He showed early great zeal in anatomy, botany, chemistry, and other branches of knowledge; and after studying in Italy, travelled to other countries for his improvement. In 1548, he was appointed professor of anatomy at Pisa, and three years after at Padua; where he also taught botany, but with less celebrity. His death happened in 1563 He distinguished himself, not only as an anatomist, but also in medicine and surgery. Douglas has characterized him as highly systematic in teaching, successful in treating diseases, and expeditious in operating. Some of the discoveries, to which he laid claim, appear to have been anticipated; as, for instance, the tubes proceeding from the uterus, though generally called after him *Fallopian*. However, he has the merit of recovering many of the observations of the ancients, which had fallen into oblivion. His "Observationes Anatomicæ," published in 1561, was one of the best works of the 16th century; in this some of the errors, which had escaped his master, Vesalius, are modestly pointed out. Many other publications, ascribed to him, were printed after his death; some of which are evidently spurious.

FALX. See *Falciform process.*

FA'MES. Hunger.

FAMES CANINA. See *Bulimia.*

FAMIGERATI'SSIMUM EMPLASTRUM. (From *famigeratus*, renowned; from *fama*, fame, and *gero*, to bear: so named from its excellence.) A plaster used in intermittent fever, made of aromatic, irritating substances, and applied to the wrists.

FAMILY. *Familia.* A term used by naturalists to express a certain order of natural productions, agreeing in the principal characters, and containing numerous individuals not only distinct from one another, but in whole sets, several members being to be collected out of the same family, all of which have the family character, and all some subordinate distinction peculiar to that whole number, or, though found in every individual of it, not found in those of any others.

It has been too common to confound the words, class, family, order, &c. in natural history; but the determinate meaning of the word family seems to be that larger order of creatures under which classes and orders are subordinate distinctions.

FA'RFARA. (From *farfarus*, the white poplar: so called because its leaves resemble those of the white poplar.) See *Tussilago farfara.*

FARI'NA. (From *far*, corn, of which it is made.) Meal, or flour. A term given to the pulverulent and glutinous part of wheat, and other seeds, which is obtained by grinding and sifting. It is highly nutritious, and consists of gluten, starch, and mucilage. See *Triticum.*

FARINA'CEA. (From *farina*, flour.) This term includes all those substances, employed as aliment, called *cerealia, legumina*, and *nuces oleosæ.*

FARINA'CEOUS. (*Farinaceus; from farina*, flour.) A term given to all articles of food which contain *farina.* See *Farina.*

FARINA'RIUM. See *Alica.*

FA'RREUS. (From *far*, corn.) Scurfy. An epithet of urine, where it deposites a branny sediment.

FA'SCIA. (From *fascis*, a bundle; because, by means of a band, materials are collected into a bundle.) 1. A bandage, fillet, or roller.

2. The tendinous expansions of muscles, which bind parts together, are termed *fasciæ.* See *Aponeurosis.*

FASCIA LATA. A thick and strong tendinous expansion, sent off from the back, and from the tendons of the glutei and adjacent muscles, to surround the muscles of the thigh. It is the thickest on the outside of the thigh and leg, but towards the inside of both becomes gradually thinner. A little below the trochanter major, it is firmly fixed to the linea aspera; and, further down, to that part of the head of the tibia that is next the fibula, where it sends off the tendinous expansion along the outside of the leg. It serves to strengthen the action of the muscles, by keeping them firm in their proper places when in action, particularly the tendons that pass over the joints where this membrane is thickest.

FASCIA'LIS. (From *fascia*, a fillet.) See *Tensor vaginæ femoris.*

FASCIA'TIO. (From *fascia*, a fillet.) The binding up any diseased or wounded part with bandages.

FASCICULARIS. (From *fascis*, a bundle.) Applied to roots which are sessile at their base, and consist of bundles of finger-like processes; as the root of the *Ophris nidus avis.*

FASCICULATUS. Fasciculate. Bundled or clustered. Applied to nerves, stems of plants, leaves, &c. See *Leaf* and *Caulis.*

FASCI'CULUS. (From *fascis*, a bundle. 1. In pharmacy, a handful.

2. In botany, a fascicule is applied to flowers on little stalks, variously inserted and subdivided, collected into a close bundle, level at the top; as in Sweet-william. It differs from,

1. A *corymb*, in the little stalks coming only from about the apex of the peduncle, and not from its whole length.

2. An *umbel*, from the stalks not coming from a common point.

3. A *cyme*, in not having its principal division umbellate.

FAT. *Adeps.* A concrete oily matter contained in the cellular membrane of animals, of a white, or yellowish colour, with little or no smell, or taste. It differs in different animals in solidity, colour, taste, &c. and likewise in the same animal at different ages. In infancy it is white, insipid, and not very solid; in the adult it is firm and yellowish, and in animals of an advanced age, its colour is deeper, its consistence various, and its taste in general stronger.

The fat appears to be useful in the animal economy principally by its physical properties; it forms a sort of elastic cushion in the orbit upon which the eye moves with facility; in the soles of the feet, and in the hips, it forms a sort of layer, which renders the pressure exerted by the body upon the skin and other soft parts less severe; its presence beneath the skin concurs in rounding the outlines, in diminishing the bony and muscular projections, and in beautifying the form; and as all fat bodies are bad conductors of caloric, it contributes to the preservation of that of the body. Full persons in general suffer little in winter by the cold.

Age, and the various modes of life, have much influence upon the developement of this fluid: very young children are generally fat. Fat is rarely abundant in the young man; but the quantity of it increases much towards the age of thirty years, particularly if the nourishment is succulent, and the life sedentary; the abdomen projects, the hips increase in size, as well as the breasts in women. The fat becomes more yellow in proportion as the age is more advanced. Fat meat is nourishing to those that have strong digestive powers. It is used externally, as a softening remedy, and enters into the composition of ointments and plasters.

"Concerning the nature of this important product of animalization, nothing definite was known, till Chevreuil devoted himself with meritorious zeal and perseverance to its investigation. He has already published in the Annales de Chimie, seven successive memoirs on the subject, each of them surpassing its predecessor in interest. We shall in this article give a brief abstract of the whole.

By dissolving fat in a large quantity of alkohol, and observing the manner in which its different portions were acted upon by this substance, and again separated from it, it is concluded that the fat is composed of an *oily substance*, which remains fluid at the ordinary temperature of the atmosphere; and of another *fatty substance* which is much less fusible. Hence it follows, that fat is not to be regarded as a simple principle, but as a combination of the above two principles, which may be separated without alteration. One of these substances melts at about 45°. the other at 100°. the same quantity of alkohol which dissolves 3.2 parts of the *oily substance*, dissolves 1.8 only of the *fatty substance:* the first is separated from the alkohol in the form of an oil; the second in that of small silky needles.

Each of the constituents of natural fat was then saponified by the addition of potassa; and an accurate description given of the compounds which were formed; and of the proportions of their constituents. The *oily substance* became saponified more readily than the *fatty substance;* the residual fluids in both cases contained the sweet oily principle; but the quantity that proceeded from the soap formed of the *oily substance*, was four or five times as much as that from the *fatty substance.* The latter soap was found to contain a much greater proportion of the *pearly matter* than the former, in the proportion of 7.5 to 2.9; the proportion of the *fluid fat* was the reverse, a greater quantity of this being found in the soap formed from the oily substance of the fat.

When the principles which constitute fat unite with potassa, it is probable that they experience a change in the proportion of their elements. This change developes at least three bodies, *margarine, fluid fat*, and *the sweet principle;* and it is remarkable, that it takes place without the absorption of any foreign substance, or the disengagement of any of the elements which are separated from each other. As this change is effected by the intermedium of the alkali, we may conclude that the newly formed principles must have a strong affinity for salifiable bases, and will in many respects resemble the acids; and, in fact, they exhibit the leading characters of acids, in reddening litmus, in decomposing the alkaline carbonates to unite to their bases, and in neutralizing the specific properties of the alkalies.

Having already pointed out the analogy between the

properties of acids and the principles into which fat is converted by means of the alkalies, the next object was to examine the action which other bases have upon fat, and to observe the effect of water, and of the cohesive force of the bases upon the process of saponification. The substances which the author subjected to experiment, were soda, the four alkaline earths, alumina, and the oxides of zinc, copper, and lead. After giving a detail of the processes which he employed with these substances respectively, he draws the following general conclusions:—Soda, barytes, strontian, lime, the oxide of zinc, and the protoxide of lead, convert fat into *margarine, fluid fat, the sweet principle, the yellow colouring principle*, and *the odorous principle*, precisely in the same manner as potassa. Whatever be the base that has been employed, the products of saponification always exist in the same relative proportion. As the above mentioned bases form with margarine and the fluid fat compounds which are insoluble in water, it follows, that the action of this liquid, as a solvent of soap, is not essential to the process of saponification. It is remarkable that the oxides of zinc and of lead, which are insoluble in water, and which produce compounds equally insoluble, should give the same results with potassa and soda,—a circumstance which proves that those oxides have a strong alkaline power. Although the analogy of magnesia to the alkalies is, in other respects, so striking, yet we find that it cannot convert fat into soap under the same circumstances with the oxides of zinc and lead.

It was found that 100 parts of hog's-lard were reduced to the completely saponified state by 16.36 parts of potassa.

The properties of spermaceti were next examined: it melts at about 112°; it is not much altered by distillation; it dissolves readily in hot alkohol, but separates as the fluid cools; the solution has no effect in changing the colour of the tincture of litmus, a circumstance, as it is observed, in which it differs from margarine, a substance which, in many respects, it resembles.—Spermaceti is capable of being saponified by potassa, with nearly the same phenomena as when we submit hogs-lard to the action of potassa, although the operation is effected with more difficulty

The author's general conclusion respecting the fatty matter of dead bodies is, that even after the lactic acid, the lactates, and other ingredients which are less essential, are removed from it, it is not a simple, ammoniacal soap, but a combination of various fatty substances with ammonia, potassa, and lime. The fatty substances which were separated from alkohol, had different melting points, and different sensible properties. It follows, from Chevreuil's experiments, that the substance which is the least fusible, has more affinity for bases than those which are more so. It is observed, that adipocere possesses the characters of a saponified fat; it is soluble in boiling alkohol in all proportions, reddens litmus, and unites readily to potassa, not only without losing its weight, but without having its fusibility or other properties changed.

Chevreuil has shown, that hog's-lard, in its natural state, has not the property of combining with alkalies; but that it acquires it by experiencing some change in the proportion of its elements. This change being induced by the action of the alkali, it follows that the bodies of the new formation must have a decided affinity for the species of body which has determined it. If we apply this foundation of the theory of saponification to the change into fat which bodies buried in the earth experience, we shall find that it explains the process in a very satisfactory manner. In reality, the fatty matter is the combination of the two adipose substances with ammonia, lime, and potassa: one of these substances has the same sensible properties with margarine procured from the soap of hog's-lard; the other, the orange-coloured oil, excepting its colour, appears to have a strong analogy with the fluid fat. From these circumstances, it is probable that the formation of the fatty matter may be the result of a proper saponification produced by ammonia, proceeding from the decomposition of the muscle, and by the potassa and lime, which proceed from the decomposition of certain salts.

The author remarks, that he has hitherto made use of periphrases when speaking of the different bodies that he has been describing, as supposing that their nature was not sufficiently determined. He now, however, conceives, that he may apply specific names to them, which will be more commodious, and, at the same time, by being made appropriate, will point out the relation which these bodies bear to each other. The following is the nomenclature which he afterward adopted:—The crystalline matter of human biliary calculi is named *cholesterine*, from the Greek word χολη, bile, and ϛερεος, solid; spermaceti is named *cetine*, from κητος, a whale; the fatty substance and the oily substance, are named respectively, *stearine* and *elaine*, from the words ϛεαρ, and ελαιον, oil; margarine, and the fluid fat obtained after saponification, are named *margaric acid* and *oleic acid*, while the term *cetic acid* is applied to what was named saponified spermaciti. The *margarates*, *oleates*, and *cetates*, will be the generic names of the soaps or combinations which these acids are capable of forming by their union with salifiable bases.

Two portions of human fat were examined, one taken from the kidney, the other from the thigh: after some time they both of them manifested a tendency to separate into two distinct substances, one of a solid, and the other of a fluid consistence: the two portions differed in their fluidity and their melting point. These variations depend upon the different proportions of stearine and elaine; for the concrete part of fat is a combination of the two with an excess of stearine, and the fluid part is a combination with an excess of elaine. The fat from the other animals was then examined, principally with respect to their melting point and their solubility in alkohol; the melting point was not always the same in the fat of the same species of animal.

Chevreuil next examines the change which is produced in the different kinds of fat respectively by the action of potassa. All the kinds of fat are capable of being perfectly saponified, when excluded from the contact of the air, in all of them there was the production of the saponified fat and the sweet principle; no carbonic acid was produced, and the soaps formed contained no acetic acid, or only slight traces of it. The saponified fats had more tendency to crystallize in needles than the fats in their natural state; they were soluble in all proportions in boiling alkohol of the specific gravity of 821. The solution, like that of the saponified fat of the hog, contained both the margaric and the oleic acids. They were less fusible than the fats from which they were formed: thus, when human fat, after being saponified, was melted, the thermometer became stationary at 95°, when the fluid began to congeal, in that of the sheep, the thermometer fell to 118.5°, and rose to 122°; in that of the ox it remained stationary at 118.5°; and in that of the jaguar at 96.5°.

The method of analysis employed was to expose the different kinds of fat to boiling alkohol, and to suffer the mixture to cool: a portion of the fat that had been dissolved was then separated in two states of combination; one with an excess of stearine was deposited, the other with an excess of elaine remained in solution. The first was separated by filtration, and by distilling the filtered fluid, and adding a little water towards the end of the operation, we obtain the second in the retort, under the form of an alkoholic aqueous fluid. The distilled alkohol which had been employed in the analysis of human fat, had no sensible odour; the same was the case with that which had served for the analysis of the fat of the ox, of the hog, and of the goose. The alkohol which had been employed in the analysis of the fat of the sheep, had a slight odour of candlegrease.

All the soaps of stearine were analyzed by the same process as the soap of the fat from which they had been extracted: there was procured from them the pearly super-margarate of potassa and the oleate; but the first was much more abundant than the second. The margaric acid of the stearines had precisely the same capacity for saturation as that which was extracted from the soaps formed of fat. The margaric acid of the stearine of the sheep was fusible at 144°, and that of the stearine of the ox at 143.5°; while the margaric acids of the hog and the goose had nearly the same fusibility with the margaric acid of the fat of these animals.

Chevreuil technically calls spermaceti, *cetine*. In the fifth memoir, in which we have an account of many of the properties of this substance, it was stated, that it is not easily saponified by potassa, but that it is converted by this reagent into a substance which is soluble in water, but has not the saccharine flavour of the sweet principle of oils; into an acid analogous to the margaric, to which the name of *cetic* was applied; and into another acid, which was conceived to be analogous to the oleic. Since he wrote the fifth memoir, the author has made the following observations on this subject:—1. That the portion of the soap of cetine which is insoluble in water, or the cetate of potassa, is in part gelatinous, and in part pearly: 2. The two kinds of crystals were produced from the cetate of potassa which had been dissolved in alkohol: 3. That the cetate of potassa exposed, under a bell glass, to the heat of a stove, produced a sublimate of a fatty matter which was not acid. From this circumstance Chevreuil was led to suspect, that the supposed cetic acid might be a combination, or a mixture of margaric acid, and of a fatty body which was not acid. He accordingly treated a small quantity of it with barytic water, and boiled the soap which was formed in alkohol; the greatest part of it was not dissolved, and the alkoholic solution, when cooled, filtered, and distilled, produced a residuum of fatty matter which was not acid. The suspicion being thus confirmed, Chevreuil determined to subject cetine to a new train of experiments. Being treated with boiling alkohol, a cetine was procured which was fusible at 120°, and a yellow fatty matter which began to become solid at 89.5°, and which at 73.5° contained a fluid oil, which was separated by filtration.—*Ure's Chem. Dic.*

FATUI'TAS. (From *fatuus*, silly.) Fatuity or foolishness.

FAU'CES. (*Faux*, pl. *fauces.*) A cavity behind the tongue, palatine arch, uvula, and tonsils; from which the pharynx and larynx proceed.

FAU'FEL. Terra japonica, or catechu.

[FAUSSE AVOINE. False oats. Indian rice. See *Zizania aquatica*. A.]

FAUX. (*Faux, cis.* f.) 1. The gorge, or mouth, or opening of the gullet.

2. Applied by botanists to the opening of the tube of monopetalous corals. See *Corolla*.

FAVA'GO AUSTRALIS. (From *favus*, a honey-comb; from its resemblance to a honey-comb.) A species of bastard sponge.

FAVOSUS. (From *favus*, a honey-comb.) Honey-comb-like. 1. Applied to some eruptive diseases; as *Lichen favosus*, the secretion in which is cellular and honey-comb-like.

2. To parts of plants, as the receptacle of the onopordium which has cells like a honey-comb.

FAVUS. 1. A honey-comb.

2. A species of achor, or foul ulcer.

FE'BRES. (The plural of *febris.*) An order in the class *Pyrexiæ*, of Cullen, characterized by the presence of pyrexia, without primary local affection.

FEBRI'CULA. (Dim. of *febris*, a fever.) A term employed to express a slight degree of symptomatic fever.

FEBRI'FUGA. (From *febrem fugare*, to drive away a fever.) The plant feverfew; less centaury.

FE'BRIFUGE. (*Febrifugus;* from *febris*, a fever, and *fugo*, to drive away.) That which possesses the property of abating the violence of any fever.

FEBRIFUGUM CRENII. Regulus of antimony.

FEBRIFUGUM OLEUM. Febrifuge oil. The flowers of antimony, made with sal-ammoniac and antimony sublimed together, and exposed to the air, when they deliquesce.

FEBRIFUGUS PULVIS. Febrifuge powder. The Germans give this name to the pulvis stypticus Helvetii. In England, a mixture of oculi cancrorum and emetic tartar, in the proportion of half a drachm and two grains, has obtained the same name; in fevers it is given in doses of gr. iii. to iv.

FEBRIFUGUS SAL. Regenerated marine salt.

FEBRIS. (*Febris, is.* f.; from *ferveo*, to burn.) A fever. A disease characterized by an increase of heat, an accelerated pulse, a foul tongue, and an impaired state of several functions of the body.

FEBRIS ALBA. See *Chlorosis*.

FEBRIS AMPHIMERINA. A quotidian fever.

FEBRIS ANGINOSA. See *Scarlatina anginosa*.

FEBRIS APHTHOSA. See *Aphtha*.

FEBRIS ARDENS. Fever attended by a very hot or burning state of the skin. A burning inflammatory fever.

FEBRIS ASSODES. A tertian fever, with extreme restlessness.

FEBRIS BULLOSA. See *Pemphigus*.

FEBRIS CACATORIA. An intermittent fever, with diarrhœa.

FEBRIS CARCERUM. The prison fever.

FEBRIS CASTRENSIS. A camp fever, generally typhus.

FEBRIS CATARRHALIS. A fever, either typhoid, nervous, or synochal, attended with symptoms of catarrh.

FEBRIS CHOLERICA. A fever, attended throughout with bilious diarrhœa.

FEBRIS CONTINUA. A continued fever. A division of the order *Febres*, in the class *Pyrexiæ*, of Cullen Continued fevers have no intermission, but exacerbations come on usually twice in one day. The genera of continued fever are:

1. *Synocha*, or inflammatory fever, known by increased heat; pulse frequent, strong, and hard; urine high-coloured; senses not much impaired. See *Synocha*.

2. *Typhus*, or putrid-tending fever, which is contagious, and is characterized by moderate heat; quick, weak, and small pulse; senses much impaired, and great prostration of strength. This genus has two species; *Typhus petechialis*, attended with petechiæ; and *Typhus icterodes*, or yellow fever; and of the former there are two varieties: *Typhus mitior*, or nervous fever; and *Typhus gravior*, or putrid fever. See *Febris nervosa*, and *Typhus*.

3. *Synochus*, or mixed fever. See *Synochus*.

FEBRIS ELODES. A fever with continual and profuse sweating.

FEBRIS EPIALA. A fever with a continual sense of coldness. See *Epialus*.

FEBRIS ERYSIPELATOSA. See *Erysipelas*.

FEBRIS EXANTHEMATICA. A fever with an eruption. See *Exanthema*.

FEBRIS FLAVA. See *Typhus*.

FEBRIS HECTICA. A genus of disease in the class *Pyrexiæ*, and order *Febris*, of Cullen. It is known by exacerbations at noon, but greater in the evening, with slight remissions in the morning, after nocturnal sweats; the urine depositing a furfuraceo-lateritious sediment; appetite good; thirst moderate. Hectic fever is symptomatic of chlorosis, scrofula, phthisis, diseased viscera, &c.

FEBRIS HUNGARICA. A species of tertian intermittent fever.

FEBRIS HYDRODES. A fever with profuse sweats.

FEBRIS INFLAMMATORIA. See *Synocha*.

FEBRIS INTERMITTENS. An intermittent fever, or ague. A division of the order *Febres*, of Cullen, in the class *Pyrexiæ*. Intermittent fevers are known by cold, hot, and sweating stages, in succession, attending each paroxysm, and followed by an intermission or remission. There are three genera of intermitting fevers, and several varieties.

1. *Quotidiana*. A quotidian ague. The paroxysms return in the morning, at an interval of about twenty-four hours.

2. *Tertiana*. A tertian ague. The paroxysms commonly come on at mid-day, at an interval of about forty-eight hours.

3. *Quartana*. A quartan ague. The paroxysms come on in the afternoon, with an interval of about seventy-two hours. The tertian ague is most apt to prevail in the spring, and the quartan in autumn.

Of the quotidian, tertian, and quartan intermittents, there are several varieties and forms; as the double tertian, having a paroxysm every day, with the alternate paroxysms, similar to one another. The double tertian, with two paroxysms every other day. The triple tertian, with two paroxysms on one day, and another on the next. The double quartan, with two paroxysms on the first day, none on the second and third, and two again on the fourth day. The double quartan, with a paroxysm on the first day, another on the second, but none on the third. The triple quartan, with three paroxysms every fourth day. The triple quartan, with a paroxysm every day, every fourth paroxysm being similar.

When these fevers arise in the spring of the year, they are called vernal; and when in the autumn, they are known by the name of autumnal. Intermittents often prove obstinate, and are of long duration in warm climates; and they not unfrequently resist every mode of cure, so as to become very distressing to the patient; and by the extreme debility which they thereby induce, often give rise to other chronic complaints.

It seems to be pretty generally acknowledged, that marsh miasmata, or the effluvia arising from stagnant water, or marshy ground, when acted upon by heat, are the most frequent exciting causes of this fever. In marshes, the putrefaction of both vegetable and animal matter is always going forward, it is to be presumed; and hence it has been generally conjectured, that vegetable and animal putrefaction imparted a peculiar quality to the effluvia arising from thence. We are not yet acquainted with all the circumstances, which are requisite to render marsh miasma productive of the intermittents; but it may be presumed that a moist atmosphere has a considerable influence in promoting its action. A watery poor diet, great fatigue, long watching, grief, much anxiety, exposure to cold, lying in damp rooms or beds, wearing damp linen, the suppression of some long-accustomed evacuation, or the recession of eruptions, have been ranked among the exciting causes of intermittents; but it is more reasonable to suppose that these circumstances act only by inducing that state of the body, which predisposes to these complaints. By some it has been imagined that an intermittent fever may be communicated by contagion; but this supposition is by no means consistent with general observation.

One peculiarity of this fever is, its great susceptibility of a renewal from very slight causes, as from the prevalence of an easterly wind, even without the repetition of the original exciting cause. It would appear that a predisposition is left in the habit, which favours the recurrence of the complaint. In this circumstance, intermittents differ from most other fevers, as it is well known, that after a continued fever has once occurred, and been removed, the person so affected is by no means so liable to a fresh attack of the disorder, as one in whom it had never taken place.

We have not yet attained a certain knowledge of the proximate cause of an intermittent fever, but a deranged state of the stomach and primæ viæ is that which is most generally ascribed.

Each paroxysm of an intermittent fever is divided into three different stages, which are called the *cold*, the *hot*, and the *sweating stages* or *fits*.

The *cold* stage commences with languor, a sense of debility and sluggishness in motion, frequent yawning and stretching, and an aversion to food. The face and extremities become pale, the features shrink, the bulk of every external part is diminished, and the skin over the whole body appears constricted, as if cold had been applied to it. At length the patient feels very cold, and universal rigors come on, with pains in the head, back, loins, and joints, nausea, and vomiting of bilious matter; the respiration is small, frequent, and anxious; the urine is almost colourless; sensibility is greatly impaired; the thoughts are somewhat confused; and the pulse is small, frequent, and often irregular. In a few instances, drowsiness and stupour have prevailed in so high a degree as to resemble coma or apoplexy; but this is by no means usual.

These symptoms abating after a short time, the second stage commences with an increase of heat over the whole body, redness of the face, dryness of the skin, thirst, pain in the head, throbbing in the temples, anxiety and restlessness; the respiration is fuller and more free, but still frequent; the tongue is furred, and the pulse has become regular, hard, and full. If the attack has been very severe, then perhaps delirium will arise.

When these symptoms have continued for some time, a moisture breaks out on the forehead, and by degrees becomes a sweat, and this, at length, extends over the whole body. As this sweat continues to flow, the heat of the body abates, the thirst ceases, and most of the functions are restored to their ordinary state. This constitutes the third stage.

It must, however, be observed, that in different cases these phenomena may prevail in different degrees, and their mode of succession vary; that the series of them may be more or less complete; and that the several stages, in the time they occupy, may be in different proportions to one another.

Such a depression of strength has been known to take place on the attack of an intermittent, as to cut off the patient at once; but an occurrence of this kind is very uncommon.

Patients are seldom destroyed in intermittents from general inflammation, or from a fulness of the vessels either of the brain or of the thoracic viscera, as happens sometimes in a continued fever; but when they continue for any length of time, they are apt to induce other complaints, such as a loss of appetite, flatulency, schirrhus of the liver, dropsical swellings, and general debility, which in the end now and then prove fatal. In warm climates, particularly, intermittents are very apt to terminate in this manner, if not speedily removed; and in some cases, they degenerate into continued fevers. When the paroxysms are of short duration, and leave the intervals quite free, we may expect a speedy recovery; but when they are long, violent, and attended with much anxiety and delirium, the event may be doubtful. Relapses are very common to this fever at the distance of five or six months, or even a year; autumnal intermittents are more difficult to remove than vernal ones, and quartans more so than the other types.

Dissections of those who have died of an intermittent, show a morbid state of many of the viscera of the thorax and abdomen; but the liver, and organs concerned in the formation of bile, as likewise the mesentery, are those which are usually most affected.

The treatment of an intermittent fever resolves itself into those means, which may be employed during a paroxysm, to arrest its progress, or to mitigate its violence; and those, which may prevent any return, and effect a permanent cure: this forms of course the more important part of the plan; but it is sometimes necessary to palliate urgent symptoms; and it is always desirable to suspend a paroxysm, if possible, not only to prevent mischief, but also that there may be more time for the use of the most effectual remedies. When therefore a fit is commencing, or shortly expected, we may try to obviate it by some of those means, which excite movements of an opposite description in the system; an emetic will generally answer the purpose, determining the blood powerfully to the surface of the body; or a full dose of opium, assisted by the pediluvium, &c.; æther also, and various stimulant remedies, will often succeed, but these may perhaps aggravate, should they not prevent the fit; the cold bath, violent exercise, strong impressions on the mind, &c. have likewise been occasionally employed with effect. Should the paroxysm have already come on, and the cold stage be very severe, the warm bath, and cordial diaphoretics in repeated moderate doses, may assist in bringing warmth to the surface: when, on the contrary, great heat prevails, the antiphlogistic plan is to be pursued; and it may be sometimes advisable, when an organ of importance is much pressed upon, to take some blood locally, or even from the general system, if the patient is plethoric and robust: and where profuse perspirations occur, acidulated drink may be exhibited, with a little wine to support the strength, keeping the surface cool at the same time. In the intermissions, in conjunction with a generous diet, moderate exercise, and other means calculated to improve the vigour of the system; tonics are the remedies especially relied upon. At the head of these we must certainly place the cinchona, which, taken largely in substance, will seldom fail to cure the disease, where it is not complicated with visceral affection: in a quotidian an ounce at least should be given between the fits, in a tertian half as much more, and in a quartan two ounces. It will be generally better to clear out the primæ viæ before this remedy is begun with; and various additions may often be required, to make it agree better with the stomach and bowels, particularly aromatics and other stimulants, aperients or small doses of opium, according to circumstances. We must not be content with the omission of a single paroxysm, but continue it till the health appears fully established. In failure of the cinchona, other vegetable tonics may be tried, as the salix, gentian, calumba, and other bitters; or the astringents, as tormentil, galls, &c.; or these variously combined with each other, or with aromatics. The mineral acids are often powerfully tonic, and the sulphuric has been of late stated to have proved very successful in the removal of this disease. Some metallic preparations are also highly efficacious, particularly the liquor arsenicalis, which, however, is too hazardous a remedy to be employed indiscriminately; it must be given in small doses two or three times a day, and its effects assiduously watched. The sulphate of zinc, and chalybeates, may be used more freely alone, or preferably joined with bitters. Where visceral disease attends, we can hardly succeed in curing the ague, till this be removed; a state of congestion, or inflammatory tendency, may require local bleeding, blistering, purging, &c.; and when there is a more fixed obstruction, particularly in the liver, the cautious use of mercury will be most likely to avail.

FEBRIS LACTEA. Milk fever, which is mostly of the synochus-type attended with much irregularity of mind, and nervousness.

FEBRIS LENTA. See *Febris nervosa*

FEBRIS LENTICULARIS. A fever, either typhus or synochus, attended by an eruption like small lentils.

FEBRIS MALIGNA. See *Typhus.*

FEBRIS MILIARIS. See *Miliaria*

FEBRIS MORBILLOSA. See *Rubeola*

FEBRIS NERVOSA. *Febris lenta nervosa.* The nervous fever. A variety of the *typhus mitior* of Cullen, but by many considered as a distinct disease. It mostly begins with loss of appetite, increased heat and vertigo; to which succeed nausea, vomiting, great languor, and pain in the head, which is variously described, by some like cold water pouring over the top, by others a sense of weight. The pulse, before little increased, now becomes quick, febrile, and tremulous; the tongue is covered with a white crust, and there is great anxiety about the præcordia. Towards the seventh or eighth day, the vertigo is increased, and tinnitus aurium, cophosis, delirium, and a dry and tremulous tongue, take place. The disease mostly terminates about the fourteenth or twentieth day. See *Typhus.*

FEBRIS NOSOCOMIORUM. The fever of hospitals, mostly the *typhus gravior.*

FEBRIS PALUSTRIS. The marsh fever

FEBRIS PESTILENS. See *Pestis.*

FEBRIS PETECHIALIS. See *Typhus.*

FEBRIS PUTRIDA. See *Typhus.*

FEBRIS REMITTENS. A remittent fever: a fever with strong exacerbations, which approach in some cases to the nature of a paroxysm of an intermittent, and which follow each other so closely as to leave very little time between. In some, there is a great secretion of bile, when it is called *a bilious* remittent; in others, there is great putrescency, when it is termed a *putrid* remittent, and so on.

FEBRIS SCARLATINA. See *Scarlatina.*

FEBRIS SYNOCHA. See *Synocha.*

FEBRIS TYPHODES. See *Typhus.*

FEBRIS URTICARIA. See *Urticaria.*

FEBRIS VARIOLOSA. See *Variola.*

FEBRIS VESICULOSA. See *Erysipelas.*

FE'CULA. See *Fæcula.*

FECUNDATION. See *Generation.*

FEL. See *Bile.*

FEL NATURÆ. See *Aloes.*

FEL-WORT. So called from its bitter taste, like bile. See *Gentiana.*

FELLI'CULUS. The gall-bladder.

FELLI'FLUA PASSIO. See *Cholera.*

Felon. See *Paronychia.*

FELSPAR. An important mineral genus, distributed by Jameson into four species: prismatic felspar; pyramidal felspar; prismato-pyramidal felspar; rhomboidal felspar.

1. The prismatic felspar has nine sub-species,

a. Adularia.
b. Glassy felspar.
c. Ice spar.
d. Common felspar.
e. Labradore felspar.
f. Compact felspar.
g. Clink-stone.
h. Earthy common spar.
i. Porcelain earth.

2. Pyramidal felspar. This embraces the scapolite and elaolite.

3. Prismato-pyramidal felspar. See *Meionite.*

4. Rhomboidal felspar. See *Nepheline.* Chiastolite and sodalite have also been annexed to this species.

[*Fesite.* Blue felspar of Stiria. A.]

FE'MEN. (*Quasi ferimen;* from *fero,* to bear: so called because it is the chief support of the body.) The thigh.

FEMINEUS. A flower is termed a female, which is furnished with the pistillum, and not with the stamina: the pistil being considered as the female generative organ.

FEMORAL. (*Femoralis;* from *femur,* the thigh.) Of or belonging to the thigh.

FEMORA'LIS ARTERIA. A continuation of the external iliac along the thigh, from Poupart's ligament to the ham.

FE'MORIS OS. The thigh-bone. A long cylindrical bone, situated between the pelvis and tibia. Its upper extremity affords three considerable processes; these are, the head, the trochanter major, and trochanter minor. The head, which forms about two-thirds of a sphere, is turned inwards, and is received into the acetabulum of the os innominatum, with which it is articulated by enarthrosis. It is covered by a cartilage, which is thick in its middle part, and thin at its edges, but which is wanting in its lower internal part, where a round spongy fossa is observable, to which the strong ligament, usually, though improperly, called the *round* one, is attached. This ligament is about an inch in length, flattish, and of a triangular shape, having its narrow extremity attached to the fossa just described, while its broader end is fixed obliquely to the rough surface near the inner and anterior edge of the acetabulum of the os innominatum, so that it appears shorter internally and anteriorly, than it does externally and posteriorly.

The head of the os femoris is supported obliquely, with respect to the rest of the bone, by a smaller part, called the *cervix,* or *neck,* which, in the generality of subjects, is about an inch in length. At its basis we observe two oblique ridges, which extend from the trochanter major to the trochanter minor. Of these ridges, the posterior one is the most prominent. Around this neck is attached the capsular ligament of the joint, which likewise adheres to the edge of the cotyloid cavity, and is strengthened anteriorly by many strong ligamentous fibres, which begin from the lower and anterior part of the ilium, and spreading broader as they descend, adhere to the capsular ligament, and are attached to the anterior oblique ridge at the bottom of the neck of the femur. Posteriorly and externally, from the basis of the neck of the bone, a large unequal protuberance stands out, which is the *trochanter major.* The upper edge of this process is sharp and pointed posteriorly, but is more obtuse anteriorly. A part of it is rough and unequal, for the insertion of the muscles; the rest is smooth, and covered with a thin cartilaginous crust, between which and the tendon of the glutæus maximus that slides over it, a large bursa mucosa is interposed. Anteriorly, at the root of this process, and immediately below the bottom of the neck, is a small process called *trochanter minor.* Its basis is nearly triangular, having its two upper angles turned towards the head of the femur and the great trochanter, while its lower angle is placed towards the body of the bone. Its summit is rough and rounded. These two processes have gotten the name of *trochanters,* from the muscles that are inserted into them being the principal instruments of the rotatory motion of the thigh. Immediately below these two processes the body of the bone may be said to begin. It is smooth and convex before, but is made hollow behind by the action of the muscles. In the middle of this posterior concave surface is observed a rough ridge, called *linea aspera,* which seems to originate from the trochanters, and extending downwards, divides at length into two branches, which terminate in the tuberosities near the condyles. At the upper part of it, blood-vessels pass to the internal substance of the bone by a hole that runs obliquely upwards.

The lower extremity of the os femoris is larger than the upper one, and somewhat flattened, so as to form two surfaces, of which the anterior one is broad and convex, and the posterior one narrower and slightly concave. This end of the bone terminates in two large protuberances, called *condyles,* which are united before so as to form a pulley, but are separated behind by a considerable cavity, in which the crural vessels and nerves are placed secure from the compression to which they would otherwise be exposed in the action of bending the leg. Of these two condyles, the external one is the largest; and when the bone is separated from the rest of the skeleton, and placed perpendicularly, the internal condyle projects less forwards, and descends nearly three-tenths of an inch lower than the external one; but in its natural situation, the bone is placed obliquely, so that both condyles are then nearly on a level with each other. At the side of each condyle, externally, there is a tuberosity, the situation of which is similar to that of the condyles of the os humeri. The two branches of the linea aspera terminate in these tuberosities, which are rough, and serve for attachment of ligaments and muscles.

FE'MUR. (*Femur, moris.* n.) The thigh.

FENE'STRA. (From φαινω, *quasi phænestra.*) A window, entry, or hole.

Fenestra ovalis. An oblong or elliptical foramen, between the cavity of the tympanum and the vestibulum of the ear. It is shut by the stapes.

Fenestra rotunda. A round foramen, leading from the tympanum to the cochlea of the ear. It is covered by a membrane in the fresh subject.

FE'NNEL. See *Anethum fœniculum.*

Fennel, hog's. See *Peucedanum.*

FE'NUGREEK. See *Trigonella fœnum græcum.*

FE'RINE. (*Ferinus*, savage or brutal.) A term occasionally applied to any malignant or noxious disease.

FERMENTA'TION. (*Fermentatio, onis.* f.; from *fermento*, to ferment.) When aqueous combinations of vegetable or animal substances are exposed to ordinary atmospherical temperatures, they speedily undergo spontaneous changes, to which the generic term of fermentation has been given. There are several circumstances required in order that fermentation may proceed: such are, 1. A certain degree of fluidity: thus, dry substances do not ferment at all. 2. A certain degree of heat. 3. The contact of air. Chemists, after Boerhaave, have distinguished three kinds of fermentation.

1. The *vinous* or *spirituous*, which affords ardent spirit.

2. The *acetous*, which affords vinegar, or acetic acid.

3. The *putrid* fermentation, or putrefaction, which produces volatile alkali.

I. The conditions necessary for vinous fermentation are: 1. A saccharine mucilage. 2. A degree of fluidity slightly viscid. 3. A degree of heat between 55 and 65 of Fahrenheit. 4. A large mass, in which a rapid commotion may be excited. When these four conditions are united, the vinous fermentation takes place, and is known by the following characteristic phenomena: 1. An intestine motion takes place. 2. The bulk of the mixture then becomes augmented. 3. The transparency of the fluid is diminished by opaque filaments. 4. Heat is generated. 5. The solid parts mixed with the liquor rise and float in consequence of the disengagement of elastic fluid. 6. A large quantity of carbonic acid gas is disengaged in bubbles. All these phenomena gradually cease in proportion as the liquor loses its sweet and mild taste, and it becomes brisk, penetrating, and capable of producing intoxication. In this manner, wine, beer, cider, &c. are made. All bodies which have undergone the spirituous fermentation are capable of passing on to the acid fermentation; but although it is probable that the acid fermentation never takes place before the body has gone through the spirituous fermentation, yet the duration of the first is frequently so short and imperceptible, that it cannot be ascertained. Besides the bodies which are proper for spirituous fermentation, this class includes all sorts of fæcula boiled in water.

II. The conditions required for the acid fermentation are, 1. A heat from 70 to 85 degrees of Fahrenheit. 2. A certain degree of liquidity. 3. The presence of atmospheric air. 4. A moderate quantity of fermentable matter. The phenomena which accompany this fermentation, are an intestine motion, and a considerable absorption of air. The transparent liquor becomes turbid, but regains its limpidity when fermentation is over. The fermented liquor now consists, in a great measure, of a peculiar acid, called the acetic acid, or vinegar. Not a vestige of spirit remains, it being entirely decomposed, but the greater the quantity of spirit in the liquor, previous to the fermentation, the greater will be the quantity of true vinegar obtained. As the ultimate constituents of vegetable matter are oxygen, hydrogen, and carbon; and of animal matter, the same three principles with azote, we can readily understand that all the products of fermentation must be merely new compounds of these three or four ultimate constituents. Accordingly, 100 parts of real vinegar, or acetic acid, are resolvable, by Gay Lussac and Thenard's analysis, into 50.224 carbon + 46.911 hydrogen and oxygen, as they exist in water, + 2.863 oxygen in excess. In like manner, wines are all resolvable into the same ultimate components, in proportions somewhat different. The aëriform results of putrefactive fermentation are in like manner found to be, hydrogen, carbon, oxygen, and azote, variously combined, and associated with minute quantities of sulphur and phosphorus. The residuary matter consists of the same principles, mixed with the saline and earthy parts of animal bodies.

Lavoisier was the first philosopher who instituted, on right principles, a series of experiments to investigate the phenomena of fermentation, and they were so judiciously contrived, and so accurately conducted, as to give results comparable to those derived from the more rigid methods of the present day. Since then, Thenard and Gay Lussac have each contributed most important researches. By the labours of these three illustrious chemists, those material metamorphoses, formerly quite mysterious, seem susceptible of a satisfactory explanation.

As sugar is a substance of uniform and determinate composition, it has been made choice of for determining the changes which arise when its solution is fermented into wine or alkohol. Lavoisier justly regarded it as a true vegetable oxide, and stated its constituents to be, 8 hydrogen, 28 carbon, and 64 oxygen, in 100 parts. By two different analyses of Berzelius, we have,

Hydrogen	6.802	6.891
Carbon	44.115	42.704
Oxygen	49.083	50.405
	100.000	100.000

Gay Lussac and Thenard's analysis gives,

Hydrogen	6.90	} 57.53 water,
Oxygen	50.63	}
Carbon	42.47	42.47
	100.00	100.00

It has been said, that sugar requires to be dissolved in at least 4 parts of water, and to be mixed with some yest, to cause its fermentation to commence. But this is a mistake. Syrup stronger than the above will ferment in warm weather, without addition. If the temperature be low, the syrup weak, and no yest added, acetous fermentation alone will take place. To determine the vinous, therefore, we must mix certain proportions of saccharine matter, water, and yest, and place them in a proper temperature.

To observe the chemical changes which occur, we must dissolve 4 or 5 parts of pure sugar in 20 parts of water, put the solution into a matrass, and add 1 part of yest. Into the mouth of the matrass a glass tube must be luted, which is recurved, so as to dip into the mercury of a pneumatic trough. If the apparatus be now placed in a temperature of from 70° to 80°, we shall speedily observe the syrup to become muddy, and a multitude of air bubbles to form all around the ferment. These unite, and attaching themselves to particles of the yest, rise along with it to the surface, forming a stratum of froth. The yesty matter will then disengage itself from the air, fall to the bottom of the vessel, to reacquire buoyancy a second time by attached air bubbles, and thus in succession. If we operate on 3 or 4 ounces of sugar, the fermentation will be very rapid during the first ten or twelve hours; it will then slacken, and terminate in the course of a few days. At this period the matter being deposited which disturbed the transparency of the liquor, this will become clear.

The following changes have now taken place: 1. The sugar is wholly, and the yest partially, decomposed. 2. A quantity of alkohol and carbonic acid, together nearly in weight to the sugar, is produced. 3. A white matter is formed, composed of hydrogen, oxygen, and carbon, equivalent to about half the weight of the decomposed ferment. The carbonic acid passes over into the pneumatic apparatus; the alkohol may be separated from the vinous liquid by distillation, and the white matter falls down to the bottom of the matrass with the remainder of the yest.

The quantity of yest decomposed is very small. 100

parts of sugar require for complete decomposition, only two and a half of that substance, supposed to be in a dry state. It is hence very probable, that the ferment, which has a strong affinity for oxygen, takes a little of it from the saccharine particles, by a part of its hydrogen and carbon, and thus the equilibrium being broken between the constituent principles of the sugar, these so react on each other, as to be transformed into alkohol and carbonic acid. If we consider the composition of alkohol, we shall find no difficulty in tracing the steps of this transformation.

Neglecting the minute products which the yest furnishes, in the act of fermentation, let us regard only the alkohol and carbonic acid. We shall then see, on comparing the composition of sugar to that of alkohol, that to transform sugar into alkohol, we must withdraw from it one volume of vapour of carbon, and one volume of oxygen, which form by their union one volume of carbonic acid gas. Finally, let us reduce the volumes into weights, we shall find, that 100 parts of sugar ought to be converted, during fermentation, into 51.55 of alkohol, and 48.45 of carbonic acid.

When it is required to preserve fermented liquors in the state produced by the first stage of fermentation, it is usual to put them into casks before the vinous process is completely ended; and in these closed vessels a change very slowly continues to be made for many months, and perhaps for some years.

But if the fermentative process be suffered to proceed in open vessels, more especially if the temperature be raised to 90 degrees, the acetous fermentation comes on. In this, the oxygen of the atmosphere is absorbed; and the more speedily in proportion as the surfaces of the liquor are often changed by lading it from one vessel to another. The usual method consists in exposing the fermented liquor to the air in open casks, the bunghole of which is covered with a tile to prevent the entrance of the rain. By the absorption of oxygen which takes place, the inflammable spirit becomes converted into an acid. If the liquid be then exposed to distillation, pure vinegar comes over instead of ardent spirit.

III. When the spontaneous decomposition is suffered to proceed beyond the acetous process, the vinegar becomes viscid and foul; air is emitted with an offensive smell; volatile alkali flies off; an earthy sediment is deposited; and the remaining liquid, if any, is mere water. This is the putrefactive process. See also *Putrefaction.*

FERME'NTUM. (*Quasi fervimentum*, from *ferveo*, to work.) Yest.

Fermentum cerevisiæ. Yest; Barm; the scum which collects on beer while fermenting, and has the property of exciting that process in various other substances. Medicinally it is antiseptic and tonic; and has been found useful internally in the cure of typhus fever attended with an obvious tendency to putrefaction in the system with petechiæ, vibices, and the like: the best way to administer it, is to mix a fluid ounce with seven of strong beer, and give three table spoonfuls to an adult every three or four hours. Externally, it is used in the fermenting cataplasm.

FERN. See *Filix* and *Polypodium.*

Fern, male. See *Polydodium filix mas.*

Fern, female. See *Pteris aquilina.*

FERNEL, John, was born at Claremont, near the end of the 15th century. He went at the age of 19 to prosecute his studies at Paris, and distinguished himself so much, that, after taking the degree of master of arts, he was chosen professor of dialectics in his college. His application then became intense, till a quartan ague obliged him to seek his native air: and on his return to Paris, he determined on the medical profession, and taught philosophy for his support, till in 1530, he took his doctor's degree. Soon after he married, and speedily got into extensive practice; and at length was made physician to the Dauphin, who afterward became Henry II. He was obliged to accompany that monarch in his campaigns, yet he still, though at the age of sixty, seldom passed a day without writing. But in 1558, having lost his wife of a fever, he did not long survive her. His works are numerous on philosophical, as well as medical subjects: of the latter, the most esteemed were his "Medicina," dedicated to Henry II., and a posthumous treatise on fevers.

Ferramentum. An instrument made of iron.

FERRO-CHYAZIC ACID. *Acidum ferro-chyazicum; chyazicum,* from the initial letters of carbon, hydrogen, and azote.) An acid obtained by Porrett by adding to a solution of ferro-cyanite of barytes, sulphuric acid just enough to precipitate the barytes. It has a pale yellow colour, no smell, and is decomposed by gentle heat or strong light, in which case hydrocyanic acid is formed, and white hydrocyanite of iron is deposited, which becomes blue by exposure.

FERRO-CYANATE. A compound of ferro-prussic acid with salifiable bases.

FERRO-CYANIC ACID. See *Ferro-prussic acid.*

FERRO-PRUSSIC ACID. *Acidum ferro-prussicum. Acidum ferro-cyanicum.* Into a solution of the amber-coloured crystals, usually called prussiates of potassa, pour hydro-sulphuret of barytes, as long as any precipitate falls. Throw the whole on a filter, and wash the precipitate with cold water. Dry it; and having dissolved 100 parts in cold water, add gradually thirty of concentrated sulphuric acid; agitate the mixture, and set it aside to repose. The supernatant liquid is ferro-prussic acid, called by Porrett, who had the merit of discovering it, ferruretted chyazic acid.

It has a pale lemon-yellow colour, but no smell. Heat and light decompose it. Hydrocyanic acid is then formed, and white ferro-prussiate of iron, which soon becomes blue. Its affinity for the bases enables it to displace acetic acid, without heat, from the acetates, and to form ferro-prussiates.

FE'RRUM. (*Ferrum, i.* neut.; the etymology uncertain.) Iron. See *Iron.*

Ferrum ammoniatum. Ammoniated iron; formerly known by the names of *flores martiales; flores salis ammoniaci martiales; ens martis; ens veneris Boylei; sal martis muriaticum sublimatum,* and lately by the title of *ferrum ammoniacale.* Take of subcarbonate of iron, muriate of ammonia, of each a pound. Mix them intimately, and sublime by immediate exposure to a strong fire; lastly, reduce the sublimed ammoniated iron to powder. This preparation is astringent and deobstruent, in doses from three to fifteen grains, or more, in the form of bolus or pills, prepared with some gum. It is exhibited in most cases of debility, in chlorosis, asthenia, menorrhagia, intermittent fevers, &c. This or some other strong preparation of iron, as the Tinct. ferri muriatis, Mr. Cline is wont to recommend in schirrhous affections of the breast. See *Tinctura ferri ammoniati.*

Ferrum tartarizatum. Tartarized iron. A tartrate of potassa and iron; formerly called *tartarus chalybeatus; mars solubilis; ferrum potabile.* Take of iron, a pound; supertartrate of potassa, powdered, two pounds; water, a pint. Rub them together; and expose them to the air in a broad glass vessel for eight days, then dry the residue in a sand bath, and reduce it to a very fine powder. Add to this powder a pint more water, and expose it for eight days longer, then dry it, and reduce it to a very fine powder. Its virtues are astringent and tonic, and it forms in solution an excellent tonic fomentation to contusions, lacerations, distortions, &c. Dose from ten grains to half a drachm.

Ferri alkalini liquor. Solution of alkaline iron. Take of iron, two drachms and a half; nitric acid, two fluid ounces; distilled water, six fluid ounces; solution of subcarbonate of potassa, six fluid ounces. Having mixed the acid and water, pour them upon the iron, and when the effervescence has ceased, pour off the clear acid solution; add this gradually, and at intervals, to the solution of subcarbonate of potassa, occasionally shaking it, until it has assumed a deep brown-red colour, and no further effervescence takes place. Lastly, set it by for six hours, and pour off the clear solution. This preparation was first described by Stael, and called tinctura martis alkalina, and is now introduced in the London Pharmacopœia as affording a combination of iron distinct from any other, and often applicable to practice. The dose is from half a drachm to a drachm.

Ferri carbonas. See *Ferri subcarbonas.*

Ferri limatura purificata. Purified iron filings. These possess tonic, astringent, and deobstruent virtues, and are calculated to relieve chlorosis and other diseases in which steel is indicated, where acidity in the primæ viæ abounds.

Ferri rubigo. See *Ferri subcarbonas.*

Ferri subcarbonas. *Ferri carbonas; Ferrum præcipitatum,* formerly called *chalybis rubigo præpa-*

rata and *ferri rubigo*. Subcarbonate of iron. Take of sulphate of iron, eight ounces; subcarbonate of soda, six ounces; boiling water, a gallon. Dissolve the sulphate of iron and subcarbonate of soda separately, each in four pints of water; then mix the solutions together and set it by, that the precipitated powder may subside; then having poured off the supernatant liquor, wash the subcarbonate of iron with hot water, and dry it upon bibulous paper in a gentle heat. It possesses mild corroborant and stimulating properties, and is exhibited with success in leucorrhœa, ataxia, asthenia, chlorosis, dyspepsia, rachitis, &c. Dose from two to ten grains.

FERRI SULPHAS. Sulphate of iron; formerly called *sal martis*, *vitriolum martis*, *vitriolum ferri*, and *ferrum vitriolatum*. Green vitriol. Take of iron, sulphuric acid, of each by weight, eight ounces; water, four pints. Mix together the sulphuric acid and water in a glass vessel, and add thereto the iron; then after the effervescence has ceased, filter the solution through paper, and evaporate it until crystals form as it cools. Having poured away the water, dry these upon bibulous paper. This is an excellent preparation of iron, and is exhibited, in many diseases, as a styptic, tonic, astringent, and anthelmintic. Dose from one grain to five grains.

[FERRILITE. *Common trap* of Kirwan. *Amorphous basalt* of Cleaveland. The *Ferrilite*, and perhaps the *Mullen stone* of Kirwan, may be referred to this variety of basalt. A.]

FERRURETTED CHYAZIC ACID. See *Ferroprussic acid.*

FERSÆ. The measles.

Fertile flower. See *Flos.*

FE'RULA. The name of a genus of plants in the Linnæan system. Class *Pentandria*; Order, *Digynia.*

FERULA AFRICANA GALBANIFERA. The galbanum plant. See *Bubon galbanum.*

FERULA ASSAFŒTIDA. The systematic name of the assafœtida plant. *Assafœtida. Hingiseh* of the Persians. *Altiht* of the Arabians. By some thought to be the σιλφιον, vel οπος σιλφιου of Dioscorides, Theophrastus, and Hippocrates. *Laser et laserpitium* of the Latins. *Ferula assafœtida—foliis alternatim sinuatis, obtusis*, of Linnæus. This plant, which affords us the assafœtida of the shops, grows plentifully on the mountains in the provinces of Chorassan and Laar, in Persia.

The process of obtaining it is as follows: the earth is cleared away from the top of the roots of the oldest plants; the leaves and stalks are then twisted away, and made into a covering, to screen the root from the sun; in this state the root is left for forty days, when the covering is removed, and the top of the root cut off transversely; it is then screened again from the sun for forty-eight hours, when the juice it exudes is scraped off, and exposed to the sun to harden. A second transverse section of the root is made, and the exudation suffered to continue for forty-eight hours, and then scraped off. In this manner it is eight times repeatedly collected in a period of six weeks. The juice thus obtained has a bitter, acrid, pungent taste, and is well known by its peculiar nauseous smell, the strength of which is the surest test of its goodness. This odour is extremely volatile, and of course the drug loses much of its efficacy by keeping. It is brought to us in large irregular masses, composed of various little shining lumps, or grains, which are partly of a whitish colour, partly reddish, and partly of a violet hue. Those masses are accounted the best which are clear, of a pale reddish colour, and variegated with a great number of elegant white tears. This concrete juice consists of two-thirds of gum, and one-third of resin and volatile oil, in which its taste and smell reside. It yields all its virtues to alkohol. Triturated with water, it forms a milk-like mixture, the resin being diffused by the medium of the gum. Distilled with water, it affords a small quantity of essential oil. It is the most powerful of all the fœtid gums, and is a most valuable remedy. It is most commonly employed in hysteria, hypochondriasis, some symptoms of dyspepsia, flatulent colics, and in most of those diseases termed nervous, but its chief use is derived from its antispasmodic effects; and it is thought to be the most powerful remedy we possess, for those peculiar convulsive and spasmodic affections, which often recur in the first of these diseases, both taken into the stomach and in the way of enema. It is also recommended as an emmenagogue, anthelmintic, anti asthmatic, and anodyne. Dr. Cullen prefers it as an expectorant to gum ammoniacum. Where we wish it to act immediately as an antispasmodic, it should be used in a fluid form, as that of tincture, from half a drachm to two drachms. When given in the form of a pill, or triturated with water, its usual dose is from five to twenty grains. When in the form of enema, one or two drachms are to be diffused in eight ounces of warm milk or water. It is sometimes applied externally as a plaster and stimulating remedy, in hysteria, &c.

FERULA MINOR. All-heal of Æsculapius. This plant is said to be detergent.

FERULA'CCA. See *Bubon galbanum.*

FEVER. See *Febris.*

FEVERFEW. See *Matricaria.*

FI'BER. (From *fiber*, extreme, because it resides in the extremities of lakes and rivers.) The beaver. See *Castor fiber.*

FIBRE. *Fibra.* A very simple filament. It is owing to the difference in the nature and arrangements of the fibres that the structure of the several parts of animals and vegetables differ: hence the barks, woods, leaves, &c. of vegetables, and the cellular structure, membranes, muscles, vessels, nerves, and, in short every part of the body, has its fibres variously constituted and arranged, so as to form these different parts.

Fibre muscular. See *Muscular fibre.*

FIBRIL. (*Fibrila*, diminutive of *fibra.*) A small thread-like fibre: applied to the little roots which are given off from radicles.

FI'BRIN. "A peculiar organic compound found both in vegetables and animals. Vauquelin discovered it in the juice of the papaw-tree. It is a soft solid, of a greasy appearance, insoluble in water, which softens in the air, becoming viscid, brown, and semi-transparent. On hot coals it melts, throws out greasy drops crackles, and evolves the smoke and odour of roasting meat. Fibrin is procured, however, in its most characteristic state from animal matter. It exists in chyle; it enters into the composition of blood; of it, the chief part of muscular flesh is formed; and hence it may be regarded as the most abundant constituent of the soft solids of animals.

To obtain it, we may beat blood as it issues from the veins with a bundle of twigs. Fibrin soon attaches itself to each stem, under the form of long reddish filaments, which become colourless by washing them with cold water. It is solid, white, insipid, without smell, denser than water, and incapable of affecting the hue of litmus or violets. When moist it possesses a species of elasticity; by desiccation it becomes yellowish, hard, and brittle. By distillation we can extract from it much carbonate of ammonia, some acetate, a fœtid brown oil, and gaseous products; while there remains in the retort a very luminous charcoal, very brilliant, difficult of incineration, which leaves, after combustion, phosphate of lime, a little phosphate of magnesia, carbonate of lime, and carbonate of soda.

Cold water has no action on fibrin. Treated with boiling water, it is so changed as to lose the property of softening and dissolving in acetic acid. The liquor filtered from it, yields precipitates with infusion of galls, and the residue is white, dry, hard, and of an agreeable taste.

When kept for some time in alkohol of 0.810, it gives rise to an adipocerous matter, having a strong and disagreeable odour. This matter remains dissolved in the alkohol, and may be precipitated by water. Æther makes it undergo a similar alteration, but more slowly. When digested in weak muriatic acid, it evolves a little azote, and a compound is formed, hard, horny, and which, washed repeatedly with water, is transformed into another gelatinous compound. This seems to be a neutral muriate, soluble in hot water; while the first is an acid muriate, insoluble even in boiling water. Sulphuric acid, diluted with six times its weight of water, has similar effects. When not too concentrated, nitric acid has a very different action on fibrin. For example, when its sp. gr. is 1.25, there results from it at first a disengagement of azote, while the fibrin becomes covered with fat, and the liquid turns yellow. By digestion of twenty-four hours, the whole fibrin is attacked, and converted into a pulverulent mass of lemon-yellow colour, which seems to be composed of a mixture of fat and fibrin, altered and intimately com bined with the malic and nitric or nitrous acids. In fact, if we put this mass on a filter, and wash it copiously with water, it will part with a portion of its acid, will preserve the property of reddening litmus, and will take an orange hue. On treating it afterward with boiling alkohol, we dissolve the fatty matter; and putting the remainder in contact with chalk and water, an effervescence will be occasioned by the escape of carbonic acid, and malate or nitrate of lime will remain in solution.

Concentrated acetic acid renders fibrin soft at ordinary temperatures, and converts it by the aid of heat into a jelly, which is soluble in hot water, with the disengagement of a small quantity of azote. This solution is colourless, and possesses little taste. Evaporated to dryness, it leaves a transparent residue, which reddens litmus paper, and which cannot be dissolved even in boiling water, but by the medium of more acetic acid. Sulphuric, nitric, and muriatic acids, precipitate the animal matter, and form acid combinations. Potassa, soda, ammonia, effect likewise the precipitation of this matter, provided we do not use too great an excess of alkali; for then the precipitated matter would be redissolved. Aqueous potassa and soda gradually dissolve fibrin in the cold, without occasioning any perceptible change in its nature; but with heat they decompose it, giving birth to a quantity of ammoniacal gas, and other usual animal products. Fibrin does not putrefy speedily when kept in water. It shrinks on exposure to a considerable heat, and emits the smell of burning horn. It is composed, according to the analysis of Gay Lussac, and Thenard, of

Carbon,	53.360	
Azote,	19.934	
Oxygen,	19.685	22.14 water.
Hydrogen,	7.021	4.56 hydrogen.

FIBROLITE. A crystallized mineral harder than quartz, of a white or gray colour, found in the Carnatic, and composed of alumina, silica, and iron.

FIBROSUS. (From *fibre*, a fibre.) Fibrous. A term frequently used in anatomy to express the texture of parts. In botany, its meaning is the same, and is applied to roots and other parts, as those of grasses, &c.

FI'BULA. (*Quasi figilula;* from *figo*, to fasten: so named because it joins together the tibia and the muscles.) A long bone of the leg, situated on the outer side of the tibia, and which forms, at its lower end, the outer ankle. Its upper extremity is formed into an irregular head, on the inside of which is a slightly concave articulating surface, which, in the recent subjects, is covered with cartilage, and receives the circular flat surface under the edge of the external cavity of the tibia. This articulation is surrounded by a capsular ligament, which is farther strengthened by other strong ligamentous fibres, so as to allow only a small motion backwards and forwards.—Externally, the head of the fibula is rough and protuberant, serving for the attachment of ligaments, and for the insertion of the biceps cruris muscle.—Immediately below it, on its inner side, is a tubercle, from which a part of the gastrocnemius internus has its origin. Immediately below this head the body of the bone begins. It is of a triangular shape, and appears as if it were slightly twisted at each end, in a different direction. It is likewise a little curved inwards and forwards. This curvature is in part owing to the action of muscles; and in part perhaps to the carelessness of nurses.—Of the three angles of the bone, that which is turned towards the tibia is the most prominent, and serves for the attachment of the interosseous ligament, which, in its structure and uses, resembles that of the forearm, and, like that, is a little interrupted above and below. The three surfaces of the bone are variously impressed by different muscles. About the middle of the posterior surface is observed a passage for the medullary vessels, slanting downwards. The lower end of the fibula is formed into a spongy, oblong head, externally rough and convex, internally smooth and covered with a thin cartilage, where it is received by the external triangular depression at the lower end of the tibia. This articulation, which resembles that of its upper extremity, is furnished with a capsular ligament, and farther strengthened by ligamentous fibres, which are stronger and more considerable than those before described. They extend from the tibia to the fibula, in an oblique direction, and are more easily discernible before than behind. Below this the fibula is lengthened out, so as to form a considerable process, called *malleolus externus*, or the outer ankle. It is smooth and covered with cartilage on the inside, where it is contiguous to the astragalus, or first bone of the foot. At the lower and inner part of this process, there is a spongy cavity, filled with fat; and a little beyond this, posteriorly, is a cartilaginous groove, for the tendons of the peroneus longus and peroneus brevis, which are here bound down by the ligamentous fibres that are extended over them.

The principal uses of this bone seem to be, to afford origin and insertion to muscles, and to contribute to the articulation of the leg with the foot.

FICA'RIA. (From *ficus*, a fig; so called from its likeness.) See *Ranunculus ficaria.*

FICA'TIO. (From *ficus*, a fig.) A tuberculous disease, near the anus and pudenda.

FICOIDE'A. *Ficoides.* Resembling a fig. A name of the house-leek. See *Sempervivum tectorium.*

FI'CUS. 1. A fleshy substance about the anus, in figure resembling a fig.

2. The name of a genus of plants in the Linnæan system. Class, *Polygamia;* Order, *Diœcia.* The fig-tree.

FICUS CARICA. The systematic name of the fig-tree. *Carica; Ficus; Ficus vulgaris; Ficus communis.* Συκη of the Greeks. French figs are, when completely ripe, soft, succulent, and easily digested, unless eaten in immoderate quantities, when they are apt to occasion flatulency, pain of the bowels, and diarrhœa. The dried fruit, which is sold in our shops, is pleasanter to the taste, and more wholesome and nutritive. They are directed in the *decoctum hordei compositum*, and in the *confectio sennæ.* Applied externally, they promote the suppuration of tumours; hence they have a place in maturating cataplasms; and are very convenient to apply to the gums, and, when boiled with milk, to the throat.

FICUS INDICA. See *Lacca.*

Fiddle-shaped. See *Leaf.*

FIDICINA'LES. (*Fidicinalis*, sc. *musculus.*) See *Lumbricales.*

FIENUS, THOMAS, was son of a physician of Antwerp, and born in 1567. After studying at Leyden and Bologna, he was invited, at the age of 26, to be one of the medical professors at Louvaine, where he took his degrees. With the exception of one year, during which he attended the Duke of Bavaria, he remained in that office till his death in 1631. Besides his great abilities in medicine and surgery, he was distinguished for his knowledge of natural history, the learned languages, and the mathematics. He has left several works: the chief of which is termed "Libri Chirurgici XII.," treating of the principal operations; it passed through many editions. His father, *John*, was author of a well-received treatise, "De Flatibus."

FIG. See *Ficus carica.*

FIGURESTONE. Bildstein. *Agalmatolite.* A massive mineral of a gray colour, or brown flesh-red, and sometimes spotted, or with blue veins; unctuous to the touch, and yielding to the nail. It comes from China, cut into grotesque figures. It differs from steatite in wanting the magnesia. It is also found in Transylvania, and in Wales.

FIGWORT. See *Ranunculus ficaria.*

FILA'GO. (From *filum*, a thread, and *ago*, to produce or have to do with, in allusion to the cottony web connected with every part of the plant.) Cud or cotton-weed; formerly used as an astringent.

FILA'MENT. (*Filamentum;* from *filum*, a thread.) 1. A term applied in anatomy to a small thread-like portion adhering to any part, and frequently synonymous with fibre. See *Fibre.*

2. The *stamen* of a flower consists of the filament, anther, and pollen. The filament is the column which supports the anther.

From its *figure* it is called,

1. *Capillary;* as in *Plantago.*
2. *Filiform;* as in *Scilla maritima.*
3. *Flat;* as in *Allium cepa.*
4. *Dilatate*, spreading laterally; as in *Ornithogalum umbellatum.*
5. *Pedicellate*, affixed transversely to a little stalk; as in *Salvia.*
6. *Bifid*, having two; as in *Stemodia.*

7. *Bifurced;* as in *Prunella.*
8. *Multifid;* as in *Carolina princeps.*
9. *Dentate;* as in *Rosmarinus officinalis.*
10. *Nicked;* as in *Allium cepa.*
11. *Lanceolate;* as in *Ornithogalum pyrenaicum.*
12. *Castrate,* the anther naturally wanting; as in *Gratiola officinalis.*
13. *Subulate;* as in *Tulipa gesneriani.*

From the *pubescence,*

1. *Barbate,* bearded; as in *Lycium.*
2. *Lanate,* woolly; as in *Verbascum thapsus.*
3. *Pilose;* as in *Anthericum frutescens.*
4. *Gland-bearing;* as in *Laurus* and *Rheum.*

From its direction,

1. *Erect;* as in *Tulipa gesneriana.*
2. *Incurved;* curved inward, and a little bent.
3. *Declinate;* as in *Hemerocalis fulva.*
4. *Connivent;* as in *Physalis alkekengi.*

From its concretion,

1. *Liberate,* free, nowhere adhering; as in *Nicotiana tabacum.*
2. *Connate,* adhering at their base; as in *Malva sylvestris,* and *Alcea rosea.*

From its insertion,

1. *Receptaculine,* inserted into the receptaculum; as in *Papaver somniferum.*
2. *Corolline,* as in *Verbascum thapsus,* and *Nerium oleander.*
3. *Calicine;* as in *Pyrus malus,* and *Mespilus germanica.*
4. *Styline;* as in the *Orchides.*
5. *Nectorine;* as in *Pancratium declinatum.*

From its length, it is said to be very *long;* as in *Plantago major:* very *short* in *Jasminum* and *Vinca:* and *unequal,* some long, some short; as in *Cheiranthus cheiri.*

FILARIA. The name of a genus of intestinal worms.

File'llum. (From *filum,* a thread; because it resembles a string.) The frænum of the penis and tongue.

File'tum. (From *filum,* a thread; named from its string-like appearance.) The frænum of the tongue and penis.

FILICES. (*Filix, cis.* f.; from *filum,* a thread.) Ferns. One of the families, or natural tribe into which the whole vegetable kingdom is divided. They are defined plants which bear their flower and fruit on the back of the leaf or stalk, which is termed *frons.*

FILI'CULA. (Dim. of *filix,* fern; a small sort of fern: or from *filum,* a thread, which it resembles.) Common maiden-hair. See *Adianthum capillus veneris.*

FILIFORMIS. Filiform, thread-like: applied to many parts of animals and vegetables from their resemblance.

FILIPE'NDULA. (From *filum,* a thread, and *pendeo,* to hang; so named because the numerous bulbs of its roots hang, as it were, by small threads.) See *Spiræa filipendula.*

Filipendula aquatica. Water-dropwort; the *Œnanthe fistulosa* of Linnæus.

Filius ante patrem. Any plant, the flower of which comes out before the leaf; as coltsfoot.

FI'LIX. (From *filum,* a thread; so called from its being cut, as it were, in slender portions, like threads.) Fern. See *Polypodium.*

Filix aculeata. See *Polypodium aculeatum.*

Filix florida. See *Osmunda regalis.*

Filix fœmina. See *Pteris aquilina.*

Filix mas. See *Polypodium filix mas.*

FILTRA'TION. (*Filtratio;* from *filtrum,* a strainer.) An operation, by means of which a fluid is mechanically separated from consistent particles merely mixed with it. It does not differ from straining.

An apparatus fitted up for this purpose is called a filter. The form of this is various, according to the intention of the operator. A piece of tow, or wool, or cotton, stuffed into the pipe of a funnel, will prevent the passage of grosser particles, and by that means render the fluid clearer which comes through. Sponge is still more effectual. A strip of linen rag wetted and hung over the side of a vessel containing a fluid, in such a manner as that one end of the rag may be immersed in the fluid, and the other end may remain without, below the surface, will act as a syphon, and carry over the clearer portion. Linen or woollen stuffs may either be fastened over the mouths of proper vessels, or fixed to a frame, like a sieve, for the purpose of filtering. All these are more commonly used by cooks and apothecaries than by philosophical chemists, who, for the most part, use the paper called cap paper, made up without size.

As the filtration of considerable quantities of fluid could not be effected at once without breaking the filter of paper, it is found requisite to use a linen cloth, upon which the paper is applied and supported.

Precipitates and other pulverulent matters are collected more speedily by filtration than by subsidence. But there are many chemists who disclaim the use of this method, and avail themselves of the latter only, which is certainly more accurate, and liable to no objection, where the powders are such as will admit of edulcoration and drying in the open air.

Some fluids, as turbid water, may be purified by filtering through sand. A large earthen funnel, or stone bottle with the bottom beaten out, may have its neck loosely stopped with small stones, over which smaller may be placed, supporting layers of gravel increasing in fineness, and lastly covered to the depth of a few inches with fine sand all thoroughly cleansed by washing. This apparatus is superior to a filtering stone, as it will cleanse water in large quantities, and may readily be renewed when the passage is obstructed, by taking out and washing the upper stratum of sand.

A filter for corrosive liquors may be constructed, on the same principles, of broken and pounded glass.—*Ure's Chem. Dict.*

FI'LTRUM. A filter, straining or filtering instrument.

FILUM. A thread or filament.

Filum arsenicale. Corrosive sublimate.

FI'MBRIA. (A fringe, *quasi finibria;* from *finis,* the extremity.) A fringe. 1. A term used by anatomists to curled membraneous productions. See *Fimbriæ.*

2. In botany, it is applied to the dentate or fringe-like ring of the operculum of mosses, by the elastic power of which the operculum is displaced. See *Peristomium.*

Fimbriæ. (*Fimbria,* a fringe. *Quasi finibria;* from *finis,* the extremity.) The extremities of the Fallopian tubes. See *Uterus.*

FINCKLE. See *Anethum fœniculum.*

Fingered leaf. See *Leaf.*

FIORITE. See *Pearl sinter.*

FIR. See *Pinus.*

Fir balsam. See *Pinus balsamea.*

Fir, Canada. See *Pinus balsamea.*

Fir, Norway spruce. See *Pinus abies.*

Fir, Scotch. See *Pinus sylvestris.*

Fir, silver. See *Pinus picea.*

FIRE. *Ignis.* A very simple and active element, the principal agent in nature to balance the power and natural effect of attraction. The most useful acceptation of the word fire comprehends *heat* and *light.* There have been several theories proposed respecting fire, but no one as yet is fully established. See *Caloric* and *Light.*

[**FFIRTH, Dr. S.** of Salem, in New-Jersey, published a dissertation on malignant fever in 1805, with an attempt to prove that yellow fever is not contagious. The experiments he tried with the matter of *black-vomit* are bold and decisive. He proves by his experiments, that neither the black-vomit, serum, nor saliva of persons labouring under yellow fever, are capable of communicating that disease. He dropped the matter of black-vomit in his eye, inoculated himself with, and even swallowed it. For the particulars of these and other experiments, see *Black-vomit.* A.]

Firmi'sium mineralium. Antimony.

FISCHER, John Andrew, son of an apothecary at Erfurt, was born in 1667. He graduated there, and was appointed in succession to several professorships; but that of pathology and the practice of medicine he did not receive till the age of 48. He acquired considerable reputation in his profession; and he had been ten years physician to the court of Mayence when he died in 1729. Among several minor works he was author of some of greater importance; as the "Consilia Medica," in three volumes; the "Responsa Practica," and a Synopsis of Medicine, facetiously termed "Ilias in Nuce."

[FISHERY, SEAL. Vessels belonging to the United States, employed in voyages for catching seals, usually pass round Cape-Horn, and visit the islands of Juan Fernandez and Massafuero. At the latter of these, seals were formerly very numerous. They are also taken at Falkland's Islands, Southern Georgia, Tristan d'Acunha, St. Paul's, and Amsterdam islands. But of late years they have been found to be much more rare. Even at Massafuero, and the islands in its vicinity, they are no longer found in that abundance which prevailed when these voyages were first undertaken.

The sea-elephant belongs to the same family with the seal. He is found on many of the uninhabited islands of the great southern ocean, particularly at Kerguelan's Land, which they frequent in great herds. They make little resistance, and of course are easily killed. Several of our vessels are said to have been engaged in their destruction. Their oil is found to be of an excellent quality; and not only answers for home consumption, but makes a valuable article of exportation. A.]

["FISHERY, WHALE. This branch of business seems to be less inviting and profitable than it formerly was. Whether this is owing to a scarcity of whales, to greater exertions of other nations, or to the inferiority of the market at home, and high duties abroad, we need not examine particularly here. The decline of the whale-fishery among the people of the United States, is probably to be ascribed to the operation of all these causes, as well as to bounties and immunities granted by some of the European powers so generously as to tempt many of our most enterprising whalemen to engage themselves and their capitals in foreign service."—*Med. Repos.*

These observations were made in 1805, since which there has been a great increase in the amount of capital, number of ships, and seamen engaged in the whale fishery from the United States. The greatest number of ships in this business are fitted out at New-Bedford in Massachusetts, the island of Nantucket, and Sag-Harbour, on the east end of Long-Island, of the state of New-York. Some few are fitted out from this city, and some from ports in Connecticut. Few or none of our vessels pursue this business in the Arctic seas. Some take the right whale on the coast of Brazil, but most of those engaged in this employment from the United States resort to the Pacific ocean, where they take both the spermaceti and the right whale.

Vessels are fitted out on shares; the owners, master, and seamen, dividing the proceeds of the voyage according to a certain ratio agreed upon before the voyage commences, and which generally lasts about two years. The success depends upon the skill and enterprise of the officers and crew, which generally consists of hardy and active young men. The greater their success the greater their share of the profits. The spermaceti-whale is the great object of their search in the Pacific, as from this animal is derived the pharmacopœial substance called *sperma ceti*. Ambergris is also occasionally found in the intestines of this whale. A.]

[FISHERY, COD. "This employment appears to be on the increase. Notwithstanding the abundance of business which might be followed on shore, in a country having so many millions of unappropriated acres, there are found plenty of people who prefer the catching of fish along the coasts of the United States, and on the Banks of Newfoundland. Government allows a bounty on the tonnage of the vessels engaged in the cod-fishery, in lieu of a drawback upon the salt used in curing the fish."—*Med. Rep.*

The cod taken along our shores and on the Banks of Newfoundland is the *Gadus morhua*, though some of the other species are also taken. On the rocky shores of Maine, the hake (*Gadus merluccius*) is abundantly taken. The fish is not so good as the Gadus morhua, but it has a very large sound from which icthyocolla, or fish glue, of a good quality, may be prepared in any quantity. A.]

FISH-GLUE. See *Ichthyocolla.*

FISSURA. A fissure. 1. That species of fracture in which the bone is slit, but not completely divided.

2. A name given to a deep and long depression in a part.

FISSURA MAGNA SYLVII. The anterior and middle lobes of the cerebrum on each side are parted by a deep narrow sulcus, which ascends obliquely backwards from the temporal ala of the os sphenoides, to near the middle of the os parietale, and this sulcus is thus called.

FISSUS. Cleft, cloven. Applied to leaves, and pods, *folia fissa*, that are, as it were, cut into fissures or straight segments. See *Leaf.*

FISTIC-NUT. See *Pistachia vera.*

FI'STULA. (*Quasi fusula:* from *fundo*, to pour out; or from its similarity to a pipe, or reed.) *Eligii morbus.* A term in surgery, applied to a long and sinuous ulcer that has a narrow opening, and which sometimes leads to a larger cavity, and has no disposition to heal.

FISTULA'RIA. (From *fistula*, a pipe, so called because its stock is hollow.) Stavesacre. See *Delphinium staphisagria.*

FIXED. In chemistry, the term fixed bodies is applied to those substances which cannot be caused to pass by a strong rarefaction from the solid or liquid state of an elastic fluid.

Fixed air. See *Carbonic acid.*

FIXITY. The property by which bodies resist the action of heat, so as not to rise in vapour.

FLAG. See *Acorus* and *Iris.*

[FLAGG, DR. JOHN, was son of the Rev. Ebenezer Flagg, the first minister of Chester, in New-Hampshire. He was graduated at Harvard University in 1761, and studied medicine under the direction of Dr. Osgood, of Andover. He commenced practice at Woburn, but in 1769 removed to Lynn, where he enjoyed the full confidence of his fellow-citizens, and acquired a high standing in his profession.

When, in 1775, the dark cloud overspread our political hemisphere, Dr. Flagg was prepared to unite in the strong measures of resistance against every encroachment upon the rights and freedom of his country. He was an active and useful member of the committee of safety, and contributed largely to the promotion of the military preparations to meet the exigencies which soon after happened. From a native modesty, he declined any appointment in the councils of the state, but was prevailed upon to accept the commission of lieutenant-colonel of militia, under the venerable Col. Timothy Pickering, which, however, he soon after resigned, that he might devote his whole attention to the practice of medicine, which he preferred to military pursuits.

He was elected a member of the Massachusetts Medical Society immediately after its incorporation, when the number of fellows was restricted to seventy in the whole commonwealth. He held a commission of justice of the peace before the revolution and after the adoption of our state constitution, till his death. The fatigues of an extensive circle of practice, and the exposures incident to a professional life, impaired his constitution, and he fell a victim to pulmonary consumption in 1793, in the 50th year of his age. A.]

FLAGELLIFORMIS. Whip-like. A term applied to a stem that is long and pliant, whip-like; as that of jasmine and blue boxthorn. See *Caulis.*

Flake-white. Oxide of bismuth.

FLA'MMULA. (Dim. of *flamma*, a fire: named from the burning pungency of its taste.) See *Ranunculus flammula.*

FLAMMULA JOVIS. See *Clematis recta.*

FLATULENT. Windy.

FLAX. See *Linum.*

Flax-leaved daphne. See *Daphne gnidium.*

Flax, purging. See *Linum catharticum.*

Flax, spurge. See *Daphne gnidium.*

FLEA-WORT. See *Plantago psyllium.*

FLE'MEN. (From *flecto*, to incline downwards.) *Flegma.* A tumour about the ankles.

FLERE'SIN. Gout.

FLESH. 1. The muscles of animals.

2. A vulgar term for all the soft parts of an animal

3. It is also applied to leaves, fruit, &c. which have the appearance or consistence of flesh.

FLE'XOR. The name of several muscles, the office of which is to bend parts into which they are inserted.

FLEXOR ACCESSORIUS DIGITORUM PEDIS. See *Flexor longus digitorum pedis.*

FLEXOR BREVIS DIGITORUM PEDIS, PERFORATUS, SUBLIMIS. A flexor muscle of the toes, situated on the foot. *Flexor brevis digitorum pedis, perforatus* of

Albinus *Flexor brevis* of Douglas. *Flexor digitorum brevis, sive perforatus pedis* of Winslow. *Perforatus, seu flexor secundi internodii digitorum pedis* of Cowper; and *Calcano sus-phalangettien commun* of Dumas. It arises by a narrow, tendinous, and fleshy beginning, from the inferior protuberance of the os calcis. It likewise derives many of its fleshy fibres from the adjacent aponeurosis, and soon forms a thick belly, which divides into four portions. Each of these portions terminates in a flat tendon, the fibres of which decussate, to afford a passage to a tendon of the long flexor, and afterward reuniting, are inserted into the second phalanx of each of the four less toes. This muscle serves to bend the second joint of the toes.

FLEXOR BREVIS MINIMI DIGITI PEDIS. *Parathenar minor* of Winslow. This little muscle is situated along the inferior surface and outer edge of the metatarsal bone of the little toe. It arises tendinous from the basis of that bone, and from the ligaments that connect it to the os cuboides. It soon becomes fleshy, and adheres almost the whole length of the metatarsal bone, at the anterior extremity of which it forms a small tendon, that is inserted into the root of the first joint of the little toe. Its use is to bend the little toe.

FLEXOR BREVIS POLLICIS MANUS. *Flexor secundi internodii* of Douglas. *Thenar* of Winslow. *Flexor primi et secundi ossis pollicis* of Cowper; and *Carpo-phalangien du pouce* of Dumas. This muscle is divided into two portions by the tendon of the flexor longus pollicis. The outermost portion arises tendinous from the anterior part of the os trapezoides and internal annular ligament. The second, or innermost, and thickest portion, arises from the same bone, and likewise from the os magnum, and os cuneiforme. Both these portions are inserted tendinous into these sesamoid bones of the thumb. The use of this muscle is to bend the second joint of the thumb.

FLEXOR BREVIS POLLICIS PEDIS. A muscle of the great toe, that bends the first joint of that part. *Flexor brevis* of Douglas. *Flexor brevis pollicis* of Cowper; and *Tarsophalangien du pouce* of Dumas. It is situated upon the metatarsal bone of the great toe, arises tendinous from the under and anterior part of the os calcis, and from the under part of the os cuneiforme externum. It soon becomes fleshy and divisible into two portions, which do not separate from each other till they have reached the anterior extremity of the metatarsal bone of the great toe, where they become tendinous, and then the innermost portion unites with the tendon of the abductor, and the outermost with that of the abductor pollicis. They adhere to the external os sesamoideum, and are finally inserted into the root of the first joint of the great toe. These two portions, by their separation, form a groove, in which passes the tendon of the flexor longus pollicis.

FLEXOR CARPI RADIALIS. A long thin muscle, situated obliquely at the inner and anterior part of the forearm, between the palmaris longus and the pronator teres. *Radialis internus* of Albinus and Winslow; and *Epitrochlo metacarpien* of Dumas. It arises tendinous from the inner condyle of the os humeri, and, by many fleshy fibres, from the adjacent tendinous fascia. It descends along the inferior edge of the pronator teres, and terminates in a long, flat, and thin tendon, which afterward becomes narrower and thicker, and, after passing under the internal annular ligament, in a groove distinct from the other tendons of the wrist, it spreads wider again, and is inserted into the fore and upper part of the metacarpal bone that sustains the fore-finger. It serves to bend the hand, and its oblique direction may likewise enable it to assist in its pronation.

FLEXOR CARPI ULNARIS. *Ulnaris internus* of Winslow and Albinus. *Epitrochli cubito carpien* of Dumas. A muscle situated on the cubit or forearm, that assists in bending the arm. It arises tendinous from the inner condyle of the os humeri, and, by a small fleshy origin, from the anterior edge of the olecranon. Between these two portions, we find the ulnar nerve passing to the forearm. Some of its fibres arise likewise from the tendinous fascia that covers the muscles of the forearm. In its descent, it soon becomes tendinous, but its fleshy fibres do not entirely disappear till it has reached the lower extremity of the ulna, where its tendon spreads a little, and after sending off a few fibres to the external and internal and annular ligaments, is inserted into the os pisiforme.

FLEXOR LONGUS DIGITORUM PEDIS PROFUNDUS PERFORANS. A flexor muscle of the toes, situated along the posterior part and inner side of the leg. *Perforans seu flexor profundus* of Douglas. *Flexor digitorum longus, sive perforans pedis*, and *perforans seu flexor tertii internodii digitorum pedis* of Cowper; and *Tibio phalangetien* of Dumas. It arises fleshy from the back part of the tibia, and, after running down to the internal ankle, its tendon passes under a kind of annular ligament, and then through a sinuosity at the inside of the os calcis. Soon after this it receives a small tendon from the flexor longus pollicis pedis, and about the middle of the foot it divides into four tendons, which pass through the slits of the flexor brevis digitorum pedis, and are inserted into the upper part of the last bone of all the less toes. About the middle of the foot, this muscle unites with a fleshy portion, which, from the name of its first describer, has been usually called *massa carnea Jacobi Sylvii*: it is also termed *Flexor accessorius digitorum pedis.* This appendage arises by a thin fleshy origin, from most part of the sinuosity of the os calcis, and likewise by a thin tendinous beginning from the anterior part of the external tubercle of that bone; it soon becomes all fleshy, and unites to the long flexor just before it divides into its four tendons. The use of this muscle is to bend the last joint of the toes.

FLEXOR LONGUS POLLICIS MANUS. *Flexor longus pollicis* of Albinus. *Flexor tertii internodii* of Douglas; *Flexor tertii internodii sive longissimus pollicis* of Cowper; and *radio-phalangetien du pouce* of Dumas. A muscle of the thumb placed at the side of the flexor longus digitorum, profundus, perforans, and covered by the extensores carpi radiales. It arises fleshy from the anterior surface of the radius, immediately below the insertion of the biceps, and is continued down along the oblique ridge, which serves for the insertion of the supinator brevis, as far as the pronator quadratus. Some of its fibres spring likewise from the neighbouring edge of the interosseous ligament. Its tendon passes under the internal annular ligament of the wrist, and, after running along the inner surface of the first bone of the thumb, between the two portions of the flexor brevis pollicis, goes to be inserted into the last joint of the thumb, being bound down in its way by the ligamentous expansion that is spread over the second bone. In some subjects we find a tendinous portion arising from the inner condyle of the os humeri, and forming a fleshy slip that commonly terminates near the upper part of the origin of this muscle from the radius. The use of this muscle is to bend the last joint of the thumb.

FLEXOR LONGUS POLLICIS PEDIS. A muscle of the great toe, situated along the posterior part of the leg. It arises tendinous and fleshy a little below the head of the fibula, and its fibres continue to adhere to that bone almost to its extremity. A little above the heel it terminates in a round tendon, which, after passing in a groove formed at the posterior edge of the astragalus, and internal and lateral part of the os calcis, in which it is secured by an annular ligament, goes to be inserted into the last bone of the great toe, which it serves to bend.

FLEXOR OSSIS METACARPI POLLICIS. *Opponens pollicis* of Innes. *Opponent pollicis manus* of Albinus. *Flexor primi internodii* of Douglas. *Antithenar sive semi-interosseus pollicis* of Winslow; and *Carpo phalangien du pouce* of Dumas. A muscle of the thumb, situated under the abductor brevis pollicis, which it resembles in its shape. It arises tendinous and fleshy from the os scaphoides, and from the anterior and inner part of the internal annular ligament. It is inserted tendinous and fleshy into the under and anterior part of the first bone of the thumb. It serves to turn the first bone of the thumb upon its axis, and at the same time to bring it inwards opposite to the other fingers.

FLEXOR PARVUS MINIMI DIGITI. *Abductor minimi digiti, Hypothenar Riolani* of Douglas. *Hypothenar minimi digiti* of Winslow; and second *carpo-phalangien du petit doigt* of Dumas. A muscle of the little finger, situated along the inner surface of the metacarpal bone of the little finger. It arises tendinous and fleshy from the hook-like process of the unciform bone, and likewise from the anterior surface of the adjacent part of the annular ligament. It terminates in a flat tendon which is connected with that of the abductor minimi digiti, and inserted into the inner and anterior part of the upper end of the first bone of the little finger. It serves to bend the little finger, and likewise to assist the abductor.

Flexor profundus perforans. *Profundus*, of Albinus. *Perforans*, of Douglas. *Perforans vulgo profundus*, of Winslow; *Flexor tertii internodii digitorum manus, vel perforatus manus*, of Cowper; and *Cubito phalangetien commun*, of Dumas. A muscle of the fingers situated on the forearm, immediately under the *perforatus*, which it greatly resembles in its shape. It arises fleshy from the external side, and upper part of the ulna, for some way downwards, and from a large portion of the interrosseous ligament. It splits into four tendons a little before it passes under the annular ligament of the wrist, and these pass through the slit in the tendons of the flexor sublimis, to be inserted into the fore and upper part of the third or last bone of all the fore-fingers, the joint of which they bend.

Flexor sublimis perforatus. This muscle, which is the *perforatus* of Cowper, Douglas, and Winslow, is, by Albinus and others, named *sublimis*. It has gotten the name of *perforatus*, from its tendons being perforated by those of another flexor muscle of the finger, called the *perforans*. They who give it the appellation of *sublimis*, consider its situation with respect to the latter, and which, instead of *perforans*, they name *profundus*. It is a long muscle, situated most commonly at the anterior and inner part of the forearm, between the palmaris longus and the flexor carpi ulnaris; but, in some subjects, we find it placed under the former of these muscles, between the flexor carpi ulnaris and the flexor carpi radialis. It arises, tendinous and fleshy, from the inner condyle of the os humeri, from the inner edge of the coronoid process of the ulna, and from the upper and forepart of the radius, down to near the insertion of the pronator teres. A little below the middle of the forearm, its fleshy belly divides into four portions, which degenerate into as many round tendons, that pass all together under the internal annular ligament of the wrist, after which they separate from each other, become thinner and flatter, and running along the palm of the hand, under the aponeurosis palmaris, are inserted into the upper part of the second bone of each finger. Previous to this insertion, however, the fibres of each tendon decussate near the extremity of the first bone, so as to afford a passage to a tendon of the perforans. Of these four tendons, that of the middle finger is the largest, that of the forefinger the next in size, and that of the little finger the smallest. The use of this muscle is to bend the second joint of the fingers.

Flexor tertii internodii. See *Flexor longus pollicis manus*.

FLEXUOSUS. Flexuous; full of turnings or windings. A stem is so named which is zigzag, forming angles alternately from right to left, and from left to right; as in *Smilax aspera*.

FLINT. A hard stone, found in beds of chalk, and in primitive, transition, secondary, and alluvial mountains. Its constituents are silica, lime, alumina, and oxide of iron.

FLINTY SLATE. Basanite. A mineral, of which there are two kinds.

1. *Common flinty slate*, of an ash-gray colour, with other colours, in flamed, striped, and spotted delineations. It is found in different parts of the great tract of clay-slate and gray-wacke which extends from St. Abb's head to Portpatrick.

2. *Lydian stone*, of a grayish-black and velvet-black colour. It is found frequently along with common flinty slate, in beds of clay-slate. It occurs in Bohemia and the Pentland hills, near Edinburgh. It is sometimes used as a touchstone for ascertaining the purity of gold and silver.

FLOATSTONE. The spongiform quartz of Jameson.

FLOCCILATION. (*Floccilatio;* from *floccus*, the nap of clothes.) Picking the bedclothes. A symptom of great danger in acute diseases.

FLORAL. (*Floralis;* from *flos*, a flower.) Belonging to a flower; as floral leaf. See *Bractea*.

[FLORA OF NORTH AMERICA. "Before the revolutionary struggle began in France, Louis 16th had patronized a botanical inquiry into the vegetable productions of North America. In the sixth volume of our Medical Repository, we gave an account of the establishments formed for that purpose, and of the *history of the oaks of North America*, published by Mr. Michaux, the botanist employed by that monarch. Since that work on the *Quercus* family was published, the great performance of Mr. Michaux on the vegetables of that extensive country generally, has made its appearance."

"The industrious author of this work had spent six years in Persia before his mission to America. He afterward passed twelve years in exploring the regions between Hudson's Bay and Carolina. In the course of the numerous excursions he made during that time through the diversified states, provinces, and territories, he collected the materials of this new and more complete synopsis of North American plants. This, he hopes, will be found to be the case, notwithstanding the prior descriptions of the plants of Canada by Cornuti; of Virginia by Clayton, aided by Gronovius; of Carolina by Catesby, with plates, as well as by Walther and Bartram; and of the more northern parts, by Marshall and Forster.

"This work is published by the author's son, the father having left it in his hands rather unfinished, when he set off on his voyage of discovery to the islands lying in the Great South Sea. We mention with concern the death of this indefatigable naturalist in 1802. He fell a victim to the zeal with which he urged his physical inquiries on the coast of Madagascar.

"The author follows the Linnæan or sexual system. In addition to the vegetables, which are indigenous in America, he has also noted the European plants growing there. The generic characters are chiefly taken from Murray's last edition of the system of vegetables. Mr. Michaux seems to have confirmed as many of the Linnæan species as he could; though, for the sake of perspicuity, he has described some of them over again. It is affirmed that the work contains no species that have not either been seen or gathered by Michaux himself. This must give to this Flora great value, and render it peculiarly interesting to the lovers of botany in the United States. Genuine descriptions recently made of the plants of the country by an actual observer, possessing remarkable skill and discernment in the practical as well as the theoretical parts of the science, cannot fail to increase the facility of its acquirement among our studious youth. To them, in particular, it will shorten the way to knowledge, and at the same time, render it much more easy and delightful.

"Particular labour has been bestowed upon the *Cyperaceæ* and Gramineæ; and all the Cryptogamia have been sedulously attended to, except the *fungi*. As respects the *Filices*, he adopts the arrangement of J. E. Smith; on the *Musci*, the system of Hedwig; and he follows the method of Acharius on the *Lichens*. Care has been taken that the genera of the same order should be assembled under the banner of affinities, and thrown into sections as far as the laws of the system would permit; so that they may be found by the inquirer and student with the greater readiness and ease.

"We consider this *Flora boreali Americana* as a most desirable addition to the natural history of our country. With this work in his hand, the botanist will be enabled to pursue his studies on the vegetables of *Fredon* (U. S.) and the adjoining regions, with additional ease and success. Though we cannot dismiss it from our notice, without expressing our regret that the author had not enriched his book with some of the synonyms from other writers, with some of the popular and trivial names, and with some little sketch of the dietetic, medicinal, and economical uses of the more distinguished species."—*Med. Repos. vol.* 8. A.]

Flores benzoes. See *Benzoic acid*.

Flores martiales. See *Ferrum ammoniatum*.

Flores salis ammoniaci. See *Ammoniæ subcarbonas*.

Flores sulphuris. See *Sulphur*.

Flores sulphuris loti. See *Sulphur lotum*.

FLORESCENTIA. (From *floresco*, to flourish or bloom.) The act of flowering, which Linnæus compares to the act of generation in animals.

FLORET. A little flower.

FLOS. (*Flos, ris. f.*; a flower.) 1. A flower. That part of a plant, for the most part beautifully coloured, and protecting the internal organs.

Every flower has parts, which are

1. *Essential*, constituting properly the flower; as the pistil, stamen, and receptacle.

2. *Less essential*, without which the flower is in some instances formed; as the *calyx*, *corolla*, and *pedunculus*.

3. *Accidental*, noticed in a few only; as the *bractea* and *nectarium*.

A flower is said to be,

1. *Complete*, when furnished with calyx and corolla; as *Nicotiana tabacum*.

2. *Incomplete*, when the calyx or corolla is wanting.

3. *Naked*, devoid of the calyx; as in *Lilium candidum*, and *Tulipa gesneriana*.

4. *Apetaloid*, without the corolla; as in *Galena Africana*, and *Saururus cernuus*.

When the stamens and pistils are both, as usual, in one flower, that flower is called *perfect*, or united; when they are situated in different flowers of the same species, they are called *separated flowers*; that which has the stamens being named the *barren* flower, as producing no fruit in itself, and that with the pistils the *fertile* one, as bearing the seed.

The flower contains the internal or genital parts of a plant:

1. The *stamen* or male genital organ.

2. The *pistillum* or female genital organ.

From their diversity, flowers are called,

1. *Male*, which have the stamina only.

2. *Female*, in which are the pistils only.

3. *Hermaphrodite*, which contain both stamens and pistils.

4. *Neuter*, naturally deficient of stamens and pistils; as the marginal flowers of the *Centaurea cyanus*, and *Jacobea*.

5. *Castrate*, when the anthers or the pistils are naturally wanting. The pistils, for example, are wanting in the *Calendula officinalis*, and in the *Viola mirabilis*, there are no anthers.

6. *Abortive*, the fecundated germens of which wither before the maturity of the fruit; as happens to the florets in the radius of the *Helianthus annuus*.

7. *Monstrous*, when the internal organs become petals, as is the case with full or double flowers.

Besides these distinctions, Linnæus's favourite division is into,

1. *Aggregate*.

2. *Compound*.

3. *Amentaceous*

4. *Glumose*, or chaffy, peculiar to the grasses.

5. The *sheathed flower*, the common receptacle of which springs from a sheath; as in *Arum*.

6. The *Umbellate*.

7. The *Cymose*. See also *Inflorescence*.

II. A term used by former chemists to whatever had a flower-like appearance, especially if obtained by sublimation, as flowers of sulphur, benjamin, zinc, &c.

Flos ferri. A radiated variety of carbonate of lime.

FLOSCULUS. A little flower. A term applied in botany to the small and numerous florets of a compound flower, which are all sessile on a common undivided receptacle, and enclosed in one contiguous calyx, or perianth.

FLOUR. The powder of the gramineous seeds.

FLOWER. See *Flos*.

FLOWER-DE-LUCE. See *Iris germanica*.

Flowers of benjamin. See *Benzoic acid.*

FLOYER, Sir John, was born at Hinters, in Staffordshire, about the year 1649, and graduated at Oxford. He then settled at Litchfield, where his attention and skill procured him extensive reputation, insomuch that he was honoured with knighthood, as a reward for his talents. He strongly advocated the use of cold bathing, particularly in chronic rheumatism, and nervous disorders: and he ascribed the increasing prevalence of consumption to the discontinuance of the practice of baptizing children by immersion. He published several works on this and other subjects; particularly an excellent treatise on the asthma, under which he himself laboured from the time of puberty, notwithstanding which he lived to be an old man. He is said to have been one of the first who reckoned the number of pulsations by a time-piece.

FLUATE. *Fluas.* A compound of the fluoric acid with salifiable bases: thus, fluate of lime, &c.

FLUCTUATION. *Fluctuatio.* A term used by surgeons, to express the undulation of a fluid; thus when pus is formed in an abscess, or when water accumulates in the abdomen, if the abscess or abdomen be lightly pressed with the fingers, the motion of fluctuation may be distinctly felt.

FLUELLIN. See *Antirrhinum elatine.*

FLUID. *Fluidus.* A fluid is that, the particles of which so little attract each other, that when poured out, it drops *guttatim*, and adapts itself in every respect to the form of the vessel containing it.

The fluids of animal bodies, and particularly those of the human body, are something very considerable in proportion to the solids; the ratio in the adult being as nine to one. Chaussier put a dead body of 120 pounds into an oven, and found it, after many days' successive desiccation, reduced to 12 pounds. Bodies found, after being buried for a long time in the burning sands of the Arabian deserts, present an extraordinary diminution of weight.

The animal fluids are sometimes contained in vessels, wherein they move with more or less rapidity; sometimes in little areolæ or spaces, where they seem to be kept in reserve; and at other times they are placed in the great cavities where they make only a temporary stay of longer or shorter duration.

The fluids of the human body are,

1. The blood.

2. The lymph.

3. The perspiratory or perspirable fluids, which comprise the liquids of cutaneous transpiration: the transpiration or exhalation of mucous membranes, as also of the synovial, serous, and cellular; of the adipose cells, the medullary membranes, the thyroid and thymus glands, &c.

4. The follicular fluid; the sebaceous secretion of the skin, the cerumen, the ropy matter from the eyelids, the mucus from the glands and follicles of that name from the tonsils, the cardiac glands, the prostate, the vicinity of the anus, and some other parts.

5. The glandular fluids; the tears, the saliva, the pancreatic fluid, the bile, the urine, the secretion from Cowper's glands, the semen, the milk, the liquid contained in the supra-renal capsules, that of the testicles, and of the mammæ of new-born infants.

6. The chyme and the chyle.

The properties of fluids, both chemical and physical, are exceedingly various. Many have some analogy to each other under these two relations; but none exhibit a perfect resemblance. The writers of all ages have attached a considerable degree of importance to their methodical arrangement; and according to the doctrine then flourishing in the schools, they have created different systems of classification. Thus, the ancients, who attributed much importance to the four elements, said that there were four principal humours, the blood, the lymph, or *pituita*, the yellow bile, the black bile, or *atra bilis;* and these four humours correspond to the four elements, to the four seasons of the year, to the four divisions of the day, and to the four temperaments. Afterward, at different periods, other divisions have been substituted to this classification of the ancients. Thus, some have made three classes of liquids:—1. the chyme and chyle; 2. the blood; 3. the humours emanating from the blood. Some authors have been content with forming two classes:—1. *primary*, alimentary, or useless fluids; 2. *secondary*, or useful. Consequently, they distinguished them into—

1. *Recrementitious*, or humours destined from their formation to the nourishment of the body.

2. *Excrementitious*, or fluids destined to be thrown off from the system;

3. Humours, which at times participate in the characters of the two former classes, and are therefore named *excremento-recrementitious*.

In later times, chemists have endeavoured to class the humours according to their intimate or component nature, and thus they have established albuminous, fibrinous, saponaeccus, watery, &c. fluids.

FLUOBORATE. A compound of the fluoboric acid with a salifiable basis.

FLUOBORIC ACID. *Acidum fluoboricum.* Probably a compound of fluorine with boron. It is a gaseous acid, and may be obtained by heating in a glass retort twelve parts of sulphuric acid with a mixture of one part of fused boracic acid, and two of fluor-spar, reduced to a very fine powder. It must be received over mercury. It combines with salifiable bases, and forms salts called *fluoborites*.

FLU'OR. Octohedral fluor of Jameson. It is divided into three sub-species, compact fluor, foliated fluor, and earthy fluor. This genus of mineral abounds in nature, formed by the combination of the fluoric acid with lime. It is called spar, because it has the spary form and fracture: fluor, because it melts very readily; and vitreous, because it has the appearance of glass, and may be fused into glass of no contemptible appearance.

FLUOR ALBUS. See *Leucorrhœa*.

FLUO'RIC ACID. (*Acidum fluoricum*, because obtained from the fluor-spar.) Hydro-fluoric acid.

"The fusible spar which is generally distinguished by the name of Derbyshire spar, consists of calcareous earth in combination with this acid. If the pure fluor, or spar, be placed in a retort of lead or silver, with a receiver of the same metal adapted, and its weight of sulphuric acid be then poured upon it, the fluoric acid will be disengaged by the application of a moderate heat. This acid gas readily combines with water; for which purpose it is necessary that the receiver should previously be half filled with that fluid.

If the receiver be cooled with ice, and no water put in it, then the condensed acid is an intensely active liquid. It has the appearance of sulphuric acid, but is much more volatile, and sends off white fumes when exposed to air. Its specific gravity is only 1.0609. It must be examined with great caution, for when applied to the skin it instantly disorganizes it, and produces very painful wounds. When potassium is introduced into it, it acts with intense energy, and produces hydrogen gas and a neutral salt; when lime is made to act upon it, there is a violent heat excited, water is formed, and the same substance as fluor-spar is produced. With water in a certain proportion, its density increases to 1.25. When it is dropped into water, a hissing noise is produced, with much heat, and an acid fluid not disagreeable to the taste is formed if the water be in sufficient quantity. It instantly corrodes and dissolves glass.

It appears extremely probable, from all the facts known respecting the fluoric combinations, that fluor-spar contains a peculiar acid matter; and that this acid matter is united to lime in the spar, seems evident from the circumstance, that gypsum or sulphate of lime is the residuum of the distillation of fluor-spar and sulphuric acid. The results of experiments on fluor-spar have been differently stated by chemists.

Some have considered fluoric acid as a compound of fluorine with hydrogen, but it seems on the whole to be the *analogy* of chlorine. But the analogy is incomplete. Certainly it is consonant to the true logic of chemical science to regard chlorine as a simple body, since every attempt to resolve it into simpler forms of matter has failed. But fluorine has not been exhibited in an insulated state like chlorine; and here therefore the analogy does not hold.

The marvellous activity of fluoric acid may be inferred from the following remarks of Sir H. Davy, from which also may be estimated in some measure the prodigious difficulty attending refined investigations on this extraordinary substance.

'I undertook the experiment of electrising pure liquid fluoric acid with considerable interest, as it seemed to offer the most probable method of ascertaining its real nature; but considerable difficulties occurred in executing the process. The liquid fluoric acid immediately destroys glass, and all animal and vegetable substances; it acts on all bodies containing metallic oxides; and I know of no substances which are not rapidly dissolved or decomposed by it, except metals, charcoal, phosphorus, sulphur, and certain combinations of chlorine. I attempted to make tubes of sulphur, of muriates of lead, and of copper containing metallic wires, by which it might be electrised, but without success. I succeeded, however, in boring a piece of horn silver in such a manner that I was able to cement a platina wire into it by means of a spirit lamp; and by inverting this in a tray of platina, filled with liquid fluoric acid, I contrived to submit the fluid to the agency of electricity in such a manner, that, in successive experiments, it was possible to collect any elastic fluid that might be produced. Operating in this way with a very weak voltaic power, and keeping the apparatus cool by a freezing mixture, I ascertained that the platina wire at the positive pole rapidly corroded, and became covered with a chocolate powder; gaseous matter separated at the negative pole, which I could never obtain in sufficient quantities to analyze with accuracy, but it inflamed like hydrogen. No other inflammable matter was produced when the acid was pure.'

If instead of being distilled in metallic vessels, the mixture of fluor-spar and oil of vitriol be distilled in glass vessels, little of the corrosive liquid will be obtained; but the glass will be acted upon, and a peculiar gaseous substance will be produced, which must be collected over mercury. The best mode of procuring this gaseous body is to mix the fluor-spar with pounded glass or quartz; and in this case the glass retort may be preserved from corrosion, and the gas obtained in greater quantities. This gas, which is called *silicated fluoric gas*, is possessed of very extraordinary properties.

It is very heavy; about 48 times denser than hydrogen. When brought into contact with water, it instantly deposites a white gelatinous substance, which is hydrate of silica; it produces white fumes when suffered to pass into the atmosphere. It is not affected by any of the common combustible bodies; but when potassium is strongly heated in it, it takes fire and burns with a deep red light; the gas is absorbed, and a fawn-coloured substance is formed, which yields alkali to water with slight effervescence, and contains a combustible body. The washings afford potassa, and a salt, from which the strong acid fluid previously described, may be separated by sulphuric acid.

If, instead of glass or silica, the fluor spar be mixed with dry vitreous boracic acid, and distilled in a glass vessel with sulphuric acid, the proportions being one part boracic acid, two fluor-spar, and twelve oil of vitriol, the gaseous substance formed is of a different kind, and is called the *fluoboric gas*. It is colourless; its smell is pungent, and resembles that of muriatic acid; it cannot be breathed without suffocation; it extinguishes combustion; and reddens strongly the tincture of turnsol. It has no manner of action on glass, but a very powerful one on vegetable and animal matter. It attacks them with as much force as concentrated sulphuric acid, and appears to operate on these bodies by the production of water; for while it carbonizes them, or evolves carbon, they may be touched without any risk of burning. Exposed to a high temperature, it is not decomposed; it is condensed by cold without changing its form. When it is put in contact with oxygen, or air, either at a high or low temperature, it experiences no change, except seizing, at ordinary temperatures, the moisture which these gases contain It becomes in consequence a liquid which emits extremely dense vapours. It operates in the same way with all the gases which contain hygrometric water. However little they may contain, it occasions in them very perceptible vapours. It may hence be employed with advantage to show whether or not a gas contains moisture.

No combustible body, simple or compound, attacks fluoboric gas, if we except the alkaline metals. Potassium and sodium, with the aid of heat, burn in this gas, almost as brilliantly as in oxygen. Boron and fluate of potassa are the products of this decomposition. It might hence be inferred, that the metal seizes the oxygen of the boracic acid, sets the boron at liberty, and is itself oxidized and combined with the fluoric acid. According to Sir H. Davy's views, the fluoboric gas being a compound of fluorine and boron, the potassium unites to the former, giving rise to the fluoride of potassium, while the boron remains disengaged.

Fluoboric gas is very soluble in water. Dr. John Davy says, water can combine with 700 times its own volume, or twice its weight, at the ordinary temperature and pressure of the air. The liquid has a specific gravity of 1.770. If a bottle containing this gas be uncorked under water, the liquid will rush in and fill it with explosive violence. Water saturated with this gas is limpid, fuming, and very caustic. By heat about one-fifth of the absorbed gas may be expelled; but it is impossible to abstract more. It then resembles concentrated sulphuric acid, and boils at a temperature considerably above 212°. It afterward condenses altogether, in *striæ*, although it contains still a very larg quantity of gas. It unites with the bases forming salt called fluoborates, none of which has been applied to any use.

The 2d part of the Phil. Transactions, for 1812, contains an excellent paper by Dr. John Davy on fluosilicic and fluoboric gases, and the combinations of the latter with ammoniacal gas. When united in equal volumes, a pulverulent salt is formed; a second volume of ammonia, however, gives a liquid compound; and a third of ammonia, which is the limit of combination, affords still a liquid; both of them curious on many accounts. 'They are,' says he, 'the first salts that have been observed liquid at the common temperature of the atmosphere. And they are additional facts in support of the doctrine of definite proportions, and of the relation of volumes.' The fluosilicic acid also unites to bases forming fluosilicates.

From the remarkable property fluoric acid possesses of corroding glass, it has been employed for etching on it, both in the gaseous state, and combined with water; and an ingenious apparatus for this purpose is given by Mr. Richard Knight, in the Philosophical Magazine, vol. xvii. p. 357.

Of the combinations of this acid with most of the bases, little is known.

Beside the fluor spar and cryolite, in which it is abundant, fluoric acid has been detected in the topaz; in wavelite, in which, however, it is not rendered sensible by sulphuric acid; and in fossil teeth and fossil ivory, though it is not found in either of these in their natural state."—*Ure's Chem. Dict.*

Fluoric acid, silicated. See *Fluoric acid.*

FLUORIDE. A combination of fluorine with a salifiable basis.

FLUORINE. The imaginary radical of fluoric acid.

FLUOSILICIC ACID. See *Fluoric acid.*

FLUX. 1. This word is often employed for *dysenteria.*

2. A general term made use of to denote any substance or mixture added to assist the fusion of metals.

FLUXION. *Fluxio.* A term mostly applied by chemists, to signify the change of metals, or other bodies, from the solid into the fluid state, by the application of heat. See *Fusion.*

FLY. *Musca.*

Fly, Spanish. See *Cantharis.*

FO'CILE. The ulna and the radius are occasionally denominated by the barbarous appellations of *focile majus* and *minus*; the tibia and fibula in the leg are also so called.

Fo'cus. A lobe of the liver.

Fodi'na. (From *fodio*, to dig.) A quarry. The labyrinth of the ear.

Fœnicula'tum lignum. A name for sassafras.

FŒNI'CULUM. (*Quasi fœnum oculorum*, the hay or herb good for the sight; so called because it is thought good for the eyes.) Fennel. See *Anethum.*

Fœniculum alpinum. The herb spignel. See *Æthusa meum.*

Fœniculum annuum. Royal cummin.

Fœniculum aquaticum. See *Phellandrium aquaticum.*

Fœniculum dulce. See *Anethum fœniculum.*

Fœniculum germanicum. See *Anethum fœniculum.*

Fœniculum marinum. Samphire.

Fœniculum orientale. See *Cuminum.*

Fœniculum porcinum. See *Peucedanum officinale.*

Fœniculum sinense. Aniseed.

Fœniculum sylvestre. Bastard spignel. See *Sseli montanum*, of Linnæus.

Fœniculum tortuosum. French hartwort. See *Seseli tortuosum.*

Fœniculum vulgare. See *Anethum fœniculum.*

FŒ'NUM. (*Fœnum, i.* n. hay.) Hay.

Fœnum camelorum. See *Juncus odoratus.*

Fœnum græcum. See *Trigonella fœnum græcum.*

Fœnum sylvestre. Wild fenugreek.

FOËSIUS, Anutius, was born at Mentz, in 1528, and received his education at Paris, where he imbibed a strong predilection for the Greek language, and particularly the works of Hippocrates. Returning to his native place about the age of 28, his talents soon procured him such extensive reputation, that several princes endeavoured to allure him to their respective courts, but without success. The practice of his profession, instead of weakening his attachment to Hippocrates, only stimulated him to a more profound study of his writings; where he found the most correct delineations of diseases, and the most important observations concerning them, made about two thousand years before. He first published an excellent Latin translation and commentary on his second book of Epidemics: then an explanation of the terms used by him, under the title of "Œconomia Hippocratis;" and, lastly, at the solicitation of the chief physicians of Europe, he undertook a complete correct edition of his works, with an interpretation and notes, which he accomplished in six years, in such a manner as to rank him among the ablest interpreters of the ancients. He was also author of a Pharmacopœia for his native city; and died in 1595.

Fœta'bulum. (From *fœteo*, to become putrid.) 1. An encysted abscess.

2. A foul ulcer.

FŒ'TUS. (From *feo*, to bring forth, according to Vossius.) *Epicyema; Epigonion.* The child enclosed in the uterus of its mother, is called a fœtus from the fifth month after pregnancy until the time of its birth. See *Ovum.*

Foliata terra. 1. Sulphur.

2. An old name of the acetate of potassa.

FOLIATIO. (From *folium*, a leaf.) The manner in which leaves are folded up in their buds. See *Vernatio.*

FOLIA'TUS. (From its resemblance to *folium*, a leaf.) Foliate, leafy.

FOLICULUS. (Diminutive of *follis*, a leather bag.) A small follicle.

FOLIOLUM. A leaflet or little leaf.

FO'LIUM. (*Folium, i.* n.; from φυλλον, the leaf of a tree.) See *Leaf.*

Folium orientale. See *Cassia senna.*

FOLLICLE. (*Folliculus*; diminutive of *follis*, a bag.) A small bag; applied to glands. See *Folliculose.*

FOLLICULOSE. (*Folliculosus*; from *folliculus*, a little bag.) A term applied to a simple gland or follicle. One of the most simple species of gland, consisting merely of a hollow vascular membrane or follicle, and an excretory duct; such are the muciparous glands, the sebaceous, &c.

FOLLI'CULUS. (Diminutive of *follis*, a bag.) 1. A little bag. See *Folliculose.*

2. In botany, a follicle is a one-valved pericarp, or seed-vessel. It has one cell, and bursts lengthwise, and bears the seeds on or near its edges, or on a receptacle parallel therewith.

From the adhesion of the seeds it is distinguished into,

1. Follicle, *with a partition*, when the seeds adhere to an intermediate dissepiment.

2. Follicle, *without a partition*, when the seeds adhere to the internal sides only.

From the number of seeds,

1. *Monosperm follicle*; as in *Orontium.*
2. *Polysperm*; as in *Asclepias syriaca.*

From the direction into,

1. *Erect*; as in *Vinca* and *Nerium.*
2. *Reflected*; as in *Plumeria.*
3. *Horizontal*; as in *Cameraria.*

Folliculis fellis. The gall-bladder.

FOMENTA'TION. *Fomentatio.* A sort of partial bathing, by applying hot flannels to any part, dipped in medicated decoctions, whereby steams are communicated to the parts, their vessels are relaxed, and their morbid action sometimes removed.

Fomes ventriculi. Hypochondriacism.

FO'MITES. A term mostly applied to substances imbued with contagion.

FONS. A fountain.

Fons pulsatilis. See *Fontanella.*

FONTANE'LLA. (Diminutive of *fons*, a fountain.) *Fons pulsatilis.* The parietal bones and the frontal do not coalesce until the third year after birth, so that, before this period, there is an obvious interstice, commonly called *mould*, and scientifically the *fontanel*, or *fons pulsatilis.* There is also a less space, occasionally, between the occipital and parietal bones, termed the *posterior fontanel.* These spaces between the bones are filled up by the dura mater, pericranium, and external integuments, so that, during birth, the size of the head may be lessened; for, at that time, the bones of the head, upon the superior part, are not only pressed nearer to each other, but they frequently lap over one another, in order to diminish the size during the passage of the head through the pelvis.

FONTI'CULUS. (Diminutive of *fons.*) An issue. An artificial ulcer formed in any part, and kept discharging, by introducing daily a pea, covered with any digestive ointment.

FORA'MEN. (From *foro*, to pierce.) A little opening.

FORAMEN CŒCUM. 1. A single opening in the basis of the cranium between the ethmoid and the frontal bone, that gives exit to a small vein.

2. The name of a hole in the middle of the tongue.

FORAMEN LACERUM IN BASI CRANII. A foramina in the basis of the cranium, through which the internal jugular vein, and the eighth pair and accessary nerves pass.

FORAMEN LACERUM ORBITALE SUPERIUS. A large opening between the greater and less wing of the sphenoid bone on each side, through which the third, fourth, first branch of the fifth, and the sixth pair of nerves, and the ophthalmic artery pass.

FORAMEN OPTICUM. The hole transmitting the optic nerve.

FORAMEN OVALE. The opening between the two auricles of the heart of the fœtus. See also *Innominatum os.*

Foramen of Winslow. An opening in the omentum. See *Omentum.*

FORAMI'NULUM OS. The ethmoid bone.

Force, vital. See *Vis vitæ.*

FO'RCEPS. (*Forceps, cipis.* f.; *quasi ferriceps*, as being the iron with which we seize any thing hot, from *ferrum*, iron, and *capio*, to take.) Pincers. A surgical instrument with which extraneous bodies, or other substances, are extracted. Also an instrument occasionally used by men midwives to bring the head of the fœtus through the pelvis.

FORDYCE, GEORGE, was born at Aberdeen, in 1736, after the death of his father, and his mother having married again, he was sent to Fouran, when about two years old, where he received his school education; and thence returned to Aberdeen, where he was made master of arts, when only fourteen. Having evinced an inclination to medicine, he was soon after sent to his uncle, Dr. John Fordyce, who practised at Uppingham, with whom he remained several years. He then studied at Edinburgh, where he graduated in 1758, having defended a thesis on catarrh: after which he went to Leyden, principally to improve himself in anatomy under Albinus. The following year he settled in London, and began to give lectures on chemistry; and, in 1764, he undertook also to teach the practice of physic, and the materia medica: these subjects occupied him nearly three hours every morning, except on Sunday, for about thirty years successively. In 1770, he was chosen physician to St. Thomas's hospital, and, six years after, a Fellow of the Royal Society: also, in 1787, he was admitted a Fellow of the College of Physicians; having been a licentiate for twenty-two years before. In 1793, he assisted in forming a small Society for the improvement of Medical and Chirurgical Knowledge, which has since published three volumes of their Transactions. He died in 1802. The countenance of Dr. Fordyce was by no means expressive of his powers of mind: he was rather negligent of his dress, and not sufficiently pleasing in his manners, to enable him to get into very extensive practice: besides, he was too fond of the pleasures of society, to which he often sacrificed the hours that should have been dedicated to sleep. The vigour of his constitution long resisted these irregularities; but at length they brought on the gout, which was followed by dropsy, and this terminated his existence. He possessed a remarkably strong memory, which enabled him to lecture without any notes, and to compose his works for publication without referring to authors, which he had before read; and his having relied too much on this faculty may help to explain the want of method and elegance, and the many inaccuracies, which appear in his writings. He was author of several publications on medical and philosophical subjects; many of which are to be found in the transactions of the societies to which he belonged. The most esteemed, and that on which he employed most labour, was a series of "Dissertations on Fever;" four of them appeared during his life, and another was left in manuscript, which has since been printed. His Treatise on Digestion, was read originally as the Gulstonian Lecture before the College of Physicians. He was the projector of the Experiments in heated rooms, of which Sir Charles Blagden gave an account.

FORDYCE, Sir WILLIAM, was born at Aberdeen in 1724. At the age of eighteen, having acquired a competent knowledge of physic and surgery, he went into the army. The support of the friends, whom he there procured, together with his own merit, soon brought him into great practice, when he afterward settled in London. The wealth, which he thus acquired, was liberally employed in acts of friendship, and in supporting useful projects; though he had some very severe losses. He wrote a Treatise on Fevers, and on the Ulcerated Sore Throat; on his entering into practice, he likewise published on the Venereal Disease. He died after a long illness in 1792.

FORENSIC. *Forensis.* Belonging to the forum, or courts of law: hence forensic medicine is that which is connected with a legal inquiry as to the cause of defect, disease, or death.

FORESKIN. See *Prepuce*

FORESTUS, or VAN FOREST, PETER, was born at Alcmaer, in 1522. He was sent to Louvain to study the law, but soon showed a strong inclination to medicine. He therefore cultivated this science at different universities in Italy, and afterward at Paris; but he graduated at Bologna. After being twelve years settled in his native town, he was invited to Delft, which was ravaged by a contagious epidemic; and being extremely successful in the treatment of this, he received a considerable pension, and was retained as the public physician for nearly thirty years. In 1575, he was prevailed upon to give the first lecture on Medicine at the opening of the University of Leyden. He spent the latter part of his life in his native city, where he died in 1597. He was a very diligent observer of diseases and showed often great judgment in anticipating the result, or in treating them successfully. He published at different periods six volumes of Medical and Surgical Cases; to one of which was added a Dissertation, exposing the fallacy and absurdity of pretending to judge of every thing by the urine. Boerhaave has highly commended his writings, which have been often reprinted.

[FORMATIONS, MINERAL. "The word *Formation* may signify a single mass of one kind of rock, more or less extensive, or a collection of mineral substances, formed by the same agent, under the same or similar circumstances; or it may convey the idea, that certain masses or collections of minerals were formed not only by the same agent, but also at the *same time.* In this latter sense, indeed, the term is almost always employed. The agent and time are to be determined by a careful examination of the external and internal relations of the whole formation."—*Cleav. Min.* A.]

FO'RMIATE. *Formias.* A compound produced by the union of the formic acid with a salifiable basis: thus, *formiate of ammonia*, &c.

FORMIC ACID. See *Formica rufa.*

FORMI'CA. (*Formica, æ.* f.; *quod ferat micas*, because of his diligence in collecting small particles of provision together.)

1. The name of a genus of insects. The ant or pismire. See *Formica rufa.*

2. The name of a black wart with a broad base, and cleft superficies, because the pain attending it resembles the biting of an ant.

3. A varicose tumour on the anus and glans penis.

FORMICA MILIARIS. Any herpetic eruption.

FORMICA RUFA. The ant or pismire. This industrious little insect contains an acid juice, and gross oil, which were supposed to possess aphrodisiac virtues. The chrysalides of this animal are said to be diuretic and carminative, and by some recommended in the cure of dropsy.

The ant also furnishes an acid called the formic, which it has been long known to contain, and occasionally to emit. It may be obtained, either by simple distillation, or by infusion of them in boiling water, and subsequent distillation of as much of the water as can be brought over without burning the residue. After this it may be purified by repeated rectifications, or by boiling to separate the impurities; or after rectification it may be concentrated by frost.

This acid has a very sour taste, and continues liquid even at very low temperatures. Its specific gravity is 1.1168 at 68°, which is much denser than acetic acid ever is.

Dobereiner has recently succeeded in forming this acid artificially. When a mixture of tartaric acid, or of cream of tartar, black oxide of magnesia and water is heated, a tumultuous action ensues, carbonic acid is evolved, and a liquid acid distils over, which, on superficial examination, was mistaken for acetic acid, but which now proves to be formic acid. This acid, mixed with concentrated sulphuric acid, is at common temperatures converted into water and carbonic oxide; nitrate of silver or of mercury converts it, when gently heated, into carbonic acid, the oxides being at the same time reduced to the metallic state. With barytes, oxide of lead, and oxide of copper, it produces compounds, having all the properties of the genuine formiates of these metals. If a portion of sulphuric acid be employed in the above process, the tartaric acid is resolved entirely into carbonic acid, water, and formic acid; and the product of the latter is much increased. The best proportions are, two parts tartaric acid, five peroxide of manganese, and five sulphuric acid diluted with about twice its weight in water.

Fo'rmix. See *Herpes exedens.*

FO'RMULA. (Diminutive of *forma*, a form.) A little form of prescriptions, such as physicians direct in extemporaneous practice, in distinction from the greater forms in pharmacopœias, &c.

Fo'rnax. A furnace.

FORNICIFORMIS. Vaulted. Applied to the nectary of some plants; as the *Symphytum officinale*, &c. See *Nectarium.*

FO'RNIX. (*Fornix*, an arch or vault.) A part of the corpus callosum in the brain is so called, because, if viewed in a particular direction, it has some resemblance to the arch of an ancient vault. It is the medullary body, composed of two anterior and two posterior crura, situated at the bottom and inside of the lateral ventricle over the third ventricle, and below the septum lucidum.

FO'SSA. (From *fodio*, to dig.) *Fovea.* A little depression or sinus. The pudendum muliebre.

Fossa amyntæ. A double-headed roller for the face.

Fossa magna. 1. The great groove of the ear.

2. The pudendum muliebre.

Fossa navicularis. 1. The cavity at the bottom of the entrance of the pudendum muliebre.

2. The great groove of the ear.

Fossa ovalis. The depression in the right auricle of the human heart, which in the fœtus opened into the other auricle, forming the foramen ovale.

Fossa pituitaria. The depression in the sella turcica of the sphenoid bone.

FO'SSIL. (*Fossilis;* from *fodio*, to dig.) Any thing dug out of the earth.

Fossil copal. Highgate resin. A semi-transparent, brittle, resinous substance, of a yellowish-brown colour; found in the bed of blue clay at Highgate, near London.

Fo'ssilus. The bone of the leg.

FOTHERGILL, John, was born in Yorkshire, in 1712, of a respectable Quaker family. After passing through an apprenticeship to an apothecary, he went to Edinburgh, where he graduated at the age of twenty-four, taking for his inaugural thesis the use of emetics. He then studied for two years at St. Thomas's Hospital, and after an excursion to the continent, settled in London in 1740, and six years after became a licentiate. His practice was for some time chiefly gratuitous; but his "Account of the Putrid Sore Throat," published in 1748, brought him speedily into reputation. He was successively elected a Fellow of the College of Physicians at Edinburgh, of the Royal Society of London, and of some other societies abroad. His early partiality to botany induced him, as his practice increased, to purchase a large piece of ground for the cultivation of rare and valuable plants, in which he spared no expense; neither did he neglect other departments of natural history. He was also an active and liberal promoter of many successful schemes for the public benefit; and particularly in instituting the school at Ackworth in Yorkshire. He was of a rather delicate constitution, but a steady temperance preserved his health, till in 1778 he had an attack of a suppression of urine, occasioned by a disease of the prostate gland; which, returning two years after, soon put a period to his existence. He had a quick and comprehensive understanding; and his pleasing address procured him general confidence, which his discretion was not apt to forfeit afterward. Besides the works already noticed, several papers of Dr. Fothergill were printed in the Philosophical Transactions, and in the Medical Observations and Inquiries: he also sent several communications to the Gentleman's Magazine, and other periodical publications.

FO'TUS. (*Fotus*, ûs. m.) See *Fomentation.*

FO'VEA. (From *fodio*, to dig.) 1. A little depression.

2. The pudendum muliebre.

3. A partial sweating-bath.

FOVEATUS. Having a little depression, or pit. Applied to the nectary of plants. See *Nectarium.*

FOX-GLOVE. See *Digitalis.*

Fox-glove, Eastern. See *Sesamum orientale.*

FRACASTORIUS, Hieronymus, was born at Verona, in 1483. He made a rapid progress in his studies, and attained early considerable excellence as a poet, philosopher, and astronomer. He was also much valued as a physician, particularly by the general of the Venetian army, whom he attended during several campaigns: but on his dying, in 1515, Fracastorius returned to his native place. He corresponded with most of the great men of his age, especially with Cardinal Bembo, to whom he dedicated his poem, "Syphilis;" which was thought worthy of comparison with the Georgics of Virgil by some of the best judges. He died in 1553; and a statue was erected to him by the town of Verona. He published also on Contagious Diseases, and several other Medical and Philosophical Subjects.

FRA'CTURE. (*Fractura;* from *frango*, to break.) *Catagma; Clasis; Clasma; Agme.* A solution of a bone into two or more fragments. A *simple* fracture is when the bone only is divided. A *compound* fracture is a division of the bone, with a laceration of the integuments, the bone mostly protruding. A fracture is also termed transverse, oblique, &c. according to its direction.

FRÆ'NULUM. (Diminutive of *frænum*, a bridle.) The cutaneous fold under the apex of the tongue, that connects the tongue to the infralingual cavity. It is sometimes, in infancy, so short as to prevent the child from sucking, when it is necessary to cut it, in order to give more room for the motion of the tongue.

FRÆ'NUM. The membraneous fold which connects the prepuce to the inferior part of the glans penis.

FRA'GARIA. (From *fragro*, to smell sweet.) The strawberry. 1. The name of a genus of plants in the Linnæan system. Class, *Icosandria;* Order, *Polygynia.*

2. The pharmacopœial name of the strawberry. See *Fragaria vesca.*

Fragaria sterilis. Barren strawberry. Astringent, seldom used.

Fragaria vesca. The systematic name of the strawberry plant. *Fragaria.* The mature fruit of the *Fragaria, fragellis reptantibus* of Linnæus, was formerly recommended in gouty and calculous affections, in consequence, it would appear, of its efficacy in removing tartar from the teeth, which it is said to do very effectually.

Fragile vitreum. An obsolete name for the fragilitas ossium.

FRAGILIS. Brittle.

FRAGI'LITAS. Brittleness.

Fragilitas ossium. Brittleness of the bones.

Fra'gmen. *Fragmentum.* A splinter of a bone.

FRA'GUM. (From *fragro*, to smell sweet.) The strawberry. See *Fragaria.*

FRAMBŒ'SIA. (From *framboise*, Fr. for a raspberry.) The yaws. A genus of disease, arranged by Cullen in the class *Cachexiæ*, and order *Impetigines.* It is somewhat similar in its nature to the lues venerea, and is endemial to the Antilles islands, as well as Africa. It appears with excrescences like mulberries growing out of the skin in various parts of the body, which discharge an ichorous fluid.

FRA'NGULA. (From *frango*, to break: so called because of the brittleness of its branches.) See *Rhamnus frangula.*

FRANKINCENSE. See *Juniperus lycia*, and *Pinus abies.*

[**Frasera Walteri.** See *American Columbo.* A.]

FRAXINE'LLA. (From *fraxinus*, the ash: so called because its leaves resemble those of the ash.) See *Dictamnus albus.*

Fraxinella, white. See *Dictamnus albus.*

FRA'XINUS. (*A fragore*, from the noise its seeds make when shaken by the wind; or from φραξις, a hedge, because of its use in forming hedges.) The ash.

1. The name of a genus of plants in the Linnæan system. Class, *Polygamia*; Order, *Diœcia.*

2. The pharmacopœial name of the ash-tree. See *Fraxinus excelsior.*

Fraxinus excelsior. The systematic name of the ash-tree. *Fraxinus.* Called also *brumelli* and *bumelia.* The bark of this tree, *Fraxinus—foliis serratis floribus apetalis* of Linnæus, when fresh, has a moderately strong bitterish taste. It possesses resolvent and diuretic qualities, and has been successfully exhibited in the cure of intermittents. The seeds are occasionally exhibited medicinally as diuretics, in the dose of a drachm. In warm climates, a sort of manna exudes from this species of fraxinus.

Fraxinus ornus. The systematic name of the tree from which manna flows. This substance is also termed *Manna Calabrina*; *Ros calabrinus*; *Acromeli*; *Alusar*; *Drysomeli.* That species which is of a rosy colour, is called *nuba. Mel aërium*, from the supposition that it descended from heaven. Manna is the condensed juice of the flowering ash, or *Fraxinus ornus—foliis ovato oblongis serratis petiolatis, floribus corollatis*, Hort. Kew. which is a native of the southern parts of Europe, particularly Sicily and Calabria. Many other trees and shrubs have likewise been observed to emit a sweet juice, which concretes upon exposure to the air, and may be considered of the manna kind, especially the *Fraxinus rotundifolia*, and *excelsior.* In Sicily these three species of fraxinus are regularly cultivated for the purpose of procuring manna, and with this view are planted on the declivity of a hill with an eastern aspect. After ten years' growth, the trees first begin to yield the manna, but they require to be much older before they afford it in any considerable quantity. Although the manna exudes spontaneously upon the trees, yet, in order to obtain it more copiously, incisions are made through the bark, by means of a sharp crooked instrument; and the season thought to be most favourable for instituting this process, is a little before the dog days commence, when the weather is dry and serene. Manna is generally distinguished into different kinds, viz. the manna in tear, the canulated and flaky manna, and the common brown or fat manna. All these varieties seem rather to depend upon their respective purity, and the manner in which they are obtained from the plant, than upon any essential difference of the drug. The best manna is in oblong pieces or flakes, moderately dry, friable, very light, of a whitish or pale yellow colour, and in some degree transparent: the inferior kinds are moist, unctuous, and brown. Manna is well known as a gentle purgative, so mild in its operation, that it may be given with safety to children and pregnant women, to the delicacy of whose frames and situations it is particularly adapted. It is esteemed a good and pleasant auxiliary to the purgative neutral salts. It sheathes acrimony, and is useful in coughs, disorders of the breast, and such as are attended with fever and inflammation, as in pleuritis, &c. It is particularly efficacious in bilious complaints, and helps the discharge of mineral waters, when they are not of themselves sufficiently active. It is apt, in large doses, to create flatulencies and gripes; both of which are prevented by a small addition of some warm carminatives. It purges in doses of from ℥j to ℥ij; but its purgative quality is much increased, and its flatulent effects prevented, by a small addition of cassia. The dose for children is from one scruple to three. It is best dissolved in whey.

Fraxinus rotundifolia. The systematic name of a tree which affords manna. See *Fraxinus ornus.*

FREIND, John, was born in 1675, at Croton, in Northamptonshire, of which his father was rector. After being educated at Westminster he went to Oxford, where he distinguished himself greatly by his classical attainments. Having for some time studied medicine, he communicated to the Royal Society some singular cases: but a work, which he published in 1703, entitled "Emmenologia," explaining the phenomena of menstruation, both natural and morbid, on mechanical principles, first brought him into notice as a physiologist and physician. In the following year, he was appointed professor of Chemistry at Oxford, but soon after went to Spain as physician to the English forces; and he took this opportunity of visiting Italy. On his return, in 1707, he was created a Doctor by diploma, and published his Chemical Lectures in Latin. In 1712, he was chosen a Fellow of the Royal Society; but soon went abroad again with the troops into Flanders. On the conclusion of the peace in the following year he settled in London, and rose to high professional reputation. In 1716, he was received as Fellow of the College of Physicians, and published the first and third books of Hippocrates on Epidemics, with a Commentary on Fevers, in nine parts; a work of great erudition and judgment. Some of his opinions having been severely attacked, he was led to defend them in a letter to Dr. Mead, entitled "De purgantibus in secundo Variolarum confluentium Febre adhibendis," 1719. A few years after this he got into parliament, and having warmly sided with the opposition, he was, in common with several persons of consequence, imprisoned on suspicion of high treason: but the minister, Sir Robert Walpole, having fallen sick, Dr. Mead refused to attend him till his friend was liberated; when he made over to him 5000 guineas, which he had received from his patients during his confinement of a few months only. While in the Tower, Dr. Freind formed the plan of his great work, "The History of Physic from Galen to the beginning of the Sixteenth Century, chiefly with regard to Practice;" which came out in two volumes within three years after. This was intended as a continuation of Le Clerc, and met with a very favourable reception; indeed it still continues to be a standard book. On the accession of George II. he was appointed physician to the Queen; and having died in July 1728, his widow and son experienced the royal protection.

Fre'na. The sockets of the teeth.

Frigera'na. A putrid fever.

FRIGIDA'RIUM. (From *frigidus*, cold.) The cold bath.

FRINGE. See *Fimbria.*

Fringed leaf. See *Leaf.*

FRONS. (*Frons, tis.* f. or m.) 1. The forehead. The part between the eyebrows and the hairy scalp.

2. (*Frons, dis*, f.) The frond, or leaf; a tree: now used by botanists to the cryptogamious plants only.

FRONTAL. (*Frontalis*; from *frons*, the forehead.) Belonging to the forehead.

Frontal bone. See *Frontis os.*

Frontal sinus. See *Frontis os.*

FRONTA'LIS. See *Occipito frontalis.*

Frontalis verus. See *Corrugator supercilii.*

FRO'NTIS OS. The frontal bone. *Os coronale*; *Os inverecundum*; *Metopon.* The external surface of this bone is smooth at its upper convex part, but below several cavities and processes are observed. At each angle of the orbits the bone juts out to from two internal and two external processes; and the ridge under the eyebrow on each side is called the superciliary process; from which the orbitar processes extend backwards, forming the upper part of the orbits; and between these the ethmoid bone is received. The nasal process is situated between the two internal angular processes. At the internal angular process is a cavity for the caruncula lachrymalis; and at the external, another for the pulley of the major oblique muscle. The foramina are three on each side; one in each superciliary ridge, through which a nerve, artery, and vein, pass to the integuments of the forehead; a second near the middle of the internal side of the orbit, called internal orbitar; the third is smaller, and lies about an inch deeper in the orbit. On the inside of the os frontis there is a ridge which is hardly perceptible at the upper part, but grows more prominent at the bottom, where the foramen cœcum appears; to this ridge the falx is attached. The frontal sinus is placed over the orbit on each side, except at this part the frontal bone is of mean thickness between the parietal and occipital; but the orbitar process is so thin as to be almost transparent.

FRUCTIFICATION. (*Fructificatio*; from *fructus*,

fruit, and *facio*, to make.) Under this term are comprehended the flowers and the fruit of a plant. It is a temporary part of plants appropriated to generation, terminating the old vegetable and beginning the new. By the parts of fructification, Sir James Smith observes, each species is perpetually renewed without limits, while all other modes of propagation are but the extension of an individual, and sooner or later terminate in its total extinction. The fructification is therefore essential to vegetables. A plant may be destitute of stem, leaves, or even roots, because if one of these parts be wanting, the others may perform its functions, but it can never be destitute of those organs by which its species is propagated.

Linnæus distinguishes seven parts of fructification, some of which are essential to the very nature of a flower or fruit; others not so indispensably necessary, and therefore are not universal.

1. The *calyx*, or flower-cup, not essential and often absent. See *Calyx*.

2. The *corolla*, or petals, likewise not essential. See *Corolla*.

3. The *stamen* or *stamina*. These are essential. See *Stamen*.

4. The *pistillum*, or *pistilla*, in the centre of the flower, consisting of the rudiments of the fruit, with one or more organs attached to them, and therefore essential. See *Pistillum*.

5. The *pericarpium*, or seed-vessel, wanting in many plants. See *Pericarpium*.

6. The *semen*, or seed, the perfecting of which is the sole end of all the other parts.

7. The *receptaculum*, which must necessarily be present in some form or other. See *Receptaculum*.

FRU'CTUS. (*Fructus*, *tûs*. m.; *à fruor*.) The fruit of a tree or plant. By this term is understood in botany, the produce of the germen, consisting of the seed-vessel and seed.

Fructus horæi. Summer fruits. Under this term are comprehended strawberries, cherries, currants, mulberries, raspberries, and the like. They possess a sweet subacid taste, and are exhibited as dietetic auxiliaries, as refrigerants, antiseptics, attenuants, and aperients. Formerly they were exhibited medicinally in the cure of putrid affections, and to promote the alvine and urinary excretions. The acid which they contain is either the tartaric, oxalic, citric, or mallic, or a mixture of two or more of them with sugar and gluten, starch, and a gelatinous substance. Considering them as an article of diet, they afford little nourishment, and are liable to produce flatulencies. To persons of a bilious constitution and rigid fibres, and where the habit is disposed naturally, or from extrinsic causes, to an inflammatory or putrescent state, their moderate and even plentiful use, is salubrious; by those of a cold inactive disposition, where the vessels are lax, the circulation languid, and the digestion weak, they should be used very sparingly. The juices extracted from these fruits by expression, contain their active qualities freed from their grosser indigestible matter. On standing, the juice ferments and changes to a vinous or acetous state. By proper addition of sugar, and by boiling, their fermentative power is suppressed, and their medicinal qualities preserved. The juices of these fruits, when purified from their fæculencies by settling and straining, may be made into syrups, with a due proportion of sugar in the usual way.

FRUIT. See *Fructus*.

Fruits, summer. See *Fructus horæi*.

[*Fruits affording spirit*. "I shall class only the several productions which afford ardent spirits, and which may be worked to advantage at this day in the form of results of late experiments in some, and a slight knowledge of others, for the benefit of future improvement and research, beginning with

"The *Apple*. The juice of this fruit (which is called cider, when expressed and fermented,) affords, by distillation, one-tenth of its weight of spirit of the first proof on Dica's hydrometer.

"The *Pear*. This fruit, when expressed as the apple, affords nearly the same result; the qualities differing, as the quality of the fruit differs, in the same ratio as the apple. Process, the same as the apple.

"The *Peach*. This fruit is cultivated in abundance throughout the United States, though in greater abundance to the southward of Pennsylvania. It affords, by distillation, about one-eighth by clear expression. Although this is seldom done, it is nevertheless the best method to procure a fine flavour, which fixes the principal value.

"Peaches intended for distilling are thrown into bins; when the ripest should be assorted out, and thrown into a trough or vat, into which persons enter and mash them with their feet. In the southern states, wooden stampers are used, as they cannot conveniently be ground in a mill, owing to the danger of the stone. This is a practice which might well be remedied, by supplying their mills with stones after the manner of a tanner's bark-mill. It would also be attended with the advantage of breaking the peach-stones, which would impart that rich aromatic bitter which its kernel possesses, and which is so highly prized in that celebrated cordial called noyeau. After being well macerated, it is thrown into vats or casks, and diluted with water, so as to prevent an empyreuma. In this state it is called mobby, and, after a thorough fermentation, it is in that state committed to the still, together with the mass. Others press it in cider-presses.

"The *Plum*. This is a fruit which is more used in culinary purposes, and for the table. But there is a kind of plum which grows plentifully in most parts of the United States, called the red plum. It is of a beautiful saffron colour, inclining to red. This fruit affords nearly the same product as the peach, and should be treated in the same manner.

"The *Cherry*. There is a variety of this fruit: that which affords the greatest quantity of spirit is the black-heart cherry, which should be treated precisely as the peach. This fruit is more valued for the aromatic flavour which it imparts to spirit, and from which is made the exhilarating water called cherry-bounce.

"The *Papaw* is a fruit resembling seed cucumber. Its pulp is of a saffron colour, nearly of the consistence of a melon, and its flavour much like custard. It is too luscious, when ripe, to be agreeable to the palate, but when boiled, green, is pleasant. It ripens about the middle of September; is a native of Kentucky, Maryland, and Pennsylvania. The tree grows from twelve to twenty-six feet high. The fruit affords, by distillation, a spirit by some highly prized, and in considerable quantities. The process is well known to the inhabitants where the fruit grows in abundance.

"The *Blackberry*, *Whortleberry*, &c. afford spirit in tolerable quantities, by expression, fermentation, and distillation.

"The *Sugar-maple* is a tree which abounds in the northern and western parts of the United States: it grows from forty to sixty feet in height. The sap is drawn in February and March: of this sap the inhabitants make large quantities of sugar. This sap, duly fermented and distilled, produces a spirit of a very superior quality, and highly esteemed. The process is simply a fermentation of the sap, and distillation in the common way.

"The *Persimmon* is a fruit so well known throughout the United States, that a description is unnecessary. This fruit is fit for distillation only after a severe frost, which instantly ripens it, when it is gathered and thrown into a cistern or cask, in which state it is easily crushed and diluted with warm water, fermented, and the whole mass committed to the still. Some strain the mass through a coarse catgut, which takes out the seeds, that are of a powerful astringent quality. This spirit is not highly esteemed.

"The *Potato*. There are two kinds of the potato; one of which is commonly called the Irish potato, and the other the sweet potato; the latter of which affords the greatest quantity by distillation. The process is the same in both, yet the sweet potato works more kindly. After being well boiled in water, (steam is the best,) they are macerated by various means (a heavy roller is the best): they are then diluted with a sufficient quantity of water, and strained through a coarse canvass, to separate the skins (this is a process, however, which may be dispensed with); they are then thrown into casks, fermented, and committed to the still. The distillation of potatoes may, in a short time, become a matter worthy of attention. At present, the negroes of Georgia and the Carolinas are the only manufacturers. The spirit is of an inferior quality, and is used by the poorer class of inhabitants but a vast field for improvement lies open.

"*Turnips*, *Parsnips*, *Carrots*, *Pumpions*, *Cashaws*, &c. afford spirit of an inferior quality, and in tolerable quantities. They are to be treated similar to the potato.

"*Grain*, of every description, affords spirits of different qualities, according to weight.

Wheat, weighing	60lbs. per bush.	affords	8 to 12	quarts.
Rye,	60	do.	10 - 14	..
Indian corn,	60	do.	10 - 14	..
Buckwheat,	—	do.	6 - 8	..
Oats,	32	do.	5 - 7	..
Barley,	45	do.	7 - 9	..
Speltz,	60	do.	9 - 13	..
Rice,	70	do.	13 - 16	..

"The spirit afforded by the distillation of rice is what is usually termed rack, or arrack. This article is imported chiefly from Bengal, and is distilled from rice, although the real and genuine arrack is distilled in the island of Goa, from the sap of a tree, drawn in the same manner as our sugar-maple.

"The *Grape*. In the United States, the cultivation of the domestic grape has but just commenced: the numerous species, however, of our wild grape, with which our forests abound, make it a matter of consideration. These being collected in sufficient quantities, when ripe, they may be treated with success, after the process of the apple, and afford a beautiful spirit, not unlike cogniac.

"*Indian Corn* (the stalk). The young stalk of the Indian corn, (which should be used about the time of earing,) like the sugar-cane of the West Indies, affords a large quantity of juice or sap by expression, which, when fermented and distilled, yields abundantly of spirit of a very superior quality. This should be broken and worked in the same manner as the sugar-cane, which is by nut-mills of iron, after the manner of our cider-mills.—*Krafft's Amer. Distiller*. A.]

FRUMENTA'CEOUS. A term applied to all such plants as have a conformity with wheat, either with respect to their fruit, leaves, or ears.

FRUTESCENTIA. (From *fructus*, fruit.) The time at which the fruit arrives at maturity.

FRUTEX. A shrub or plant, which rises with a woody durable stem, but never arrives at the height, or has the appearance of an *arbor*, or tree.

FU'CUS. The name of a genus of plants in the Linnæan system. Class, *Cryptogamia*; Order, *Algæ*.

Fucus digitatus. This fucus grows upon stones and rocks in the sea near the shore. It has several plain, long leaves or sinuses springing from a round stalk, in the manner of fingers when extended. It affords soda.

Fucus esculentus. Edible fucus. Hudson has made this a distinct species, but Linnæus included it under his saccharinus. It grows plentifully in the sea near the shores of Scotland, and also those of Cumberland. It has a broad, plain, simple, sword-shaped leaf, springing from a pinnated stalk.

Fucus helminthocorton. See *Corallina corsicana*.

Fucus palmatus. Handed fucus. This grows in the sea, and consists of a thin-lobed leaf like a hand.

Fucus saccharinus. Sea-belts; so called from the supposed resemblance of its leaves to a belt or girdle. It grows upon rocks and stones by the sea-shore. The leaves are very sweet, and when washed and hung up to dry, will exude a substance like sugar, from whence it was named.

Fucus vesiculosus. The systematic name of the sea-oak. Sea wreck. *Quercus marina*. This sea-weed, the *Fucus—fronde plana dichotoma costata integerrima, vesiculis axillaribus geminis, terminalibus tuberculatis*, of Linnæus, is said to be a useful assistant to sea-water, in the cure of disorders of the glands. Burnt in the open air, and reduced to a black powder, it forms the æthiops vegetabilis, which, as an internal medicine, is similar to burnt sponge.

FULCRUM. A prop or support. This term is applied by Linnæus, not only to those organs of vegetables correctly so denominated, such as tendrils, but also to various other appendages to the herbage of a plant, none of which are universal or essential, nor is there any one plant furnished with them all. Sir James Smith prefers the English term *appendage*, for these organs in general, to *props*, because the latter applies only to one of them.

The greater *props*, or *fulcra* of vegetables are the roots, trunks, and branches.

To the *less* are referred,

1. The *petiolus*, or petiole, which is the fulcrum of the leaf.

2. *Cirrus*, the tendril. See *Cirrus*.

3. The *stolo*, or sucker; a filament, or underground bud, protruded from the root, and sending off radicles into the earth, pushes up a stem resembling the parent plant; as in the strawberry, and *Syringa vulgaris*.

4. *Sarmentum*, the runner, which gives off from the stem, and radicates on that which is nearest to it; as does the *Hedera helix*, or ivy.

The *fulcra of a flower* are the peduncle, scape, and receptacle.

FULI'GO. (*Quasi fumiligo*; from *fumus*, smoke.) *Araxos*; *Asoper*; *Asuoli*. Soot. Wood-soot, *fuligo ligni*, or the condensed smoke from burning wood, has a pungent, bitter, and nauseous taste, and is resolved by chemical analysis into a volatile alkaline salt, an empyreumatic oil, a fixed alkali, and an insipid earth. The tincture prepared from this substance, *tinctura fuliginis*, is recommended as a powerful antispasmodic in hysterical affections.

[FULLER, Dr. Samuel, one of the memorable planters of Plymouth, who came over with the first settlers, in 1620. He was the first regularly-educated physician that visited New-England. He did not confine his benevolent offices to the inhabitants of New-Plymouth, and to the aboriginals of the country, but readily gave his assistance to the people of Naumkeak (Salem) and Charlestown, after Mr. Endicott came to that part of Massachusetts Bay. Several of the people died of the 'scurvy, and other distempers,' and many were subjected to diseases arising from unwholesome diet, and want of proper accommodations. Having no physician among themselves, it was fortunate for those planters that Plymouth could supply them with one so well qualified as Dr. Fuller, who visited them at the request of Governor Endicott, and met with great success in his practice. He visited Salem first in 1628, and again in 1629, on account of the sickness introduced there by the newly-arrived ships. When he arrived at Plymouth, from Salem, Governor Endicott wrote to Governor Bradford a letter of thanks, speaking highly in praise of the physician, and also expressing his hearty concurrence with their church at Plymouth, its form and discipline: from which it is evident that the conversation of Dr. Fuller had some effect upon his religious opinions, for there was a difference of sentiment before this interview, and a jealousy, lest the Plymouth church should exercise a jurisdiction over the church in Salem.

In his medical character, and for his Christian virtues and unfeigned piety, Dr. Fuller was held in the highest estimation, and was resorted to as a father and wise counsellor during the perils of his day. He was finally one of several heads of families who died of a fever, which prevailed in Plymouth in the summer of 1633, and was most deeply lamented by all the colonists."—*Thatch. Med. Biog*. A.]

FULLERS' EARTH. An earth found in large beds in Buckinghamshire and Surrey, composed of silica, alumine, magnesia, lime, muriate of soda, a trace of potassa, and oxide of iron. See *Earth, Fuller's*.

["FULTON, Robert. Notwithstanding the various unsuccessful projects of propelling boats by means of steam-enginery, Mr. Robert Fulton has had the courage to undertake and construct one at New-York, upon a plan of his own, and his success is undoubted. His boat is upwards of 140 feet long, and about 15 feet wide, resembling a batteau of large dimensions. The engine is upon the plan of Watt & Boulton's latest improvement, and is a most complete piece of machinery. The power is applied to the water in which the boat moves, by means of wheels, with only eight arms, revolving on their axis. When the piston makes 20 strokes in a minute, these are turned with a motion brisk enough to stem the currents both of the East and North rivers, at the rate of four miles and more in an hour. She draws but a few inches of water. She actually made a voyage to Albany and back again in 100 hours, or a little more than four days, and she promises to be of the greatest service in working her way against the streams of rivers, such as the Mississippi, and others that have no tides."—*Med. Repos*. vol. xi.

The preceding notice of Fulton's first experiment with his rough-constructed steamboat, was published in the summer of 1807, in the New-York Medical Repository. The writer of this article was on board during the first trial, and observed the anxiety and joy of Mr. Fulton at the prospect before him. The vessel moved from the dock in the eastern part of the city of New-York, and was steered into the North or Hudson river, opposite Hoboken, where she was anchored, and after remaining there a while, returned to the place of starting. On the next day, Mr. Fulton proceeded to ascend the Hudson river, and, as stated above, was 100 hours in going to Albany and returning thence to New-York, a distance of 300 miles, or nearly that, being on an average less than four miles an hour. This boat was afterward fitted up as a packet-boat for passengers, and called the *Car of Neptune*. The next summer (1808) another boat was constructed upon a better model, and her speed surpassed the first. Some alteration or improvement was made in every subsequent boat constructed under the direction of Mr. Fulton, until the time of his death, (in Feb. 1815), when his boats went from New-York to Albany in about 20 hours, making an average of more than seven miles an hour. Since his death further improvements have been made in the construction of steamboats and their machinery, so that some of them make the trip from New-York to Albany by daylight, and some have made the passage down the river from Albany to New-York, in the extremely short period of twelve hours, making an average speed of more than twelve miles an hour. It is the opinion of some that further improvements will take place, and that the same distance will be run in nine or ten hours.

Mr. Fulton has the merit of being the first engineer who made a practical and successful application of steam-power to the propulsion of vessels through the water. He claimed no more. He used Watt & Boulton's steam engine, and modified it to suit his wishes, and the object he had in view; and having succeeded beyond his own most sanguine expectations, and to the astonishment of all his countrymen, he has died and left a legacy of incalculable value to his country and the whole civilized world. Others had indeed engaged in similar experiments, but without success. He was the master spirit who pointed out the true method, and succeeding engineers have profited by his experience; and steamboats now navigate the rivers, bays, and lakes of the United States, in greater numbers than in any other country.

Robert Fulton was a native of Pennsylvania, and by profession a portrait-painter. He became acquainted with Robert Livingston in Paris, while residing there as Minister of the United States near the French government. Their views corresponding on the feasibility of constructing a steamboat, Mr. Fulton was patronized by the minister, whose wealth enabled him to make all the necessary advances towards accomplishing this object. He was so far successful as to put a boat in rapid motion on the river Seine; and after this prelude to his future success, he returned to his native country, and constructed his first boat in 1807, as above stated, from which has emanated all the steamboats now in use in this country and Europe. A.]

FULMINA'TION. *Fulminatio.* Detonation. A quick and lively explosion of bodies, such as takes place with fulminating gold, fulminating powder, and in the combustion of a mixture of inflammable gas and vital air.

FUMA'RIA. (From *fumus*, smoke, from its juice, when dropped into the eye, producing the same sensations as smoke.)

1. The name of a genus of plants in the Linnæan system. Class, *Diadelphia*; Order, *Decandria*. Fumitory.

2. The pharmacopœial name of the common fumitory. See *Fumaria officinalis*.

FUMARIA BULBOSA. *Aristolochia fabacea.* The root of this plant, *Fumaria—caule simplici, bracteis longitudine florum*, of Linnæus, was formerly given to restore suppressed menses, and as an anthelmintic.

FUMARIA OFFICINALIS. The systematic name of the fumitory. *Fumaria; Fumus terræ; Capnos; Herba melancholifuga.* The leaves of this indigenous plant, *Fumaria—pericarpiis monospermis racemosis, caule diffuso*, of Linnæus, are directed for medicinal use by the Edinburgh college; they are extremely succulent, and have no remarkable smell, but a bitter, somewhat saline taste. The infusion of the dried leaves, or the expressed juice of the fresh plant, is esteemed for its property of clearing the skin of many disorders of the leprous kind.

FUMIGA'TION. (*Fumigatio*; from *fumus*, smoke.) The application of fumes, to destroy contagious miasmata or effluvia. The most efficacious substance for this purpose is chlorine; next to it the vapour of nitric acid; and, lastly, that of the muriatic. The fumes of heated vinegar, burning sulphur, or the smoke of exploded gunpowder, deserve little confidence as antiloimics. The air of dissecting rooms should be nightly fumigated with chlorine, whereby their atmosphere would be more wholesome and agreeable during the day.

FUMITORY. See *Fumaria*.

FUMUS. Smoke.

FUNCTION. See *Action*.

FUNGI. (The plural of *fungus*.) An order of the class *Cryptogamia* of Linnæus's system. They cannot probably be said to have any herbage; their substance is fleshy; their parts of fructification are in form of very small capsules buried in their fleshy substance. These seminiferous capsules are on the surface, or in plates, and are called *lamellæ*, or gills, pores, or prickles, and they burst, as in the algæ.

A fungus or mushroom affords the following parts.

1. *Pileus*, the hat, which is the round upper part, or head.

2. The *Umbo*, the knob, or boss, or more prominent part in the centre of the hat.

3. *Lamellæ*, the gills, or membraneous parts on the under side. These are peculiar to the *Agarici*.

4. The *pores*, or small punctures on the under surface, observed only in the genus *Boletus*.

5. *Echini*, or *Aculei*, elevated points on the upper surface of the pileus, noticed in the genus *Hydra* only.

6. *Verrucæ*, warts, observed on the inferior surface.

7. *Stipes*, the stem supporting the hat.

8. *Volva*, the wrapper, or covering, of a membraneous texture, surrounding the stem, and concealing the parts of fructification, and in due time bursting all around, forming a ring upon the stalk; as in *Agaricus campestris*. Linnæus also uses this term for the more fleshy external covering of some other fungi, which is scarcely raised out of the ground, and enfolds the whole plant when young.

9. *Annulus*, the ring, or slender membrane surrounding the stem.

The varieties of the *pileus*, or hat, are,

1. *Planus*, flat.
2. *Convexus*; as in *Boletus bovinus*.
3. *Concavus*; as in *Octospora*.
4. *Umbonatus*, umbo or navel-like; as in *Agaricus conspurcatus*.
5. *Campanulatus*; as in *Agaricus fimitarius*
6. *Viscidus*, viscid.
7. *Dimidiatus*, half round; as in *Agaricus niveus*.
8. *Squamosus*, covered with coloured scales; as in *Agaricus procerus*.
9. *Squarrosus*, having stiff elevated scales; as in *Agaricus conspurcatus*.

The varieties of the *lamellæ* are,

1. *Equal*; as in *Agaricus crinitus*.
2. *Unequal*.
3. *Branched*, when several run into one; as in *Merulius cantharellus*.
4. *Decurrent*, proceeding down the stem.
5. *Venous*, so small that they appear like elevated veins.
6. *Dimidiate*, half round; as in *Agaricus muscarius*.
7. *Labyrinth-like*; as in *Agaricus quercinus*

The varieties of the *volva* are,

1. *Simple*.
2. *Double*.
3. *Stellate*, cut several times; as in *Lycopodium stellatum*.

The varieties of the *annulus* are,

1. *Erect*, loose above, and fixed below; as in *Agaricus conspurcatus*.
2. *Inverse*, fixed above, free, and bell-like below; as in *Agaricus Mappa*.
3. *Sessile*, fixed only laterally
4. *Mobile*; as in *Agaricus antiquatus*.
5. *Persistent*, remaining after the perfect formation of the plant.

6. *Evanescent*, disappearing after the complete evolution of the fungus.

7. *Arachnoid*, resembling a slender white web.

The varieties of the *stipes* or stem.

1. *Annulate*, having a ring.
2. *Naked*, without any.
3. *Squamose*, scaly.
4. *Bulbous;* as in *Agaricus separatus*.
5. *Filiform;* as in *Agaricus crinitus*.

FUNGIC ACID. *Acidum fungicum*. The expressed juice of the *boletus juglandis*, *boletus pseudo-igniarius*, the *phallus impudicus*, *merulius cantharellus*, or the *peziza nigra*, being boiled to coagulate the albumen, then filtered, evaporated to the consistence of an extract, and acted on by pure alkohol, leaves a substance which is called *Fungic acid*.

It is a colourless, uncrystallizable, and deliquescent mass, of a very sour taste. The fungates of potassa and soda are uncrystallizable; that of ammonia forms regular six-sided prisms; that of lime is moderately soluble, and is not affected by the air; that of barytes is soluble in fifteen times its weight of water, and crystallizes with difficulty; that of magnesia appears in soluble granular crystals. This acid precipitates from the acetate of lead a white flocculent fungate, which is soluble in distilled vinegar. When insolated, it does not affect solution of nitrate of silver; but the fungates decompose this salt.

FUNGIN. The fleshy part of mushrooms deprived by alkohol and water of every thing soluble.

FU'NGUS. 1. Proud-flesh. A term in surgery to express any luxuriant formation of flesh on an ulcer.

2. In morbid anatomy it is applied to a disease of the structure of a part which enlarges, is soft, and excrescential.

3. The name of an order of plants in the Linnæan system, belonging to the *Cryptogamia* class.

FUNGUS HÆMATODES. See *Hæmatoma*.

FUNGUS IGNIARIUS. See *Boletus igniarius*.

FUNGUS LARICIS. See *Boletus laricis*.

FUNGUS MELITENSIS. See *Cynomorium*.

FUNGUS ROSACEUS. See *Bedeguar*.

FUNGUS SALICIS. The willow fungus. See *Boletus suaveolens*.

FUNGUS SAMBUCINUS. See *Peziza auricula*.

FUNGUS VINOSUS. The dark cobweb-like fungus, which vegetates in dry cellars, where wine, ale, and the like are kept.

FUNI'CULUS. (*Funiculus;* diminutive of *funis*, a cord.) A little cord.

FUNICULUS UMBILICALIS. See *Umbilical cord*.

The funiculus of a seed is a little filament by which the immature seed adheres to the receptacle, seen in *Pisum sativum* and *Lundria annua*.

FU'NIS A rope or cord.

FUNIS UMBILICALIS. See *Umbilical cord*

FUNNEL-SHAPED. See *Infundibuliformis*.

FURCA. A fork or species of armature of plants See *Aculeus*.

FURCE'LLA INFERIOR. The ensiform cartilage

FU'RCULA. The clavicle.

FU'RFUR. 1. Bran.

2. A disease of the skin, in which the cuticle keeps falling off in small scales like bran.

FURFURA'CEOUS. (*Furfuraceus;* from *furfur*, bran.) A term applied to the bran-like sediment occasionally deposited in the urine.

FURNACE. *Furnus*. The furnaces employed in chemical operations are of three kinds:

1. The *evaporatory furnace*, which has received its name from its use; it is employed to reduce substances into vapour by means of heat, in order to separate the more fixed principles from those which are more volatile.

2. The *reverberatory furnace*, which name it has received from its construction, the flame being prevented from rising; it is appropriated to distillation.

3. The *forge furnace*, in which the current of air is determined by bellows.

FU'ROR. Fury, rage.

FUROR UTERINUS. (From *furo*, to be mad, and *uterus*, the womb.) See *Nymphomania*.

FURU'NCULUS. (From *furo*, to rage: so named from its heat and inflammation before it suppurates.) *Dothein* of Paracelsus. *Chiadus; Chioli*. A bile. An inflammation of a subcutaneous gland, known by an inflammatory tumour that does not exceed the size of a pigeon's egg.

Fusible metal. A combination of three parts of lead, with two of tin, and five of bismuth. It melts at 197° Fahr.

FUSIBILITY. The property by which metals and minerals assume the fluid state.

FUSIFORMIS. Fusiform. Spindleshaped or tapering. Applied to parts of plants, as roots, &c. which penetrate perpendicularly into the earth; as the carrot, parsnip, radish, &c.

FUSION. (*Fusio;* from *fundo*, to pour out.) A chemical process, by which bodies are made to pass from the solid to the fluid state, in consequence of the application of heat. The chief objects susceptible of this operation are salts, sulphur, and metals. Salts are liable to two kinds of fusion; the one, which is peculiar to saline matters, is owing to water contained in them, and is called *aqueous fusion;* the other, which arises from the heat alone, is known by the name of *igneous fusion*.

FUSUS. (From *fundo*, to pour out.) Poured out. Applied by Dr. Good to a species of purging, *diarrhœa fusa*, in which the fæces are loose, copious, and of a bright yellow colour.

G

GABIA'NUM OLEUM. See *Petroleum rubrum*.

GABI'REA. A fatty kind of myrrh, mentioned by Dioscorides.

GADOLINATE. A hard black-coloured semitransparent mineral from Sweden, composed of silica, yttria, oxide of cerum, and oxide of iron.

GADUS. The name of a genus of fishes, of the jugular tribe. The following species are brought to the European markets for the use of the table.

GADUS CILIARIS. The Baltic torsk. The Icelanders prepare it by salting and drying, when it becomes an article of commerce, under the name of *Tetteling*. Its flesh is white, tender, and well flavoured.

GADUS MORHUA. The cod-fish. This well-known fish in our markets, abounds in the northern seas. Its flesh is white, tender, and delicious. When salted, it is also well flavoured, and in general esteem.

GADUS ÆGLEFINUS. The haddock. An inhabitant of the northern seas of Europe. The larger ones are much esteemed during the winter; the smaller ones for summer use. They are of easy digestion. Salted and dried they are eaten at breakfast as a delicacy.

GADUS MINUTUS. Very small, never exceeding six or seven inches in length. It is found in the Mediterranean in great abundance, where it is called a *capelau*, or officier.

GADUS MERLANGUS. The whiting. A delicate white fish in great abundance in the Irish seas and German Ocean.

GADUS POLLACIUS. The whiting pollack, found on the rocky coasts of Britain, and other parts of Europe, and is in great esteem for the table.

GADUS CARBONARIUS. The coal-fish. Very abundant on the rocky coasts of the northern parts of this island, about the Orkneys, and the coast of Yorkshire, where they become two and three feet long, and constitute the chief support of the poor.

GADUS MERLUCCIUS. The hake. A native of the North and Mediterranean seas, not much eaten, except by the poor when dried. when it is called poor John, or stock-fish.

GADUS MOLVA. The ling. This grows to the length of five or six feet. It is not so good as the *morhua*, when fresh; but dried and salted, is much esteemed, and is the common food of the poor in Cornwall, where it is prepared for exportation.

Gadus lota. The burbot. The flesh of this is considered delicious and of easy digestion.

Gadus brosme. The torsk. This swarms in the seas about the Shetland islands, and forms a considerable article of commerce, either dried, or salted, or packed in barrels.

[Most of the fishes belonging to the genus *Gadus*, are edible. Of the preceding enumerated species three of them are common to the waters of the United States, as the *Gadus morhua*, *Gadus æglefinus*, and *Gadus merluccius*. Besides these, there are found on the stalls of the fishermen in the markets of New-York the following species, viz. *Gadus callarias*, *Gadus tomcodus*, *Gadus blennoides*, *Gadus purpureus*, *Gadus tenuis*, *Gadus longipes*, and *Gadus punctatus*. Of these different species, all of which are used as food, the *Gadus morhua*, or bank cod, and the *Gadus callarias*, are the most abundant, and most esteemed. The *Gadus merluccius*, or hake, is remarkable for its large sound, or swimming-bladder, which is prepared and dried for sale, and forms excellent *icthyocolla;* (which see.) A.]

GALA'CTIA. (From γαλα, *lac*, milk; or γαλακτινος, *lacteus*, milky.) *Galactirrhœa*. 1. An excess or overflowing of the milk.

2. The name of a genus of diseases, Class *Genetica;* Order, *Cenotica*, of Good's Nosology. Mislactation. It comprehends five species, viz. *Galactia prœmatura; defectura; depravata; erratica; virorum.*

Galactina. (From γαλα, milk.) Aliment prepared of milk.

GALACTIRRHŒ'A. (From γαλα, milk, and ρεω, to flow.) See *Galactia*.

Galacto'des. (From γαλα, milk.) In Hippocrates it signifies both milk-warm and a milky colour.

GALACTO'PHORUS. (From γαλα, milk, and φερω, to bring or carry.) 1. That which has the property of increasing the secretion of the milk.

2. The excretory ducts of the glands of the breasts of women, which terminate in the papilla, or nipple, are so called, because they bring the milk to the nipple.

GALACTOPOIE'TIC. (*Galactopoieticus;* from γαλα, milk, and ποιεω, to make.) Milk-making, the faculty of making milk: applied to particular foods, plants, &c.

GALACTOPO'SIA. (From γαλα, milk, and πινω, to drink.) The method of curing diseases by a milk diet.

GALA'NGA. (Perhaps its Indian name.) See *Maranta* and *Kæmpferia*.

Galanga major. See *Kæmpferia galanga*.

Galanga minor. See *Maranta Galanga*.

GALANGAL. See *Maranta Galanga*.

Galangal, English. See *Cyperus longus*.

GALBANUM. (From *chalbanah*, Heb.) See *Bubon galbanum*.

Ga'lbeum. A medical bracelet worn by the Romans.

GA'LBULUS. (The name of the nut, or little round ball of the cypress-tree.) Gærtner applies this term, the classical name of the cypress fruit, which is a true *strobilus*, to a globular spurious berry with three or more seeds formed by the coalescing of a few scales, of a fertile catkin become succulent, which happens in the Juniper.—*Smith*.

Galbulus. (From *galbus*, yellow.) When the skin of the body is naturally yellow.

GA'LDA. A gum-resin, mentioned by old writers, but totally forgot in the present day, and not to be obtained. Externally, it is of a brown colour, but white within, of a hard lamellated structure, and smells and tastes somewhat like elemi. When burnt it gives out an agreeable odour. It was formerly used as a warm stimulating medicine, and applied in plasters as a strengthener.

GA'LEA. (From γαλη, a cat, of the skin of which it was formerly made.) A helmet. 1. In anatomy, the amnios is so called, because it surrounds the fœtus like a helmet

2. In surgery; a bandage for the head.

3. A species of headache is so called, when it surrounds the head like a helmet.

4. In botany it is applied to upper arched lip of ringent and personate corols. See *Corolla*.

GALEANTHRO'PIA. (This term seems to be from γαλη, a cat, and ανθρωπος, a man.) It is a species of madness, in which a person imagines himself to be a cat, and imitates its manners.

GA'LEGA. (From γαλα, milk: so named because it increases the milk of animals which eat it.) 1. The name of a genus of plants in the Linnæan system. Class, *Diadelphia;* Order, *Decandria*.

2. The pharmacopœial name of the *Ruta capraria*. See *Galega officinalis*.

Galega officinalis. The systematic name of the goat's rue. *Galega. Ruta capraria.* From the little smell and taste of this plant, *Galega leguminibus strictis, erectis; foliolis lanceolatis, striatis, nudis*, of Linnæus, it may be supposed to possess little virtues. In Italy, the leaves are eaten among salads.

Galegæ. A species of senna from the East Indies. The *cassia tora* of Linnæus.

GALE'NA. (From γαλειν, to shine.) The name of an ore formed by the combination of lead with sulphur. A native sulphuret of lead ore.

GALE'NIC. That practice of medicine which conforms to the rules of Galen, and runs much upon multiplying herbs and roots in the same composition, was long called Galenical medicine, after the manner of Galen. It is opposed to chemical medicine, which, by the force of fire, and a great deal of art, fetches out the virtues of bodies, chiefly mineral, into a small compass.

Gale'nium. (From γαληνη, galena.) A cataplasm; in the composition of which was the galena. In Paulus Ægineta it is considered as anodyne.

GALENUS, Claudius, was born at Pergamus, in Asia Minor, in 131. His father, Nicon, having instructed him in the rudiments of knowledge, sent him to attend the best schools of philosophy. Galen soon displayed his judgment by selecting what appeared most rational from the different sects; but he totally rejected the Epicurean system, which was then in fashion. About the age of 17, he began his attachment to the science of medicine, over which he was destined to preside for many centuries with oracular authority. During his youth, he travelled much, that he might converse with the most intelligent physicians of the age, and inform himself concerning the drugs brought from other countries. He resided several years at Alexandria, which was then the great resort of men of science, and the best school of medicine in the world. At the age of 28, returning to his native place, he met with distinguished success in practice; but four years after he attempted to establish himself at Rome. Here he encountered much opposition from his professional brethren, who stigmatized him as a theorist, and even as a dealer in magic; and though he gained the esteem of several men of learning and rank, yet wanting temper and experience sufficient to maintain a successful contest with a numerous and popular party, he was obliged to return to Pergamus within five years, under the pretence of avoiding the plague, which then raged at Rome. He was, however, soon after sent for to attend the emperors Marcus Aurelius and Lucius Verus, of whom the latter died; and the former conceived so high an opinion of Galen, that subsequently, during his German expedition, he committed his two sons to the care of that physician. These princes were seized with fevers, in which Galen having prognosticated a favourable issue, contrary to the opinion of all his colleagues, and having accordingly restored them to health, he attained an eminence of reputation, which enabled him to defy the power, and finally to ruin the credit, of his former opponents. It is not certain whether he continued at Rome till his death, nor at what precise period this occurred; but Fabricius asserts that he attained the age of 70, which corresponds to the 7th year of Severus; and his writings appear to indicate, that he was still in that city in the early part of this emperor's reign. The greatest part of Galen's life was spent in the zealous pursuit of knowledge, and especially of every thing which might have the least connexion with medicine, and he is said to have composed about 750 different essays on such subjects. He appears, however, to have been too much elated with the consciousness of his superior endowments, and to have behaved rather contemptuously towards his brethren; which may have inflamed their opposition to him. The chief object in his writing appears to be to illustrate those of Hippocrates, which he thought succeeding physicians had misunderstood or misrepresented: in this he has displayed great acuteness and learning, though he has not much increased the stock of practical information.

His example, too, had the unfortunate effect of introducing a taste for minute distinctions and abstract speculations; while the diligent observation of nature, which distinguished the father of medicine, fell into neglect. We must therefore regret that the splendour of Galen's talents so completely dazzled his successors, that, until about the middle of the 17th century, his opinion bore almost undivided sway. Numerous editions of his works, in the original Greek, or translated into Latin, have been printed in modern times.

GALEO'BDOLON. (From γαλεη, *felis*, and βδολος, *crepitus*.) See *Galeopsis*.

GALEO'PSIS. (From καλος, good, and οψις, vision: so called because it was thought good for the sight, or from γαλη, a cat, and οψις, aspect; the flowers gaping like the open mouth of that animal.) *Galeobdolon*. See *Lamium album*.

GALERI'CULUM APONEUROTICUM. A name in old writings for the tendinous expansion which lies over the pericranium.

Galipot. See *Barras*.

GA'LIUM. (From γαλα, milk; some species having the property of coagulating milk.) 1. The name of a genus of plants in the Linnæan system. Class, *Tetrandria*; Order, *Monogynia*.

2. The pharmacopœial name of the herb cheese-rennet, or ladies' bedstraw. See *Galium verum*.

3. A name for madder.

GALIUM ALBUM. The greater ladies' bedstraw. See *Galium mollugo*.

GALIUM APARINE. The systematic name of the goose-grass, and cleavers' bees. Cleavers; Goose-share; Hayriff. *Aparine*; *Philanthropus*; *Ampelocarpus*; *Omphalocarpus*; *Ixus*; *Asparine*; *Asperula*. This plant is common in our hedges and ditches: *Galium—foliis octonis lanceolatis carinatis scabris retrorsum aculeatis, geniculis venosis, fructu hispido*, of Linnæus. The expressed juice has been given with advantage as an aperient and diuretic in incipient dropsies; but the character in which it has of late been chiefly noticed, is that of a remedy against cancer. A tea-cupful, internally, gradually increased to half a pint, two or three times a day, and the herb applied, in cataplasm, externally, has been said to cure cancers. Such beneficial results are not confirmed by the experience of others.

GALIUM MOLLUGO. The systematic name of the greater ladies' bedstraw. *Galium album*. *Galium—foliis octonis, ovato-linearibus, subserratis, patentissimis, mucronatis; caule flaccido, ramis patentibus* of Linnæus. This herb, with its flowers, is used medicinally. Five ounces or more of the expressed juice, taken every evening upon an empty stomach, is said to cure epilepsy.

GALIUM VERUM. The systematic name of the true ladies' bed-straw, or cheese-rennet. *Galium* of the pharmacopœias. The tops of this plant, *Galium—foliis octonis, linearibus, sulcatis; ramis floriferis, brevibus*, of Linnæus, were long used as an efficacious medicine in the cure of epilepsy; but, in the practice of the present day, they are abandoned. Indeed, from the sensible qualities of the plant, little can be expected. The leaves and flowers possess the property of curdling milk; it is on that account styled cheese-rennet.

GALL. See *Bile*.

GALL SICKNESS. (See *Febris remittens*.) A popular name for the remitting fever occasioned by marsh miasmata, in the Netherlands, and which proved so fatal to thousands of the English soldiers after the capture of Walcheren in the year 1809. Dr. Lind informs us, that at Middleburg, the capital of Walcheren, a sickness generally reigns towards the latter end of August or the beginning of September, which is always most violent after hot summers. It commences after the rains which fall in the end of July; the sooner it begins the longer it continues, and it is only checked by the coldness of the weather. Towards the end of August and the beginning of September, it is a continual burning fever, attended with a vomiting of bile, which is the *gall-sickness*. This fever, after continuing three or four days, intermits and assumes the form of a double tertian; leaving the patient in a fortnight or perhaps sooner. Strangers, that have been accustomed to breathe a dry, pure air, do not recover so quickly. Foreigners in indigent circumstances, such as the Scots and German soldiers, who were garrisoned in the adjacent places, were apt, after those fevers, to have a swelling in the legs, and a dropsy; of which many died.

These diseases are the same with the double tertians common within the tropics. Such as are seized with the gall sickness, have at first some flushes of heat over the body, a loss of appetite, a white, foul tongue, a yellow tinge in the eyes, and a pale colour of the lips. Such as live well, drink wine, and have warm clothes and a good lodging, do not suffer so much during the sickly season as the poor people; however, these diseases are not infectious, and seldom prove mortal to the natives.

Sir John Pringle observes, that the prevailing epidemic of autumn, in all marshy countries, is a fever of an intermitting nature, commonly of a tertian form, but of a bad kind; which, in the dampest places and worst seasons, appears as a double tertian, a remitting, or even an ardent fever. But, however these may vary in their appearance, according to the constitution of the patient and other circumstances, they are all of a similar nature. For though, in the beginning of the epidemic, when the heat, or rather the putrefaction in the air, is the greatest, they assume a continued or a remitting form; yet, by the end of autumn, they usually terminate in regular intermittents.

But although in the gall sickness there is both a redundance and a depravation of the bile, still the disease cannot, with justice, be said to originate wholly from that cause. It is certain, however, that the disease may be continued, and the symptoms aggravated by an increased secretion and putrefaction of the bile, occasioned by the fever. In proportion to the coolness of the season, or the height and dryness of the ground, this disease is milder, remits and intermits more freely, and removes further from the nature of a continued fever. The higher ranks of people in general are the least liable to the diseases of the marshes; for such countries require dry houses, apartments raised above the ground, moderate exercise, without labour, in the sun, or evening damps; a just quantity of fermented liquors, plenty of vegetables and fresh meats. Without such helps, not only strangers but the natives themselves are sickly, especially after hot and close summers. The hardiest constitutions are very little excepted more than others; and hence the British in the Netherlands have always been subject to this fever.

By this disease, the British troops were harassed throughout the war, from 1743 to 1747. It appeared in the month of August, 1743: the paroxysms came on in the evening, with great heat, thirst, a violent headache, and often a delirium. These symptoms lasted most of the night, but abated in the morning, with an imperfect sweat; sometimes with an hæmorrhage of the nose, or looseness. The stomach, from the beginning, was disordered with a nausea and sense of oppression; frequently with a bilious and offensive vomiting. If evacuations were either neglected or too sparingly used, the patient fell into a continued fever, and sometimes grew yellow, as in jaundice. When the season was further advanced, this fever was attended with a cough, rheumatic pains, and sizy blood. The officers, being better accommodated than the common men, and the cavalry, who had cloaks to keep them warm, were not so subject to it; and others, who belonged to the army, but lay in quarters, were least of all affected; and the less in proportion to their being exposed to heats, night damps, and the other fatigues of the service. In this manner did the remitting fever infest the army for the remaining years of the war: and that exactly in proportion to their distance from the marshy places, of which we have several notable instances in Pringle's observations.

GALL-BLADDER. *Vesicula fellis*. An oblong membraneous receptacle, situated under the liver, to which it is attached in the right hypochondrium. It is composed of three membranes, a common, fibrous, and villous. Its use is to retain the bile which regurgitates from the hepatic duct, there to become thicker, more acrid, and bitter, and to send it through the cystic duct, which proceeds from its neck into the ductus communis choledochus, to be sent on to the duodenum.

GALL-STONE. *Calculus biliosus*. Biliary concretion. Hard concrete bodies, formed in the gall bladder of animals. Of these there are four different kinds.

1. The first has a white colour, and when broken presents crystalline plates, or striæ, brilliant and white like mica, and having a soft, greasy feel. Sometimes its colour is yellow or greenish; and it has constantly a nucleus of inspissated bile. Its specific gravity is inferior to that of water: Gren found the specific gravity of one 0.803. When exposed to a heat considerably greater than that of boiling water, this crystallized calculus softens and melts, and crystallizes again when the temperature is lowered. It is altogether insoluble in water, but hot alkohol dissolves it with facility. Alkohol, of the temperature of 167°, dissolves one-twentieth of its weight of this substance; but alkohol, at the temperature of 60°, scarcely dissolves any of it. As the alkohol cools, the matter is deposited in brilliant plates, resembling talc or boracic acid. It is soluble in oil of turpentine. When melted, it has the appearance of oil, and exhales the smell of melted wax; when suddenly heated, it evaporates altogether in a thick smoke. It is soluble in pure alkalies, and the solution has all the properties of a soap. Nitric acid also dissolves it; but it is precipitated unaltered by water.

This matter, which is evidently the same with the crystals Cadet obtained from bile, and which he considered as analogous to sugar of milk, has a strong resemblance to spermaceti. Like that substance, it is of an oily nature, and inflammable; but it differs from it in a variety of particulars. Since it is contained in bile, it is not difficult to see how it may crystallize in the gall-bladder if it happen to be more abundant than usual; and the consequence must be a gall-stone of this species. Fourcroy found a quantity of the same substance in the dried human liver. He called it *adipocere*.

2. The second species of biliary calculus is of a round or polygonal shape, often of a gray colour externally, and brown within. It is formed of concentric layers of a matter, which seems to be inspissated bile; and there is usually a nucleus of the white crystalline matter at the centre. For the most part, there are many of this species of calculus in the gall-bladder together; indeed, it is frequently filled with them. The calculi belonging to this species are often light and friable, and of a brownish-red colour. The gall-stones of oxen, used by painters, belong to this species. These are also adipocere.

3. The third species of calculi are most numerous of all. Their colour is often deep brown or green; and when broken, a number of crystals of the substance resembling spermaceti are observable, mixed with inspissated bile. The calculi belonging to these three species are soluble in alkalies, in soap ley, in alkohol, and in oils.

4. Concerning the fourth species of gall-stone, very little is known with accuracy. Dr. Saunders tells us, that he has met with some gall-stones insoluble both in alkohol and oil of turpentine; some of which do not flame, but become red, and consume to ashes like charcoal. Haller quotes several examples of similar calculi. Gall-stones often occur in the inferior animals, particularly in cows and hogs; but the biliary concretions of these animals have not hitherto been examined with much attention.

Gall-stones often lie quiet; so that until dissection after death, some are never known to exist; but when they are prevented from passing through the gall-ducts, they obstruct the passage of the bile into the intestines, and produce also many inconvenient symptoms, particularly the jaundice.

The diagnostics of this disorder are generally very obscure and uncertain: for other causes produce the same kind of symptoms as those which occur in this disease. The usual symptoms are a loss of appetite, a sense of fulness in the stomach, sickness, and vomiting, languor, inactivity, sleepiness; and, if the obstruction continues for a time, there is wasting of the flesh; yellowness of the eyes, skin, and urine; whitish stools; a pain in the pit of the stomach; while the pulse remains in its natural state. The pain excited by an obstruction of the gall-ducts, in consequence of gall-stones passing through them, and this not affecting the pulse, is considered as the leading pathognomonic symptom. This pain, in some, is extremely acute, in others there is only a slight uneasiness felt about the region of the liver; but its particular seat is the gall-duct, just where it enters the duodenum. In some patients there is no yellowness of the skin; in others it exists for several months. There is no disease more painful than this, in some instances; it is as frequent as any other affection of the liver; it admits of much relief from medicine, and is not immediately dangerous to the patient. See *Icterus*.

GA'LLA. (From *Gallus*, a river in Bithynia.) A gall. See *Quercus cerris*.

GALLA TURCICA. See *Quercus cerris*.

[" GAL'LÆ. *Galls*. Most species of the oak, when stimulated by the puncture of an insect, and the deposition of its egg, produce a kind of spherical excrescence, which serves as the habitation and food of the young larva when hatched. These excrescences are known by the general name of galls, and are produced on various parts of the trees by different insects of the genera *Cynips*, and *Diplolepsis*. The best galls, and those which predominate in commerce, are brought from Smyrna, Aleppo, and the neighbouring countries. The Edinburgh College considers them as produced on the *Quercus Cerris*, a tree growing in the south of Europe. The French travoller, Olivier, informs us, that the Asiatic galls are the product of a species of oak, which he names *Quercus infectoria*, and that the puncturing insect is the *Diplolepsis gallæ tinctoriæ* of Geoffroy. Both the insect and the gall have been observed in France.

Good galls are round, of a dark colour, and studded with tubercles. They are of various sizes, under that of a cherry. They are hard, brittle, and exhibit an irregular and partly resinous fracture. Their taste is highly astringent, and somewhat bitter and acrid. Those which have been perforated by the insect are of an inferior quality, their central portion being consumed The *chemical* constituents, which give to galls their chief value, are tannin and gallic acid. Besides these, they contain, according to Davy, extractive mucilage; according to Bronchi, a concrete, volatile oil; and according to Braconnot, another acid, which he calls *ellagic* acid. Chemists, however, are not agreed as to their entire composition. It is obvious, that the presence or absence of the larva, as well as its stage of growth, must materially affect the analysis.

Most metallic salts produce precipitates with infusion of galls, consisting of the metallic oxides, tannin, and gallic acid. It is questionable how far the astringency of the galls is affected by such combinations. The sulphuric and muriatic acids, lime water, and the alkaline carbonates, also, occasion precipitates. Gelatin and starch combine immediately with the tannin of the galls.

Galls are among the most powerful vegetable astringents. They are sometimes given internally, in *doses* of a scruple; but their chief medical use is as a local remedy in the form of gargles, and in the *ointment;* which see. On account of the purple or black colour, which they strike with salts of iron, they are extensively consumed in dying and ink-making. For the latter purpose, no substitute can be safely used instead of them."—*Big. Mat. Med.* A.]

GALLIC ACID. *Acidum gallicum.* An acid found in vegetable substances possessing astringent properties, but most abundantly in the excrescences termed galls, whence it derives its name. It may be obtained by macerating galls in water, filtering, and suffering the liquor to stand exposed to the air. It will grow mouldy, be covered with a thick glutinous pellicle, abundance of glutinous flocks will fall down, and, in the course of two or three months, the sides of the vessel will appear covered with small yellowish crystals, abundance of which will likewise be found on the under surface of the supernatant pellicle. These crystals may be purified by solution in alkohol, and evaporation to dryness.

Or muriate of tin may be added to the infusion of galls, till no more precipitate falls down; the excess of oxide of tin remaining in the solution, may then be precipitated by sulphuretted hydrogen gas, and the liquor will yield crystals of gallic acid by evaporation.

A more simple process, however, is to boil an ounce of powdered galls in sixteen ounces of water to eight, and strain. Dissolve two ounces of alum in water, precipitate the alumina by carbonate of potassa; and after edulcorating it completely by repeated ablutions, add it to the decoction, frequently stirring the mixture with a glass rod. The next day filter the mixture, wash the precipitate with warm water, till this will no longer blacken sulphate of iron; mix the washings with the filtered liquor, evaporate, and the gallic acid will be obtained in fine needled crystals.

These crystals obtained in any of these ways, however, are contaminated with a small portion of extractive matter; and to purify them they may be placed in a glass capsule in a sand-heat, and sublimed into another capsule inverted over this, and kept cool.

The gallic acid placed on a red-hot iron, burns with flame, and emits an aromatic smell, not unlike that of benzoic acid. It is soluble in 20 parts of cold water, and in three parts at a boiling heat. It is more soluble in alkohol, which takes up an equal weight if heated, and one-fourth of its weight cold.

It has an acido-astringent taste, and reddens tincture of litmus. It does not attract humidity from the air.

This acid, in its combinations with the salifiable bases, presents some remarkable phenomena. If we pour its aqueous solution by slow degrees into lime, barytes, or strontites water, there will first be formed a greenish-white precipitate. As the quantity of acid is increased, the precipitate changes to a violet hue, and eventually disappears. The liquid has then acquired a reddish tint. Among the salts, those only of black oxide and red oxide of iron, are decomposed by the pure gallic acid. It forms a blue precipitate with the first, and a brown with the second. But when this acid is united with tannin, it decomposes almost all the salts of the permanent metals.

Concentrated sulphuric acid decomposes and carbonizes it; and the nitric acid converts it into malic and oxalic acids.

United with barytes, strontian, lime, and magnesia, it forms salts of a dull yellow colour, which are little soluble, but more so if their base be in excess. With alkalies it forms salts that are not very soluble in general.

Its most distinguishing characteristic is its great affinity for metallic oxides, so as, when combined with tannin, to take them from powerful acids. The more readily the metallic oxides part with their oxygen, the more they are alterable by the gallic acid. To a solution of gold, it imparts a green hue; and a brown precipitate is formed, which readily passes to the metallic state, and covers the solution with a shining golden pellicle. With nitric solution of silver, it produces a similar effect. Mercury it precipitates of an orange-yellow; copper, brown; bismuth, of a lemon colour; lead, white; iron, black. Platina, zinc, tin, cobalt, and manganese, are not precipitated by it.

The gallic acid is of extensive use in the art of dying, as it constitutes one of the principal ingredients in all the shades of black, and is employed to fix or improve several other colours. It is well known as an ingredient in ink.

GA'LLICUS. Belonging to the French: applied to the venereal disease. See *Lues venerea*.

GALLINA'GO. (Diminutive of *gallus*, a cock.) 1. The woodcock.

2. An eminence within the prostate gland is called *caput callinaginis*, from its fancied resemblance to a woodcock's head.

GALLI'TRICHIS. Corrupted from *callitrichis*, or *callitrichum*. See *Callitriche*.

GA'LLIUM. See *Galium*.

GA'LVANISM. A professor of anatomy, in the university of Bologna, named *Galvani*, was one day making experiments on electricity in his elaboratory: near the machine were some frogs that had been flayed, the limbs of which became convulsed every time a spark was drawn from the apparatus. Galvani, surprised at this phenomenon, made it a subject of investigation, and discovered that metals, applied to the nerves and muscles of these animals, occasioned powerful and sudden contractions, when disposed in a certain manner. He gave the name of animal electricity to this order of new phenomena, from the analogy that he considered existing between these effects and those produced by electricity.

The name animal electricity has been superseded, notwithstanding the great analogy that exists between the effects of electricity and those of Galvanism, in favour of the latter term; which is not only more applicable to the generality of the phenomena, but likewise serves to perpetuate the memory of the discoverer.

In order to give rise to Galvanic effects in animal bodies, it is necessary to establish a communication between two points of one series of nervous and muscular organs. In this manner a circle is formed, one arch of which consists of the animal parts, rendered the subject of experiment, while the other arch is composed of excitatory instruments, which generally consist of several pieces, some placed under the animal parts called supporters, others destined to establish a communication between the latter, are called conductors. To form a complete Galvanic circle, take the thigh of a frog, deprived of its skin; detach the crural nerve, as far as the knee; put it on a piece of zinc; put the muscles of the leg on a piece of silver; then finish the excitatory arch, and complete the Galvanic circle by establishing a communication by means of the two supporters; by means of iron or copper-wire, pewter or lead. The instant that the communicators touch the two supporters, a part of the animal arch formed by the two supporters will be convulsed. Although this disposition of the animal parts, and of Galvanic instruments, be most favourable to the developement of the phenomena, yet the composition of the animal and excitatory arch may be much varied. Thus contractions are obtained, by placing the two supporters under the nerve, and leaving the muscle out of the circle, which proves that nerves essentially constitute the animal arch.

It is not necessary for nerves to be entire in order to produce contractions. They take place whether the organs be tied or cut through, provided there exists a simple contiguity between the divided ends. This proves that we cannot strictly conclude what happens in muscular action, from that which takes place in Galvanic phenomena; since, if a nerve be tied or divided, the muscles on which this is distributed lose the power of action.

The cuticle is an obstacle to Galvanic effects; they are always feebly manifested in parts covered by it. When it is moist, fine, and delicate, the effect is not entirely interrupted. Humboldt, after having detached the cuticle from the posterior part of the neck and back, by means of two blisters, applied plates of metal to the bare cutis, and, at the moment of establishing a communication, he experienced sharp prickings, accompanied with a sero-sanguineous discharge.

If a plate of zinc be placed under the tongue, and a flat piece of silver on its superior surface, on making them touch each other, an acerb taste will be perceived, accompanied with a slight trembling.

The excitatory arch may be constructed with three, two, or even one metal only, with alloys, amalgams, or other metallic or mineral combinations, carbonated substances, &c. It is observed that metals which are in general the most powerful excitors, induce contractions so much the more as they have an extent of sur face. Metals are all more or less excitants; and it is observed that zinc, gold, silver, pewter, are of the highest rank; then copper, lead, nickel, antimony, &c.

Galvanic susceptibility, like muscular irritability, is exhausted by too long continued exercise, and is recruited by repose. Immersion of nerves and muscles in alkohol and opiate solutions diminishes, and even destroys, this susceptibility, in the same manner, doubtless, as the immoderate use of these substances in the living man blunts, and induces paralysis in muscular action. Immersion in oxymuriatic acid restores the fatigued parts, to be again acted on by the stimulus. Animals killed by the repeated discharge of an electric battery, acquire an increase of Galvanic susceptibility; and this property subsists unchanged in animals destroyed by submersion in mercury, pure hydrogen gas, azote, and ammonia; and finally, it is totally annihilated in animals suffocated by the vapour of charcoal.

Galvanic susceptibility is extinct in the muscles of animals of warm blood, in proportion as vital heat is dissipated; sometimes even when life is terminated in convulsions, contractility cannot be put into action, although warmth be not completely gone, as though the vital property were consumed by the convulsion, amidst which the animals had expired. In those of cold blood, on the contrary, it is more durable. The thighs of frogs, long after being separated from every thing, and even to the instant of incipient putrefaction, are influenced by Galvanic stimuli; doubtless, because irritability, in these animals, is less intimately connected with respiration, and life more divided among the different organs, which have less occasion to act on each other for the execution of its phenomena. The Galvanic chain does not produce sensible actions (that is, contractions,) until the moment it is completed, by establishing a communication with the parts constituting it. During the time it is complete, that is, throughout the whole space of time that the communication remains established, every thing remains tranquil; nevertheless, Galvanic influence is not suspended: in fact, excitability is evidently increased, or diminished, in muscles that have been long continued in the Galvanic chain, according to the difference of the reciprocal situation of the connecting metals.

If silver has been applied to nerves, and zinc to muscles, the irritability of the latter increases in proportion to the time they have remained in the chain. By this method, the thighs of frogs have been revivified in some degree, and afterward become sensible to stimuli, that before had ceased to act on them. By distributing the metals in an inverse manner, applying zinc to nerves and silver to muscles, an effect absolutely contrary is observed; and the muscles that possess the most lively irritability when placed in the chain, seem to be rendered entirely paralytic if they remain long in this situation.

This difference evidently depends on the direction of the Galvanic fluid, determined towards the muscles or nerves, according to the manner in which these metals are disposed, and this is of some importance to be known for the application of Galvanic means to the cure of diseases.

Galvanic Pile.—Volta's apparatus is as follows:—

Raise a pile, by placing a plate of zinc, a flat piece of wet card, and a plate of silver, successively; then a second piece of zinc, &c. until the elevation is several feet high; for the effects are greater in proportion to its height; then touch both extremities of the pile, at the same instant, with one piece of iron wire; at the moment of contact, a spark is excited from the extremities of the pile, and luminous points are often perceived at different heights, where the zinc and silver come into mutual contact. The zinc end of this pile appears to be negatively electrified; that formed by the silver, on the contrary, indicates marks of positive electricity.

If we touch both extremities of the pile, after having dipped our hands into water, or, what is better, a saline solution, a commotion, followed by a disagreeable prickling in the fingers and elbow, is felt.

If we place in a tube filled with water, and hermetically closed by two corks, the extremities of two wires of the same metal which are in contact at the other extremity, one with the summit, the other with the base of the pile; these ends, even when separated only by the space of a few lines, experience evident changes at the instant the extremities of the pile are touched; the wire in contact with that part of the pile composed of silver becomes covered with bullæ of hydrogen gas; that which touches the extremity formed by zinc, becomes oxidized, or gives off oxygen gas. Fourcroy attributes this phenomenon to the decomposition of water by the Galvanic fluid, which abandons the oxygen to the metal that touches the positive extremity of the pile; then conducts the other gas invisibly to the end of the other wire there to be disengaged.

Galvanic Trough.—This is a much more convenient apparatus. Plates of two metals, commonly zinc and copper, are fastened together, and cemented into a wooden trough, so as to form a number of cells; or earthenware troughs with partitions being procured, the metals connected by a slip, are suspended over these, so that in each cell, except at the ends, there is a plate of each metal; then a diluted acid, (usually the sulphuric, nitric, or muriatic mixed with from twelve to twenty parts of water,) is poured into the trough. It is necessary that the metals be placed in the same order throughout, or one series will counteract another. The zinc end becomes negative, the copper positive; and the power is in proportion to the number of the series: and several such troughs may be connected together, so as to form a most powerful apparatus.

From the number of experiments of Davy, many new and important facts have been established, and Galvanism has been found one of the most powerful agents in chemistry: by its influence, platina wire has been melted; gold, silver, copper, and most of the metals, have easily been burnt; the fixed alkalies, and many of the earths, have been made to appear as consisting of a metallic base, and oxygen; compound substances, which were before extremely difficult to decompose, are now, by the aid of Galvanism, easily resolved into their constituents.

The Galvanic influence has been considered by some practitioners as likely to increase the nervous influence in paralyzed and debilitated states of the muscular system, and many ingenious ways of applying it have been resorted to; but it does not seem to have been useful. Dr. Ure's observations and experiments on this subject and on Galvanism are highly interesting The following account of them is extracted from his Chemical Dictionary. "Many experiments," he observes, "have been performed, in this country and abroad, on the bodies of criminals, soon after their execution. Vassali, Jullo, and Rossi, made an ample set, on several bodies decapitated at Turin. They paid particular attention to the effect of Galvanic electricity on the heart, and other involuntary muscles: a subject of much previous controversy. Volta asserted, that these muscles are not at all sensible to this electric power. Fowler maintained, that they were affected; but with difficulty and in a slight degree. This opinion was confirmed by Vassali; who further showed, that the muscles of the stomach and intestines might thus also be excited. Aldini, on the contrary, declared, that he could not affect the heart by his most powerful Galvanic arrangements."

Most of the above experiments were however made either without a voltaic battery, or with piles, feeble in comparison with those now employed. Those indeed performed on the body of a criminal, at Newgate, in which the limbs were violently agitated; the eyes opened and shut; the mouth and jaws worked about, and the whole face thrown into frightful convulsions, were made by Aldini, with, I believe a considerable series of voltaic plates.

A circumstance of the first moment, in my opinion, has been too much overlooked in experiments of this kind,—that a muscular mass through which the Galvanic energy is directly transmitted, exhibits very weak contractile movements, in comparison with those which can be excited by passing the influence along the principal nerve of the muscle. Inattention to this important distinction, I conceive to be the principal source of the slender effects hitherto produced in such experiments on the heart, and other muscles, independent of the will. It ought also to be observed, that too little distinction has been made between the positive and negative poles of the battery; though there are good reasons for supposing, that their powers on muscular contraction are by no means the same.

According to Ritter, the electricity of the positive pole augments, while the negative diminishes, the actions of life. Tumefaction of parts is produced by the former; depression by the latter. The pulse of the hand, he says, held a few minutes in contact with the positive pole, is strengthened; that of the one in contact with the negative is enfeebled: the former is accompanied with a sense of heat; the latter with a feeling of coldness. Objects appear to a positively electrified eye, larger, brighter, and red; while to one negatively electrified, they seem smaller, less distinct, and bluish,—colours indicating opposite extremities of the prismatic spectrum. The acid and alkalines tastes, when the tongue is acted on in succession by the two electricities, are well known, and have been ingeniously accounted for by Sir H. Davy, in his admirable Bakerian lectures. The smell of oxymuriatic acid, and of ammonia, are said by Ritter to be the opposite odours, excited by the two opposite poles; as a full body of sound and a sharp tone are the corresponding effects on the ears. These experiments require verification.

Consonant in some respects, though not in all, with these statements, are the doctrines taught by a London practitioner, experienced in the administration of medical electricity. He affirms, that the influence of the electrical fluid of our common machines, in the cure of diseases, may be referred to three distinct heads; first, the form of *radii*, when projected from a point positively electrified; secondly, that of a star, or the negative fire, concentrated on a brass ball; thirdly, the Leyden explosion. To each of these forms he assigns a specific action. The first acts as a sedative, allaying morbid activity; the second as a stimulant; and the last has a deobstruent operation, in dispersing chronic tumours. An ample narrative of cases is given in confirmation of these general propositions. My own experience leads me to suppose, that the negative pole of a Voltaic battery gives more poignant sensations than the positive.

The most precise and interesting researches on the relation between Voltaic electricity and the phenomena of life, are those contained in Dr. Wilson Philip's Dissertations in the Philosophical Transactions, as well as in his experimental Inquiry into the Laws of the Vital Functions, more recently published.

In his earlier researches he endeavoured to prove, that the circulation of the blood, and the action of the involuntary muscles, were independent of the nervous influence. In a late paper, read in January, 1816, he showed the immediate dependence of the secretory functions on the nervous influence.

The eighth pair of nerves distributed to the stomach, and subservient to digestion, were divided by incisions in the necks of several living rabbits. After the operation, the parsley which they ate remained without alteration in their stomachs; and the animals, after evincing much difficulty of breathing, seemed to die of suffocation. But when in other rabbits, similarly treated, the Galvanic power was transmitted along the nerve, below its section, to a disc of silver, placed closely in contact with the skin of the animal, opposite to its stomach, no difficulty of breathing occurred. The Voltaic action being kept up for twenty-six hours, the rabbits were then killed, and the parsley was found in as perfectly digested a state, as that in healthy rabbits fed at the same time; and their stomachs evolved the smell peculiar to that of a rabbit during digestion. These experiments were several times repeated with similar results.

Hence it appears that the Galvanic energy is capable of supplying the place of the nervous influence, so that, while under it, the stomach, otherwise inactive, digests food as usual. I am not, however, willing to adopt the conclusion drawn by its ingenious author, that the identity of Galvanic electricity and nervous influence is established by these experiments.' They clearly show a remarkable analogy between these two powers, since the one may serve as a substitute for the other. It might possibly be urged by the anatomist, that as the stomach is supplied by twigs of other nerves, which communicate under the place of Dr. Philip's section of the *par vagum*, the Galvanic fluid may operate merely as a powerful stimulus, exciting those slender twigs to perform such an increase of action, as may compensate for the want of the principal nerve. The above experiments were repeated on dogs, with like results; the battery never being so strong as to occasion painful shocks.

The removal of dyspnœa, as stated above, led him to try Galvanism as a remedy in asthma. By transmitting its influence from the nape of the neck to the pit of the stomach, he gave decided relief in every one of twenty-two cases, of which four were in private practice, and eighteen in the Worcester Infirmary. The power employed varied from ten to twenty-five pairs.

The general inferences deduced by him from his multiplied experiments, are, that Voltaic electricity is capable of effecting the formation of the secreted fluids, when applied to the blood in the same way in which the nervous influence is applied to it; and that it is capable of occasioning an evolution of caloric from arterial blood. When the lungs are deprived of the nervous influence, by which their function is impeded, and even destroyed, when digestion is interrupted, by withdrawing this influence from the stomach, these two vital functions are renewed by exposing them to the influence of a Galvanic trough. 'Hence,' says he, 'Galvanism seems capable of performing all the functions fo the nervous influence in the animal economy; but obviously it cannot excite the functions of animal life, unless when acting on parts endowed with the living principle.'

These results of Dr. Philip have been recently confirmed by Dr. Clarke Abel, of Brighton, who employed, in one of the repetitions of the experiments, a comparatively weak, and in the other a considerable power of Galvanism. In the former, although the Galvanism was not of sufficient power to occasion evident digestion of the food, yet the efforts to vomit, and the difficulty of breathing, constant effects of dividing the eighth pair of nerves, were prevented by it. These symptoms recurred when it was discontinued, and vanished on its reapplication. 'The respiration of the animal,' he observes, 'continued quite free during the experiment, except when the disengagement of the nerves from the tin-foil rendered a short suspension of the Galvanism necessary during their readjustment.' The nongalvanized rabbit breathed with difficulty, wheezed audibly, and made frequent attempts to vomit.' In the latter experiment, in which the greater power of Galvanism was employed, digestion went on as in Dr. Philip's experiments.—*Jour. Sc.* ix.

Gallois, an eminent French physiologist, had endeavoured to prove, that the motion of the heart depends entirely upon the spinal marrow, and immediately ceases when the spinal marrow is removed or destroyed. Dr. Philip appears to have refuted this notion by the following experiments. Rabbits were rendered insensible by a blow on the occiput; the spinal marrow and brain were then removed, and the respiration kept up by artificial means; the motion of the heart, and the circulation, were carried on as usual. When spirit of wine or opium was applied to the spinal marrow or brain, the rate of the circulation was accelerated.

A middle-sized, athletic, and extremely muscular man, about thirty years of age, was the subject of the following highly interesting experiments. He was suspended from the gallows nearly an hour, and made no convulsive struggle after he dropped; while a thief, executed along with him, was violently agitated for a considerable time. He was brought to the anatomical theatre of our university in about ten minutes after he was cut down. His face had a perfectly natural aspect, being neither livid nor tumefied; and there was no dislocation of his neck.

Dr. Jeffray, the distinguished professor of anatomy, having on the preceding day requested me (says Dr. Ure) to perform the Galvanic experiments, I sent to his theatre, with this view, next morning, my *minor* Voltaic battery, consisting of 270 pairs of four-inch plates, with wires of communication, and pointed metallic rods with insulating handles, for the more commodious application of the electric power. About five minutes before the police officers arrived with the body, the battery was charged with a dilute nitro-sulphuric acid, which speedily brought it into a state of intense action. The dissections were skilfully executed by Mr. Marshal, under the superintendence of the professor.

Exp. 1. A large incision was made into the nape of the neck, close below the *occiput*. The posterior half of the *atlas vertebra* was then removed by bone forceps, when the spinal marrow was brought into view. A profuse flow of liquid blood gushed from the wound, inundating the floor. A considerable incision was at the same time made in the left hip, through the great gluteal muscle, so as to bring the sciatic nerve into sight; and a small cut was made in the heel. From neither of these did any blood flow. The pointed rod connected with one end of the battery, was now placed in contact with the spinal marrow, while the other rod was applied to the sciatic nerve. Every muscle of the body was immediately agitated with convulsive movements, resembling a violent shuddering from cold. The left side was most powerfully convulsed at each renewal of the electric contact. On moving the second rod from the hip to the heel, the knee being previously bent, the leg was thrown out with such violence as nearly to overturn one of the assistants, who in vain attempted to prevent its extension.

Exp. 2. The left phrenic nerve was now laid bare at the outer edge of the *sterno-thyroideus* muscle, from three to four inches above the clavicle; the cutaneous incision having been made by the side of the sterno-cleido mastoideus. Since this nerve is distributed to the diaphragm, and since it communicates with the heart through the eighth pair, it was expected, by transmitting the Galvanic power along with it, that the respiratory process would be renewed. Accordingly, a small incision having been made under the cartilage of the seventh rib, the point of the one insulating rod was brought into contact with the great head of the diaphragm, while the other point was applied to the phrenic nerve in the neck. This muscle, the main agent of respiration, was instantly contracted, but with less force than was expected. Satisfied, from ample experience on the living body, that more powerful effects can be produced in Galvanic excitation, by leaving the extreme communicating rods in close contact with the parts to be operated on, while the electric chain or circuit is completed by running the end of the wires along the top of the plates in the last trough of either pole, the other wire being steadily immersed in the last cell of the opposite pole, I had immediate recourse to this method. The success of it was truly wonderful. Full, nay, laborious breathing, instantly commenced. The chest heaved, and fell; the belly was protruded, and again collapsed, with the relaxing and retiring diaphragm. This process was continued, without interruption, as long as I continued the electric discharges.

In the judgment of many scientific gentlemen who witnessed the scene, this respiratory experiment was perhaps the most striking ever made with a philosophical apparatus. Let it also be remembered, that for full half an hour before this period, the body had been well nigh drained of its blood, and the spinal marrow severely lacerated. No pulsation could be perceived meanwhile at the heart or wrist; but it may be supposed, that but for the evacuation of the blood,—the essential stimulus of that organ,—this phenomenon might also have occurred.

Exp. 3. The supra-orbital nerve was laid bare in the forehead, as it issues through the supra-ciliary *foramen*, in the eyebrow: the one conducting rod being applied to it, and the other to the heel, most extraordinary grimaces were exhibited every time that the electric discharges were made, by running the wire in my hand along the edges of the last trough, from the 220th to the 270th pair of plates: thus fifty shocks, each greater than the preceding one, were given in two seconds. Every muscle in his countenance was simultaneously thrown into fearful action; rage, horror, despair, anguish, and ghastly smiles, united their hideous expression in the murderer's face, surpassing far the wildest representations of a Fuseli or a Kean. At this period several of the spectators were forced to leave the apartment from terror or sickness, and one gentleman fainted.

Exp. 4. The last Galvanic experiment consisted in transmitting the electric power from the spinal marrow to the ulnar nerve, as it passes by the internal condyle at the elbow: the fingers now moved nimbly, like those of a violin performer; an assistant, who tried to close the fist, found the hand to open forcibly, in spite of his efforts. When the one rod was applied to a slight incision in the tip of the forefinger, the fist being previously clenched, that finger extended instantly; and from the convulsive agitation of the arm, he seemed to point to the different spectators, some of whom thought he had come to life.

About an hour was spent in these operations.

In deliberating on the above Galvanic phenomena, we are almost willing to imagine, that if, without cutting into and wounding the spinal marrow and blood-vessels in the neck, the pulmonary organs had been set a-playing at first, (as I proposed,) by electrifying the phrenic nerve, (which may be done without any dangerous incision,) there is a probability that life might have been restored. This event, however little desirable with a murderer, and perhaps contrary to law, would yet have been pardonable in one instance, as it would have been highly honourable and useful to science. From the accurate experiments of Dr. Philip it appears, that the action of the diaphragm and lungs is indispensable towards restoring the suspended action of the heart and great vessels, subservient to the circulation of the blood.

It is known, that cases of deathlike lethargy, or suspended animation, from disease and accidents, have occurred, where life has returned, after longer interruption of its functions than in the subject of the preceding experiments. It is probable, when apparent death supervenes from suffocation with noxious gases, &c. and when there is no organic læsion, that a judiciously directed Galvanic experiment will, if any thing will, restore the activity of the vital functions The plans of administering Voltaic electricity, hitherto pursued in such cases, are, in my humble apprehension, very defective. No advantage, we perceive, is likely to accrue from passing electric discharges across the chest, directly through the heart and lungs. On the principles so well developed by Dr. Philip, and now illustrated on Clydesdale's body, we should transmit along the channel of the nerves, that substitute for nervous influence, or that power which may perchance awaken its dormant faculties. Then, indeed, fair hopes may be formed of deriving extensive benefit from Galvanism; and of raising this wonderful agent to its expected rank among the ministers of health and life to man.

I would, however, beg leave to suggest another nervous channel, which I conceive to be a still readier and more powerful one, to the action of the heart and lungs, than the phrenic nerve. If a longitudinal incision be made, as is frequently done for aneurism, through the integuments of the neck at the outer edge of the *sterno-mastoideus* muscle, about half way between the clavicle and angle of the lower jaw; then, on turning over the edge of this muscle, we bring into view the throbbing carotid, on the outside of which, the *par vagum*, and great sympathetic nerve, lie together in one sheath. Here, therefore, they may both be directly touched and pressed by a blunt metallic conductor. These nerves communicate directly, or indirectly, with the phrenic; and the superficial nerve of the heart is sent off from the sympathetic.

Should, however, the phrenic nerve be taken, that of the left side is the preferable of the two. From the position of the heart, the left phrenic differs a little in its course from the right. It passes over the *pericardium*, covering the *apex* of the heart.

While the point of one metallic conductor is applied to the nervous cords above described, the other knob ought to be firmly pressed against the side of the person, immediately under the cartilage of the seventh rib. The skin should be moistened with a solution of common salt, or, what is better, a hot saturated solution of sal-ammoniac, by which means, the electric energy will be more effectually conveyed through the cuticle so as to complete the Voltaic chain.

To lay bare the nerves above described, requires, as I have stated, no formidable incision, nor does it demand more anatomical skill, or surgical dexterity, than every practitioner of the healing art ought to possess. We should always bear in mind, that the subject of experiment is at least insensible to pain; and that life is at stake, perhaps irrecoverably gone. And assuredly, if we place the risk and difficulty of the operations in competition with the blessings and glory consequent on success, they will weigh as nothing, with the intelligent and humane. It is possible, indeed, that two small brass knobs, covered with cloth moistened with solution of sal ammoniac, pressed above and below, on the place of the nerve, and the diaphragmatic region, may suffice, without any surgical operation: it may first be tried.

Immersion of the body in cold water accelerates greatly the extinction of life arising from suffocation; and hence less hopes need be entertained of recovering drowned persons after a considerable interval, than when the vital heat has been suffered to continue with little abatement. None of the ordinary practices judiciously enjoined by the Humane Society, should ever on such occasions be neglected. For it is surely culpable to spare any pains which may contribute, in the slightest degree, to recall the fleeting breath of man to its cherished mansion.

My attention has been again particularly directed to this interesting subject, by a very flattering letter which I lately received from the learned Secretary of the Royal Humane Society.

In the preceding account, I had accidentally omitted to state a very essential circumstance relative to the electrization of Clydesdale. The paper indeed was very rapidly written, at the busiest period of my public prelections, to be presented to the society, as a substitute for the essay of an absent friend, and was sent off to London the morning after it was read.

The positive pole or wire connected with the zinc end of the battery, was that which I applied to the nerve; and the negative, or that connected with the copper end, was that which I applied to the muscles. This is a matter of primary importance, as the following experiments will prove.

Prepare the posterior limbs of a frog for Voltaic electrization, leaving the crural nerves connected, as usual, to a detached portion of the spine. When the excitability has become nearly exhausted, plunge the limbs into the water of one wine-glass, and the crural nerves with their pendent portion of spine, into that of the other. The edges of the two glasses should be almost in contact. Then taking a rod of zinc in one hand, and a rod of silver (or a silver tea-spoon) in the other, plunge the former into the water of the limbs' glass, and the latter into that of the nerves' glass, without touching the frog itself, and gently strike the dry parts of the bright metals together. Feeble convulsive movements, or mere twitching of the fibres, will be perceived at every contact. Reverse now the position of the metallic rods, that is, plunge the zinc into the nerves' glass, and the silver into the other. On renewing the contact of the dry surfaces of the metal now, very lively convulsions will take place; and if the limbs are skilfully disposed in a narrowish conical glass, they will probably spring out to some distance. This interesting experiment may be agreeably varied in the following way, with an assistant operator: let that person seize, in the moist fingers of his left hand, the spine and nervous cords of the prepared frog; and in those of the right hand, a silver rod; and let the other person lay hold of one of the limbs with his right hand, while he holds a zinc rod in the moist fingers of the left. On making the metallic contact, feeble convulsive twitchings will be perceived as before. Holding still the frog as above, let them merely exchange the pieces of metal. On renewing the contacts now, lively movements will take place, which become very conspicuous, if one limb be held nearly horizontal, while the other hangs freely down. At each touch of the Voltaic pair, the drooping limb will start up, and strike the hand of the experimenter.

It is evident, therefore, that for the purposes of resuscitating dormant irritability of nerves, or contractility of their subordinate muscles, the positive pole must be applied to the former, and the negative to the latter."—*Ure's Chemical Dictionary.*

GAMA'NDRA. See *Stalagmitis.*

GAMBI'ENSE GUMMI. See *Kino.*

GAMBOGE. See *Stalagmitis.*

GAMBO'GIA. See *Cambogia* and *Stalagmitis.*

GAMBO'GIUM. See *Stalagmitis.*

GAMBOI'DEA. See *Stalagmitis.*

GA'MMA. (From the letter Γ, *gamma*, which it resembles.) A surgical instrument for cauterizing a hernia.

GAMPHE'LE. (From γαμψος, crooked.) The cheek. The jaw.

GA'NGAMON. (From γαγγαμη, a fishing-net, which it was said to resemble.) 1. A name of the omentum.

2. Some call the contexture of nerves about the navel by this name.

GA'NGLION. (Γαγγλιον, a knot.) A knot. 1. In anatomy it is applied to a natural knot-like enlargement in the course of a nerve.

2. In surgery it is an encysted tumour, formed in the sheath of a tendon, and containing a fluid like the white of an egg. It most frequently occurs on the back of the hand or foot.

GA'NGRENE. (Γαγγραινα; from γραω, to feed upon: so named from its eating away the flesh.) *Gangrena.* See *Mortification.*

GA'RAB. An Arabic name for the disorder of the eyes. See *Ægylops.*

GARCI'NIA. (So called in honour of Dr. Garcin, who accurately described it.) The name of a genus of plants in the Linnæan system. Class *Dodecandria;* Order, *Monogynia.*

GARCINIA MANGOSTANA. The systematic name of the mangosteen tree. The mangosteen is a fruit about the size of an orange, which grows in great abundance on this tree in Java and the Molucca islands. According to the concurring testimonies of all travellers, it is the most exquisitely flavoured, and the most salubrious of all fruits, it being such a delicious mixture of the tart and sweet. The flesh is juicy, white, almost transparent, and of a more delicate and agreeable flavour than the richest grape. It is eaten in almost every disorder, and the dried bark is used medicinally in dysenteries and tenesmus, and a strong decoction of it is much esteemed as a gargle in ulcerated sore throats.

GA'RGALE. Γαργαλη. *Gargalos; Gargalismos.* Irritation, or stimulation.

GARGA'REON. (Hebrew.) The uvula, or glandulous body, which hangs down into the throat.

GA'RGARISM. See *Gargarisma.*

GARGARI'SMA. (*Gargarisma, atis.* n.; and *Gargarismus, i.* m.; and *Gargarismum, i.* n.; from γαργαριζω, to gargle.) A gargle, or wash for the throat.

GARGARISMUM. See *Gargarisma.*

GA'RGATHUM. A bed on which lunatics, &c. were formerly confined.

GARGLE. See *Gargarisma.*

GARLIC. See *Allium.*

GARNET. Professor Jameson divides this mineral genus into three species: the pyramidal garnet, dodecahedral garnet, and prismatic garnet.

1. The *Pyramidal* contains three sub-species; Vesuvian, Egeran, Gehlenite.

2. The *Dodecahedral* contains nine sub-species; Pyreneite, Grossulare, Melanite, Pyrope, Garnet, Allochroite, Colophonite, Cinnamon-stone, Helvin.

3. The *Prismatic;* the grenatite. Of the garnet proper, there are two species:

1. The precious or noble garnet.

2. The common garnet.

GARNET, THOMAS, was born in 1766, at Casterton in Westmoreland. After serving his time to a surgeon and apothecary, he went to study at Edinburgh, where he took his degree at twenty-two, and then attended the London hospitals for two years. In 1790 he settled at Bradford, and began to give private lectures on Philosophy and Chemistry; and here he wrote his Treatise on the Horley Green Spa. But in the following year he removed to Knaresborough, and soon after published an Analysis of the different Waters of Harrowgate, which place he visited during the summer season. About this period he formed the design of going to America; but while waiting to take his passage at Liverpool, he was solicited to deliver some lectures there, which were so favourably received, that he was induced to repeat his course at various other places; and at length the professorship at Anderson's Institution in Glasgow was offered him, where he began lecturing in 1796. Two years after he made a tour to the Highlands, of which he subsequently published an account. On the formation of the Royal Institution in London, he was invited by Count Rumford to become the lecturer there; he accepted the appointment, and the room was crowded with persons of the first distinction and fashion. He then turned his thoughts more seriously to the practice of his profession, as likely to afford the most permanent support; but his prospects were cut short by death about the middle of the year 1802. A posthumous volume, entitled "Zoonomia," was published for the benefit of his family.

GA'RON. Γαρον. A kind of pickle prepared of fish; at first it was made from a fish, which the Greeks call *Garos;* but the best was made from mackarel. Among the moderns, *garum* signifies the liquor in which fish is pickled.

GAROU. See *Daphne gnidium.*

GARROPHY'LLUS. See *Eugenia caryophyllata.*

GARROTI'LLO. (From *garottar*, to bind closely Spanish.) A name of the cynanche maligna, from its sense of strangulation, as if the throat were bound with a cord.

GAS. (From *Gascht*, German, an eruption of wind.) *Gaz.* Elastic fluid; Aëriform fluid. This term is applied to all permanently elastic fluids, simple or compound, except the atmosphere, to which the term *air* is appropriated.

Some of the gases exist in nature without the aid of art, and may therefore be collected; others, on the contrary, are only producible by artificial means.

All gases are combinations of certain substances, reduced to the gaseous form by the addition of caloric. It is, therefore, necessary to distinguish in every gas, the matter of heat which acted the part of a solvent, and the substance which forms the basis of the gas.

Gases are not contained in those substances from which we obtain them in the state of gas, but owe their formation to the expansive property of caloric.

Formation of Gases.—The different forms under which bodies appear, depend upon a certain quantity of caloric, chemically combined with them. The very formation of gases corroborates this truth. Their production totally depends upon the combination of the particular substances with caloric; and though called permanently elastic, they are only so because we cannot so far reduce their temperature, as to dispose them to part with it; otherwise they would undoubtedly become fluid or solid.

Water, for instance, is a solid substance in all degrees below 32° of Fahrenheit's scale; above this temperature it combines with caloric, and becomes a fluid. It retains its liquid state under the ordinary pressure of the atmosphere, till its temperature is augmented to 212°. It then combines with a larger portion of caloric, and is converted, *apparently*, into gas, or at least into elastic vapour; in which state it would continue, if the temperature of our atmosphere was above 212°. Gases are therefore *solid substances, between* the particles of which a repulsion is established by the quantity of caloric.

But as in the gaseous water or steam, the caloric is retained with but little force, on account of its quitting the water when the vapour is merely exposed to a lower temperature, we do not admit steam among the class of gases, or permanently elastic aëriform fluids. In gases, caloric united by a very forcible affinity, and no diminution of temperature, or increase of pressure, that has ever yet been effected, can separate it from them. Thus the air of our atmosphere, in the most intense cold, or when very strongly compressed, still remains in the aëriform state; and hence is derived the essential character of gases, namely, *that they shall remain aëriform, under all variations of pressure and temperature.*

In the modern nomenclature, the name of every substance existing in the aëriform state, is derived from its supposed solid base; and the term gas is used to denote its existence in this state.

In order to illustrate the formation of gases, or to show in what manner caloric is combined with them, the following experiment may serve. Put into a retort, capable of holding half a pint of water, two ounces of muriate of soda (common salt): pour on it half its weight of sulphuric acid, and apply the heat of a lamp; a great quantity of gas is produced, which might be collected and retained over mercury. But to serve the purpose of this experiment, let it pass through a glass receiver, having two openings, into one of which the neck of the retort passes, while, from the other, a bent tube proceeds, which ends in a vessel of water. Before closing the apparatus, let a thermometer be included in the receiver, to show the temperature of the gas. It will be found that the mercury in the thermometer will rise only a few degrees: whereas the water in the vessel which receives the bent tube, will soon become boiling hot.

Explanation.—Common salt consists of muriatic acid, united to soda; on presenting sulphuric acid to this union, a decomposition takes place, especially when assisted by heat. The sulphuric acid unites by virtue of its greater affinity to the soda, and forms sulphate of soda, or Glauber's salt; the muriatic acid becomes therefore disengaged, and takes the gaseous form in which it is capable of existing at the common temperature. To trace the caloric during this experiment, as was our object, we must remark, that it first flows from the lamp to the disengaged muriatic acid, and converts it into gas; but the heat thus expended is chemically united, and therefore not appreciable by the thermometer. The caloric, however, is again evolved, when the muriatic acid gas is condensed by the water, with which it forms liquid muriatic acid.

In this experiment we therefore trace caloric in a chemical combination producing gas; and from this union we again trace it in the condensation of the gas, producing sensible heat.

Such, in general, is the cause of the formation and fixation of gases. It may be further observed, that each of these fluids loses or suffers the disengagement of different quantities of heat, as it becomes more or less solid in its new combination, or as that combination is capable of retaining more or less specific heat.

The discovery of aëriform gaseous fluids has occasioned the necessity of some peculiar instruments, by means of which those substances may be conveniently collected and submitted to examination. The principal ones for that purpose are styled the *pneumatic apparatus.*

The *pneumatic trough* is made either of wood or strong sheet iron, tinned, japanned, or painted. A trough of about two feet long, sixteen inches wide, and fifteen high, has been found to be sufficient for most experiments. Two or three inches below its brim, a horizontal shelf is fastened, in dimension about half or one-third part of the width of the trough. In this shelf are several holes: these holes must be made in the centre of a small excavation, shaped like a funnel, which is formed in the lower part of the shelf.

This trough is filled with water sufficient to cover the shelf to the height of an inch.

The use of this shelf is to support receivers, jars, or bell-glasses, which, being previously filled with water, are placed invertedly, their open end turned down upon the above-mentioned holes, through which the gases, conveyed there and directed by means of the funnel-shaped excavations, rise in the form of air-bubbles into the receiver.

When the gaseous fluids are capable of being absorbed by water, as is the case with some of them, the trough must be filled with mercury. The price and gravity of this fluid make it an object of convenience and economy, that the trough should be smaller than when water is used.

A mercurial trough is best cut in marble, free-stone, or a solid block of wood. A trough about twelve inches long, three inches wide, and four deep, is sufficient for all private experiments.

Method of collecting gases, and transferring them from one vessel to another.—If we are desirous of transmitting air from one vessel to another, it is necessary that the vessel destined to receive it be full of water, or some fluid heavier than air. For that purpose, take a wide-mouthed bell-glass, or receiver; plunge it under the water in the trough, in order to fill it; then raise it with the mouth downwards, and place it on the shelf of the trough, so as to cover one or more of the holes in it.

It will now be full of water, and continue so as long as the mouth remains below the surface of the fluid in the cistern; for, in this case, the water is sustained in the vessel by the pressure of the atmosphere, in the same manner as the mercury is sustained in the barometer. It may without difficulty be imagined, that if common air (or any other fluid resembling common air in lightness and elasticity) be suffered to enter the inverted vessel filled with water, it will rise to the upper part, on account of its levity, and the surface of the water will subside. To exemplify this, take a glass, or any other vessel, in that state which is usually called *empty*, and plunge it into the water with its mouth downwards; scarce any of it will enter the glass, because its entrance is opposed by the elasticity of the included air; but if the vessel be turned with its mouth upwards, it immediately fills, and the air rises in bubbles to the surface. Suppose this operation be performed under one of the jars or receivers, which are filled with water, and placed upon the perforated shelf, the air will ascend in bubbles as before, but, instead of escaping, it will be caught in the upper part of the jar, and expel part of the water it contains.

In this manner we see that air may be emptied out of one vessel into another by a kind of inverted pouring, by which means it is made to ascend from the lower to the upper vessel. When the receiving vessel has a narrow neck, the air may be poured, in a similar manner, through an inverted funnel, inserted in its mouth.

If the air is to be transferred from a vessel that is stopped like a bottle, the bottle must be unstopped, with its orifice downwards in the water; and then inclined in such a manner that its neck may come under the perforated excavation of the shelf. The gas will escape from the bottle, and passing into the vessel destined to receive it, will ascend in it in the form of bubbles.

In whatever manner this operation is performed, the necessity of the excavation in the lower part of the shelf may be readily conceived. It is, as mentioned before, destined to collect the gas which escapes from the vessel, and direct it in its passage towards the vessel adapted to receive it. Without this excavation, the gas, instead of proceeding to the place of its destination, would be dispersed and lost, unless the mouth of the receiving vessel were large

The vessels, or receivers, for collecting the disengaged gases, should be glass cylinders, jars, or bell-glasses of various sizes; some of them should be open at both ends, others should be fitted with necks at the top, ground perfectly level, in order that they may be stopped by ground flat pieces of metal, glass, slate, &c.; others should be furnished with ground stoppers. Some should be graduated into cubic inches, and subdivided into decimal or other equidistant parts. Besides these, common glass-bottles, tumblers, &c. may be used.

Classification of Gases.—All the elastic aëriform fluids with which we are hitherto acquainted, are generally divided, by systematic writers, into two classes, namely: those that are *respirable* and *capable of maintaining combustion*, and those that are *not respirable* and *incapable of maintaining combustion.* This division, indeed, has its advantage, but the term respirable, in its physiological application, has been very differently employed by different writers. Sometimes by the respirability of a gas has been meant its power of supporting life, when repeatedly applied to the blood in the lungs. At other times all gases have been considered respirable which were capable of introduction into the lungs by voluntary efforts, without any relation to their vitality. In the last case, the word respirable seems to us most properly employed, and in this sense it is here used.

Non-respirable gases are those which, when applied to the external organs of respiration, stimulate the muscles of the epiglottis in such a manner as to keep it perfectly close on the glottis; thus preventing the smallest particle of gas from entering into the bronchia, in spite of voluntary exertions.

Of respirable gases, or those which are capable of being taken into the lungs by voluntary efforts, only one has the power of uniformly supporting life, namely, atmospheric air; other gases, when respired, sooner or later impair the health of the human constitution, or perhaps occasion death; but in different modes.

Some gases effect *no positive* change in the blood; animals immersed in it die of a disease produced by the privation of atmospheric air, analogous to that occasioned by their submersion in water.

Others again produce *some positive* change in the blood, as appears from the experiments of Dr. Beddoes and Sir Humphrey Davy. They seem to render it incapable of supplying the nervous and muscular fibres with principles essential to sensibility and irritability. These gases, therefore, destroy animal life on a different principle.

It is obvious, therefore, that the above classification is not very precise, but capable of misleading the student without proper explanation.

Gas, azotic. See *Nitrogen.*

Gas, carbonic acid. See *Carbonic acid.*

Gas, heavy carbonated hydrogen. See *Carburetted hydrogen gas.*

Gas, hepatic. See *Hydrogen gas, sulphuretted.*

Gas, hydrogen. See *Hydrogen.*

Gas, light carbonated hydrogen See *Carburetted hydrogen gas.*

Gaseous oxide of carbon. See *Carbon, gaseous oxide of.*

GA'STRIC. (*Gastricus;* from γαςηρ, the stomach.) Appertaining to the stomach.

Gastric artery. *Arteria gastrica.* The right or greater gastric artery, is a branch of the hepatic; the left, or smaller, a branch of the splenic.

Gastric juice. *Succus gastricus.* A fluid separated by the stomach. See *Digestion.*

Gastrinum. Potassa.

GASTRI'TIS. (From γαςηρ, the stomach.) Inflammation of the stomach. A genus of disease in the class *Pyrexiæ*, and order *Phlegmasiæ* of Cullen. It is known by pyrexia, anxiety, heat, and pain in the epigastrium, increased when any thing is taken into the stomach, vomiting, hiccup, pulse small and hard, and prostration of strength. There are two species:

1. *Gastritis phlegmonodea*, with acute pain and severe fever.

2. *Gastritis erythematica*, when the pain and fever are slighter, with an erysipelatous redness appearing in the fauces.

Gastritis is produced by acrid substances of various kinds, such as arsenic, corrosive sublimate, &c. taken into the stomach, as likewise by food of an improper nature; by taking large draughts of any cold liquor when the body is much heated by exercise, or dancing, and by repelled exanthemata and gout. Besides these, it may arise from an inflammation of some of the neighbouring parts being communicated to the stomach.

The erysipelatous gastritis arises chiefly towards the close of other diseases, marking the certain approach to dissolution, and being unaccompanied with any marks of general inflammation, or by any burning pain in the stomach.

The symptoms of phlegmonous gastritis, as observed above, are a violent burning pain in the stomach, with great soreness, distention, and flatulency; a severe vomiting, especially after any thing is swallowed, whether it be liquid or solid; most distressing thirst; restlessness, anxiety, and a continual tossing of the body, with great debility, constant watching, and a frequent, hard, and contracted pulse. In some cases, severe purging attends.

If the disease increases in violence, symptoms of irritation then ensue; there is a great loss of strength, with faintings; a short and interrupted respiration; cold, clammy sweats, hiccups, coldness of the extremities, an intermittent pulse, and the patient is soon cut off.

The event of gastritis is seldom favourable, as the person is usually either suddenly destroyed by the violence of the inflammation, or else it terminates in suppuration, ulceration, or gangrene.

If the symptoms are very mild, and proper remedies have been employed at an early period of the disease, it may, however, terminate in resolution, and that in the course of the first, or, at farthest, the second week

Its termination in suppuration may be known by the symptoms, although moderate, exceeding the continuance of this period, and a remission of pain occurring, while a sense of weight and anxiety still remain; and, on the formation of an abscess, cold shiverings ensue, with marked exacerbations in the evening, which are followed by night sweats, and other symptoms of hectic fever; and these at length prove fatal, unless the pus is thrown up by vomiting, and the ulcer heals.

Its tendency to gangrene may be dreaded, from the violence of its symptoms not yielding to proper remedies early in the disease; and, when begun, it may be known by the sudden cessation of the pain; by the pulse continuing its frequency, but becoming weaker; and by delirium, with other marks of increasing debility ensuing.

Fatal cases of this disease show, on dissection, a considerable redness of the inner coat of the stomach, having a layer of coagulable lymph lining its surface. They likewise show a partial thickening of the substance of the organ, at the inflamed part, the inflammation seldom extending over the whole of it. Where ulceration has taken place, the ulcers sometimes are found to penetrate through all its coats, and sometimes only through one or two of them.

The cure is to be attempted by copious and repeated bleedings, employed at an early period of the disease, not regarding the smallness of the pulse, as it usually becomes softer and fuller after the operation: also several leeches should be applied to the epigastrium, followed by fomentations, or the hot bath; after which a large blister will be proper. The large intestines may be in some measure evacuated by a laxative clyster; but scarcely any internal medicine can be borne by the stomach, till the violence of the disease is much abated; we may then try magnesia, or other mild cathartic, to clear out the canal effectually. Where acrid substances have been taken, mucilaginous drinks may be freely exhibited, to assist their evacuation and sheathe the stomach; otherwise only in small quantity: and, in the former case, according to the nature of the poison, other chemical remedies may come in aid, but ought never to be too much relied upon. Should suppuration occur, little can be done beyond avoiding irritation, and supporting strength by a mild farinaceous diet, and giving opium occasionally to relieve pain.

GASTRO. Names compounded with this word have some connexion with the stomach.

GASTROCE'LE. (From γαςηρ, the stomach, an κηλη, a tumour.) A hernia of the stomach, occasioned by a protrusion of that viscus through the abdominal parietes. See *Hernia ventriculi.*

GASTROCNE'MIUS. (From $\gamma\alpha\varsigma\eta\rho$, the stomach, and $\kappa\nu\eta\mu\eta$, the leg.) The calf or belly of the leg.

GASTROCNEMIUS EXTERNUS. *Gemellus.* An extensor muscle of the foot, situated immediately under the integuments at the back part of the leg; sometimes called *gemellus*: this latter name is adopted by Albinus. Winslow describes it as two muscles, which he calls *gastrocnemii*; and Douglas considers this and the following as a *quadriceps*, or muscle with four heads, to which he gives the name of *extensor tarsi suralis*. It is called *bi femoro calcanien* by Dumas. The gastrocnemius externus arises by two distinct heads. The first, which is the thickest and longest of the two, springs by a strong thick tendon from the upper and back part of the inner condyle of the os femoris, adhering strongly to the capsular ligament of the joint, between which and the tendon is a considerable *bursa mucosa*. The second head arises by a thinner and shorter tendon from the back part of the outer condyle of the os femoris. A little below the joint, their fleshy bellies unite in a middle tendon, and below the middle of the tibia they cease to be fleshy, and terminate in a broad tendon, which, a little above the lower extremity of the tibia, unite with that of the gastrocnemius internus, to form one round tendon, sometimes called *chorda magna*, but commonly *tendo Achillis*.

GASTROCNEMIUS INTERNUS. *Tibio peronei calcanien* of Dumas. This, which is situated immediately under the last described muscle, is sometimes named *soleus*, on account of its shape, which resembles that of the sole-fish. It arises by two heads. The first springs by tendinous and fleshy fibres from the posterior part of the head of the fibula, and for some way below it. The second arises from an oblique ridge at the upper and posterior part of the tibia, which affords origin to the inferior edge of the popliteus, continuing to receive fleshy fibres from the inner edge of the tibia for some way down. This muscle, which is narrow at its origin, spreads wider, as it descends, as far as its middle; after which it becomes narrower again, and begins to grow tendinous, but its fleshy fibres do not entirely disappear till it has almost reached the extremity of the tibia, a little above which it unites with the last described muscle, to form the *tendo Achillis*. This thick round chord is inserted into the lower and posterior part of the os calcis, after sliding over a cartilaginous surface on that bone, to which it is connected by a tendinous sheath that is furnished with a large *bursa mucosa*.

Both the gastrocnemii have the same use, viz. that of extending the foot, by drawing it backwards and downwards.

GASTROCO'LIC. (*Gastrocolicus*; from $\gamma\alpha\varsigma\eta\rho$, the stomach, and $\kappa\omega\lambda o\nu$, the colon.) A term applied to a vein which proceeds from the stomach to the colon.

GASTRODY'NIA. (From $\gamma\alpha\varsigma\eta\rho$, the stomach, and $o\delta\upsilon\nu\eta$, pain.) Pain in the stomach.

GASTRO-EPIPLOIC ARTERY. *Arteria gastrico-epiploica.* The branch of the greater gastric artery that runs to the epiploon.

GASTRORAPHY. (*Gastroraphe*; from $\gamma\alpha\varsigma\eta\rho$, the stomach, and $\rho\alpha\phi\eta$, a suture.) The sewing of wounds of the abdomen.

GASTROTO'MIA. (From $\gamma\alpha\varsigma\eta\rho$, the belly, and $\tau\epsilon\mu\nu\omega$, to cut.) The operation of cutting open the belly.

GAU'BIUS, JEROME DAVID, a celebrated Dutch physician, was a pupil of the illustrious Boerhaave at Leyden, where he graduated in 1725, and about ten years after he became professor there, and taught with great applause for a period of forty years. His reputation was extended all over Europe by several valuable publications, particularly by his "Institutiones Pathologiæ Medicinalis," and his "Adversaria;" which contributed not a little to the improvement both of the theory and practice of medicine. In another work, he treated ably of the medical regulation of the mind: and he printed also a very elegant little book "De Methodo concinnandi formulas Medicamentorum." He died in 1780, in the seventy-sixth year of his age.

GAULE. See *Myrica gale*.

["GAULTHERIA. *Partridge berry.* The *gaultheria procumbens* is a well known creeping evergreen, found in woody and mountainous tracts throughout the United States. Its taste is astrigent and aromatic, and has been compared to that of orange flowers. It exactly resembles that of black birch (betula lenta). The medical properties of this plant are not unlike those of cinnamon, being a warm, aromatic, astringent, particularly useful in the secondary stage of diarrhœa. It is popularly considered an emmenagogue. The dose may be one or two scruples, but a tincture and infusion are more convenient forms. The volatile oil of this article is officinal."—*Bigel. Mat. Med* A.]

["GAYLUSSACITE. This name has recently been given to a new metal obtained from a species of pyrites found in South America, of which the following account has been received by Dr. Mitchill, together with a specimen of the substance in a crystalline form.

"The pyrites is obtained from a small lake in the province of Merida de Columbia, being the upper coat of a substratum of strong mineral alkali, called *urao*, much used by the lower class of the natives of Columbia, mixed with an extract of tobacco, and then called *chimoo*. The alkali produces to the government a rental of from 50,000 to 60,000 dollars per annum. The mineral is at the bottom of the lake, about three fathoms under water. Several Indians are employed by the government to dive and extract it, which they do by means of small crowbars. They are paid about two reales per pound for it, and the government afterward sell it at one dollar. The situation of the lake is about ten leagues west of the city of Merida, called Lagunillas. The pyrites are there called *espejuelas*, and have been analyzed in Paris, and found to contain a metal hitherto unknown, and now called Gaylussacite, from the celebrated French chemist of that name."—A.]

GAZ. (From *gascht*, a German word which means an eruption of wind.) See *Gas*.

GEHLENITE. A mineral substance allied to Vesuvian, found along with calcareous spar in the Tyrol.

GEISO'MA. (From $\gamma\epsilon\iota\sigma o\nu$, the eaves of the house.) *Geison.* The prominent parts of the eyebrows, which hang over the eyes like the eaves of a house.

GEI'SON. See *Geisoma*.

GELA'SINOS. (From $\gamma\epsilon\lambda\alpha\omega$, to laugh.) An epithet for the middle fore-teeth, because they are shown in laughter.

GELA'SMUS. (From $\gamma\epsilon\lambda\alpha\omega$, to laugh.) The Sardonic laugh. See *Sardonic laugh*.

GE'LATIN. Gelly, or jelly. An animal substance soluble in water, but not in alkohol: capable of assuming a well-known elastic or tremulous consistence, by cooling, when the water is not too abundant, and liquifiable again, by increasing its temperature. This last property remarkably distinguishes it from albumen, which becomes consistent by heat. It is precipitated in an insoluble form by tannin, and it is this action of tannin on gelatin that is the foundation of the art of tanning leather.

Jellies are very common in our kitchens; they may be extracted from all the parts of animals, by boiling them in water. Hot water dissolves a large quantity of this substance. Acids likewise dissolve them, as do likewise more particularly the alkalies. Jelly, which has been extracted without long decoction, possesses most of the characters of vegetable mucilage; but it is seldom obtained without a mixture of albumen.

Jellies, in a pure state, have scarcely any smell or remarkable taste. By distillation, they afford an insipid and inodorous phlegm, which easily putrefies. A stronger heat causes them to swell up, become black, and emit a fœtid odour, accompanied with white acrid fumes. An impure volatile alkali, together with empyreumatic oil, then passes over, leaving a spongy coal, not easily burned, and containing common salt and phosphate of lime.

The jelly of various animal substances is prepared for the use of seafaring persons under the name of portable soup. The whole art of performing this operation consists in boiling the meat, and taking the scum off, as usual, until the soup possesses the requisite flavour. It is then suffered to cool, in order that the fat may be separated. In the next place, it is mixed with five or six whites of eggs, and slightly boiled. This operation serves to clarify the liquid, by the removal of opaque particles, which unite with the white of egg at the time it becomes solid by the heat, and are consequently removed along with it. The liquor is then to be strained through flannel, and evaporated on the water-bath, to the consistence of a very thick paste; after which it is spread, rather thin, upon a smooth stone, then cut into cakes, and, lastly, dried in a stove, until it becomes brittle. These cakes may be kept four or five years, if defended from moisture. When intended to be used, nothing more is required to be done than to dissolve a sufficient quantity in boiling water, which by that means becomes converted into soup.

Jelly is also found in vegetables, as ripe currants, and other berries mixed with an acid.

GELA'TIO. (From *gelo*, to freeze.)

1. Freezing.

2. That rigidity of the body which happens in a catalepsy, as if the person were frozen.

GEM. This word is used to denote a stone which is considered as precious; as the diamond, ruby, sapphire, topaz, chrysolite, beryl, emerald, &c.

GEME'LLUS. (From *geminus*, double, having a fellow.) See *Gastrocnemius* and *Gemini*.

GEMINI. *Gemelli* of Winslow. Part of the *marsupialis* of Cowper. *Ischio spini trochanterien* of Dumas. A muscle of the thigh, which has been a subject of dispute among anatomists since the days of Vesalius. Some describe it as two distinct muscles; and hence the name it has gotten of *gemini*. Others contend that it ought to be considered as a single muscle. The truth is, that it consists of two portions, which are united together by a tendinous and fleshy membrane, and afford a passage between them to the tendon of the obdurator internus, which they enclose as it were in a purse. These two portions are placed under the glutæus maximus, between the ischium and the great trochanter.

The superior portion, which is the shortest and thickest of the two, rises fleshy from the external surface of the spine of the ischium; and the inferior, from the tuberosity of that bone, and likewise from the posterior sacro-ischiatic ligament. They are inserted, tendinous and fleshy, into the cavity at the root of the great trochanter. Between the two portions of this muscle, and the termination of the obturator internus, there is a small *bursa mucosa*, connected to both, and to that part of the capsular ligament of the joint which lies under the gemini.

This muscle assists in rolling the os femoris outwards, and prevents the tendon of the obturator internus from slipping out of its place while that muscle is in action.

GEMMA. 1. A precious stone or gem.

2. In botany this term is now applied exclusively to the buds on the stems of plants. The ancients used the terms *germen* and *oculus* to denote those buds which contain the rudiments of branches and leaves, and *gemma* those in which flowers only are contained; but by the moderns, *germen* has been applied to denote the rudiment of the fruit, or as a generic term for all buds.—*Thompson*.

A *gemma* or bud contains the rudiments of a plant, or of part of a plant, for a while in a latent state, till the time of the year, and other circumstances, favour their evolution. In the bud, therefore, the vital principle is dormant. Buds of trees or shrubs, destined for cold countries, are formed in the course of the summer in the bosoms of their leaves, and are generally solitary; but in the *Lonicera cærulea*, or blue-berried honey-suckle, they grow one under another for three successive seasons.

The buds of the plane-tree, *Platanus*, are concealed in the footstalk, which must be removed before they can be seen, and which they force off by their increase; so that no plant can have more truly and necessarily deciduous leaves.

Shrubs in general have no buds, neither have the trees of hot climates.

Buds are various in their forms, but very uniform in the same species, or even genus. They consist of scales closely enveloping each other, and enfolding the embryo plant or branch. Externally they have often an additional guard of gum, resin, or woolliness, against wet or cold. The horse-chesnut affords a fine example of large and well-formed buds.

The contents of buds are different, even in different species of the same genus, as willows. The buds of some produce leaves only, others flowers, while in other species the same bud bears both leaves and flowers. Different causes, depending on the soil or situation, seem in one case to generate leaf-buds, in another flower-buds. In general, whatever checks the luxuriant production of leaf-buds, favours the formation of flowers and seeds.—*Smith*.

Gems are found in all trees and shrubs in temperate climates. In the majority of instances they are visible from the first, in which case they are *axillary*, that is, seated in the axillæ of the leaves, or the angle which the upper part of the footstalk of the leaf makes with the surface of the stem; but in some instances, as the sumachs and planes, they are *latent*, being hid within the base of the footstalk, and never seen until the fall of the leaf. Gems are however sometimes protruded from the trunk, long after it has ceased to produce leaves, as in the case of adventitious buds; they are also situated on roots, and on tubers, but in these cases they are usually denominated *oculi*, or *eyes*.

Annual plants are supposed to be furnished with gems; but although they are devoid of covered gems, yet their lateral shoots proceed from naked buds which immediately spread into foliage.

The relative position of *axillary* gems is necessarily regulated by that of the leaf, and therefore we find them,

1. *Opposite*, or placed exactly on the same line on opposite sides of the stem or the branch.

2. *Alternate*, or placed alternately, although on opposite sides; and,

3. *Spiral*, that is, placed round the stem or branch in such a manner that a cord wound in a spiral manner round it would touch each gem. They are said to be *simple* or *solitary*, when one gem only is seen in the axilla of each leaf, as in the greater number of instances; and *aggregate*, when, as in some plants, two, three, or even more are protruded at the same time: thus we find two in the *Sambucus nigra*, or common elder; three in the *Aristolochia sipho*, or broad-leaved birth-wort; and many in the *Zanthoxylum fraxineum*, or toothache tree.

Du Hamel first noticed the fact, that stems and branches furnished with alternate axillary gems have generally one *terminal* gem only; and those with opposite have generally three terminal gems.

The gems on most trees and shrubs rise with a broad base from the surface where they are protruded, and consequently being in close contact with it, are said to be *sessile*; but they are distant or stalked on some, as the common alder, on which they are supported on a short footstalk, and are termed *pedicillatæ*, or stalked.

Gems differ very considerably in the number and characters of the enclosing scales, their contents, the folding up of the leaves within them, and the manner in which they are evolved in the spring.

a. The scales differ in size and texture, even in the same gem; in the gems of different plants, they differ also in number and in the nature of their coverings; some gems are entirely destitute of scales; as those of annual plants, and many perennials of tropical climates. The scales in some instances are besmeared with a resinous matter; in others they are entirely free from any moist exudation, but are smooth and polished, being covered with a dry gummy varnish: or they are externally hairy or enveloped in a velvety down.

Gems are arranged into three species:

1. *Gemmæ foliiferæ*, leaf gems.
2. *Gemmæ floriferæ*, flower gems.
3. *Gemmæ mixtæ*, mixed gems.

The *Amygdalus persica*, or peach-tree, the *Daphne mezereum*, and many other plants, afford examples of distinct leaf and flower gems; the *Syringa vulgaris* and *Æsculus hippocastanum*, of mixed gems; and the pear and apple trees of both leaf and mixed gems.

The leaves, as has already been mentioned, are variously folded up so as to occupy the smallest possible space in the gem. This regulates the expansion of the leaves when the gem opens in spring, and it is invariably the same in individual plants of the same species. This process is termed *foliation*, and the figures which the leaves assume at the time have received different appellations.—*Thompson*.

1. *Foliatio involuta*, involute, in which each internal margin of the leaf is rolled inwards; as in *Humulus lupulus* and *Nymphæa lutea*.

2. *F. revoluta*, revolute, in which the lateral margins are rolled outwards; as in willows, and *Rumex patientia*.

3. *F. obvoluta*, obvolute, in which one leaf, doubled lengthways, embraces within its doubling one half of the other leaf, folded in the same manner; as in *Salvia officinalis*, and *Dipsacus communis*.

4. *F. convoluta*, convolute, in which the leaf is rolled lengthwise in a spiral manner, one margin forming the axis round which the other turns; as in *Prunus domestica*, and *Prunus armeniaca*, the cabbage, grasses, &c.

5. *F. equitans*, equitant, in which the leaf is so folded that the two sides deeply embrace the opposite leaf, which in its turn encloses the one opposed to it, and so on to the centre of the bud: this is beautifully exemplified in the *Hemarocallis*, or day-lily, and *Syringa vulgaris*.

6. *F. conduplicata*, in which the two sides of the leaf lie parallel to each other; as in *Fagus sylvatica* and *Quercus robur*.

7. *F. plicata*, plaited, the leaf being folded up like a fan; as in *Betula alba*, and *Alchemilla vulgaris*.

8. *F. reclinata*, reclinate, turned down, the leaf hanging down and wrapped round the footstalk; as in *Aconitum* and *Arum*.

9. *F. circinata*, circinal, in which the leaf is rolled from the apex to the base; as in all ferns.

As the gems open, the leaves gradually unfold themselves, and assume their natural forms; but the opening of the bud does not, in every instance, immediately set free the leaves, for in some gems each leaf is separately enclosed in a membraneous cover.

GEMMACEUS. A term used by botanists to a flower-stalk which grows out of a leaf-bud, as is seen in the *Berberis vulgaris*.

GEMMATIO. (From *gemma*, a bud.) A term used by Linnæus expressive of the origin, form, &c. of buds.

Gemu'rsa. (From *gemo*, to groan: so called from the pain it was said to occasion in walking.) The name of an excrescence between the toes.

Genei'as. (From γενυς, the cheek.)

1. The downy hairs which first cover the cheek.

2. The name of a bandage mentioned by Galen, which covers the cheek, and comes under the chin.

GENERATION. (*Generatio;* from γεινομαι, to beget.) Many ingenious hypotheses have been instituted by physiologists to explain the mystery of generation; but the whole of our knowledge concerning it appears to be built upon the phenomena it affords, and may be seen in the works of Haller, Buffon, Cruickshanks, and Haighton. It is a sexual action, performed in different ways in most animals; many of them have different sexes and require conjunction: such are the human species, quadrupeds, and others. The females of quadrupeds have a matrix, separated into two cavities, *uterus bicornis*, and a considerable number of teats; they have no menstrual flux; most of them bear several young at a time, and the period of their gestation is generally short. The generation of birds is very different. The males have a strong genital organ, which is often double. The vulva in the females is placed behind the anus; the ovaries have no matrices, and there is a duct for the purpose of conveying the egg from the ovarium into the intestines: this passage is called the oviduct. The eggs of pullets have exhibited unexpected facts to physiologists, who examined the phenomena of incubation. The most important discoveries are those of the immortal Haller, who found the chicken perfectly formed in eggs which were not fecundated. There is no determinate conjunction between fishes; the female deposites her eggs on the sands, over which the male passes, and emits its seminal fluid, doubtless for the purpose of fecundating them; these eggs are hatched after a certain time. The males of several oviparous quadrupeds have a double or forked organ. Insects exhibit all the varieties which are observed in other animals: there are some, indeed the greater number, which have the sexes in two separate individuals; among others, the reproduction is made either with or without conjunction, as in the vine-fretter; one of these insects, confined alone beneath a glass, produces a great number of others. The organ of the male in insects is usually armed with two hooks to seize the female: the place of these organs is greatly varied; with some, it is at the upper part of the belly, near the chest, as in the female dragon-fly; in others, it is at the extremity of the *antenna*, as in the male spider. Most worms are hermaphrodite; each individual has both sexes. Polypi, with respect to generation, are singular animals; they are reproduced by buds or offsets: a bud is separated from each vigorous polypus, which is fixed to some neighbouring body, and grows: polypi are likewise found on their surface, in the same manner as branches issue from plants. These are the principal modes of generation in animals. In the human species, which engages our attention more particularly, the phenomena are as follow:

The part of the male, in the act of reproduction, is to deposite the semen in the vagina, at a greater or less distance from the orifice of the uterus.

The function which the female discharges is much more obscure; some feel, at this moment, very strong voluptuous sensations; others appear entirely insensible; while others, again, experience a sensation which is very painful. Some of them pour out a mucous substance in considerable abundance, at the instant of the most vivid pleasure: while, in the greater part, this phenomenon is entirely wanting. In all these respects, there is, perhaps, no exact resemblance between any two females.

These different phenomena are common to the most frequent acts of copulation, that is, to those which do not produce impregnation, as well as those which are effective.

The most recent opinion is, that the uterus during impregnation opens a little, draws in the semen by aspiration, and directs it to the ovarium by means of the Fallopian tubes, the fimbriated extremity of which closely embraces that organ.

The contact of the semen determines the rupture of one of the vesicles, and the fluid that passes from it, or the vesicle itself, passes into the uterus, where the new individual is to be developed.

However satisfactory this explanation may appear it is purely hypothetical, and even contrary to the experiments of the most exact observers.

In the numerous attempts made upon animals, by Harvey, DeGraaf, Valisneri, &c. the semen has never been perceived in the cavity of the uterus; much less has it been seen in the Fallopian tube at the surface of the ovarium. It is quite the same with the motion which the Fallopian tube is supposed to have in embracing the circumference of the ovarium: it has never been proved by experiment. Even if one should suppose that the semen penetrates into the uterus at the moment of coition, which is not impossible, though it has not been observed, it would still be very difficult to comprehend how the fluid could pass into the Fallopian tubes, and arrive at the ovarium. The uterus in the empty state is not contractible; the uterine orifice of the Fallopian tubes is extremely narrow, and these canals have no known sensible motion.

On account of the difficulty of conceiving the passage of the semen to the ovarium, some authors have imagined that this matter is not carried there, but only the vapour which exhales from it, or the *aura seminalis*. Others think that the semen is absorbed in the vagina, passes into the venous system, and arrives at the ovaria by the arteries. The phenomena which accompany the fecundation of women are, then, nearly unknown. An equal obscurity rests on the fecundation of other mammiferous females. Nevertheless, it would be more easy to conceive a passage of the semen to the ovaria in these, since the uterus and the Fallopian tubes possess a peristaltic motion like that of the intestines. Fecundation, however, taking place by the contact of the semen with the ova, in fishes, reptiles, and birds, it is not very likely that nature employs any other mode for the *mammifera;* it is necessary, then, to consider it as very probable, that, either at the instant of coition, or at a greater or a less time afterward, the semen arrives at the ovarium, where it exerts more especially its action upon the vessels most developed.

But, even should it be out of doubt that the semen arrives at the vesicles of the ovarium, it would still remain to be known how its contact animates the germ contained in it. Now, this phenomenon is one of those on which our senses, and even our mind, have to hold: it is one of those impenetrable mysteries of which we are, and, perhaps, shall ever remain ignorant.

We have, however, on this subject, some very ingenious experiments of Spallanzani, which have removed the difficulty as far as it seems possible.

This philosopher has proved, by a great number of trials, 1st, that three grains of semen, dissolved in two pounds of water, are sufficient to give to it the fecundating virtue; 2d, that the spermatic animalcula are not necessary to fecundation, as Buffon and other authors have thought; 3d, that the *aura seminalis*, or seminal vapour, has no fecundating property; 4th, that a bitch can be impregnated by the mechanical injection of semen into her vagina, &c. &c.

It is thus necessary to consider as conjectural what authors say about the general signs of fecundation. At the instance of conception, the woman feels, it is said, a universal tremor, continued for some time, accompanied by a voluptuous sensation; the features are discomposed, the eyes lose their brilliancy, the pupils are dilated, the visage pale, &c. No doubt, impregnation is sometimes accompanied by these signs; but many mothers have never felt them, and reach even the third month of their pregnancy without suspecting their situation."—*Magendie's Physiology.*

Fecundation having thus taken place, a motion is induced in the vivified ovum, which ruptures the tender vesicle that contains it; the fimbriæ of the Fallopian tube then grasp and convey it into the tube, which, by its peristaltic motion, conducts it into the cavity of the uterus, there to be evolved and brought to maturity, and, at the expiration of nine months, to be sent into the world.

Generation, organs of. The parts subservient to generation in a woman are divided into external and internal. The external parts are the *mons veneris*, the *labia*, the *perinæum*, the *clitoris*, and the *nymphæ*. To these may be added the *meatus urinarius*, or orifice of the urethra. The *hymen* may be esteemed the barrier between the external and internal parts. The internal parts of generation are the *vagina* and *uterus*, and its appendages.

The parts which constitute the organs of generation in men, are the *penis*, *testes*, and *vesiculæ seminales*.

GENICULATUS. Geniculate; bent like the knee: applied to the culm or straw of grasses; as in *Alopecuris geniculatus*.

GENIO. (From γενειον, the chin.) Names compounded of this word belong to muscles which are attached to the chin.

Genio-hyo-glossus. (From γενειον, the chin, υοειδες, the os hyoides, and γλωσσα, the tongue; so called from its origin and insertion.) *Genio glossus* of some authors. The muscle which forms the fourth layer between the lower jaw and os hyoides. It arises from a rough protuberance in the inside of the middle of the lower jaw; its fibres run like a fan, forwards, upwards, and backwards, and are inserted into the tip, middle, and root of the tongue, and base of the os hyoides, near its corner. Its use is to draw the tip of the tongue backwards into the mouth, the middle downwards, and to render its back concave. It also draws its root and the os hyoides forwards, and thrusts the tongue out of the mouth.

Genio-hyoideus. (From γενειον, the chin, and υοειδες, the os hyoides; so called from its origin in the chin, and its insertion in the os hyoides.) The muscle which contitutes the third layer between the lower jaw and os hyoides. It is a long, thin, and fleshy muscle, arising tendinous from a rough protuberance at the inside of the chin, and growing somewhat broader and thicker as it descends backward to be inserted by very short tendinous fibres into both the edges of the base of the os hyoides. It draws the os hyoides forwards to the chin.

Geniopharyngæ'us. See *Constrictor pharyngis superior.*

Genipi album. See *Artemisia rupestris.*

Genipi verum. The plant directed for medicinal purposes under this title, is the *Achillea—foliis pinnatis, pinnis simplicibus, glabris, punctatis*, of Haller. It has a very grateful smell, and a very bitter taste, and is exhibited in Switzerland, in epilepsy, diarrhœa, and debility of the stomach.

GENI'STA. (From *genu*, a knee; so called from the inflection and angularity of its twigs.) 1. The name of a genus of plants in the Linnæan system. Class, *Diadelphia*; Order, *Decandria*.

2. The pharmacopœial name of the common broom. See *Spartium scoparium.*

Genista canariensis. This tree was supposed to afford the lignum Rhodium, which is now known to be an aspalathus. See *Aspalathus canariensis.*

Genista spinosa indica. *Bahel schulli.* An Indian tree, a decoction of the roots of which is diuretic. The leaves, boiled and sprinkled in vinegar, have the same effect, according to Ray.

Genista tinctoria. The systematic name of *Chamæpartium*, or Dyer's broom.

GENITALE. (From *gigno*, to beget.) The membrum virile. See *Penis.*

Genita'lium. (From *genitale*, the membrum virile.) A disease of the genital parts.

GENITICA. (From γεινομαι, *gignor*.) The name of a class of diseases, in Good's Nosology, embracing diseases of the sexual function. It has three orders, viz. *Cenotica*, *Orgastica*; *Carpotica*.

Genitu'ra. (From *gigno*.) 1. The male seed.

2. The membrum virile.

Ge'non. (From γενυ, the knee.) A moveable articulation like that of the knee.

["Genesee oil. This is a variety of petroleum found in various parts of the United States, sometimes abundantly, as in *Kentucky*, *Ohio*, the western parts of *Pennsylvania*, and in *New-York*, at Seneca lake, &c. It usually floats on the surface of springs, which, in many cases, are known to be in the vicinity of coal. It is sometimes called Seneca or Genesee oil."—*Cleav. Min.* A.]

GENSING. See *Panax.*

GENTIA'NA. (From *Gentius*, king of Illyria, who first used it.) 1. The name of a genus of plants in the Linnæan system. Class, *Pentandria*; Order, *Digynia*. Gentian.

2. The pharmacopœial name of the gentian root. See *Gentiana lutea.*

Gentiana alba. See *Laserpitium latifolium.*

Gentiana centaurium. Less centaury was so called in the Linnæan system; but it is now *Chironia centaurium.*

Gentiana lutea. The systematic name of the officinal gentian. *Gentiana rubra.* Felwort. The gentian met with in the shops is the root of the *gentiana—corollis subquinquefidis rotatis verticillatis, calycibus spathaceis*, of Linnæus; and is imported from Switzerland and Germany. It is the only medicinal part of the plant, has little or no smell, but to the taste manifests great bitterness, on which account it is in general use as a tonic, stomachic, anthelmintic, antiseptic, emmenagogue, and febrifuge. The officinal preparations of this root are the *infusum gentianæ compositum*, and *tinctura gentianæ composita*, of the London Pharmacopœia; and the *infusum amarum*, *vinum amarum*, *tinctura amara*, of the Edinburgh Pharmacopœia; and the *extractum gentianæ* is ordered by both.

Gentiana rubra. See *Gentiana lutea.*

["Gentiana catesbœi. *Blue gentian.* Of various native species of gentian, which our country affords; this approaches most nearly to the officinal plant in bitterness. Its virtue appears to reside chiefly in an extractive principle, soluble in water and alkohol. It has also a little resin. Like the imported gentian, it is an active tonic, invigorating the stomach, and giving relief in complaints arising from indigestion. It appears to possess much reputation in the Southern States, to which its growth is principally confined."—*Bigel. Mat. Med.* A.]

Gentianine. The bitter principle of the Gentian root.

["The discovery of this immediate principle, presents a circumstance so singular as to merit being related.

"M. Henry, chief of central pharmacy, and M. Caventou, were occupied at the same time, and without the knowledge of each other, on the analysis of gentian. They arrived at results so much alike, that having communicated their labours to each other, they perceived that they seemed to have acted in concert, and resolved to publish them in common.

"*Preparation of gentianine.* The powder of gentian is treated with cold ether. After forty-eight hours, a tincture is obtained of a greenish yellow;—this tincture filtered, poured into an open vase, and exposed to heat, will become, by cooling, if the liquor is sufficiently concentrated, a yellow crystalline mass, with a very perceptible taste and smell of gentian.

"This mass is treated with alkohol until it ceases taking a citron tinge. The washings are reunited and exposed to a mild heat; the yellow crystalline mass reappears, which, upon evaporation, becomes concentrated, and of a very strong bitterness.

"Resumed by feeble alkohol, it is redissolved in part, with the exception of a certain quantity of oily matter

"This last alkoholic solution, besides the bitter principle of the gentian, contains an acid substance, and the odorous matter of gentian.

"By evaporating this liquor to dryness, soaking the matter in water, adding a little washed and calcined magnesia, boiling and evaporating with a vapour bath, the greatest part of the odorous matter of the gentian is expelled; the acidity disappears by means of the magnesia, and the yellow bitter principle remains in part free and in part combined with the magnesia, to which it communicates a beautiful yellow colour. Then by boiling this magnesia with ether, the greater part of this bitter principle is taken up, which is obtained pure and alone by evaporation. If it be wished to separate the greatest part of the bitter principle, which remains fixed in the magnesia, and which the ether could not take up, it must be treated with oxalic acid, in a quantity sufficient to produce acidity. This acid unites with the magnesia, and sets free the bitter principle, which is retaken by the means already pointed out.

"*Properties of gentianine.* The gentianine is yellow, inodorous, with the aromatic bitterness of the gentian very strong, and which is increased very much when it is dissolved in an acid.

"It is very soluble in ether and alkohol, and is separated by spontaneous evaporation, in the form of very small yellow crystalline needles. It is much less soluble in cold water, which it renders, however, very bitter; boiling water dissolves more.

"The dilute alkalies deepen very much its colour, and dissolve it a little more than water alone.

"Acids lighten its yellow colour in a very evident manner. Its solutions are almost colourless with sulphuric and phosphoric acid, and yellowish with acids more feeble, such as the acetic acid. Concentrated sulphuric acid carbonizes it and destroys its bitterness.

"Gentianine, exposed in a glass tube to the heat of boiling mercury, is sublimed in the form of small yellow crystalline needles. One part is decomposed.

"*Action of gentianine on man and other animals.* Some which I made, taught me that gentianine has no poisonous qualities. Several grains of this substance injected into the veins, produce no apparent effect. I myself swallowed two grains dissolved in alkohol, and only experienced an extreme bitterness, and a slight feeling of warmth at the stomach

"*Mode of employing gentianine.* The tincture is the preparation which should be most frequently used. It may be prepared from the following formula:

Tincture of gentianine. ℞. Alkohol at 24°, 1 ounce.
Gentianine, 5 grains.

"This tincture replaces with success the elixir of gentian, and is employed in the same circumstances:

Syrup of gentianine ℞. syrup of sugar, 1 pound.
Gentianine, 16 grains.

"This is one of the best bitters which can be used in scrofulous affections."—*Magendie's Formulary.* A.]

GE'NU. The knee.

GENU'GRA. (From γενυ, the knee, and αγρα, a seizure.) A name in Paracelsus for the gout in the knee.

GENUS. (From γενος, a family.) By this term is understood, in natural history, a certain analogy of a number of species, making them agree together in the number, figure, and situation of their parts; in such a manner, that they are easily distinguished from the species of any other genus, at least by some one article. This is the proper and determinate sense of the word genus, whereby it forms a subdivision of any class, or order of natural beings, whether of the animal, vegetable, or mineral kingdoms, all agreeing in certain common and distinct characters.

GEODES. A kind of ætites, the hollow of which contains only loose earth, instead of a nodule.

GEOFFRÆ'A. (Named in honour of Dr. Geoffroy.) *Geoffroya.* 1. The name of a genus of plants in the Linnæan system. Class, *Diadelphia;* Order, *Decandria.*

2. The pharmacopœial name of the cabbage bark-tree. See *Geoffræa inermis.*

GEOFFRÆA INERMIS. The systematic name of the cabbage bark-tree, or worm bark-tree. *Geoffræa—foliis lanceolatis of* Swartz. It has a mucilaginous and sweetish taste, and a disagreeable smell. According to Dr. Wright of Jamaica, it is powerfully medicinal as an anthelmintic.

GEOFFRÆA JAMAICENSIS. The systematic name of the bastard cabbage-tree, or bulgewater-tree. *Geoffroya—inermis foliolis lanceolatis*, of Swartz. The bark is principally used in Jamaica, and with great success, as a vermifuge.

GEOFFRÆA SURINAMENSIS. The systematic name of a tree, the bark of which is esteemed as an anthelmintic.

GEOFFROY, STEPHEN FRANCIS, was born at Paris, in 1672. After giving him an excellent general education, his father, who was an apothecary, sent him to study his own profession at Montpelier; where he attended the several lectures. On his return to Paris, having already acquired considerable reputation, he was appointed to attend the Duke de Tallard, on his embassy to England, in 1698. Here he was very favourably received, and elected a member of the Royal Society: and he afterward visited Holland and Italy. His attention was chiefly directed to natural history and the materia medica, his father wishing him to succeed to his establishment at Paris: however, he became ambitious of the higher branch of the profession, and at length graduated in 1704. His reputation rapidly increased; and he was called in consultation even by the most distinguished practitioners. In 1709 he was appointed to the professorship of medicine on the death of Tournefort. He then undertook to deliver to his pupils a complete History of the Materia Medica, divided into mineral, vegetable, and animal substances; the first part of which he finished, and about half of the second: this was afterward published from his papers, in Latin, in three octavo volumes. In 1712 he was made professor of chemistry in the king's garden; and 14 years after, dean of the faculty. In this office he was led into some active disputes; whence his health, naturally delicate, began to decline; and he died in the beginning of 1731. Nothwithstanding his illness, however, he completed a work, which had been deemed necessary by preceding deans, but never accomplished; namely, a Pharmacopœia, which was published under the name of "Code Medicamentaire de la Faculté de Paris."

GEOGNOSY. The same as geology.

GEOLOGY. (*Geologia;* from γη, the earth, and λογος, a discourse.) A description of the structure of the earth. This study may be divided, like most others, into two parts; observation and theory. By the first we learn the relative positions of the great rocky or mineral aggregates that compose the crust of our globe; through the second, we endeavour to penetrate into the causes of these collocations. A valuable work was some time since published, comprehending a view of both parts of the subject, by Mr. Greenough, to which the reader is referred for much instruction, communicated in a very lively manner.

Very recently the world has been favoured with the first part of an excellent view of this science by Messrs. Conybeare and Phillips, in their "Outlines of the Geology of England and Wales;" from which work, the following brief sketch of the subject is taken: The *Traité de Geognosie* of D'Aubuisson bears a high character on the continent.

WERNER'S *Table of the different Mountain Rocks, from Jameson.*

CLASS I.—*Primitive rocks.*

1. Granite.
2. Gneiss.
3. Mica-slate.
4. Clay-slate.
5. Primitive limestone.
6. Primitive trap.
7. Serpentine.
8. Porphyry.
9. Syenite.
10. Topaz-rock.
11. Quartz-rock.
12. Primitive flinty-slate.
13. Primitive gypsum.
14. White stone.

CLASS II.—*Transition rocks.*

1. Transition lime-stone.
2. Transition trap.
3. Greywacke
4. Transition flinty-slate.
5. Transition gypsum.

CLASS III.—*Floetz rocks.*

1. Old red sandstone, or first sandstone formation.
2. First or oldest floetz limestone.
3. First or oldest floetz gypsum.
4. Second or variegated sandstone formation.
5. Second floetz gypsum.
6. Second floetz limestone.
7. Third floetz limestone.

8 Rocksalt formation.
9. Chalk formation.
10. Floetz-trap formation.
11. Independent coal formation.
12. Newest floetz-trap formation.

CLASS IV.—*Alluvial rocks.*

1. Peat.
2. Sand and gravel.
3. Loam.
4. Bog-iron ore.
5. Nagelfluh.
6. Calc-tuff.
7. Calc-sinter.

CLASS V.—*Volcanic rocks.*

Pseudo-volcanic rocks.

1. Burnt clay.
2. Porcelain jasper.
3. Earth slag.
4. Columnar clay ironstone.
5. Polier, or polishing slate.

True volcanic rocks.

1. Ejected stones and ashes.
2. Different kinds of lava.
3. The matter of muddy eruptions.

The primitive rocks lie undermost, and never contain any traces of organized beings imbedded in them. The transition rocks contain comparatively few organic remains, and approach more nearly to the chemical structure of the primitive, than the mechanical of the secondary rocks. As these transition rocks were taken by Werner from among those which, in his general arrangement, were called secondary, the formation of that class made it necessary to abandon the latter term. To denote the mineral masses reposing in his transition series, he accordingly employed the term floetz rocks, from the idea that they were generally stratified in planes nearly horizontal, while those of the older strata were inclined to the horizon at considerable angles. But this holds good with regard to the structure of those countries which are comparatively low; in the Jura chain, and on the borders of the Alps and Pyrenees, Werner's floetz formations are highly inclined. Should we therefore persist in the use of this term, says Mr. Conybeare, we must prepare ourselves to speak of vertical beds of floetz, (*i. e.* horizontal), limestone, &c. As the inquiries of geologists extended the knowledge of the various formations, Werner, or his disciples, found it necessary to subdivide the bulky class of floetz rocks into floetz and newest floetz, thus completing a fourfold enumeration. Some writers have bestowed the term *tertiary* on the newest floetz rocks of Werner. The following synoptical view of geological arrangement is given by the Rev. Mr. Conybeare.

CHARACTER.	PROPOSED NAMES.	WERNERIAN NAMES	OTHER WRITERS.
1. Formations (chiefly of *sand* and *clay*) above the chalk.	*Superior order.*	Newest floetz class.	Tertiary class.
2. Comprising, a. Chalk. b. Sands and clay, *beneath the chalk.* c. Calcareous freestones (*oolites*) and argillaceous beds. d. *New red sandstone, conglomerate, and magnesian limestone.*	*Supermedial order.*	Floetz class.	Secondary class.
3. Carboniferous rocks, comprising, a. *Coal measures.* b. *Carboniferous limestone.* c. *Old red sandstone.*	*Medial order.*	Sometimes referred to the preceding, sometimes to the succeeding class, by writers of these schools; very often the coal measures are referred to the former, the subjacent limestone and sandstone to the latter.	
4. *Roofing slate*, &c. &c.	*Submedial order.*	Transition class.	Intermediate class.
5. *Mica slate, gneiss, granite*, &c.	*Inferior order.*	Primitive class.	Primitive class.

In all these formations, from the lowest to the highest, we find a repetition of rocks and beds of similar chemical composition; *i. e.* siliceous, argillaceous, and calcareous, but with a considerable difference in texture; those in the lowest formations being compact and often crystalline, while those in the highest and most recent are loose and earthy. These repetitions form what the Wernerians call formation suites. We may mention,

1*st.* The *limestone suite.* This exhibits, in the inferior or primitive order, crystalline marbles; in the two next, or transition and carboniferous orders, compact and subcrystalline limestones (Derbyshire limestone); in the supermedial or floetz order, less compact limestone (lias), calcareous freestone (Portland and Bath stone), and chalk; in the superior or newest floetz order, loose earthy limestones.

2*d.* The *argillaceous suite* presents the following gradations; clay-slate, shale of the coal-measures, shale of the lias, clays alternating in the oolite series, and that of the sand beneath the chalk; and, lastly, clays above the chalk.

3*d.* The *siliceous suite* may (since many of the sandstones of which it consists present evident traces of felspar and abundance of mica, as well as grains of quartz, and since mica is more or less present in every bed of sand) perhaps deserves to have granite placed at its head, as its several members may possibly have been derived from the detritus of that rock: it may be continued thus; quartz rock and transition sandstone, old red sandstone, millstone-grit, and coal-grits, new red sandstone, sand and sandstone beneath the chalk, and above the chalk. In all these instances a regular diminution in the degree of consolidation may be perceived in ascending the series.

["*A Geological Nomenclature for North America, founded upon Geological Surveys, by Amos Eaton, Professor in the Rensellaer School at Troy, N. Y.*

Classes of Rocks.

CLASS 1. *Primitive Rocks;* being those which contain no organic relics nor coal See Fig. 1, 2, 3, 4, 5, and 6.

CLASS 2. *Transition Rocks;* being those which contain no animal remains, but radiated and molluscous—the latter more than one valved, or one valved and chambered. See Fig. 7, 8, 9, 10, 11, and 12.

CLASS 3. *Secondary Rocks;* being those which contain in some localities, one valved molluscous animal remains, *not chambered.* They embrace most of those remains found in transition rocks also; and the upper secondary rocks contain oviparous vertebral remains. See Fig. 13, 14, 15, 16, 17, 18, and 19.

CLASS 4. *Superincumbent Rocks;* being those hornblende rocks, which overlay others without any regular order of superposition, supposed to be of volcanic origin. See Fig. 20.

Classes of Detritus.

CLASS 5. *Alluvial Detritus;* being those masses of detritus, which have been washed into their present situation. See Fig. 21, 22, 23, and 24.

CLASS 6. *Analluvial Detritus;* being those masses of detritus, which have not been washed from places where they were first formed by the disintegration of rocks. See Fig. 25 and 26.

GEOLOGICAL NOMENCLATURE

CASE OF SPECIMENS. CLASSES 2 & 1.	GENERAL STRATA and SUBDIVISIONS.	VARIETIES.	IMBEDDED and DISSEMINATED.
12 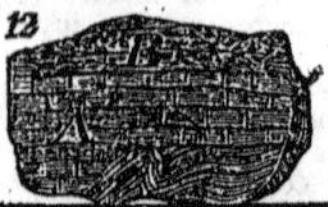	SECOND GRAY-WACKE. B. *Rubble.* A. *Compact.*	Red sandy, (old red sand ?) Horne-slate. Grind-stone.	Manganese. Anthracite.
11 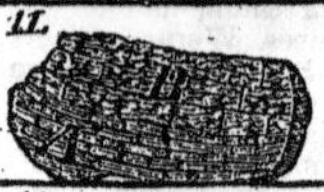	METALLIFEROUS LIMEROCK. B. *Shelly.* A. *Compact.*	Birdseye marble.	
10 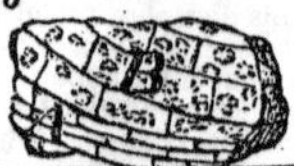	CALCIFEROUS SANDROCK. B. *Geodiferous* A. *Compact.*	Quartzose. Sparry. Oolitic.	Semi-opal. Anthracite. Barytes. Concentric concretions.
9 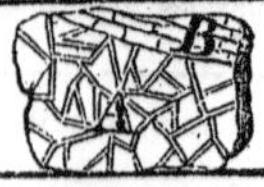	SPARRY LIMEROCK. B. *Slaty.* A. *Compact.*	Checkered rock.	Chlorite. Calc spar.
8 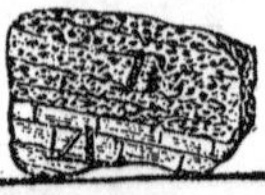	FIRST GRAY-WACKE.* B. *Rubble.* A. *Compact.*	Chloritic.	Milky quartz. Calc spar. Anthracite.
7 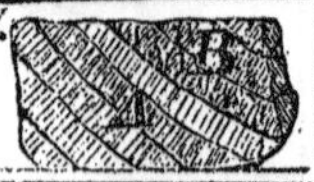	ARGILLITE. B. *Wacke Slate.* A. *Clay Slate.*	Chloritic. Glazed. Roof-slate. Red. Purple.	Flinty slate. Anthracite. Striated quartz. Milky quartz. Chlorite.
6 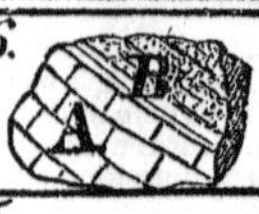	GRANULAR LIMEROCK. B. *Sandy.* A. *Compact.*	Verd-antique. Dolomite. Statuary marble.	Tremolite. Serpentine. Chromate of iron.
5 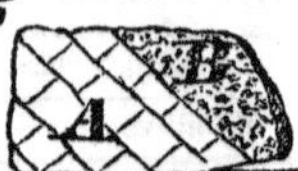	GRANULAR QUARTZ. B. *Sandy.* A. *Compact.*	Ferruginous. Yellowish. Translucent.	Manganese. Hematite.
4 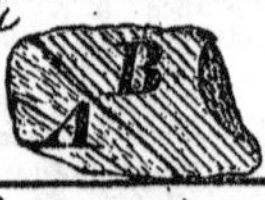	TALCOSE SLATE. B. *Fissile.* A. *Compact.*	Chloritic.	Octahedral crystals of iron ore. Chlorite.
3 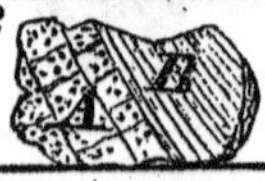	HORNBLENDE ROCK. B. *Slaty.* A. *Granitic.*	Greenstone. Gneissoid. Porphyritic. Sienitic.	Granite. Actynolite. Augite.
2 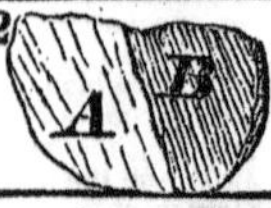	MICA-SLATE. B. *Fissile.* A. *Compact.*		Staurotide. Sappare. Garnet.
1 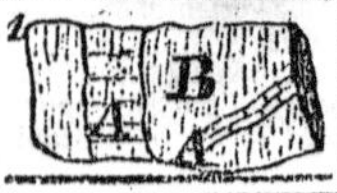	GRANITE. B. *Slaty* (gneiss). A. *Crystalline.*	Sandy. Porphyritic. Graphic.	Shorl. Plumbago. Steatite. Diallage.

* No. 8. (Second Gray-Wacke) is a secondary rock, and embraces the Anthracite coal of the Lehigh river, in Pennsylvania.

CASE OF SPECIMENS. Classes 4 & 3.	GENERAL STRATA and SUBDIVISIONS.	VARIETIES.	IMBEDDED and DISSEMINATED.
20. 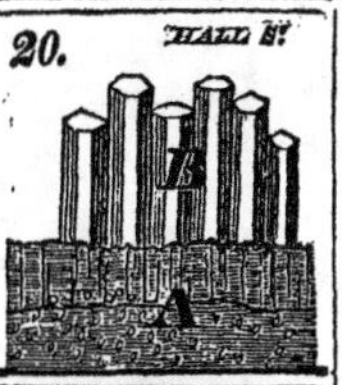 HALL ST	Basalt. B. *Greenstone trap* (columnar). A. *Amygdaloid* (cellular).	Granular Compact Toadstone.	Amethyst. Calcedony. Prehnite. Zeolite. Opal.
19. 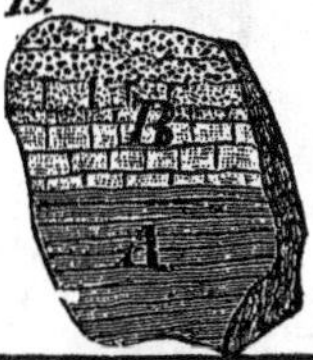	Third Graywacke.* B. *Pyritiferous grit.* A. *Pyritiferous slate.*	Conglomerate (breccia). Calcareous grit. Red sandstone, (old red sandstone?) Red-wacke. Argillaceous.	Grindstone. Hornstone? Honeslate. Bituminous shale and coal. Fibrous barytes.
18. 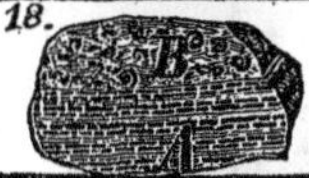	Cornitiferous Limerock. B. *Shelly.* A. *Compact.*		Hornstone.
17. 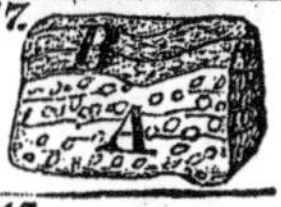	Geodiferous Limerock. B. *Sandy.* A. *Swinestone.*	Fœtid.	Snow-gypsum. Strontian. Zinc. Fluor spar.
16 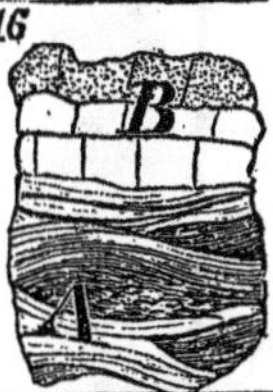	Lias. B. *Calciferous grit.* A. *Calciferous slate.*	Shell grit. Argillaceous. Conchoidal.	Shell limestone. Vermicular. Water cement. Gypsum.
15 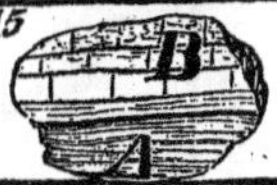	Ferriferous Rock. B. *Sandy.* A. *Slaty.*	Conglomerate. Green. Blue.	Argillaceous iron ore (reddle).
14 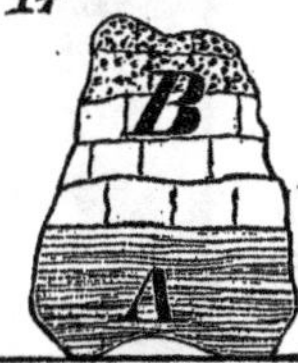	Saliferous Rock. B. *Sandy.* A. *Marl-slate.*	Conglomerate Gray-band. Red-sandy. Gray slate. Red slate.	Salt, or salt springs
13 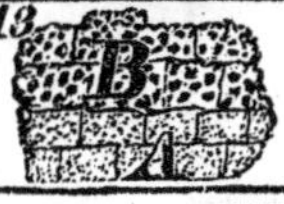	Millstone Grit. B. *Conglomerate.* A. *Sandy.*		Coal?

* No 19. (Third Graywacke) is overlaid by Oolite, in the State of Ohio. It is the upper secondary of Bakewell

NOMENCLATURE OF DETRITUS

CASE OF SPECIMENS. CLASSES 6 & 5.	GENERAL DEPOSITES AND SUBDIVISIONS.	VARIETIES.	IMBEDDED AND DISSEMINATED SUBSTANCES.
26. 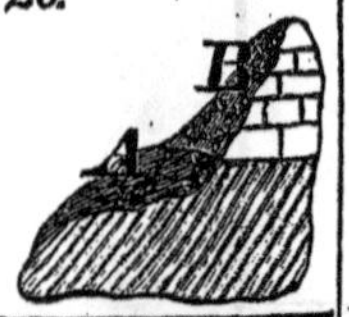	SUPERFICIAL ANALLUVION. B. *Granulated* (from graywacke). A. *Clay-loam* (from argillite).		Various boulders. Pebbles.
25 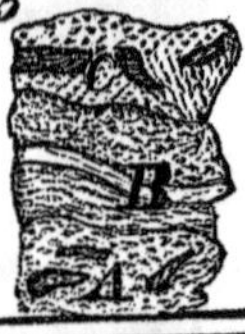	STRATIFIED ANALLUVION. C. *Lias.* B. *Ferriferous.* A. *Saliferous.*		Gypsum. Shell limestone. Reddle.
24. 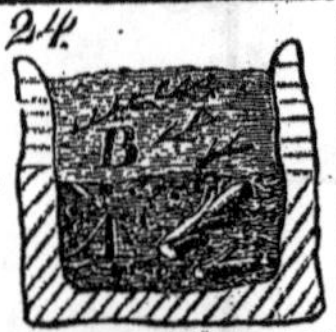	POST-DILUVION. B. *Sediment.* A. *Pebbles* (in the rocky bed of a river).		Various boulders. Trees and herbs. Fish bones and shells. Works of art.
23 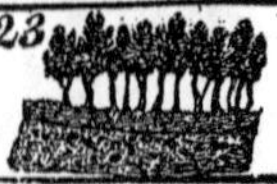	ULTIMATE DILUVION (on crag in old forests).	Yellowish gray. Grayish yellow.	
22 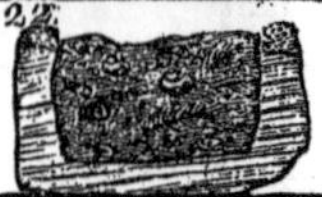	DILUVION (in an antediluvial trough).	Quicksand. Gravel. Vegetable mould.	Boulders. Trees and leaves. Bones and shells. No works of art.
21. 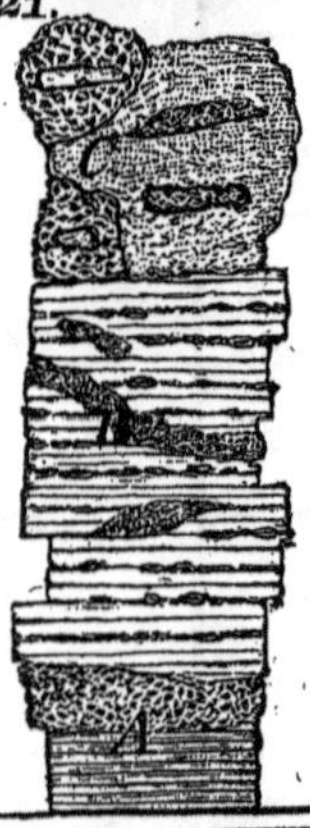	ANTEDILUVION, OR UPPER TERTIARY.* C. *Marine*, or *Bagshot, sand, and crag.* B. *Marly clay.* A. *Plastic clay.*	Quicksand. Yellow sand. Hardpan. Brick earth.	Pudding-stone. Buhrstone. Bog ore. Shell-marl. Indurated marl Septaria?

* No. 21. (Antediluvion) is the genuine tertiary formation in New Jersey, along the bay of Amboy. Professor Eaton has recently reviewed most of the territory upon which his synopsis was founded. He now says that all strata may be arranged under *five series*, each comprising *three formations:* the first series according with the primitive class, the second with the transition, the third with the lower secondary, the fourth with the upper secondary, and the fifth with the tertiary; that the lower formation of every series is carboniferous, the middle one quartzose, the upper one calcareous. In the course of a year, this view of the subject will probably be published, illustrated by a geological map of the State of New York. A prodeomus of these series will appear in Silliman's Journal.

DEFINITIONS* OF NAMES ARRANGED IN THE SYNOPSIS.

Names under the Primitive Class.

1. **Granite**, is an aggregate of angular masses of quartz, felspar, and mica. *Subdivisions.*—It is called *chrystalline* (granite proper) when the felspar and quartz present a crystalline, not a slaty, form. It is called *slaty* (gneiss) when the mica is so interposed in layers as to present a slaty form. *Varieties.*—It is *graphic* when the felspar is in a large proportion, and the quartz is arranged in oblong masses, so as to present an appearance resembling Chinese letters. It is *porphyritic* when spotted with cuboid blocks of felspar. This variety is peculiar to the slaty division.

2 **Mica-Slate**, is an aggregate of grains of quartz and scales of mica. Subdivisions.—*Compact*, when the slaty laminæ are so closely united, that it will present a uniform smooth face when cut transversely. *Fissile*, when the laminæ separate readily by a blow upon its surface.

3. **Hornblende Rock**,† is an aggregate, not basaltic, consisting wholly, or in part, of hornblende and felspar. Subdivisions.—*Granitic*, when it presents the appearance of crystalline granite with hornblende substituted for mica. *Slaty*, when of a rifty or tabular structure. Varieties.—*Gneisseoid*, when it resembles slaty granite (gneiss) with scales of hornblende substituted for mica. *Greenstone*, when of a pretty uniform green colour, and containing but a small proportion of felspar, generally of a slaty structure. *Porphyritic*, when spotted with cuboid blocks of felspar. *Sienitic*, when speckled with small irregular masses of felspar.

4. **Talcose Slate**, is an aggregate of grains of quartz and scales of mica and talc.‡ Subdivisions.—*Compact*, having the laminæ so closely united that a transverse section may be wrought into a smooth face. When the quartzose particles are very minute and in a large proportion, it is manufactured into scythe-whetstones, called Quinnebog stones. *Fissile*, when the laminæ separate readily by a blow upon the surface. Varieties.—*Chloritic*, when coloured green by chlorite. In some localities the chlorite seems to form beds; or rather the rock passes into an aggregate consisting of quartz, mica, talc, and a large proportion of chlorite. Vast beds of pure chlorite are embraced in this rock on Deerfield river, in Florida, Mass.

5. **Granular Quartz**, consists of grains of quartz united without cement. Subdivisions.—*Compact*, when it consists of fine grains, so as to appear almost homogeneous; generally in large rhomboidal blocks. *Sandy*, when the grains are so slightly attached as to be somewhat friable. Varieties.—*Translucent*, when it is so compact and homogeneous as to transmit light. *Yellow*, when slightly tinged with iron (probably a carbonate). *Ferruginous*, when an aggregate of minute crystals, strongly coloured yellow or red with the carbonate or peroxyde of iron. There is a remarkable locality two miles north of Bennington village, in Vermont. Large masses may be found consisting of six-sided crystals, with six-sided pyramids on both ends.

6. **Granular Limestone**, consists of glimmering grains of carbonate of lime united without cement. Subdivisions.—*Compact*, when it consists of grains of nearly pure carbonate of lime, so closely united that it will take a polish. *Sandy*, when grains of quartz are aggregated with the grains of carbonate of lime, but so loosely as to be somewhat friable. Varieties.—*Dolomite*, when it consists in part of magnesia, and is friable. *Verd-antique*, when it is variegated in colour by the presence of serpentine, giving it more or less of a clouded green.

Names under the Transition Class.

7. **Argillite**, is a slate rock of an aluminous character and nearly homogeneous, always consisting of tables or laminæ whose direction forms a large angle with the general direction of the rock. Subdivisions.—*Clay Slate*, when the argillite is nearly destitute of all grittiness, and contains no scales of mica or talc. *Wacke Slate*, when it is somewhat gritty and contains glimmering scales of mica or talc. Varieties.—*Roof Slate*, when the slate is susceptible of division into pieces suitable for roofing houses and for ciphering slate. *Glazed Slate*, when the natural cleavages are lined with a black glazing. This variety contains anthracite coal and marine organic relics.

8. **First Graywacke**, is an aggregate of angular grains of quartzose sand, united by an argillaceous cement, apparently disintegrated clay slate, and is never above the calciferous sandrock. Subdivisions.—*Compact*, when the grains are so fine and united so compactly, as to be suitable for quarrying. *Rubble*, when the grains, or a part of them, are too large for quarrying. This division is often very hard, and sometimes contains felspar, and has the appearance of coarse granite; though some of the largest pebbles are generally rounded. It is often coloured green with chlorite. Every kind of first graywacke is almost horizontal—being a little elevated at the edge next to the primitive rocks only.

9. **Sparry Limerock**, consists of carbonate of lime intermediate in texture between granular and compact; and is traversed by veins of calcareous spar. Subdivisions.—*Compact*, when the masses or blocks, between the veins of spar, are sufficiently homogeneous and uniform to receive a polish. *Slaty*, when the rock is in slaty tables or laminæ, with transverse veins of calcareous spar. This rock is often cut into very small irregular blocks by the spar, which gives it the name of checkered rock.

10. **Calciferous Sandrock**, consists of fine grains of quartzose sand and of carbonate of lime, united without cement, or with an exceeding small proportion. Subdivisions.—*Compact*, when the rock is uniform, or nearly so, without cells or cavities. *Geodiferous* when it contains numerous geodes, or curvilinear cavities; which are empty or filled with calc spar, quartz crystals, barytes, anthracite, or other mineral substances different from the rock. Varieties.—*Oolitic*, when it consists in part of oolite, of a dark colour, and harder than the kind which is common in the lias or oolitic formation of Europe.

11. **Metalliferous Limerock**, consists of carbonate of lime in a homogeneous state, or in a state of petrifactions. Subdivisions.—*Compact*, when it contains but few petrifactions, and is susceptible of a polish. *Shelly*, when it consists of petrifactions, mostly of bivalve molluscous animals. Variety.—*Birdseye marble*, when the natural layers are pierced transversely with cylindrical petrifactions, so as to give the birds eye appearance when polished.

12. **Second Graywacke**, scarcely distinguished from first graywacke, excepting by its relative position, being always above calciferous sandrock. Subdivisions.—*Compact*, when in blocks or slaty, consisting of fine grains. *Rubble*, when it consists of, or contains large rounded pebbles. The rubble of second graywacke is in a much smaller proportion than in first graywacke. Varieties.—*Red sandy*, when it passes into red sandstone, which formation occurs in a few localities. *Hone-slate*, when soft, and suitable for setting a fine edge. *Grind-stone*, when the quartzose particles are sharp-angular.

Names under the Secondary Class.

13. **Millstone Grit**, is a coarse, hard aggregate of sharp-angular quartzose sand or pebbles; mostly without any cement, always gray or rusty gray. Subdivisions.—*Sandy*, when it contains few or no pebbles. *Conglomerate*, when it consists chiefly of rounded pebbles.

14. **Saliferous Rock**, consists of red, or bluish-gray, sand or clay-marle, or both. The grains of sand are mostly somewhat rounded, and all the varieties of this rock, in some localities, form the floor of salt mines and salt springs. Subdivisions.—*Marle-slate*, when the rock is soft, slaty, and contains minute grains of carbonate of lime. *Sandy*, when it is in solid blocks or layers, consisting of red or bluish-gray quartzose sand. Varieties.—*Gray-band*, the uppermost layers of bluish-gray sandrock. *Conglomerate*, (breccia) consisting chiefly of rounded pebbles, red, gray, or

* Every rock consists, *essentially*, of one, two, or three, of the following nine homogeneous minerals. These are called the *geological alphabet;* and every student must procure and familiarize himself with a specimen of each, before he commences the study of geology—quartz, felspar, mica, talc, hornblende, argillite, limestone, gypsum, chlorite. He should procure also a specimen of iron pyrites, hornstone, calc spar, reddle-ore, bog-ore, glance coal, bituminous coal.

† I believe M'Clure first applied this general name, to all the varieties of primitive hornblende rock.

‡ That a small proportion of talc scales should serve to distinguish this rock from mica-slate, would scarcely satisfy a mere cabinet student. But the travelling geologist will acknowledge its importance. See Taghconnuc and Saddle mountains, and the same range along the west side of the Green mountains to Canada.

rust-colour, as under the superincumbent rocks at Mount Holyoke, the Palisades, on the Hudson river, &c.

15. FERRIFEROUS ROCK, is a soft, slaty, argillaceous, or a hard, sandy, siliceous rock, embracing red argillaceous iron ore. Subdivisions.—*Slaty*, consists of green, or bluish-green, smooth soft slate, generally immediately under the layer of red argillaceous iron ore. *Sandy*, consists of a gray, or rusty-gray, aggregate of quartzose sandrock, in compact blocks or layers, overlaying or embracing red argillaceous iron ore. Variety.—*Conglomerate*, consists of rounded pebbles, cemented together by carbonate or oxide of iron, or adhering without cement.

16. LIAS, consists of rounded grains of quartzose sand, clay-slate, and sometimes partly of other aluminous compounds, of a dark or light-gray colour, aggregated with fine grains of carbonate of lime. Subdivisions.—*Calciferous slate*, when it is of a slaty texture, and the argillaceous and calcareous constituents predominate. *Calciferous grit*, when it is in blocks or thick layers, and the quartzose sand, or sharp grit, predominates. Varieties.—*Conchoidal*, when the slaty kind is separated into small divisions, somewhat of a lenticular form, by natural conchoidal cleavages. *Shell grit*, when the gritty variety consists, in part, of petrifactions of quartzose sand.

17. GEODIFEROUS LIMEROCK, (lowest of the oolitic formation of Europe,) consists of carbonate of lime, combined with a small proportion of argillite or quartz, in a compact state, mostly fœtid, and always containing numerous geodes. Subdivisions.—*Swinestone*, when it contains very little or no quartzose sand, is irregular in structure, fœtid and abounds in geodes. *Sandy*, when it contains quartzose sand, is stratified, scarcely fœtid, and contains but few geodes.

18. CORNITIFEROUS LIMEROCK, (included in the oolitic formation of Europe,) consists of carbonate of lime, embracing hornstone. Subdivisions.—*Compact*, when the rock is close-grained; and it generally contains hornstone in layers. *Shelly*, when it consists of shells, and contains hornstone in nodules or irregular masses.

19. THIRD GRAYWACKE, (well-known to be embraced in the oolitic formation of Europe; but contains no oolite,) having the character of first and second graywacke in general; but differing in containing much iron pyrites, fine grains of carbonate of lime, in larger or smaller proportion, and in having the quartzose grains mostly rounded.—Subdivisions.—*Pyritiferous slate*, when the rock has a slaty structure, and is in thin laminæ or in blocks or thick layers. *Pyritiferous grit*, when the rock has a siliceous or gritty structure, containing a large proportion of quartzose sand or pebbles. Varieties.—*Red sandstone*, and *red wacke*, when the gray rock passes into a dirty orange, and thence into a red siliceous sandrock. This has been called old red sandstone; but I do not believe that such a general stratum is admissible. *Conglomerate*, (breccia) when the rock consists chiefly of rounded pebbles, of a light-red, grayish red, or rust colour.

Names under the Superincumbent Class.

20. BASALT, is a hornblende rock, not primitive, probably of volcanic origin. Subdivisions.—*Amygdaloid*, when amorphous, of a compact texture, but containing cellules, empty or filled. *Greenstone trap*, when of a columnar structure, or in angular blocks, often coarse-grained. Variety.—*Toadstone*, when the amygdaloid has a warty appearance, and resembles slag.

Names under the Alluvial Class.

21. ANTEDILUVION, OR UPPER TERTIANS, when the detritus is in layers, so situated that it must have been deposited from water, while standing over it at a great depth, in nearly a quiescent state. As we have no chalk in North America, and as no tertiary rocks have hitherto been ascertained, this grand division may all be referred to detritus. Subdivisions.—*Plastic clay*, when it will not effervesce with acids; being destitute of carbonate of lime. *Marly clay*, when the clay contains fine grains of carbonate of lime, sufficient to effervesce strongly with acids. *Marine, or Bagshot, sand* and *crag*, when it consists of quartzose sand, nearly pure, or combined with a little loam, it is called marine sand; when it passes into a gravelly formation, often containing pudding-stone, beds of clay, &c., it is called *crag*. Variety.—*Hard-pan*, when the crag consists of gravel, strongly cemented by clay.

22. DILUVION, consists of a confused mixture of gravel, sand, clay, loam, plants, shell-animals, &c. so situated, that it must have been deposited from water, in a state of forcible and violent action. To make its character perfectly evident, it must be so situated, that the elevation of the water, sufficient for making the deposite, could not have been effected by any existing cause.

23. ULTIMATE DILUVION, a thin deposite of yellowish-gray loam, reposing on crag or some other substance in ancient uncultivated forest grounds. It is so situated, that it could not have been produced by the disintegration of *any* stratum in the vicinity, nor by water when running with much velocity. It appears to have been deposited from waters greatly elevated, and which had been rendered turbid by violent action, but had become almost quiescent. It may be considered as the last settlings of a deluge.

24. POST-DILUVION, when the detritus is so arranged that coarse pebbles appear towards the source of the waters which deposited them, and fine sediment more remote.

Names under the Analluvial Class.

25. STRATIFIED ANALLUVION, is the detritus formed by the disintegration of rock strata, which remains in the situation formerly occupied by the rocks, retaining the same order of superposition. Subdivisions.—These take the names, and retain the essential characters, of the original rocks; as *saliferous*, *ferriferous*, *lias*, *&c.*

26. SUPERFICIAL ANALLUVION, is the detritus formed by the disintegration of the exposed surfaces of all rocks, and remains on or near the place of disintegration. Subdivisions.—*Clay-loam*, when the detritus is fine and adhesive. *Granulated*, when in coarse grains, or friable. The character of the soil depends on the character of the rock disintegrated.

Remarks.

1. *The upper part of every general rock-stratum, is either more fissile or more loose and siliceous, than the under part.* This affords a natural character for making the two-fold divisions adopted in this nomenclature.

2. *The upper surface of every general rock-stratum in our district, is destitute of a superimposed rocky covering, for a great distance.* This affords a very natural guide for the limit of general strata.

3. *By general strata is meant, those deposites of rocks and detritus, which constitute the exterior visible rind of the earth, of nearly equal importance.* They may be distinguished from each other by essential characters. The most conclusive is *relative position*—the next in importance is the *contents*—the last is *the constituents.* For example, we know the third graywacke as the uppermost rock in the regular series of superposition—we know the ferriferous rock from its embracing the argillaceous peroxyde of iron—we know the granite from its consisting of quartz, feldspar, and mica.

4. *The words upper and lower are applied, without reference to degree of elevation.* A stratum is said to be geologically the lowest, or oldest, when it is nearest to the centre of the range of *granite* towards which it inclines.

5. *General strata may be very naturally subdivided, are subject to variations in character, and contain beds.* Numerous minerals not essential to their respective characters, are found in them in the state of veins and of dissemination. They appear to have become hard, while the strata containing them were in a soft state; for their forms are always impressed in them.

6. *All strata have their peculiar associates and contents.* Therefore a knowledge of strata enables us to foretell the probable discovery of useful minerals. Geology, then, embraces the "Science of Mining."

7. The bassetting, or out-cropping sides of transition and secondary rocks, at and near the edges approaching primitive rocks, present more of a primitive aspect, and contain fewer petrifactions, than other parts of the same rocks. A.]

GERA'NIS. (From γερανος, a crane: so called from its supposed resemblance to an extended crane.) A bandage for a fractured clavicle.

GERA'NIUM. (From γερανος, a crane: so called because its pistil is long like the bill of a crane.) Class, *Monadelphia;* Order, *Decandria.* The name of a genus of plants in the Linnæan system. Geranium or crane's-bill.

GERANIUM BATRACHIOIDES. See *Geranium pratense.*

GERANIUM COLUMBINUM. See *Geranium rotundifolium.*

GERANIUM MOSCHATUM. The adstringent property of this plant has induced practitioners to exhibit it in cases of debility and profluvia.

GERANIUM PRATENSE. The systematic name of the crow foot crane's-bill. *Geranium batrachioides.* A plant which possesses adstringent virtues, but in a slight degree.

GERANIUM ROBERTIANUM. Stinking crane's-bill. Herb Robert. This common plant has been much esteemed as an external application in erysipelatous inflammations, cancer, mastodynia, and old ulcers, but is now deservedly fallen into disuse.

GERANIUM ROTUNDIFOLIUM. The systematic name of the dove's-foot. *Geranium columbinum.* This plant is slightly astringent.

GERANIUM SANGUINARIUM. See *Geranium sanguineum.*

GERANIUM SANGUINEUM. The systematic name of the *Geranium sanguinarium.* Bloody crane's-bill. The adstringent virtues ascribed to this plant do not appear to be considerable.

["GERANIUM MACULATUM. Crane's-bill. The *Geranium maculatum* is a native (American) plant, common about woods and fences, and conspicuous for its large purple flowers in May and June.

"The root is horizontal, nearly as large as the little finger, tortuous, and full of knobs. To the taste it is a pure and powerful astringent. It abounds with tannin, which is imparted in great quantities both to the tincture and watery solution, and appears to be the basis of its medicinal efficacy.

"It is applicable to all the purposes of vegetable astringents, being surpassed by very few articles of that class. In various debilitating discharges, particularly from the bowels, it has afforded relief, when the disease has been of a nature to require astringent medicines. In apthous eruptions, and ulcerations of the mouth and throat, a strong decoction has been found beneficial as a gargle. A dose of the powder is twenty or thirty grains, and of a saturated tincture from one to two fluid drachms. The extract of this root is a very powerful astringent, and may be substituted for kino and catechu."—*Big. Mat. Med.* A.]

GERM. See *Corculum.*

GERMANDER. See *Teucrium chamædrys.*

Germander water. See *Teucrium Scordium.*

GERMEN. This is the rudiment of the young fruit and seed, and is found at the bottom of the pistil. See *Pistillum.* It appears under a variety of shapes and sizes.

From its figure it is called,

1. *Globose;* as in *Rosa eglantaria*, and *cinnamomea.*

2. *Oblong;* as in *Stellaria biflora.*

3. *Ovate;* as in *Rosa canina*, and *alba.*

From its situation, it is distinguished into,

1. *Superior*, when internal between the corolla; as in *Prunus.*

2. *Inferior*, below and without the corolla; as in *Galanthus nivalis.*

3. *Pedicellate*, upon a footstalk; as in the *Euphorbia.*

It is of great moment, for botanical distinctions, to observe whether it be superior, above the bases of the calyx, or below.

GERMINATION. *Germinatio.* The vital developement of a seed, when it first begins to grow.

GEROCO'MIA. (From γερων, an aged person, and κομεω, to be concerned about.) That part of medicine which regards the regimen and treatment of old age.

GERONTOPO'GON. (From γερων, an old man, and πωγων, a beard; so called because its downy seed, while enclosed in the calyx, resembles the beard of an aged man.) The herb old man's beard, a species of tragopogon.

GERONTO'XON. (From γερων, an old person, and τοξον, a dart.) 1. A small ulcer, like the head of a dart, appearing sometimes in the cornea of old persons.

2. The socket of a tooth.

GEROPO'GON. See *Gerontopogon.*

GESNER, CONRAD, was born at Zurich, in 1516. His father was killed in the civil war, and left him in such poverty, that he was obliged to become a servant at Strasburg. His master allowed him to devote some time to study, in which he made great progress; and having acquired a little money, he went to Paris, where he improved rapidly in the classics and rhetoric, and then turned his attention to philosophy and medicine. But he was soon compelled to return to his native country, and teach the languages, &c. for a livelihood. This enabled him afterward to resume his medical studies at Montpelier, and he graduated at Basil in 1540. He then settled in his native city, where he was appointed professor of philosophy, which office he discharged with great reputation for twenty-four years. He had an early predilection for botany, which led him to cultivate other parts of natural history; he was the first collector of a museum, and acquired the character of being the greatest naturalist since Aristotle. He also founded and supported a botanic garden, had numerous drawings and wood engravings made of plants, and appears to have meditated a general work on that subject. He likewise discovered the only true principles of botanical arrangement in the flower and fruit. Though of a feeble and sickly constitution, he traversed the Alps, and even sometimes plunged into the waters in search of plants: he also carefully studied their medical properties, and frequently hazarded his life by experiments on himself; indeed he was at one time reported to have been killed by the root of doronicum. His other occupations prevented his entering very extensively into practice, but his enlarged views rendered him successful; and the profits of his profession enabled him to support the great expense of his favourite pursuits. He gave also many proofs of liberal and active friendship. He died of the plague, in 1565. His chief works are his "Historiæ Animalium," in three folio volumes, with wood cuts; and a pharmacopœia, entitled "De Secretis Remediis Thesaurus," which passed through many editions.

Gestation, uterine. See *Pregnancy.*

GE'UM. 1. The name of a genus of plants in the Linnæan system. Class, *Icosandria;* Order, *Polygynia.*

2. The pharmacopœial name of the two following species of this genus.

GEUM RIVALE. The root is the part directed for medicinal uses. It is inodorous, and imparts an austere taste. In America it is in high estimation in the cure of intermittents, and is said to be more efficacious than the Peruvian bark. Diarrhœas and hæmorrhages are also stopped by its exhibition.

GEUM URBANUM. The systematic name of the herb bennet, or avens. *Caryophyllata; Herba benedicta; Caryophyllus vulgaris; Garyophylla; Janamunda; Geum—floribus erectis, fructibus globosis villosis, aristis uncinatis nudis, foliis lyratis*, of Linnæus. The root of this plant has been employed as a gentle styptic, corroborant, and stomachic. It has a mildly austere, somewhat aromatic taste, and a very pleasant smell, of the clove kind. It is also esteemed on the Continent as a febrifuge.

GIBBUS. Gibbous; swelled; applied to leaves when swelled on one side or both, from excessive abundance of pulp; as in the *Aloe retusa.*

GIDDINESS. See *Vertigo.*

GILBERT, WILLIAM, was born at Colchester, in 1540. After studying at Cambridge, he went abroad for improvement, and graduated at some foreign university. He returned with a high character for philosophical and chemical knowledge, and was admitted into the college of physicians in London, where he settled about the year 1573. He was so successful in his practice, that he was at length made first physician to Queen Elizabeth, who allowed him a pension to prosecute philosophical experiments. He died in 1603, leaving his books, apparatus, and minerals, to the college of physicians. His capital work on the magnet was published three years before his death; it is not only the earliest complete system on that subject, but also one of the first specimens of philosophy founded upon experiments; which method the great Lord Bacon afterward so strenuously recommended.

Gilead, balsam. See *Amyris gileadensis.*

GILLIFLOWER. See *Dianthus caryophyllus.*

["GILLENIA TRIFOLIATA. The Gillenia trifoliata is a native, perennial plant, more generally known to cultivators of the American Materia Medica by the Linnæan name of *Spiræa trifoliata.* It grows in and about woods, in light soil, throughout most parts of the Union, excepting the eastern states.

"The root is much branched and knobby. It consists of a woody portion, invested with a thick bark, which, when dry, is brittle, and very bitter to the taste. The predominant soluble ingredients appear to be, a bitter extractive matter and resin. When boiled in water, it imparts to it a beautiful red wine-colour, and an intensely bitter taste. The tincture deposites an abundant resinous precipitate on the addition of water.

"This article is one of the most prominent indigenous emetics, resembling ipecacuanha in its operation, but requiring a large dose. It sometimes fails to produce vomiting, especially if the portion used has become old. Thirty grains of the bark of the root, recently dried and powdered, are a suitable dose for an emetic. In doses so small as not to excite nausea, it has been thought useful as a tonic. The *Gillenia stipulacea*, of the western states, possesses properties similar to those of this species."—*Bigelow's Mat. Med.* A.]

GIN. *Spiritus Juniperi.* Geneva. Hollands. The name of a spirit distilled from malt or rye, which afterward undergoes the same process, a second time, with juniper-berries. This is the original and most wholesome state of the spirit; but it is now prepared without juniper-berries, and is distilled from turpentine, which gives it something of a similar flavour. The consumption of this article, especially in the metropolis, is immense, and the consequences are pernicious to the health of the inhabitants.

GINGER. See *Zingiber.*

GI'NGIBER. See *Zingiber.*

Gingibra'chium. (From *gingivæ*, the gums, and *brachium*, the arm.) A name for the scurvy, because the gums, arms, and legs, are affected with it.

Gingi'dium. A species of *Daucus.*

Gi'ngihil. See *Zingiber.*

Gingipe'dium. (From *gingivæ*, the gums, and *pes*, the foot.) A name for the scurvy, because the gums, arms, and legs are affected.

GINGI'VÆ. (From *gigno*, to beget; because the teeth are, as it were, born in them.) The gums. See *Gums.*

GI'NGLYMUS. (Γιγγλυμος, a hinge.) The hinge-like joint. A species of diarthrosis or moveable connexion of bones, which admits of flexion and extension, as the knee-joint, &c.

GI'NSENG. An Indian word. See *Panax quinquefolium.*

Gir. Quick-lime.

Gi'rmir. Tartar.

GITHAGO. A name used by Pliny, for the *Lolium*, or darnel-grass.

GIZZARD. The stomach of poultry. Those from white flesh, have long been considered in France as medicinal. They have been recommended in obstructions of the urinary passages, complaints of the bladder, and nephritic pains; but particularly as a febrifuge. Bouillon Lagrange considers its principal substance as oxygenated gelatine, with a small quantity of extractive matter.

Glabe'lla. (From *glaber*, smooth; because it is without hair.) The space between the eyebrows.

GLABER. Glabrous; Smooth; applied to stems, leaves, seeds, &c. of plants, and opposed to all kinds of hairiness and pubescence; as in the stem of the *Euphorbia peplus*, and the seeds of *Galium montanum.*

GLACIES. Ice.

GLADI'OLUS. (Diminutive of *gladius*, a sword; so named from the sword-like shape of its leaf.) The name of a genus of plants in the Linnæan system. Class, *Triandria;* Order, *Monogynia.*

Gladiolus luteus. See *Iris pseudacorus.*

Gla'ma. Γλαμα. The sordes of the eye.

GLAND. *Glans. Glandula.* I. In anatomy, an organic part of the body, composed of blood-vessels, nerves, and absorbents, and destined for the secretion or alteration of some peculiar fluid. The glands of the human body are divided, by anatomists, into different classes, either according to their structure, or the fluid they contain. According to their fabric, they are distinguished into four classes:

1. Simple glands.
2. Compounds of simple glands.
3. Conglobate glands.
4. Conglomerate glands.

According to their fluid contents, they are more properly divided into,

1. Mucous glands.
2. Sebaceous glands.
3. Lymphatic glands.
4. Salival glands.
5. Lachrymal glands.

1. *Simple glands* are small hollow follicles, covered with a peculiar membrane, and having a proper excretory duct, through which they evacuate the liquor contained in their cavity. Such are the mucous glands of the nose, tongue, fauces, trachea, stomach, intestine, and urinary bladder, the sebaceous glands about the anus, and those of the ear. These simple glands are either dispersed here and there, or are contiguous to one another, forming a heap in such a manner that they are not covered by a common membrane, but each hath its own excretory duct, which is never joined to the excretory duct of another gland. The former are termed solitary simple glands, the latter aggregate or congregate simple glands.

2. *The compound glands* consist of many simple glands, the excretory ducts of which are joined in one common excretory duct; as the sebaceous glands of the face, lips, palate, and various parts of the skin, especially about the pubes.

3. *Conglobate*, or, as they are also called, *lymphatic glands*, are those into which lymphatic vessels enter, and from which they go out again: as the mesenteric, lumbar, &c. They have no excretory duct, but are composed of a texture of lymphatic vessels connected together by cellular membrane: they are the largest in the fœtus.

4. *Conglomerate glands* are composed of a congeries of many simple glands, the excretory ducts of which open into one common trunk: as the parotid gland, thyroid gland, pancreas, and all the salival glands. Conglomerate glands differ but little from the compound glands, yet they are composed of more simple glands than the compound.

The excretory duct of a gland is the duct through which the fluid of the gland is excreted. The vessels and nerves of glands always come from the neighbouring parts, and the arteries appear to possess a high degree of irritability. The use of the glands is to separate a peculiar liquor, or to change it. The use of the conglobate glands is unknown.

II. In botany, Linnæus defines it, a little tumour discharging a fluid.

From their situation they are said to be,

1. *Foliares*, when on the surface of the leaf; as in the *Gossypium religiosum*, which has one gland on the leaf; and *Gossypium barbadense*, the leaves of which have three.

2. *Petiolares*, when in the footstalk; as in *Prunus cerasus.*

3. *Corollares.* The claw of the corolla of the *Berberis vulgaris* has two glands.

4. *Filamentares*, in the filaments; as in *Dictamnus albus.*

From their adhesion,

1. *Glandula sessilis*, without any peduncle; as in *Prunus cerasus.*

2. *Glandula pedicillata*, furnished with a peduncle; as in *Drosera.*

Glands are abundant on the stalk and calyx of the moss-rose, and between the serratures of the leaf of the *Salix pentandria;* on the footstalks of the *Viburnum opulus*, and various species of passion-flower. The liquor discharged is resinous and fragrant.

GLANDORP, Matthias Louis, was born at Cologne, in 1595. Soon after commencing his medical pursuits, he went to Padua, which had at that time great reputation. He improved so much in anatomy under Spigelius, that he was deemed competent to give public demonstrations: and he took his degree in 1618. He settled in Bremen, whence his family originated; and he was so successful in practice, that he was raised to the most honourable offices. He was physician to the archbishop, and to the republic, when he died in 1640. He left several works, with plates, containing many important observations on anatomy, &c. The principal are his "Speculum Chirurgorum," and a Treatise on Issues and Setons. He was very partia. to the use of the actual cautery, even in the most common disorders.

GLA'NDULA. (A diminutive of *glans*, a gland.) A small gland. See *Gland.*

GLANDULA LACHRYMALIS. See *Lachrymal gland.*

GLANDULÆ MYRTIFORMES. See *Carunculæ myrtiformes.*

GLANDULÆ PACCHIONIÆ. A number of small, oval, fatty substances, not yet ascertained to be glandular, situated under the dura mater, about the sides of the longitudinal sinus. Their use is not known.

GLANDULOSOCA'RNEUS. An epithet given by Ruysch to some excrescences, which he observed in the bladder.

GLANDULOSUS. Glandular. 1. In anatomy, having the appearance, structure, or function of a gland.

2. In botany, applied to leaves which have little glandiform elevations; as the bay-leaved willow, and *Hypericum montanum.*

GLANS. A gland, or nut. See *Gland.*

GLANS PENIS. The very vascular body that forms the apex of the penis. The posterior circle is termed the *corona glandis.* See *Corpus spongiosum urethræ.*

GLANS UNGUENTARIA. See *Guilandina moringa.*

GLASS. This substance was formerly employed by surgeons, when roughly powdered, to destroy opacities of the cornea.

Glass of antimony. See *Antimony.*

Glass-wort, snail-seeded. See *Salsola kali.*

GLA'STUM. (*Quasi callastum;* from *Callia,* who first used it.) The herb woad. See *Isatis tinctoria.*

Glauber's salt. A sulphate of soda. It is found native in Bohemia, and is the produce of art. See *Sodæ sulphas.*

GLAUBERITE. A native crystallized salt, composed of dry sulphate of lime, and dry sulphate of soda, found in rock salt at Villarubra in Spain.

GLAUCEDO. (From γλαυκος, bluish, or greenish tint.) See *Glaucoma.*

GLAU'CIUM. (So named from its glaucous or sea-green colour. The name of a genus of plants in the Linnæan system. Class, *Polyandria;* Order, *Monogynia.*) The horned poppy.

GLAUCO'MA. (From γλαυκος, blue; because of the eye becoming of a blue, or sea-green colour.) *Glaucedo; Glaucosis; Apoglaucosis.* 1. An opacity of the vitreous humour. It is difficult to ascertain, and is only to be known by a very attentive examination of the eye.

2. A species of cataract. See *Cataract.*

GLAUCO'SIS. See *Glaucoma.*

GLAUCUS. (Γλαυκος, sea-green.) Stems are called glaucous which are clothed with a fine sea-green mealiness, which easily rubs off; as in *Chlora perfoliata.*

GLECO'MA. (From γληχων, the name of a plant in Dioscorides.) Class, *Didynamia;* Order, *Gymnospermia.* The name of a genus of plants in the Linnæan system. Ground-ivy.

GLECOMA HEDERACEA. The systematic name of the ground-ivy, or gill. *Hedera terrestris. Glecoma—foliis reniformibus crenatis,* of Linnæus. This indigenous plant has a peculiar strong smell, and a bitterish somewhat aromatic taste. It is one of those plants which was formerly much esteemed for possessing virtues that, in the present age, cannot be detected. In obstinate coughs, it is a favourite remedy with the poor.

GLE'CHON. (Γληχων.) Pennyroyal.

GLECHONI'TES. (From γληχων, pennyroyal.) Wine impregnated with pennyroyal.

GLEET. In consequence of the repeated attacks of gonorrhœa, and the debility of the part occasioned thereby, it not unfrequently happens, that a gleet, or constant small discharge takes place, or remains behind, after all danger of infection is removed. Mr. Hunter remarks, that it differs from gonorrhœa in being *uninfectious,* and in the discharge consisting of globular particles, contained in a slimy mucus, instead of serum. It is unattended with pain, scalding in making of water, &c.

GLE'NE. Γληνη. Strictly signifies the cavity or socket of the eye; but by some anatomists is also used for that cavity of a bone which receives another within it.

GLE'NOID. (*Glenoides;* from γληνη, a cavity, and ειδος, resemblance.) The name of articulate cavities of bones.

GLEU'CINUM. (From γλευκος, must.) An ointment, in the preparation of which was must.

GLEU'XIS. (From γλευκυς, sweet.) A sweet wine.

GLIADINE. See *Gluten.*

GLI'SCERE. To increase gradually, properly as fire does; but, by physical writers, is sometimes applied to the natural heat and increase of spirits; and by others to the exacerbation of fevers which return periodically.

GLISCHRO'CHOLOS. (From γλισχρος, viscid, and χολη, the bile.) Viscid bilious excrement.

GLISCRA'SMA. (From γλισχραινω, to become glutinous.) Viscidity.

GLISOMA'RGO. White chalk.

GLISSON, FRANCIS, was born in Dorsetshire, 1597. He studied at both the English universities; but took his degree of doctor in Cambridge, where he was made Regius professor of Physic, which office he held about forty years. He settled, however, to practise in London, and became a Fellow of the College in 1635; four years after which he was chosen reader of Anatomy, and distinguished himself much by his lectures "De Morbis Partium," which he was requested to publish. During the civil wars he retired to Colchester, where he practised with great credit; and was there during the siege of that town by the Parliamentary forces. He was one of the members of the society which, about the year 1645, held weekly meetings in London to promote Natural Philosophy: and which having removed to Oxford during the troubles, was augmented after the Restoration, and became ultimately the present Royal Society. He was afterward several years president of the College of Physicians, and died at the advanced age of eighty. He left the following valuable works: 1. A Treatise on the Rickets. 2. The Anatomy of the Liver, which he described much more accurately than any one before, and particularly the capsule of the Vena Portarum, which has since been named after him. 3. A large metaphysical treatise "De Natura Substantiæ Energetica," after the manner of Aristotle. 4. A Treatise on the Stomach, Intestines, &c., a well-arranged and comprehensive work, with various new observations, which came out the year before his death.

Glisson's Capsule. See *Capsule of Glisson.*

GLOBATE. See *Gland.*

GLOBOSUS. Globose. A root is so called which is rounded, and gives off radicles in every direction; as that of the *Cyclamen europeum.* The receptacle of the *Cephalanthus* and *Nauclea,* are so called from their form.

GLOBULA'RIA. (From *globus,* a globe: so called from the shape of its flower.) The French daisy.

GLOBULA'RIA ALYPUM. The leaves of this plant are used in some parts of Spain in the cure of the venereal disease. It is said to act also as a powerful but safe cathartic.

GLO'BUS. A ball.

GLOBUS HYSTERICUS. The air rising in the œsophagus, and prevented by spasm from reaching the mouth, is so called by authors, because it mostly attends hysteria, and gives the sensation of a ball ascending in the throat.

GLOCHIS. (Γλωχις, *cuspis teli.*) A pointed hair. A sharp point: used in botany to a bristle-like pubescence, which is turned backwards at its point into many straight teeth.

GLO'MER. A clue of thread. A term mostly applied to glands.

GLOMERATE. A gland is so called which is formed of a glomer of sanguineous vessels, having no cavity, but furnished with an excretory duct; as the lachrymal and mammary glands

GLOMERULUS. In botany, a smal tuft, or *capitulum,* mostly in the axilla of the peduncle.

GLOSSA'GRA. (From γλωσσα, the tongue, and αγρα, a seizure.) A violent pain in the tongue.

GLO'SSO. (From γλωσσα, the tongue.) Names compounded with this word belong to muscles, nerves, or vessels, from their being attached, or going to the tongue.

GLOSSO-PHARYNGEAL NERVES. The ninth pair of nerves. They arise from the processes of the cerebellum, which run to the medulla spinalis, and terminate by numerous branches in the muscles of the tongue and pharynx.

GLOSSO-PHARYNGEUS. See *Constrictor pharyngeus superior.*

GLOSSO-STAPHYLINUS. See *Constrictor isthmi faucium.*

GLOSSOCA'TOCHOS. (From γλοσσα, tongue, and κατεχω, to hold.) An instrument in P. Ægineta for depressing the tongue. A spatula linguæ. The ancient glossocatochus was a sort of forceps, one of the blades of which served to depress the tongue, while the other was applied under the chin.

GLOSSOCE'LE. (From γλωσσα, the tongue, and κηλη, a tumour.) An extrusion of the tongue.

GLOSSOCOMA. A retraction of the tongue.

GLOSSOCOMI'ON. (From γλωσσα, a tongue, and κομεω, to guard.) By this was formerly meant a case for the tongue, for a hautboy; but the old surgeons, by metaphor, use it to signify an instrument, or case, for containing a fractured limb.

GLO'TTA. (Γλωττα, the tongue.) The tongue.

GLO'TTIS. (From γλωττα, the tongue.) The superior opening of the larynx at the bottom of the tongue.

GLUCINA. (From γλυκυς, which signifies sweet, because it gives that taste to the salts in forms.) The name of an earth, for the discovery of which we are indebted to Vauquelin, who found it, in 1795, in the Aigue-marine or beryl, a transparent stone, of a green colour, and in the emerald of Peru. It exists combined with silex, alumine, lime, and oxide of iron, in the one; and with the same earths, and oxide of chrome, in the other. It has lately been discovered in the gadolinite by Mr. Ekeberg.

Glucina is white, light, and soft to the touch. It is insipid, and adheres to the tongue; and is infusible by itself in the fire. Its specific gravity is 2.967. It is soluble in alkalies and their carbonates, and in all the acids except the carbonic and phosphoric, and forms with them saccharine and slightly astringent salts. It is exceedingly soluble in sulphuric acid used to excess. It is fusible with borax, and forms with it a transparent glass. It absorbs one-fourth of its weight of carbonic acid. It decomposes sulphate of alumine. It is not precipitated by the hydro-sulphurets nor by prussiate of potassa, but by all the succinates. Its affinity for the acids is intermediate between magnesia and alumine.

To obtain this earth, reduce some beryl to an impalpable powder, fuse it with three times its weight of potassa, and dissolve the mass in muriatic acid. Separate the silex by evaporation and filtration, and decompose the remaining fluid by adding carbonate of potassa; redissolve the deposite when washed in sulphuric acid, and by mingling this solution with sulphate of potassa, alum will be obtained, which crystallizes.

Then mix the fluid with a solution of carbonate of ammonia, which must be used in excess; filter and boil it, and a white powder will gradually fall down, which is glucine.

GLUE. An inspissated jelly made from the parings of hides and other offals, by boiling them in water, straining through a wicker basket, suffering the impurities to subside, and then boiling it a second time. The articles should first be digested in lime water, to cleanse them from grease and dirt; then steeped in water, stirring them well from time to time; and, lastly, laid in a heap, to have the water pressed out, before they are put into the boiler. Some recommend, that the water should be kept as nearly as possible to a boiling heat, without suffering it to enter into ebullition. In this state it is poured into flat frames or moulds, then cut into square pieces when congealed, and afterward dried in a coarse net. It is said to improve by age; and that glue is reckoned the best, which swells considerably without dissolving by three or four days' infusion in cold water, and recovers its former dimensions and properties by drying. Shreds or parings of vellum, parchment, or white leather, make a clear and almost colourless glue.

GLUMA. (*Gluma, à glubendo;* a husk of corn.) The husk. The peculiar calyx of grasses and grass-like plants, of a chaffy texture, formed of little concave leaflets which are called *valves.* To the husk belongs the *arista,* the *beard* or *awn.* See *Arista.*

The gluma is,

1. *Univalve,* in *Loilum perenne.*
2. *Bivalve,* in most grasses.
3. *Trivalved* in *Panicum miliaceum.*
4. *Many-valved,* in *Uniola paniculata.*
5. *Coloured,* otherwise than green; as in *Holcus bicolor.*

From the number of flowers the husk contains, it is called,

1. *Gluma uniflora,* one-flowered; as in *Panicum.*
2. *G. biflora,* with two; as in *Aira.*
3. *G. multiflora,* having many; as in *Poa* and *Avena.*

From the external appearance, the gluma is termed,

1. *Glabrous,* smooth; as in *Holcus laxus.*
2. *Hispid,* briskly; as in *Secale orientale.*
3. *Striate,* as in *Holcus striatus.*
4. *Villose;* as in *Holcus sorgham, Holcus saccharatus,* and *Bromus purgans.*
5. *Ciliate,* fringed; as in *Bromus ciliatus.*
6. *Beardless;* as in *Briza* and *Poa.*
7. *Awned;* as in *Hordeum.*

GLUMOSUS. A flower is so called, which is aggregate, and has a glumous or husky calyx.

GLUTEAL. Belonging to the buttocks.

GLUTEAL ARTERY. A branch of the internal iliac artery.

GLU'TEN. (*Quasi geluten;* from *gelo,* to congeal.) See *Glue.*

GLUTEN, ANIMAL. This substance constitutes the basis of the fibres of all the solid parts. It resembles in its properties the gluten of vegetables.

GLUTEN, VEGETABLE. If wheat-flower be made into a paste, and washed in a large quantity of water, it is separated into three distinct substances: a mucilaginous saccharine matter, which is readily dissolved in the liquor, and may be separated from it by evaporation; starch, which is suspended in the fluid, and subsides to the bottom by repose; and gluten, which remains in the hand, and is tenacious, very ductile, somewhat elastic, and of a brown-gray colour. The first of these substances does not essentially differ from other saccharine mucilages. The second, namely, the starch, forms a gluey fluid by boiling in water, though it is scarcely, if at all, acted upon by that fluid when cold. Its habitudes and products with the fire, or with nitric acid, are nearly the same as those of gum and of sugar. It appears to be as much more remote from the saline state than gum, as gum is more remote from that state than sugar.

The vegetable gluten, though it existed before the washing in the pulverulent form, and has acquired its tenacity and adhesive qualities from the water it has imbibed, is nevertheless totally insoluble in this fluid. It has scarcely any taste. When dry, it is semitransparent, and resembles glue in its colour and appearance. If it be drawn out thin, when first obtained, it may be dried by exposure to the air: but if it be exposed to warmth and moisture while wet, it putrefies like an animal substance. The dried gluten applied to the flame of a candle, crackles, swells, and burns, exactly like a feather, or piece of horn. It affords the same products by destructive distillation as animal matters do; is not soluble in alkohol, oils, or æther; and is acted upon by acids and alkalies, when heated. According to Rouelle, it is the same with the caseous substance of milk.

Gluten of Wheat.—Taddey, an Italian chemist, has lately ascertained that the gluten of wheat may be decomposed into two principles, which he has distinguished by the names, *gliadine* (from γλια, gluten,) and *zimome* (from ζυμη, ferment.) They are obtained in a separate state by kneading the fresh gluten in successive portions of alkohol, as long as that liquid continues to become milky, when diluted with water The alkohol solutions being set aside, gradually deposite a whitish matter, consisting of small filaments of gluten, and become perfectly transparent. Being now left to slow evaporation, the gliadine remains behind, of the consistence of honey, and mixed with a little yellow resinous matter, from which it may be freed by digestion in sulphuric æther, in which gliadine is not sensibly soluble. The portion of the gluten not dissolved by the alkohol is the *zimome.*

Properties of Gliadine.—When dry, it has a straw-yellow colour, slightly transparent, and in thin plates, brittle, having a slight smell, similar to that of honey-comb, and, when slightly heated, giving out an odour similar to that of boiled apples. In the mouth, it becomes adhesive, and has a sweetish and balsamic taste. It is pretty soluble in boiling alcohol, which loses its transparency in proportion as it cools, and then retains only a small quantity in solution. It forms a kind of varnish in those bodies to which it is applied. It softens, but does not dissolve in cold distilled water. At a boiling heat it is converted into froth, and the liquid remains slightly milky. It is specifically heavier than water.

The alkoholic solution of gliadine becomes milky when mixed with water, and is precipitated in white flocks by the alkaline carbonates. It is scarcely affected by the mineral and vegetable acids. Dry gliadine dissolves in caustic alkalies and in acids. It swells upon red-hot coals, and then contracts in the manner of animal substances. It burns with a pretty lively flame, and leaves behind it a light spongy charcoal, difficult to incinerate. Gliadine, in some respects, approaches the properties of resins; but differs from them in being insoluble in sulphuric æther. It is very sensibly affected by the infusion of nut-galls. It is capable of itself of undergoing a slow fermentation, and produces fermentation in saccharine substances.

From the flour of barley, rye, or oats, no gluten can be extracted as from that of wheat, probably because they contain too small a quantity.

The residue of wheat which is not dissolved in alkohol, is called *zimome.* If this be boiled repeatedly in alkohol, it is obtained pure.

Zimome thus purified has the form of small globules, or constitutes a shapeless mass, which is hard, tough, destitute of cohesion, and of an ash-white colour. When washed in water, it recovers part of its viscosity, and becomes quickly brown, when left in contact with the air. It is specifically heavier than water. Its mode of fermenting is no longer that of gluten; for when it purifies it exhales a fœtid urinous odour. It dissolves completely in vinegar, and in the mineral acids at a boiling temperature. With caustic potassa, it combines and forms a kind of soap. When put into lime water, or into the solutions of the alkaline carbonates, it becomes harder, and assumes a new appearance without dissolving. When thrown upon red-hot coals, it exhales an odour similar to that of burning hair or hoofs, and burns with flame.

Zimome is to be found in several parts of vegetables. It produces various kinds of fermentation, according to the nature of the substance with which it comes in contact.

GLUTE'US. (From γλουτος, the buttocks.) The name of some muscles of the buttocks.

GLUTEUS MAXIMUS. *Gluteus magnus* of Albinus. *Glutæus major* of Cowper; and *Ilio sacro femoral* of Dumas. A broad radiated muscle, on which we sit, is divided into a number of strong fasciculi, is covered by a pretty thick aponeurosis derived from the *fascia lata*, and is situated immediately under the integuments. It arises fleshy from the outer lip of somewhat more than the posterior half of the spine of the ilium, from the ligaments that cover the two posterior spinous processes; from the posterior sacro-ischiatic ligament; and from the outer sides of the os sacrum and os coccygis. From these origins the fibres of the muscle run towards the great trochanter of the os femoris, where they form a broad and thick tendon, between which and the trochanter there is a considerable *bursa mucosa.* This tendon is inserted into the upper part of the *linea aspera*, for the space of two or three inches downwards; and sends off fibres to the fascia lata, and to the upper extremity of the vastus externus. This muscle serves to extend the thigh, by pulling it directly backwards; at the same time it draws it a little outwards, and thus assists in its rotatory motion. Its origin from the coccyx seems to prevent that bone from being forced too far backwards.

GLUTEUS MEDIUS. *Ilio trochanterien* of Dumas. The posterior half of this muscle is covered by the gluteus maximus, which it greatly resembles in shape; but the anterior and upper part of it is covered only by the integuments, and by a tendinous membrane which belongs to the fascia lata. It arises fleshy from the outer lip of the anterior part of the spine of the ilium, from part of the posterior surface of that bone, and likewise from the fascia that covers it. From these origins its fibres run towards the great trochanter, into the outer and posterior part of which it is inserted by a broad tendon. Between this tendon and the trochanter there is a small thin *bursa mucosa.* The uses of this muscle are nearly the same as those of the gluteus maximus; but it is not confined, like that muscle, to rolling the os femoris outwards, its anterior portion being capable of turning that bone a little inwards. As it has no origin from the coccyx, it can have no effect on that bone.

GLUTEUS MINIMUS. *Glutæus minor* of Albinus and Cowper; and *Ilio ischii trochanterien* of Dumas. A radiated muscle, is situated under the gluteus medius. In adults, and especially in old subjects, its outer surface is usually tendinous. It arises fleshy between the two semicircular ridges we observe on the outer surface of the ilium, and likewise from the edge of its great niche. Its fibres run, in different directions, towards a thick flat tendon, which adheres to a capsular ligament of the joint, and is inserted into the fore and upper part of the great trochanter. A small *bursa mucosa* may be observed between the tendon of this muscle and the trochanter. This muscle assists the two former in drawing the thigh backwards and outwards, and in rolling it. It may likewise serve to prevent the capsular ligament from being pinched in the motions of the joint.

GLU'TIA. (From γλουτος, the buttocks.) The buttocks. See *Nates*

GLUTTU'PATENS. (From *gluttus*, the throat, and *pateo*, to extend.) The stomach, which is an extension of the throat.

GLU'TUS. (Γλουτος; from γλοιος, filthy.) The buttock. See *Nates*.

GLYCA'SMA. (From γλυκυς, sweet.) A sweet medicated wine.

GLYCYPI'CROS. (From γλυκυς, sweet, and πικρος, bitter: so called from its bitterish-sweet taste.) See *Solanum dulcamara.*

GLYCYRRHI'ZA. (From γλυκυς, sweet, and ριζα, a root.) 1. The name of a genus of plants in the Linnæan system. Class, *Diadelphia;* Order, *Decandria.*

2. The pharmacopœial name of liquorice. See *Glycyrrhiza glabra.*

GLYCYRRHIZA ECHINATA. This species of liquorice is substituted in some places for the root of the *glabra.*

GLYCYRRHIZA GLABRA. The systematic name of the officinal liquorice. *Glycyrrhiza; leguminibus glabris, stipulis nullis, foliolo impari petiolato.* A native of the south of Europe, but cultivated in Britain. The root contains a great quantity of saccharine matter, joined with some proportion of mucilage, and hence it has a viscid sweet taste. It is in common use as a pectoral or emollient, in catarrhal defluxions on the breast, coughs, hoarsenesses, &c. Infusions, or the extract made from it, which is called *Spanish liquorice*, afford likewise very commodious vehicles for the exhibition of other medicines; the liquorice taste concealing that of unpalatable drugs more effectually than syrups or any of the sweets of the saccharine kind.

GLYCYSA'NCON. (From γλυκυς, sweet, and αγκων, the elbow: so called from its sweetish taste, and its inflections, or elbows at the joints.) A species of southern wood.

GNAPHA'LIUM. (From γναφαλον, cotton: so named from its soft downy surface.) 1. The name of a genus of plants in the Linnæan system. Class, *Syngenesia;* Order, *Polygamia superflua.*

2. The pharmacopœial name of the herb cotton weed. See *Gnaphalium dioicum.*

GNAPHALIUM ARENARIUM. The flowers of this plant, as well as those of the gnaphalium stœchas, are called, in the pharmacopœias, *flores elichrysi.* See *Gnaphalium stœchas.*

GNAPHALIUM DIOICUM. The systematic name of the *pes cati. Gnaphalium albinum.* Cotton weed. The flores gnaphalii of the pharmacopœias, called also *flores hispidulæ, seu pedis cati*, are the produce of this plant. They are now quite obsolete, but were formerly used as astringents, and recommended in the cure of hooping-cough, phthisis pulmonalis, and hæmoptysis.

GNAPHALIUM STŒCHAS. The systematic name of Goldilocks. *Elichrysum; Stœchas citrina.* The flowers of this small downy plant are warm, pungent, and bitter, and said to possess aperient and corroborant virtues.

GNA'THUS. (From γναπτω, to bend; so called from their curvature.) 1. The jaw, or jaw-bones.

2. The cheek.

GNEISS. A compound rock, consisting of felspar, quartz, and mica, disposed in slates, from the preponderance of the mica scales.

Gni'dius. A term applied by Hippocrates, and others since, to some medicinal precepts wrote in the island of Gnidos.

Goat's-rue. See *Galega.*

Goat's-thorn. See *Astragalus verus.*

GOAT-WEED. See *Œgopodium.*

GOUT-WEED. See *Œgopodium podagraria.*

GODDARD, Jonathan, was born at Greenwich, in 1617. After studying at Oxford, and travelling for improvement, he graduated at Cambridge, and settled to practise in London. He was elected a Fellow of the College of Physicians in 1646, and, the following year, appointed Lecturer on Anatomy. He formed a Society for Experimental Inquiry, which met at his house; and he was very assiduous in promoting its objects. Having gained considerable reputation, and sided with the popular party, he was appointed by Cromwell chief physician to the army, and attended him in some of his expeditions. Cromwell then made him warden of Merton College, Oxford, afterward sole representative of that university in the short parliament, in 1653, and in the same year one of the Council of State. On the Restoration, being driven from Oxford, he removed to Gresham College, where he had been chosen Professor of Physic. Here he continued to frequent those meetings, which gave birth to the Royal Society, and he was nominated one of the first council of that institution. He was an able and conscientious practitioner; and was induced, partly from the love of experimental chemistry, but principally from doubting the competency of apothecaries, to prepare his own medicines: in which, however, finding numerous obstacles, he published "A Discourse, setting forth the unhappy Condition of the Practice of Physic in London;" but this was of no avail. Two papers of his appeared in the Philosophical Transactions, and many others in Birch's History of the Royal Society. He died in 1674, of an apoplectic stroke.

GOELICKE, Andrew Offon, a German physician, acquired considerable reputation in the beginning of the eighteenth century, as a medical professor, and especially as an advocate of the doctrines of Stahl. He left several works which relate principally to the History of Anatomy, &c., particularly the "Historia Medicinæ Universalis," which was published in six different portions, between the years 1717 and 1720.

Goitre. See *Bronchocele.*

GOLD. *Aurum.* A metal found in nature only in a metallic state; most commonly in grains, ramifications, leaves, or crystals, rhomboidal, octahedral, or pyramidal. Its matrix is generally quartz, sandstone, siliceous schistus, &c. It is found also in the sands of many rivers, particularly in Africa, Hungary, and France, in minute irregular grains, called *gold dust.* Native gold, found in compact masses, is never completely pure; it is alloyed with silver, or copper, and sometimes with iron and tellurium. The largest piece of native gold that has been hitherto discovered in Europe, was found in the county of Wicklow, in Ireland. Its weight was said to be twenty-two ounces, and the quantity of alloy it contained was very small. Several other pieces, exceeding one ounce, have also been discovered at the same place, in sand, covered with turf, and adjacent to a rivulet.

Gold is also met with in a particular sort of argentiferous copper pyrites, called, in Hungary, *Gelf.* This ore is found either massive, or crystallized in rhomboids, or other irregular quadrangular or polygonal masses. It exists likewise in the sulphurated ores of Nigaya in Transylvania. These all contain the metal called tellurium. Berthollet, and other French chemists, have obtained gold out of the ashes of vegetables.

GOLD-CUP. See *Ranunculus.*

GOLDEN-ROD. See *Solidago virga aurea.*

Golden maidenhair. See *Polytrichum commune.*

GOLDILOCKS. See *Gnaphalium stœchas*

[Goldthread. See *Coptis trifolia.* A.]

GOMPHI'ASIS. (From γομφος, a nail.) *Gomphiasmus.* A disease of the teeth, when they are loosened from the sockets, like nails drawn out of the wood.

Gomphia'smus. See *Gomphiasis.*

Go'mphioi. (From γομφος, a nail: so called because they are as nails driven into their sockets.) The dentes molares, or grinding teeth.

Gompho'ma. See *Gomphosis.*

GOMPHO'SIS. (From γομφοω, to drive in a nail.) *Gomphoma.* A species of immoveable connexion of bones, in which one bone is fixed in another, like a nail in a board, as the teeth in the alveoli of the jaws.

GONA'LGIA. See *Gonyalgia.*

GONA'GRA. (From γονυ, the knee, and αγρα, a seizure.) The gout in the knee.

GO'NE. (γονη.) 1. The seed.

2. In Hippocrates it is the uterus.

GONG. Tam-tam. A species of cymbal which produces a very loud sound when struck. It is an alloy of about eighty parts of copper with twenty of tin.

GONGRO'NA. (From γογγρος, a hard knot.) 1. The cramp.

2. A knot in the trunk of a tree.

3. A hard round tumour of the nervous parts; but particularly a bronchocele, or other hard tumour of the neck.

Gongy'lion. (From γογγυλος, round.) A pill.

GONIOMETER. An instrument for measuring the angles of crystals.

GONOI'DES. (From γονη, seed, and ειδος, form.) Resembling seed. Hippocrates often uses it as an epithet for the excrements of the belly, and for the contents of the urine, when there is something in them which resembles the seminal matter.

GONORRHŒ'A. (From γονη, the semen, and ρεω, to flow; from a supposition of the ancients, that it was a seminal flux.) A genus of disease in the class *Locales,* and order *Apocenoses,* of Dr. Cullen's arrangement, who defines it a preternatural flux of fluid from the urethra in males, with or without libidinous desires. Females, however, are subject to the same complaint in some forms. He makes four species, viz.

1. *Gonorrhœa pura* or *benigna;* a puriform discharge from the urethra, without dysuria, or lascivious inclination, and not following an impure connexion.

2. *Gonorrhœa impura, maligna, syphilitica, virulenta;* a discharge resembling pus, from the urethra, with heat of urine, &c., after impure coition, to which often succeeds a discharge of mucus from the urethra, with little or no dysury, called a gleet. This disease is also called *Fluor albus malignus Blennorrhagia,* by Swediaur. In English, a *clap,* from the old French word *clapises,* which were public shops, kept and inhabited by single prostitutes, and generally confined to a particular quarter of the town, as is even now the case in several of the great towns in Italy. In Germany, the disorder is named *tripper,* from dripping; and in French, *chaudpisse,* from the heat and scalding in making water.

No certain rule can be laid down with regard to the time that a clap will take before it makes its appearance, after infection has been conveyed. With some persons it will show itself in the course of three or four days, while, with others, there will not be the least appearance of it before the expiration of some weeks. It most usually is perceptible, however, in the space of from six to fourteen days, and in a male, begins with an uneasiness about the parts of generation, such as an itching in the glans penis, and a soreness and tingling sensation along the whole course of the urethra; soon after which, the person perceives an appearance of whitish matter at its orifice, and also some degree of pungency upon making water.

In the course of a few days, the discharge of matter will increase considerably; will assume, most probably, a greenish or yellowish hue, and will become thinner, and lose its adhesiveness; the parts will also be occupied with some degree of redness and inflammation, in consequence of which the glans will put on the appearance of a ripe cherry, the stream of urine will be smaller than usual, owing to the canal being made narrower by the inflamed state of its internal membrane, and a considerable degree of pain, and scalding heat will be experienced on every attempt to make water.

Where the inflammation prevails in a very high degree, it prevents the extension of the urethra, on the taking place of any erection, so that the penis is, at that time, curved downwards, with great pain, which is much increased, if attempted to be raised towards the belly, and the stimulus occasions it often to be erected, particularly when the patient is warm in bed, and so deprives him of sleep, producing, in some cases, an involuntary emission of semen.

In consequence of the inflammation, it sometimes happens that, at the time of making water, owing to the rupture of some small blood-vessel, a slight hæmorrhage ensues, and a small quantity of blood is voided. In consequence of inflammation, the prepuce likewise becomes often so swelled at the end, that it cannot be drawn back, which symptom is called a phimosis; or, that being drawn behind the glans, it cannot be returned, which is known by the name of paraphimosis. Now and then, from the same cause, little hard swellings arise on the lower surface of the penis, along the course of the urethra, and these perhaps suppurate and form into fistulous sores.

The adjacent parts sympathizing with those already affected, the bladder becomes irritable, and incapable of retaining the urine for any length of time, which gives the patient a frequent inclination to make water, and he feels an uneasiness about the scrotum, perinæum, and fundament. Moreover, the glands of the groins grow indurated and enlarged, or perhaps the testicles become swelled and inflamed, in consequence of which he experiences excruciating pains, extending from the seat of the complaint up into the small of the back; he gets hot and restless, and a small symptomatic fever arises.

Where the parts are not occupied by much inflammation, few or none of the last-mentioned symptoms will arise, and only a discharge with a slight heat or scalding in making water will prevail.

If a gonorrhœa be neither irritated by any irregularity of the patient, nor prolonged by the want of timely and proper assistance, then, in the course of about a fortnight, or three weeks, the discharge, from having been thin and discoloured at first, will become thick, white, and of a ropy consistence; and from having gradually begun to diminish in quantity, will at last cease entirely, together with every inflammatory symptom whatever; whereas, on the contrary, if the patient has led a life of intemperance and sensuality, has partaken freely of the bottle and high-seasoned meats, and has, at the same time, neglected to pursue the necessary means, it may then continue for many weeks or months; and, on going off, may leave a weakness or gleet behind it, besides being accompanied with the risk of giving rise, at some distant period, to a constitutional affection, especially if there has been a neglect of proper cleanliness; for where venereal matter has been suffered to lodge between the prepuce and glans penis for any time, so as to have occasioned either excoriation or ulceration, there will always be danger of its having been absorbed.

Another risk, arising from the long continuance of a gonorrhœa, especially if it has been attended with inflammatory symptoms, or has been of frequent recurrence, is the taking place of one or more strictures in the urethra. These are sure to occasion a considerable degree of difficulty, as well as pain, in making water, and, instead of its being discharged in a free and uninterrupted stream, it splits into two, or perhaps is voided drop by drop. Such affections become, from neglect, of a most serious and dangerous nature, as they not unfrequently block up the urethra, so as to induce a total suppression of urine.

Where the gonorrhœa has been of long standing, warty excrescences are likewise apt to arise about the parts of generation, owing to the matter falling and lodging thereon; and they not unfrequently prove both numerous and troublesome.

Having noticed every symptom which usually attends on gonorrhœa, in the male sex, it will only be necessary to observe, that the same heat and soreness in making water, and the same discharge of discoloured mucus, together with a slight pain in walking, and an uneasiness in sitting, take place in females as in the former; but as the parts in women, which are most apt to be affected by the venereal poison, are less complex in their nature, and fewer in number, than in men, so of course the former are not liable to many of the symptoms which the latter are; and, from the urinary canal being much shorter, and of a more simple form, in them than in men, they are seldom, if ever, incommoded by the taking place of strictures.

With women, it indeed often happens, that all the symptoms of a gonorrhœa are so very slight, they experience no other inconvenience than the discharge except perhaps immediately after menstruation, at which period, it is no uncommon occurrence for them to perceive some degree of aggravation in the symptoms.

Women of a relaxed habit, and such as have had frequent miscarriages, are apt to be afflicted with a disease known by the name of fluor albus, which it is often difficult to distinguish from gonorrhœa virulenta, as the matter discharged in both is, in many cases, of the same colour and consistence. The surest way of forming a just conclusion, in instances of this nature, will be to draw it from an accurate investigation, both of the symptoms which are present and those which have preceded the discharge; as likewise from the concurring circumstances, such as the character and mode of life of the person, and the probability there may be of her having had venereal infection conveyed to her by any connexion in which she may be engaged.

Not long ago, it was generally supposed that gonorrhœa depended always upon ulcers in the urethra, producing a discharge of purulent matter; and such ulcers do, indeed, occur in consequence of a high degree of inflammation and suppuration; but many dissections of persons, who have died while labouring under a gonorrhœa, have clearly shown that the disease may, and often does, exist without any ulceration in the urethra, so that the discharge which appears is usually of a vitiated mucus, thrown out from the mucous follicles of the urethra. On opening this canal, in recent cases, it usually appears red and inflamed; its mucous glands are somewhat enlarged, and its cavity is filled with matter to within a small distance from its extremity. Where the disease has been of long continuance, its surface all along, even to the bladder, is generally found pale and relaxed, without any erosion.

3. *Gonorrhœa laxorum, libidinosa;* a pellucid discharge from the urethra, without erection of the penis, but with venereal thoughts while awake.

4. *Gonorrhœa dormientium. Oneirogonos.* When, during sleep, but dreaming of venereal engagements, there is an erection of the penis, and a seminal discharge.

Gonorrhœa balani. A species of gonorrhœa affecting the glans penis only.

GONYA'LGIA. (From γονυ, the knee, and αλγος, pain.) *Gonialgia; Gonalgia.* Gout in the knee.

GOOSE. *Anser.* The *Anser domesticus*, or tame goose.

GOOSE-FOOT. See *Chenopodium.*

GOOSE-GRASS. See *Galium aparine.*

GO'RDIUS. 1. The name of a genus of the Order *Vermes*, of animals.

2. The gordius, or hair-tail worm, of old writers, which is the *seta equina* found in stagnant marshes and ditches in Lapland, and other places.

Gordius medinensis. The systematic name of a curious animal. See *Medinensis vena.*

GORGONIA. The name of a genus of corals.

Gorgonia nobilis. The red coral.

GOSSY'PIUM. (From *gotne*, whence *gottipium*, Egyptian.) 1. The name of a genus of plants in the Linnæan system. Class, *Monadelphia;* Order, *Polyandria.*

2. The pharmacopœial name of the cotton-tree. See *Gossypium herbaceum.*

Gossypium herbaceum. The systematic name of the cotton-plant. *Gossypium; Bombax. Gossypium—foliis quinquelobis subtus eglandulosis, caule herbaceo*, of Linnæus. The seeds are directed for medicinal use in some foreign pharmacopœias; and are administered in coughs, on account of the mucilage they contain. The cotton, the produce of this tree, is well known for domestic purposes.

[Besides the *Gossypium herbaceum*, there are other species, producing cotton-wool, some of which is of a fawn-colour, found in Peru, and used by the natives of the country. Which of the following species it is, we have not been able to ascertain. Persoon, in his *Synopsis Plantarum*, gives the ten following species of Gossypium, viz.

1. Gossypium herbaceum.
2. .. indicum.
3. .. micranthum.
4. .. arboreum.
5. .. vitifolium.

6. Gossypium hirsutum.
7. .. religiosum.
8. .. latifolium.
9. .. barbadense.
10. .. peruvianum. A.]

Goulard's Extract. A saturated solution of acetate of lead. See *Plumbi acetatis liquor.*

GOULSTON, Theodore, was born in Northamptonshire. After studying medicine at Oxford, he practised for a time with considerable reputation at Wymondham, of which his father was rector. Having taken his doctor's degree in 1610, he removed to London, and became a fellow of the College of Physicians. He was much esteemed for classical and theological learning, as well as in his profession. He died in 1632, and bequeathed £200 to purchase a rent-charge for maintaining an annual Pathological Lecture, to be read at the college by one of the four junior doctors. He translated and wrote learned notes on some of the works of Aristotle and Galen; of which the latter were not published till after his death.

GOURD. See *Cucurbita.*

Gourd, bitter. See *Cucumis colocynthis*

GOUT. See *Arthritis*, and *Podagra.*

Gout stone. See *Chalk stone.*

GRAAF, Reinier de, was born at Schoonhove, in Holland, 1641. He studied physic at Leyden, where he made great progress, and at the age of twenty-two published his treatise "De Succo Pancreatico," which gained him considerable reputation. Two years after he went to France, and graduated at Angers; he then returned to his native country, and settled at Delft, where he was very successful in practice; but he died at the early age of thirty-two. He published three dissertations relative to the organs of generation in both sexes; upon which he had a controversy with Swammerdam.

GRA'CILIS. (So named from its smallness.) *Rectus interior femoris, sive gracilis interior* of Winslow. *Sous pubio creti tibial* of Dumas. A long, straight, and tender muscle, situated immediately under the integuments, at the inner part of the thigh. It arises by a broad and thin tendon, from the anterior part of the ischium and pubis, and soon becoming fleshy, descends nearly in a straight direction along the inside of the thigh. A little above the knee, it terminates in a slender and roundish tendon, which afterward becomes flatter, and is inserted into the middle of the tibia, behind and under the sartorius. Under the tendons of this and the rectus, there is a considerable *bursa mucosa*, which on one side adheres to them and to the tendon of the semitendinosus, and on the other to the capsular ligament of the knee. This musle assists in bending the thigh and leg inwards.

GRÆCUS. The trivial name of some herbs found in or brought from Greece.

GRAFTING. Budding and inoculating is the process of uniting the branches or buds of two or more separate trees. The bud or branch of one tree, accompanied by a portion of its bark, is inserted into the bark of another, and the tree which is thus engrafted upon is called the stock. By this mode different kinds of fruits, pears, apples, plums, &c., each of which is only a variety accidentally raised from seed, but no further perpetuated in the same manner, are multiplied; buds of the kind wanted to be propagated, being engrafted on so many stalks of a wild nature.

GRA'MEN. (*Gramen, inis.* n.) Grass. Any kind of grass-like herb.

Gramen arundinaceum. See *Calamagrostis.*

Gramen caninum. See *Triticum repens.*

Gramen crucis cyperioidis. *Gramen ægyptiacum.* Egyptian cock's-foot grass, or grass of the cross. The roots and plants possess the same virtues as the dog's grass, and are serviceable in the earlier stages of dropsy. They are supposed to correct the bad smell of the breath, and to relieve nephritic disorders, colics, &c., although now neglected.

Gramia. The sordes of the eyes.

GRAMMATITE. See *Tremolite.*

Gra'mme. (From γραμμη, a line: so called from its linear appearance.) The iris of the eye.

Granadi'lla. (Diminutive of *granado*, a pomegranate, Spanish: so called because at the top of the flower there are points, like the grains of the pomegranate.) The passion-flower, the fruit of which is said to possess refrigerating qualities.

GRANATITE. See *Grenatite.*

Granatri'stum. A bile or carbuncle.

GRANATUM. (From *granum*, a grain, because it is full of seed.) The pomegranate. See *Punica granatum.*

Grande'balæ. (*Quod in grandioribus ætate nascantur*, because they appear in those who are advanced in years.) The hairs under the arm-pits.

Grandinosum os. The *os cuboides.*

GRA'NDO. (*Grando, inis. f. Quod similitudinem granorum habeat*, because it is in shape and size like a grain of seed.)

1. Hail.

2. A moveable tumour on the margin of the eyelid is so called, from its likeness to a hail-stone.

GRANITE. A compound rock consisting of quartz, felspar, and mica, each crystallized, and cohering by mutual affinity without any basis or cement.

GRANULA'TION. (*Granulatio;* from *granum*, a grain.) 1. In surgery: The little grainlike fleshy bodies which form on the surfaces of ulcers and suppurating wounds, and serve both for filling up the cavities, and bringing nearer together and uniting their sides, are called granulations.

Nature is supposed to be active in bringing parts as nearly as possible to their original state, whose disposition, action, and structure, have been altered by accident, or disease; and after having, in her operations for this purpose, formed pus, she immediately sets about forming a new matter upon surfaces, in which there has been a breach of continuity. This process is called *granulating* or *incarnation*; and the substance formed is called *granulations.* The colour of healthy granulations is a deep florid red. When livid, they are unhealthy, and have only a languid circulation. Healthy granulations, on an exposed or flat surface, rise nearly even with the surface of the surrounding skin, and often a little higher; but when they exceed this, and take on a growing disposition, they are unhealthy, become soft, spongy, and without any disposition to form skin. Healthy granulations are always prone to unite to each other, so as to be the means of uniting parts.

2. In chemistry: The method of dividing metallic substances into grains or small particles, in order to facilitate their combination with other substances, and sometimes for the purpose of readily subdividing them by weight.

GRANULATUS. Granulated, Applied to ulcers and to parts of plants. A root is so called which is jointed; as that of the *Oxalis acetocella.*

GRA'NUM. (*Granum, i.* n.) A grain or kernel.

Granum cnidium. See *Daphne mezereum.*

Granum infectorium. Kermes berries.

Granum kermes. Kermes berries.

Granum moschi. See *Hibiscus abelmoschus*

Granum paradisi. See *Amomum.*

Granum regium. The castor-oil seed.

Granum tiglii. See *Croton tiglium.*

Granum tinctoriæ. Kermes berries.

GRAPHIC ORE. An ore of tellurium.

GRAPHIOI'DES. (From γραφις, a pencil, and ειδος, a form.) 1. The styliform process of the os temporis.

2. A process of the ulna.

3. The digastricus was formerly so called from its supposed origin from the above-mentioned process of the temporal bone

GRAPHITE. Rhomboidal graphite of Jameson, or plumbago, or black-lead, of which he gives two subspecies, the scaly and compact.

Gra'ssa. Borax.

GRATI'OLA. (Diminutive of *gratia*, so named from its supposed admirable qualities.) Hyssop.

1. The name of a genus of plants in the Linnæan system. Class, *Diandria:* Order, *Monogynia.*

2. The pharmacopœial name of the hedge-hyssop. See *Gratiola officinalis.*

Gratiola officinalis. The systematic name of the hedge-hyssop. *Digitalis minima; Gratia dei; Gratiola centauriodes.* This exotic plant, the *Gratiola;—foliis lanceolatis, serratis, floribus pedunculatis*, of Linnæus, is a native of the south of Europe; but is raised in our gardens. The leaves have a nauseous bitter taste, but no remarkable smell; they purge and vomit briskly in the dose of half a drachm of the dry herb, or of a drachm infused in wine or water

This plant, in small doses, has been commonly employed as a cathartic and diuretic in hydropical diseases; and instances of its good effects in ascites and anasarca are recorded by many respectable practitioners. Gesner and Bergius found a scruple of the powder a sufficient dose, as in this quantity it frequently excited nausea or vomiting; others have given it to half a drachm, two scruples, a drachm, and even more.

An extract of the root of this plant is said to be more efficacious than the plant itself, and exhibited in the dose of half a drachm, or drachm, in dysenteries, produces the best effect. We are also told by Kostrzewski that in the hospitals at Vienna, three maniacal patients were perfectly recovered by its use; and in the most confirmed cases of lues venerea, it effected a complete cure; it usually acted by increasing the urinary, cutaneous, or salivary discharges.

GRAVE'DO. (From *grăvis*, heavy.) A catarrh, or cold, with a sense of heaviness in the head.

GRAVEL. See *Calculus*.

[Gravel root. See *Eupatorium purpureum*. A.]

GRAVITY. A term used by physical writers to denote the cause by which all bodies move toward each other, unless prevented by some other force or obstacle.

Gravity, specific. The density of the matter of which any body is composed, compared to the destiny of another body, assumed as the standard. This standard is pure distilled water, at the temperature of 60° F. To determine the specific gravity of a solid, we weigh it, first in air, and then in water. In the latter case, it loses of its weight a quantity precisely equal to the weight of its own bulk of water; and hence, by comparing this weight, with its total weight, we find its specific gravity. The rule, therefore, is, Divide the total weight by the *loss* of weight in water, the quotient is the specific gravity. If it be a liquid or a gas, we weigh it in a glass or other vessel of known capacity; and dividing that weight by the weight of the same bulk of water, the quotient is, as before, the specific gravity.

["GREEN, Thomas. The family of Green has made itself remarkable, in the medical profession, by its humble and singular origin. The subject of this notice, the medical ancestor of the family, was born in Malden, and was one of the first settlers of Leicester, county of Worcester, Massachusetts. He received his first medical impressions, and impulse, from a book, given him by a surgeon of a British ship, who resided a few months at his father's, and took an interest in his vigorous and opening intellect. His outfit, for the wilderness, consisted of his gun, his axe, his book, his sack, and his cow. His first habitation was built by nature, its roof composed of a shelving rock. Here he passed the night in sound repose, after the labour of the day, in felling and clearing the forest. Soon after he began his settlement, he was attacked by a fever. Foreseeing the difficulties which must attend his situation, without a friendly hand to administer even the scanty necessaries of life, he had the precaution to tie a young calf to his cabin, formed under the rock. By this stratagem he was enabled to obtain sustenance from the cow, as often as she returned to give nourishment to her young. In this manner he derived his support for some weeks. By the aid of his book, and the knowledge of simples, a proficiency in which he early acquired by an intercourse with the Indians, he was soon enabled to prescribe successfully for the simple maladies of his fellow-settlers. By practice, from the necessity of the case, as well as from choice, he acquired theory and skill, and soon rose to great reputation. Thus, from fortuitous circumstances, and an humble beginning, the name of Green has attained its present eminence in the medical profession "—*Thach. Med. Biog.* A.]

["GREEN, Dr. John, (senior,) son of the above mentioned, was born at Leicester, in the year 1736. By the aid of his father, he early became a physician, and settled at Worcester. He married a daughter of Brigadier Ruggles, of Hardwick, and became the father of a large family. Not satisfied, as too many are, with the limited means of knowledge which necessarily fell to his lot, he afforded his children the best education in his power. He was extensively employed, and distinguished himself for his tenderness and fidelity. He inherited a taste and skill in botany, with his profession, from his father. In his garden were to be found the useful plant, the healing herb, and the grateful fruit; which either his humanity bestowed on the sick, or his hospitality on his friends. He died, November 29th, 1799, aged 63 years.—*Thach. Med. Biog.* A.]

["GREEN, Dr. John, (junior,) son of the preceding, was born A. D. 1763. Descended from ancestors who made the art of healing their study, Dr. Green was easily initiated in the school of physic; and, from his childhood, the natural bias of his mind led him to that profession, which, through life, was the sole object of his ardent pursuit. To be distinguished as a physician, was not his chief incentive. To assuage the sufferings of humanity, by his skill, was a higher motive of his benevolent mind. Every duty was performed with delicacy and tenderness. With these propensities, aided by a strong, inquisitive, and discriminating mind, he attained to a pre-eminent rank among the physicians and surgeons of our country To this sentiment of his worth, correctly derived from witnessing his practice on others, a more feeling tribute is added by those who have experienced his skill; for so mild was his deportment, so soothing were his manners, and so indefatigable was his attention, that he gained the unbounded confidence of his patients, and the cure was in a good measure performed before medicine was administered. To those who were acquainted with Dr. Green, the idea, that "*some men are born physicians*," was not absurd; for he not only possessed an innate mental fitness for the profession, but was constitutionally formed to bear its fatigues and privations. Few men, of his age, have had such extensive practice, or endured a greater variety of fatigue, or have been so often deprived of stated rest and refreshment. It is worthy of remark, that in all the variety of duty, incident to his calling, he was never known to yield to the well-intended proffer of that kind of momentary refreshment, so ready at command, and so often successfully pressed upon the weary, exhausted, and incautious physician.

"The firmness and equanimity of his mind, which were conspicuous in all the exigencies of life, forsook him not in death. With Christian resignation, he "*set his house in order*," knowing he "*must die and not live.*" In perfect possession of his intellectual faculties, with a mind calm and collected, he spent the last moments of life performing its last duties, with the sublime feelings of a philosopher and Christian. And when, by an examination of his pulse, he found the cold hand of death pressing hard upon him, he bade a calm adieu to his attending physicians, whom he wished should be the sole witnesses of nature's last conflict. Placing himself in the most favourable posture for an easy exit, he expressed a hope that his fortitude would save his afflicted family and friends from the distress of hearing a dying groan. His hope was accomplished! He died, August 11th, 1808, aged 45 years. At his request, his body was examined. The cause of death was found in the enlargement, and consequent flaccidity, of the aorta."—*Thacher's Med. Biog.* A.]

GREEN EARTH. Mountain green. A mineral of a celandine green colour, found in Saxony, Verona, and Hungary.

GREEN SICKNESS. See *Chlorosis*.

Green vitriol. Sulphate of iron.

GREENSTONE. A rock of the *trap* formation, consisting of a hornblend, and felspar, both in the state of grains or small crystals. See *Diabase*.

GREGORY, John, was born in 1725, his father being professor of medicine at King's College, Aberdeen: after studying under whom, he went to Edinburgh, Leyden, and Paris. At the age of 20, he was elected professor of philosophy at Aberdeen, and was made doctor of medicine. In the year 1756 he was chosen professor of medicine on the death of his brother James, who had succeeded his father in that chair But about nine years after he went to Edinburgh; and was appointed professor of the practice of medicine there, Dr. Rutherford having resigned in his favour The year following, on the death of Dr. White, he was nominated first physician to the king for Scotland. He also enjoyed very extensive practice, prior to his death in 1773. He published, in 1765, "A Comparative View of the State and Faculties of Man with those of the Animal World," which contains many just and original remarks, and was very favourably received. Five years after his "Observations on the Duties and Offices of a Physician, &c.," given in his introductory lectures, were made public surreptitiously; which induced him to print them in a more correct form. The work has been greatly admired. His last publication, "Elements of the Practice of Physic" was intended as a syllabus to his lectures; but he did not live to complete it.

GRENATITE. Prismatoidal garnet.

GRESSU'RA. (From *gradior*, to proceed.) The perinæum which goes from the pudendum to the anus.

GREW, NEHEMIAH, was born at Coventry; where, after graduating at some foreign university, he settled in practice. He there formed the idea of studying the anatomy of plants. His first essay on this subject was communicated to the Royal Society in 1670, and met with great approbation: whence he was induced to settle in London, and two years after became a fellow of that society; of which he was also at one period secretary. In 1680 he was made an honorary fellow of the College of Physicians. He is said to have attained considerable practice, and died in 1711. His 'Anatomy of Vegetable Roots and Trunks," is a large collection of original and useful facts; though his theories have been invalidated by subsequent discoveries. He had no correct ideas of the propulsion or direction of the sap; but he was one of the first who adopted the doctrine of the sexes of plants; nor did even the principles of methodical arrangement entirely escape his notice. In 1681, he published a descriptive catalogue of the Museum of the Royal Society; to which were added some lectures on the comparative anatomy of the stomach and intestines. Another publication was entitled "Cosmographia Sacra, or a Discourse of the Universe; as it is the Creature and Kingdom of God." His works were soon translated into French and Latin: but the latter very incorrectly

GREYWACKE. A mountain formation, consisting of two similar rocks, which alternate with, and pass into each other, called greywacke, and greywacke-slate.

GRIAS. (A name mentioned by Apuleius.) The name of a genus of plants. Class, *Polyandria;* Order, *Monogynia.*

GRIAS CAULIFLORA. The systematic name of the tree, the fruit of which is the anchovy pear. The inhabitants of Jamaica esteem it as a pleasant and cooling fruit.

GRIE'LUM. A name formerly applied to parsley and smallage.

GRIPHO'MENOS. (From γριφος, a net; because it surrounds the body as with a net.) Applied to pains which surround the body at the loins.

GROMWELL. See *Lithospermum.*

GROSSULARE. A mineral of an asparagus-green colour, of the garnet genus.

GROSSULA'RIA. (Diminutive of *grossus*, an unripe fig; so named because its fruit resembles an unripe fig.) The gooseberry, or gooseberry-bush. See *Ribes.*

GROTTO DEL CANE. (The Italian for the dogs' grotto.) A grotto near Naples, in which dogs are suffocated. The carbonic acid gas rises about eighteen inches. A man therefore is not affected, but a dog forcibly held in, or that cannot rise above it, is soon killed, unless taken out. He is recovered by plunging him in an adjoining lake.

Ground ivy. See *Glecoma hederacea.*

Ground liverwort. See *Lichen caninus.*

Ground-nut. See *Bunium bulbocastanum.*

Ground-pine. See *Teucrium chamæpitys.*

GROUNDSEL. See *Senecio vulgaris.*

GRUINALES. (From *grus*, a crane.) The name of an order of plants in Linnæus's Fragments of a Natural Method, consisting of geranium, or crane's-bill genus principally.

GRU'TUM. A hard, white tubercle of the skin, resembling in size and appearance a millet-seed.

GRYLLUS. The name of an extensive genus of insects, including the grasshoppers, and the locust of the Scriptures.

GRYLLUS VERRUCIVORUS. The wart-eating grasshopper. It has green wings, spotted with brown, and is caught by the common people in Sweden to destroy warts, which they do, by biting off the excrescence and discharging a corrosive liquor on the wound.

GRYPHO'SIS. (From γρυποω, to incurvate.) A disease of the nails, which turn inwards, and irritate the soft parts below.

GUAI'ACUM. (From the Spanish *Guayacan*, which is formed from the Indian *Hoaxacum.*) 1. The name of a genus of plants in the Linnæan system. Class, *Decandria;* Order, *Monogynia.*

2. The pharmacopœial name of the officinal guaiacum. See *Guaiacum officinale.*

GUAIACUM OFFICINALE. This tree, *Guaiacum—foliis bijugis, obtusis* of Linnæus, is a native of the West Indian islands. The wood, gum, bark, fruit, and even the flowers, have been found to possess medicinal qualities. The wood, which is called *Guaiacum Americanum; Lignum vitæ; Lignum sanctum; Lignum benedictum; Palus sanctus,* is brought principally from Jamaica, in large pieces of four or five hundred weight each, and from its hardness and beauty is used for various articles of turnery-ware. It scarcely discovers any smell, unless heated, or while rasping, in which circumstances it yields a light aromatic one: chewed, it impresses a slight acrimony, biting the palate and fauces. The gum, or rather resin, is obtained by wounding the bark in different parts of the body of the tree, or by what has been called jagging. It exudes copiously from the wounds, though gradually; and when a quantity is found accumulated upon the several wounded trees, hardened by exposure to the sun, it is gathered and packed up in small kegs for exportation: it is of a friable texture, of a deep greenish colour, and sometimes of a reddish hue; it has a pungent acrid taste, but little or no smell, unless heated. The *bark* contains less resinous matter than the wood, and is consequently a less powerful medicine, though in a recent state it is strongly cathartic. "The *fruit*," says a late author, "is purgative, and, for medicinal use, far excels the bark. A decoction of it has been known to cure the venereal disease, and even the yaws in its advanced stage, without the use of mercury." The *flowers*, or blossoms, are laxative, and in Jamaica are commonly given to the children in the form of syrup. It is only the wood and resin of guaiacum which are now in general medicinal use in Europe; and as the efficacy of the former is supposed to be derived merely from the quantity of resinous matter which it contains, they may be considered indiscriminately as the same medicine. Guaiacum was first introduced into the materia medica soon after the discovery of America; and previous to the use of mercury in the lues venerea, it was the principal remedy employed in the cure of that disease: its great success brought it into such repute, that it is said to have been sold for seven gold crowns a pound: but notwithstanding the very numerous testimonies in its favour, it often failed in curing the patient, and was at length entirely superseded by mercury; and though it be still occasionally employed in syphilis, it is rather with a view to correct other diseases in the habit, than for its effects as an anti-venereal. It is now more generally employed for its virtues in curing gouty and rheumatic pains, and some cutaneous diseases. Dr. Woodville and others frequently conjoined it with mercury and soap, and in some cases with bark or steel, and found it eminently useful as an alterative. In the pharmacopœia it is directed in the form of mixture and tincture: the latter is ordered to be prepared in two ways, *viz.* with rectified spirit, and the aromatic spirit of ammonia. Of these latter compounds, the dose may be from two scruples to two drachms; the gum is generally given from six grains to twenty, or even more, for a dose, either in pills or in a fluid form, by means of mucilage or the yelk of an egg. The decoctum lignorum (Pharm. Edinb.) of which guaiacum is the chief ingredient, is commonly taken in the quantity of a pint a day.

As many writers of the sixteenth century contended that guaiacum was a true specific for the venereal disease, and the celebrated Boerhaave maintained the same opinion, the following observations are inserted: Mr. Pearson mentions, that when he was first intrusted with the care of the Lock Hospital, 1781, Mr. Bromfield and Mr. Williams were in the habit of reposing great confidence in the efficacy of a decoction of guaiacum wood. This was administered to such patients as had already employed the usual quantity of mercury; but who complained of nocturnal pains, or had gummata, nodes, ozæna, and other effects of the venereal virus, connected with secondary symptoms, as did not yield to a course of mercurial frictions. The diet consisted of raisins, and hard biscuit; from two to four pints of the decoction were taken every day; the hot bath was used twice a week; and a dose of antimonial wine and laudanum, or Dover's powder, was commonly taken every evening. Constant confinement to bed was not deemed necessary; neither was exposure to the vapour of burning spirit, with a view of exciting perspiration, often practised; as only a moist state of the skin was desired. This treatment was sometimes of singular advantage to those whose health had sustained injury from the disease, long confinement, and mercury. The strength increased; bad ulcers healed; exfoliations were completed; and these anomalous symptoms which would have been exasperated by mercury, soon yielded to guaiacum.

Besides such cases, in which the good effects of guaiacum made it be erroneously regarded as a specific for the lues venerea, the medicine was also formerly given, by some, on the first attack of the venereal disease. The disorder being thus benefited, a radical cure was considered to be accomplished: and though frequent relapses followed, yet, as these partly yielded to the same remedy, its reputation was still kept up. Many diseases also, which got well, were probably not venereal cases. Pearson seems to allow, that in syphilitic affections, it may indeed operate like a true antidote, suspending, for a time, the progress of certain venereal symptoms, and removing other appearances altogether; but he observes that experience has evinced, that the unsubdued virus yet remains active in the constitution.

Pearson has found guaiacum of little use in pains of the bones, except when it proved sudorific; but that it was then inferior to antimony or volatile alkali. When the constitution has been impaired by mercury and long confinement, and there is a thickened state of the ligaments, or periosteum, or foul ulcers still remaining, Pearson says, these effects will often subside during the exhibition of the decoction; and it will often suspend, for a short time, the progress of certain secondary symptoms of the lues venera; for instance, ulcers of the tonsils, venereal eruptions, and even nodes. Pearson, however, never knew one instance in which guaiacum eradicated the virus; and he contends, that its being conjoined with mercury neither increases the virtue of this mineral, lessens its bad effects, nor diminishes the necessity of giving a certain quantity of it. Pearson remarks that he has seen guaiacum produce good effects in many patients, having cutaneous diseases, the ozæna, and scrofulous affections of the membranes and ligaments.

GUILA'NDINA. (Named after Guilandus, a Prussian, who travelled in Palestine, Egypt, Africa, and Greece, and succeeded Fallopius in the botanical chair at Padua. He died in 1589.) The name of a genus of plants. Class, *Decandria*; Order, *Monogynia*.

Guilandina bonduc. The systematic name of the plant, the fruit of which is called *Bonduch indorum*. Molucca or bezoar nut. It possesses warm, bitter, and carminative virtues.

Guilandina moringa. This plant, *Guilandina—inermis, foliis subpinnatis, foliolis inferioribus ternatis* of Linnæus, affords the ben-nut and the lignum nephriticum.

1. *Ben nux; Glans unguentaria; Balanus myrepsica; Coatis.* The oily acorn, or ben-nut. A whitish nut, about the size of a small filberd, of a roundish triangular shape, including a kernel of the same figure, covered with a white skin. They were formerly employed to remove obstructions of the primæ viæ. The oil afforded by simple pressure, is remarkable for its not growing rancid in keeping, or, at least, not until it has stood for a number of years; and on this account, it is used in extricating the aromatic principles of such odoriferous flowers as yield little or no essential oil in distillation. The unalterability of this oil would render it the most valuable substance for cerates, or liniments, were it sufficiently common. It is actually employed for this purpose in many parts of Italy.

2. *Lignum nephriticum.* Nephritic wood. It is brought from America in large, compact, ponderous pieces, without knots, the outer part of a whitish, or pale yellowish colour, the inner of a dark brown or red. When rasped, it gives out a faint aromatic smell. It is never used medicinally in this country, but stands high in reputation abroad, against difficulties of making urine, nephritic complaints, and most disorders of the kidneys and urinary passages.

GUINEA PEPPER. See *Capsicum annuum*.

Guinea-worm. See *Medinensis vena*.

GUINTERIUS, John, was born in 1487, at Andernach, in Germany. He was of obscure birth, and his real name was said to have been Winther. He showed very early a great zeal for knowledge, and at the age of 12 went to Utrecht to study; but he had to struggle with great hardships, supported partly by his own industry, partly by the bounty of those who commiserated his situation. At length, having given striking proofs of his talents, he was appointed professor of Greek at Louvain. But his inclination being to medicine, he went to Paris in 1525; where he was made doctor five years after. He was appointed physician to the king, and practised there during several years; giving also lectures on anatomy. His reputation had reached the north of Europe; and he received the most advantageous offers to repair to the court of Denmark. But in 1537 he was compelled by the religious disturbances to retire into Germany. At Strasburgh he was received with honour by the magistrates, and had a chair assigned him by the faculty; he also practised very extensively and successfully; and at length letters of nobility were conferred upon him by the emperor. He lived, however, only twelve years to enjoy these honours, having died in 1574. His works are numerous, consisting partly of translations of the best ancient physicians, but principally of commentaries and illustrations of them.

GUM. I. *Gummi.* The mucilage of vegetables. It is usually transparent, more or less brittle when dry, though difficultly pulverable; of an insipid, or slightly saccharine taste; soluble in, or capable of combining with, water in all proportions, to which it gives a gluey adhesive consistence, in proportion as its quantity is greater. It is separable, or congulates by the action of weak acids; it is insoluble in alkohol, and in oil; and capable of the acid fermentation, when diluted with water. The destructive action of fire causes it to emit much carbonic acid, and converts it into coal without exhibiting any flame. Distillation affords water, acid, a small quantity of oil, a small quantity of ammonia, and much coal.

These are the leading properties of gums, rightly so called; but the inaccurate custom of former times applied the term gum to all concrete vegetable juices, so that in common we hear of gum copal, gum sandarach, and other gums, which are either pure resins, or mixtures of resins with the vegetable mucilage.

The principal gums are, 1. The common gums, obtained from the plum, the peach, the cherry-tree, &c. 2. Gum Arabic, which flows naturally from the acacia in Egypt, Arabia, and elsewhere. This forms a clear transparent mucilage with water. 3. Gum Seneca, or Senegal. It does not greatly differ from gum Arabic: the pieces are larger and clearer; and it seems to communicate a higher degree of the adhesive quality to water. It is much used by calico-printers and others The first sort of gums are frequently sold by this name, but may be known by their darker colour. 4. Gum adragant, or tragacanth. It is obtained from a small plant, a species of astragalus, growing in Syria, and other eastern parts. It comes to us in small white contorted pieces, resembling worms. It is usually dearer than other gums, and forms a thicker jelly with water.

Willis has found, that the root of the common bluebell, *Hyacinthus non scriptus*, dried and powdered, affords a mucilage possessing all the qualities of that from gum Arabic. The roots of the vernal squill, white lily, and orchis, equally yield mucilage. Lord Dundonald has extracted a mucilage also from lichens.

Gums treated with nitric acid afford the saclactic, malic, and oxalic acids.

II. *Gingiva.* The very vascular and elastic substance that covers the alveolar arches of the upper and under jaws, and embraces the necks of the teeth.

Gum acacia. See *Acacia vera.*

Gum arabic. See *Acacia vera.*

Gum, elastic. See *Caoutchouc.*

GUM-BILE. See *Parulis.*

GU'MMA. A strumous tumour on the periosteum of a bone.

GUMMI. (*Gummi*, n. *indeclin.*) See *Gum.*

GUMMI ACACIÆ. See *Acacia vera.*
GUMMI ACANTHINUM. See *Acacia vera.*
GUMMI ARABICUM. See *Acacia vera.*
GUMMI CARANNÆ. See *Caranna.*

GUMMI CERASORUM. The juices which exude from the bark of cherry-trees. It is very similar to gum Arabic, for which it may be substituted.

GUMMI CHIBOU. A spurious kind of gum elemi, but little used.

GUMMI COURBARIL. An epithet sometimes applied to the juice of the *Hymenæa courbaril.* See *Anime.*

GUMMI EUPHORBII. See *Euphorbia.*
GUMMI GALDA. See *Galda.*
GUMMI GAMBIENSE. See *Kino.*
GUMMI GUTTÆ. See *Stalagmitis.*
GUMMI HEDERÆ. See *Hedera helix.*
GUMMI JUNIPERINUM. See *Juniperus communis.*
GUMMI KIKEKUNEMALO. See *Kikekunemalo.*
GUMMI KINO. See *Kino.*
GUMMI LACCA. See *Lacca.*
GUMMI LAMAC. See *Acacia vera.*
GUMMI LUTEA. See *Botany Bay.*
GUMMI MYRRHA. See *Myrrha.*
GUMMI RUBRUM ASTRINGENS GAMBIENSE. See *Kino.*
GUMMI SAGAPENUM. See *Sagapenum.*
GUMMI SCORPIONIS. See *Acacia vera.*
GUMMI SENEGA. See *Acacia vera.*
GUMMI SENEGALENSE. See *Mimosa Senegal.*
GUMMI SENICA. See *Acacia vera.*
GUMMI THEBAICUM. See *Acacia vera.*
GUMMI TRAGACANTHÆ. See *Astragalus.*

GUM-RE'SIN. *Gummi resina.* Gum-resins are the juices of plants that are mixed with resin, and an extractive matter, which has been taken for a gummy substance. They seldom flow naturally from plants, but are mostly extracted by incision in the form of white, yellow, or red fluids, which dry more or less quickly. Water, spirit of wine, wine, or vinegar, dissolve them only in part according to the proportion they contain of resin or extract. Gum-resins may also be formed by art, by digesting the parts of vegetables containing the gum-resin in diluted alkohol, and then evaporating the solution. For this reason most tinctures contain gum-resin. The principal gum-resins employed medicinally are aloes, ammoniacum, assafœtida, galbanum, cambogia, guaiacum, myrrha, olibanum, opoponax, sagapenum, sarcocolla, scammonium, and styrax.

GUNDELIA. (The name given by Tournefort in honour of his companion and friend, Andrew Gundelscheimer, its discoverer, in the mountains of Armenia.) A genus of plants. Class, *Syngenesia;* Order, *Polygamia segregata.*

GUNDELIA TOURNIFORTII. The young shoots of this plant are eaten by the Indians but the roots are emetic.

GU'TTA. (*Gutta, æ.* f.) 1. A drop. Drops are uncertain forms of administering medicines, and should never be trusted to. The shape of the bottle or of its mouth, from whence the drops fall, as well as the consistence of the fluid, occasion a considerable difference in the quantity administered. See *Minimum.*

2. A name of apoplexy, from a supposition that its cause was a drop of blood falling from the brain upon the heart.

GUTTA GAMBA. See *Stalagmitis.*

GUTTA NIGRA. The black drop, occasionally called the Lancashire, or the Cheshire drop. A secret prepreparation of opium said to be more active than the common tincture, and supposed to be less injurious, as seldom followed by headache.

GUTTA OPACA. A name for the cataract.

GUTTA SERENA. (So called by the Arabians.) See *Amaurosis*

GUTTÆ ROSACEÆ. Red spots upon the face and nose.

GU'TTURAL. Belonging to the throat.

GUTTURAL ARTERY. The superior thyroideal artery. The first branch of the external carotid.

GYMNA'STIC. (*Gymnasticus;* from γυμνος, naked, performed by naked men in the public games.) This term is applied to a method of curing diseases by exercise, or that part of physic which treats of the rules that are to be observed in all sorts of exercises, for the preservation of health. This is said to have been invented by one Herodicus, born at Salymbria, a city of Thrace; or, as some say, at Leutini, in Sicily. He was first master of an academy where young gentlemen came to learn warlike and manly exercises; and observing them to be very healthful on that account, he made exercise become an art in reference to the recovering of men out of diseases, as well as preserving them from them, and called it *Gymnastic,* which he made a great part of his practice. But Hippocrates, who was his scholar, blames him sometimes for his excesses with this view. And Plato exclaims against him with some warmth, for enjoining his patients to walk from Athens to Megara, which is about 25 miles, and to come home on foot as they went, as soon as ever they had but touched the walls of the city.

GYMNOCARPI. The second division in Persoon's arrangement of mushrooms, such as bear seeds embedded in an appropriate, dilated, exposed membrane, denominated *hymenium,* like *helvella,* in which that part is smooth and even; *boletus,* in which it is porous; and the vast genus *agaricus,* in which it consists of gills.

GYMNOSPERMIA. (From γυμνος, naked, and σπερμα, a seed.) The name of an order of the class *Didynamia,* of the sexual system of plants, embracing such as have added to the didynamial character, four naked seeds.

GYNÆ'CIA. (From γυνη, a woman.) The menses, and also the lochia.

GYNÆ'CIUM. (From γυνη, a woman.)

1. A seraglio.
2. The *pudendum muliebre.*
3. A name for *antimony.*

GYNÆCOMA'NIA. (From γυνη, a woman, and μανια, madness.) That species of insanity that arises from love.

GYNÆCOMY'STAX. (From γυνη, a woman, and μυςταξ, a beard.) The hairs on the female pudendum.

GYNÆCOMA'STON. (From γυνη, a woman, and μαςος, a breast.) An enormous increase of the breasts of women.

GYNANDRIA. (From γυνη, a woman, and ανηρ, a man, or husband.) The name of a class in the sexual system of plants. It contains those hermaphrodite flowers, the stamina of which grow upon the pistil, so that the male and female organs are united, and do not stand separate as in other hermaphrodite flowers.

GYPSATA. (From *gypsum,* a saline body consisting of sulphuric acid and lime.) Dr. Good denominates a species of purging *diarrhœa gypsata,* in which the digestions are liquid, serous, and compounded of earth of lime.

GYPSUM. A genus of minerals, composed of lime and sulphuric acid, containing, according to Jameson, two species: the prismatic and the axifrangible.

1. *Prismatic* gypsum, or *anhydrite,* has five sub-species: sparry anhydrite, scaly anhydrite, fibrous anhydrite, convoluted anhydrite, compact anhydrite. See *Anhydrite.*

2. *Axifrangible* gypsum contains six sub-species: sparry gypsum, foliated, compact, fibrous, scaly foliated, and earthy gypsum

H

[HAARKIES. Werner's name for the capillary pyrites of Jameson, and the Nickel natif of Haüy. Native nickel. A.]

HABE'NA. A bridle. A bandage for keeping the lips of wounds together, made in the form of a bridle.

HACUB. See *Gundelia tournefortii.*

HÆMAGO'GA. (From αιμα, blood, and αγω, to bring off) Medicines which promote the menstrual and hæmorrhoidal discharges.

HÆMALO'PIA. (From αιμα, blood, and οπ7ομαι, to see.) A disease of the eyes, in which all things appear of a red colour. A variety of the *Pseudoblepsis imaginaria.*

HÆ'MALOPS. (From αιμα, blood, and ωψ, the face.) 1. A red or livid mark in the face or eye.

2. A blood-shot eye.

HÆMA'NTHUS. (From αιμα, blood, and ανθος, a flower, so called from its colour.) The blood-flower.

HÆMATE'MESIS. (From αιμα, blood, and εμεω, to vomit.) *Vomitus cruentus.* A vomiting of blood is readily to be distinguished from a discharge from the lungs, by its being usually preceded by sense of weight, pain, or anxiety in the region of the stomach; by its being unaccompanied by any cough; by the blood being discharged in a very considerable quantity; by its being of a dark colour, and somewhat grumous; and by its being mixed with the other contents of the stomach.

The disease may be occasioned by any thing received into the stomach, which stimulates it violently or wounds it; or may proceed from blows, bruises, or any other cause capable of exciting inflammation in this organ, or of determining too great a flow of blood to it; but it arises more usually as a symptom of some other disease (such as a suppression of the menstrual, or hæmorrhoidal flux, or obstructions in the liver, spleen, and other viscera) than as a primary affection. It is seldom so profuse as to destroy the patient suddenly, and the principal danger seems to arise, either from the great debility which repeated attacks of the complaint induce, or from the lodgment of blood in the intestines, which by becoming putrid might occasion some other disagreeable disorder.

This hæmorrhage, being usually rather of a passive character, does not admit of large evacuations. Where it arises, on the suppression of the menses, in young persons, and returns periodically, it may be useful to anticipate this by taking away a few ounces of blood; not neglecting proper means to help the function of the uterus. In moderate attacks, particularly where the bowels have been confined, the infusion of roses and sulphate of magnesia may be employed: if this should not check the bleeding, the sulphuric acid may be exhibited more largely, or some of the more powerful astringents and tonics, as alum, tincture of muriate of iron, decoction of bark, or superacetate of lead. Where pain attends, opium should be given freely, taking care that the bowels be not constipated; and a blister to the epigastrium may be useful. If depending on scirrhous tumours, these must be attacked by mercury, hemlock, &c. In all cases the food should be light, and easy of digestion; but more nourishing as the patient is more exhausted.

HÆMATICA. The name of a class of diseases in Good's Nosology, of the sanguineous system. Its orders are, *Pyretica, Phlegotica, Exanthematica, Dysthetica.*

HÆMATIN. The colouring matter of logwood, and according to Chevreuil, a distinct vegetable substance. See *Hæmatoxylon.*

HÆMATI'TES. (From αιμα, blood: so named from its property of stopping blood, or from its colour.) *Lapis hæmatites.* An elegant iron ore called bloodstone. Finely levigated, and freed from the grosser parts by frequent washings with water, it has been long recommended in hæmorrhages, fluxes, uterine obstructions, &c. in doses of from one scruple to three or four.

HÆMATI'TINUS. (From αιμα7ι7ης, the bloodstone.) An epithet of a collyrium, in which was the bloodstone.

HÆMATOCE'LE. (From αιμα, blood, and κηλη, a tumour.) A swelling of the scrotum, or spermatic cord proceeding from or caused by blood. The distinction of the different kinds of hæmatocele, though not usually made, is absolutely necessary towards rightly understanding the disease; the general idea, or conception of which, appears to Pott to be somewhat erroneous, and to have produced a prognostic which is ill founded and hasty. According to this eminent surgeon, the disease, properly called hæmatocele, is of four kinds; two of which have their seat within the tunica vaginalis testis; one within the albuginea; and the fourth in the tunica communis or common cellular membrane, investing the spermatic vessels.

In the passing an instrument, in order to let out the water from a hydrocele of the vaginal coat, a vessel is sometimes wounded, which is of such size, as to tinge the fluid pretty deeply at the time of its running out: the orifice becoming close, when the water is all discharged, and a plaster being applied, the blood ceases to flow from thence, but insinuates itself partly into the cavity of the vaginal coat, and partly into the cells of the scrotum; making in the space of a few hours, a tumour nearly equal in size to the original hydrocele. This is one species.

It sometimes happens in tapping a hydrocele, that although the fluid discharged by that operation be perfectly clear and limpid, yet in a very short space of time (sometimes in a few hours,) the scrotum becomes as large as it was before, and palpably as full of a fluid. If a new puncture be now made, the discharge, instead of being limpid (as before,) is either pure blood or very bloody. This is another species; and, like the preceding, confined to the tunica vaginalis.

The whole vascular compages of the testicle is sometimes very much enlarged, and at the same time rendered so lax and loose, that the tumour produced thereby has, to the fingers of an examiner, very much the appearance of a swelling composed of a mere fluid, supposed to be somewhat thick, or viscid. This is in some measure a deception; but not totally so: the greater part of the tumefaction is caused by the loosened texture of the testes; but there is very frequently a quantity of extravasated blood also. If this be supposed to be a hydrocele, and pierced, the discharge will be mere blood. This is a third kind of hæmatocele; and very different, in all its circumstances, from the two preceding: the fluid is shed from the vessels of the glandular part of the testicle, and contained within the tunica albuginea.

The fourth consists in a rupture of, and an effusion of blood, from a branch of the spermatic vein, in its passage from the groin to the testicles. In which case, the extravasation is made into the tunica communis, or cellular membrane, investing the spermatic vessels.

Each of these species, Pott says, he has seen so distinctly, and perfectly, that he has not the smallest doubt concerning their existence, and of their difference from each other.

HÆMATO'CHYSIS. (From αιμα, blood, and χεω, to pour out.) A hæmorrhage or flux of blood.

HÆMATO'DES. (From αιμα, blood, and ειδος, appearance: so called from the red colour.) 1. An old name for the bloody crane's-bill. See *Geranium sanguineum.*

2. A fungus, which has somewhat the appearance of blood. See *Hæmatoma.*

HÆMATO'LOGY. (*Hæmatologia;* from αιμα, blood, and λογος, a discourse.) The doctrine of the blood.

HÆMATOMA. (From αιμα, blood.) *Fungus hæmatodes.* The bleeding fungus. Spongoid inflammation of Burns. This disease has been described also under the names of soft cancer and medullary sarcoma. It assumes a variety of forms, and attacks most parts of the body, but particularly the testicle, eye, breast, and the extremities. It begins with a soft enlargement or tumour of the part, which is extremely elastic, and in some cases very painful; as it increases, it often has the feel of an encysted tumour, and at length becomes irregular, bulging out here and there, and in sinuates itself between the neighbouring parts, and forms a large mass, if under an aponeurotic expansion. When it ulcerates it bleeds, shoots up a mass of a bloody fungus, and then shows its decided character if unknown before. Most of the medicines which have been employed against cancerous diseases have been unprofitably exhibited against hæmatoma; as alteratives, both vegetable and mineral; tonics and narcotics. Extirpation, when practicable, is the only cure.

HÆMATOMPHALOCE'LE. (From αιμα, blood, ομφαλος, the navel, and κηλη, a tumour.) A tumour about the navel, from an extravasation of blood. A species of ecchymosis.

HÆMATOPEDE'SIS. (From αιμα, blood, and πεδαω, a leap.) The leaping of the blood from a wounded artery.

HÆMATO'SIS. (From αιμα, blood.) A hæmorrhage or flux of blood.

HÆMATO'XYLON. (From αιμα, blood, and ξυλον, wood: so called from the red colour of its wood.) The name of a genus of plants in the Linnæan system. Class, *Decandria*; Order, *Monogynia*.

HÆMATOXYLON CAMPECHIANUM. The systematic name of the logwood-tree. *Acacia Zeylonica.* The part ordered in the Pharmacopœia, is the wood, called *Hæmatoxyli lignum; Lignum campechense; Lignum campechianum; Lignum campescanum; Lignum indicum; Lignum sappan.* Logwood. It is of a solid texture and of a dark red colour. It is imported principally as a substance for dying, cut into junks and logs of about three feet in length; of these pieces the largest and thickest are preserved, as being of the deepest colour. Logwood has a sweetish sub-adstringent taste, and no remarkable smell; it gives a purplish red tincture both to watery and spirituous infusions, and tinges the stools, and sometimes the urine, of the same colour. It is employed medicinally as an adstringent and corroborant. In diarrhœas it has been found peculiarly efficacious, and has the recommendation of some of the first medical authorities; also in the latter stages of dysentery, when the obstructing causes are removed; to obviate the extreme laxity of the intestines usually superinduced by the repeated dejections. In the form of a decoction the proportion is two ounces to 2lb. of fluid, reduced by boiling to one. An extract is ordered in the pharmacopœias. The dose from ten to forty grains. The colouring principle of this root is called *hemetin.* On the watery extract of logwood, digest alkohol for a day, filter the solution, evaporate, add a little water, evaporate gently again, and then leave the liquid at rest. Hematin is deposited in small crystals, which, after washing with alkohol, are brilliant, and of a reddish-white colour. Their taste is bitter, acrid, and slightly astringent.

Hematin forms an orange-red solution with boiling water, becoming yellow as it cools, but recovering, with increase of heat, its former hue. Excess of alkali converts it first to purple, then to violet, and, lastly, to brown: in which state the hematin seems to be decomposed. Metallic oxides unite with hematin, forming a blue-coloured compound. Gelatin throws down reddish flocculi. Peroxide of tin, and acid, merely redden it.

HÆMATO'XYLUM. See *Hæmatoxylon.*

HÆMATU'RIA. (From αιμα, blood, and ουρον, urine.) The voiding of blood with urine. This disease is sometimes occasioned by falls, blows, bruises, or some violent exertion, such as hard riding and jumping; but it more usually arises, from a small stone lodged either in the kidney or ureter, which by its size or irregularity wounds the inner surface of the part it comes in contact with; in which case the blood discharged is most usually somewhat coagulated, and the urine deposites a sediment of a dark brown colour, resembling the grounds of coffee.

A discharge of blood by urine, when proceeding from the kidney or ureter, is commonly attended with an acute pain in the back, and some difficulty of making water, the urine which comes away first, being muddy and high coloured, but towards the close of its flowing, becoming transparent and of a natural appearance. When the blood comes immediately from the bladder, it is usually accompanied with a sense of heat and pain at the bottom of the belly.

The voiding of bloody urine is always attended with some danger, particularly when mixed with purulent matter When it arises in the course of any malignant disease, it shows a highly putrid state of the blood, and always indicates a fatal termination.

The appearances to be observed on dissection will accord with those usually met with in the disease which has given rise to the complaint.

When the disease has resulted from a mechanical injury in a plethoric habit, it may be proper to take blood, and pursue the general antiphlogistic plan, open ing the bowels occasionally with castor oil, &c. When owing to calculi, which cannot be removed, we must be chiefly content with palliative measures, giving alkalies or acids according to the quality of the urine; likewise mucilaginous drinks and clysters; and opium, fomentations, &c. to relieve pain; uva ursi also has been found useful under these circumstances; but more decidedly where the hæmorrhage is purely passive; in which case also some of the terebinthate remedies may be cautiously tried; and means of strengthening the constitution must not be neglected.

HÆMO'DIA. (From αιμωδεω, to stupefy.) A painful stupor of the teeth, caused by acrid substances touching them.

HÆMO'PTOE. (From αιμα, blood, and πτυω, to spit up.) The spitting of blood. See *Hæmoptysis.*

HÆMO'PTYSIS. (From αιμα, blood, and πτυω, to spit.) *Hæmoptoe.* A spitting of blood. A genus of disease arranged by Cullen in the class *Pyrexiæ*, and order *Hæmorrhagiæ*. It is characterized by coughing up florid or frothy blood, preceded usually by heat or pain in the chest, irritation in the larynx, and a saltish taste in the mouth. There are five species of this disease.

1. *Hæmoptysis plethorica*, from fulness of the vessels.
2. *Hæmoptysis violenta*, from some external violence.
3. *Hæmoptysis phthisica*, from ulcers corroding the small vessels.
4. *Hæmoptysis calculosa*, from calculous matter in the lungs.
5. *Hæmoptysis vicaria*, from the suppression of some customary evacuation.

It is readily to be distinguished from hæmatemesis as in this last, the blood is usually thrown out in considerable quantities; and is, moreover, of a darker colour, more grumous, and mixed with the other contents of the stomach; whereas blood proceeding from the lungs is usually in small quantity, of a florid colour, and mixed with a little frothy mucus only.

A spitting of blood arises most usually between the ages of sixteen and twenty-five, and may be occasioned by any violent exertion either in running, jumping, wrestling, singing loud, or blowing wind-instruments; as likewise by wounds, plethora, weak vessels, hectic fever, coughs, irregular living, excessive drinking, or a suppression of some accustomed discharge, such as the menstrual or hæmorrhoidal. It may likewise be occasioned by breathing air which is too much rarefied to be able properly to expand the lungs.

Persons in whom there is a faulty proportion, either in the vessels of the lungs, or in the capacity of the chest, being distinguished by a narrow thorax and prominent shoulders, or who are of a delicate make and sanguine temperament, seem much predisposed to this hæmorrhage; but in these, the complaint is often brought on by the concurrence of the various occasional and exciting causes before mentioned.

A spitting of blood is not, however, always to be considered as a primary disease. It is often only a symptom, and in some disorders, such as pleurisies, peripneumonies, and many fevers, often arises, and is the presage of a favourable termination.

Sometimes it is preceded, as has already been observed, by a sense of weight and oppression at the chest, a dry tickling cough, and some slight difficulty of breathing. Sometimes it is ushered in with shiverings, coldness at the extremities, pains in the back and loins, flatulency, costiveness, and lassitude. The blood which is spit up is generally thin, and of a florid red colour; but sometimes it is thick, and of a dark or blackish cast; nothing, however, can be inferred from this circumstance, but that the blood has lain a longer or shorter time in the breast, before it was discharged

An hæmoptoe is not attended with danger, where no symptoms of phthisis pulmonalis have preceded or accompanied the hæmorrhage, or where it leaves behind no cough, dyspnœa, or other affection of the lungs; nor is it dangerous in a strong healthy person, of a sound constitution; but when it attacks persons of a weak lax fibre, and delicate habit, it may be difficult to remove it.

It seldom takes place to such a degree as to prove fatal at once; but when it does, the effusion is from some large vessel. The danger, therefore, will be in proportion as the discharge of blood comes from a large vessel, or a small one.

When the disease proves fatal, in consequence of the rupture of some large vessels, there is found, on dissection, a considerable quantity of clotted blood in the lungs, and there is usually more or less of an inflammatory appearance at the ruptured part. Where the disease terminates in pulmonary consumption, the same morbid appearances are to be met with as described under that particular head.

In this hæmorrhage, which is mostly of the active kind, the antiphlogistic regimen must be strictly observed; particularly avoiding heat, muscular exertion, and agitation of the mind; and restricting the patient to a light, cooling, vegetable diet. Acidulated drink will be useful to quench the thirst, without so much liquid being taken. Where the blood is discharged copiously, but no great quantity has been lost already, it will be proper to attempt to check it by bleeding freely, if the habit will allow: and sometimes, where there is pain in the chest, local evacuations and blisters may be useful. The bowels should be well cleared with some cooling saline cathartic, which may be given in the infusion of roses. Digitalis is also a proper remedy, particularly where the pulse is very quick, from its sedative influence on the heart and arteries. Antimonials in nauseating doses have sometimes an excellent effect, as well by checking the force of the circulation, as by promoting diaphoresis; calomel also might be added with advantage; and opium, or other narcotic, to relieve pain and quiet cough, which may perhaps keep up the bleeding. Emetics have, on some occasions, been successful; but they are not altogether free from danger. In protracted cases, internal astringents are given, as alum, kino, &c. but their effects are very precarious: the superacetate of lead, however, is perhaps the most powerful medicine, especially combined with opium, and should always be resorted to in alarming or obstinate cases, though as it is liable to occasion colic and paralysis, its use should not be indiscriminate; but it acts probably rather as a sedative than astringent. Sometimes the application of cold water to some sensible part of the body, producing a general refrigeration, will check the bleeding. When the discharge is stopped, great attention to regimen is still required, to obviate its return, with occasional evacuations: the exercise of swinging, riding in an easy carriage, or on a gentle horse, or especially sailing, may keep up a salutary determination of the blood to other parts: an occasional blister may be applied, where there are marks of local disease, or an issue or seton perhaps answer better. Should hæmoptysis occasionally exhibit rather the passive character, evacuations must be sparingly used, and tonic medicines will be proper, with a more nutritious diet.

HÆMORRHAGIA. (From αιμα, blood, and ῥηγνυμι, to break out.) A hæmorrhage, or flow of blood.

HÆMORRHA'GIÆ. Hæmorrhages, or fluxes of blood. The name of an order in the class *Pyrexiæ* of Cullen's Nosology is so called. It is characterized by pyrexia with a discharge of blood, without any external injury; the blood on venæsection exhibiting the buffy coat. The order *Hæmorrhagiæ* contains the following genera of diseases, viz. epistaxis, hæmoptysis, (of which phthisis is represented as a sequel,) hæmorrhois, and menorrhagia.

HÆMORRHOI'DAL. (*Hæmorrhoidalis;* the name of the vessels which are the seat of the hæmorrhoids or piles.) 1. Of or belonging to the hæmorrhoidal vessels.

2. The trivial name of some plants which were supposed to be efficacious against piles; as *Carduus hæmorrhoidales*, &c.

Hæmorrhoidal arteries. *Arteriæ hæmorrhoidales.* The arteries of the rectum are so called: they are sometimes two, and at other times three in number. 1. The upper hæmorrhoidal artery, which is the great branch of the lower mesenteric continued into the pelvis 2 The middle hæmorrhoidal, which sometimes comes off from the hypogastric artery, and very often from the pudical artery. It is sometimes wanting. 3 The lower or external hæmorrhoidal is almost always a branch of the pudical artery, or that artery which goes to the penis.

Hæmorrhoidal veins. *Venæ Hæmorrhoidales.* These are two. 1. The external, which evacuates itself into the vena iliaca interna.

2. The internal, which conveys its blood into the vena portæ.

HÆMO'RRHOIS. (From αιμα, blood, and ρεω, to flow.) *Aimorrhois.* The piles. A genus of disease in the class *pyrexiæ*, and order *Hæmorrhagiæ* of Cullen. They are certain excrescences or tumours arising about the verge of the anus, or the inferior part of the intestinum rectum; when they discharge blood, particularly upon the patient's going to stool, the disease is known by the name of *bleeding piles;* but when there is no discharge, it is called *blind piles.* The rectum, as well as the colon, is composed of several membranes connected to each other by an intervening cellular substance; and as the muscular fibres of this intestine always tend, by their contraction, to lessen its cavity, the internal membrane, which is very lax, forms itself into several rugæ, or folds. In this construction nature respects the use of the part, which occasionally gives passage to, or allows the retention of, the excrements, the hardness and bulk of which might produce considerable lacerations, if this intestine were not capable of dilatation. The arteries and veins subservient to this part are called hæmorrhoidal, and the blood that returns from hence is carried to the meseraic veins. The intestinum rectum is particularly subject to the hæmorrhoids, from its situation, structure, and use; for while the course of the blood is assisted in almost all the other veins of the body, by the distention of the adjacent muscles, and the pressure of the neighbouring parts, the blood in the hæmorrhoidal veins, which is to ascend against the natural tendency of its own weight, is not only destitute of these assistances, but is impeded in its passage: for, first, the large excrements which lodge in this intestine dilate its sides, and the different resistances which they form there are so many impediments obstructing the return of the blood; not in the large veins, for they are placed along the external surface of the intestine, but in all the capillaries which enter into its composition. Secondly, as often as these large excrements, protruded by others, approached near the anus, their successive pressure upon the internal coats of the intestine, which they dilate, drives back the blood into the veins, and for so long suspends its course; the necessary consequence of which is, a distention of the veins in proportion to the quantity of blood that fills them. Thirdly, in every effort we make, either in going to stool, or upon any other occasion, the contraction of the abdominal muscles, and the diaphragm pressing the contents of the abdomen downwards, and these pressing upon the parts contained in the pelvis, another obstruction is thereby opposed, to the return of the blood, not only in the large veins, but also in the capillaries, which, being of too weak a texture to resist the impulse of the blood that always tends to dilate them, may hereby become varicose.

The dilatation of all these vessels is the *primary cause* of the hæmorrhoids; for the internal coat of the intestine, and the cellular membrane which connects that to the muscular coat, are enlarged in proportion to the distention of the vessels of which they are composed. This distention, not being equal in every part, produces separate tumours in the gut, or at the verge of the anus, which increases according as the venal blood is obstructed in them, or circulates there more slowly.

Whatever, then, is capable of retarding the course of the blood in the hæmorrhoidal veins, may occasion this disease. Thus, persons that are generally costive, who are accustomed to sit long at stool, and strain hard; pregnant women, or such as have had difficult labours: and likewise persons who have an obstruction in their liver, are for the most part afflicted with the piles; yet every one has not the hæmorrhoids, the different causes which are mentioned above being not common to all, or at least not having in all the same effects. When the hæmorrhoids are once formed, they seldom disappear entirely, and we may judge of those within the rectum by those which, being at the verge of the anus, are plainly to be seen. A small pile, that has been painful for some days, may cease to be so, and dry up; but the skin does not afterward retain its former firmness, being more lax and wrinkled, like the empty skin of a grape. If this external pile swells and sinks again several times, we may perceive, after each return, the remains of each pile, though shrivelled and decayed, yet still left larger than before. The case is the same with those that are situated within the rectum; they may happen indeed never to return again, if the cause that produced them is removed; but it is probable that the excrements in passing out occasion a return of the swelling, to which the external ones are less liable: for the internal piles make a sort of knots or tumours in the intestine, which straightening the passage, the excrements in passing out, occasion irritations there that are more or less painful in proportion to the efforts which the person makes in going to stool; and it is thus these tumours become gradually larger. The hæmorrhoids are subject to many variations; they may become inflamed from the above irritations to which they are exposed, and this inflammation cannot always be removed by art. In some, the inflammation terminates in an abscess, which arises in the middle of the tumour, and degenerates into a fistula. These piles are very painful till the abscess is formed. In others, the inflammation terminates by induration of the hæmorrhoid, which remains in a manner scirrhous. These never lessen, but often grow larger. This scirrhus sometimes ulcerates, and continually discharges a sanies, which the patient perceives by stains on his shirt, and by its occasioning a very troublesome itching about the verge of the anus. These kinds of hæmorrhoids sometimes turn cancerous. There are some hæmorrhoids, and those of different sizes, which are covered with so fine a skin as frequently to admit blood to pass through. This fine skin is only the internal coat of the rectum, greatly attenuated by the varicose distention of its vessels. The hæmorrhage may proceed from two causes, namely, either from an excoriation produced by the hardness of the excrements, or from the rupture of the tumefied vessels, which break by their too great distention. In some of these, the patient voids blood almost every time he goes to stool; in others not so constantly. We sometimes meet with men who have a periodical bleeding by the piles, not unlike the menses in women; and as this evacuation, if moderate, does not weaken the constitution, we may infer that it supplies some other evacuation which nature either ceases to carry on, or does not furnish in due quantity; and hence also we may explain why the suppression of this discharge, to which nature had been accustomed, is frequently attended with dangerous diseases. The hæmorrhoids are sometimes distended to that degree as to fill the rectum, so that if the excrements are at all hard they cannot pass. In this case the excrements force the hæmorrhoids out of the anus to procure a free passage, consequently the internal coat of the rectum, to which they are connected, yields to extension, and upon examining these patients immediately after having been at stool, a part of the internal coat of that gut is perceived. A difficulty will occur in the return of these, in proportion to their size, and as the verge of the anus is more or less contracted. If the bleeding piles come out in the same manner upon going to stool, it is then they void most blood, because the verge of the anus forms a kind of ligature above them. The treatment of this complaint will vary much, according to circumstances. When the loss of blood is considerable, we should endeavour to stop it by applying cold water, or ice; or some astringent, as a solution of alum, or sulphate of zinc: but a more certain way is making continued pressure on the part. At the same time internal astringents may be given; joined with opium, if much pain or irritation attend. Care must be taken, however, to avoid constipation: and in all cases patients find benefit from the steady use of some mild cathartic, procuring regular loose motions. Sulphur is mostly resorted to for this purpose; and, especially in combination with supertartrate of potassa, tamarinds, &c. in the form of electuary, usually answers very well; likewise castor oil is an excellent remedy in these cases. Should the parts be much inflamed, leeches may be applied near the anus, and cold saturnine lotions used; sometimes, however, fomenting with the decoction of poppy will give more relief; where symptomatic fever attends, the antiphlogistic regimen must be strictly observed, and besides clearing the bowels, antimonials may be given to promote diaphoresis. Where the tumours are considerable and flaccid, without inflammation, powerful astringent or even stimulant applications will be proper, together with similar internal medicines; and the part should be supported by a compress kept on by a proper bandage. An ointment of galls is often very useful, with opium, to relieve pain; and some of the liquor plumbi subacetatis may be farther added, if there be a tendency to inflammation. In these cases of relaxed piles of some standing, the copaiba frequently does much good, both applied locally and taken internally, usually keeping the bowels regular; also the celebrated Ward's paste, a medicine of which the active ingredient is black pepper. Sometimes where a large tumour has been formed by extravasated blood, subsequently become organized, permanent relief can only be obtained by extirpating this.

HÆMOSTA'SIA. (From αιμα, blood, and ιςημι, to stand.) A stagnation of blood.

HÆMOSTA'TICA. (From αιμα, blood, and ςαω, to stop.) Medicines which stop hæmorrhages. See *Styptics*.

HAEN, ANTHONY DE, was born in Leyden, in 1704, and became one of the distinguished pupils of the celebrated Boerhaave. After graduating at his native place, he settled at the Hague, where he practised with considerable reputation for nearly 20 years. Baron Van Swieten, being acquainted with the extent of his talents, invited him to Vienna, to assist in the plan of reform, which the empress had consented to support in the medical faculty of that capital. De Haen accordingly repaired thither in 1754, was made professor of the practice of medicine, and fully answered the expectation which had been formed of him. He undertook a system of clinical education, as the best method of forming good physicians: the result of this was the collection of a great number of valuable observations, which were published in successive volumes of a work, entitled, "Ratio Medendi in Nosocomio Practico," amounting ultimately to 16. He left also several other works, as On the Division of Fevers, &c., and died at the age of 72. He was generally an enemy to new opinions and innovations in practice, which led him into several controversies; particularly against variolous inoculation, and the use of poisonous plants in medicine: but he exhibited much learning and practical knowledge.

HAGIOSPE'RMUM. (From αγιος, holy, and σπερμα, seed: so called from its reputed virtues.) Wormseed.

HAGIO'XYLUM. (From αγιος, holy, and ξυλον, wood: so named because of its medical virtues.) Guaiacum.

HAIR. See *Capillus*.

[HAIR SALT. The *Haar salz*, (or hair salt,) of Werner, formerly supposed to be a variety of alum, is, according to Klaproth, a mixture of the sulphates of magnesia and iron.—*Cleav. Min.* A.]

HALA'TIUM. (From αλς, salt.) A clyster, composed chiefly of salt.

Halberd-shaped leaf. See *Leaf*.

[HALB-OPAL. This is the *Semi-opal* of Jameson, and Cleaveland. The other synonymes are *La demi-opale* of Brochant; *Silex résinite* of Brogniart; *Quartz résinite commune* of Haüy: all these being the same as the *Halb-opal* of Werner. "This variety is a little harder than the precious opal, and is easily broken. Its fracture is imperfectly conchoidal with large cavities, or nearly even, usually more or less glistening and a little resinous, but sometimes nearly dull. The edges of the conchoidal fracture, and those of the fragments, are usually very sharp. It is more or less translucent, sometimes only in a slight degree at the edges, and some specimens are semitransparent." *Cleav. Min.* A.]

HALCHE'MIA. (From αλς, salt, and χεω, to pour out.) The art of fusing salts

HALELÆ'UM. (From αλς, salt, and ελαιον, oil.) A medicine composed of salt and oil.

HALICA'CABUM. (From αλς, the sea, and κακαβος, night-shade: so called because it grows upon the banks of the sea.) See *Physalis alkekengi*.

HA'LIMUS. (From αλιμος, belonging to the sea.) The *Atriplex halimus* of Linnæus or sea-purslain, said to be antispasmodic.

HALINI'TRUM. (From αλς, the sea, and νιτρον, nitre.) Nitre, or rather rock salt.

HA'LITUS. (From *halito*, to breathe out.) A vapour

HALLER, Albert, was born at Berne, where his father was an advocate, in 1709. He displayed, at a very early age, extraordinary marks of industry and talents. He was intended for the church, but having lost his father when only thirteen, he soon after determined upon the medical profession. Having studied a short time at Tubingen, he was attracted to Leyden by the reputation of Boerhaave, to whom he has expressed his obligations in the most affectionate terms; but he took his degree at the former place, when about seventeen years of age. He soon after visited England and France; then returning to his native country, first acquired a taste for botany, which he pursued with great zeal, making frequent excursions to the neighbouring mountains. He also composed a "Poem on the Alps," and other pieces, which were received with much applause. Having settled in his native city, about 1730, he began to give lectures on anatomy, but with indifferent success; and some detached pieces on anatomy and botany having gained him considerable reputation abroad, he was invited by George II., in 1736, to become professor in the university, which he had recently founded at Gottingen. He accepted this advantageous offer, and, though his arrival was rendered melancholy by the loss of a beloved wife, from some accident which occurred in the journey, he commenced at once the duties of his office with great zeal; he encouraged the most industrious of his pupils to institute an experimental investigation on some part of the animal economy, affording them his assistance therein. He was likewise himself indefatigable in similar researches, during the seventeen years which he spent there, having in view a grand reform in physiology, which his writings ultimately effected, dissipating the metaphysical and chemical jargon, whereby it was before obscured. He procured the establishment of a botanic garden, an anatomical theatre, a school for surgery and for midwifery, with a lying-in hospital, and other useful institutions at that university. He received also many honourable testimonies of his fame, being chosen a member of the Royal Societies of Stockholm and London, made physician and counsellor to George II., and the emperor conferred on him the title of Baron; which, however, he declined, as it would not have been esteemed in his native country. To this he returned in 1753, and during the remainder of his life discharged various important public offices there. He ultimately received every testimony of the general estimation in which he was held; the learned societies of Europe, as well as several sovereigns, vying with each other in conferring honours upon him. His constitution was delicate, and impatience of pain, or interruption to his studies, led him to use violent remedies when ill; however, by temperance and activity, he reached an advanced age, having died towards the end of 1777. He was one of the most universally informed men in modern times. He spoke with equal facility the German, French, and Latin languages; and read all the other tongues of Europe, except the Sclavonic; and there was scarcely any book of reputation, with which he was not acquainted. His own works were extremely numerous, on anatomy, physiology, pathology, surgery, botany, &c., besides his poems and political and religious publications. The principal are, 1. His large work on the Botany of Switzerland, in 3 vols. folio, with many plates; 2. Commentaries on Boerhaave's Lectures, 7 vols. octavo; 3. Elements of Physiology, 8 vols. quarto, a work of the greatest merit; 4. His "Bibliotheca," or Chronological Histories of Authors, with brief Analyses; 2 vols. quarto on Botany, two on Surgery, two on Anatomy, and four on the Practice of Medicine, displaying an immense body of research.

HALLUCINA'TIO. (From *hallucinor*, to err.) An erroneous imagination.

Halmyro'des. (From αλμυρος, salted.) A term applied to the humours; it means acrimonious. It is also applied to fevers which communicate such an itching sensation as is perceived from handling salt substances.

HA'LO. (From αλος, an area or circle.) The red circle surrounding the nipple, which becomes somewhat brown in old people, and is beset with many sebaceous glands.

Hama'lgama. See *Amalgam.*

HAMOSUS. Hooked. Applied to the bristly pubescence of seeds and plants; as the pericarpe of the *Arctium lappa;* the seeds of *Daucus muricatus,* and *Alisma cordifolia.*

HAMPSTEAD. A village near to London, where there is an excellent chalybeate water, not inferior to that of Tunbridge-wells in any respect, except being nearer to the metropolis.

HA'MULUS. (Diminutive of *hamus*, a hook.) A term in anatomy, applied to any hook-like process, as the hamulus of the pterygoid process of the sphenoid bone.

HA'MUS. A hook. A species of pubescence of plants formed of bristles, bent at their point into a hook; as in *Rumex tuberosus, Caucalis daucoides*, and *Galium aparine*, &c.

HAND. *Manus.* The hand is composed of the carpus or wrist, metacarpus, and fingers. The *arteries* of the hand are the palmary arch, and the digital arteries. The veins are the digital, the cephalic of the thumb, and the salvatella. The nerves are the cutaneous, externus, and internus.

Harde'sia. See *Lapis Hibernicus.*

HARE. See *Lepus timidus.*

HARE-LIP. *Lagocheilus; Lagostoma; Labium leporinum.* A fissure or longitudinal division of one or both lips. Children are frequently born with this kind of malformation, particularly of the upper lip. Sometimes the portions of the lip which ought be united, have a considerable space between them; in other instances they are not much apart. The cleft is occasionally double, there being a little lobe, or small portion of the lip, situated between the two fissures. Every species of the deformity has the same appellation of hare-lip, in consequence of the imagined resemblance which the part has to the upper lip of a hare.

The fissure commonly affects only the lip itself. In many cases, however, it extends along the bones of the palate, even as far as the uvula. Sometimes these bones are totally wanting: sometimes they are only divided by a fissure.

Such a malformation is always peculiarly afflicting. In its least degree, it constantly occasions considerable deformity; and when it is more marked, it frequently hinders infants from sucking, and makes it indispensable to nourish them by other means. When the lower lip alone is affected, which is more rarely the case, the child can neither retain its saliva, nor learn to speak, except with the greatest impediment. But when the fissure pervades the palate, the patient not only never articulates perfectly, but cannot masticate nor swallow, except with great difficulty, on account of the food readily getting up into the nose.

HARMO'NIA. (From αρω, to fit together.) Harmony. A species of synarthrosis, or immoveable connexion of bones, in which bones are connected together by means of rough margins, not dentiform: in this manner most of the bones of the face are connected together.

HARMOTOME. See *Cross-stone.*

HARRIS, Walter, was born at Gloucester about the year 1651. He took the degree of bachelor of physic at Oxford, but, having embraced the Roman Catholic religion, he was made doctor at some French university. He settled in London in 1676, and two years after, to evade the order that all Catholics should quit the metropolis, he publicly adopted the Protestant Faith. His practice rapidly augmented, and on the accession of William III. he was appointed his physician in ordinary. He died in 1725. His principal work, "De Morbis Acutis Infantum," is said to have been published at the suggestion of the celebrated Sydenham: it passed through several editions. He left also a Treatise on the Plague, and a collection of medical and surgical papers, which had been read before the College of Physicians.

HARROGATE. The villages of High and Low Harrogate are situate in the centre of the county of York, adjoining the town of Knaresborough. The whole of Harrogate, in particular, has long enjoyed considerable reputation, by possessing two kinds of very valuable springs: and, some years ago, the chalybeate was the only one that was used internally, while the sulphureous water was confined to external use. At present, however, the latter is employed largely as an internal medicine.

The sulphureous springs of Harrogate are four in number of the same quality, though different in the degree of their powers. This water, when first taken up, appears perfectly clear and transparent, and sends forth a few air bubbles, but not in any quantity. It possesses a very strong sulphureous and fœtid smell, precisely like that of a damp rusty gun barrel, or bilge-water. To the taste it is bitter, nauseous, and strongly saline, which is soon borne without any disgust. In a few hours of exposure this water loses its transparency, and becomes somewhat pearly, and rather greenish to the eye; its sulphureous smell abates, and at last the sulphur is deposited in the form of a thin film, on the bottom and sides of the vessel in which it is kept. The volatile productions of this water show carbonic acid, sulphuretted hydrogen, and azotic gas.

The sensible effects which this water excites, are often a headache and giddiness on being first drunk, followed by a purgative operation, which is speedy and mild, without any attendant gripes: and this is the only apparent effect the exhibition of this water displays.

The diseases in which this water is used are numerous, particularly of the alimentary canal, and irregularity of the bilious secretions. Under this water the health, appetite, and spirits improve; and, from its opening effects, it cannot fail to be useful in the costive habit of hypochondriasis. But the highest recommendation of this water has been in cutaneous diseases, and for this purpose it is universally employed, both as an internal medicine, and an external application: in this united form, it is of particular service in the most obstinate and complicated forms of cutaneous affections; nor is it less so in states and symptoms supposed connected with worms, especially with the round worm and ascarides, when taken in such a dose as to prove a brisk purgative; and in the latter case also, when used as a clyster, the ascarides being chiefly confined to the rectum, and, therefore, within the reach of this form of medicine. From the union of the sulphureous and saline ingredients, the benefit of its use has been long established in hæmorrhoidal affections.

A course of Harrogate waters should be conducted so as to produce sensible effects on the bowels; half a pint taken in the morning, and repeated three or four times, will produce it, and its nauseating taste may be corrected by taking a dry biscuit, or a bit of coarse bread after it. The course must be continued, in obstinate cases, a period of some months, before a cure can be expected.

HARTFELL. The name of a place near Moffat, in Scotland. It has a mineral water which contains iron dissolved by the sulphuric acid, and is much celebrated in scrofulous affections, and cutaneous diseases. It is used no less as an external application, than drank internally. The effects of this water, at first, are some degree of drowsiness, vertigo, and pain in the head, which soon go off, and this may be hastened by a slight purge. It produces generally a flow of urine, and an increase of appetite. It has acquired much reputation also in old and languid ulcers, where the texture of the diseased part is very lax, and the discharge profuse and ill conditioned.

The dose of this water is more limited than that of most of the mineral springs which are used medicinally. It is of importance in all cases, and especially in delicate and irritable habits, to begin with a very small quantity, for an over-dose is apt to be very soon rejected by the stomach, or to occasion griping and disturbance in the intestinal canal; and it is never as a direct purgative that this water is intended to be employed. Few patients will bear more that an English pint in the course of the day; but this quantity may be long continued. It is often advisable to warm the water for delicate stomachs, and this may be done without occasioning any material change in its properties.

HARTLEY, David, was born in 1705, son of a clergyman in Yorkshire. He studied at Cambridge, and was intended for the church, but scruples about subscribing to the 39 Articles led him to change to the medical profession; for which his talents and benevolent disposition well qualified him. After practising in different parts of the country, he settled for some time in London, but finally went to Bath, where he died in 1757. He published some tracts concerning the stone, especially in commendation of Mrs. Stephens's medicine, and appears to have been chiefly instrumental in procuring her a reward from Parliament; yet he is said to have died of the disease after taking about two hundred pounds of soap, the principal ingredient in that nostrum. Some other papers were also written by him; but the principal work, upon which his fame securely rests, is a metaphysical treatise, entitled 'Observations on Man, his Frame, his Duty, and his Expectations." The doctrine of vibration, indeed, on which he explained sensation, is merely gratuitous; but his Disquisitions on the Power of Association, and other mental Phenomena, evince great subtlety and accuracy of research.

HARTSHORN. See *Cornu.*

Hartshorn shavings. See *Cornu*

HART'S-TONGUE. See *Asplenium scholopendrium.*

HART-WORT. See *Laserpitium siler.*

Hart-wort of Marseilles. See *Seseli tortuosum.*

HARVEY, William, the illustrious discoverer of the circulation of the blood, was born at Folkstone, in Kent, in 1578. After studying four years at Cambridge, he went abroad at the age of 19, visited France and Germany, and then fixed himself at Padua, which was the most celebrated medical school in Europe, where he was created Doctor in 1602. On returning to England he repeated his graduation at Cambridge, and settled in London: he became a Fellow of the College of Physicians in 1603, and soon after physician to St. Bartholomew's hospital. In 1615 he was appointed Lecturer on Anatomy and Surgery to the College, which was probably the more immediate cause of the publication of his grand discovery. He appears to have withheld his opinions from the world, until reiterated experiment had confirmed them, and enabled him to prove the whole in detail, with every evidence of which the subject will admit. The promulgation of this important doctrine brought on him the most unjust opposition, some condemning it as an innovation, others pretending that it was known before; and he complained that his practice materially declined afterward: however, he had the satisfaction of living to see the truth fully established. He likewise received considerable marks of royal favour from James and Charles I., to whom he was appointed physician; and the latter particularly assisted his inquiries concerning generation, by the opportunity of dissecting numerous females of the deer kind in different stages of pregnancy. During the civil war, when he retired to Oxford, his house in London was pillaged, and many valuable papers, the result of several years labour, destroyed. He published his first work on the circulation in 1628, at Frankfort, as the best means of circulating his opinions throughout Europe; after which he found it necessary to write two "Exercitations" in refutation of his opponents. In 1651 he allowed his other great work, "De Generatione Animalium," to be made public, leading to the inference of the universal prevalence of oval generation. In the year following he had the gratification of seeing his bust in marble, with a suitable inscription recording his discoveries, placed in the hall of the College of Physicians, by a vote of that body, and he was soon after chosen President, but declined the office on account of his age and infirmities. In return he presented to the College an elegantly furnished convocation room, and a museum filled with choice books and surgical instruments. He also gave up his paternal estate of 56 pounds per annum for the institution of an annual feast, at which a Latin oration should be spoken in commemoration of the benefactors of the College, &c. He died in 1658. A splendid edition of his works was printed in 1766, by the College, in quarto, to which a Latin life of the author was prefixed, written by Dr. Laurence.

HASTATUS. Spear, or halberd-shaped. Applied to a triangular leaf, hollowed out at the base and sides, but with spreading lobes; as in *Rumex acetocella* and *Solanum dulcamara.*

Hatchet-shaped. See *Dolabriformis.*

HAUYNE. A blue-coloured mineral found imbedded in the basalt rock of Albaco and Frescate, which Jameson thinks is allied to the azure stone. So named after Haüy, the celebrated French mineralogist.

Hay, camel's. See *Juncus odoratus.*

HEAD. See *Caput.*

HEARING. *Auditus.* "The hearing is a function intending to make known to us the vibratory motion of bodies.

Sound is to the hearing what light is to the sight. Sound is the result of an impression produced upon the ear by the vibratory motion impressed upon the atoms of the body by percussion, or any other cause. This word signifies also the vibratory motion itself. When the atoms of a body have been thus put in motion, they communicate it to the surrounding elastic bodies: these communicate it in the same manner, and so the vibratory motion is often continued to a great distance. In general, only elastic bodies are capable of producing and propagating sound; but for the most part solid bodies produce it, and the air is generally the medium by which it reaches the ear.

There a e three things distinguished in sound, *intensity*, *tone*, and *timbre*, or *expression*. The intensity of sound depends on the extent of the vibrations.

The tone depends on the number of vibrations which are produced in a given time, and, in this respect, sound is distinguished into *acute* and *grave*. The grave sound arises from a small number of vibrations, the acute from a great number.

The gravest sound which the air is capable of perceiving, is formed of thirty-two vibrations in a second. The most acute sound is formed of twelve thousand vibrations in a second. Between these two limits are contained all the distinguishable sounds; that is, those sounds of which the ear can count the vibration. Noise differs from distinguishable sound in so much as the ear cannot distinguish the number of vibrations of which it is composed.

A distinguishable sound, composed of double the number of vibrations of another sound, is said to be its octave. There are intermediate sounds, between these two, which are seven in number, and which constitute the *diatonic scale*, or gamut: they are distinguished by the names, *ut*, *re*, *mi*, *fa*, *sol*, *la*, *si*.

When the sonorous body is put in motion by percussion, there is at first heard a sound very distinct, more or less intense, more or less acute, &c., according as it may happen; this is the fundamental sound; but with a little attention other sounds can be perceived. These are called harmonic sounds. This can be easily perceived in touching the strings of an instrument.

The *timbre*, or expression of sound, depends on the nature of the sonorous body.

Sound is propagated through all elastic bodies. Its rapidity is variable according to the body which propagates it. The rapidity of sound in the air is a thousand one hundred and thirty English feet. It is still more rapidly transmitted by water, stone, wood, &c. Sound loses its force in a direct proportion to the square of the distance; this happens at least in the air. It may also become more intense as it proceeds; as happens when it passes through very elastic bodies, such as metals, wood, condensed air, &c. All sorts of sounds are propagated with the same rapidity, without being confounded one with another.

It is generally supposed that sound is propagated in right lines, forming cones, analogous to those of light, with this essential difference, however, that, in sonorous cones, the atoms have only a motion of oscillation, while those of the cones of light have a real transitive motion.

When sound meets a body that prevents its passage, it is reflected in the same manner as light, its angle of reflection being equal to the angle of incidence. The form of the body which reflects sound, has similar influence upon it. The slowness with which sound is propagated, produces certain phenomena, for which we can easily account. Such is the phenomenon of echo, of the mysterious chamber, &c.

Apparatus of Hearing.—There are in the apparatus of hearing a number of organs, which appear to concur in that function by their physical properties; and behind them, a nerve for the purpose of receiving and transmitting impressions.

The apparatus of hearing is composed of the outer, middle, and internal ear; and of the acoustic nerve.

The auricle collects the sonorous radiations, and directs them towards the meatus externus; in proportion as it is large, elastic, prominent from the head, and directed forward. Boerhaave supposed he had proved by calculation, that all the sonorous radiations (or pulsations) which fall upon the external face of the pinna, are, ultimately, directed to the auditory passage. This assertion is evidently erroneous, at least for those pinnæ in which the *antihelix* is more projecting than the *helix*. How could those rays arrive at the concha, which fall upon the posterior surface of the antihelix? The pinna is not indispensable to the hearing; for, both in men and in the animals, it may be removed without any inconvenience beyond a few days.

The *Meatus auditorius* transmits the sound in the same manner as any other conduit, partly by the air it contains, and partly by its parietes, until it arrives at the membrane of the tympanum. The hairs, and the cerumen with which it is provided at the entrance, are intended to prevent the introduction of sand, dust, insects, &c.

The *Membrane of the Tympanum* receives the sound which has been transmitted by the meatus auditorius. In what circumstances is it stretched by the internal muscle of the malleus? Or when is it relaxed by the contraction of the anterior muscle of the malleus?—All our knowledge on this subject is merely conjectural. An opening made in this membrane does not much impair the faculty of hearing. As this membrane is dry and elastic, it ought to transmit the sound very well, both to the air contained in the tympanum, and to the chain of little bones. The chorda tympani cannot fail to participate in the vibrations of the membrane, and transmit impressions to the brain. The contact of any foreign body upon the membrane is very painful, and a violent noise also gives great pain. The membrane of the tympanum may be torn, or even totally destroyed, without deranging the hearing in any sensible degree.

The *Cavity of the Tympanum* transmits the sounds from the external to the internal ear. The transmission of sound by the tympanum happens—1st, By the chain of bones which has a particular action upon the membrane of the *fenestra ovalis*. 2d, By the air which fills it, and which acts upon the whole petrous portion, but particularly upon the membranum of the *fenestra ovalis*. 3d, By its sides.

The *Eustachian Tube* renews the air in the tympanum; being destroyed, it is said to cause deafness.

The notion of its being capable of carrying sound to the internal ear is erroneous; there is nothing to support this assertion: it permits the air to pass in cases when the *tympanum* is struck by violent sounds, and it permits the renewal of that which fills the *tympanum*, and the mastoid cells. The air in the *tympanum* being much rarefied, is very suitable for diminishing the intensity of the sounds it transmits.

The use of the *mastoid cells* is not well known; it is supposed that they help to augment the intensity of the sound that arises in the cavity. If they produce this effect it ought to be rather from the vibrations of the partitions which separate the cells than from the air which they contain. Sound may arrive in the *tympanum* by another way than the external meatus; the shocks received by the bones of the head are directed towards the temples, and perceived by the ear. It is well known that the movement of a watch is heard distinctly when it is placed in contact with the teeth.

We know little of the *functions* of the internal ear; we can only imagine that the sonorous vibrations are propagated in different modes, but principally by the membrane of the *fenestra ovalis*, by that of the *fenestra rotunda*, and by the internal partition of the *tympanum;* that the liquor of Cotunnius ought to suffer vibrations which are transmitted to the acoustic nerve. It may be conceived how necessary it is that this liquid should give way to those vibrations which are too intense, and which might injure this nerve. Possibly, in his case, it flows into the aqueducts of the *cochlea* and of the vestibule, which, in this respect, would *tube.*
have a great deal of analogy with the *Eustachian*

The internal *gyri* of the *cochlea* ought to receive the vibrations principally by the membrane of the *fenestra ovalis;* the vestibule, by the chain of bones; the semicircular canals, by the sides of the *tympanum*, and perhaps by the mastoid cells, which frequently extend beyond the canals. But the aid which is given to the hearing by each separate part of the internal ear is totally unknown.

The osseo-membraneous partition, which separates the *cochlea* into two parts, has given rise to an hypothesis which no one now admits.

The impressions are received and transmitted to the brain by the *acoustic nerve;* the brain perceives them with more or less facility and exactness in different individuals. Many people have a false ear, which means that they do not distinguish sounds perfectly.

There is no explanation given of the action of the acoustic nerve and of the brain in hearing.

In order to be heard, sounds must be within certain limits of intensity. Too strong a sound hurts us, while one too weak produces no sensation. We can perceive a great number of sounds at once. Sounds, particularly appreciable sounds, combined, and succeeding each other in a certain manner, are a source of agreeable sensations. It is in such combinations, for the production of this effect, that music is employed. On the contrary, certain combinations of sound produce a disagreeable impression; the ear is hurt by very acute sounds. Sounds which are very intense and very grave, hurt excessively the membrane of the *tympanum*. By the absence of the liquor of *Cotunnius*, the hearing is destroyed. When a sound has been of long duration, we still think we hear it, though it may have been some time discontinued.

We receive two impressions, though we perceive only one. It has been said that we use only one ear at once, but this notion is erroneous.

When the sound comes more directly to the one ear, it is in reality distinguished with more facility by that one, than by the other: therefore in this case we employ only one ear; and when we listen with attention to a sound which we do not hear exactly, we place ourselves so that the rays may enter directly into the concha; but when it is necessary to determine the direction of the sound, that is, the point whence it proceeds, we are obliged to employ both ears, for it is only by comparing the intensity of the two impressions, that we are capable of deciding from whence the sound proceeds. Should we shut one ear perfectly close, and cause a slight noise to be made, in a dark place, at a short distance, it would be utterly impossible to determine its direction; in using both ears this could be determined. In these cases the eye is of great use, for even in using both ears it is frequently impossible to tell in the dark from whence a sound comes. By the sound we may also estimate the distance of the body from which it proceeds: but in order to judge exactly in this respect we ought to be perfectly acquainted with the nature of the sound, for without this condition the estimation is always erroneous. The principle upon which we judge is, that an intense sound proceeds from a body which is near, while a feeble sound proceeds from a body at a distance: if it happen that an intense sound comes from a distant body while a feeble sound proceeds from a body which is near, we fall into acoustic errors. We are generally very subject to deception with regard to the point whence a sound comes: sight and reason are of great use in assisting our judgment.

The different degree of convergence, and divergence, of the sonorous rays, do not seem to have any influence on the hearing, neither are they modified in their course, except for the purpose of making them enter into the ear in greater quantity: it is to produce this effect that speaking trumpets are used for those who do not hear well. Sometimes it is necessary to diminish the intensity of sounds: in this case a soft and scarcely elastic body is placed in the external meatus." —*Magendie's Physiology*.

HEART. *Cor*. A hollow muscular viscus, situated in the cavity of the pericardium for the circulation of the blood. It is divided externally into a *base*, or its broad part; a *superior* and an *inferior surface*, and an *anterior* and *posterior* margin. Internally, it is divided into a *right* and *left ventricle*. The situation of the heart is oblique, not transverse; its base being placed on the right of the bodies of the vertebræ, and its apex obliquely to the sixth rib on the left side; so that the left ventricle is almost posterior, and the right anterior. Its inferior surface lies upon the diaphragm. There are two cavities adhering to the base of the heart, from their resemblance called *auricles*. The right auricle is a muscular sac, in which are four *apertures*, two of the venæ cavæ, an opening into the right ventricle, and the opening of the coronary vein. The left is a similar sac, in which there are five *apertures*, viz. those of the four pulmonary veins, and an opening into the left ventricle. The cavities in the heart are called *ventricles*: these are divided by a fleshy septum, called *septum cordis*, into a right and left. Each ventricle has two *orifices*; the one auricular, through which the blood enters, the other arterious, through which the blood passes out. These four orifices are supplied with *valves*, which are named from their resemblance; those at the arterior orifices are called the *semilunar*; those at the orifice of the right auricle, *tricuspid*; and those at the orifice of the left auricle, *mitral*. *The valve of Eustachius* is situated at the termination of the vena cava inferior, just within the auricle. The substance of the heart is muscular; its exterior fibres are longitudinal, its middle transverse, and its interior oblique. The internal superfices of the ventricles and auricles of the heart are invested with a strong and smooth membrane, which is extremely irritable. The vessels of the heart are divided into *common* and *proper*. The *common* are, 1. The *aorta*, which arises from the left ventricle. 2. The *pulmonary artery*, which originates from the right ventricle. 3. The four pulmonary veins, which terminate in the left auricle. 4. The two *venæ cavæ*, which evacuate themselves into the right auricle. The *proper vessels are*, 1. The *coronary arteries*, which arise from the aorta, and are distributed on the heart. 2. The *coronary veins*, which return the blood into the right auricle. The *nerves* of the heart are branches of the eighth and great intercostal pairs. The heart of the fœtus differs from that of the adult, in having a *foramen ovale*, through which the blood passes from the right auricle to the left.

Heart-shaped. See *Cordatus*.

HEART'S EASE. See *Viola tricolor*

HEAT. See *Caloric*.

HEAT, ABSOLUTE. This term is applied to the whole quantity of caloric, existing in a body in chemical union.

HEAT, ANIMAL. "An inert body which does not change its position, being placed among other bodies, very soon assumes the same temperature, on account of the tendency of caloric to an equilibrium. The body of man is very different: surrounded by bodies hotter than itself, it preserves its inferior temperature as long as life continues; being surrounded with bodies of a lower temperature, it maintains its temperature more elevated. There are, then, in the animal economy, two different and distinct properties, the one of producing heat, the other of producing cold. We will examine these two properties. Let us first see how heat is produced.

The respiration appears to be the principal, or at least the most evident source of animal heat. In fact, experience demonstrates that the heat of the blood increases nearly a degree in traversing the lungs; and as it is distributed to all parts of the body from the lungs, it carries the heat every where into the organs; for we have also seen that the heat of the veins is less than that of the arteries.

This developement of heat in the respiration appears, as we have already said, to proceed from the formation of carbonic acid, whether it takes place directly in the lungs, or happens afterward in the arteries, or in the parenchyma of the organs. Some very good experiments of Lavoisier, and De Laplace, lead to this conclusion: they placed animals in a *calorimeter*, and compared the quantity of acid formed by the respiration, with the quantity of heat produced in a given time: except a very small proportion, the heat produced was that which would have been occasioned by the quantity of carbonic acid which was formed.

It has also been proved by the experiments of Brodie, Thillage, and Legallois, that if the respiration of an animal is incommoded, either by putting it in a fatiguing position, or in making it respire artificially, its temperature lowers, and the quantity of carbonic acid that it forms becomes less. In diseases when the respiration is accelerated, the heat increases, except in particular circumstances. The respiration is then a focus in which caloric is developed.

In considering for an instant only this source of heat in the economy, we see that the caloric must be distributed to the different parts of the body in an unequal manner; those farthest from the heart, those that receive least blood, or which cool more rapidly, must generally be colder than those that are differently disposed.

This difference partly exists. The extremities are

colder than the trunk; sometimes they present only 89° or 91° F., and often much less, while the cavity of the thorax is about 104° F.: but the extremities have a considerable surface relative to their mass; they are farther from the heart, and receive less blood than most of the organs of the trunk.

On account of the extent of their surface and distance from the heart, the feet and hands would probably have a temperature still lower than that which is peculiar to them, if these parts did not receive a greater proportional quantity of blood. The same disposition exists for all the exterior organs that have a very large surface, as the nose, the pavilion of the ear, &c.: their temperature is also higher than their surface and distance from the heart would seem to indicate.

Notwithstanding the providence of nature, those parts that have large surfaces lose their caloric with greater facility; and they are not only habitually colder than the others, but their temperature often becomes very low: the temperature of the feet and hands in winter is often nearly as low as 32° F. It is on this account we expose them so willingly to the heat of our fires.

Among other means that we instinctively employ to remedy or prevent coldness, are motion, walking, running, leaping, which accelerate the circulation; pressure, shocks upon the skin, which attract a great quantity of blood into the tissue of this membrane. Another equally effective means consists in diminishing the surface in contact with the bodies that deprive us of caloric. Thus we bend the different parts of the limbs upon each other, we apply them forcibly to the trunk when the exterior temperature is very low. Children and weak persons often take this position when in bed. In this respect it would be very proper that young children should not be confined too much in their swathing clothes to prevent them from thus bending themselves. Our clothes preserve the heat of our bodies; for the substance of which they are formed being bad conductors of caloric, they prevent that of the body from passing off.

According to what has been said, the combination of the oxygen of the air with the carbon of the blood is sufficient for the explanation of most of the phenomena presented by the production of animal heat; but there are several which, if real, could not be explained by this means. Authors worthy of credit have remarked, that, in certain local diseases, the temperature of the diseased place rises several degrees above that of the blood, taken at the left auricle. If this is so, the continual renewal of the arterial blood is not sufficient to account for this increase of heat.

This second source of heat must belong to the nutritive phenomena which take place in the diseased part.

There is nothing forced in this supposition; for most of the chemical combinations produce elevations of temperature, and it cannot be doubted that both in the secretions and in the nutrition, combinations of this sort take place in the organs.

By means of these two sources of heat, life can be maintained though the external temperature is very low, as that of winter in countries near the pole, which descends sometimes to — 42° F. Generally such an excessive cold is not supported without great difficulty, and it often happens that the parts most easily cooled are mortified: many of the military suffered these accidents in the wars of Russia. Nevertheless, as we easily resist a temperature much lower than our own, it is evident that we are possessed of the faculty of producing heat to a great degree.

The faculty of producing cold, or, in more exact terms, of resisting foreign heat, which has a tendency to enter our organs, is more confined. In the torrid zone, it has happened that men have died suddenly, when the temperature has approached 122° F.

But this property is not less real, though limited. Banks, Blagden, and Fordyce, having exposed themselves to a heat of nearly 260°, they found that their bodies had preserved nearly their own temperature. More recent experiments of Berger and Delaroche have shown that by this cause the heat of the body may rise several degrees: for this to take place it is only necessary that the surrounding temperature should be a little elevated. Having both placed themselves in a stove of 120°, their temperature rose nearly 6.8° F. Delaroche having remained sixteen minutes in a dry stove at 176°, his temperature rose 9° F.

Franklin, to whom the physical and moral sciences are indebted for many important discoveries, and a great many ingenious views, was the first who discovered the reason why the body thus resists such a strong heat. He showed that this effect was due to the evaporation of the cutaneous and pulmonary transpiration, and that in this respect the bodies of animals resemble the porous vases called *alcarrazas*. These vessels, which are used in hot countries, allow the water that they contain to sweat through them; their surface is always humid, and a rapid evaporation takes place, which cools the liquid they contain.

In order to prove this important result, Delaroche placed animals in a hot atmosphere that was so saturated with humidity that no evaporation could take place. These animals could not support a heat but a little greater than their own without perishing, and they became heated, because they had no longer the means of cooling themselves. Thus, there is no doubt that the cutaneous and pulmonary evaporation are the causes which enable man and animals to resist a strong heat. This explanation is also confirmed by the considerable loss of weight that the body suffers after having been exposed to a great heat.

According to these facts it is evident that the authors who have represented animal heat as fixed, have been very far from the truth. To judge exactly of it, it would be necessary to take into account the surrounding temperature and humidity; the degree of heat of different parts ought to be considered, and the temperature of one part ought not to be determined by that of another.

We have few correct observations upon the temperature proper to the body of man; the latest are due to Edwards and Gentil. These authors observed that the most suitable place for judging of the heat of the body is the armpit. They noticed nearly 2½ degrees of difference between the heat of a young man and that of a young girl: the heat of her hand was a little less than 97½°, that of the young man was 98.4°. The same person observed great differences of heat in the different temperaments. There are also diurnal variations; the temperature may change about two or three degrees from morning to evening.—*Ure's Chem. Dict.*

HEAT, FREE. If the heat which exists in any substance be from any cause forced in some degree to quit that substance, and to combine with those that surround it, then such heat is said to be free, or sensible, until the equilibrium is restored.

HEAT, LATENT. When any body is in equilibrium with the bodies which surround it with respect to its heat, that quantity which it contains is not perceptible by any external sign, or organ of sense, and is termed combined caloric, or latent heat.

Heat, sensible. See *Heat, free.*

Heavy carbonated hydrogen. See *Carburetted hydrogen.*

HEAVY SPAR. Baryte. A genus of minerals, divided by Professor Jameson into four species.

1. *Rhomboidal* baryte, or *Witherite.* This is a carbonate of barytes; and is found in Cumberland and Durham.

2. *Prismatic* baryte, or *heavy spar*, a sulphate; found also in Cumberland and Durham.

3. *Diprismatic baryte*, or *strontianite.* A carbonate of barytes; found in Strontian, in Argyleshire.

4. *Axifrangible baryte*, or *Celestine.* A sulphate of strontites, with about two per cent. of sulphate of barytes: found near Edinburgh, in Inverness-shire, and Bristol.

Heavy inflammable air. See *Carburetted hydrogen gas.*

HEBERDEN, WILLIAM, was born in London in 1710, and graduated at Cambridge, where he afterward practised during ten years, and gave lectures on the Materia Medica. During this period he published a little Tract, entitled "Antitheriaca," condemning the complication of certain ancient Formulæ of Medicines. In 1748, he removed to London, having previously been elected a fellow of the College of Physicians; and he was shortly after admitted into the Royal Society. He soon rose to considerable reputation and practice in his profession. At his suggestion "the Medical Transactions of the College of Physicians," first appeared in 1768; and four other volumes have since been published at different periods. Dr. Heberden contributed some valuable papers to this work, especially on the Angina Pectoris, a disease not before described; and on Chicken Pox, which he first accurately distinguished from Small Pox. Some other papers of his appeared in the Philosophical Transactions. As he advanced in years he began to relax from the fatigue of practice: and in 1782 he drew up the result of his experience in a volume of "Commentaries," written in Latin, the great excellence of which is its style. He reserved it for publication, however, till after his death, which did not happen till 1801.

HECTIC. (*Hecticus*; from εξις, habit.) See *Febris Hectica.*

HE'DERA. (From *hæreo*, to stick, because it attaches itself to trees and old walls.) The name of a genus of plants in the Linnæan system. Class, *Pentandria*; Order, *Monogynia.* The ivy.

HEDERA ARBOREA. See *Hedera Helix.*

HEDERA HELIX. *Hedera arborea.* The ivy. The leaves of this tree have little or no smell, but a very nauseous taste. Haller informs us, that they are recommended in Germany against the atrophy of children. By the common people of this country they are sometimes applied to running sores, and to keep issues open. The berries were supposed by the ancients to have a purgative and emetic quality; and an extract was made from them by water, called by Quercetanus *extractum purgans.* Later writers have recommended them in small doses as alexipharmic and sudorific; it is said, that in the plague at London, the powder of them was given in vinegar, or white wine, with good success. It is from the stalk of this tree that a resinous juice, called *Gummi hederæ*, exudes very plentifully in warm climates. It is imported from the East Indies, though it may be collected from trees in this country. It is brought over in hard compact masses, externally of a reddish brown colour, internally of a bright brownish yellow, with reddish specks or veins. It has a strong, resinous, agreeable smell, and an adstringent taste. Though never used in the practice of the present day, it possesses corroborant, astringent, and antispasmodic virtues.

HEDERA TERRESTRIS. See *Glecoma.*

HEDERACEÆ. (From *hedera*, the ivy.) The name of an order of plants in Linnæus's Fragments of a Natural Method, consisting of the ivy and a few other genera which in their form and appearance resemble it.

Hedge hyssop. See *Gratiola officinalis.*

Hedge mustard. See *Erysimum officinale.*

Hedge mustard, stinking. See *Erysimum Alliaria.*

HE'DRA. 1. The anus.

2. Excrement.

3. A fracture

HEDYO'SMOS. Mint.

HEISTER, LAURENCE, was born at Frankfort on the Maine in 1683. After studying in different German universities, and serving sometime as an army-surgeon, he graduated at Leyden: and in 1709 was appointed physician general to the Dutch Military Hospital. The next year he became professor of anatomy and surgery at Altorf: and having distinguished himself greatly by his lectures and writings, he received in 1720 a more advantageous appointment at Helmstadt, under the Duke of Brunswick, as physician, Aulic counsellor, and professor of medicine; in which he continued, notwithstanding an invitation to Russia from the Czar Peter, till the period of his death in 1758. He was author of several esteemed works, particularly a Compendium of Anatomy, which became very popular, being remarkable for its conciseness and clearness. "His Institutions of Surgery," also gained him great credit; being translated into Latin, and most of the modern languages of Europe. Another valuable practical work was entitled "Medical, Surgical, and Anatomical Cases and Observations." He had some taste for botany also, which he taught at Helmstadt, and considerably enriched the garden there; but he unfortunately became an antagonist of the celebrated Linnæus, not properly appreciating the excellence of the system of that eminent naturalist.

HELCO'MA. Ulceration.

HELCONIA. (From ελκος, an ulcer.) An ulcer in the external or internal superficies of the cornea, known by an excavation and oozing of purulent matter from the cornea.

HELCY'DRION. (From ελκος, an ulcer, and υδωρ, water.) *Helcydrium.* A moist ulcerous pustule.

HELCY'STER. (From ελκω, to draw.) An instrument for extracting the fœtus.

HELE'NIUM. (From *Helene*, the island where it grew.) See *Inula helenium.*

HELIANTHUS. (From ηλιος, the sun; and ανθος, a flower. This name originated from the resemblance which its broad golden disk and ray bear to the sun, and is rendered further appropriate by its having the power of constantly presenting its flowers to that luminary.) The name of a genus of plants. Class, *Syngenesia*; Order, *Polygamia frustranea.* The sun-flower.

HELIANTHUS ANNUUS. The systematic name of the *Corona solis*, and *chimalatus.* The seeds have been made into a nutritious bread. The whole plant when young is boiled and eaten in some countries, as being aphrodisiac.

HELIANTHUS TUBEROSUS. Jerusalem artichoke. Although formerly in estimation for the table, this root is now neglected, it being apt to produce flatulency and dyspepsia.

HELICA'LIS MAJOR. See *Helicis major.*

HELICA'LIS MINOR. See *Helicis minor.*

HE'LICIS MAJOR. A proper muscle of the ear, which depresses the part of the cartilage of the ear into which it is inserted; it lies upon the upper or sharp point of the helix, or outward ring, arising from the upper and acute part of the helix anteriorly, and passing to be inserted into its cartilage a little above the tragus.

HELICIS MINOR. A proper muscle of the ear, which contracts the fissure of the ear; it is situated below the helicis major, upon part of the helix. It arises from the inferior and anterior part of the helix, and is inserted into the crus of the helix, near the fissure in the cartilage opposite to the concha.

HELIOTROPE. A sub-species of rhomboidal quartz.

HELIOTROPIUM. (Ἡλιοτροπιον τω μεγα, of Dioscorides; from ηλιος, the sun, and τροπη, a turning or inclination: because, says that ancient writer, it turns its leaves round with the declining sun.) The name of a genus of plants. Class, *Pentandria*; Order, *Monogynia.*

HELIOTRO'PII SUCCUS. See *Croton tinctorium.*

HE'LIX. (Ελιξ, from ειλω, to turn about.) The external circle or border of the outer ear, that curls inwards.

HELIX HORTENSIS. The garden snail.

HELLEBORA'STER. (From ελλεβορος, hellebore.) See *Helleborus fœtidus.*

HELLEBORE. See *Helleborus.*

Hellebore, black. See *Helleborus niger.*

Hellebore, white. See *Veratrum album.*

HELLE'BORUS. (Ελλεβορος: παρα το τη βορα ελλειν, because it destroys, if eaten.) The name of a genus of plants in the Linnæan system. Class *Polyandria*; Order, *Polygynia.* Hellebore.

HELLEBORUS ALBUS. See *Veratrum album.*

HELLEBORE FŒTIDUS. Stinking Hellebore, or bear's-foot. *Helleboraster. Helleborus—caule multifloro folioso, foliis pedatis*, of Linnæus. The leaves of this indigenous plant are recommended by many as possessing extraordinary anthelmintic powers. The smell of the recent plant is extremely fœtid, and the taste is bitter and remarkably acrid, insomuch that, when chewed, it excoriates the mouth and fauces. It commonly operates as a cathartic, sometimes as an emetic, and in large doses proves highly deleterious.

HELLEBORUS NIGER. Black hellebore, or Christmas rose. *Melampodium. Helleborus—scapo subbiflore subnudo, foliis pedatis*, of Linnæus. The root of this exotic plant is the part employed medicinally: its taste, when fresh, is bitterish, and somewhat acrid: it also emits a nauseous acrid smell: but, being long kept, both its sensible qualities and medicinal activity suffer very considerable diminution. The ancients esteemed it as a powerful remedy in maniacal cases. At present it is exhibited principally as an alterative, or, when given in a large dose, as a purgative. It often proves a very powerful emmenagogue in plethoric habits, where steel is ineffectual, or improper. It is also recommended in dropsies, and some cutaneous diseases.

HELMET-FLOWER. See *Anthora.*

HELMI'NTHAGOGUE. (*Helminthagogus*, from ελμινς, a worm, and αγω, to drive out.) Whatever destroys and expels worms. See *Anthelmintic.*

HELMINTHIA. The name of a genus of diseases

Class, *Cœliaca;* Order, *Enterica*, in Good's Nosology. Invermination, worms. It has three species, viz. *Helminthia alvi, podicis, erratica.*

HELMINTHI'ASIS. (Ελμινθιασις; from ελμινς, which signifies any species of worm.) A disease in which worms, or the larvæ of worms, are bred under the skin, or some external part of the body. It is endemial to Martinique, Westphalia, Transylvania, and some other places.

HELMINTHOCO'RTON. See *Corallina corsicana.*

HELMONT, JOHN BAPTIST VAN, was born of a noble family at Brussels in 1577. He exhibited very early proofs of superior abilities, and soon became convinced how much hypothesis was ranked under the name of science and philosophy in books; he seems to have perceived the necessity of experiment and induction in the discovery of real knowledge; but did not methodize his ideas sufficiently, to pursue that plan with its full advantage. After taking his degree at Louvain he travelled during ten years, and in this period acquired some practical knowledge of chemistry. On his return in 1609 he married a noble lady of large fortune, which enabled him to pursue his researches into the three kingdoms of nature with little interruption. He declined visiting patients, but gave gratuitous advice to those who went to consult him; and he boasts of having cured several thousands annually. He continued his investigations with astonishing diligence during thirty years, and made several discoveries in chemistry; among which were certain articles possessed of considerable activity on the human body. This confirmed his opposition to the Galenical school, the absurd hypotheses, and inert practice of which he attacked with great warmth and ability. Indeed he contributed greatly to overturn their influence; but from a desire to explain every thing on chemical principles, he substituted doctrines equally gratuitous or unintelligible. He published various works from time to time, which brought him considerable reputation, and he was repeatedly invited to Vienna; but he preferred continuing in his laboratory. He died in 1644.

HELO'DES. (From ελος, a marsh.) A term applied to fevers generated from marsh miasma.

HELO'SIS. (From ειλω, to turn.) An eversion or turning up of the eyelids.

HELVINE. A sub-species of dodecahedral garnet.

HE'LXINES. (From ελκω, to draw: so called because it sticks to whatever it touches.) Pellitory of the wall.

HEMALO'PIA. Corruptly written for hæmalopia.

HEMATIN. The colouring principle of logwood. See *Hæmatoxylon campechianum.*

HEMATU'RIA. See *Hæmaturia.*

HEMERALO'PIA. (From ημερα, the day, and ωψ, the eye.) A defect in the sight, which consists in being able to see in the daytime, but not in the evening. The following is Scarpa's description of this curious disorder. Hemeralopia, or *nocturnal blindness*, is properly nothing but a kind of imperfect periodical amaurosis, most commonly sympathetic with the stomach. Its paroxysms come on towards the evening, and disappear in the morning. The disease is endemic in some countries, and epidemic, at certain seasons of the year, in others. At sunset, objects appear to persons affected with this complaint as if covered with an ash-coloured veil, which gradually changes into a dense cloud, which intervenes between the eyes and surrounding objects. Patients with hemeralopia, have the pupil, both in the day and nighttime, more dilated, and less moveable than it usually is in healthy eyes. The majority of them, however, have the pupil more or less moveable in the daytime, and always expanded and motionless at night. When brought into a room faintly lighted by a candle, where all the bystanders can see tolerably well, they cannot discern at all, or in a very feeble manner, scarcely any one object; or they only find themselves able to distinguish light from darkness, and at moonlight their sight is still worse. At daybreak they recover their sight, which continues perfect all the rest of the day till sunset.

["According to M. Dujardin, this term is derived from ἡμέρα, the day, ἀλαος, blind, and ωψ, the eye; and in its right signification is therefore inferred to be *diurna cæcitudo*, or *day blindness.* In the same sense, Dr. Hillary and Dr Heberden, have employed the term "*Hemeralopia* then, which is of very rare occurrence, stands in opposition to the *nyctalopia* of the ancients, or *night-blindness.* Numerous modern writers, however, have used these terms in the contrary sense; considering the hemeralopia, as denoting sight during the day, and blindness in the night; and nyctalopia as expressing night-seeing, (owl-sight, as the French call it,) and blindness during the daytime."—*Cooper's Sur. Dic.* A.]

HEMERALOPS. (From ημερα, the day, and ωψ, the eye.) One who can see but in the daytime.

HEMICERAU'NIOS. (From ημισυς, half, and κειρω, to cut: so called because it was cut half way down.) A bandage for the back and breast.

HEMICRA'NIA. (From ημισυς, half, and κρανιον, the head.) A pain that affects only one side of the head. It is generally nervous or hysterical, sometimes bilious; and in both cases sometimes comes at a regular period, like an ague. When it is accompanied by a strong pulsation like that of a nail piercing the part, it is denominated *clavus.*

HEMIO'PSIA. (From ημισυς, half, and ωψ, an eye.) A defect of vision, in which the person sees the half, but not the whole of an object.

HEMIPA'GIA. (From ημισυς, half, and παγιος, fixed.) A fixed pain on one side of the head. See *Hemicrania.*

HEMIPLE'GIA. (From ημισυς, half, and πλησσω, to strike.) A paralytic affection of one side of the body. See *Paralysis.*

HEMLOCK. See *Conium maculatum.*

HEMLOCK-DROPWORT. See *Œnanthe crocata.*

Hemlock, water. See *Cicuta virosa.*

Hemorrhage from the lungs. See *Hæmoptysis.*

Hemorrhage from the nose. See *Epistaxis.*

Hemorrhage from the stomach. See *Hæmatemesis.*

Hemorrhage from the urinary organs. See *Hæmaturia.*

Hemorrhage from the uterus. See *Menorrhagia.*

HEMP. See *Cannabis.*

HEMP-AGRIMONY. See *Eupatorium cannabinum.*

Hemp, water. See *Eupatorium.*

HENBANE. See *Hyoscyamus.*

HE'PAR. (*Hepar, atis.* n. Ηπαρ, the liver.) See *Liver.*

HEPAR SULPHURIS. Liver of sulphur. A sulphuret made either with potassa or soda. See *Sulphuretum potassæ.*

HEPAR UTERINUM. The placenta.

HEPATA'LGIA. (From ηπαρ, the liver, and αλγος, pain.) Pain in the liver.

HEPATIC. (*Hepaticus;* from ηπαρ, the liver.) Belonging to the liver.

Hepatic air. See *Hydrogen sulphuretted.*

HEPATIC ARTERY. *Arteria hepatica.* The artery which nourishes the substance of the liver. It arises from the cœliac, where it almost touches the point of the *lobulus Spigelii.* Its root is covered by the pancreas; it then turns a little forwards, and passes under the pylorus to the porta of the liver, and runs between the biliary ducts and the vena portæ, where it divides into two large branches, one of which enters the right, and the other the left lobe of the liver. In this place it is enclosed along with all the other vessels in the capsule of Glisson.

HEPATIC DUCT. *Ductus hepaticus.* The trunk of the biliary pores. It runs from the sinus of the liver towards the duodenum, and is joined by the cystic duct, to form the ductus communis choledochus. See *Biliary duct.*

HEPATIC VEINS. See *Vein*, and *Vena portæ.*

HEPATICA. (From ηπαρ, the liver: so called because it was thought to be useful in diseases of the liver.) See *Marchantia polymorpha.*

HEPATICA NOBILIS. See *Anemone hepatica.*

HEPATICA TERRESTRIS. See *Marchantia polymorpha.*

HEPATIRRHŒ'A. (From ηπαρ, the liver, and ρεω, to flow.) 1. A purging with bilious evacuations.

2. A diarrhœa, in which portions of flesh, like liver are voided.

HEPATITE. Fœtid, straight, lamellar, heavy spar. A variety of lamellar barytes, containing a small quantity of sulphur, in consequence of which, when it is heated or rubbed, it emits a fœtid sulphureous odour.

HEPATI'TIS. (From ηπαρ, the liver.) *Inflammatio hepatis.* An inflammation of the liver. A genus of disease in the class *Pyrexiæ*, and order *Phlegmasiæ* of Cullen, who defines it "febrile affection, attended with tension and pain of the right hypochondrium, often pungent, like that of a pleurisy, but more frequently dull, or obtuse, a pain at the clavicle and at the top of the shoulder of the right side; much uneasiness in lying down on the left side: difficulty of breathing; a dry cough, vomiting, and hiccup."

Besides the causes producing other inflammations, such as the application of cold, external injuries from contusions, blows, &c. this disease may be occasioned by certain passions of the mind, by violent exercise, by intense summer heats, by long-continued intermittent and remittent fevers, and by various solid concretions in the substance of the liver. In warm climates this viscus is more apt to be affected with inflammation than perhaps any other part of the body, probably from the increased secretion of bile which takes place when the blood is thrown on the internal parts, by an exposure to cold; or from the bile becoming acrid, and thereby exciting an irritation in the part. Hepatitis has generally been considered of two kinds; one the *acute*, the other *chronic*.

The *acute* species of hepatitis comes on with a pain in the right hypochondrium, extending up to the clavicle and shoulder; which is much increased by pressing upon the part, and is accompanied with a cough, oppression of breathing, and difficulty of lying on the left side; together with nausea and sickness, and often with a vomiting of bilious matter. The urine is of a deep saffron colour, and small in quantity; there is oss of appetite, great thirst, and costiveness, with a strong, hard, and frequent pulse; and when the disease has continued for some days, the skin and eyes become tinged of a deep yellow. When the inflammation is in the cellular structure or substance of the liver, it is called by some *hepatitis parenchymatosa*, and when the gall-bladder which is attached to this organ, is the seat of the inflammation, it has been called *hepatitis cystica*.

The *chronic* species is usually accompanied with a morbid complexion, loss of appetite and flesh, costiveness, indigestion, flatulency, pains in the stomach, a yellow tinge of the skin and eyes, clay-coloured stools, high-coloured urine, depositing a red sediment and ropy mucus; an obtuse pain in the region of the liver, extending to the shoulder, and not unfrequently with a considerable degree of asthma.

These symptoms are, however, often so mild and insignificant as to pass almost unnoticed; as large abscesses have been found in the liver upon dissection, which in the person's lifetime had created little or no inconvenience, and which we may presume to have been occasioned by some previous inflammation.

Hepatitis, like other inflammations, may end in resolution, suppuration, gangrene, or scirrhus, but its termination in gangrene is a rare occurrence.

The disease is seldom attended with fatal consequences of an immediate nature, and is often carried off by hæmorrhage from the nose, or hæmorrhoidal vessels, and likewise by sweating, by a diarrhœa, or by an evacuation of urine, depositing a copious sediment. In a few instances, it has been observed to cease on the appearance of erysipelas, in some external part.

When suppuration takes place, as it generally does, before this forms an adhesion with some neighbouring part, the pus is usually discharged by the different outlets with which this part is connected, as by coughing, vomiting, purging, or by an abscess breaking outwardly; but, in some instances, the pus has been discharged into the cavity of the abdomen, where no such adhesion had been formed.

On dissection, the liver is often found much enlarged, and hard to the touch; its colour is more of a deep purple than what is natural, and its membranes are more or less affected by inflammation. Dissections likewise show that adhesions to the neighbouring parts often take place, and large abscesses, containing a considerable quantity of pus, are often found in its substance.

The treatment of this disease must be distinguished, as it is of the acute, or of the chronic form. In acute hepatitis, where the symptoms run high, and the constitution will admit, we should, in the beginning, bleed freely from the arm; which it will seldom be necessary to repeat, if carried to the proper extent at first in milder cases, or where there is less power in the system, the local abstraction of blood, by cupping or leeching, may be sufficient. We should next give calomel alone, or combined with opium, and followed up by infusion of senna with neutral salts, jalap, or other cathartic, to evacuate bile, and thoroughly clear out the intestines. When, by these means, the inflammation is materially abated, we should endeavour to promote diaphoresis by suitable medicines, assisted by the warm bath; a blister may be applied; and the antiphlogistic regimen is to be duly enforced. But the discharge of bile, by occasional doses of calomel, must not be neglected: and where the alvine evacuations are deficient in that secretion, it will be proper to push this, or other mercurial preparation, till the mouth is in some measure affected. In India this is the remedy chiefly relied upon, and exhibited often in much larger doses than appear advisable in more temperate climates. Should the disease proceed to suppuration, means must be used to support the strength; a nutritious diet, with a moderate quantity of wine, and decoction of bark, or other tonic medicine: fomentations or poultices will also be proper to promote the discharge externally; but when any fluctuation is perceptible, it is better to make an opening, lest it should burst inwardly. In the chronic form of the disease, mercury is the remedy chiefly to be relied upon; but due caution must be observed in its use, especially in scrofulous subjects. It appears more effectual in restoring the healthy action of the liver, when taken internally: but if the mildest forms, though guarded by opium, or rather sedative, cannot so be borne, the ointment may be rubbed in. In the meantime, calumba, or other tonic, with antacids, and mild aperients, as rhubarb, to regulate the state of the primæ viæ, will be proper. Where the system will not admit the adequate use of mercury, the nitric acid is the most promising substitute. An occasional blister may be required to relieve unusual pain; or where this is very limited and continued, an issue, or seton may answer better. The strength must be supported by a light nutritious diet; and gentle exercise with warm clothing, to maintain the perspiration steadily, is important, in the convalescent state: more especially a sea voyage in persons long resident in India has often appeared the only means of restoring perfect health.

Hepatitis parenchymatosa. Inflammation of the substance of the liver.

Hepatitis peritonæalis. Inflammation in the peritonæum covering the liver.

HEPATOCE'LE. (From ηπαρ, the liver, and κηλη, a tumour.) A hernia, in which a portion of the liver protrudes through the abdominal parietes.

Hepato'rium. The same as *Eupatorium.*

Hephæ'stias. (From Ηφαιςος, Vulcan, or fire.) A drying plaster of burnt tiles.

Hepi'alus. (From ηπιος, gentle.) A mild quotidian fever.

HEPTA'NDRIA. (From επτα, seven, and ανηρ, a man, or husband.) The name of a class in the sexual system of plants, consisting of such hermaphrodite flowers as have seven stamens.

Heptapha'rmacum. (From επ7α, seven, and φαρμακον, medicine.) A medicine composed of seven ingredients, the principal of which were cerusse, litharge, wax, &c.

HEPTAPHY'LLUM. (From επ7α, seven, and φυλλον, a leaf: so named because it consists of seven leaves.) See *Tormentilla erecta.*

Heptaple'urum. (From επ7α, seven, and πλευρα, a rib: so named from its having seven ribs upon the leaf.) The herb plantain. See *Plantago major.*

HERA'CLEA. 1. Water hoarhound.

2. The common wild marjoram received a trivial name from its growing in abundance in Heraclea See *Origanum vulgare.*

HERA'CLEUM. (From *Heraclea*, the city near which it grows; or from Ἡρακλης, Hercules, being the plant sacred to him.) The name of a genus of plants in the Linnæan system. Class, *Pentandria;* Order, *Digynia.*

Heracleum gummiferum. This species is supposed by Wildenow to afford the gum ammoniacum. See *Ammoniacum.*

Heracleum spondylium. *Branca ursina Germa-*

nica; Spondylium. Cow-parsnip. All-heal. *Hera cleum—foliolis pinnatifidis, lævibus; floribus uniformibus* of Linnæus. The plant which is directed by the name of *Branca ursina* in foreign pharmacopœias. In Siberia it grows extremely high, and appears to have virtues in the cure of dysentery which the plants of this country do not possess.

["The *Heracleum Lanatum* is one of our largest native umbellate plants, growing frequently to the height of a man, with a stalk more than an inch in thickness. Its taste is strong and acrid. The bruised root or leaves, externally applied, excite rubefaction. Internally used, this article has been recommended in epilepsy. It appears to me to possess a virose character, and should be used with caution, especially when gathered from a watery or damp situation"—*Big. Mat. Med.* A.]

HERB-BENNET. See *Geum urbanum.*

HERB-OF-GRACE. See *Gratiola.*

HERB-MASTICH. See *Thymus mastichina.*

Herb-trinity. See *Anemone hepatica.*

HERBA. An herb. A plant is properly so called which bears its flower and fruit once only, and then with its root wholly perishes. There are two kinds: *annuals,* which perish the same year; and *biennials,* which have their leaves the first year, and their flowers and fruit the second, and then die away.

By the term *herba,* Linnæus denominates that portion of every vegetable which arises from the root, and is terminated by the fructification.

HERBA BRITANNICA. See *Rumex hydrolapathum.*

HERBA MILITARIS. See *Achillæa millefolium.*

HERBA SACRA. See *Verbena trifoliata.*

HERBA TRINITATIS. See *Anemone hepatica.*

HERBACEUS. Herbaceous. Plants are so considered which have succulent stems or stalks, and die down to the root every year.

HERBARIUM. A collection of dried or preserved plants; called also *Hortus siccus*

HERCULES'S ALL-HEAL. See *Laserpitium chironium.*

HERCULES BOVII. Gold and mercury dissolved in a distillation of copperas, nitre, and sea-salt.

HERE'DITARY. (From *hæres,* an heir.) A disease, or predisposition to a disease, which is transferred from parents to their children.

HERMA'PHRODITE. (*Hermaphroditus;* from Ἑρμης, Mercury, and Αφροδιτη, Venus, *i. e.* partaking of both sexes.) 1. The true hermaphrodite of the ancients was, the man with male organs of generation, and the female stature of body, that is, narrow chest and large pelvis; or the woman with female organs of generation, and the male stature of body, that is, broad chest and narrow pelvis. The term is now, however, used to express any *lusus naturæ* wherein the parts of generation appear to be a mixture of both sexes

2. In botany, an hermaphrodite flower is one which contains both the male and female organs, for the production of the fruit, within the same calyx and petals.

HERME'TIC. (From Ἑρμης, Mercury.) In the language of the ancient chemists, Hermes was the father of chemistry, and the hermetic seal was the closing the end of a glass vessel while in a state of fusion, according to the usage of chemists.

HERMODACTYL. See *Hermodactylus.*

HERMODA'CTYLUS. (Ἑρμοδακτυλος. Etymologists have always derived this word from Ἑρμης, Mercury, and δακτυλος, a finger. It is, however, probably named from *Hermus,* a river in Asia, upon whose banks it grows, and δακτυλος, a date, which it is like.) *Anima articulorum.* The root of a species of colchicum, not yet ascertained, but supposed to be the *Colchicum illyricum* of Linnæus, of the shape of a heart, flattened on one side, with a furrow on the other, of a white colour, compact and solid, yet easy to cut or powder. This root, which has a viscous, sweetish, farinaceous taste, and no remarkable smell, is imported from Turkey. Its use is totally laid aside in the practice of the present day. Formerly the roots were esteemed as cathartics, which power is wanting in those that reach this country

HE'RNIA. (From ἑρνος, a branch; from its protruding out of its place.) A rupture. Surgeons understand, by the term *hernia,* a tumour formed by the protrusion of some of the viscera of the abdomen out of that cavity into a kind of sac, composed of the portion of peritoneum, which is pushed before them. However, there are certainly some cases which will not be comprehended in this definition; either because the parts are not protruded at all, or have no hernial sac. The places in which these swellings most frequently make their appearance, are the groin, the navel, the labia pudendi, and the upper and forepart of the thigh; they do also occur at every point of the anterior part of the abdomen; and there are several less common instances, in which hernial tumours present themselves at the foramen ovale, in the perinæum, in the vagina, at the ischiatic notch, &c. The parts which, by being thrust forth from the cavity, in which they ought naturally to remain, mostly produce herniæ, are either a portion of the omentum, or a part of the intestinal canal, or both together. But the stomach, the liver, the spleen, uterus, ovaries, bladder, &c. have been known to form the contents of some hernial tumours. From these two circumstances of situations and contents, are derived all the different appellations by which herniæ are distinguished. If a portion of intestine only forms the contents of the tumour, it is called *enterocele;* if a piece of omentum only, *epiplocele;* and if both intestine and omentum contribute to the formation of a tumour, it is called *entero-epiplocele.* When the contents of a hernia are protruded at the abdominal ring, but only pass as low as the groin, or labium pudendi, the case receives the name of *bubonocele,* or *inguinal hernia;* when the parts descend into the scrotum, it is called an *oscheocele* or *scrotal hernia.* The *crural,* or *femoral hernia,* is the name given to that which takes place below Poupart's ligament. When the bowels protrude at the navel, the case is named an *exomphalos,* or *umbilical hernia;* and *ventral* is the epithet given to the swelling, when it occurs at any other promiscuous part of the front of the abdomen. The *congenital rupture* is a very particular case, in which the protruded viscera are not covered with a common hernial sac of peritoneum, but are lodged in the cavity of the tunica vaginalis, in contact with the testicle; and, as must be obvious, it is not named, like hernia in general, from its situation, or contents, but from the circumstances of its existing from the time of birth.

When the hernial contents lie quietly in the sac, and admit of being readily put back into the abdomen, it is termed a *reducible hernia:* and when they suffer no constriction, yet cannot be put back, owing to adhesions, or their large size in relation to the aperture, through which they have to pass, the hernia is termed *irreducible.* An *incarcerated,* or *strangulated* hernia, signifies one which not only cannot be reduced, but suffers constriction: so that, if a piece of intestine be protruded, the pressure to which it is subjected stops the passage of its contents onward towards the anus, makes the bowel inflame, and brings on a train of most alarming and often fatal consequences.

The general symptoms of a hernia, which is reducible and free from strangulation, are—an indolent tumour at some point of the parietes of the abdomen; most frequently descending out of the abdominal ring, or from just below Poupart's ligament, or else out of the navel; but occasionally from various other situations. The swelling mostly originates suddenly, except in the circumstances above related; and it is subject to a change of size, being smaller when the patient lies down upon his back, and larger when he stands up, or draws in his breath. The tumour frequently diminishes when pressed, and grows large again when the pressure is removed. Its size and tension often increase after a meal, or when the patient is flatulent. Patients with hernia, are apt to be troubled with colic, constipation, and vomiting in consequence of the unnatural situation of the bowels. Very often, however, the functions of the viscera seem to suffer little or no interruption.

If the case be an *enterocele,* and the portion of the intestine be small, the tumour is small in proportion; but though small, yet, if the gut be distended with wind, inflamed, or have any degree of stricture made on it, it will be tense, resist the impression of the finger, and give pain upon being handled. On the contrary if there be no stricture, and the intestine suffers no degree of inflammation, let the prolapsed piece be of what length it may, and the tumour of whatever size, yet the tension will be little, and no pain will attend the handling of it; upon the patient's coughing, it will feel as if it was blown into; and, in general, it will be found very easily returnable. A guggling noise is often made when the bowel is ascending.

If the hernia be an *epiplocele*, or one of the omental kind, the tumour has a more flabby and a more unequal feel, it is in general perfectly indolent, is more compressible, and (if in the scrotum) is more oblong and less round than the swelling occasioned in the same situation by an intestinal hernia; and, if the quantity be large, and the patient an adult, it is, in some measure, distinguishable by its greater weight.

If the case be an *entero-epiplocele*, that is, one consisting of both intestine and omentum, the characteristic marks will be less clear than in either of the simple cases; but the disease may easily be distinguished from every other one, by any body in the habit of making the examination.

Hernia cerebri. *Fungus cerebri.* This name is given to a tumour which every now and then rises from the brain, through an ulcerated opening in the dura mater, and protrudes through a perforation in the cranium, made by the previous application of the trephine.

Hernia congenita. (So called because it is, as it were, born with the person.) This species of hernia consists in the adhesion of a protruded portion of intestine or omentum to the testicle, after its descent into the scrotum. This adhesion takes place while the testicle is yet in the abdomen. Upon its leaving the abdomen, it draws the adhering intestine, or omentum, along with it into the scrotum, where it forms the hernia congenita.

From the term *congenital*, we might suppose that this hernia always existed at the time of birth. The protrusion, however, seldom occurs till after this period, on the operation of the usual exciting causes of hernia in general. The congenital hernia does not usually happen till some months after birth; in some instances not till a late period. Hey relates a case, in which a hernia congenita was first formed in a young man, aged sixteen, whose right testis had, a little while before the attack of the disease, descended into the scrotum. It seems probable that, in cases of hernia congenita, which actually take place when the testicle descends into the scrotum before birth, the event may commonly be referred, as observed above, to the testicle having contracted an adhesion to a piece of intestine, or of the omentum, in its passage to the ring. Wrisberg found one testicle which had not passed the ring, adhering, by means of a few slender filaments, to the omentum, just above this aperture, in an infant that died a few days after birth.

Excepting the impossibility of feeling the testicle in hernia congenita, as we can in most cases of bubonocele, (which criterion Mr. Samuel Cooper, in his Surgical Dictionary, observes Mr. Pott should have mentioned,) the following account is very excellent. "The appearance of a hernia, in very early infancy, will always make it probable that it is of this kind; but in an adult, there is no reason for supposing his rupture to be of this sort, but his having been afflicted with it from his infancy; there is no external mark, or character, whereby it can be certainly distinguished from the one contained in a common hernial sac; neither would it be of any material use in practice, if there was."

Hernia cruralis. Femoral hernia. The parts composing this kind of hernia are always protruded under Poupart's ligament, and the swelling is situated towards the inner part of the bend of the thigh. The rupture descends on the side of the femoral artery and vein, between these vessels and the os pubis. Females are particularly subject to this kind of rupture in consequence of the great breadth of their pelvis, while in them the inguinal hernia is rare. It has been computed, that nineteen out of twenty married women, afflicted with hernia, have this kind; but that not one out of a hundred unmarried females, or out of the same number of men, have this form of the disease. The situation of the tumour makes it liable to be mistaken for an enlarged inguinal gland; and many fatal events are recorded to have happened from the surgeon's ignorance of the existence of the disease. A gland can only become enlarged by the gradual effects of inflammation; the swelling of a crural hernia comes on in a momentary and sudden manner; and, when strangulated, occasions the train of symptoms described in the account of the hernia incarcerata, which symptoms an enlarged gland could never occasion. Such circumstances seem to be sufficiently discriminative: though the feel of the two kinds of swelling is often not in itself enough to make the surgeon decided in his opinion A femoral hernia may be mistaken for a bubonocele, when the expanded part of the swelling lies over Poupart's ligament. As the taxis and operation for the first case ought to be done differently from those for the latter, the error may lead to very bad consequences. The femoral hernia, however, may always be discriminated, by the neck of the tumour having Poupart's ligament above it. In the bubonocele, the angle of the pubes is behind and below this part of the sac; but in the femoral hernia, it is on the same horizontal level, a little on the inside of it.

Until very lately, the stricture, in cases of femoral hernia, was always supposed to be produced by the lower border of the external oblique muscle, or as it is termed, Poupart's ligament. A total change of surgical opinion on this subject has, however, latterly taken place, in consequence of the accurate observations first made in 1768, by Gimbernat, surgeon to the king of Spain. In the crural hernia, (says he,) the aperture through which the parts issue is not formed by two bands, (as in the inguinal hernia,) but it is a foramen, almost round, proceeding from the internal margin of the crural arch, (Poupart's ligament,) near its insertion into the branch of the os pubis. between the bone and the iliac vein, so that, in this hernia, the branch of the os pubis is situated more internally than the intestine, and a little behind; the vein externally, and behind; and the internal border of the arch before. Now it is this border which always forms the strangulation.

Hernia flatulenta. A swelling of the side, caused by air that has escaped through the pleura: an obsolete term.

Hernia gutturis. Bronchocele, or tumour of the bronchial gland.

Hernia humoralis. See *Orchitis.*

Hernia incarcerata. Incarcerated hernia. Strangulated hernia, or a hernia with stricture. The symptoms are a swelling in the groin, &c. resisting the impression of the fingers. If the hernia be of the intestinal kind, it is generally painful to the touch, and the pain is increased by coughing, sneezing, or standing upright. These are the very first symptoms, and, if they are not relieved, are soon followed by others; viz. a sickness at the stomach, a frequent retching, or inclination to vomit, a stoppage of all discharge per anum, attended with frequent hard pulse, and some degree of fever. These are the first symptoms; and if they are not appeased by the return of the intestine, that is, if the attempts made for this purpose do not succeed, the sickness becomes more troublesome, the vomiting more frequent, the pain more intense, the tension of the belly greater, the fever higher, and a general restlessness comes on, which is very terrible to bear. When this is the state of the patient, no time is to be lost; a very little delay is now of the utmost consequence; and if the one single remedy, which the disease is now capable of, be not administered immediately, it will generally baffle every other attempt. This remedy is the operation whereby the parts engaged in the stricture may be set free. If this be not now performed, the vomiting is soon exchanged for a convulsive hiccup, and a frequent gulping up of bilious matter: the tension of the belly, the restlessness and fever, having been considerably increased for a few hours, the patient suddenly becomes perfectly easy, the belly subsides, the pulse, from having been hard, full, and frequent, becomes low languid, and generally interrupted; and the skin, especially that of the limbs, cold and moist; the eyes have now a languor and glassiness, a lack lustre not easy to be described: the tumour of the part disappears, and the skin covering it sometimes changes its natural colour for a livid hue; but whether it keeps or loses its colour, it has an emphysematous feel, a crepitus to the touch, which will easily be conceived by all who have attended to it, but is not easy to convey an idea of by words. This crepitus is the too sure indicator of gangrenous mischief within. In this state, the gut either goes up spontaneously or is returned with the smallest degree of pressure; a discharge is made by stool, and the patient is generally much pleased at the ease he finds; but this pleasure is of short duration, for the hiccup and the cold sweats continuing and increasing, with the addition of spasmodic rigours and subtultus tendinum, the tragedy soon finishes.

HERNIA INGUINALIS. *Bubonocele.* Inguinal hernia. *The hernia inguinalis* is so called because it appears in both sexes at the groin. It is one of the divisions of hernia, and includes all those herniæ in which the parts displaced pass out of the abdomen through the ring, that is, the arch formed by the aponeurosis of the musculus obliquus externus in the groin, for the passage of the spermatic vessels in men, and the round ligament in women. The parts displaced that form the hernia, the part into which they fall, the manner of the hernia being produced, and the time it has continued, occasion great differences in this disorder. There are three different parts that may produce a hernia in the groin, viz., one or more of the intestines, the epiploon, and the bladder. That which is formed by one or more of the intestines, was called, by the ancients, *enterocele.* The intestine which most frequently produces the hernia, is the *ilium:* because, being placed in the iliac region, it is nearer the groin than the rest: but notwithstanding the situation of the other intestines, which seems not to allow of their coming near the groin, we often find the jejunum, and frequently also a portion of the colon and cæcum, included in the hernia. It must be remembered, that the mesentery and mesocolon are membranous substances, capable of extension, which, by little and little, are sometimes so far stretched by the weight of the intestines, as to escape with the ilium, in this species of hernia. The hernia made by the epiploon, is called *epiplocele;* as that caused by the epiploon and any of the intestines together, is called *entero epiplocele.* The hernia of the bladder is called *crytocele.* Hernia of the bladder is uncommon, and has seldom been known to happen but in conjunction with some of the other viscera. When the parts, having passed through the abdominal rings, descend no lower than the groin, it is called an incomplete hernia; when they fall into the scrotum in men, or into the *labia pudendi* in women, it is then termed complete.

The marks of discrimination between some other diseases and inguinal hernia are these:—

The disorders in which a mistake may possibly be made, are the circocele, bubo, hydrocele, and hernia humoralis, or inflamed testicle.

For an account of the manner of distinguishing circocele from a bubonocele, see *Circocele.*

The circumscribed incompressible hardness, the situation of the tumour, and its being free from all connexion with the spermatic process, will sufficiently point out its being a bubo, at least while it is in a recent state; and when it is in any degree suppurated, he must have a very small share of the *tactus eruditus* who cannot fee the difference between matter, and either a piece of intestine or omentum.

The perfect equality of the whole tumour, and freedom and smallness of the spermatic process above it, the power of feeling the spermatic vessels, and the vas deferens in that process; its being void of pain upon being handled, the fluctuation of the water, the gradual formation of the swelling, its having begun below and proceeded upwards, its not being affected by any posture or action of the patient, nor increased by his coughing or sneezing, together with the absolute impossibility of feeling the testicle at the bottom of the scrotum, will always, to an intelligent person, prove the disease to be hydrocele.

Pott, however, allows that there are some exceptions in which the testicle cannot be felt at the bottom of the scrotum, in cases of hernia. In recent bubonoceles, while the hernial sac is thin, has not been long, or very much distended, and the scrotum still preserves a regularity of figure, the testicle may almost always be easily felt at the inferior and posterior part of the tumour. But in old ruptures, which have been long, down, in which the quantity of contents is large, the sac considerably thickened, and the scrotum of an irregular figure, the testicle frequently cannot be felt; neither is it in general easily felt in the *congenital hernia,* for obvious reasons.

In the *hernia humoralis,* the pain in the testicle, its enlargement, the hardened state of the epididymus, and the exemption of the spermatic cord from all unnatural fulness, are such marks as cannot easily be mistaken; not to mention the generally preceding gonorrhœa. But if any doubt still remains of the true nature of the disease, the progress of it from above downwards, its different state and size in different postures, particularly lying and standing, together with its descent and ascent, will, if duly attended to, put it out of all doubt that the tumour is a *true hernia.*

When an inguinal hernia does not descend through the abdominal ring, but only into the canal for the spermatic cord, it is covered by the aponeurosis of the external oblique muscle, and the swelling is small and undefined.

Now and then, the testicle does not descend into the scrotum till a late period. The first appearance of this body at the ring, in order to get into its natural situation, might be mistaken for that of a hernia, were the surgeon not to pay attention to the absence of the testicle from the scrotum, and the peculiar sensation occasioned by pressing the swelling.

HERNIA INTESTINALIS. A rupture caused by the protrusion of a portion of the intestine. See *Hernia inguinalis.*

HERNIA ISCHIATICA. A rupture at the ischiatic notch. This is very rare. A case, however, which was strangulated, and undiscovered till after death, is related in Sir A. Cooper's second part of his work on hernia. The disease happened in a young man aged 27. On opening the abdomen, the ilium was found to have descended on the right side of the rectum into the pelvis; and a fold of it was protruded into a small sac, which passed out of the pelvis at the ischiatic notch. The intestine was adherent to the sac at two points; the strangulated part, and about three inches on each side, were very black. The intestines towards the stomach, were very much distended with air, and here and there had a livid spot on them. A dark spot was even found on the stomach itself, just above the pylorus. The colon was exceedingly contracted, as far as its sigmoid flexure. A small orifice was found in the side of the pelvis, in front of, but a little above the sciatic nerve, and on the forepart of the pyriformis muscle. The sac lay under the glutæus maximus muscle, and its orifice was before the internal iliac artery, below the obturator artery, but above the vein.

HERNIA LACHRYMALIS. When the tears pass through the puncta lachrymalia, but stagnate in the succulus lachrymalis, the tumour is styled *hernia lachrymalis* with little propriety or precision. It is with equal impropriety called, by Anel, *a dropsy of the lachrymal sac.* If the inner angle of the eye is pressed, and an aqueous humour flows out, the disease is the *fistula lachrymalis.*

HERNIA MESENTERICA. Mesenteric hernia. If one of the layers of the mesentery be torn by a blow, while the other remains in its natural state, the intestines may insinuate themselves into the aperture and form a kind of hernia. The same consequences may result from a natural deficiency in one of these layers. Sir A. Cooper relates a case, in which all the small intestines, except the duodenum, were thus circumstanced. The symptoms during life were unknown.

HERNIA MESOCOLICA. Mesocolic hernia. So named by Sir A. Cooper, when the bowels glide between the layers of the mesocolon. Every surgeon should be aware that the intestines may be strangulated from the following causes: 1. Apertures in the omentum, mesentery, or mesocolon, through which the intestine protrudes. 2. Adhesions, leaving an aperture, in which a piece of intestine becomes confined. 3. Membranous bands at the mouth of hernial sacs, which becoming elongated by the frequent protrusion and return of the viscera, surround the intestine, so as to strangulate them within the abdomen when returned from the sac.

HERNIA OMENTALIS. *Epiplocele.* A rupture of the omentum; or a protrusion of the omentum through apertures in the integuments of the belly. Sometimes, according to Sharpe, so large a quantity of the omentum hath fallen into the scrotum, that its weight, drawing the stomach and bowels downwards, hath excited vomiting, inflammation, and symptoms similar to those of the incarcerated hernia.

HERNIA PERINEALIS. Perineal hernia. In men, the parts protrude between the bladder and rectum; in women, between the rectum and vagina. The hernia does not project so as to form an external tumour; and, in men, its existence can only be distinguished by examining in the rectum. In women, it may be detected both from this part and the vagina.

HERNIA PHRENICA. Phrenic hernia. The abdominal viscera are occasionally protruded through the diaphragm, either through some of the natural apertures in this muscle, or deficiencies, or wounds, and lacerations in it. The second kind of case is the most frequent. Morgagni furnishes an instance of the first. Two cases related by Dr. Macauley, and two others published by Sir A. Cooper, are instances of the second sort. And another case has been lately recorded by the latter gentleman, affording an example of the third kind. Hildanus, Paré, Petit, Schenck, &c. also mention cases of phrenic hernia.

HERNIA PUDENDALIS. Pudendal hernia. This is the name assigned by Sir A. Cooper, to that which descends between the vagina and ramus ischii, and forms an oblong tumour in the labium, traceable within the pelvis, as far as the os uteri. Sir A. C. thinks this case has sometimes been mistaken for a hernia of the foramen ovale.

HERNIA SCROTALIS. *Hernia Oschealis. Oscheocele.* Paracelsus calls it *Crepatura.* When the omentum, the intestine, or both, descend into the scrotum, it has these appellations; when the omentum only, it is called *epiploscheocele.* It is styled a perfect rupture in contradistinction to a bubonocele, which is the same disorder; but the descent is not so great. The hernia scrotalis is distinguished into the true and false; in the former, the omentum or intestine, or both, fall into the scrotum; in the latter, an inflammation, or a fluid, causes a tumour in this part, as in hernia humoralis, or hydrocele. Sometimes sebaceous matter is collected in the scrotum; and this hernia is called *steatocele.*

HERNIA THYROIDEALIS. *Hernia foraminis ovalis.* Thyroideal hernia. In the anterior and upper part of the obturator ligament there is an opening, through which the obturator artery, vein, and nerve proceed, and through which occasionally a piece of omentum or intestine is protruded, covered with a part of the peritonæum, which constitutes the hernial sac.

HERNIA UMBILICALIS. *Epiploomphalon; Omphalocele; Exomphalos; Omphalos;* and when owing to flatulency, *Pneumatomphalos.* The exomphalos, or umbilical rupture, is so called from its situation, and has, like other herniæ, for its general contents, a portion of intestine, or omentum, or both. In old umbilical ruptures, the quantity of omentum is sometimes very great. Mr. Ranby says, that he found two ells and a half of intestine in one of these, with about a third part of the stomach, all adhering together. Gay and Nourse found the liver in the sac of an umbilical hernia; and Bohnius says that he did also. But whatever are the contents, they are originally contained in the sac, formed by the protrusion of the peritoneum.

In recent and small ruptures, this sac is very visible; but in old and large ones, it is broken through at the knot of the navel, by the pressure and weight of the contents, and is not always to be distinguished; which is the reason why it has by some been doubted whether this kind of rupture has a hernial sac or not.

Infants are very subject to this disease, in a small degree, from the separation of the funiculus; but in general they either get rid of it as they gather strength, or are easily cured by wearing a proper bandage. It is of still more consequence to get this disorder cured in females, than in males; that its return, when they are become adult and pregnant, may be prevented as much as possible; for at this time it often happens, from the too great distention of the belly, or from unguarded motion when the parts are upon the stretch.

Dr. Hamilton has met with about two cases annually for the space of seventeen years, of umbilical hernia, which strictly deserve the name of *congenital* umbilical hernia. The funis ends in a sort of bag, containing some of the viscera, which pass out of the abdomen through an aperture in the situation of the navel. The swelling is not covered with skin, so that the contents of the hernia can be seen through the then distended covering of the cord. The disease is owing to a preternatural deficiency in the abdominal muscles, and the hope of cure must be regulated by the size of the malformation and quantity of viscera protruded.

HERNIA UTERI. *Hysterocele.* Instances have occurred of the uterus being thrust through the rings of the muscles; but this is scarcely to be discovered, unless in a pregnant state, when the strugglings of a child would discover the nature of the disease. In that state, however, it could scarcely ever occur. It is the *cerexis* of Hippocrates.

HERNIA VAGINALIS. *Elytrocele.* Vaginal hernia. A tumour occurs within the os externum of the vagina. It is elastic, but not painful. When compressed, it readily recedes, but is reproduced by coughing, or even without this, when the pressure is removed. The inconveniences produced are an inability to undergo much exercise or exertion; for every effort of this sort brings on a sense of bearing down. The vaginal hernia protrudes in the space left between the uterus and rectum. This space is bounded below by the peritoneum, which membrane is forced downwards, towards the perinæum; but being unable to protrude further in that direction, is pushed towards the back part of the vagina. These cases probably are always intestinal. Some herniæ protrude at the anterior part of the vagina.

HERNIA VARICOSA. See *Circocele.*

HERNIA VENTOSA. See *Pneumatocele.*

HERNIA VENTRALIS. *Hypogastrocele.* The ventral hernia may appear at almost any point of the anterior part of the belly, but is most frequently found between the recti muscles. The portion of intestine, &c. &c. is always contained in a sac made by the protrusion of the peritonæum. Sir A. Cooper imputes its causes to the dilatation of the natural foramina, for the transmission of vessels, to congenital deficiencies, lacerations, and wounds of the abdominal muscles, or their tendons In small ventral herniæ, a second fascia is found beneath the superficial one; but in large ones the latter is the only one covering the sac.

HERNIA VENTRICULI. *Gastrocele.* A ventral rupture caused by the stomach protruding through some part of the abdominal parietes. It rarely occurs, but it does it generally at or near the navel.

HERNIA VESICALIS. *Hernia cystica; Cystocele.* The urinary bladder is liable to be thrust forth, from its proper situation, either through the openings in the oblique muscle, like the inguinal hernia, or under Poupart's ligament, in the same manner as the femoral.

This is not a very frequent species of hernia, but does happen, and has as plain and determined a character as any other.

HERNIA'RIA. (From *hernia*, a rupture: so called from its supposed efficacy in curing ruptures.) The name of a genus of plants in the Linnæan system. Class, *Pentandria;* Order, *Digynia.* Rupture-wort.

HERNIA GLABRA. The systematic name of the rupture-wort. *Herniaria.* This plant, though formerly esteemed as efficacious in the cure of hernias, appears to be destitute, not only of such virtues, but of any other. It has no smell nor taste.

HERNIO'TOMY. (*Herniotomia;* from *hernia*, and τεμνω, to cut.) The operation to remove the strangulated part in cases of incarcerated herniæ.

HE'RPES. From ἑρπω, to creep; because it creeps and spreads about the skin.) Tetter. A genus of disease in the class *Locales*, and order *Dialyses* of Cullen, distinguished by an assemblage of numerous little creeping ulcers, in clusters, itching very much, and difficult to heal, but terminating in furfuraceous scales.

Bell, in his Treatise on Ulcers, arranges the herpes among the cutaneous ulcers, and says, that all the varieties of importance may be comprehended in the four following species:

1. *Herpes farinosus*, or what may be termed the *dry tetter*, is the most simple of all the species. It appears indiscriminately in different parts of the body, but most commonly on the face, neck, arms and wrists, in pretty broad spots and small pimples. These are generally very itchy, though not otherwise troublesome; and, after continuing a certain time, they at last fall off in the form of a white powder, similar to fine bran, leaving the skin below perfectly sound; and again returning in the form of a red efflorescence, they fall off, and are renewed as before.

2. *Herpes pustulosus.* This species appears in the form of pustules, which originally are separate and distinct, but which afterward run together in clusters. At first, they seemed to contain nothing but a thin watery serum, which afterward turns yellow, and, exuding over the whole surface of the part affected, it at last dries into a thick crust, or scab; when this falls off, the skin below frequently appears entire, with only a slight degree of redness on its surface; but on some occasions, when the matter has probably been more acrid,

upon the scab falling off, the skin is found slightly excoriated. Eruptions of this kind appear most frequently on the face, behind the ears, and on other parts of the head; and they occur most commonly in children.

3. *Herpes miliaris.* The miliary tetter. This breaks out indiscriminately over the whole body; but more frequently about the loins, breast, perinæum, scrotum, and inguina, than in other parts. It generally appears in clusters, though sometimes in distinct rings, or circles, of very minute pimples, the resemblance of which to the millet-seed has given rise to the denomination of the species. The pimples are at first, though small, perfectly separate, and contain nothing but a clear lymph, which, in the course of this disease, is excreted upon the surface, and there forms into small distinct scales; these, at last, fall off, and leave a considerable degree of inflammation below, and still continues to exude fresh matter, which likewise forms into cakes, and so falls off as before. The itching, in this species of complaint, is always very troublesome; and the matter discharged from the pimples is so tough and viscid, that every thing applied to the part adheres, so as to occasion much trouble and uneasiness on its being removed.

4. *Herpes exedens,* the eating and corroding tetter (so called from its destroying or corroding the parts which it attacks,) appears commonly, at first, in the form of several small painful ulcerations, all collected into larger spots, of different sizes and of various figures, with always more or less of an erysipelatous inflammation. These ulcers discharge large quantities of a thin, sharp, serous matter, which sometimes forms into small crusts, that in a short time fall off; but most frequently the discharge is so thin and acrid as to spread along the neighbouring parts, where it soon produces the same kind of sores. Though these ulcers do not, in general, proceed farther than the cutis vera, yet sometimes the discharge is so very penetrating and corrosive as to destroy the skin, cellular substance, and, on some occasions, even the muscles themselves. It is this species that should be termed the *depascent,* or *phagedenic* ulcer, from the great destruction of parts which it frequently occasions. See *Phagedæna.*

Herpes ambulativa. A species of erysipelas which moves from one part to another.

Herpes depascens. The same as herpes exedens. See *Herpes.*

Herpes esthiomenos. Herpes destroying the skin by ulceration.

Herpes farinosus. See *Herpes.*

Herpes ferus. An erysipelas.

Herpes indica. A fiery, itchy herpes, peculiar to India.

Herpes miliaris. See *Herpes.*

Herpes periscelis. The shingles. See *Erysipelas phlyctænodes.*

Herpes pustulosus. See *Herpes.*

Herpes serpigo. The ring-worm.

Herpes siccus. The dry, mealy tetter

Herpes zoster. Shingles encircling the body. See *Erysipelas.*

HERPETIC. Relating to Herpes

He'rpeton. (From ἑρπεω, to creep.) A creeping pustule, or ulcer.

HESPERIDEÆ. (From *Hesperides,* whose orchards, according to the poets, produced golden apples.) Golden or precious fruit. The name of an order of plants in Linnæus's Fragments of a Natural Method, consisting of plants which have rigid evergreen leaves; odorous and polyandrous flowers; as the myrtle, clove, &c.

[" The *Heuchera Cortusa* of Michaux, is a native plant, growing in woods, from New-England to Carolina. The root is one of the strongest vegetable astringents. As such, it has been employed in various complaints, to which astringents are adapted, and favourable reports are made of its operation. Hitherto it has been more known as an external application than as an internal remedy."—*Big. Mat. Med.* A.]

HEWSON, William, was born at Hexham, in 1739. After serving an apprenticeship to his father, he came to London at the age of twenty, and resided with Mr. John Hunter, attending also the lectures of Dr. Hunter. His assiduity and skill were so conspicuous, that he was appointed to superintend the dissecting room, when the former went abroad with the army in 1760. He then studied a year at Edinburgh, and in 1762 he became associated with Dr. Hunter in delivering the anatomical lectures, and he was afterward allowed an apartment in Windmill-street. Here he pursued his anatomical investigations, and his experimental inquiries into the properties of the blood, of which he published an account in 1771. He also communicated to the Royal Society several papers concerning the lymphatic system in birds and fishes, for which he received the Copleyan medal, and was soon after elected a fellow of that body. He began a course of lectures alone in 1772, having quitted Dr Hunter two years before, and soon became very popular. In 1774, he published his work on the Lymphatic System. But not long after, his life was terminated by a fever, occasioned by a wound received in dissecting a morbid body, in the thirty-fifth year of his age.

HEXAGY'NIA. (From ἑξ, six, and γυνη, a woman, or wife.) The name of an order of plants in the sexual system, which, besides the classic character, have six females or pistils.

HEXA'NDRIA. (From ἑξ, six, and ανηρ, a man, or husband.) The name of a class of plants in the sexual system, consisting of plants with hermaphrodite flowers that are furnished with six stamens of an equal length.

Hexapha'rmacum. (From ἑξ, six, and φαρμακον, a medicine.) Any medicine in the composition of which are six ingredients.

Hibe'rnicus lapis. See *Lapis hibernicus.*

HIBI'SCUS. (From ιβις, a stork, who is said to chew it, and inject it as a clyster.) The name of a genus of plants in the Linnæan system. Class, *Monadelphia;* Order, *Polyandria.*

Hibiscus abelmoschus. The systematic name of the plant, the seeds of which are called musk-seed; *Abelmoschus; Granum moschi; Moschus Arabum; Ægyptia moschata; Bamia moschata; Alcea; Alcea Indica; Alcea Ægyptiaca villosa; Abrette; Abelmosch; Abelmusk.* The plant is indigenous in Egypt, and in many parts of both the Indies. These seeds have the flavour of musk. The best comes from Martinico. By the Arabians, they are esteemed cordial, and are mixed with their coffee, to which they impart their fragrance. In this country they are used by the perfumers.

HICCUP. *Singultus.* A spasmodic affection of the diaphragm, generally arising from irritation produced by acidity in the stomach, error of diet, &c.

HIDRO'A. (From ιδρως, sweat.) A pustular disease, produced by sweating in hot weather.

HIDRO'CRISIS. (From ιδρως, sweat, and κρινω, to judge.) A judgment formed from the sweat of the patient.

HIDRO'NOSOS. (From ιδρως, sweat, and νοσος, a disease.) The sweating sickness.

HIDROPY'RETUS. (From ιδρως, sweat, and πυρετος, a fever.) Sweating fever.

HIDRO'TICA. (From ιδρως, sweat.) Medicines which cause perspiration.

HIDROTOPOIE'TICA. (From ιδρως, sweat, and ποιεω, to make.) Sudorifics.

HI'ERA. (From ιερος, holy; and from ιεραξ, a hawk.) Holy. Also applied to some plants which hawks are said to be fond of.

Hiera picra. (From ιερος, holy, and πικρος, bitter. Holy bitter.) *Pulvis aloeticus,* formerly called *hiera logadii,* made in the form of an electuary with honey. It is now kept in the form of dry powder, prepared by mixing Socotorine aloes, one pound, with three ounces of white canella.

Hierabo'tane. (From ιερος, holy, and βοτανη, an herb: so called from its supposed virtues.) See *Verbena trifoliata.*

Hieraca'ntha. (From ιεραξ, a hawk, and ανθος, a flower: so named because it seizes passengers as a hawk does its prey.) A sort of thistle.

HIERA'CIUM. (From ιεραξ, a hawk: so called because hawks feed upon it, or because it was said that hawks applied the juice of it to cleanse their eyes.) The name of a genus of plants in the Linnæan system. Class, *Syngenesia;* Order, *Polygamia equalis.* Hawk-weed.

Hieracium pilosella. The systematic name of the mouse-ear, *Auricula muris; Pilosella; Myosotis; Hieraculum.* This common plant contains a bitter lactescent juice, which has a slight degree of astringeney. The roots are more powerful than the leaves. They are very seldom used in this country.

HIERA'CULUM. See *Hieracium.*

HIERA'NOSOS. (From ιερος, holy, and νοσος, a disease: so called because it was supposed to be that disorder which our Saviour cured in those who were said to be possessed of devils.) The epilepsy.

HIERA'TICUM. (From ιερος, holy.) A poultice for the stomach, so named from its supposed divine virtues.

Highgate resin. See *Fossil copal.*

HIGHMORE, NATHANIEL, was born at Fordingbridge, in Hampshire, in 1613. After graduating at Oxford, he settled at Sherborne, where he obtained considerable reputation in practice, and died in 1684. He pursued the study of anatomy with zeal, though with limited opportunities of dissection; and his name has been attached to a part, though not originally discovered by him, namely, the Antrum Maxillare, which had been before mentioned by Casserius. His principal work is "Corporis humani Disquisitio anatomica," printed at the Hague in 1651, with figures, chiefly from Vesalius. He also published two dissertations on Hysteria and Hypochondriasis; and a history of Generation.

Highmore's antrum. See *Antrum of Highmore.*

HIGUE'RO. The calabash-tree, the fruit of which is said to be febrifuge.

HILDA'NUS. See *Fabricius, William.*

HILUM. The scar, or point by which the seed is attached to its seed-vessel or receptacle, and through which alone life and nourishment are conveyed for the perfecting of its internal parts. Consequently all those parts must be intimately connected with the inner surface of this scar, and they are all found to meet there, and to divide or divaricate from that point, more or less immediately. In describing the form or various external portions of any seed, the *hilum* is always to be considered as the base. When the seed is quite ripe, the communication through this channel is interrupted, it separates from the parent plant without injury, a scar being formed on each. Yet the hilum is so far capable of resuming its former nature, that the moisture of the earth is imbibed through it, previous to germination.—*Smith.*

HIMANTO'SIS. (From ιμας, a thong of leather.) A relaxation of the uvula, when it hangs down like a thong.

HI'MAS. A relaxation of the uvula.

HIN. *Hindisch. Hing.* Assafœtida.

HIP. The ripe fruit of the dog-rose. They are chiefly used as a sweetmeat, or in a preserved state. See *Confectio rosæ caninæ.*

HIPPOCAMPUS. (Ιπποκαμπος, the name of a sea insect which has a head like that of the horse, and tail like the καμπη, or *eruca.*) 1. The sea-horse.

2. Some parts are so called from their supposed resemblance. See *Cerebrum.*

HIPPOCA'STANUM. (From ιππος, a horse, and καςανον, a chesnut: so called from its size.) See *Æsculus hippocastanum.*

HIPPOCRATES, usually called the father of physic, was born in the island of Cos, about 460 years before Christ. He is reckoned the 18th lineal descendant from Æsculapius, the profession of medicine having been hereditarily followed in that family, under whose direction the Coan school attained its high degree of eminence, and by the mother's side he is said to have descended from Hercules. Born with these advantages, and stimulated by the fame of his ancestors, he devoted himself zealously to the cultivation of the healing art. Not content with the empirical practice, which was derived from his predecessors, he studied under Herodicus, who had invented the gymnastic medicine, as well as some other philosophers. But he appears to have judged carefully for himself, and to have adopted only those principles, which seemed founded in sound reason. He was thus enabled to throw light on the deductions of experience, and clear away the false theories with which medicine had been loaded by those who had no practical knowledge of diseases, and bring it into the true path of observation, under the guidance of reason. Hence the physicians of the rational or dogmatic sect always acknowledged him as their leader. The events of his life are involved in much obscurity and fable. But he appears to have travelled much, residing at different places for some time, and practising his profession there. He died at Larissa, in Thessaly, at a very advanced age, which is variously stated from 85 to 109 years. He left two sons, Thessalus and Draco, who followed the same profession, and a daughter, married to his favourite pupil Polybus, who arranged and published his works; and he formed many other disciples. He acquired a high reputation among his countrymen, which has descended to modern times; and his opinions have been respected as oracles, not only in the schools of medicine, but even in the courts of law. He has shared with Plato the title of divine: statues and temples have been erected to his memory, and his altars covered with incense, like those of Æsculapius himself. Indeed, the qualifications and duties required in a physician, were never more fully exemplified than in his conduct, and more eloquently described than by his pen. He is said to have admitted no one to his instructions without the solemnity of an oath, in which the chief obligations are, the most religions attention to the advantages of the sick, the strictest chastity, and inviolable secrecy concerning matters which ought not to be divulged. Besides these characteristics, he displayed great simplicity, candour, and benevolence, with unwearied zeal, in investigating the progress and nature of disease, and in administering to their cure. The books attributed to him amount to 72; of which, however, many are considered spurious, and others have been much corrupted. The most esteemed, and generally admitted genuine, are the essay "On Air, Water, and Situation," the first and third books of "Epidemics," that on "Prognostics," the "Aphorisms," the treatise "On the Diet in acute Diseases," and that "On Wounds of the Head." He wrote in the Ionic dialect, in a pure but remarkably concise style. He was necessarily deficient in the knowledge of anatomy, as the dissection of human bodies was not then allowed; whence his Physiology also is, in many respects, erroneous: but he, in a great measure, compensated this by unceasing observation of diseases, whereby he attained so much skill in pathology and therapeutics, that he has been regarded as the founder of medical science: and his opinions still influence the healing art in a considerable degree. He diligently investigated the several causes of diseases, but especially their symptoms, which enabled him readily to distinguish them from each other: and very few of those noticed by him are now unknown, mostly retaining even the same names. But he is more remarkably distinguished by his Prognostics, which have been comparatively little improved since founded upon various appearances in the state of the patient, but especially upon the excretions. His attention seems to have been directed chiefly to these in consequence of a particular theory. He supposed that there are four humours in the body, blood, phlegm, yellow and black bile, having different degrees of heat or coldness, moisture or dryness, and that to certain changes in the quantity or quality of these, all diseases might be referred; and farther, that in acute disorders a concoction of the morbid humours took place, followed by a critical discharge, which he believed to happen, especially on certain days. But he seems to have paid little, if any, attention to the state of the pulse. He advanced another opinion, which has since very generally prevailed, that there is a principle, or power in the system, which he called Nature, tending to the preservation of health, and the removal of disease. He, therefore, advised practitioners carefully to observe and promote the efforts of nature, at the same time correcting morbid states by their opposites, and endeavouring to bring back the fluids into their proper channels. The chief part of his treatment at first was a great restriction of the diet; in very acute diseases merely allowing the mouth to be moistened occasionally for three or four days, and only a more plentiful dilution during a fortnight, provided the strength would bear it; afterward a more substantial diet was directed, but hardly any medicines, except gentle emetics, and laxatives, or clysters. Where these means failed, very active purgatives were employed, as hellebore, elaterium, &c. or sometimes the sudorific regimen, or garlic and other diuretics. He seems cautious in the use of narcotics, but occasionally had recourse to some of the preparations of lead, copper, silver, and iron. He bled freely in cases of extreme pain or inflammation, sometimes opening two veins at once, so as to produce fainting; and also took blood often by cupping, but preferably from a remote part, with a view of producing a revulsion. Where medicines fail, he recommends the knife, or even fire, as a last resource, and he advises trepanning, in cases of violent headache. But he wishes the more difficult operations of surgery to be performed only by particular persons, who might thereby acquire more expertness.

HIPPOCRATIC. Relating to Hippocrates. See *Facies hippocratica.*

HIPPOLA'PATHUM. (From ἱππος, a horse, and λαπαθον, the lapathum.) A species of lapathum; so named from its size. See *Rumex patientia.*

HIPPOMA'RATHRUM. (From ἱππος, a horse, and μαραθρον, fennel: so named from its size.) See *Peucedanum silaus.*

HIPPOSELI'NUM. (From ἱππος, a horse, and σελινον, purslane; so named because it resembles a large kind of purslane.) See *Smyrnaum olusatrum.*

HIPPU'RIS. (From ἱππος, a horse, and ουρα, a tail.) 1. Some herbs are thus named because they resemble a horse's tail.

2. The name of a genus of plants in the Linnæan system. Class, *Monandria;* Order, *Monogynia.* Mare's tail.

HIPPURUS VULGARIS. The systematic name of the horse's or mare's tail. *Equisetum; Cauda equina.* It possesses astringent qualities, and is frequently used by the common people as tea in diarrhœas and hæmorrhages. The same virtues are also attributed to the *Equisetum arvense, fluviatile, limosum,* and other species, which are directed indiscriminately by the term *Equisetum.*

HIPPUS. (From ἱππος, a horse; because the eyes of those who labour under this affliction are continually twinkling and trembling, as is usual with those who ride on horseback.) A repeated dilatation and alternate constriction of the pupil, arising from spasm, or convulsion of the iris.

HIR. (From χειρ, the hand.) The palm of the hand.

HIRA. (From *hir*, the palm of the hand; because it is usually found empty.) The intestinum jejunum.

HIRCUS. *Tragus.* The goat.

HIRCUS BEZOARTICUS. (*Quasi hirtus;* from his shaggy hair.) The goat which affords the oriental bezoar.

HI'RQUUS. (From ἑρκος, a hedge; because it is hedged in by the eyelash.) The angle of the eye.

HIRSUTIES. A trivial name in Good's Nosology for a species of disease in which hair grows in extraneous parts, or superfluously in parts where it naturally grows. *Trichosis hirsuties.*

HIRSUTUS. Hairy: applied to leaves, petals, seeds, &c. of plants; as the petals of the *Menyanthes trifoliata* and *Asclepias crispa:* the seeds of the *Scandix trichosperma.*

HI'RTUS. (A contraction of *hirsutus.*) Hairy: applied to stems of plants, as that of the *Cirastium alpinum.*

HIRU'DO. (*Quasi haurudo;* from *haurio*, to draw out: so named from its greediness to suck blood.) See *Leech.*

HIRUDO MEDICINALIS. See *Leech.*

HIRUNDINA'RIA. (From *hirundo*, the swallow: so called from the resemblance of its pods to a swallow.) Swallowwort, or asclepias. See *Lysimachia nummularia* and *Asclepias vincetoxicum.*

HIRU'NDO. (*Ab hærendo;* from its sticking its nest to the eaves of houses.)

1. The swallow.

2. The cavity in the bend of the arm.

HISPI'DULA. (From *hispidus*, rough: so named from the rough, woolly surface of its stalks.) See *Gnaphalium.*

HISPIDUS. Bristly: applied to stems, seeds, &c. of plants. The *Borago officinalis* is a good example of the *Caulus hispidus:* the seeds of the *Daucus carota*, and *Galium boreale.*

HOARHOUND. See *Marrubium.*

HODGES, NATHANIEL, son of the Dean of Hereford, was born at Kensington, and graduated at Oxford in 1659. He then settled in London, and continued there during the plague, when most other physicians deserted their post. He was twice taken ill, but by timely remedies recovered. He afterward published an authentic account of the disease, which appears to have destroyed 68,596 persons in the year 1665. It is to be regretted, that a person who had performed such an important and dangerous service to his fellow-citizens should have died in prison, confined for debt, in 1684

HOFFMANN, FREDERIC, was born at Halle, in Saxony, 1660. Having lost his parents from an epidemic disease, he went to study medicine at Jena, where he graduated in 1681. The year following he published an excellent tract, "De Cinnabari Antimonii," which gained him great applause, and numerous pupils to attend a course of chemical lectures, which he delivered there. He then practised his profession for two years at Minden with very good success; and after travelling to Holland and England, where he received many marks of distinction, he was appointed, on his return in 1685, physician to the garrison, and subsequently to Frederic William, Elector of Brandenburgh, and the whole principality of Minden. He was, however, induced to settle, in 1688, as public physician at Halberstadt; where he published a treatise, "De Insufficiencia Acidi et Viscidi." A university being founded at Halle, by Frederic III., afterward first King of Prussia, Hoffman was appointed, in 1693, primary Professor of Medicine, and composed the Statutes of that institution, and recommended Stahl as his colleague. He was most active in his professional duties; and by the eloquence and learning displayed in his lectures and publications, he extended his own reputation, and that of the new university. He was admitted into the scientific societies at Berlin, Petersburgh, and London; and had the honour of attending many of the German courts as physician. Haller asserts that he acquired great wealth by the sale of various chemical nostrums. He examined many of the mineral waters in Germany, particularly those of Seidlitz, which he first introduced to public notice in 1717. The year after he commenced the publication of his "Medicina Rationalis Systematica," which was received with great applause by the faculty in various parts of Europe, and is said to have occupied him nearly twenty years. He also published two volumes of "Consultations," and three books of select chemical observations. In 1727, he was created Count Palatine, by the Prince of Swartzenburgh, whom he carried through a dangerous disease. About seven years after, he attended Frederic William, King of Prussia, and is said by dignified remonstrance to have secured himself against the brutal ruedness shown by that monarch to those about him; he was ultimately distinguished with great honours, and invited strongly to settle at Berlin, but declined it on account of his advanced age. He continued to perform his duties at Halle till 1742, in which year he died. Hoffman was a very voluminous writer. His works have been collected in six folio volumes, printed at Geneva. They contain a great mass of valuable practical matter, partly original, but detailed in a prolix manner, and intermixed with much hypothesis. He has the merit, however, of first turning the attention of practitioners to the morbid affections of the nervous system, instead of framing mere mechanical or chemical theories; but he did not carry the doctrine to its fullest extent, and retained some of the errors of the humoral pathology. He pursued the study of chemistry and pharmacy with considerable ardour; but his practice was cautious, particularly in advanced age, trusting much to vegetable simples.

[HOFFMAN'S ANODYNE LIQUOR. Formerly so called; now known by the name of compound spirit of Sulphuric ether. A.]

Hog's fennel. See *Peucedanum.*

[*Hog-tooth spar.* A variety of calcareous spar. A.]

HO'LCIMOS. (From ἑλκω, to draw.) It sometimes means a tumour of the liver.

HO'LCUS. 1. The name of a genus of plants in the Linnæan system. Class, *Polygamia;* Order, *Monœcia.*

2. The Indian millet-seed, which is said to be nutritive.

HOLCUS SORGUM Guinea corn.

HOLERACEUS. See *Oleraceous.*

[HOLYOKE, DR. EDWARD. This beloved and venerated man was born at Marblehead, Mass. in 1728. The house in which he was born is still standing. He was graduated at Harvard University in 1746, and settled in this place in 1749, where he has ever since, for a period of 80 years, resided, useful, beloved and honoured. He was married, the first time in 1755, and a second time in 1759. He had by the second marriage 12 children, of whom only two survive. His only child by his first wife died in infancy He has lived in his mansion-house, in Essex-street, for the last 60 years, and at one period of his practice, he has stated that there was not a dwelling-house in Salem which he had not visited professionally. For a long period he nearly engrossed the medical practice of the place, and is known to have made a hundred professional visits in a day. This was in May or June of 1783, at which time the measles prevailed epidemically. He passed his long life in almost uninterrupted health, without any of those accidents and dangers which his skill was exerted to remedy and remove in others, and his old age has been almost without infirmity, and literally without decrepitude. Who that saw him does not recollect his firm and elastic step and his cheerful looks on the day of his hundredth anniversary? To much *exercise* and great *temperance* he was disposed to attribute his health and advanced age. And when to these causes we add those of pious opinions, virtuous practices, and a calm, cheerful, and contented spirit, we shall have disclosed much of the secret of his corporeal advantages. Of his temperance we are induced to make one remark, that it was not a system of rules in diet and regimen, but a temperance of *moderate desires*. He enjoyed all the bounties of Providence with remarkable appetency, but his well-regulated mind always saved him from excessive indulgence. Of his exercise some idea may be formed by a computation which he made a short time before his decease, that he had walked in the course of his practice, a distance which would reach three times round the globe. He died in 1829. A.]

Hollow leaf. See *Concavus*.

HOLLY. See *Ilex*.

Holly, knee. See *Ruscus*.

Holly, sea. See *Eryngium*.

HOLMI'SCUS. (Dim. of ολμος, a mortar.)

1. A small mortar.

2. The cavity of the large teeth, because they pound the food as in a mortar.

HOLMITE. A new mineral composed of lime, carbonic acid, alumina, silica, oxide of iron, and water.

HOLOPHLY'CTIDES. (From ολος, whole, and φλυκ7ις, a pustule.) Little pimples all over the body.

HOLO'STES. See *Holosteus*.

HOLO'STEUM. See *Holosteus*.

HOLO'STEUS. (From ολος, whole, and ος εον, a bone) Glue-bone. See *Osteocolla*.

HOLOTO'NICUS. (From ολος, whole, and τεινω, to stretch.) A term formerly applied to diseases accompanied with universal convulsion, or rigour.

HOLY THISTLE. See *Centaurea benedicta*.

HOLYWELL. There is a mineral water at this place arranged under the class of simple cold waters, remarkable for its purity. It possesses similar virtues to that of Malvern. See *Malvern water*.

HO'MA. An anasarcous swelling.

Homberg's phosphorus. Ignited muriate of lime.

Homberg's salt. See *Boracic acid*.

HOMOGENEOUS. (*Homogeneus*; from ομος, like, and γενος, a kind.) Uniform, of a like kind or species, of the same quality. A term used in contradistinction to *heterogeneous*, when the parts of the body are of different qualities.

HOMOPLA'TA. (From ωμος, the shoulder, and πλα7α, the blade.) See *Scapula*.

HONEY. See *Mel*.

HONEY-STONE. Mellite. Crystalhartz of Mohs. Pyramidal honey-stone of Jameson. This is of a honey colour, distinctly crystallized, and occurs on bituminous wood and earth coal, and is usually accompanied with sulphur at Artern, in Thuringia.

HONEY-SUCKLE. See *Lonicera periclymenum*.

Hooded leaf. *Cucullatus*.

HOOPING-COUGH. See *Pertussis*.

HOP. See *Humulus lupulus*.

HOPLOCHRI'SMA. (From οπλον, a weapon, and χρισμα, a salve.) A salve which was ridiculously said to cure wounds by consent; that is, by anointing the instrument with which the wound was made.

HORDE'OLUM. (Diminutive of *hordeum*, barley.) A little tumour on the eyelids, resembling a barley-corn. A stye. Scarpa remarks, the stye is strictly only a little bile, which projects from the edge of the eyelids, mostly near the great angle of the eye. This little tumour, like the furunculus, is of a dark red colour, much inflamed, and a great deal more painful than might be expected, considering its small size. The latter circumstance is partly owing to the vehemence of the inflammation producing the stye, and partly to the exquisite sensibility and tension of the skin, which covers the edge of the eyelids. On this account, the hordeolum very often excites fever and restlessness in delicate, irritable constitutions; it suppurates slowly and imperfectly; and, when suppurated, has no tendency to burst.

The stye, like other furunculous inflammations, forms an exception to the general rule, that the best mode in which inflammatory swellings can end, is resolution; for whenever a furunculous inflammation extends so deeply as to destroy any of the cellular substance, the little tumour can never be resolved, or only imperfectly so. This event, indeed, would rather be hurtful, since there would still remain behind a greater or smaller portion of dead cellular membrane; which, sooner or later, might bring on a renewal of the stye in the same place as before, or else become converted into a hard indolent body, deforming the edge of the eyelid.

HO'RDEUM. (*Ab horrore aristæ*; from the unpleasantness of its beard to the touch.) 1. The name of a genus of plants in the Linnæan system. Class *Triandria*; Order, *Digynia*. Barley.

2. The pharmacopœial name of the common barley See *Hordeum vulgare*.

HORDEUM CAUSTICUM. See *Cevadilla*.

HORDEUM DISTICHON. This plant affords the barley in common use. See *Hordeum vulgare*.

HORDEUM PERLATUM. See *Hordeum vulgare*.

HORDEUM VULGARE. The systematic name of the common barley. The seed called barley, is obtained from several species of *hordeum*, but principally from the *vulgare*, or common or Scotch barley, and the *distichon*, or *hordeum gallicum vel mundatum*, or French barley, of Linnæus. It is extremely nutritious and mucilaginous, and in common use as a drink, when boiled, in all inflammatory diseases and affections of the chest, especially where there is cough or irritation about the fauces. A decoction of barley with gum, is considered a useful diluent and demulcent in dysury and strangury; the gum mixing with the urine, sheaths the urinary canal from the acrimony of the urine. Among the ancients, decoctions of barley, κριθη, were the principal medicine, as well as aliment, in acute diseases. Barley is freed from its shells in mills, and in this state called Scotch and French barley. In Holland, they rub barley into small round grains, somewhat like pearls, which is therefore called *pearl barley*, or *hordeum perlatum*.

HORIZONTALIS. Horizontal: applied to leaves, roots, &c. which spread in the greatest possible degree; as the leaves of *Gentiana campestris*, and roots of the *Laserpitium prutenicum*.

HO'RMINUM. (From ορμαω, to incite: named from its supposed qualities of provoking venery.) See *Salvia sclarea*.

HORN. An animal substance chiefly membraneous, composed of coagulated albumen, with a little gelatin, and about a half per cent. of phosphate of lime. The horns of the buck and hart are of a different nature, being intermediate between bone and horn. See *Cornu*.

Horn silver. A chloride of silver.

HORNBLENDE. A sub-species of straight-edged augite. There are three varieties of it:

1. *Common hornblende*, which is of a greenish black colour: is an essential ingredient of the mountain rocks, syenite and green-stone, and occurs frequently in granite, gneiss, &c. It is found abundantly in the British isles, and on the Continent.

2. *Hornblende slate*, of a colour intermediate between green and black. It occurs in beds of gneiss in many parts of Scotland, England, and the Continent.

3. *Basaltic hornblende*, of a velvet black colour. It is found imbedded in basalt, along with olivine and augite, at Arthur's Seat, near Edinburgh, and in basaltic rocks of England, Ireland, and the Continent.

HORNSTONE. Professor Jameson's ninth sub species of rhomboidal quartz.

HORRIPILA'TIO. Horripilation. (From *horror*

and *pilus*, a hair.) A shuddering or a sense of creeping in different parts of the body. A symptom of the approach of fever.

Horse-chesnut. See *Æsculus hippocastanum.*

Horse-radish. See *Cochlearia armoracia.*

HORSE-TAIL. See *Hippurus vulgaris.*

HORSTIUS, GREGORY, was born at Torgau, in 1578. After studying in different parts of Germany and Switzerland, he graduated at Basil in 1606, and was soon after appointed to a medical professorship at Wittenburg. But two years after he received a similar appointment at Giessen, and was made chief physician of Hesse; where he attained considerable reputation in his profession. In 1722 he went to Ulm, on an invitation from the magistracy as public physician and president of the college; where his learning, skill, and humanity, procured him general esteem. He died in 1636. His works were collected by his sons in three folio volumes.

HO'RTUS. (From *orior*, to rise, as being the place where vegetables grow up.) 1. A garden.

2. The genitals of a woman, which is the repository of the human semen.

HORTUS SICCUS. A collection of dried plants

HOUNDS-TONGUE. See *Cynoglossum.*

HOUSE-LEEK. See *Sempervivum tectorum.*

HUBER, JOHN JAMES, was born at Basle in 1707, and graduated there at the age of 26, after studying under the celebrated Haller and other able teachers. Two years after he was appointed physician to the Court of Baden Dourlach. He materially assisted Haller in his work on the Botany of Switzerland, and was consequently invited by him in 1738 to be dissector at Gottingen.

He speedily rose to considerable reputation there, and received different public appointments. He had likewise the honour of being elected into the most celebrated of the learned societies in Europe. He died in 1778. The chief objects of his research were the spinal marrow, and the nerves originating from it: he also inquired into the supposed influence of the imagination of the mother on the fœtus, and into the cause of miscarriages.

[HULL, DR. AMOS G. This gentleman is a living practitioner of physic and surgery in the city of New-York. He has paid particular attention to the cure of Reducible Hernia, and has succeeded beyond all other surgeons in the cure of this frequent complaint. Practitioners have most usually directed their patients to *apply a truss.* Dr. Hull, however, in attending more particularly and personally to the adaptation of trusses to different kinds of Reducible Hernia, found that they were all made upon erroneous principles. He has accordingly invented a truss differing from all preceding trusses, and it has the general approbation of practitioners in this country, for its simplicity and superior utility. He has improved upon those he first made, and he now calls it his *improved hinge and pivot* Truss, for an account of which see article, TRUSS. A.]

HULME, NATHANIEL, was born at Halifax, in Yorkshire, 1732, and bred to the profession of a surgeon-apothecary. After serving some time in the navy, he graduated at Edinburgh in 1765. He then settled in London, and was soon after appointed physician to the General Dispensary, the first institution of that kind established in the metropolis. About the year 1775 he was elected physician to the Charter-house. In 1807 he died, in consequence of a severe bruise by a fall. He was author of several dissertations on scurvy, puerperal fever, &c. He also made a series of experiments on the light spontaneously emitted from various bodies, published in the Philosophical Transactions: and he was one of the editors of the London Practice of Physic.

HUMECTA'NTIA. (From *humecto*, to make moist.) Medicines which are supposed capable of softening by making the solids of the body moist.

HUMERAL. *Humeralis.* Belonging to the humerus or arm.

HUMERAL ARTERY. *Arteria humeralis.* Brachial artery. The axillary artery, having passed the tendon of the great pectoral muscle, changes its name to the brachial or humeral artery, which name it retains in its course down the arm to the bend, where it divides into the radial and ulnar arteries. In this course it gives off several muscular branches, three of which only deserve attention: 1. *The arteria profunda superior*, which goes round the back of the arm to the exterior muscle, and is often named the upper muscular artery. 2. Another like it, called *arteria profunda inferior*, or the lower muscular artery. 3. *Ramus anastomoticus major*, which anastomoses round the elbow with the branches of the ulnar artery.

HUMERALIS MUSCULUS. See *Deltoides.*

HU'MERUS. (From ωμος, the shoulder.)

1. The arm, as composed of hard and soft parts, from the shoulder to the forearm.

2. The shoulder.

3. The bone of the arm, or *os humeri, os brachii.* A long cylindrical bone, situated between the scapula and forearm. Its upper extremity is formed somewhat laterally and internally, into a large, round, and smooth head, which is admitted into the glenoid cavity of the scapula. Around the basis of this head is observed a circular fossa, deepest anteriorly and externally, which forms what is called the neck of the bone, and from the edge of which arises the capsular ligament, which is further strengthened by a strong membraneous expansion, extending to the upper edge of the glenoid cavity, and to the coracoid process of the scapula; and likewise by the tendinous expansions of the muscles, inserted into the head of the humerus. This capsular ligament is sometimes torn in luxation, and becomes an obstacle to the easy reduction of the bone. The articulating surface of the head is covered by a cartilage, which is thick in its middle part, and thin towards its edges; by which means it is more convex in the recent subject than in the skeleton. This upper extremity, besides the round smooth head, affords two other smaller protuberances. One of these, which is the largest of the two, is of an irregular oblong shape, and is placed at the back of the head of the bone, from which it is separated by a kind of groove, that makes a part of the neck. This tuberosity is divided, at its upper part, into three surfaces; the first of these, which is the smallest and uppermost, serves for the insertion of the supraspinatus muscle; the second or middlemost, for the insertion of the infraspinatus; and the third, which is the lowest and hindmost, for the insertion of the teres minor. The other smaller tuberosity is situated anteriorly, between the larger one and the head of the humerus, and serves for the insertion of the subscapularis muscle. Between these two tuberosities there is a deep groove for lodging the tendinous head of the biceps brachii; the capsular ligament of the joint affording here a prolongation, thinner than the capsule itself, which covers and accompanies this muscle to its fleshy portion, where it gradually disappears in the adjacent cellular membrane. Immediately below its neck, the os humeri begins to assume a cylindrical shape, so that here the body of the bone may be said to commence. At its upper part is observed a continuation of the groove for the biceps, which extends downward, about the fourth part of the length of the bone in an oblique direction. The edges of this groove are continuations of the greater and smaller tuberosities, and serve for the attachment of the pectoralis, latissimus dorsi, and teres major muscles. The groove itself is lined with a glistening substance like cartilage, but which seems to be nothing more than the remains of tendinous fibres. A little lower down, towards the external and anterior side of the middle of the bone, it is seen rising into a rough ridge for the insertion of the deltoid muscle. On each side of this ridge the bone is smooth and flat, for the lodgment of the brachialis internus muscle; and behind the middle part of the outermost side of the ridge is a channel, for the transmission of vessels into the substance of the bone. A little lower down, and near the inner side of the ridge, there is sometimes seen such another channel, which is intended for the same purpose. The os humeri, at its lower extremity, becomes gradually broader and flatter, so as to have this end nearly of a triangular shape. The bone, thus expanded, affords two surfaces, of which the anterior one is the broadest, and somewhat convex; and the posterior one narrower and smoother. The bone terminates in four large processes, the two outermost of which are called *condyles*, though not designed for the articulation of the bone. These condyles, which are placed at some distance from each other, on each side of the bone, are rough and irregular protuberances, formed for the insertion of muscles and ligaments, and differ from each other in size and shape. The external

condyle, when the arm is in the most natural position, is found to be placed somewhat forwarder than the other. The internal condyle is longer, and more protuberant, than the external. From each of these processes a ridge is continued upwards, at the side of the bone. In the interval between the two condyles are placed the two articulating processes, contiguous to each other, and covered with cartilage. One of these, which is the smallest, is formed into a small, obtuse, smooth head, on which the radius plays. This little head is placed near the external condyle, as a part of which it has been sometimes described. The other, and larger process, is composed of two lateral protuberances and a middle cavity, all of which are smooth and covered with cartilage. From the manner in which the ulna moves upon this process, it has gotten the name of *trochlea*, or pulley. The sides of this pulley are unequal; that which is towards the little head, is the highest of the two; the other, which is contiguous to the external condyle, is more slanting, being situated obliquely from within outwards, so that when the forearm is fully extended, it does not form a straight line with the os humeri, and, for the same reason, when we bend the elbow, the hand comes not to the shoulder, as it might be expected to do, but to the forepart of the breast. There is a cavity at the root of these processes, on each of the two surfaces of the bone. The cavity on the anterior surface is divided by a ridge into two, the external of which receives the end of the radius, and the internal one lodges the coronoid process of the ulna in the flexions of the forearm. The cavity on the posterior surface, at the basis of the pulley, is much larger, and lodges the olecranon when the arm is extended. The internal structure of the os humeri is similar to that of other long bones. In newborn infants, both the ends of the bone are cartilaginous, and the large head, with the two tubercles above, and the condyles, with the two articulating processes below, become epiphyses before they are entirely united to the rest of the bone.

HU'MILIS. (From *humi*, on the ground: so named because it turns the eye downwards, and is expressive of humility.) See *Rectus inferior oculi.*

HUMITE. A mineral of a reddish brown colour found near Naples, and named by Count Bournon in honour of Sir Abraham Hume, a distinguished cultivator of mineralogy.

HU'MOR. (*Ab humo*, from the ground; because moisture springs from the earth.) Humour, a general name for any fluid of the body except the blood.

Humor vitreus. The vitreous humour of the eye, which takes its name from the resemblance to melted glass, is less dense than the crystalline but more than the aqueous humour; it is very considerable in the human eye, and seems to be formed by the small arteries that are distributed in cells of the *hyaloid* membrane; it is heavier than common water, slightly albuminous and saline.

HUMOUR. See *Humor.*

Humour, aqueous. See *Aqueous humour.*

Humour, vitreous. See *Humor vitreus.*

Humours of the Eye. See *Eye.*

HUMULIN. The narcotic principle of the fruit of the hop. See *Humulus.*

HU'MULUS. (From *humus*, the ground: so named because, without factitious support, it creeps along the ground.) The name of a genus of plants in the Linnæan system. Class, *Diœcia;* Order, *Pentandria.* The hop.

Humulus lupulus. The systematic name of the hop-plant. *Lupulus; Convolvulus perennis.* The hop is the floral leaf or bractea of this plant: it is dried and used in various kinds of strong beer. Hops have a bitter taste, less ungrateful than most of the other strong bitters, accompanied with some degree of warmth and aromatic flavour, and are highly intoxicating. The hop-flower also exhales a considerable quantity of its narcotic power in drying; hence those who sleep in the hop-houses are with difficulty roused from their slumber. A pillow stuffed with these flowers is said to have laid our late monarch to sleep when other remedies had failed. The young sprouts, called hop-tops, if plucked when only a foot above the ground, and boiled, are eaten, like asparagus, and are a wholesome delicacy. The active or narcotic principle of the hop, is called *humulin.*

HUNGER. *Fames.* "The want of solid aliments is characterized by a peculiar sensation in the region of the stomach, and by a general feebleness, more or less marked. This feeling is generally renewed after the stomach has been for some time empty; it is variable in its intensity and its nature in different individuals, and even in the same individual. In some its violence is excessive, in others it is scarcely felt; some never feel it, and eat only because the hour of repast is come. Many persons perceive a drawing, a pressure more or less painful in the epigastric region, accompanied by yawnings, and a particular noise, produced by the gases contained in the stomach, which becomes contracted. When this want is not satisfied it increases, and may become a severe pain: the same takes place with the sensation of weakness and general fatigue, which is felt, and which may increase, so as to render the motions difficult, or even impossible.

Authors distinguish in hunger, local phenomena, and general phenomena.

This distinction is good in itself, and may be useful for study; but have not mere gratuitous suppositions been described as local or general phenomena of hunger, the existence of which was rendered probable by this theory? This point of physiology is one of those in which the want of direct experiment is the most strongly felt.—The pressure and contraction of the stomach are considered among the local phenomena of hunger: 'the sides of that viscus,' it is said, 'become thicker; it changes its form and situation, and draws the duodenum a little towards it; its cavity contains saliva mixed with air, mucosities, bile, which has regurgitated in consequence of the dragging of the duodenum; the quantity of these humours increases in the stomach in proportion as hunger is of longer continuation. The cystic bile does not flow into the duodenum; it collects in the gall-bladder, and it becomes abundant and black according to the continuance of abstinence. A change takes place in the order of the circulation of the digestive organs; the stomach receives less blood, perhaps on account of the flexion of these vessels, which is then greater; perhaps by the compression of the nerves, in consequence of this confinement, the influence of which upon the circulation will then be diminished. On the other hand, the liver, the spleen, the epiploon, receive more, and perform the office of *diverticula:* the liver and the spleen, because they are less supported when the stomach is empty, and then present a more easy access to the blood; and the epiploon, because the vessels are then less *flexuous*,' &c. The most of these data are mere conjectures, and nearly devoid of proof. After twenty-four, forty-eight, and even sixty hours of complete abstinence, Dr. Magendie says he never saw the contraction and pressure of the stomach of which some authors speak: this organ has always presented to him very considerable dimensions, particularly in its splenic extremity; it was only after the fourth and fifth day that it appeared to return upon itself, to diminish much in size, and slightly in position; even these effects are not strongly marked unless fasting has been very strictly observed.

Bichât thinks that the pressure sustained by the empty stomach is equal to that which it supports when distended by aliments, since, says he, the sides of the abdomen are compressed in proportion as the volume of the stomach diminishes. The contrary of this may be easily proved by putting one or two fingers into the abdominal cavity, after having made an incision in its sides; it will then be easily seen that the pressure sustained by the viscera, is, in a certain degree, in direct proportion to the distention of the stomach; if the stomach is full, the finger will be stronger pressed, and the viscera will press outward to escape through the opening; if it is empty, the pressure will be very trifling, and the viscera will have little tendency to pass out from the abdominal cavity. It must be understood that in this experiment the pressure exerted by the abdominal muscle, when they are relaxed, ought not to be confounded with that which they exert when contracted with force. Also, when the stomach is empty, all the reservoirs contained in the abdomen are more easily distended by the matters which remain some time in them. Perhaps this is the principal reason why bile then accumulates in the gall-bladder. With regard to the presence of bile in the stomach, that some persons regard as the cause of hunger, unless in certain sickly cases bile does not enter it, though it continues to flow into the small intestine.

The quantity of mucus that the cavity of the stomach presents is so much greater in proportion to the prolongation of abstinence.

Relatively to the quantity of blood which goes to the stomach when empty, in proportion to the volume of its vessels, and the mode of circulation which then exists, the general opinion is that it receives less of this fluid than when it is full of aliments; but, far from being in this respect in opposition with the other abdominal organs, this disposition appears to be common to all the organs contained in the abdomen.

To the general phenomena of hunger is ascribed a weakness and diminution of the action of all the organs; the circulation and the respiration become slow, the heat of the body lowers, the secretions diminish, the whole of the functions are exerted with more difficulty. The absorption alone is said to become more active, but nothing is strictly demonstrated in this respect.

Hunger, appetite itself, which is only its first degree, ought to be distinguished from that feeling which induces us to prefer one sort of food to another, from that which causes us, during a repast, to choose one dish rather than another, &c.

These feelings are very different from real hunger, which expresses the true wants of the economy; they in a great measure depend on civilization, on habits, and certain ideas relative to the properties of aliments. Some of them are in unison with the season, the climate, and then they are equally legitimate as hunger itself; such is that which inclines us to a vegetable regimen in hot countries, or during the heats of summer.

Certain circumstances render hunger more intense, and cause it to return at nearer intervals; such as a cold and dry air, winter, spring, cold baths, dry frictions upon the skin, exercise on horseback, walking, bodily fatigue, and generally all the causes that put the action of the organs in play, and accelerate the nutritive process with which hunger is essentially connected. Some substances, being introduced into the stomach, excite a feeling like hunger, but which ought not to be confounded with it.

There are causes which diminish the intensity of hunger, and which prolong the periods at which it habitually manifests itself; among this number are the inhabiting of hot countries, and humid places, rest of the body and mind, depressing passions, and indeed all the circumstances that interrupt the action of the organs, and diminish the activity of nutrition. There are also substances which, being brought into the digestive canals, prevent hunger, or cause it to cease, as opium, hot drinks, &c.

With respect to the cause of hunger, it has been, by turns, attributed to the providence of the vital principle, to the frictions of the sides of the stomach against each other, to the dragging of the liver upon the diaphragm, to the action of bile upon the stomach, to the acrimony and acidity of the gastric juice, to fatigue of the contracted fibres of the stomach, to compression of the nerves of this viscus, &c. &c.

Hunger arises, like all other internal sensations, from the action of the nervous system; it has no other seat than this system itself, and no other causes than the general laws of organization. What very well proves the truth of this assertion is, that it sometimes continues though the stomach is filled with food; that it cannot be produced though the stomach has been some time empty; lastly, that it is so subject to habit as to cease spontaneously after the habitual hour of repast is over. This is true not only of the feeling which takes place in the region of the stomach, but also of the general weakness that accompanies it, and which, consequently, cannot be considered as real, at least in the first instant in which it is manifested."

HUNTER, William, was born in 1718, at Kilbride in Scotland. He was educated for the church at Glasgow; but feeling scruples against subscription, and having become acquainted with the celebrated Cullen, he determined to pursue the medical profession. After living three years with that able teacher, who then practised as a surgeon-apothecary at Hamilton, he went to Edinburgh in November, 1740; and in the following summer came to London with a recommendation to Dr. James Douglas, who engaged him to assist in his dissections, and superintend the education of his son. He was also enabled by that physician's liberality to attend St. George's Hospital, and other teachers; but death deprived him of so valuable a friend within a year. However, he remained in the family, and prosecuted his studies with great zeal. In 1743, he communicated to the Royal Society a paper on the structure and diseases of articulating cartilages, which was much admired. He now formed the design of teaching anatomy; and, after encountering some difficulties, commenced by giving a course on the operations of surgery to a society of navy surgeons in lieu of Mr. Samuel Sharpe. At first he felt considerable solicitude in speaking in public; but gradually this wore off, and he evinced a remarkable facility in expressing himself with perspicuity and elegance. He gave so much satisfaction, that he was requested to extend the plan to anatomy, which he began accordingly in 1746. His success was considerable, but having somewhat embarrassed himself at first by assisting his friends, he was obliged to adopt proper caution in lending money; which, with his talents, industry, and economy, enabled him to acquire an ample fortune. In 1748, he accompanied his pupil, young Douglas, on a tour, and having seen the admirable injections of Albinus at Leyden, he was inspired with a strong emulation to excel in that branch. On his return, he relinquished the profession of surgery, and devoted himself to midwifery, to which his person and manners well adapted him; and having been appointed to the Middlesex and British lying-in hospitals, as well as favoured by other circumstances, he made a rapid advance in practice. In 1750 he obtained a doctor's degree from Glasgow, and was afterward often consulted as a physician, in cases which required peculiar anatomical skill. Six years after, he was admitted a licentiate of the College in London; and also a member of the society, by which the "Medical Observations and Inquiries" were published. He enriched that work with many valuable communications; particularly an account of the disease, since called Aneurismal Varix, a case of emphysema, with practical remarks, wherein he showed the fat to be deposited in distinct vesicles; and some observations on the retroversion of the uterus: and, on the death of Dr. Fothergill, he was chosen president of that society. In 1762 he published his "Medical Commentaries," in which he laid claim, with much asperity, to several anatomical discoveries, especially relative to the absorbent system, in opposition to the second Monro, of Edinburgh. He was extremely tenacious of his rights in this respect, and would not allow them to be infringed, even by his own brother. It must be very difficult, and of little importance, to decide such controversies; especially as the principal points concerning the absorbent system had been stated as early as 1726, in a work printed at Paris by M. Noguez. About the same period, the queen being pregnant, Dr. Hunter was consulted; and, two years after, he was appointed her physician extraordinary. In 1767 he was chosen a Fellow of the Royal Society, to which he communicated some papers; and, in the year following, he was appointed, by the king, Professor of Anatomy to the Royal Academy, on its first institution; he was also elected into the Society of Antiquaries, and some respectable foreign associations. In 1775 he published a splendid work, which had occupied him for 24 years previously, "The Anatomy of the Gravid Uterus," illustrated by plates, admirable for their accuracy, as well as elegance; among other improvements, the membrana decidua reflexa, discovered by himself, was here first delineated. He drew up a detailed description of the figures; which was published after his death by his nephew, Dr. Baillie. Another posthumous publication, deservedly much admired, was the "Two Introductory Lectures" to his anatomical course. As his wealth increased, he formed the noble design of establishing an anatomical school; and proposed to government, on the grant of a piece of ground, to build a proper edifice and endow a perpetual professorship: but this not being acceded to, he set about the establishment in Great Windmill-street, where he collected a most valuable museum of anatomical preparations, subjects of natural history, scarce books, coins, &c. to which an easy access was always given. He continued to lecture and practise till near the period of his death, in 1783. He bequeathed the use of his museum, for thirty years, to Dr. Baillie; after which it was to belong to the University of Glasgow.

HUNTER, John, was born ten years after his brother William. His early education was much neglected, and his temper injured, through his mother's indulgence. At a proper age he was put under a relation, a carpenter and cabinet-maker, who failed in his business. Hearing, at this period, of his brother's success, he applied to become his assistant, and accordingly came to London in the autumn of 1748. He made such proficiency in dissection, that he was capable of undertaking the demonstrations in the following season. During the summer he attended the surgical practice at different hospitals; and, in 1756, he was appointed house-surgeon at St. George's. He had been admitted by his brother to a partnership in the lectures the year before. After labouring about ten years with unexampled ardour in the study of human anatomy, he turned his attention to that of other animals, with a view to elucidate physiology. His health was so much impaired by these pursuits, that, in 1760, he went abroad as surgeon on the staff, and thus acquired a knowledge of gun-shot wounds. On his return, after three years, he settled in London as a surgeon, and gave instructions in dissection and the performance of operations; and he continued, with great zeal, his researches into comparative anatomy and natural history. Several papers were communicated by him to the Royal Society, of which he was elected a member in 1767. About this time, by his brother's interest, he was appointed one of the surgeons at St. George's Hospital; and his professional reputation was rapidly increasing. In 1771 he published the first part of his work on the teeth, displaying great accuracy of research: and, two years after, he began a course of lectures on the principles of surgery. He fell short of his brother in methodical arrangement, and facility of expressing his ideas, and indeed adopted a peculiar language, perhaps in part from the deficiency of his education; but he certainly brought forward many ingenious speculations in physiology and pathology, and suggested some important practical improvements, particularly the operation for popliteal aneurism. In 1776 he was appointed surgeon-extraordinary to the king; and soon after received marks of distinction from several foreign societies. His emoluments increasing, he took a large house in Leicester-square, and built a spacious museum, which he continued to store with subjects in comparative anatomy, at a very great expense. The post of Deputy-Surgeon General to the Army was conferred upon him in 1786; and, in the same year, his great work on the venereal disease appeared, which will ever remain a monument of his extraordinary sagacity and talent for observation. He also published, at this period, "Observations on the Animal Economy," chiefly composed of papers already printed in the Philosophical Transactions. In 1790 he was appointed Inspector-General of Hospitals, and Surgeon-General to the Army; when he resigned his lectures to Mr. Home, whose sister he had married. He had been for two years before labouring under symptoms of organic disease about the heart, which were aggravated by any sudden exertion or agitation of his mind; these increased progressively, and, in October 1793, while at the hospital, being vexed by some untoward circumstance, he suddenly expired. He left a valuable treatise on the blood, inflammation, and gun-shot wounds, which was published soon after, with a life prefixed, by his brother-in-law. His museum was directed to be offered to the purchase of government: it was bought for 15,000*l.* and presented to the College of Surgeons, on condition of their opening it to public inspection, and giving a set of lectures annually, explanatory of its contents. The preparations are arranged so as to exhibit all the gradations of nature, from the simplest state of animated existence up to man, according to the different functions. It comprehends also a large series of entire animals, skeletons of almost every genus, and other subjects of natural history.

HURTSICKLE. (So called because it is troublesome to cut down, and sometimes notches the sickle.) See *Centaurea cyanus.*

HUSK. See *Gluma.*

HUXHAM, John, was born about the end of the 17th century, and practised as a physician, with considerable reputation, at Plymouth, where he died in 1768 His writings display great learning and talent for observation. He kept a register of the weather and prevailing diseases for nearly thirty years, which was published in Latin, in three volumes. He was early elected into the Royal Society, and communicated several papers on pathology and morbid anatomy. But his fame rests chiefly upon his "Essay on Fevers," which went through several editions; a dissertation being afterward added on the malignant sore throat.

HYACINTH. 1. A sub-species of pyramidal zircon. It comes from Ceylon, and is much esteemed as a gem.

2. See *Hyacinthus.*

HYACI'NTHUS. (Said by the poets to be named from the friend of Apollo, who was turned into this flower.) The name of a genus of plants. Class, *Hexandria;* Order, *Monogynia.*

Hyacinthus muscari. *Muscari.* The systematic name of the musk-grape flower, which, according to Ray, possesses emetic and diuretic qualities.

Hyacinthus non scriptus. Hare-bells. The systematic name of the blue-bells, so common in our hedges in spring. The roots are bulbous; the flowers agreeably scented. Galen considered the root as a remedy in jaundice. It is ranked among the astringents, but of very inferior power.

HYALITE. A transparent siliceous stone, which is often cut into ring-stones, found near Frankfort on the Maine.

HYALO'IDES. (*Membrana hyaloides;* from ὑαλος, glass, and ειδος, likeness.) *Membrana arachnoidea.* Capsule of the vitreous humour. The transparent membrane enclosing the vitreous humour of the eye.

HYBERNACULUM. This is defined by Linnæus to be a part of the plant which protects the embryo herb from external injuries.

An organic body which sprouts from the surface of different parts of a plant, enclosing the rudiments of the new shoot, and which is capable of evolving a new individual perfectly similar to the parent. This is a modification of the definition of Gærtner.—*Thompson*

Hyboma. A gibbosity of the spine.

HYBRID. (*Hybrida,* from ὑβρις, an injury; because its nature is tainted.) A monstrous production of two different species of animals or plants. In the former it is called mongrel, or mule. Neither the animal nor the seeds of hybrid plants propagate their species.

HYDA'RTHRUS. (From ὑδωρ, water, and αρθρον, a joint.) *Hydarthron. Hydarthros. Spina ventosa* of the Arabian writers, Rhazes and Avicenna. White-swelling. The white-swelling, in this country, is a peculiarly common and exceedingly terrible disease. The varieties of white-swelling are very numerous, and might usefully receive particular appellations. Systematic writers have generally been content with a distinction into two kinds, viz. *rheumatic* and *scrofulous* The last species of the disease they also distinguish into such tumours as primarily affect the bones, and then the ligaments and soft parts; and into other cases, in which the ligaments and soft parts become diseased before there is any morbid affection of the bones.

These divisions, Mr. Samuel Cooper, in his Treatise on the Diseases of the Joints, proves to be not sufficiently comprehensive; and the propriety of using the term *rheumatic* he thinks to be very questionable.

The knee, ankle, wrist, and elbow, are the joints most subject to white-swellings. As the name of the disease implies, the skin is not at all altered in colour. In some instances, the swelling yields, in a certain degree, to pressure; but it never pits, and is almost always sufficiently firm to make an uninformed examiner believe that the bones contribute to the tumour. The pain is sometimes vehement from the very first in other instances, there is hardly the least pain in th beginning of the disease. In the majority of scrofulous white-swellings, let the pain be trivial or violent it is particularly situated in one part of the joint, viz either *the centre of the articulation,* or the *head of the tibia,* supposing the knee affected. Sometimes the pain continues without interruption; sometimes there are intermissions; and in other instances the pain recurs at regular times, so as to have been called by some writers, periodical. Almost all authors describe the patient as suffering more uneasiness in the diseased part, when he is warm, and particularly when he is in this condition in bed.

At the commencement of the disease in the majority

of instances, the swelling is very inconsiderable, or there is even no visible enlargement whatever. In the little depressions, naturally situated on each side of the patella, a fulness first shows itself, and gradually spreads all over the affected joint.

The patient, unable to bear the weight of his body on the disordered joint, in consequence of the great increase of pain thus created, gets into the habit of only touching the ground with his toes: and the knee being generally kept a little bent in this manner, soon loses the capacity of becoming extended again. When white-swellings have lasted a while, the knee is almost always found in a permanent state of flexion. In scrofulous cases of this kind, pain constantly precedes any appearance of swelling; but the interval between the two symptoms differs very much in different subjects.

The morbid joint, in the course of time, acquires a vast magnitude. Still the integuments retain their natural colour, and remain unaffected. The enlargement of the articulation, however, always seems greater than it really is, in consequence of the emaciation of the limb both above and below the disease.

An appearance of blue distended veins, and a shining smoothness, are the only alterations to be noticed in the skin covering the enlarged joint. The shining smoothness seems attributable to the distention, which obliterates the natural furrows and wrinkles of the cutis. When the joint is thus swollen, the integuments cannot be pinched up into a fold, as they could in the state of health, and even in the beginning of the disease.

As the distemper of the articulation advances, collections of matter form about the part, and at length burst. The ulcerated openings sometimes heal up; but such abscesses are generally followed by other collections, which pursue the same course. In some cases, these abscesses form a few months after the first affection of the joint; on other occasions, several years elapse, and no suppuration of this kind makes its appearance.

Such terrible local mischief must necessarily produce constitutional disturbance. The patient's health becomes gradually impaired; he loses both his appetite and natural rest and sleep; his pulse is small and frequent; and obstinate debilitating diarrhœa and profuse nocturnal sweats ensue. Such complaints are sooner or later followed by dissolution, unless the constitution be relieved in time, either by the amendment or removal of the diseased part. In different patients, however, the course of the disease, and its effects upon the system, vary very much in relation to the rapidity with which they occur.

Rheumatic white-swellings are very distinct diseases from the *scrofulous distemper* of large joints. In the first, the pain is said never to occur without being attended with swelling. Scrofulous white-swellings, on the other hand, are always preceded by a pain, which is particularly confined to one point of the articulation. In rheumatic cases, the pain is more general, and diffused over the whole joint.

With respect to the particular causes of all such white-swellings as come within the class of rheumatic ones, little is known. External irritation, either by exposure to damp or cold, or by the application of violence, is often concerned in bringing on the disease; but very frequently no cause of this kind can be assigned for the complaint. As for scrofulous white-swellings, there can be no doubt that they are under the influence of a particular kind of constitution, termed a *scrofulous* or *strumous* habit. In this sort of temperament, every cause capable of exciting inflammation, or any morbid and irritable state of a large joint, may bring such disorder as may end in the severe disease of which we are now speaking.

In a man of a sound constitution, an irritation of the kind alluded to might only induce common healthy inflammation of the affected joint.

In scrofulous habits, it also seems probable that the irritation of a joint is much more easily produced than in the other constitutions; and no one can doubt that, when once excited in scrofulous habits, it is much more dangerous and difficult of removal than in other patients.

HYDATID. (*Hydatis*; from ὑδωρ, water. 1. A very singular animal, formed like a bladder, and distended with an aqueous fluid. These animals are sometimes formed in the natural cavities of the body, as the abdomen and ventricles of the brain, but more frequently in the liver, kidney, and lungs, where they produce diseased actions of those viscera. Cullen arranges these affections in the class *Locales*, an order *Tumores*. If the vires naturæ medicatrices are not sufficient to effect a cure, the patient mostly falls a sacrifice to their ravages. Dr. Baillie gives the following interesting account of the hydatids, as they are sometimes found in the liver:—'There is no gland in the human body in which hydatids are so frequently found as the liver, except the kidneys, where they are still more common. Hydatids of the liver are usually found in a cyst, which is frequently of considerable size, and is formed of very firm materials, so as to give to the touch almost the feeling of cartilage. This cyst, when cut into, is obviously laminated, and is much thicker in one liver than another. In some livers it is not thicker than a shilling, and in others it is near a quarter of an inch in thickness. The laminæ which compose it are formed of a white matter, and on the inside there is a lining of a pulpy substance, like the coagulable lymph. The cavity of the cyst, I have seen, in one instance, subdivided by a partition of this pulpy substance. In a cyst may be found one hydatid, or a greater number of them. They lie loose in the cavity, swimming in a fluid; or some of them are attached to the side of the cyst. They consist of a round bag, which is composed of a white, semi-opaque, pulpy matter, and contain a fluid capable of coagulation. Although the common colour of hydatids be white, yet I have occasionally seen some of a light amber colour. The bag of the hydatid consists of two laminæ, and possesses a good deal of contractile power. In one hydatid this coat, or bag, is much thicker and more opaque than in another; and even in the same hydatid, different parts of it will often differ in thickness. On the inside of a hydatid, smaller ones are sometimes found, which are commonly not larger than the heads of pins, but sometimes they are even larger in their size than a gooseberry. These are attached to the larger hydatid, either at scattered irregular distances, or so as to form small clusters; and they are also found floating loose in the liquor of the larger hydatids. Hydatids of the liver are often found unconnected with each other; but sometimes they have been said to enclose each other in a series, like pill-boxes. The most common situation of hydatids of the liver is in its substance, and enclosed in a cyst; but they are occasionally attached to the outer surface of the liver, hanging from it, and occupying more or less of the general cavity of the abdomen. The origin and real nature of these hydatids are not fully ascertained; it is extremely probable, however, that they are a sort of imperfect animalcules. There is no doubt at all, that the hydatids in the livers of sheep are animalcules; they have been often seen to move when taken out of the liver and put into warm water; and they retain this power of motion for a good many hours after a sheep has been killed. The analogy is great between hydatids in the liver of a sheep and those of the human subject. In both, they are contained in strong cysts, and in both they consist of the same white pulpy matter. There is undoubtedly some difference between them in simplicity of organization; the hydatid in the human liver being a simple uniform bag, and the hydatid in that of a sheep having a neck and mouth appendant to the bag. This difference need be no considerable objection to the opinion above stated. Life may be conceived to be attached to the most simple form of organization. In proof of this, hydatids have been found in the brains of sheep, resembling almost exactly those in the human liver, and which have been seen to move and therefore are certainly known to be animalcules. The hydatids of the human liver, indeed, have not, as far as I know, been found to move when taken out of the body and put into warm water; were this to have happened, no uncertainty would remain. It is not difficult to see a good reason why there will hardly occur any proper opportunity of making this experiment. Hydatids are not very often found in the liver, because it is not a very frequent disease there; and the body is allowed to remain for so long a time after death before it is examined, that the hydatids must have lost their living principle, even if they were animalcules, and it appears even more difficult to account for their production, according to the common theory of generation, than for that of intestinal worms We do not get rid of the difficulty by asserting, that the hydatids in the human liver are not living animals, because in sheep they are certainly such, where the difficulty of accounting for their production is precisely the same."

2. The name of a tumour, the contents of which is a water-like fluid.

HYDERUS. (From υδερος, *ley-drops;* from υδωρ, water.) An increased flow of urine.

HY'DRAGOGUE. (*Hydragogus;* from υδωρ, water, and αγω, to drive out.) Medicines are so termed which possess the property of increasing the secretions or excretions of the body so as to cause the removal of water from any of its cavities, such as cathartics, &c.

HYDRARGYRATUS. Of or belonging to mercury.

HYDRA'RGYRUM. (Υδραργυρος; from υδωρ, water, and αργυρος, silver: so named from its having a resemblance to fluid silver.) *Hydrargyrus.* The name in the London Pharmacopœia, and other works, for mercury. See *Mercury.*

HYDRARGYRUM PRÆCIPITATUM ALBUM. White precipitated mercury. *Calx hydrargyri alba.* Take of oxymuriate of mercury, half a pound; muriate of ammonia, four ounces; solution of subcarbonate of potassa, half a pint; distilled water, four pints. First dissolve the muriate of ammonia, then the oxymuriate of mercury, in the distilled water, and add thereto the solution of subcarbonate of potassa. Wash the precipitated powder until it becomes tasteless; then dry it. It is only used externally, in the form of ointment, as an application in some cutaneous affections.

HYDRARGYRUM PURIFICATUM. Purified mercury. *Argentum vivum purificatum.* Take of mercury, by weight, six pounds; iron filings, a pound. Rub them together, and distil the mercury from an iron retort, by the application of heat to it. Purified quicksilver is sometimes administered in its metallic state, in doses of an ounce or more, in constipation of the bowels.

HYDRARGYRUS ACETATUS. *Mercurius acetatus; Pilulæ Keyseri.* By this preparation of mercury, the celebrated Keyser acquired an immense fortune in curing the venereal disease. It is an acetate of mercury, and therefore termed *hydrargyri acetas* in the new chemical nomenclature. The dose is from three to five grains. Notwithstanding the encomium given to it by some, it does not appear to be so efficacious as some other preparations of mercury.

HYDRARGYRUM CUM CRETA. Mercury with chalk. *Mercurius alkalizatus.* Take of purified mercury, by weight, three ounces; prepared chalk, five ounces. Rub them together, until the metallic globules disappear. This preparation is milder than any other mercurial, except the sulphuret, and does not so easily act upon the bowels; it is therefore used largely by many practitioners, and possesses alterative properties in cutaneous and venereal complaints, in obstructions of the viscera, or of the prostate gland, given in the dose of ℈ss to ʒss, two or three times a day.

HYDRARGYRUS PHOSPHORATUS. This remedy has been observed to heal inveterate venereal ulcers in a very short time, nay, in the course of a very few days, particularly those about the pudenda. In venereal inflammations of the eyes, chancres, rheumatisms, and chronic eruptions, it has proved of eminent service. Upon the whole, if used with necessary precaution, and in the hands of a judicious practitioner, it is a medicine mild and gentle in its operation. The cases in which it deserves the preference over other mercurial preparations, are these: in an inveterate stage of syphilis, particularly in persons of torpid insensible fibres; in cases of exostosis, as well as obstructions in the lymphatic system; in chronic complaints of the skin. The following is the formula. ℞. Hydrargyri phosphorati, gr. iv. Corticis cinnamomi in pulverem triti, gr. xiv. Sacchari purif. ʒss. Misce. The whole to be divided into eight equal parts, one of which is to be taken every morning and evening, unless salivation takes place, when it ought to be discontinued. Some patients, however, will bear from one to two grains of the phosphate of quicksilver, without inconvenience.

HYDRARGYRUS PRECIPITATUS CINEREUS. This preparation is an oxide of mercury, and nearly the same with the *hydrargyri oxydum cinereum* of the London pharmacopœia. It is used as an alterative in cases of pains arising from an admixture of rheumatism with syphilis. It may be substituted for the hydrargyrus sulphuratus ruber, in fumigating ozæna, and venereal ulcerated sore throat, on account of its not yielding any vapour offensive to the patient.

HYDRARGYRUS VITRIOLATUS. *Turpethum minerale; Mercurius emeticus flavus; Sulphas hydrargyri.* Formerly this medicine was in more general use than in the present day. It is a very powerful and active alterative when given in small doses. Two grains act on the stomach so as to produce violent vomitings. is recommended as an errhine in cases of amaurosis In combination with antimony it acts powerfully on the skin.

HYDRARGYRI NITRICO-OXYDUM. *Nitrico-oxydum hydrargyri; Hydrargyrus nitratus ruber; Mercurius corrasivus ruber; Mercurius præcipitatus corrosivus.* Nitric oxide of mercury. Red precipitate. Take of purified mercury, by weight, three pounds of nitric acid, by weight, a pound and a half: of distilled water two pints. Mix in a glass vessel, and boil the mixture in a sand-bath, until the mercury be dissolved, the water also evaporated, and a white mass remain. Rub this into powder, and put it into another shallow vessel, then apply a moderate heat, and raise the fire gradually, until red vapour shall cease to rise This preparation is very extensively employed by surgeons as a stimulant and escharotic, but its extraordinary activity does not allow of its being given internally. Finely levigated and mixed with common cerates, it is an excellent application to indolent ulcers, especially those which remain after burns and scalds, and those in which the granulations are indolent and flabby. It is also an excellent caustic application to chancres.

HYDRARGYRI OXYDUM CINEREUM. *Oxydum hydrargyri nigrum.* The gray or black oxide of mercury. It has received several names; *Æthiops per se; Pulvis mercurialis cinereus; Mercurius cinereus; Turpethum nigrum; Mercurius præcipitatus niger.* Take of submuriate of mercury, an ounce; limewater, a gallon. Boil the submuriate of mercury in the limewater, constantly stirring, until a gray oxide of mercury is separated. Wash this with distilled water, and then dry it. The dose from gr. ii. to x. There are four other preparations of this oxide in high estimation:

One made by rubbing mercury with mucilage of gum-arabic. Plenk, of Vienna, has written a treatise on the superior efficacy of this medicine. It is very troublesome to make; and does not appear to possess more virtues than some other mercurial preparations. Another made by triturating equal parts of sugar and mercury together. The third, composed of honey or liquorice and purified mercury. The fourth is the blue mercurial ointment. All these preparations possess anthelmintic, antisyphilitic, alterative, sialagogue, and deobstruent virtues, and are exhibited in the cure of worms, syphilis, amenorrhœa, diseases of the skin, chronic diseases, obstructions of the viscera, &c.

HYDRARGYRI OXYDUM NIGRUM. See *Hydrargyri oxydum cinereum.*

HYDRARGYRI OXYDUM RUBRUM. *Oxydum hydrargyri rubrum; Hydrargyrus calcinatus.* Red oxide of mercury. Take of purified mercury by weight a pound. Pour the mercury into a glass matrass, with a very narrow mouth and broad bottom. Apply a heat of 600° to this vessel, without stopping it, until the mercury has changed into red scales: then reduce these to a very fine powder. The whole process may probably require an exposure of six weeks. This preparation of mercury is given with great advantage in the cure of syphilis. Its action, however, is such, when given alone, on the bowels, as to require the addition of opium, which totally prevents it. It is also given in conjunction with opium and camphire, as a diaphoretic, in chronic pains and diseases of long continuance. It is given as an alterative and diaphoretic from gr. ss. to ii. every night, joined with camphor and opium, each gr. one-fourth or one-half. It is violently emetic and cathartic in the dose of gr. iv. to gr. v.

HYDRARGYRI OXYMURIAS. *Oxymurias hydrargyri; Hydrargyrus muriatus.* Oxymuriate of mercury. Take of purified mercury by weight two pounds, sulphuric acid by weight thirty ounces, dried muriate of soda four pounds. Boil the mercury with the sulphuric acid in a glass vessel until the sulphate of mercury shall be left dry. Rub this, when it is cold, with the muriate of soda in an earthen-ware mortar: then sublime it in a glass cucurbit, increasing the heat gradually. An extremely acrid and violently poisonous preparation.

Given internally in small doses properly diluted, and never in the form of pill, it possesses antisyphilitic and alterative virtues. Externally, applied in form of lotion, it facilitates the healing of venereal sores, and cures the itch. In gargles for venereal ulcers in the throat, the oxymuriate of mercury gr. iii. or iv. barley decoction ℔j., honey of roses ℥ij., proves very serviceable; also in cases of tetters, from gr. v. to gr. x. in water ℔j.; and for films and ulcerations of the cornea, gr. i. to water ℥iv.

Mr. Pearson remarks, that "when the sublimate is given to cure the primary symptoms of syphilis, it will sometimes succeed; more especially, when it produces a considerable degree of soreness of the gums, and the common specific effects of mercury in the animal system. But it will often fail of removing even a recent chancre; and where that symptom has vanished during the administration of corrosive sublimate, I have known, says he, a three months' course of that medicine fail of securing the patient from a constitutional affection. The result of my observation is, that simple mercury, calomel or calcined mercury, are preparations more to be confided in for the cure of primary symptoms, than corrosive sublimate. The latter will often check the progress of secondary symptoms very conveniently, and I think it is peculiarly efficacious in relieving venereal pains, in healing ulcers of the throat, and in promoting the desquamation of eruptions. Yet even in these cases it never confers permanent benefit; for new symptoms will appear during the use of it; and on many occasions it will fail of affording the least advantage to the patient from first to last. I do, sometimes, indeed, employ this preparation in venereal cases; but it is either at the beginning of a mercurial course, to bring the constitution under the influence of mercury at an early period, or during a course of inunction, with the intention of increasing the action of simple mercury. I sometimes also prescribe it after the conclusion of a course of friction, to support the mercurial influence in the habit, in order to guard against the danger of a relapse. But on no occasion whatever do I think it safe to confide in this preparation singly and uncombined for the cure of any truly venereal symptoms."

A solution of it is ordered in the pharmacopœia, termed *Liquor hydrargyri oxymuriatis*. Solution of oxymuriate of mercury. Take of oxymuriate of mercury, eight grains; distilled water, fifteen fluid ounces; rectified spirit, a fluid ounce. Dissolve the oxymuriate of mercury in the water, and add the spirit.

This solution is directed in order to facilitate the administration of divisions of the grain of this active medicine. Half an ounce of it contains one-fourth of a grain of the salt. The dose is from one drachm to half an ounce.

Hydrargyri submurias. *Submurias hydrargyri*. Submuriate of mercury. *Calomelas*. Calomel. Take of oxymuriate of mercury, a pound; purified mercury, by weight nine ounces. Rub them together until the metallic globules disappear, then sublime; take out the sublimed mass, and reduce it to powder, and sublime it in the same manner twice more successively. Lastly, bring it into the state of very fine powder by the same process which has been directed for the preparation of chalk. Submuriate, or mild muriate of mercury, is one of the most useful preparations of mercury. As an anti-venereal it is given in the dose of a grain night and morning, its usual determination to the intestines being prevented, if necessary, by opium. It is the preparation which is perhaps most usually given in the other diseases in which mercury is employed, as in affections of the liver, or neighbouring organs, in cutaneous diseases, chronic rheumatism, tetanus, hydrophobia, hydrocephalus, and febrile affections, especially those of warm climates. It is employed as a cathartic alone, in doses from v. to xii. grains, or to promote the operation of other purgatives. Its anthelmintic power is justly celebrated; and it is perhaps superior to the other mercurials in assisting the operation of diuretics in dropsy. From its specific gravity it ought always to be given in the form of a bolus or pill.

Hydrargyri sulphuretum nigrum. *Hydrargyrus cum sulphure*. Æthiop's mineral. Take of purified mercury, sublimed sulphur, each a pound, by weight. Rub them together, till the metallic globules disappear. Some suppose that the mercury is oxidized in this process, but that is not confirmed by the best experiments. The mercury, by this admixture of the sulphur, is deprived of its salivating power, and may be administered with safety to all ages and constitutions, as an anthelmintic and alterative.

Hydrargyri sulphuretum rubrum. Red sulphuret of mercury. *Hydrargyrus sulphuratus ruber; Minium purum; Minium Græcorum; Magnes epilepsiæ; Atzemafor; Amnion; Azamar*. Vitruvius calls it *anthrax*. A red mineral substance composed of mercury combined with sulphur. It is either native or factitious. The native is an ore of quicksilver moderately compact, and of an elegant striated red colour. It is found in the dutchy of Deuxponts, in the Palatinate, in Spain, South America, &c. It is called native vermilion, and cinnabar in flowers. The factitious is thus prepared: "Take of purified mercury, by weight forty ounces; sublimed sulphur, eight ounces. Having melted the sulphur over the fire, mix in the mercury, and as soon as the mass begins to swell, remove the vessel from the fire, and cover it with considerable force to prevent inflammation; then rub the mass into powder, and sublime." This preparation is esteemed a mild mercurial alterative, and given to children in small doses. Hoffman greatly recommends it as a sedative and antispasmodic. Others deny that cinnabar, taken internally, has any medicinal quality; and their opinion is grounded on the insolubility of it in any menstruum. In surgery its chief and almost only use is in the administration of quicksilver by fumigation. Thus employed it has proved extremely serviceable in venereal cases. Ulcers and excrescences about the pudendum and anus in women, are particularly benefited by it; and in these cases it is most conveniently applied by placing a red hot heater at the bottom of a night stool-pan, and after sprinkling on it a few grains of the red sulphuret of quicksilver, placing the patient on the stool. To fumigate ulcers in the throat, it is necessary to receive the fumes on the part affected, through the tube of a funnel. By enclosing the patient naked in a box, it has on some occasions been contrived to fumigate the whole body at once, and in this way the specific powers of the quicksilver have been very rapidly excited.

This mode of curing the lues venerea is spoken of as confirmed; and the subject has of late years been revived in a treatise by Sabonette, and by trials made in Bartholomew's hospital.

Mr. Pearson, from his experiments on mercurial fumigation, concludes, that where checking the progress of the disease suddenly is an object of great moment, and where the body is covered with ulcers or large and numerous eruptions, and in general to ulcers, fungi, and excrescences, the vapour of mercury is an application of great efficacy and utility; but that it is apt to induce a ptyalism rapidly, and great consequent debility, and that for the purpose of securing the constitution against a relapse, as great a quantity of mercury must be introduced into the system, by inunction, as if no fumigation had been employed.

HYDRATE. Hydroxure. Hydro-oxide. A compound of oxygen, in a definite proportion, with water.

HYDRELÆ'UM. (From υδωρ, water, and ελαιον, oil.) A mixture of oil and water.

HYDRENTEROCE'LE. (From υδωρ, water, εντερον, an intestine, and κηλη, a tumour.) A hydrocele, or dropsy of the scrotum, attended with a rupture.

HYDRIODATE. A salt consisting of the hydriodic acid, combined in a definite proportion with an oxide.

HYDRIODIC ACID. *Acidum hydriodicum*. A gaseous acid in its insulated state. "If four parts of iodine be mixed with one of phosphorus, in a small glass retort, applying a gentle heat, and adding a few drops of water from time to time, a gas comes over, which must be received in the mercurial bath. Its specific gravity is 4.4; 100 cubic inches, therefore, weigh 134.2 grs. It is elastic and invisible, but has a smell somewhat similar to that of muriatic acid. Mercury after some time decomposes it, seizing its iodine, and leaving its hydrogen, equal to one-half the original bulk, at liberty. Chlorine, on the other hand, unites to its hydrogen, and precipitates the iodine. From these experiments, it evidently consists of vapour of iodine and hydrogen, which combine in equal volumes, without change of their primitive bulk. Hydriodic acid is partly decomposed at a red-heat, and the decomposition is complete if it be mixed with oxygen. Water is formed, and iodine separated.

We can easily obtain an aqueous hydriodic acid very economically, by passing sulphuretted hydrogen gas through a mixture of water and iodine in a Woolfe's bottle. On heating the liquid obtained, the excess of sulphur flies off, and leaves liquid hydriodic acid. At temperatures below 262°, it parts with its water; and becomes of a density = 1.7. At 262° the acid distils over. When exposed to the air, it is speedily decomposed, and iodine is evolved. Concentrated sulphuric and nitric acids also decompose it. When poured into a saline solution of lead, it throws down a fine orange precipitate. With solution of peroxide of mercury, it gives a red precipitate; and with that of silver, a white precipitate insoluble in ammonia. Hydriodic acid may also be formed, by passing hydrogen over iodine at an elevated temperature.

The compounds of hydriodic acid with the salifiable bases may be easily formed, either by direct combination, or by acting on the basis in water, with iodine. The latter mode is most economical. Upon a determinate quantity of iodine, pour solution of potassa or soda, till the liquor ceases to be coloured. Evaporate to dryness, and digest the dry salt in alkohol of the specific gravity 0.810, or 0.820. As the iodate is not soluble in this liquid, while the hydriodate is very soluble, the two salts easily separate from each other. After having washed the iodate two or three times with alkohol, dissolve it in water; and neutralize it with acetic acid. Evaporate to dryness, and digest the dry salt in alkohol, to remove the acetate. After two or three washings, the iodate is pure. As for the alkohol containing the hydriodate, distil it off, and then complete the neutralization of the potassa, by means of a little hydriodic acid separately obtained. Sulphurous and muriatic acids, as well as sulphuretted hydrogen, produce no change on the hydriodates, at the usual temperature of the air.

Chlorine, nitric acid, and concentrated sulphuric, instantly decompose them, and separate the iodine.

With solution of silver, they give a white precipitate insoluble in ammonia; with the pernitrate of mercury, a greenish-yellow precipitate; with corrosive sublimate, a precipitate of a fine orange-red, very soluble in an excess of hydriodate; and with nitrate of lead, a precipitate of an orange-yellow colour. They dissolve iodine, and acquire a deep reddish-brown colour.

Hydriodate of potassa, or in the dry state, *iodide of potassium*, yields crystals like sea-salt, which melt and sublime at a red-heat. This salt is not changed by being heated in contact with air. 100 parts of water at 64°, dissolve 143 of it. It consists of 15.5 iodine, and 5 potassium.

Hydriodate of soda, called in the dry state *iodide of sodium*, may be obtained in pretty large flat rhomboidal prisms. It consists, when dry, of 15.5 iodine + 3 sodium.

Hydriodate of barytes crystallizes in fine prisms, similar to muriate of strontites. In its dry state, it consists of 15.5 iodine + 8.75 barium.

The *hydriodates of lime* and *strontites* are very soluble; and the first exceedingly deliquescent.

Hydriodate of ammonia results from the combination of equal volumes of ammoniacal and hydriodic gases; though it is usually prepared by saturating the liquid acid with ammonia. It is nearly as volatile as sal ammoniac; but it is more soluble and more deliquescent. It crystallizes in cubes.

Hydriodate of magnesia is formed by uniting its constituents together; it is deliquescent, and crystallizes with difficulty.—It is decomposed by a strong heat.

Hydriodate of zinc is easily obtained, by putting iodine into water with an excess of zinc, and favouring their action by heat. When dried it becomes an iodide.

All the hydriodates have the property of dissolving abundance of iodine; and thence they acquire a deep reddish-brown colour. They part with it on boiling, or when exposed to the air after being dried."

HYDRO-CHLORIC ACID. Muriatic acid; a compound of chlorine and hydrogen. See *Muriatic acid.*

HYDRO-CYANIC ACID. See *Prussic acid.*

HYDRO-FLUORIC ACID. *Acidum hydrofluoricum.* This is procured by distilling, in lead or silver, a mixture of one part of the purest fluor spar, in fine powder, with two of sulphuric acid. The heat required is not considerable; sulphate of lime remains in the retort, and a highly acrid and corrosive liquid passes over, which requires the assistance of ice for its condensation.

HYDRO-SULPHURIC ACID. The aqueous solution of sulphuretted hydrogen, is so called by Gay Lussac.

HYDRO-SULPHUROUS ACID. When three volumes of sulphuretted hydrogen gas and two of sulphurous acid gas, both dry, are mixed together over mercury, they are condensed into a solid orange-yellow body, which Dr. Thompson calls hydro-sulphurous acid.

HYDRO'A. (From υδωρ, water.) A watery pustule.

HYDROCARBONATE. See *Carburetted hydrogen gas.*

HYDROCA'RDIA. (From υδωρ, water, and καρδια, the heart.) *Hydrocordis. Hydrops pericardii.* Dropsy of the heart. Dropsy of the pericardium. A collection of fluid in the pericardium, which may be either coagulable lymph, serum, or a puriform fluid. It produces symptoms similar to those of hydrothorax, with violent palpitation of the heart, and mostly an intermittent pulse. It is incurable.

HYDROCE'LE. (From υδωρ, water, and κηλη, a tumour.) The term *hydrocele*, used in a literal sense, means any tumour produced by water; but surgeons have always confined it to those which possess either the membranes of the scrotum, or the coats of the testicle and its vessels. The first of these, viz. that which has its seat in the membranes of the scrotum, anasarca integumentorum, is common to the whole bag, and to all the cellular substance which loosely envelopes both the testes. It is, strictly speaking, only a symptom of a disease, in which the whole habit is most frequently more or less concerned, and very seldom affects the part only. The latter, or that which occupies the coats immediately investing the testicle and its vessels, hydrocele tunica vaginalis, is absolutely local, very seldom affects the common membrane of the scrotum, generally attacks one side only; and is frequently found in persons who are perfectly free from all other complaints.

The anasarca integumentorum retains the impression of the finger. The vaginal hydrocele has an undulating feel.

The hydrocele of the tunica vaginalis testis is a morbid accumulation of the water separated on the internal surface of the tunica vaginalis, to moisten or lubricate the testicle.

From its first appearance, it seldom disappears or diminishes, but generally continues to increase, sometimes rapidly, at others more slowly. In some it grows to a painful degree of distention in a few months: in others, it continues many years with little disturbance. As it enlarges, it becomes more tense, and is sometimes transparent; so that if a candle is held on the opposite side, a degree of light is perceived through the whole tumour; but the only certain distinction is the fluctuation, which is not found when the disease is a hernia of the omentum, or intestines, or an inflammatory or scirrhous tumour of the testicle.

HYDROCELE CYSTATA. Encysted hydrocele of the spermatic cord, resembles the common hydrocele; but the tumour does not extend to the testicle, which may be felt below or behind it, while, in the hydrocele of the vaginal coat, when large, the testicle cannot be discovered. In this disease, also, the penis is not buried in the tumour. Sometimes the fluid is contained in two distinct cells; and this is discovered by little contractions in it. It is distinguished from the anasarcous hydrocele by a sensible fluctuation, and the want of the inelastic pitting; from hernia, by its beginning below, from its not receding in a horizontal position, and not enlarging by coughing and sneezing.

HYDROCELE FUNICULI SPERMATICI, or hydrocele of the spermatic cord. Anasarcous hydrocele of the spermatic cord sometimes accompanies ascites, and, at other times, it is found to be confined to the cellular substance, in or about the spermatic cord. The causes of this disease may be obstructions in the lymphatics, leading from the part, in consequence of scirrhous affections of the abdominal viscera, or the pressure of a truss applied for the cure of hernia

When the affection is connected with anasarca in other parts, it is then so evident as to require no particular description. When it is local it is attended with a colourless tumour in the course of the spermatic cord, soft and inelastic to the touch, and unaccompanied with fluctuation. In an erect position of the body, it is of an oblong figure; but when the body is recumbent, it is flatter, and somewhat round. Generally it is no longer than the part of the cord which lies in the groin; though sometimes it extends as far as the testicle, and even stretches the scrotum to an uncommon size. By pressure a great part of the swelling can always be made to recede into the abdomen. It instantly, however, returns to its former situation, on the pressure being withdrawn.

Hydrocele peritonæi. The common dropsy of the belly.

Hydrocele spinalis. A watery swelling on the vertebræ.

HYDROCE'PHALUS. (From ὑδωρ, water, and κεφαλη, the head.) *Hydrocephalum; Hydrencephalus.* Dropsy of the brain. Dropsy of the head. A genus of disease arranged by Cullen in the class *Cachexiæ*, and order *Intumescentiæ*. It is distinguished by authors into external and internal:

1. *Hydrocephalus externus*, is a collection of water between the membranes of the brain.

2. *Hydrocephalus internus*, is when a fluid is collected in the ventricles of the brain, producing dilatation of the pupils, apoplexy, &c. See *Apoplexia.* It is sometimes of a chronic nature, when the water has been known to increase to an enormous quantity, effecting a diastasis of the bones of the head, and an absorption of the brain.

Pain in the head, particularly across the brow, stupor, dilatation of the pupils, nausea, vomiting, preternatural slowness of the pulse, and convulsions, are the pathognomonic symptoms of this disease, which have been laid down by the generality of writers.

Hydrocephalus is almost peculiar to children, being rarely known to extend beyond the age of twelve or fourteen; and it seems more frequently to arise in those of a scrofulous and rickety habit than in others. It is an affection which has been observed to pervade families, affecting all or the greater part of the children at a certain period of their life; which seems to show that, in many cases, it depends more on the general habit, than on any local affection or accidental cause.

The disease has generally been supposed to arise in consequence either of injuries done to the brain itself, by blows, falls, &c. from scirrhous tumours or excrescences within the skull, from original laxity or weakness in the brain, or from general debility and an impoverished state of the blood.

With respect to its proximate cause, very opposite opinions are still entertained by medical writers, which, in conjunction with the equivocal nature of its symptoms, prove a source of considerable embarrassment to the young practitioner. Some believe it to be inflammatory, and bleed largely.

Dr. Withering observes, that in a great many cases, if not in all, congestion, or slight inflammation, are the precursors to the aqueous accumulation.

Dr. Rush thinks that, instead of its being considered an idiopathic dropsy, it should be considered only as an effect of a primary inflammation or congestion of blood in the brain. It appears, says he, that the disease, in its first stage, is the effect of causes which produce a less degree of that inflammation which constitutes phrenitis; and that its second stage is a less degree of that effusion which produces serous apoplexy in adults. The former partakes of the nature of the chronic inflammation of Dr. Cullen, and the asthenic inflammation of Dr. Brown.—There are others, again, who view the subject in a very different light. Dr. Darwin supposes inactivity, or torpor of the absorbent vessels of the brain, to be the cause of hydrocephalus internus; but he confesses, in another part of his work, that the torpor of the absorbent vessels may often exist as a secondary effect.

Dr. Whytt, who has published an ingenious treatise on the disease, observes, the immediate cause of every kind of dropsy is the same; viz. such a state of the parts as makes the exhalent arteries throw out a greater quantity of fluids than the absorbents can take up From what he afterward mentions, he evidently considers this state as consisting in debility.

As many cases are accompanied with an increased or inflammatory action of the vessels of the brain, and others again are observed to prevail along with general anasarca, it seems rational to allow, that hydrocephalus is, in some instances, the consequence of congestion, or slight inflammation of the brain; and that, in others, it arises either from general debility or topical laxity. In admitting these as incontrovertible facts, Dr. Thomas is, at the same time, induced to suppose, that the cases of it occurring from mere debility are by no means frequent.

The great analogy subsisting between the symptoms which are characteristic of inflammation, and those which form the first stage of the acute species of hydrocephalus, (for the disease, as already observed, has been divided into the chronic and acute by some writers,) together with the good effects often consequent on blood-letting, and the inflammatory appearance which the blood frequently exhibits, seems to point out strong proof of the disease being, in most instances, an active inflammation, and that it rarely occurs from mere debility, as a primary cause.

The progress of the disorder has, by some, been divided into three stages.

When it is accompanied by an increased or inflammatory action of the brain, as not uncommonly happens, its first stage is marked with many of the symptoms of pyrexia, such as languor, inactivity, loss of appetite, nausea, vomiting, parched tongue, hot, dry skin, flushing of the face, headache, throbbing of the temporal arteries, and quickened pulse; which symptoms always suffer an exacerbation in the evening, but towards morning become milder.

When it is unaccompanied by any inflammatory action of the brain, many of these appearances are not to be observed. In these cases, it is marked by a dejection of countenance, loss of appetite, pains over the eyes, soreness of the integuments of the cranium to the touch, propensity to the bed, aversion to being moved, nausea, and costiveness. The disease, at length, makes a remarkable transition, which denotes the commencement of its second stage. The child screams out, without being able to assign any cause; its sleep is much disturbed; there is a considerable dilatation of the pupils of the eyes, without any contraction on their being exposed to light: lethargic torpor, with strabismus, or perhaps double vision ensues, and the pulse becomes slow and unequal.

In the third stage, the pulse returns again to the febrile state, becoming uncommonly quick and variable; and coma, with convulsions, ensue. When the accumulation of water is very great, and the child young, the sutures recede a considerable way from each other, and the head, towards the end, becomes much enlarged.

When recoveries have actually taken place in hydrocephalus, we ought probably to attribute more to the efforts of nature than to the interference of art. It is always to be regarded as of difficult cure.

An accumulation of water in the ventricles of the brain, is one of the most common appearances to be observed on dissection. In different cases this is accumulated in greater or less quantities. It sometimes amounts only to a few ounces, and occasionally to some pints. When the quantity of water is considerable, the fornix is raised at its anterior extremity, in consequence of its accumulation, and an immediate opening of communication is thereby formed between the lateral ventricles. The water is of a purer colour and more limpid than what is found in the dropsy of the thorax, or abdomen. It appears, however, to be generally of the same nature with the water that is accumulated in these cavities. In some instances, the water in hydrocephalus contains a very small proportion of coagulable matter, and in others it is entirely free from it.

When the water is accumulatad to a very large quantity in the ventricles, the substance of the brain appears to be a sort of pulpy bag, containing a fluid. The skull, upon such occasions, is very much enlarged in its size, and altered in its shape; and it appears exceedingly large in proportion to the face. On removing the scalp, the bones are found to be very thin, and there are frequently broad spots of membrane in the bone. These appearances are, however, only to be observed where the disease has been of some years' continuance.

In some cases, where the quantity of water collected is not great, the substance of the brain has appeared to be indurated, and in others softened. At times, the organ has been found gorged with blood: collections also of a viscid tenacious matter have been discovered in cysts, upon its external surface, and tumours have been found attached to its substance.

The treatment must be prompt and active to give a tolerable chance of success. The general indications are, in the first stage, to lessen the inflammatory action, afterward to promote absorption. Should the patient be about the age of puberty, of a plethoric habit, and the symptoms run high at the beginning, it will be proper to take some blood, especially from the temporal artery, or the jugular vein; but, if younger, or the disease more advanced, a sufficient quantity may be withdrawn by leeches, applied to the temples, or in the direction of the sutures. The bowels must then be thoroughly evacuated by some active cathartic, as they are usually very torpid, calomel with scammony, or jalap, for example; and, in the progress of the complaint, this function must be kept up with some degree of activity. For this purpose, calomel may be given in divided doses, or some other mercurial preparation, which may not run off too rapidly, producing mere watery stools, but regularly clear out the bowels, as well as the liver, and promote the other secretions. Besides, mercury is the most powerful remedy in rousing the absorbents, and some of the most remarkable cures of this disease, even at an advanced period, have been affected by it: whence it would be advisable, where the disease was proceeding rapidly, and particularly if the bowels were irritable, to use mercurial frictions, that the system might be sooner affected. Another very important step, after clearing the bowels, is to apply some evaporating lotion assiduously to the scalp, previously shaved; and the antiphlogistic regimen should be steadily observed. Diaphoretics will generally be proper, assisted by the warm bath; and diuretics on some occasions may be useful; but digitalis, which has been recommended on this ground, seems more likely to avail by lessening arterial action. Blisters may be applied to the temples, behind the ears, or to the nape of the neck, each perhaps successively: and dressed with savine cerate occasionally, to increase the discharge, and irritation externally: issues appear not so likely to prove beneficial. Errhines may farther contribute to obviate internal effusion. Electricity has been proposed to rouse the absorbents to the second stage; but its efficacy, and even propriety, is very doubtful. Should the progress of the complaint be fortunately arrested, the strength must be established by a nutritious diet, and tonic medicines; taking care to keep the bowels in good order, and the head cool: an issue, under these circumstances, may be a very useful remedy.

HYDROCEPHALUS ACUTUS. See *Hydrocephalus*.

HYDROCEPHALUS EXTERNUS. Water between the brain and its membranes.

HYDROCEPHALUS INTERNUS. Water in the ventricles of the brain.

HYDROCO'TYLE. (From υδωρ, water, and κοτυλη, the cotula.) 1. The name of a genus of plants in the Linnæan system. Class, *Pentandria*; Order, *Digynia*.

2. The name, in some pharmacopœias, for the common marsh or water cotula, or pennywort, which is said to possess acrid qualities.

HYDROCY'STIS. (From υδωρ, water, and κυςις, a vesicle.) An encysted dropsy.

HY'DROGEN. (*Hydrogenium*; from υδωρ, water, and γινομαι, to become, or γεννаω, to produce, because with oxygen it produces water.) Base of *inflammable air*.

Hydrogen is a substance not perceptible to our sensations in a separate state; but its existence is not at all the less certain. Though we cannot exhibit it experimentally uncombined, we can pursue it while it passes out of one combination into another; we cannot, indeed, arrest it on its passage, but we never fail to discover it, at least if we use the proper chemical means, when it presents itself to our notice in a new compound.

Hydrogen, as its name expresses, is one of the constituent elements of water, from which it can alone be procured. Its existence was unknown till lately. It is plentifully distributed in nature, and acts a very considerable part in the process of the animal and vegetable economy. It is one of the ingredients in the varieties of bitumen, oils, fat, ardent spirits, æther, and, in fact, all the proximate, component parts of animal and vegetable bodies. It forms a constituent part of all animal and vegetable acids. It is one of the constituents of ammonia and of various other compound gases.

It possesses so great an affinity for caloric, that i can only exist separately in the state of gas; it is consequently impossible to procure it in the concrete or liquid state, independent of combination.

Solid hydrogen, therefore, united to caloric and light, forms HYDROGEN GAS.

Properties of Hydrogen Gas.

This gas, which was commonly called inflammable air, was discovered by Cavendish in the year 1768, or rather he first obtained it in a state of purity, and ascertained its more important properties, though it had been noticed long before. The famous philosophical candle attests the antiquity of this discovery.

Hydrogen gas, like oxygen gas, is a triple compound, consisting of the ponderable base of hydrogen, caloric, and light. It possesses all the mechanical properties of atmospheric air. It is the lightest substance whose weight we are able to estimate: when in its purest state, and free from moisture, it is about fourteen times lighter than atmospheric air. It is not fitted for respiration; animals, when obliged to breathe in it, die almost instantaneously. It is decomposed by living vegetables, and its basis becomes one of the constituents of oil, resin, &c. It is inflammable, and burns rapidly when kindled, *in contact with atmospheric air or oxygen gas*, by means of the electric spark, or by an inflamed body; and burns, when pure, with a yellowish lambent flame: but all burning substances are immediately extinguished when immersed in it. It is therefore, incapable of supporting combustion. It is not injurious to growing vegetables. It is unabsorbable by most substances; water absorbs it very sparingly It is capable of dissolving carbon, sulphur, phosphorus, arsenic, and many other bodies. When its basis combines with that of oxygen gas, water is formed; with nitrogen it forms ammonia. It does not act on earthy substances.

Method of obtaining Hydrogen Gas.—A ready method of obtaining hydrogen gas consists in subjecting water to the action of a substance which is capable of decomposing this fluid.

1. For this purpose, let sulphuric acid, previously diluted with four or five times its weight of water, be poured on iron filings, or bits of zinc, in a small retort, or gas-bottle, called a pneumatic flask, or proof; as soon as the diluted acid comes in contact with the metal, a violent effervescence takes place, and hydrogen gas escapes without external heat being applied. It may be collected in the usual manner over water, taking care to let a certain portion escape on account of the atmospheric air contained in the disengaging vessels.

The production of hydrogen gas in the above way is owing to the decomposition of water. The iron, or zinc, when in contact with this fluid, in conjunction with sulphuric acid, has a greater affinity to oxygen than the hydrogen has; the oxygen, therefore, unites to it, and forms an oxide of that metal which is instantly attacked and dissolved by the acid; the other constituent part of the water, the hydrogen, is set free, which, by uniting with caloric, assumes the form of hydrogen gas. The oxygen is, therefore, the bond of union between the metal and the acid.

The hissing noise, or effervescence, observable during the process, is owing to the rapid motion excited in the mixture by means of the great number of air-bubbles quickly disengaged and breaking at the surface of the fluid.

We see, also, in this case, that *two* substances exert an attraction, and are even capable of decomposing jointly a *third*, which neither of them is able to do singly; *viz.* if we present sulphuric acid alone, or iron or zinc alone, to water, they cannot detach the oxygen from the hydrogen of that fluid; but, if both are applied, a decomposition is instantly effected. This experiment, therefore, proves that the agency of chemical affinity between two or more bodies may lie dormant, until it is called into action by the interposition of another body, which frequently exerts no energy upon any of them in a separate state. Instances of this kind were formerly called *predisposing affinities*.

2. Iron, in a red heat, has also the property of decomposing water, by dislodging the oxygen from its combination with hydrogen, in the following manner:—

Let a gun-barrel, having its touch-hole screwed up, pass through a furnace, or large crucible perforated for that purpose, taking care to incline the barrel at the narrowest part; adjust to its upper extremity a retort charged with water, and let the other extremity terminate in a tube introduced under a receiver in the pneumatic trough. When the apparatus is thus disposed, and well luted, bring the gun-barrel to a red heat, and, when thoroughly red-hot, make the water in the retort boil; the vapour, when passing through the red-hot tube, will yield hydrogen gas abundantly. In this experiment, the oxygen of the water combines with the iron at a red heat, so as to convert it into an oxide, and the caloric applied combines with the hydrogen of the water, and forms hydrogen gas. It is, therefore, the result of a double affinity, that of the oxygen of the water for the metal; and that of its hydrogen for caloric.

The more caloric is employed in the experiment of decomposing water by means of iron, &c. the sooner is the water decomposed.

Hydrogen gas, combined with carbon, is frequently found in great abundance in mines and coal-pits, where it is sometimes generated suddenly, and becomes mixed with the atmospheric air of these subterraneous cavities. If a lighted candle be brought in, this mixture often explodes, and produces the most dreadful effects. It is called by miners, *fire damp*. It generally forms a cloud in the upper part of the mine, on account of its levity, but does not mix there with atmospheric air, unless some agitation takes place. The miners frequently set fire to it with a candle, lying at the same time flat on their faces to escape the violence of the shock. An easier and more safe method of clearing the mine, is by leading a long tube through the shaft of it, to the ash-pit of a furnace; by this means the gas will be conducted to feed the fire.

Sir Humphrey Davy has invented a valuable instrument called a *safety lamp*, which will enable the miners to convey a light into such impure air without risk. This is founded on the important discovery, made by him, that flame is incapable of passing through minute apertures in a metallic substance, which yet are pervious to air; the reason of which appears to be, that the ignited gas, or vapour, is so much cooled by the metal in its passage as to cease being luminous.

Hydrogen gas, in whatever manner produced, *always* originates from water, either in consequence of a preceding decomposition, by which it had been combined in the state of solid or fixed hydrogen, with one of the substances employed, or from a decomposition of water actually taking place during the experiment.

There are instances recorded of a vapour issuing from the stomach of dead persons which took fire on the approach of a candle. We even find accounts, in several works, of the combustion of living human beings, which appeared to be spontaneous. Dr. Swediaur has related some instances of porters at Warsaw, who having drunk abundantly of spirit, fell down in the street, with the smoke issuing out of their mouths; and people came to their assistance, saying they would take fire; to prevent which, they made them drink a great quantity of milk, or used a more singular expedient, by causing them to swallow the urine of the bystanders, immediately on its evacuation.

However difficult it may be to give credit to such narratives, it is equally difficult to reject them entirely, without refusing to admit the numerous testimonies of men, who were, for the most part, worthy of credit. *Citizen Lair* has collected all the circumstances of this nature which he found dispersed in different books, and has rejected those which did not appear to be supported by respectable testimony, to which he has added some others related by persons still living. These narratives are nine in number; they were communicated to the Philomathic Society, at Paris, and inserted in the bulletin Thermidor, An. 5, No. 29. The cause of this phenomenon has been attributed to a developement of hydrogen gas taking place in the stomachs of these individuals.

Lair believes that the bodies of these people were not burned perfectly spontaneously, but it appeared to be owing to some very slight external cause, such as the fire of a candle, taper, or pipe.

HYDROGEN GAS, SELENIURETTED. This gas is colourless. It reddens litmus. Its density has not been determined by experiment. Its smell resembles, at first, that of sulphuretted hydrogen gas; but the sensation soon changes, and another succeeds, which is at once pungent, astringent, and painful. The eyes become almost instantly red and inflamed, and the sense of smelling entirely disappears. A bubble of the size of a little pea is sufficient to produce these effects. Of all the bodies derived from the inorganic kingdom, seleniuretted hydrogen is that which exercises the strongest action on the animal economy. Water dissolves this gas; but in what proportions is not known. This solution disturbs almost all the metallic solutions, producing black or brown precipitates, which assume, on rubbing with polished hæmatites, a metallic lustre. Zinc, manganese, and cerium, form exceptions. They yield flesh-coloured precipitates, which appear to be hydro-seleniurets of the oxides, while the others, for the most part, are merely metallic seleniurets.

HYDROGEN, SULPHURETTED. Sulphuretted hydrogen gas possesses the properties of an acid; for, when absorbed by water, its solution reddens vegetable blues; it combines also with alkalies, earths, and with several metallic oxides. Sulphuretted hydrogen, combined with any base, forms a *hydro-sulphuret*, which may be also called an *hepatule*, to distinguish it from an *hepar*, which is the union of sulphur singly with a base. Sulphuretted hydrogen gas possesses an extremely offensive odour, resembling that of putrid eggs. It kills animals, and extinguishes burning bodies. When in contact with oxygen gas, or atmospheric air, it is inflammable. Mingled with nitrous gas, it burns with a yellowish green flame. It is decomposed by ammonia, by oxymuriatic acid gas, and by sulphurous acid gas. It has a strong action on the greater number of metallic oxides. Its specific gravity is about 1.18 when pure. It is composed, according to Thomson, of sixteen parts of sulphur, and one of hydrogen. It has the property of dissolving a small quantity of phosphorus.

Sulphuretted hydrogen gas may be obtained in several ways:—

1. Take dry sulphuret of potassa, put it into a tubulated retort, lodged in a sand-bath, or supported over a lamp; direct the neck of the retort under a receiver placed in the pneumatic trough; then pour gradually upon the sulphuret diluted sulphuric or muriatic acid; a violent effervescence will take place, and sulphuretted hydrogen gas will be liberated. When no more gas is produced spontaneously, urge the mixture with heat, by degrees, till it boils, and gas will again be liberated abundantly.

The water made use of for receiving it, should be heated to about 80° or 90°; at this temperature it dissolves little of the gas; whereas, if cold water be made use of, a much greater quantity of it is absorbed.

Explanation.—Though sulphur makes no alteration on water, which proves that sulphur has less attraction for oxygen than hydrogen has, yet if sulphur be united to an alkali, this combination decomposes water whenever it comes in contact with it, though the alkali itself has no attraction either for oxygen or hydrogen.

The formation of this gas explains this truth. On adding the sulphuret of potassa to the water, this fluid becomes decomposed, part of the sulphur robs it of its oxygen; and forms with it sulphuric acid; this generated acid unites to part of the alkali, and forms sulphate of potassa. The liberated hydrogen dissolves another part of the sulphur, and forms with it sulphuretted hydrogen, the basis of this gas, which is retained by the separated portion of the alkali. The sulphuric or muriatic acid, added now, extricates it from the alkali, and makes it fly off in the form of gas.

Diluted muriatic acid seems best adapted for the production of sulphuretted hydrogen gas from alkaline sulphurets. If nitric acid be made use of, it must be much diluted. Sulphuric acid yields little gas, unless assisted by heat. When the proportion of sulphur in the sulphuret exceeds that of the alkali, the dense sulphuric acid, poured upon it, emits sulphurous acid gas. All the rest of the acids may be made use of for decomposing the sulphurets.

2. When iron and sulphur are united together, they

afford a large quantity of sulphuretted hydrogen gas, on submitting them to the action of heat, in contact with diluted muriatic acid.

Melt together, in a crucible, equal parts of iron filings and sulphur; the product is a black brittle mass, called sulphuret of iron. Reduce this to powder, and put it, with a little water, into a tubulated retort; add diluted muriatic acid, and apply a gentle heat, till no more gas is disengaged. The philosophy of this experiment is analogous to the former. Part of the oxygen of the water unites to part of the sulphur, and forms sulphuric acid; another part oxidizes the iron, which, dissolved by the acid, forms sulphate of iron: the hydrogen of the water unites to another part of the sulphur, and forms sulphuretted hydrogen, which becomes gaseous by the addition of caloric.

3. Sulphuretted hydrogen gas may also be obtained by heating an alkaline sulphuret, with the addition of water, without the aid of an acid. In this case, the water is also decomposed; its hydrogen unites with part of the sulphur, and forms sulphuretted hydrogen; the oxygen of the water unites with another part of the sulphur, and produces sulphuric acid, which joins to the alkali and forms a sulphate. The sulphuretted hydrogen becomes disengaged by heat in the gaseous form.

4. Sulphuretted hydrogen gas may be obtained by passing hydrogen gas through sulphur, in a state of fusion.

For this purpose, put sulphur into a gun-barrel, or Wedgewood's tube, and place it across a furnace; fit to the lower extremity a bent glass tube, which goes under a receiver placed in the pneumatic trough, and adapt to the upper extremity a tubulated retort, or other apparatus proper for producing hydrogen gas. The sulphur must then be heated, and, when melted. the hydrogen gas evolved must be made to pass over it, which, in this manner, will dissolve part of the sulphur, and become converted into sulphuretted hydrogen gas.

5. It may likewise be procured in the following direct manner: let a small quantity of sulphur be enclosed in a jar full of hydrogen gas, and melt it by means of a burning-glass. This method does not succeed except the hydrogen gas be as dry as possible, for its affinity to sulphur is weakened in proportion to its moisture.

6. The method, however, which affords it purest, is by treating sulphuret of antimony with diluted muriatic acid. The explanation is similar to the preceding processes.

Hydrogen, carburetted. See *Carburetted hydrogen gas.*

Hydrogen, percarburetted. See *Carburetted hydrogen gas.*

Hydrogen, subcarburetted. See *Carburetted hydrogen gas.*

Hydrogen, phosphuretted. See *Phosphorus.*

Hydrogen, subphosphuretted. See *Phosphorus.*

Hydrogen gas, heavy, carbonated. See *Carbonated hydrogen gas.*

Hydrogen gas, light, carbonated. See *Carburetted hydrogen gas.*

HYDROGURET. See *Uret.*

Hydroguret of carbon. See *Carburetted hydrogen gas.*

HYDROLA'PATHUM. (From υδωρ, water, and λαπαθον, the dock.) See *Rumex hydrolapathum.*

HYDRO'MELI. (From υδωρ, water, and μελι, honey.) *Mulsum; Aqua Mulsa; Melicratum; Braggat; Hydromel.* Water impregnated with honey. After it is fermented, it is called vinous hydromel, or mead.

HYDROTHIONIC ACID. See *Sulphuretted hydrogen.*

HYDROMETER. (*Hydrometer;* from υδωρ, water, or fluid, and μετρον, a measure.) The best method of weighing equal quantities of corrosive volatile fluids, to determine their specific gravities, appears to consist in enclosing them in a bottle with a conical stopper, in the side of which stopper a fine mark is cut with a file. The fluid being poured into the bottle, it is easy to put in the stopper, because the redundant fluid escapes through the notch, or mark, and may be carefully wiped off. Equal bulks of water, and other fluids, are by this means weighed to a great degree of accuracy, care being taken to keep the temperature as equal as possible, by avoiding any contact of the bottle with the hand, or otherwise. The bottle itself shows with much precision, by a rise or fall of the liquid in the notch of the stopper, whether any such change have taken place.

The hydrometer of Fahrenheit consists of a hollow ball, with a counterpoise below, and a very slender stem above, terminating in a small dish. The middle, or half length of the stem, is distinguished by a fine line across. In this instrument every division of the stem is rejected, and it is immersed in all experiments to the middle of the stem, by placing proper weights in the little dish above. Then, as the part immersed is constantly of the same magnitude, and the whole weight of the hydrometer is known, this last weight, added to the weights in the dish, will be equal to the weight of fluid displaced by the instrument, as all writers on hydrostatics prove. And, accordingly, the sp. gravities for the common form of the tables will be had by the proportion:

As the whole weight of the hydrometer and its load, when adjusted in distilled water,
Is to the number 1000, &c.
So is the whole weight when adjusted in any other fluid
To the number expressing its specific gravity.

The hydrometers, or *pese-liqueurs*, of Baumé, though in reality comparable with each other, are subject in part to the defect, that their results, having no independent numerical measure, require explanation to those who do not know the instruments.

HYDROME'TRA. (From υδωρ, water, and μητρα, the womb.) *Hydrops uteri.* Dropsy of the womb. A genus of disease in the class *Cachexiæ*, and order *Intumescentiæ*, of Cullen. It produces a swelling of the hypogastric region, slowly and gradually increasing, resembling the figure of the uterus, yielding to, or fluctuating on pressure; without ischury or pregnancy. Sauvages enumerates seven species. It must be considered as a very rare disease, and one that can with difficulty be ascertained.

HYDRO'MPHALUM. (From υδωρ, water, and ομφαλος, the navel.) A tumour of the navel, containing water.

HYDRO'NOSOS. (From υδωρ, water, and νοσος, a disease.) The sweating sickness. See *Ephidrosis.*

HYDRO-OXIDE. See *Hydrate.*

HYDROPEDE'SIS. (From υδωρ, water, and πηδαω, to break out.) A breaking out into a violent sweat.

HYDROPHANE. *Oculus mundi.* A variety of opal, which has the property of becoming transparent on immersion in water.

HYDROPHO'BIA. (From υδωρ, water, and φοβεω, to fear.) *Rabies canina; Cynanthropia; Cynolesia.* Canine madness. This disease arises in consequence of the bite of a rabid animal, as a dog or cat, and sometimes spontaneously. It is termed hydrophobia, because persons that are thus bitten dread the sight or the falling of water when first seized. Cullen has arranged it under the class *Neuroses*, and order *Spasmi*, and defines it a loathing and great dread of drinking any liquids, from their creating a painful convulsion of the pharynx, occasioned most commonly by the bite of a mad animal.

There are two species of hydrophobia.

1. *Hydrophobia rabiosa*, when there is a desire of biting.

2. *Hydrophobia simplex*, when there is not a desire of biting.

Dr. James observes, that this peculiar affection properly belongs to the canine genus, viz. dogs, foxes, and wolves; in which animals only it seems to be innate and natural, scarcely ever appearing in any others, except when communicated from these. When a dog is affected with madness, he becomes dull, solitary, and endeavours to hide himself, seldom barking, but making a murmuring noise, and refusing all kinds of meat and drink. He flies at strangers; but, in this stage, he remembers and respects his master; his head and tail hang down; he walks as if overpowered by sleep; and a bite, at this period, though dangerous, is not so apt to bring on the disease in the animal bitten as one inflicted at a later period. The dog at length begins to pant; he breathes quickly and heavily; his tongue hangs out; his mouth is continually open, and discharges a large quantity of froth. Sometimes he walks slowly, as if half asleep, and then runs suddenly but not always directly forward. At last he forgets his master; his eyes have a dull, watery, red appearance: he grows thin and weak, often falls down, gets up and attempts to fly at every thing, becoming very soon quite furious. The animal seldom lives in this latter state longer than thirty hours; and it is said, that his bites toward the end of his existence, are the most dangerous. The throat of a person suffering hydrophobia is always much affected; and, it is asserted, the nearer the bite to this part the more perilous.

Hydrophobia may be communicated to the human subject from the bites of cats, cows, and other animals, not of the canine species, to which the affection has been previously communicated. However, it is from the bites of those domestic ones, the dog and cat, that most cases of hydrophobia originate. It does not appear that the bite of a person affected can communicate the disease to another; at least the records of medicine furnish no proof of this circumstance.

In the human species, the general symptoms attendant upon the bite of a mad dog, or other rabid animal, are, at some indefinite period, and occasionally long after the bitten part seems quite well; a slight pain begins to be felt in it, now and then attended with itching, but generally resembling a rheumatic pain. Then come on wandering pains, with an uneasiness and heaviness, disturbed sleep, and frightful dreams, accompanied with great restlessness, sudden startings, and spasms, sighing, anxiety, and a love for solitude. These symptoms continuing to increase daily, pains begin to shoot from the place which was wounded, all along up to the throat with a straitness and sensation of choking, and a horror and dread at the sight of water, and other liquids, together with a loss of appetite and tremor. The person is, however, capable of swallowing any solid substance with tolerable ease; but the moment that any thing in a fluid form is brought in contact with his lips, it occasions him to start back with much dread and horror, although he labours perhaps under great thirst at the time.

A vomiting of bilious matter soon comes on, in the course of the disease, and an intense hot fever ensues, attended with continual watching, great thirst, dryness and roughness of the tongue, hoarseness of the voice, and the discharge of a viscid saliva from the mouth, which the patient is constantly spitting out; together with spasms of the genital and urinary organs, in consequence of which the evacuations are forcibly thrown out. His respiration is laborious and uneasy, but his judgment is unaffected; and, as long as he retains the power of speech, his answers are distinct.

In some few instances, a severe delirium arises, and closes the tragic scene; but it more frequently happens, that the pulse becomes tremulous and irregular, that convulsions arise, and that nature being at length exhausted, sinks under the pressure of misery.

The appearances to be observed, on dissection in hydrophobia, are unusual aridity of the viscera and other parts; marks of inflammation in the fauces, gula, and larynx; inflammatory appearances in the stomach, and an accumulation or effusion of blood in the lungs. Some marks of inflammation are likewise to be observed in the brain, consisting in a serous effusion on its surface, or in a redness of the pia mater; which appearances have also presented themselves in the dog.

In some cases of dissection, not the least morbid appearance has been observed, either in the fauces, diaphragm, stomach, or intestines. The poison has, therefore, been conceived by some physicians to act upon the nervous system, and to be so wholly confined to it, as to make it a matter of doubt whether the qualities of the blood are altered or not. There is no known cure for this terrible disease: and the only preventive to be relied upon is the complete excision of the bitten part, which should be performed as soon as possible; though it may perhaps not be too late any time before the symptoms appear.

HYDROPHOSPHOROUS ACID. See *Phosphorous acid.*

HYDROPHTHA'LMIA. From υδωρ, water, and οφθαλμος, the eye.) *Hydrophthalmium.* There are two diseases, different in their nature and consequence, thus termed. The one is a mere anasarcous or œdematous swelling of the eyelid. The other, the true hydrophthalmia, is a swelling of the bulb of the eye, from too great a collection of vitreous or aqueous humours.

HYDROPHTHA'LMIUM. (From υδωρ, water, and οφθαλμος, the eye.) See *Hydrophthalmia.*

HYDROPHTORIC ACID. *Acidum hydrophtoricum.* (From υδωρ, water, and φθοριος, destructive.) Ampére's name for the base of the fluoric acid, called by Davy, *fluorine.* See *Hydro-fluoric acid.*

HYDROPHYSOCE'LE. (From υδωρ, water, φυση, flatulence, and κηλη, a tumour.) A swelling formed of water and air. It was applied to a hernia, in the sac of which was a fluid and air.

HYDRO'PICA. (From υδρωψ, the dropsy.) Medicines which relieve or cure dropsy.

HYDRO'PIPER. (From υδωρ, water, and πεπερι, pepper: so called from its biting the tongue like pepper, and growing in marshy places.) See *Polygonum hydropiper.*

HYDROPNEUMOSA'RCA. (From υδωρ, water, πνευμα, wind, and σαρξ, flesh.) A tumour of air, water, and solid substances.

HYDROPOI'DES. (From υδρωψ, a dropsy, and ειδος, likeness.) Serous or watery, formerly applied to liquid and watery excrements.

HY'DROPS. (*Hydrops, pis.* m.; from υδωρ, water.) Dropsy. A preternatural collection of serous or watery fluid in the cellular substance, or different cavities of the body. It receives different appellations, according to the particular situation of the fluid.

When it is diffused through the cellular membrane, either generally or partially, it is called *anasarca.* When it is deposited in the cavity of the cranium, it is called *hydrocephalus;* when in the chest, *hydrothorax,* or *hydrops pectoris;* when in the abdomen, *ascites.* In the uterus, *hydrometra,* and within the scrotum, *hydrocele.*

The causes of these diseases are a family disposition thereto, frequent salivations, excessive and long-continued evacuations, a free use of spirituous liquors, (which never fail to destroy the digestive powers,) scirrhosities of the liver, spleen, pancreas, mesentery and other abdominal viscera; preceding diseases, as the jaundice, diarrhœa, dysentery, phthisis, asthma, gout, intermittents of long duration, scarlet fever, and some of the exanthemata; a suppression of accustomed evacuations, the sudden striking in of eruptive humours, ossification of the valves of the heart, polypi in the right ventricle, aneurism in the arteries, tumours making a considerable pressure on the neighbouring parts, permanent obstruction in the lungs, rupture of the thoracic duct, exposure for a length of time to a moist atmosphere, laxity of the exhalants, defect in the absorbents, topical weakness, and general debility.

Hydrops articuli. A white swelling of a joint is sometimes so called.

Hydrops cystieus. A dropsy enclosed in a bag, or cyst.

Hydrops genu. An accumulation of synovia, or serum, within the capsular ligament of the knee.

Hydrops ad matulam. Diabetes.

Hydrops medullæ spinalis. See *Hydrorachitis* and *Spina bifida.*

Hydrops ovarii. A dropsy of the ovarium. See *Ascites.*

Hydrops pectoris. See *Hydrothorax.*

Hydrops pericardii. See *Hydrocardia.*

Hydrops pulmonum. Water in the cellular interstices of the lungs.

Hydrops scroti. See *Hydrocele.*

Hydrops uteri. See *Hydrometra.*

Hydropy'retus. (From υδωρ, water, and πυρετος, fever.) A sweating fever.

HYDRORACHI'TIS. (From υδωρ, water, and ραχις, the spine.) A fluctuating tumour, mostly situated on the lumbar vertebræ of new-born children. It is a genus of disease in the class *Cachexiæ,* and order *Intumescentiæ,* of Cullen, and is always incurable. See *Spina bifida.*

Hydroro'satum. A drink made of water, honey, and the juice of roses.

HYDROSA'CCHARUM. (From υδωρ, water, and σακχαρον, sugar.) A drink made of sugar and water.

HYDROSA'RCA. (From υδωρ, water, and σαρξ, the flesh.) See *Anasarca.*

HYDROSARCOCE'LE. (From υδωρ, water, σαρξ, the flesh, and κηλη, a tumour.) Sarcocele, with an effusion of water into the cellular membrane.

HYDROSELENIC ACID. The best process which

we can employ for procuring this acid, consists in treating the seleniuret of iron with the liquid muriatic acid. The acid gas evolved must be collected over mercury. As in this case a little of another gas, condensible neither by water nor alkaline solutions, appears, the best substance for obtaining absolutely pure hydroselenic acid would be seleniuret of potassium.

HYDROSELI'NUM. (From υδωρ, water, and σελινον, purslane.) A species of purslane growing in marshy places.

HYDROSULPHURET. *Hydrosulphuretum.* A compound of sulphuretted hydrogen with a salifiable basis.

HYDROSULPHURE'TUM STIBII LUTEUM. See *Antimonii sulphuretum præcipitatum.*

HYDROSULPHURETUM STIBII RUBRUM. *Kermes mineralis.* A hydro-sulphuret of antimony formerly in high estimation as an expectorant, sudorific, and antispasmodic, in difficult respiration, rheumatism, diseases of the skin and glands.

HYDROTHIONIC ACID. Some German chemists distinguish sulphuretted hydrogen by this name on account of its properties resembling those of an acid.

HYDROTHO'RAX. (From υδωρ, water, and θωραξ, the chest.) *Hydrops thoracis; Hydrops pectoris.* Dropsy of the chest. A genus of disease in the class *Cachexiæ*, and order *Intumescentiæ*, of Cullen. Difficulty of breathing, particularly when in a horizontal posture; sudden startings from sleep, with anxiety, and palpitations of the heart; cough, paleness of the visage, anasarcous swellings of the lower extremities, thirst, and a scarcity of urine, are the characteristic symptoms of hydrothorax; but the one which is more decisive than all the rest is a fluctuation of water being perceived in the chest, either by the patient himself or his medical attendant, on certain motions of the body.

The causes which give rise to the disease, are pretty much the same with those which are productive of the other species of dropsy. In some cases, it exists without any other kind of dropsical affection being present; but it prevails very often as a part of more universal dropsy.

It frequently takes place to a considerable degree before it becomes very perceptible; and its presence is not readily known, the symptoms, like those of hydrocephalus, not being always very distinct. In some instances, the water is collected in both sacs of the pleura; but, at other times, it is only in one. Sometimes it is lodged in the pericardium alone; but, for the most part, it only appears there when, at the same time, a collection is present in one or both cavities of the thorax. Sometimes the water is effused in the cellular texture of the lungs, without any being deposited in the cavity of the thorax. In a few cases, the water that is collected is enveloped in small cysts, of a membraneous nature, known by the name of hydatides, which seem to float in the cavity; but more frequently they are connected with, and attached to, particular parts of the internal surface of the pleura.

Hydrothorax often comes on with a sense of uneasiness at the lower end of the sternum, accompanied by a difficulty of breathing which is much increased by any exertion, and which is always most considerable during night, when the body is in a horizontal posture. Along with these symptoms there is a cough, that is at first dry, but which, after a time, is attended with an expectoration of thin mucus. There is likewise a paleness of the complexion, and an anasarcous swelling of the feet and legs, together with a considerable degree of thirst and a diminished flow of urine. Under these appearances, we have just grounds to suspect that there is a collection of water in the chest; but if the fluctuation can be perceived, there can then remain no doubt as to the reality of its presence.

During the progress of the disease, it is no uncommon thing for the patient to feel a numbness, or degree of palsy, in one or both arms, and to be more than ordinarily sensible to cold. With regard to the pulse, it is usually quick at first, but, towards the end, becomes irregular and intermitting.

Our prognostic in hydrothorax must, in general, be unfavourable, as it has seldom been cured, and, in many cases, will hardly admit even of alleviation, the difficulty of breathing continuing to increase, until the action of the lungs is at last entirely impeded by the quantity of water deposited in the chest. In some cases, the event is suddenly fatal; but in others, it is preceded, for a few days previous to death, by a spitting of blood.

Dissections of this disease show that, in some cases, the water is either collected in one side of the thorax, or that there are hydatides formed in some particular part of it; but they more frequently discover water in both sides of the chest, accompanied by a collection in the cellular texture and principal cavities of the body. The fluid is usually of a yellowish colour; possesses properties similar to serum, and, with respect to its quantity, varies very much, being from a few ounces to several quarts. According to the quantity, so are the lungs compressed by it; and, where it is very considerable, they are usually found much reduced in size. When universal anasarca has preceded the collection in the chest, it is no uncommon occurrence to find some of the abdominal viscera in a scirrhous state.

The treatment of this disease must be conducted on the same general plan as that of anasarca. Emetics, however, are hazardous, and purgatives do not afford so much benefit; but the bowels must be kept regular, and other evacuating remedies may be employed in conjunction with tonics. Squill has been chiefly resorted to, as being expectorant as well as diuretic; but its power is usually not great, unless it be carried so far as to cause nausea, which cannot usually be borne to any extent. Digitalis is more to be relied upon; but it will be better to conjoin them, adding, perhaps, some form of mercury; and employing at the same time other diuretics, as the supertartrate or acetate of potassa, juniper berries, &c. Where febrile symptoms attend, diaphoretics will probably be especially serviceable, as the pulvis ipecacuanhæ compositus, or antimonials, in small doses; which last may also promote expectoration. Blisters to the chest will be proper in many cases, particularly should there be any pain or other mark of inflammatory action. Myrrh seems to answer better than most other tonics, as more decidedly promoting expectoration; or the nitric acid may be given, increasing the secretion of urine, as well as supporting the strength. The inhalation of oxygen gas is stated to have been in some instances singularly beneficial. Where the fluid is collected in either of the sacs of the pleura, the operation of paracentesis of the thorax may afford relief under urgent symptoms, and, perhaps, contribute to the recovery of the patient.

HYDROXURE. See *Hydrate.*

HYDRURET. A compound of hydrogen with a metal. See *Uret.*

HYGEIA. *Hygieia.* The goddess of health. One of the four daughters of Esculapius. She often accompanies her father in the monuments of him now remaining, and appears like a young woman, commonly holding a serpent in one hand, and a patera in the other. Sometimes the serpent drinks out of the patera; sometimes he twines about the whole body of the goddess.

HYGIE'NE. (From υγιαινω, to be well.) *Hygiesis.* Modern physicians have applied this term to that division of *therapeia* which treats of the diet and non naturals of the sick.

HYGIE'SIS. See *Hygiene.*

HY'GRA. (From υγρος, humid.) An ancient term for liquid plasters.

HYGREMPLA'STRUM. (From υγρος, moist, and εμπλαςρον, a plaster.) A liquid plaster.

HYGROBLEPHA'RICUS. (From υγρος, humid, and βλεφαρον, the eyelid.) Applied to the emunctory ducts in the extreme edge, or inner part of the eyelid

HYGROCIRSOCE'LE. (From υγρος, moist, κιρσος, a varix, and κηλη, a tumour.) Dilated spermatic veins, or circocele, with dropsy of the scrotum.

HYGROCOLLY'RIUM. (From υγρος, liquid, and κολλυριον, a collyrium.) A collyrium composed of liquids

HYGRO'LOGY. (*Hygrologia*; from υγρος, a humour or fluid, and λογος, a discourse.) The doctrine of the fluids.

HYGRO'MA. (Υγρωμα; from υγρος, a liquid.) An encysted tumour, the contents of which are either serum or a fluid-like lymph. It sometimes happens that these tumours are filled with hydatids. Hygromatous tumours require the removal of the cyst, or the destruction of its secreting surface

HYGRO'METER. (*Hygrometrum;* from $\upsilon\gamma\rho\acute{o}\varsigma$, moist, and $\mu\epsilon\tau\rho o\nu$, a measure.) Hygrometer. An instrument to measure the degrees of moisture in the atmosphere. It also means an infirm part of the body, affected by moisture of the atmosphere.

HYGROMY'RUM. (From $\upsilon\gamma\rho o\varsigma$, moist, and $\mu\upsilon\rho o\nu$, a liquid ointment.) A liquid ointment.

HYGROSCO'PIC. Substances which have the property of absorbing moisture from the atmosphere. See *Atmosphere.*

HYGROPHO'BIA. See *Hydrophobia.*

HY'LE. ('Υλη, matter.) The materia medica, or matter of any kind that comes under the cognizance of a medical person.

HY'MEN. (From *Hymen*, the god of marriage, because this membrane is supposed to be entire before marriage, or copulation.) The hymen is a thin membrane, of a semilunar or circular form, placed at the entrance of the vagina, which it partly closes. It has a very different appearance in different women, but it is generally, if not always, found in virgins, and is very properly esteemed the test of virginity, being ruptured in the first act of coition. The remnants of the hymen are called the carunculæ myrtiformes. The hymen is also peculiar to the human species. There are two circumstances relating to the hymen which require medical assistance. It is sometimes of such a strong ligamentous texture, that it cannot be ruptured, and prevents the connexion between the sexes. It is also sometimes imperforated, wholly closing the entrance into the vagina, and preventing any discharge from the uterus; but both these cases are extremely rare. If the hymen be of an unnaturally firm texture, but perforated, though perhaps with a very small opening, the inconveniences thence arising will not be discovered before the time of marriage, when they may be removed by a crucial incision made through it, taking care not to injure the adjoining parts.

The imperforation of the hymen will produce its inconveniences when the person begins to menstruate. For the menstruous fluid, being secreted from the uterus at each period, and not evacuated, the patient suffers much pain from the distention of the parts, many strange symptoms and appearances are occasioned, and suspicions injurious to her reputation are often entertained. In a case of this kind, for which Dr. Denman was consulted, the young woman, who was twenty-two years of age, having many uterine complaints, with the abdomen enlarged, was suspected to be pregnant, though she persevered in asserting the contrary, and had never menstruated. When she was prevailed upon to submit to an examination, the circumscribed tumour of the uterus was found to reach as high as the navel, and the external parts were stretched by a round soft substance at the entrance of the vagina, in such a manner as to resemble that appearance which they have when the head of a child is passing through them; but there was no entrance into the vagina. On the following morning an incision was carefully made through the hymen, which had a fleshy appearance, and was thickened in proportion to its detention. Not less than four pounds of blood, of the colour and consistence of tar, were discharged; and the tumefaction of the abdomen was immediately removed. Several stellated incisions were afterward made through the divided edges, which is a very necessary part of the operation: and care was taken to prevent a reunion of the hymen till the next period of menstruation, after which she suffered no inconvenience. The blood discharged was not putrid or coagulated, and seemed to have undergone no other change after its secretion, but what was occasioned by the absorption of its more fluid parts. Some caution is required when the hymen is closed in those who are in advanced age, unless the membrane be distended by the confined menses; as Dr. Denman once saw an instance of inflammation of the peritonæum being immediately produced after the operation, of which the patient died as in the true puerperal fever; and no other reason could be assigned for the disease.

The carunculæ myrtiformes, by their elongation and enlargement, sometimes become very painful and troublesome.

HYMENÆA. (From *Hymen*, the god of marriage; because, as Linnæus informs us, its younger leaves cohere together in pairs, throughout the night.) The name of a genus of plants. Class, *Decandria;* Order, *Monogynia.*

HYMENÆA COURBARIL. The systematic name of the locust-tree which affords the resin called *gum anime*, which is now fallen into disuse, and is only to be found in the collections of the curious.

HYMENIUM. (From $\upsilon\mu\eta\nu$, a membrane.) The dilated exposed membrane of gymnocarpous mushrooms, in which the seed is placed. See *Gymnocarpi.*

HYMENODES. (From $\upsilon\mu\eta\nu$, a membrane, and $\epsilon\iota\delta o\varsigma$, likeness.) An old term for such urine as is found to be full of little films and pellicles. Hippocrates applies it also to the menstrual discharge when mixed with a tough viscid phlegm.

HYO. Names compounded of this word belong to muscles which originate from, or are inserted into, or connected with, the os hyoides; as *Hyo-glossus, Hyo-pharyngeus, Genio-hyo-glossus*, &c.

HYO-GLOSSUS. *Cerato-glossus* of Douglas and Cowper. *Basio-cerato-chondro-glossus* of Albinus. *Hyo-chondro-glosse* of Dumas. A muscle situated at the sides, between the os hyoides and the tongue. It arises from the basis, but chiefly from the corner of the os hyoides, running laterally and forwards to the tongue, which it pulls inward and downward.

HYOI'DES OS. (From the Greek letter υ, and $\epsilon\iota\delta o\varsigma$, likeness: so named from its resemblance.) This bone, which is situated between the root of the tongue and the larynx, derives its name from its supposed resemblance to the Greek letter υ, and is, by some writers, described along with the parts contained in the mouth. Ruysch has seen the ligaments of the bone so completely ossified, that the os hyoides was joined to the temporal bones by anchylosis. In describing this bone, it may be distinguished into its body, horns, and appendices. The body is the middle and broadest part of the bone, so placed that it may be easily felt with the finger in the forepart of the throat. Its forepart, which is placed toward the tongue, is irregularly convex, and its inner surface, which is turneds towards the larynx, is unequally concave. The *cornua*, or horns, which are flat, and a little bent, are considerably longer than the body of the bone, and may be said to form the sides of the υ. These horns are thickest near the body of the bone. At the extremity of each is observed a round tubercle, from which a ligament passes to the thyroid cartilage. The appendices, or smaller horns, *cornua minora*, as they are called by some writers, are two small processes, which, in their size and shape, are somewhat like a grain of wheat. They rise up from the articulations of the cornua, with the body of the bone, and are sometimes connected with the styloid process on each side, by means of a ligament. It is not unusual to find small portions of bone in these ligaments; and Ruysch, as we have already observed, has seen them completely ossified. In the fœtus, almost the whole of the bone is in a cartilaginous state, excepting a small point of a bone in the middle of its body, and in each of its horns. The appendices do not begin to appear till after birth, and usually remain cartilaginous many years. The os hyoides serves to support the tongue, and affords attachment to a variety of muscles, some of which perform the motions of the tongue, while others act on the larynx and fauces.

HYOPHARYNGE'US. (From $\upsilon o\epsilon\iota\delta\epsilon\varsigma$, the hyoid bone, and $\phi\alpha\rho\acute{\upsilon}\gamma\zeta$, the pharynx.) A muscle so called from its origin in the os hyoides, and its insertion in the pharynx.

HYOPHTHA'LMUS. (From $\upsilon\varsigma$, a swine, and $o\phi\theta\alpha\lambda\mu o\varsigma$, an eye: so named from the supposed resemblance of its flower to a hog's eye.) Hogs-eye plant. Most probably the *Buphthalmum spinosum* of Linnæus.

HYOSCIANIA. A new vegetable alkali extracted by Dr. Brande from henbane. See *Hyoscyamus niger*

HYOSCY'AMUS. (From $\upsilon\varsigma$, a swine, and $\kappa\upsilon\alpha\mu o\varsigma$, a bean: so named because hogs eat it as a medicine, or it may be because the plant is hairy and bristly, like a swine.)

1. The name of a genus of plants in the Linnæan system. Class, *Pentandria;* Order, *Monogynia.*

2. The pharmacopœial name of the henbane. See *Hyoscyamus niger.*

HYOSCYAMUS ALBUS. This plant, a native of the south of Europe, possesses similar virtues to the hyoscyamus niger.

HYOSCYAMUS LUTEUS. A species of tobacco, the *Nicotiana rustica* of Linnæus.

Hyoscyamus niger. The systematic name of common or black henbane, called also *Faba suilla; Apollinaris altercum; Agone; Altercangenon; Hyoscyamus —foliis amplexicaulibus sinuatis, floribus sessilibus* of Linnæus. The leaves of this plant, when recent, have a slightly fœtid smell, and a mucilaginous taste; when dried, they lose both taste and smell, and part also of their narcotic power. The root possesses the same qualities as the leaves, and even in a more eminent degree. Henbane resembles opium in its action, more than any other narcotic dose. In a moderate dose it increases at first the strength of the pulse, and occasions some sense of heat, which are followed by diminished sensibility and motion; in some cases, by thirst, sickness, stupor, and dimness of vision. In a larger quantity it occasions profound sleep, hard pulse, and sometimes fierce delirium, ending in coma, or convulsions, with a remarkable dilatation of the pupil, distortion of the countenance, a weak tremulous pulse, and eruption of petechiæ. On dissection, gangrenous spots have been found on the internal surface of the stomach. Its baneful effects are best counteracted by a powerful emetic, and by drinking largely of the vegetable acids.

Henbane has been used in various spasmodic and painful diseases, as in epilepsy, hysteria, palpitation, headache; paralysis, mania, and scirrhus. It is given in the form of the inspissated juice of the fresh leaves, the dose of which is from one to two grains; which requires to be gradually increased. It is sometimes employed as a substitute for opium, where the latter, from idiosyncrasy, occasions any disagreeable symptom. The henbane also is free from the constipating quality of the opium.

Dr. Brande has extracted a new alkali from this plant, which he calls *hyoscianía*. It crystallizes in long prisms, and when neutralized by sulphuric or nitric acid, forms characteristic salts.

Hyothyroi'des. (From υοειδες, the hyoid bone, and θυροειδης, the thyroid cartilage.) A muscle named from its origin in the hyoid bone, and insertion in the thyroid cartilage.

Hypa'ctica. (From υπαγω, to subdue.) Medicines which evacuate the fæces.

Hypalei'ptrum. (From υπαλειφω, to spread upon.) A spatula for spreading ointments with.

Hype'lata. (From υπελαω, to move.) Medicines which purge.

HYPERÆTHE'SIS. (From υπερ, and αισθανομαι, to feel.) Error of appetite, whether by excess or deficiency.

HYPERCATHA'RSIS. (From υπερ, *supra*, over or above, and καθαιρω, to purge.) *Hyperinesis; Hyperinos*. An excessive purging from medicines.

Hypercorypho'sis. (From υπερ, above, and κορυφη, the vertex.) A prominence or protuberance. Hippocrates calls the lobes of the liver and lungs *Hypercoryphoses*.

HYPE'RCRISIS. (Ὑπερκρισις; from υπερ, over or above, and κρινω, to separate.) A critical excretion above measure; as when a fever terminates in a looseness, the humours may flow off faster than the strength can bear, and therefore it is to be checked.

HYPERE'MESIS. (From υπερ, in excess, and εμεω, to vomit.) An excessive evacuation by vomiting.

HYPEREPHIDRO'SIS. (From υπερ, excess, and ιδρως, sweat.) Immoderate sweating.

HYPE'RICUM. (From υπερ, over, and εικων, an image or spectre: so named because it was thought to have powerover and to drive away evil spirits.) 1. The name of a genus of plants in the Linnæan system. Class, *Polyadelphia;* Order, *Polyandria*. St. John's wort.

2. The pharmacopœial name of, the common St. John's wort. See *Hypericum perfoliatum*.

Hypericum bacciferum *Caa-opia; Arbuncula gummifera Braziliensis*. A juice exudes from the wounded bark of this plant, in the Brazils, which, in a dry state, resembles camboge, but is rather darker.

Hypericum coris. *Coris lutea; Coris legitima cretica*. Bastard St. John's wort. The seeds are diuretic, emmenagogue, and antispasmodic.

Hypericum perfoliatum. The systematic name of the St. John's wort, called also *fuga dæmonum;* and *androsæmum. Hypericum perforatum—floribus trigynis, caule ancipiti, foliis obtusis pellucido-punctatis*, of Linnæus. This indigenous plant was greatly esteemed by the ancients, internally in a great variety of diseases, and externally as an anodyne and discutient, but is now very rarely used. The flowers were formerly used in our pharmacopœia, on account of the great proportion of resinous oily matter, in which the medical efficacy of the plant is supposed to reside, but are now omitted.

Hypericum saxatile. *Hypericoides*. The seeds are said to be diuretic and antispasmodic.

HYPERI'NA. (From υπερ, in excess, and ινεω, to evacuate.) Medicines which purge excessively.

Hyperine'sis. See *Hypercatharsis*.

Hyperi'nos. See *Hypercatharsis*.

Hypero'a. (From υπερ, above, and ωον, the top of a house.) The palate.

Hyperopharyngæ'us. (From υπερ, above, and φαρυγξ, the pharynx.) A muscle named from its situation above the pharynx.

HYPEROSTO'SIS. (From υπερ, upon, and ωον, a bone.) See *Exostosis*.

Hypero'um. (From υπερ, above, and ωον, the roof or palate.) A foramen in the upper part of the palate.

Hyperoxymuriate of potassa. See *Murias potassæ oxygenatus*

Hyperoxymuriatic acid. See *Chlorine*.

HYPEROXYMURIATE. A salt now called a chlorate.

HYPERSARCO MA. (From υπερ, in excess, and σαρξ, flesh.) *Hypersarcosis*. A fleshy excrescence. A polypus.

Hypersarco'sis. See *Hypersarcoma*.

HYPERSTENE. Labrador schiller spar. Found in Labrador, Greenland, and Isle of Skye. It has a beautiful copper colour when cut and polished into rings, brooches, &c.

Hyperydro'sis. (From υπερ, in excess, and υδωρ, water.) A great distention of any part, from water collected in it.

Hype'xodos. (From υπο, under, and εξοδος, passing out.) A flux of the belly.

HYPNO'BATES. (From υπνος, sleep, and βαινω, to go.) *Hypnobatasis*. One who walks in his sleep See *Oneirodynia*.

HYPNOLO'GIA. (From υπνος, sleep, and λογος, a discourse.) A dissertation, or directions for the due regulation of sleeping and waking.

HYPNOPOIE'TICA. (From υπνος, sleep, and ποιεω, to cause.) Medicines which procure sleep. See *Anodyne*.

HYPNO'TIC. (*Hipnoticus*; from υπνος, sleep.) See *Anodyne*.

HYPO-SULPHITE. A sulphuretted sulphite.

HYPOÆ'MA. (From υπο, under, and αιμα, blood; because the blood is under the cornea.) An effusion of red blood into the chambers of the eye.

Hypocaro'des. (From υπο, and καρος, a carus.) *Hypocarothis*. One who labours under a low degree of carus.

Hypocatha'rsis. (From υπω, under, and καθαιρω, to purge.) It is when a medicine does not work so much as expected, or but very little. Or a slight purging, when it is a disorder.

HYPOCAU'STRUM. (From υπο, under, and καιω, to burn.) A stove, hot house, or any such like contrivance, to preserve plants from cold air.

Hypocerchna'leon. (From υπο, and κερχνος, an asperity of the fauces.) A stridulous kind of asperity of the fauces.

Hypocheo'menos. (From υπο, under, and χεω, to pour.) One who labours under a cataract.

Hypochloro'sis. (From υπο, and χλωρωσις, the green-sickness.) A slight degree of chlorosis.

HYPOCHO'NDRIAC. (From υπο, under, and χονδρος, a cartilage.) 1. Belonging to the hypochondria.

2. A person affected with lowness of spirits. See *Hypochondriasis*

Hypochondriac regions. *Regiones hypochondriacæ; Hypochondria*. The spaces in the abdomen that are under the cartilages of the spurious ribs on each side of the epigastrium.

HYPOCHONDRI'ASIS. (From υποχονδριακος, one who is hipped.) *Hypochondriacus morbus; Affectio hypochondriaca; Passio hypochondriaca*. The hypochondriac affection, vapours, spleen, &c. A genus of disease in the class *Neuroses*, and order *Adynamiæ*, of Cullen, characterized by dyspepsia, languor, and want of energy; sadness and fear from uncertain causes, with a melancholic temperament.

The state of mind peculiar to hypochondriacs is thus described by Cullen;—"A langour, listlessness, or want of resolution and activity, with respect to all undertakings; a disposition to seriousness, sadness, and timidity, as to all future events, and apprehension of the worst or most unhappy state of them; and, therefore, often upon slight grounds, and apprehension of great evil. Such persons are particularly attentive to the state of their own health, to every the smallest change of feeling in their bodies: and from any unusual sensation, perhaps of the slightest kind, they apprehend great danger, and even death itself. In respect to these feelings and fears, there is commonly the most obstinate belief and persuasion." He adds, "that it is only when the state of mind just described is joined with indigestion, in either sex, somewhat in years, of a melancholic temperament, and a firm and rigid habit, that the disease takes the name of *Hypochondriacism.*"

The seat of the hypochondriac passions is in the stomach and bowels; for, first these parts are disordered, then the others suffer from the connexion. The causes are, sorrow, fear, or excesses of any of the passions; too long continued watching; irregular diet. Those habitually disposed to it (and these causes have little effect in other constitutions,) have generally a sallow or brown complexion, and a downcast look; a rigidity of the solids, and torpor of the nervous system. Whatever may occasion nervous disorders in general, may also be the cause of this.

The signs of this complaint are so various, that to describe them is to describe almost every other disease; but, in general, there is an insurmountable indolence, dejected spirits, dread of death, costiveness, a slow and somewhat difficult inspiration, flatulencies in the prima viæ, and various spasmodic affections. It is seldom fatal; but if neglected, or improperly treated, may bring on incurable melancholy, jaundice, madness, or vertigo, palsy, and apoplexy.

On dissections of hypochondriacal persons, some of the abdominal viscera (particularly the liver and spleen) are usually found considerably enlarged. In some few instances, effusion and a turgescence of the vessels have been observed in the brain.

This being a disease of a mixed description, the treatment must be partly corporeal, partly mental; but it has been too often neglected, as merely imaginary, and their complaints met by argument or raillery, which, however, can only weaken their confidence in the practitioner. It may be very proper to inform them, that their disorder is not so dangerous as they suppose, and may be removed by suitable remedies; but to tell them they ail nothing, is absurd. In reality, medicine is often of much service; and though others have been cured chiefly by amusements, country air, and exercise, it by no means follows, that their disorder was only in the imagination. In so far as dyspeptic symptoms appear, these must be encountered by the remedies pointed out under that head; antacids, aperients, &c. Sometimes emetics, or drastic cathartics, have produced speedy relief; but they are too debilitating to be often employed. The bowels will be better regulated by milder remedies, as castor oil, senna, aloes, (unless they are subject to hæmorrhoids,) and the like; and magnesia may at the same time correct acidity; but if the liver be torpid, some mercurial preparation will be of more avail. Flatulence and spasmodic pains may be relieved by aromatics, ether, the fœtid gum resins, musk, valerian, &c. but severe and obstinate pain, or high irritation, will be best attacked by opium: it is important, however, to guard against the patient getting into the habitual use of this remedy. Occasionally, mild tonics appear useful, especially chalybeate waters; and tepid bathing, with friction, gentle exercise, and warm clothing, are important to keep up the function of the skin. The diet should be light, and sufficiently nutritious; but moderation must be enjoined to those who have been accustomed to indulge too much in the luxuries of the table: and, in all cases, those articles which are ascescent, flatulent, or difficult of digestion, must be avoided. Malt liquors do not usually agree so well as wine or spirits, considerably diluted; but these stimuli should never be allowed unnecessarily. The mental treatment required will be such as is calculated to restore the strength, and correct the aberrations of the judgment. When any false association of ideas occurs, the best mode of removing it is, by keeping up a continued train of natural associated impressions of superior force, which may amuse the mind, and moderately exercise, without exhausting it. A variety of literary recreations and diversions, especially in the open air, with agreeable company, will be therefore advisable: frequently changing the scene, taking them to watering places, and adopting other expedients, to prevent them from dwelling too much upon their own morbid feelings.

HYPOCHO'NDRIUM. (From υπο under, and χονδρος, a cartilage.) That part of the body which lies under the cartilages of the spurious ribs.

HYPO'CHYMA. (From υπο, and χοω, to pour; because the ancients thought that the opacity proceeded from something running under the crystalline humour.) A cataract.

HYPOCI'STIS. (From υπο, under, and κιςος, the cistus.) See *Asarum hypocistis* and *Cytinus hypocistis.*

Hypocle'pticum. (From υπο, under, and κλεπτω, to steal.) A chemical vessel for separating liquors, particularly the essential oil of any vegetable from the water; and named because it steals, as it were, the water from the oil.

Hypocoelon. (From υπο, under, and κοιλον, a cavity.) The cavity under the lower eyelid.

Hypocopho'sis. A trifling degree of deafness.

Hypocra'nium. (From υπο, under, and κρανιον, the skull.) A kind of abscess, so called because seated under the cranium, between it and the dura mater.

HYPOCRATERIFORMIS. (From υπο, χρατηρ, a cup, goblet, or salver, and *forma*, likeness.) Hypocrateriform, salver-shaped; applied to leaves so shaped, as those of the *Primula.*

Hypodei'ris. In Rufus Ephesius, it is the extremity of the forepart of the neck.

Hypode'rmis. (From υπο, under, and δερμα, the skin.) 1. The skin over the clitoris, which covers it like a prepuce.

2. The clitoris.

Hypo'desis. (From υπο, under, and δεω to bind.) *Hypodesmus.* An underswathe, or bandage.

HYPO'GALA. (From υπο, under, and γαλα, milk; because it is a milk-like effusion under the cornea.) A collection of white humour, like milk, in the chambers of the eye. There are two species of this disease; the one takes place, it is said, from a deposition of the milk, as is sometimes observed in women who suckle, the other from a depression of the milky cataract.

HYPOGA'STRIC. (From υπο, under, and γαςηρ, the stomach.) Belonging to the hypogastria. See *Hypogastrium.*

Hypogastric arteries. Of or belonging to the hypogastrium. See *Iliac arteries.*

Hypogastric region. See *Hypogastrium.*

HYPOGA'STRIUM. (From υπο, under, and γαςηρ, the stomach.) *Regio hypogastrica.* The region of the abdomen that reaches from above the pubes to within three fingers' breadth of the navel.

HYPOGASTROCE'LE. (From υπογαςριον, the hypogastrium, and κηλη, a tumour.) A hernia, in the hypogastric region.

HYPOGLO'SSIS. (From υπο, under, and γλωσσα, the tongue.) The under part of the tongue, which adheres to the jaw.

HYPOGLO'SSUS. (From υπο, under, and γλωσσα, the tongue.) A nerve which goes to the under part of the tongue.

HYPOGLO'TTIDES. (From υπο, under, and γλωτ7α, the tongue.) They are a kind of lozenge to be held under the tongue until they are dissolved.

HYPOGLU'TIS. (From υπο, under, and γλουτος, the nates.) It is the fleshy part under the nates towards the thigh. Some say it is the flexure of the coxa, under the nates.

Hypo'mia. (From υπο, under, and ωμος, shoulder.) In Galen's Exegesis, it is the part subjacent to the shoulder.

HYPONITRIC ACID. See *Nitric acid.*

HYPONITROUS ACID. Pernitrous acid. "It appears from the experiments of Gay Lussac, that there exists an acid, formed of 100 azote and 150 oxygen. When into a test tube filled with mercury, we pass up from 500 to 600 volumes of deutoxide of azote, a little alkaline water, and 100 parts of oxygen gas, we obtain an absorption of 500, proceeding from the condensation of the 100 parts of oxygen with 400 of deutoxide of azote. Now these 400 parts are composed of 200 azote and 200 oxygen; consequently, the new acid is composed of azote and oxygen, in the ratio of 100 to 150, as we have said above. It is the same acid, according to Gay Lussac, which is produced on leaving for a long time a strong solution of potassa in contact with deutoxide of azote. At the end of three months he found that 100 parts of deutoxide of azote were reduced to 25 of protoxide of azote, and that crystals of *hyponitrite (pernitrite)* were formed.

Hyponitrous acid (called *pernitrous* by the French chemists) cannot be insulated. As soon as we lay hold, by an acid, of the potassa with which it is associated, it is transformed into deutoxide of azote, which is disengaged, and into nitrous or nitric acid, which remains in solution."

HYPO'NOMOS. (From υπονομος, a phagedenic ulcer.) 1. A subterraneous place.

2. A deep phagedenic ulcer.

HYPOPE'DIUM. (From υπο, under, and πους, the foot.) A cataplasm for the sole of the foot.

HYPO'PHORA. (From υποφερομαι, to be carried or conveyed underneath.) A deep fistulous ulcer.

HYPOPHOSPHOROUS ACID. This acid was lately discovered by Dulong. Pour water on the phosphuret of barytes, and wait till all the phosphuretted hydrogen be disengaged. Add cautiously to the filtered liquid dilute sulphuric acid, till the barytes be all precipitated in the state of sulphate. The supernatant liquid is hypophosphorous acid, which should be passed through a filter. This liquid may be concentrated by evaporation, till it become viscid. It has a very sour taste, reddens vegetable blues, and does not crystallize. It is probably composed of 2 primes of phosphorus $= 3 + 1$ of oxygen. Dulong's analysis approaches to this proportion. He assigns, but from rather precarious *data*, 100 phosphorus to 37.44 oxygen. The hypophosphites have the remarkable property of being all soluble in water; while many of the phosphates and phosphites are insoluble.

HYPOPHTHA'LMION. (From υπο, under, and οφθαλμος, the eye.) The part under the eye which is subject to swell in a cachexy, or dropsy.

HYPO'PHYSIS. (From υπο, under, and φυω, to produce.) A disease of the eyelids, when the hairs grow so much as to irritate and offend the pupil.

HYPO'PYUM. (From υπο, under, and πυον, pus; because the pus is under the cornea.) *Hypopion; Pyosis; Abscessus oculi.* An accumulation of a glutinous yellow fluid, like pus, which takes place in the anterior chamber of the aqueous humour, and frequently also in the posterior one, in consequence of severe, acute ophthalmy, particularly the internal species. This viscid matter of the hypopyum, is commonly called pus; but Scarpa contends, that it is only coagulating lymph. The symptoms portending an extravasation of coagulable lymph in the eye, or an hypopyum, are the same as those which occur in the highest stage of violent acute ophthalmy, viz. prodigious tumefaction of the eyelids; the same swelling and redness as in chemosis; burning heat and pain in the eye; pains in the eyebrow, and nape of the neck; fever, restlessness, aversion to the faintest light, and a contracted state of the pupil.

HYPORI'NION. (From υπο, under, and ριν, the nose.) A name for the parts of the upper lip below the nostrils.

HYPOSA'RCA. (From υπο, under, and σαρξ, flesh.) *Hyposarcidios.* A collection of fluid or air in the cellular membrane

HYPOSPADIÆ'OS. (From υπο, under, and σπαω, to draw.) The urethra terminating under the glans.

HYPOSPATHI'SMUS. (From υπο, under, and σπαθη, a spatula.) The name of an operation formerly used in surgery, for removing defluxions in the eyes. It was thus named from the instrument with which it was performed.

HYPOSPHA'GMA. (From υπο, under, and σφαζω, to kill.) *Aposphagma.* An extravasation of blood in the tunica adnata of the eye, from external injury.

HYPOSPLE'NIA. (From υπο, under, and σπλην, the spleen.) A tumour under the spleen.

HYPOSTA'PHYLE. (From υπο, and σταφυλη, the uvula.) Relaxation of the uvula.

HYPO'STASIS. (From υφιστημι, to subside.) A sediment, as that which is occasionally let down from urine.

HYPOSULPHUREOUS ACID. "In order to obtain hyposulphureous acid, Herschel mixed a dilute solution of hyposulphite of strontites with a slight excess of dilute sulphuric acid, and, after agitation, poured the mixture on three filters. The first was received into a solution of carbonate of potassa, from which it expelled carbonic acid gas. The second portion being received successively into nitrates of silver and mercury, precipitated the metals copiously in the state of sulphurets, but produced no effect on solutions of copper, iron, or zinc. The third, being tasted, was acid, astringent, and bitter. When fresh filtered, it was clear; but it became milky on standing, depositing sulphur, and colouring sulphureous acid. A moderate exposure to air, or a gentle heat, caused its entire decomposition."

HYPOSULPHURIC ACID. "Gay Lussac and Welther have recently announced the discovery of a new acid combination of sulphur and oxygen, intermediate between sulphureous and sulphuric acids, to which they have given the name of hyposulphuric acid. It is obtained by passing a current of sulphureous acid gas over the black oxide of manganese. A combination takes place; the excess of the oxide of manganese is separated by dissolving the hyposulphate of manganese in water. Caustic barytes precipitates the manganese, and forms with the new acid a very soluble salt, which, freed from excess of barytes by a current of carbonic acid, crystallizes regularly, like the nitrate or muriate of barytes. Hyposulphate of barytes being thus obtained, sulphuric acid is cautiously added to the solution, which throws down the barytes, and leaves the hyposulphuric acid in the water. This acid bears considerable concentration under the receiver of the air-pump. It consists of five parts of oxygen to four of sulphur. The greater number of the hyposulphates, both earthy and metallic, are soluble, and crystallize; those of barytes and lime are unalterable in the air.

Hyposulphuric acid is distinguished by the following properties:—

1*st*, It is decomposed by heat into sulphurous and sulphuric acids.

2*d*, It forms soluble salts with barytes, strontites, lime, lead, and silver.

3*d*, The hyposulphates are all soluble.

4*th*, They yield sulphurous acid when their solutions are mixed with acids, only if the mixture becomes hot of itself, or be artificially heated.

5*th*, They disengage a great deal of sulphurous acid at a high temperature, and are converted into neutral sulphates."

HYPO'THENAR. (From υπο, under, and θεναρ, the palm of the hand.) 1. A muscle which runs on the inside of the hand.

2. That part of the hand which is opposite to the palm.

HYPO'THESIS. An opinion, or a system of general rules, founded partly on fact but principally on conjecture. A theory explains every fact, and every circumstance connected with it; an hypothesis explains only a certain number, leaving some unaccounted for, and others in opposition to it.

HYPO'THETON. (From υπο, under, and τιθημι, to put.) A suppository, or medicine introduced into the rectum, to procure stools.

HYPO'XYLON. (From υπο, and ξυλον, wood. A species of *clavaria*, which grows under old wood.

HYPOZO'MA. (From υπο and ζωννυμι, to bind round.) The diaphragm.

HYPSIGLO'SSUS. (From υψιλοειδες, the hyoid bone and γλωσσα, the tongue.) A muscle named from its origin in the os hyoides, and its insertion in the tongue.

HYPSILOI'DES. 1. The *Os hyoides.*

2. The hyoglossus muscle.

HYPTIA'SMOS. (From υπτιαζω, to lie with the face upwards.) A supine decubiture, or a nausea, with inclination to vomit.

HYPU'LUS. (From υπο, under, and ουλη, a cicatrix.) An ulcer under a cicatrix.

HYSSOP. See *Hyssopus.*

Hyssop hedge. See *Gratiola.*

HYSSOPI'TES. (From υσσωπος, hyssop.) Wine impregnated with hyssop.

HYSSO'PUS. (Ὑσσωπος; from *Azob*, Hebrew.) 1. The name of a genus of plants in the Linnæan system. Class, *Didynamia;* Order, *Gymnospermia.* Hyssop.

2. The pharmacopœial name of the common hyssop. See *Hyssopus officinalis.*

Hyssopus capitata. Wild thyme.

Hyssopus officinalis. The systematic name of the common hyssop. *Hyssopus—spicis secundis, foliis lanceolatis* of Linnæus. This exotic plant is esteemed as an aromatic and stimulant, but is chiefly employed as a pectoral, and has long been thought useful in humoral asthmas, coughs, and catarrhal affections; for this purpose, an infusion of the leaves, sweetened with honey, or sugar, is recommended to be drank as tea.

HY'STERA. (From υςερος, behind: so called because it is placed behind the other parts.) The womb. See *Uterus.*

HYSTERA'LGIA. (From υςερα, the womb, and αλγος, pain.) A pain in the womb.

HYSTE'RIA. (From υςερα, the womb, from which the disease was supposed to arise.) *Passio hysterica.* Hysterics. Dr. Cullen places this disease in the class *Neuroses*, and order *Spasmi.* There are four species:

1. *Hysteria chlorotica*, from a retention of the menses.

2. *Hysteria à leucorrhœa*, from a fluor albus.

3. *Hysteria à menorrhagia*, from an immoderate flow of the menses.

4. *Hysteria libidinosa*, from sensual desires.

The complaint appears under such various shapes, imitates so many other diseases, and is attended with such a variety of symptoms, which denote the animal and vital functions to be considerably disordered, that it is difficult to give a just character or definition of it; and it is only by taking an assemblage of all its appearances, that we can convey a proper idea of it to others. The disease attacks in paroxysms, or fits. These are sometimes preceded by dejection of spirits, anxiety of mind, effusion of tears, difficulty of breathing, sickness at the stomach, and palpitations at the heart; but it more usually happens, that a pain is felt on the left side, about the flexure of the colon, with a sense of distention advancing upwards, till it gets into the stomach, and removing from thence into the throat, it occasions, by its pressure, a sensation as if a ball was lodged there, which by authors has been called *globus hystericus.* The disease having arrived at this height, the patient appears to be threatened with suffocation, becomes faint, and is affected with stupor and insensibility; while, at the same time, the trunk of the body is turned to and fro, the limbs are variously agitated; wild and irregular actions take place in alternate fits of laughter, crying, and screaming: incoherent expressions are uttered, a temporary delirium prevails, and a frothy saliva is discharged from the mouth. The spasms at length abating, a quantity of wind is evacuated upwards, with frequent sighing and sobbing, and the woman recovers the exercise of sense and motion without any recollection of what has taken place during the fit; feeling, however, a severe pain in her head, and a soreness over her whole body. In some cases, there is little or no convulsive motion, and the person lies seemingly in a state of profound sleep, without either sense or motion. Hiccup is a symptom which likewise attends, in some instances, on hysteria; and now and then it happens, that a fit of hysteria consists of this alone. In some cases, of this nature, it has been known to continue for two or three days, during which it frequently seems as if it would suffocate the patient, and proceeds, gradually weakening her, till it either goes off or else occasions death by suffocation: but this last is extremely rare. Besides hiccup, other slight spasmodic affections sometimes wholly form a fit of hysteria, which perhaps continue for a day or two, and then either go off of themselves, or are removed by the aid of medicine. In some cases the patient is attacked with violent pain in the back, which extend from the spine to the sternum, and at length become fixed upon the region of the stomach, being evidently of a spasmodic nature, and often prevailing in so high a degree as to cause clammy sweats, a pale cadaverous look, coldness of the extremities, and a pulse hardly perceptible.

Hysteric affections occur more frequently in a single state of life than in the married; and usually between the age of puberty and that of thirty-five years; and they make their attack oftener about the period of menstruation than at any other.

They are readily excited in those who are subject to them, by passions of the mind, and by every considerable emotion, especially when brought on by surprise; hence, sudden joy, grief, fear, &c. are very apt to occasion them. They have also been known to arise from imitation and sympathy.

Women of a delicate habit, and whose nervous system is extremely sensible, are those who are most subject to hysteric affections; and the habit which predisposes to their attacks, is acquired by inactivity and a sedentary life, grief, anxiety of mind, a suppression or obstruction of the menstrual flux, excessive evacuations, and a constant use of a low diet, or of crude unwholesome food.

Hysteria differs from hypochondriasis in the following particulars, and, by paying attention to them, may always readily be distinguished from it:—Hysteria attacks the sanguine and plethoric; comes on soon after the age of puberty; makes its onset suddenly and violently, so as to deprive the patient of all sense and voluntary motion: is accompanied with the sensation of a ball rising upwards in the throat, so as to threaten suffocation; is attended usually with much spasmodic affection; is more apt to terminate in epilepsy than in any other disease; and, on dissection, its morbid appearances are confined principally to the uterus and ovaria.

The reverse happens in hypochondriasis. It attacks the melancholic; seldom occurs till after the age of thirty-five; comes on gradually; is a tedious disease, and difficult to cure; exerts its pernicious effects on the membraneous canal of the intestines, as well by spasms as wind; is more apt to terminate in melancholy, or a low fever, than in any other disease; and, on dissection, exhibits its morbid effects principally on the liver, spleen, and pancreas, which are often found in a diseased state.

Another very material difference might be pointed out between these two diseases, which is, that hysteria is much relieved by advancing in age, whereas hypochondriasis usually becomes aggravated.

The two diseases have often been confounded together; but, from considering the foregoing circumstances, it appears that a proper line of distinction should be drawn between them.

The hysteric passion likewise differs from a syncope, as in this there is an entire cessation of the pulse, a contracted face, and a ghastly countenance; whereas, in the uterine disorder, there is often something of a colour, and the face is more expanded; there is likewise a pulse, though languid; and this state may continue some days, which never happens in a syncope.

It also differs from apoplexy, in which the abolition of sense and voluntary motion is attended with a sort of snoring, great difficulty of breathing, and a quick pulse; which do not take place in hysteria.

It differs from epilepsy, in that this is supposed to arise in consequence of a distention of the vessels of the brain: whereas, in hysteria, the spasmodic and convulsive motions arise from a turgescence of blood in the uterus, or in other parts of the genital system.

However dreadful and alarming any hysteric fit may appear, still it is seldom accompanied with danger, and the disease never terminates fatally, unless it changes into epilepsy, or that the patient is in a very weak reduced state.

The indications in this disease are, 1. To lessen the violence of the fits. 2. To prevent their return by obviating the several causes. Where the attack is slight, it may be as well to leave it in a great measure to have its course. But where the paroxysm is severe, and the disease of no long standing, occurring in a young plethoric female, as is most frequent, and especially from suppression of the menses, a liberal abstraction of blood should be made, and will often afford speedy relief. If this step do not appear advisable, and the disorder be rather connected with the state of the primæ viæ, an emetic may check its progress, if the patient can be got to swallow during a remission of the convulsions. At other times the application of cold water to the skin more or less extensively; strong and disagreeable odours, as hartshorn, burnt feathers, &c. rubbing the temples with æther; antispasmodics, particularly opium, by the mouth or in glyster: the pedivavium, &c. may be resorted to according to the state of the patient. During the intervals, we must endeavour to remove any observable predisposition; in the plethoric, by a spare diet, exercise, and occasional purgatives; in those who are weakly, and rather deficient in blood, by proper nourishment, with chalybeates, or other tonic medicines. The state of the uterine function must be particularly attended to, as well as that of the primæ viæ; those cathartics are to be preferred which are not apt to occasion flatulence, nor pa[illegible] larly irritate the rectum, unless where the menses are interrupted, when the aloetic preparations may claim a preference; and the perspiration should be maintained by warm clothing, particularly to the feet, with the prudent use of the cold bath. The mind ought also to be occupied by agreeable and useful pursuits, and regular hours will tend materially to the restoration of the general health.

HYSTERIA'LGES. (From υςερα, the womb, and αλγος, pain.) 1. An epithet for any thing that excites pain in the uterus.

2. Hippocrates applies this word to vinegar.

3. The pains which resemble labour-pains, generally called *false pains*.

HYSTERI'TIS. (From υςερα, the womb.) *Metritis*. Inflammation of the womb. A genus of disease in the class *Pyrexiæ*, and order *Phlegmasiæ*, of Cullen; characterized by fever, heat, tension, tumour, and pain in the region of the womb; pain in the os uteri, when touched, and vomiting.

In natural labours, as well as those of a laborious sort, many causes of injury to the uterus, and the peritonæum which covers it, will be applied. The long continued action of the uterus on the body of the child, and the great pressure made by its head on the soft parts, will further add to the chance of injury. Besides these, an improper application of instruments, or an officiousness of the midwife in hurrying the labour, may have contributed to the violence. To these causes may be added exposure to cold, by taking the woman too early out of bed after delivery, and thereby throwing the circulating fluids upon the internal parts, putting a stop to the secretion of milk, or occasioning a suppression of the lochia.

An inflammation of the womb is sometimes perfectly distinct, but is more frequently communicated to the peritonæum, Fallopian tubes, and ovaria; and having once begun, the natural functions of the organ become much disturbed, which greatly adds to the disease. It is oftener met with in women of a robust and plethoric habit than in those of lax fibres and a delicate constitution, particularly where they have indulged freely in food of a heating nature, and in the use of spirituous liquors. It never prevails as an epidemic, like puerperal fever, for which it has probably often been mistaken; and to this we may, with some reason, ascribe the difference in the mode of treatment which has taken place among physicians.

An inflammation of the uterus shows itself usually about the second or third day after delivery, with a painful sensation at the bottom of the belly, which gradually increases in violence, without any kind of intermission. On examining externally, the uterus appears much increased in size, is hard to the feel, and on making a pressure upon it, the patient experiences great soreness and pain. Soon afterward there ensues an increase in heat over the whole of the body, with pains in the head and back, extending into the groins, rigors, considerable thirst, nausea, and vomiting. The tongue is white and dry, the secretion of milk is usually much interrupted, the lochia are greatly diminished, the urine is high-coloured and scanty; the body is costive and the pulse hard, full, and frequent

These are the symptoms which usually present themselves when the inflammation does not run very high, and is perfectly distinct; but when it is so extensive as to affect the peritonæum, those of irritation succeed, and soon destroy the patient.

Uterine inflammation is always attended with much danger, particularly where the symptoms run high, and the proper means for removing them have not been timely adopted. In such cases, it may terminate in [illegible]uration, scirrhus, or gangrene.

[illegible] rigors, succeeded by flushings of the face, quickness and weakness of the pulse, great depression of strength, delirium, and the sudden cessation of pain and soreness in the region of the abdomen, denote a fatal termination. On the contrary, the ensuing of a gentle diarrhœa, the lochial discharge returning in due quantity and quality, the secretion of milk recommencing, and the uterus becoming gradually softer and less tender to the touch, with an abatement of heat and thirst, prognosticate a favourable issue.

When shiverings attack the patient, after several days' continuance of the symptoms, but little relief can be afforded by medicine, the event being generally fatal. In this case, the woman emaciates and loses her strength, becomes hectic, and sinks under colliquative sweating, or purging.

Upon opening the bodies of women who have died of this disease, and where it existed in a simple state, little or no extravasated fluid is usually to be met with in the cavity of the abdomen. In some instances, the peritonæal surfaces have been discovered free from the disease; while in others, that portion which covers the uterus and posterior part of the bladder, has been found partially inflamed. The inflammation has been observed, in some cases, to extend to the ovaria and Fallopian tubes, which, when cut open, are often loaded with blood. The uterus itself usually appears of a firm substance, but is larger than in its natural state, and, when cut into, a quantity of pus is often found. Gangrene is seldom, if ever, to be met with.

HYSTEROCE'LE. (From υςερα, the womb, and κηλη, a tumour.) A hernia of the womb. This is occasioned by violent muscular efforts, by blows on the abdomen at the time of gestation, and also by wounds and abscesses of the abdomen which permit the uterus to dilate the part. Ruysch relates the case of a woman, who, becoming pregnant after an ulcer had been healed in the lower part of the abdomen, the tumid uterus descended into a dilated sac of the peritonæum in that weakened part, till it hung, with the included fœtus, at her knees. Yet when her full time was come, the midwife reduced this wonderful hernia, and, in a natural way, she was safely delivered of a son.

HY'STERON. (From υςερος, afterward; so named because it comes immediately after the fœtus.) The placenta.

HYSTEROPHY'SA. (From υςερα, the womb, and φυσα, flatus.) A swelling, or distention of the womb from a collection of air in its cavity.

HYSTERO'TOMY. (*Hysterotomia*; from υςερα, the womb, and τεμνω, to cut.) See *Cæsarian operation*.

HYSTEROTOMATOCIA. See *Cæsarian operation*.

HYSTEROPTO'SIS. (From υςερα, the womb, and πιπτω, to fall.) A bearing down of the womb.

HYSTRICI'ASIS. (From υςριξ, a hedge-hog, or porcupine.) A disease of the hairs, in which they stand erect, like porcupine quills. An account of this rare disease is to be seen in the *Philosophical Transactions*, No. 424.

HY'STRICIS LAPIS. See *Bezoar hystricis*.

HYSTRI'TIS See *Hysteritis*.

IATRALEI'PTES. (From ιατρος, a physician, and αλειφω, to anoint.) One who undertakes to cure distempers by external unction and friction: Galen makes mention of such in his time, particularly one Diotas; and Pliny informs us, that this practice was first introduced by Prodicus of Selymbria, who was a disciple of Æsculapius.

IATROCHY'MICUS. (From ιατρος, a physician, and χυμια, chemistry.) *Chymiater.* A chemical physician, who cures by means of chemical medicines.

IATROLI'PTICE. (From ιατρος, a physician, and αλειφω, to anoint.) The method of curing diseases by unction and friction.

IATROPHY'SICUS. (From ιατρος, physician, and φυσις, nature.) An epithet bestowed on some writings which treat of physical subjects with relation to medicine.

IBE'RIS. (So named from Iberia, the place of its natural growth.) 1. The name of a genus of plants in the Linnæan system. Class, *Tetradynamia;* Order, *Siliculosa.*

2. The pharmacopœial name of the *Sciatica cresses.* See *Lepidium iberis.*

IBIRA'CE. See *Guaiacum.*

I'BIS. Ιβις. A bird much like our kingfisher, taken notice of by the Egyptians, because, when it was sick, it used to inject with its long bill the water of the Nile into its fundament, whence Langius, lib. ii. ep. ii. says they learned the use of clysters.

IBI'SCUS. (From ιβις, the stork, who was said to chew it and inject it as a clyster.) Marshmallow.

IBI'XUMA. (From ιβισκος, the mallow, and ιξος, glue: so named from its having a glutinous leaf, like the mallow.) *Saponaria arbor.* The soap tree, probably the *Sapindus saponaria* of Linnæus.

ICE. *Glacies.* Water made solid by the application of cold. It is frequently applied by surgeons to resolve external inflammatory diseases, to stop hæmorrhages, and constringe relaxed parts.

Iceland spar. A calcareous spar.

I'CHOR. (Ιχωρ.) A thin, aqueous, and acrid discharge.

I'CTHYA. (Ιχθυα, a fish-hook; from ιχθυς, a fish.) 1. The skin of the *Squatina*, or monkfish.

2. The name of an instrument like a fish-hook, for extracting the fœtus.

ICHTHYASIS. See *Ichthyosis.*

ICHTHYOCO'LLA. (From ιχθυς, a fish, and κολλα, glue.) *Colla piscium.* Isinglass. Fish-glue. This substance is almost wholly gelatin; 100 grains of good dry isinglass containing rather more than 98 of matter soluble in water.

Isinglass is made from certain fish found in the Danube, and the rivers of Muscovy Willoughby and others inform us, that it is made of the sound of the Beluga; and Neumann, that it is made of the Huso Germanorum, and other fish, which he has frequently seen sold in the public markets of Vienna. Jackson remarks, that the sounds of cod, properly prepared, afford this substance; and that the lakes of America abound with fish from which the very finest sort may be obtained.

Isinglass receives its different shapes in the following manner: the parts of which it is composed, particularly the sounds, are taken from the fish while sweet and fresh, slit open, washed from their slimy *sordes*, divested of a very thin membrane which envelopes the sound, and then exposed to stiffen a little in the air. In this state, they are formed into rolls about the thickness of a finger, and in length according to the intended size of the staple: a thin membrane is generally selected for the centre of the roll, round which the rest are folded alternately, and about half an inch of each extremity of the roll is turned inwards.

Isinglass is best made in the summer, as frost gives it a disagreeable colour, deprives it of weight, and impairs its gelatinous principles.

Isinglass boiled in milk forms a mild nutritious jelly, and is thus sometimes employed medicinally. This, when flavoured by the art of the cook, is the blancmanger of our tables A solution of isinglass in water, with a very small proportion of some balsam, spread on black silk, is the court-plaster of the shops.

[That variety of the codfish called the Hake, and known to naturalists as the *Gadus Merluccius*, has a very large sound or swimming bladder, which affords ichthyocolla in abundance. In 1824, a quantity was presented to the New-York Lyceum of Natural History for their inspection, and a committee of that learned body made the following report on the subject:

"The *Isinglass*, or *Ichthyocolla*, made by Mr. William Hall, at the Isle of Shoals, which was presented by him, for examination, at the last sitting of the Lyceum, has been submitted to several experiments by the committee. It proved more pure than the Russian isinglass, with which it was compared, possesses greater solubility, and exhibits more tenacity; and its solution resists longer the process of putrefaction; but it retains to a peculiar degree the unpleasant flavour peculiar to fish.

The result of the experiment induces the committee to recommend the article as a valuable acquisition to our domestic manufactures. It is found excellent in clarifying liquors, and merits the particular attention of brewers; it is valuable in preparing leather, rendering it soft and pliable, and deserves to be employed in cotton manufactories for glazing, and starching generally. In its present state, however, it would not be agreeable as an article in the preparation of food; it might be, if deprived of the fishy smell.

The form of the ichthyocolla from the Isle of Shoals, is far preferable to that of foreign manufacture. The peculiar shape of the isinglass from the Muscovy rivers was probably adopted to conceal and disguise the real substance, and to preserve the monopoly; but now, as the subterfuge is no longer necessary, it is acknowledged to answer every purpose more effectually in its native state. In the rolled or curled form, it is more apt to retain oily particles and exuvia of insects between the membranes, that frequently contaminate the liquor for whose clarification it is employed. The sounds of the Cod (gadus morhua) and Ling (gadus molva) have long been used by Newfoundland and Iceland fishermen, and bear a strong resemblance to those of the genus Accipenser; the Huso (or Beluga) which family has always supplied Muscovy (to which country we are originally indebted for it) with this article of commerce. Mr. Hall, alone, as far as we know, employs the Hake (gadus merluccius) and he offers his isinglass at $4,000 a ton, nearly one quarter less than we pay for the foreign, of which 100 tons are every year imported. If the manufacture succeeds, of which (*with capital and zeal*) we little doubt, it will save yearly from 80 to $100,000 to our citizens; at the same time it opens to them a field of enterprise which will yield annually from 4 to $5,000, and which must increase with the growth of our country.

In concluding, we may remark, that Mr. Hall employs the mode described in the 63d volume of the Transactions of the Royal Society of London, but without previously salting the sounds.

J. VAN RENSSELAER.
J. E. DE KAY.
SAMUEL AKERLY.

☞ Mr. Hall observes that the unpleasant smell of the isinglass can be entirely extracted by three weeks exposure to the night-air, after finished."—*From the Statesman, Jan. 9th, 1824.*]

ICHTHYOPHTHAL'MITE. Fish eyestone. See *Apophyllite.*

ICHTHYO'SIS. (From ιχθυα, the scale of a fish; from the resemblance of the scales to those of a fish.) *Ichthyasis.* A genus of diseases of the second order of Dr. Willan's disease of the skin. The characteristic of ichthyosis is a permanently harsh, dry, scaly, and in some cases, almost horny texture of the integuments of the body, unconnected with internal disorder Psoriasis and Lepra differ from this affection, in being but partially diffused, and in having deciduous scales.

The arrangement and distribution of the scales in ichthyosis are peculiar. Above and below the olecranon on the arm, says Dr. Willan, and in a similar situation with respect to the patella on the thigh and leg, they are small, rounded, prominent, or papillary, and of a black colour; some of the scaly papillæ have a short, narrow neck, and broad irregular tops. On some part of the extremities, and on the trunk of the body, the scales are flat and large, often placed like tiling, or in the same order as scales on the back of a fish; but, in a few cases, they have appeared separate, being intersected by whitish furrows. There is usually in this complaint a dryness and roughness of the soles of the feet; sometimes a thickened and brittle state of the skin in the palms of the hands, with large painful fissures, and on the face an appearance of the scurf rather than of scales. The inner part of the wrist, the hams, the inside of the elbow, the furrow along the spine, the inner and upper part of the thigh, are perhaps the only portions of the skin always exempt from the scaliness. Patients affected with ichthyosis are occasionally much harassed with inflamed pustules, or with large painful biles on different parts of the body; it is also remarkable, that they never seem to have the least perspiration or moisture of the skin. This disease did not, in any case, appear to Dr. Willan to have been transmitted hereditarily; nor was more than one child from the same parents affected with it. Dr. Willan never met with an instance of the horny rigidity of the integuments, *Ichthyosis cornea*, impeding the motion of the muscles or joints. It is, however, mentioned by authors as affecting the lips, prepuce, toes, fingers, &c. and sometimes as extending over nearly the whole body.

ICOSA'NDRIA. (From εικοσι, twenty, and ανηρ, a man, or husband.) The name of a class of plants in the sexual system of Linnæus, consisting of those which have hermaphrodite flowers furnished with twenty or more stamina that are inserted into the inner side of the calyx, or petals, or both. By this last circumstance is this class distinguished from *Polyandria.*

ICTERI'TIA. (From *icterus*, the jaundice.) 1. An eruption of yellowish spots.

2. A yellow discoloration of the skin.

I'CTERUS. (Named from its likeness to the plumage of the golden thrush, of which Pliny relates, that if a jaundiced person looks on one, the bird dies, and the patient recovers.) *Morbus arcuatus*, or *arquatus; Aurigo; Morbus regius; Morbus leseoli.* The jaundice. A genus of disease in the class *Cachexiæ*, and order *Impetigines*, of Cullen; characterized by yellowness of the skin and eyes; fæces white, and urine of a high colour. There are six species:—

1. *Icterus calculosus*, acute pain in the epigastric region, increasing after eating: gall-stones pass by stool.
2. *Icterus spasmodicus*, without pain, after spasmodic diseases and passions of the mind.
3. *Icterus mucosus*, without either pain, gall-stones, or spasm, and relieved by the discharge of tough phlegm by stool.
4. *Icterus hepaticus*, from an induration in the liver.
5. *Icterus gravidarum*, from pregnancy, and disappearing after delivery.
6. *Icterus infantum*, of infants.

It takes place most usually in consequence of an interrupted excretion of bile, from an obstruction in the ductus communis choledochus, which occasions its absorption into the blood-vessels. In some cases it may, however, be owing to a redundant secretion of the bile. The causes producing the first species are, the presence of biliary calculi in the gall-bladder and its ducts; spasmodic constriction of the ducts themselves; and, lastly, the pressure made by tumours in adjacent parts; hence jaundice is often an attendant symptom on a scirrhosity of the liver, pancreas, &c., and on pregnancy.

Chronic bilious affections are frequently brought on by drinking freely, but more particularly by spirituous liquors; hence they are often to be observed in the debauchee and the drinker of drams. They are likewise frequently met with in those who lead a sedentary life; and who indulge much in anxious thoughts.

A slight degree of jaundice often proceeds from the redundant secretion of bile; and a bilious habit is therefore constitutional to some people, particularly to those who reside long in a warm climate.

By attending to the various circumstances and symptoms which present themselves, we shall in general be able to ascertain, with much certainty, the real nature of the cause which has given rise to the disease.

We may be assured by the long continuance of the complaint, and by feeling the liver and other parts externally, whether or not it arises from disease of the liver, pancreas, or adjacent parts.

Where passions of the mind induce the disease, without any hardness or enlargement of the liver, or adjacent parts, and without any appearance of calculi in the fæces, or on dissection after death, we are naturally induced to conclude that the disorder was owing to a spasmodic affection of the biliary ducts.

Where gall-stones are lodged in the ducts, acute lancinating pains will be felt in the region of the parts, which will cease for a time, and then return again; great irritation at the stomach and frequent vomiting will attend, and the patient will experience an aggravation of the pain after eating. Such calculi are of various sizes, from a pea to that of a walnut; and, in some cases, are voided in a considerable number, being, like the gall, of a yellowish, brownish, or green colour.

The jaundice comes on with languor, inactivity, loathing of food, flatulence, acidities in the stomach and bowels, and costiveness. As it advances in its progress, the skin and eyes become tinged of a deep yellow; there is a bitter taste in the mouth, with frequent nausea and vomiting; the urine is very high coloured; the stools are of a gray or clayey appearance, and a dull obtuse pain is felt in the right hypochondrium, which is much increased by pressure. Where the pain is very acute, the pulse is apt to become hard and full, and other febrile symptoms to attend.

The disease, when of long continuance, and proceeding from a chronic affection of the liver, or other neighbouring viscera, is often attended with anasarcous swellings, and sometimes with ascites: also scorbutic symptoms frequently supervene.

Where jaundice is recent, and is occasioned by concretions obstructing the biliary ducts, it is probable that, by using proper means, we may be able to effect a cure; but where it is brought on by tumours of the neighbouring parts, or has arisen in consequence of other diseases attended with symptoms of obstructed viscera, our endeavours will most likely not be crowned with success. Arising during a state of pregnancy, it is of little consequence, as it will cease on parturition.

On opening the bodies of those who die of jaundice, the yellow tinge appears to pervade even the most interior part of the body; it is diffused throughout the whole of the cellular membrane, in the cartilages and bones, and even the substance of the brain is coloured with it. A diseased state of the liver, gall-bladder, or adjacent viscera, is usually to be met with.

The *Icterus infantum*, or yellow gum, is a species of jaundice which affects children, at or soon after their birth, and which usually continues for some days. It has generally been supposed to arise from the meconium, impacted in the intestines, preventing the flow of bile into them. The effects produced by it are languor, indolence, a yellow tinge of the skin, and a tendency to sleep, which is sometimes fatal, where th child is prevented from sucking.

The indications in this disease are, 1. To palliate urgent symptoms. 2. To remove the cause of obstruction to the passage of the bile into the duodenum: this is the essential part of the treatment; but the means will vary according to circumstances. When there are appearances of inflammation, of which perhaps the jaundice is symptomatic, or both produced by a gall-stone, the means explained under the head of hepatitis will be proper. If there be severe spasmodic pain, as is usual when a gall-stone is passing, the liberal use of opium and the warm bath will probably relieve it. After which, in all instances, where there is reason for supposing an obstructing cause within the duct, a nauseating emetic, or brisk cathartic, would be the most likely to force it onward: emetics, however, are hardly advisable, except in recent cases without inflammation; and calomel, seeming to promote the discharge of bile more than other cathartics, may be given in a large dose with or after the opium. Several remedies have been recommended, on the idea that they may dissolve gall-stones; which, however, is hardly probable, unless they should have advanced to the end of the common duct: the fixed alkalies, ether with oil of turpentine, raw eggs, &c. come under this head; though the alkalies may be certainly beneficial by correcting acidity, which usually results from a deficient supply of bile to the intestines; and possibly alter the secretion of the liver so much as to prevent the formation of more concretions. When the complaint arises from scirrhous tumours, mercury is the remedy most likely to afford relief, particularly should the liver itself be diseased: but it must be used with proper caution, and hemlock, or other narcotic, may sometimes enable the system to bear it better. Where this remedy is precluded, nitric acid promises to be the best substitute, the taraxacum appears by no means so much to be depended upon. In all tedious cases the strength must be supported by the vegetable bitters, or other tonics, and a nutritious diet, easy of digestion: there is often a dislike of animal food; and a craving for acids, which mostly may be indulged; indeed, when scorbutic symptoms attended, the native vegetable acids have been sometimes very serviceable. The bowels must be kept regular, and the other secretions promoted, to get rid of the bile diffused in the system; as well as to obviate febrile or inflammatory action. When accumulations of hardened fæces induce the complaint, or in the icterus infantum, cathartics may be alone sufficient to afford relief: and, in that of pregnant females, we must chiefly look to the period of delivery.

Icterus albus. The white jaundice. Chlorosis is sometimes so called.

I'CTUS. 1. A stroke or blow.

2. The pulsation of an artery.

3. The sting of a bee, or other insect.

IDÆ'US. (From ιδη, a mountain in Phrygia, their native place.) A name of the peony and blackberry.

IDE. This terminal is affixed to oxygen, chlorine, and iodine, when they enter into combination with each other, or with simple combustibles or metals in proportions not forming an acid, thus *ox-ide* of chlorine, *ox-ide* of nitrogen, *chlor-ide* of sulphur, *iod-ide* of iron.

IDE'OLOGY. (*Ideologia;* from ιδεα, a thought, and λογος, a discourse.) The doctrine or study of the understanding. "Whatever be the number and the diversity of the phenomena which belong to human intelligence, however different they appear from the other phenomena of life, though they evidently depend on the soul, it is absolutely necessary to consider them as the result of the action of the brain, and to make no distinction between them and the other phenomena that depend on the actions of that organ. The functions of the brain are absolutely subject to the same laws as the other functions; they develope and go to decay in the progress of age; they are modified by habit, sex, temperament, and individual disposition; they become confused, weakened, or elevated in diseases; the physical injuries of the brain weaken or destroy them; in a word, they are not susceptible of any explanation more than the other actions of the organ; and setting aside all hypothetical ideas, they are capable of being studied only by observation and experience.

We must also be cautious in imagining that the study of the functions of the brain is more difficult than that of the other organs, and that it appertains peculiarly to metaphysics. By keeping close to observation, and avoiding carefully any theory, or conjecture, this study becomes purely physiological, and perhaps it is easier than the most part of the other functions, on account of the facility with which the phenomena can be produced and observed. The innumerable phenomena which form the intellect of man, are only modifications of the faculty of perception. If they are examined attentively, this truth, which is well illustrated by modern metaphysicians, will be found very clear.

There are four principal modifications of the faculty of perception.

1st. *Sensibility*, or the action of the brain, by which we receive impressions, either from within or from without.

2d. The *Memory*, or the faculty of reproducing impressions, or sensations formerly received.

3d. The faculty of perceiving the relations which sensations have to each other, or the *Judgment*.

4th The *Desires*, or the *Will*.

The study of the understanding, from whatever cause, is not at present an essential part of physiology; the science which treats particularly of it is *Ideology* Whoever may wish to acquire an extensive knowledge on this interesting subject, should consult the works of Bacon, Locke, Condillac, Cabanis, and especially the excellent book of Destutt Tracy, entitled "Elements of Ideology."

IDIOCRA'SIA. See *Idiosyncrasy*.

IDIOPA'THIC. (*Idiopathicus;* from ιδιος, peculiar, and παθος, an affection.) A disease which does not depend on any other disease, in which respect it is opposed to a systematic disease, which is dependen on another.

IDIOSY'NCRASY. (*Idiosyncrasia*, from ιδιος, peculiar, συν, with, and κρασις, a temperament.) A peculiarity of constitution, in which a person is affected by certain agents, which, if applied to a hundred other persons, would produce no effect: thus some people cannot see a finger bleed without fainting; and thus violent inflammation is induced on the skin of some persons, by substances that are perfectly innocent to others.

Idiot'ropia. (From ιδιος, peculiar, and τρεπω, to turn.) The same as *Idiosyncrasia*.

IDOCRASE. See *Vesuvian*.

IGASURIC ACID. *Acidum Igusaricum*. Pelletier and Caventou, in their elegant researches in the *faba Sancti Ignatii, et nux vomica*, having observed that these substances contained a new vegetable base (strychnine) in combination with an acid, sought to separate the latter, in order to determine its nature. It appeared to them to be new, and they called it igasuric acid, from the Malay name by which the natives designate in the Indies the *faba Sancti Ignatii*. This bean, according to these chemists, is composed of igasurate of strychnine, a little wax, a concrete oil, a yellow colouring matter, gum, starch, bassorine, and vegetable fibre.

To extract the acid, the rasped bean must be heated in ether, in a digester, with a valve of safety. Thus the concrete oil, and a little igasurate of strychnine, are dissolved out. When the powder is no longer acted on by the ether, they subject it, at several times, to the action of boiling alkohol, which carries off the oil which had escaped the ether, as also wax, which is deposited on cooling, some igasurate of strychnine, and colouring matter. All the alkoholic decoctions are united, filtered, and evaporated. The brownish-yellow residuum is diffused in water; magnesia is now added, and the whole is boiled together for some minutes. By this means, the igasurate is decomposed, and from this decomposition there results free strychnine, and a sub-igasurate of magnesia, very little soluble in water. Washing with cold water removes almost completely the colouring matter, and boiling alkohol then separates the strychnine, which falls down as the liquid cools. Finally, to procure igasuric acid from the sub-igasurate of magnesia, which remains united to a small quantity of colouring matter, we must dissolve the magnesian salt in a great body of boiling distilled water; concentrate the liquor, and add to it acetate of lead, which immediately throws down the acid in the state of an igasurate of lead. This compound is then decomposed, by transmitting a current of sulphuretted hydrogen through it, diffused in 8 or 10 times its weight of boiling water.

This acid, evaporated to the consistence of syrup, and left to itself, concretes in hard and granular crystals. It is very soluble in water, and in alkohol. Its taste is acid and very styptic. It combines with the alkaline and earthy bases, forming salts soluble in water and alkohol. Its combination with barytes is very soluble, and crystallizes with difficulty, and mushroom-like. Its combination with ammonia, when perfectly neutral, does not form a precipitate with the salts of silver, mercury, and iron; but it comports itself with the salts of copper in a peculiar manner, and which seems to characterize the acid of *strychnos* (for the same acid is found in *nux vomica*, and in snake-wood, *bois de couleuvre*): this effect consists in the decomposition of the salts of copper, by its ammoniacal compound. These salts pass immediately to a green colour, and gradually deposite a greenish-white salt, of very sparing solubility in water. The acid of *strychnos* seems thus to resemble meconic acid; but it differs essentially from it, by its action with salts of iron, which immediately assume a very deep red colour with the meconic acid; an effect not produced by the acid of *strychnos*. The authors, after all, do not positively affirm this acid to be new and peculiar.

IGNA'TIA. (So named by Linnæus, because the seeds are known in the materia medica by the name of Saint Ignatius's beans.) The name of a genus of plants. Class, *Pentandria;* Order, *Monogynia.*

Ignatia amara. The systematic name of the plant which affords St. Ignatius's bean; *Faba indica; Faba Sancti Ignatii; Faba febrifuga.* These beans are of a roundish figure, very irregular and uneven, about the size of a middling nutmeg, semi-transparent, and of a hard, horny texture. They have a very bitter taste, and no considerable smell. They are said to be used in the Philippine islands in all diseases, acting as a vomit and purgative. Infusions are given in the cure of intermittents, &c.

Ignatii faba. See *Ignatia amara.*

IGNATIUS'S BEAN. See *Ignatia amara.*

I'GNIS. Fire. 1. Van Helmont, Paracelsus, and other alchemists, applied this term to what they considered as universal solvents.

2. In medicine, the older writers used it to express several diseases characterized by external redness and heat.

Ignis calidus. A hot fire: a gangrene: also a violent inflammation, just about to degenerate into a gangrene, were formerly so called by some.

Ignis fatuus. A luminous appearance or flame, frequently seen in the night in different country places, and called in England *Jack with a lantern*, or *Will with the wisp.* It seems to be mostly occasioned by the extrication of phosphorus from rotting leaves and other vegetable matters. It is probable, that the motionless ignes fatui of Italy, which are seen nightly on the same spot, are produced by the slow combustion of sulphur, emitted through clefts and apertures in the soil of that volcanic country.

Ignis frigidus. A cold fire. A sphacelus was so called, because the parts that are so affected become as cold as the surrounding air.

Ignis persicus. A name of the erysipelas, also of the carbuncle. See *Anthrax.*

Ignis rotæ. Fire for fusion. It is when a vessel, which contains some matter for fusion, is surrounded with live, *i. e.* red-hot, coals.

Ignis sacer. A name of erysipelas, and of a species of herpes.

Ignis sapientium. Heat of horse-dung.

Ignis sancti antonii. See *Erysipelas.*

Ignis sylvaticus. See *Impetigo.*

Ignis volagrius. See *Impetigo.*

Ignis volaticus. See *Erysipelas.*

I'kan radix. A somewhat oval, oblong, compressed root, brought from China. It is extremely rare, and would appear to be the root of some of the orchis tribe.

I'laphis. A name in Myrepsus for the burdoch. See *Arctium lappa.*

I'lech. By this word, Paracelsus seems to mean a first principle.

I'leon cruentum. Hippocrates describes it in lib. De Intern. Affect. In this disease, as well as in the scurvy, the breath is fœtid, the gums recede from the teeth, hæmorrhages of the nose happen, and sometimes there are ulcers in the legs, but the patient can move about.

I'LEUM. (From ειλεω, to turn about; from its convolutions.) *Ileum intestinum.* The last portion of the small intestines, about fifteen hands' breadth in length, which terminates at the valve of the cæcum. See *Intestine.*

ILEUS. See *Iliac passion.*

I'LEX. (The name of a genus of plants in the Linnæan system. Class, *Tetrandria;* Order, *Tetragynia.*) The holly.

Ilex aquifolium. The systematic name of the common holly. *Aquifolium.* The leaves of this plant, *Ilex—foliis ovatis acutis spinosis*, of Linnæus, have been known to cure intermittent fevers; and an infusion of the leaves, drank as tea, is said to be a preventive against the gout.

Ilex cassine. *Cassina; Apalachine gallis.* This tree grows in Carolina; the leaves resemble those of senna, blackish when dried, with a bitter taste, and aromatic smell. They are considered as stomachic and stimulant. They are sometimes used as expectorants; and when fresh are emetic.

I'LIA. (The plural of *Ile*, ειλη.)

1. The flanks, or that part in which are enclosed the small intestines.

2. The small intestines.

I'LIAC. (*Iliacus;* from *ileum intestinum.*) Belonging to the ilium; an intestine so called.

Iliac arteries. *Arteriæ iliacæ.* The arteries so called are formed by the bifurcation of the aorta, near the last lumbar vertebra. They are divided into *internal* and *external.* The *internal iliac*, also called the *hypogastic artery*, is distributed in the fœtus into six and in the adult into five branches, which are divided about the pelvis, viz. the little iliac, the gluteal, the ischiatic, the pudical, and the obturatory; and in the fœtus, the umbilical. The *external iliac* proceeds out of the pelvis through Poupart's ligament, to form the femoral artery.

Iliac passion. (Ειλεος, ιλεος, ειλειος, is described as a kind of nervous colic, the seat of which is the ilium.) *Passio iliaca; Volvulus; Miserere mei; Convolvulus; Chordapsus; Tormentum.* A violent vomiting, in which the fæcal portion of the food is voided by the mouth. It is produced by many morbid conditions of the bowels, by inflammatory affections of the abdominal viscera, and by herniæ.

Iliac region. The side of the abdomen, between the ribs and the hips.

ILI'ACUS. The name of muscles, regions, or diseases, situated near to, or connected with, parts about the ilia or flanks.

Iliacus internus. *Iliacus* of Winslow. *Iliaco trachanten* of Dumas. A thick, broad, and radiated muscle, which is situated in the pelvis, upon the inner surface of the ilium. It arises fleshy from the inner lip of the ilium, from most of the hollow part, and likewise from the edge of that bone, between its anterior superior spinous process and the acetabulum. It joins with the psoas magnus, where it begins to become tendinous, and passing under the ligamentum Fallopii, is inserted in common with that muscle. The tendon of this muscle has been seen distinct from that of the psoas, and, in some subjects, it has been found divided into two portions. The iliacus internus serves to assist the psoas magnus in bending the thigh, and in bringing it directly forwards.

ILI'ADUM. *Iliadus.* The first matter of all things, consisting of mercury, salt, and sulphur. These are Paracelsus's three principles. His *iliadus* is also a mineral spirit, which is contained in every element, and is the supposed cause of diseases.

Ilia'ster. Paracelsus gives this name to the occult virtue of nature, whence all things have their increase.

ILI'NGOS. (From ιλιγξ, a vortex.) A giddiness, in which all things appear to turn round, and the eyes grow dim.

Ili'scus. Avicenna says, it is madness caused by love.

I'LIUM OS. (From *ilia*, the small intestines; so named because it supports the ilia.) The haunch-bone. The superior portion of the os innominatum, which, in the fœtus, is a distinct bone. See *Innominatum os.*

ILLA. See *Ula.*

ILLE'CEBRA. (From ειλεω, to turn; because its leaves resemble worms.) See *Sedum acre.*

ILLI'CIUM. (*Illicium, ab illiciendo;* denoting an enticing plant, from its being very fragrant and aromatic.) The name of a genus of plants in the Linnæan system. Class, *Polyandria;* Order, *Polygynia.*

Illicium anisatum. The systematic name of the yellow-flowered aniseed-tree: the seeds of which are called the star aniseed. *Anisum stellatum; Anisum stinense; Semen badian.* They are used with the same views as those of the *Pimpinella anisum.* The same tree is supposed to furnish the aromatic bark, called *cortex anisi stellati*, or *cortex lavola.*

ILLO'SIS. (From ιλλος, the eye.) A distortion of the eyes.

Illutame'ntum. An ancient form of an external medicine, like the *Ceroma*, with which the limbs of wrestlers, and others delighting in like exercises, were rubbed, especially after bathing; an account of which may be met with in Bactius De Thermis.

Illuta'tio. (From *in*, and *lutum*, mud.) Illutation. A besmearing any part of the body with mud, and renewing it as it grows dry, with a view of heating, drying, and discussing. It was chiefly done with the mud found at the bottom of mineral springs.

I'llys. (From ιλλος, the eye.) A person who squints, or with distorted eyes.

I'lys. (From ιλυς, mud.) 1. The fæces of wine. An obsolete term.

2. The sediment in stools which resemble fæces of wine.

3. The sediments in urine, when it resembles the same.

Imbeci'llitas oculorum. Celsus speaks of the *Nyctalopia* by this name.

Imbibi'tio. (From *imbibo*, to receive into.) An obsolete term. In chemistry for a kind of cohobation, when the liquor ascends and descends upon a solid substance, till it is fixed therewith.

IMBRICATUS. Imbricated: like tiles upon a house. A term applied to leaves as those of the *Euphorbia paralia*.

IMMERSUS. Immersed: plunged under water—*folia immersa*: leaves which are naturally under the water, and are different from those which naturally float. See *Leaf*.

It is remarked by Linnæus, that aquatic plants have their lower, and mountainous ones their upper, leaves most divided, by which they better resist the action of the stream in one case, and of the wind in the other.

Imme'rsus. A term given by Bartholine, and some other anatomists to the *Subscapularis* muscle, because it was hidden, or, as it were, sunk.

IMPA'TIENS. (From *in*, not, and *patior*, to suffer; because its leaves recede from the hand with a crackling noise, as impatient of the touch, or from the great elasticity of the sutures of its seed vessel which is completely impatient of the touch, curling up with the greatest velocity, and scattering round the seeds, the instant any extraneous body comes in contact with it.) The name of a genus of plants. Class, *Pentandria*; Order, *Monogynia*.

IMPERATO'RIA. (From *impero*, to overcome: so named because its leaves extend and overwhelm the less herbs which grow near it.) 1. The name of a genus of plants in the Linnæan system. Class, *Pentandria*; Order, *Monogynia*.

2. The pharmacopœial name of the master-wort. See *Imperatoria ostruthium*.

Imperatoria ostruthium. The systematic name of the master-wort. *Imperatoria*; *Magistrantia*. The roots of this plant are imported from the Alps and Pyrenees, notwithstanding it is indigenous to this island: they have a fragrant smell, and a bitterish pungent taste. The plant, as its name imports, was formerly thought to be of singular efficacy; and its great success, it is said, caused it to be distinguished by the name of *divinium remedium*. At present, it is considered merely as an aromatic, and consequently is superseded by many of that class which possess superior qualities.

IMPETI'GINES. (The plural of *impetigo*; from *impeto*, to infest.) An order in the class *Cachexiæ* of Cullen, the genera of which are characterized by cachexia deforming the external parts of the body with tumours, eruptions, &c.

IMPETI'GO. *Ignis sylvaticus*; *Ignis volagrius*. A disease of the skin, variously described by authors, but mostly as one in which several red, hard, dry, prurient spots arise in the face and neck, and sometimes all over the body, and disappear by furfuraceous or tender scales.

Impetum faciens. See *Vis vitæ*.

IMPETUSA. Force or motion.

I'mpia herba. (From *in*, not, and *pius*, good; because it grows only on barren ground.) A name given to cudweed. See *Gnaphalium*.

IMPLICATED. Celsus, Scribonius, and some others, call those parts of physic so, which have a necessary dependence on one another; but the term has been more significantly applied, by Bellini, to fevers, where two at a time afflict a person, either of the same kind, as a double tertian; or, of different kinds, as an intermittent tertian, and a quotidian, called a *Semitertian*.

Implu'vium. (From *impluo*, to shower upon.) 1. The shower-bath.

2. An embrocation.

IMPOSTHUMA. A term corrupted from *impostem* and *apostem*. An abscess.

IMPREGNA'TION. *Impregnatio* See *Conception* and *Generation*.

INANI'TIO. (From *inanio*, to empty.) Inanition Applied to the body or vessels, it means emptiness; applied to the mind, it means a defect of its powers.

INCANTA'TION. *Incantatio*; *Incantamentum*. A way of curing diseases by charms, defended by Paracelsus, Helmont, and some other chemical enthusiasts.

INCANUS. Hoary. Applied to stems which are covered with a kind of scaly mealiness, as that of the *Artemisia absinthium*, and *Atriplex portulacoides*.

Ince'ndium. (From *incendo*, to burn.) A burning fever, or heat.

Ince'nsio. 1. A burning fever.

2. A hot inflammatory tumour.

Incerni'culum. (From *incerno*, to sift.)

1. A strainer, or sieve.

2. A name for the pelvis of the kidney, from its office as a strainer.

Incide'ntia. (From *incido*, to cut.) Medicines which consist of pointed and sharp particles, as acids, and most salts, which are said to incide or cut the phlegm, when they break it, so as to occasion its discharge.

INCINERA'TION. (From *incinero*, to reduce to ashes.) *Incineratio*. The combustion of vegetable and animal substances, for the purpose of obtaining their ashes or fixed residue.

INCISI'VUS. (From *incido*, to cut.) A name given to some muscles, &c.

Incisivus inferior. See *Levator labii inferioris*.

Incisivus lateralis. See *Levator labii superioris alæque nasi*.

Incisivus medius. See *Depressor labii superioris alæque nasi*.

INCI'SOR. (*Dentes incisores*; from *incido*, to cut, from their use in cutting the food.) The four front teeth of both jaws are called incisors, because they cut the food. See *Teeth*.

INCISO'RIUM. (From *incido*, to cut.) A table whereon a patient is laid for an operation.

Incisorium foramen. A name of the foramen, which lies behind the dentes incisores of the upper jaw.

INCISUS. (From *incido*, to cut.) Cut. A term applied in botany, synonymously with *dissectus*, to leaves; as those of the *Geranium dissectum*.

INCONTINE'NTIA. (From *in*, and *contineo*, to contain.) Inability to retain the natural evacuations. Hence we say, incontinence of urine, &c.

Incrassa'ntia. (*Incrassans*; from *incrasso*, to make thick.) Medicines which thicken the fluids.

I'NCUBUS. (From *incubo*, to lie upon; because the patient fancies that something lies upon his chest.) See *Oneirodynia*.

INCURVUS. Curved inwards: applied to leaves; as in *Erica empetrifolia*.

INCUS. (A smith's anvil: from *incudo*, to smite upon: so named from its likeness in shape to an anvil.) The largest and strongest of the bones of the ear in the tympanum. It is divided into a body and two crura. Its body is situated anteriorly, is rather broad and thick, and has two eminences and two depressions, both covered with cartilage, and intended for the reception of the head of the malleus. Its shorter crus extends no farther than the cells of the mastoid apophysis. Its longer crus, together with the manubrium of the malleus, to which it is connected by a ligament, is of the same extent as the shorter; but its extremity is curved inwards, to receive the os orbiculare, by the intervention of which it is united with the stapes.

I'NDEX. (From *indico*, to point out; because it is generally used for such purposes.) The forefinger

Indian arrow-root. See *Maranta.*

Indian cress. See *Tropæolum majus.*

Indian date-plum. See *Diospyros lotus*

Indian leaf. See *Laurus cassia.*

Indian pink. See *Spigelia.*

Indian-rubber. See *Caoutchouc.*

Indian wheat. See *Zea mays.*

"Indian tobacco. Lobelia. The *Lobelia inflata* is an annual American plant, found in a great variety of soils throughout the United States.

It is lactescent, like many others of its genus. When chewed it communicates to the mouth a burning, pungent sensation, which remains long in the fauces, resemblin the effect of green tobacco. The plant con tains caoutchouc, extractive, and an acrid principle, which is present in the tincture, decoction, and distilled water.

The lobelia is a prompt emetic, attended with narcotic effects during its operation. If a leaf or capsule be held in the mouth for a short time, it brings on giddiness, headache, a trembling agitation of the whole body, sickness, and finally vomiting. These effects are analogous to those which tobacco produces in the unaccustomed. If swallowed in substance, it excites speedy vomiting, accompanied with distressing and long-continued sickness, and even with dangerous symptoms, if the dose be large. On account of the violence of its operation, it is probable that this plant will never come in use for the common purpose of an emetic. It is, however, entitled to notice as a remedy in asthma and some other pulmonary affections. It produces relief in asthmatic cases, sometimes without vomiting, but more frequently after discharging the contents of the stomach. On account of the harshness of its operation, it is reluctantly resorted to by patients, who expect relief from any milder means. It, however, certainly relieves some cases, in which other emetic substances fail. In small doses the lobelia is found a good expectorant for pneumonia, in its advanced stages, and for catarrh. In rheumatism it has also been found of service.

The strength of the lobelia varies with its age, and other circumstances. In some instances, a grain will produce vomiting. The tincture is most frequently given in asthma, in *doses* of about a fluid drachm."—*Big. Mat. Med.* A.]

[INDIAN TURNIP. *Dragon root.* Arum. "The *Arum triphyllum* is an American plant, growing in damp, shady situations, and sometimes called *Indian Turnip*, and *Wake robin*. The root is large and fleshy, consisting chiefly of fœcula, which it affords, without taste or smell, in the form of a white delicate powder. In its recent state, this root, and in fact every part of the plant, is violently acrid, and almost caustic. Applied to the tongue, or to any secreting surface, it produces an effect like that of Cayenne pepper, but far more powerful, so as to leave a permanent soreness for many hours. Its action does not readily extend through the cuticle, since the bruised root may be worn upon the skin till it becomes dry, without occasioning pain or rubefaction. The acrimony of this plant resides in a highly volatile principle, which is driven off by heat, and gradually disappears in drying. It is not communicated to water, alkohol, nor oil, but may be obtained in the form of an inflammable gas or vapour, by boiling the plant under an inverted receiver, filled with water. Arum is too violently acrid to be a safe medicine in its recent state, though it has sometimes been given with impunity. The dried root, while it retains a slight portion of acrimony, is sometimes grated in milk, and given as a carminative and diaphoretic."—*Big. Mat. Med.* A.]

INDIA'NA RADIX. Ipecacuanha.

I'NDICA CAMOTES. Potatoes.

INDICANT. (*Indicans;* from *indico*, to show.) That from which the indication is drawn, which is in reality the proximate cause of a disease.

Indicating days Critical days.

INDICA'TION. (*Indicatio;* from *indico*, to show.) An indication is that which demonstrates in a disease what ought to be done. It is three-fold: preservative, which preserves health; curative, which expels a present disease; and vital, which respects the powers and reasons of diet. The scope from which indications are taken, or determined, is comprehended in this distich:

——Ars, ætas, regio, complexio, virtus,
Mos et symptoma, repletio, tempus, et usus.

INDICATOR. (From *indico*, to point: so named from its office of extending the index, or forefinger) An extensor muscle of the forefinger, situated chiefly on the lower and posterior part of the forearm. *Extensor indicis* of Cowper. *Extensor secundii internodii indicis proprius, vulgo indicator* of Douglas; and *Cubitosus phalangettien de l'index* of Dumas. It arises, by an acute fleshy beginning, from the middle of the posterior part of the ulna; its tendon passes under the same ligament with the extensor digitorum communis, with part of which it is inserted into the posterior part of the forefinger.

INDICUM LIGNUM. Logwood

INDICUS MORBUS. The venereal disease.

INDI'GENOUS. (*Indigenus; indigena ab indu, i. e. in et geno, i. e. gigno*, to beget.) Applied to diseases, plants, and other objects which are peculiar to any country.

INDIGO. A blue colouring matter extracted from the *Indigofera tinctoria*. Anil, or the indigo plant.

INDIGOFERA. (From *indigo*, and *fero*, to bear.) The name of a genus of plants. Class, *Diadelphia;* Order, *Decandria.*

INDIGOFERA TINCTORIA. The systematic name of the plant which affords indigo.

INDUCIUM. (From *induco*, to cover or draw over.) A covering. 1. A shirt.

2. The name of the amnios from its covering the fœtus like a shirt.

3. Wildenow and Swart's name for the involucrum, or thin membraneous covering of the fructification of ferns.

Its varieties are,

1. *Inducium planum*, flat; as in the genus *Polypodium.*

2. *I. peltatum*, connected with the seed by a filament or stalk; as in *Aspidium filixmas.*

3. *I. corniculatum*, round and hollow, as in *Equisetum.*

INDURA'NTIA. (From *induro*, to harden.) Medicines which harden.

INEQUALIS. Unequal. Applied to a leaf when the two halves are unequal in dimensions and the base end parallel; as in *Eucalyptus resinifera.*

INERMIS. (From *in*, priv. and *arma.*) Unarmed opposed, in designating leaves, to such as are spinous.

INE'SIS. (From ινάω, to evacuate.) *Inethus.* An evacuation of the humours.

INFECTION. See *Contagion.*

INFERNAL. A name given to a caustic, *lapis infernalis*, from its strong burning property. See *Argenti nitras.*

INFIBULA'TIO. (From *infibulo*, to button together.) An impediment to the retraction of the prepuce.

INFLAMMABLE. Chemists distinguish by this term such bodies as burn with facility, and flame in an increased temperature.

Inflammable air. See *Hydrogen gas.*

Inflammable air, heavy. See *Carburetted hydrogen gas.*

INFLAMMATION. (*Inflammatio, onis.* f.; from *inflammo*, to burn.) *Phlogosis; Phlegmasia.* A disease characterized by heat, pain, redness, attended with more or less of tumefaction and fever. Inflammation is divided into two species, viz. phlegmonous and erysipelatous.

Besides this division, inflammation is either acute or chronic, local or general, simple or complicated with other diseases.

1. *Phlegmonous inflammation* is known by its bright red colour, tension, heat, and a circumscribed, throbbing, painful tumefaction of the part; tending to suppuration. Phlegmon is generally used to denote an inflammatory tumour, situated in the skin or cellular membrane. When the same disease affects the viscera, it is usually called phlegmonous inflammation.

2. *Erysipelatous inflammation* is considered as an inflammation of a dull red colour, vanishing upon pressure, spreading unequally, with a burning pain, the tumour scarcely perceptible, ending in vesicles, or desquamation. This species of inflammation admits of a division into erythema, when there is merely an affection of the skin, with very little of the whole system; and erysipelas, when there is general affection of the system.

The fever attending erysipelatous inflammation is generally synochus or typhus, excepting when it affects very vigorous habits, and then it may be synocha. The fever attending phlegmonous inflammation is almost always synocha. Persons in the prime of life, and in full vigour with a plethoric habit of body, are most liable to the attacks of a phlegmonous inflammation; whereas those advanced in years, and those of a weak habit or body, irritable, and lean, are most apt to be attacked with erysipelatous inflammation.

Phlegmonous inflammation terminates in resolution, suppuration, gangrene, and scirrhus, or induration. Resolution is known to be about to take place when the symptoms gradually abate; suppuration, when the inflammation does not readily yield to proper remedies the throbbing increases, the tumour points externally, and rigors come on. Gangrene is about to take place, when the pain abates, the pulse sinks, and cold perspirations come on. Schirrhus, or induration, is known by the inflammation continuing a longer time than usual; the tumefaction continues, and a considerable hardness remains. This kind of tumour gives little or no pain, and, when it takes place, it is usually the sequel of inflammation affecting glandular parts. It sometimes, however, is accompanied with lancinating pains, ulcerates, and becomes cancerous.

Erythematous inflammation terminates in resolution, suppuration, or gangrene. The symptoms of inflammation are accounted for in the following way:—

The redness arises from the dilatation of the small vessels, which become sufficiently large to admit the red particles in large quantities; it appears also to occur, in some cases, from the generation of new vessels. The swelling is caused by the dilatation of the vessels, the plethoric state of the arteries and veins, the exudation of coagulable lymph into the cellular membrane, and the interruption of absorption.

In regard to the augmentation of heat, as the thermometer denotes very little increase of temperature, it appears to be accounted for from the increased sensibility of the nerves, which convey false impressions to the sensorium. The pain is occasioned by a deviation from the natural state of the parts, and the unusual condition into which the nerves are thrown. The throbbing depends on the action of the arteries.

Blood taken from a person labouring under active inflammation, exhibits a yellowish white crust on the surface; this is denominated the buffy coriaceous, or inflammatory coat. This consists of a layer of coagulable lymph, almost destitute of red particles. Blood, in this state, is often termed sizy. The colouring part of the blood is its heaviest constituent; and, as the blood of a person labouring under inflammation is longer coagulating than healthy blood, it is supposed that the red particles have an opportunity to descend to a considerable depth from the surface before they become entangled. The buffy coat of blood is generally the best criterion of inflammation; there are a few anomalous constitutions in which this state of blood is always found; but these are rare.

The occasional and exciting causes of inflammation are very numerous: they, however, may generally be classed under external violence, produced either by mechanical or chemical irritation, changes of temperature, and stimulating foods. Fever often seems to be a remote cause; the inflammation thus produced is generally considered as critical. Spontaneous inflammation sometimes occurs when no perceptible cause can be assigned for its production. Scrofula and syphilis may be considered as exciting causes of inflammation.

With regard to the proximate cause, it has been the subject of much dispute. Galen considered phlegmon to be produced by a superabundance of the humor sanguineus. Boerhaave referred the proximate cause to an obstruction in the small vessels, occasioned by a lentor of the blood. Cullen and others attributed it rather to an affection of the vessels than a change of the fluids.

The proximate cause, at the present period, is generally considered to be a morbid dilatation, and increased action of such arteries as lead and are distributed to the inflamed part.

Inflammation of the bladder. See *Cystitis.*
Inflammation of the brain. See *Phrenitis.*
Inflammation of the eyes. See *Ophthalmia.*
Inflammation of the intestines. See *Enteritis.*
Inflammation of the kidneys. See *Nephritis.*
Inflammation of the liver. See *Hepatitis.*
Inflammation of the lungs. See *Pneumonia.*
Inflammation of the peritonæum. See *Peritonitis.*
Inflammation of the pleura. See *Pleuritis.*
Inflammation of the stomach. See *Gastritis.*
Inflammation of the testicle. See *Orchitis.*
Inflammation of the uterus. See *Hysteritis.*

INFLA'TIO. (From *inflo*, to puff up.) A windy swelling. See *Pneumatosis.*

INFLA'TIVA. (*Inflativus;* from *inflo*, to puff up with wind.) Medicines or food which cause flatulence.

INFLATUS. Inflated. In botany applied to vesiculated parts, which naturally contain only air; as *legumen inflatum*, seen in *Astragalus vesicarius*, and the distended and hollow perianths of the *Cucubalus behen*, and *Physalis alkekengi* in fruit.

INFLEXUS. Curved inwards; synonymous to *incurvus*, as applied to leaves, petals, &c. See *Incurvus.* The petals of the *Pimpinella*, and *Chærophyllum*, are described as *inflexa.*

INFLORESCENCE. (*Inflorescentia;* from *infloresco*, to flower or blossom.) A term used by Linnæus to express the particular manner in which flowers are situated upon a plant, denominated by preceding writers, *modus florendi*, or manner of flowering.

It is divided into *simple*, when solitary, and *compound*, when many flowers are placed together in one place.

The first affords the following distinctions.

1. *Flos pedunculatus*, furnished with a stalk; as in *Gratiolus* and *Vinca.*
2. *F. sessilis*, adhering to the plant without a flower stalk; as in *Daphne mezerium*, and *Zinia pauciflora*
3. *F. caulinus*, when on the stem.
4. *F. rameus*, when on the branch.
5. *F. terminalis*, when on the apex of the stem, or branch; as *Paris quadrifolia*, and *Chrysanthemum leucanthemum.*
6. *F. axillaris*, in the axilla; as in *Convallaria multiflora.*
7. *F. foliaris*, on the surface of the leaf; as in *Phyllanthus.*
8. *F. radicalis*, on the root; as *Carlina acaulis*, *Crocus*, and *Colchicum*
9. *F. latitans*, concealed in a fleshy receptacle; as in *Ficus carica.*

Again, it is said to be,

1. *Alternate;* as in *Polyanthes tuberosa.*
2. *Opposite;* as in *Passiflora hirsuta.*
3. *Unilateral*, hanging all to one side; as *Erica herbacea*, and *Silene amœna.*
4. *Solitary;* as in *Campanula speculum*, and *Carduus tuberosus.*

The second, or compound inflorescence, has the following kinds:

1. The *verticillus*, or whirl.
2. The *capitulum*, or tuft.
3. The *spica*, or spike.
4. The *racemus*, or cluster.
5. The *corymbos*, or corymb.
6. The *umbella*, or umbel.
7. The *cyma*, or cyme.
8. The *fasciculus*, or fascicle.
9. The *panicula*, or panicle.
10. The *thyrsus*, or bunch.
11. The *spadix*, or sheath.
12. The *amentum*, or catkin.

INFLUE'NZA. (The Italian word for influence.) The disease is so named because it was supposed to be produced by a peculiar influence of the stars. See *Catarrhus a contagione.*

INFRASCAPULA'RIS (From *infra*, beneath, and *scapula*, the shoulder-blade.) A muscle named from its position beneath the scapula. See *Subscapularis.*

INFRASPINA'TUS. (From *infra*, beneath, and *spina*, the spine.) A muscle of the humerus, situated on the scapula. It arises fleshy, from all that part of the dorsum scapulæ which is below its spine; and from the spine itself, as far as the cervix scapulæ. The fibres run obliquely towards a tendon in the middle of a muscle, which runs forwards, and adheres to the capsular ligament. It is inserted by a flat, thick tendon, into the upper and outer part of the large protuberance on the head of the os humeri. Its use is to roll the os humeri outwards, to assist in raising and supporting it when raised, and to pull the ligament from between the bones. This muscle and the supra spinatus are covered by an aponeurosis, which extends between the costæ, and edges of the spine of the scapula, and gives rise to many of the muscular fibres.

INFUNDIBULIFORMIS. Funnel-shaped. Applied to the corolla of plants; as in *Pulmonaria.*

INFUNDI'BULUM. (From *infundo*, to pour in.) 1. A canal that proceeds from the vulva of the brain to the pituitary gland in the sella turcica.

2. The beginnings of the excretory duct of the kidney, or cavities into which the urine is first received, from the secretory cryptæ, are called *infundibula.*

INFUSION. (*Infusum;* from *infundo*, to pour in.) *Infusio.* A process that consists in pouring water of any required degree of temperature on such substances as have a loose texture, as thin bark, wood in shavings, or small pieces, leaves, flowers, &c. and suffering it to stand a certain time. The liquor obtained by the above process is called an *infusion*. The following are among the most approved infusions.

INFU'SUM. See *Infusion*.

INFUSUM ANTHEMIDIS. Infusion of chamomile. Take of chamomile-flowers, two drachms; boiling-water, half a pint. Macerate for ten minutes in a covered vessel, and strain. For its virtues, see *Anthemis nobilis*.

INFUSUM ARMORACIÆ COMPOSITUM. Compound infusion of horse-radish. Take of fresh horse-radish root, sliced, mustard-seeds, bruised, of each one ounce; boiling water, a pint. Macerate for two hours, in a covered vessel, and strain; then add compound spirit of horse-radish, a fluid ounce. See *Cochlearia armoracia*.

INFUSUM AURANTII COMPOSITUM. Compound infusion of orange-peel. Take of orange-peel, dried, two drachms; lemon-peel, fresh, a drachm; cloves, bruised, half a drachm; boiling water, half a pint. Macerate for a quarter of an hour, in a covered vessel, and strain. See *Citrus aurantium*.

INFUSUM CALUMBÆ. Infusion of calumba. Take of calumba-root, sliced, a drachm; boiling water, half a pint. Macerate for two hours, in a covered vessel, and strain. See *Calumba*.

INFUSUM CARYOPHYLLORUM. Infusion of cloves. Take of cloves, bruised, a drachm; boiling water, half a pint. Macerate for two hours, in a covered vessel, and strain. See *Eugenia caryophyllata*.

INFUSUM CASCARILLÆ. Infusion of cascarilla. Take of cascarilla bark, bruised, half an ounce; boiling water, half a pint. Macerate for two hours, in a covered vessel, and strain. See *Croton cascarilla*.

INFUSUM CATECHU COMPOSITUM. Compound infusion of catechu. Take of extract of catechu, two drachms and a half; cinnamon bark, bruised, half a drachm; boiling water, half a pint. Macerate for an hour, in a covered vessel, and strain. See *Acacia catechu*.

INFUSUM CINCHONÆ. Infusion of cinchona. Take of lance-leaved cinchona bark, bruised, half an ounce; boiling water, half a pint. Macerate for two hours, in a covered vessel, and strain. See *Cinchona*.

INFUSUM CUSPARIÆ. Infusion of cusparia. Take of cusparia bark, bruised, two drachms; boiling water, half a pint. Macerate for two hours, in a covered vessel, and strain. See *Cusparia febrifuga*.

INFUSUM DIGITALIS. Infusion of fox-glove. Take of purple fox-glove leaves, dried, a drachm; boiling water, half a pint. Macerate for four hours, in a covered vessel, and strain; then add spirit of cinnamon, half a fluid ounce. See *Digitalis purpurea*.

INFUSUM GENTIANÆ COMPOSITUM. Compound infusion of gentian. Take of gentian-root, sliced, orange-peel, dried, of each a drachm; lemon-peel, fresh, two drachms; boiling water, twelve fluid ounces. Macerate for an hour, in a covered vessel, and strain. See *Gentiana lutea*.

INFUSUM LINI. Infusion of linseed. Take of linseed, bruised, an ounce; liquorice-root, sliced, half an ounce; boiling water, two pints. Macerate for two hours, near the fire, in a covered vessel, and strain. See *Linum usitatissimum*.

INFUSUM QUASSIÆ. Infusion of quassia. Take of quassia wood, a scruple; boiling water, half a pint. Macerate for two hours and strain. See *Quassia amara*.

INFUSUM RHEI. Infusion of rhubarb. Take of rhubarb-root, sliced, a drachm; boiling water, half a pint. Macerate for two hours, and strain. See *Rheum*.

INFUSUM ROSÆ. Take of the petals of red rose, dried, half an ounce; boiling water, two pints and a half; dilute sulphuric acid, three fluid drachms; double-refined sugar, an ounce and a half. Pour the water upon the petals of the rose in a glass vessel; then add the acid, and macerate for half an hour. Lastly, strain the infusion, and add the sugar to it. See *Rosa Gallica*.

INFUSUM SENNÆ. Infusion of senna. Take of senna-leaves, an ounce and a half; ginger-root, sliced, a drachm; boiling water, a pint. Macerate for an hour, in a covered vessel, and strain the liquor. See *Cassia senna*.

INFUSUM SIMAROUBÆ. Infusion of simarouba. Take of simarouba bark bruised, half a drachm; boiling water, half a pint. Macerate for two hours, in a covered vessel, and strain. See *Quassia simarouba*.

INFUSUM TABACI. Infusion of tobacco. Take of tobacco-leaves, a drachm; boiling water, a pint. Macerate for an hour, in a covered vessel, and strain. See *Nicotiana*.

INGENHOUZ, JOHN, was born at Breda, in 1730 Little is known of his early life; but in 1767, he came to England to learn the Suttonian method of inoculation. In the following year he went to Vienna, to inoculate some of the imperial family, for which service he received ample honours; and shortly after performed the same operation on the Grand Duke of Tuscany, when he returned to this country, and spent the remainder of his life in scientific pursuits. In 1779, he published "Experiments on Vegetables," discovering their great power of purifying the air in sunshine, but injuring it in the shade and night. He was also author of several papers in the Philosophical Transactions, being an active member of the Royal Society. He died in 1799.

INGLUVIES. 1. Gluttony.

2. The claw, crop, or gorge of a bird.

INGRASSIAS, JOHN PHILIP, was born in Sicily, and graduated at Padua in 1537 with singular reputation; whence he was invited to a professorship in several of the Italian schools; bnt he gave the preference to Naples, where he distinguished himself greatly by his learning and judgment. At length he returned to his native island, and settled in Palermo, where he was also highly esteemed; and in 1563 made first physician to that country by Philip II. of Spain, to whom it then belonged. This office enabled him to introduce excellent regulations into the medical practice of the island, and when the plague raged there in 1575, the judicious measures adopted by him arrested its progress; whence the magistrates decreed him a large reward, of which, however, he only accepted a part, and applied that to religious uses. He died in 1580, at the age of 70. He cultivated anatomy with great assiduity, and is reckoned one of the improvers of that art, especially in regard to the structure of the cranium, and the organ of hearing. He is said also to have discovered the seminal vesicles. He published several works, particularly an account of the plague, and a treatise, "De Tumoribus præter Naturam," which is chiefly a commentary on Avicenna, but is deserving of notice, as containing the first modern description of Scarlatina, under the name of Rossalia; and perhaps the first account of varicella, which he called crystalli. But his principal work was published by his nephew, in 1603, entitled, "Commentaries on Galen's Book concerning the Bones."

INGRAVIDATION. (From *ingravidor*, to be great with child.) The same as impregnation, or going with child.

I'NGUEN. (*Inguen, inis.* n.) The groin. The lower and lateral part of the abdomen, above the thigh.

INGUINAL. *Inguinalis.* Appertaining to the groin.

Inguinal hernia. See *Hernia*.

Inguinal ligament. See *Poupart's ligament*.

INHUMATION. (From *inhumo*, to put into the ground.) The burying a patient in warm or medicated earth. Some chemists have fancied thus to call that kind of digestion which is performed by burying the materials in dung, or in the earth.

I'NION. (From ἰς, a nerve; as being the place where nerves originate.) The occiput. Blancard says it is the beginning of the spinal marrow; others say it is the back part of the neck.

INJACULA'TIO. (From *injaculor*, to shoot into.) So Helmont calls a disorder which consists of a violent spasmodic pain in the stomach, and an immobility of the body.

INJE'CTION. (*Injectio*; from *injicio*, to cast into. A medicated liquor to throw into a natural or preter natural cavity of the body by means of a syringe.

INNOMINA'TUS. (From *in*, priv., and *nomen*, a name.) Some parts of the body are so named: thus, the pelvic bones, which in the young subject are three in number, to which names were given, become one in the adult, which was without a name; an artery from the arch of the aorta, and the fifth pair of nerves, because they appeared to have been forgotten by the older anatomists.

INNOMINATA ARTERIA. The first branch given off by the arch of the aorta. It soon divides into the right carotid and right subclavian arteries.

Innominati nervi. The fifth pair of nerves. See *Trigemini.*

Innominatum os. (So called because the three bones of which it originally was formed grew together, and formed one complete bone, which was then left nameless.) A large irregular bone, situated at the side of the pelvis. It is divided into three portions, viz. the iliac, ischiatic, and pubic, which are usually described as three distinct bones.

The *os ilium*, or haunch-bone, is of a very irregular shape. The lower part of it is thick and narrow; its superior portion is broad and thin, terminating in a ridge, called the *spine* of the ilium, and more commonly known by the name of the *haunch*. The spine rises up like an arch, being turned somewhat outward, and from this appearance, the upper part of the pelvis, when viewed together, has not been improperly compared to the wings of a phæton. This spine, in the recent subject, appears as if tipped with cartilage; but this appearance is nothing more than the tendinous fibres of the muscles that are inserted into it. Externally, this bone is unequally prominent, and hollowed for the attachment of muscles; and internally, at its broadest forepart, it is smooth and concave. At its lower part, there is a considerable ridge on its inner surface. This ridge, which extends from the os sacrum, and corresponds with a similar prominence, both on that bone and the ischium, forms, with the inner part of the ossa pubis, what is called the brim of the pelvis. The whole of the internal surface, behind this ridge, is very unequal. The os ilium has likewise a smaller surface posteriorly, by which it is articulated to the sides of the os sacrum. This surface has, by some, been compared to the human ear, and, by others, to the head of a bird: but neither of these comparisons seem to convey any just idea of its form or appearance. Its upper part is rough and porous; lower down it is more solid. It is firmly united to the os sacrum by a cartilaginous substance, and likewise by very strong ligamentous fibres, which are extended to that bone from the whole circumference of this irregular surface. The spine of this bone, which is originally an epiphysis, has two considerable tuberosities, one anteriorly, and the other posteriorly, which is the largest of the two. The ends of this spine too, from their projecting more than the parts of the bone below them, are called spinal processes. Before the anterior spinal process, the spine is hollowed, where part of the Sartorius muscle is placed; and below the posterior spinal process, there is a very large niche in the bone, which, in the recent subject, has a strong ligament stretched over its lower part, from the os sacrum to the sharp-pointed process of the ischium; so that a great hole is formed, through which pass the great sciatic nerve and the posterior crural vessels under the pyriform muscle, part of which is likewise lodged in this hole. The lowest, thickest, and narrowest part of the ilium, in conjunction with the other two portions of each os innominatum, helps to form the acetabulum for the os femoris.

The *os ischium*, or hip-bone, which is the lowest of the three portions of each os innominatum, is of a very irregular figure, and usually divided into its body, tuberosity, and ramus. The body externally forms the inferior portion of the acetabulum, and sends a sharp-pointed process backward, called the spine of the ischium. This is the process to which the ligament is attached, which was just now described as forming a great foramen for the passage of the sciatic nerve. The tuberosity is large and irregular, and is placed at the inferior part of the bone, giving origin to several muscles. In the recent subject, it seems covered with a cartilaginous crust; but this appearance, as in the spine of the ilium, is nothing more than the tendinous fibres of the muscles that are inserted into it. This tuberosity, which is the lowest portion of the trunk, supports us when we sit. Between the spine and the tuberosity is observed a sinuosity, covered with a cartilaginous crust, which serves as a pulley, on which the obturator muscle plays. From the tuberosity, the bone, becoming narrower and thinner, forms the ramus, or branch, which, passing forwards and upwards, makes, with the ramus of the os pubis, a large hole, of an oval shape, the *foramen magnum ischii*, which affords, through its whole circumference, attachment to muscles. This foramen is more particularly noticed in describing the os pubis.

The *os pubis* or share-bone, which is the smallest of the three portions of the os innominatum, is placed at the upper and forepart of the pelvis, where the two ossa pubis meet, and are united to each other by means of a very strong cartilage, which constitutes what is called the *symphysis pubis*. Each os pubis may be divided into its body, angle, and ramus. The body, which is the outer part, is joined to the os ilium. The angle comes forward to form the symphisis, and the ramus is a thin apophysis, which, uniting with the ramus of the ischium, forms the *foramen magnum ischii*, or *thyroideum*, as it has been sometimes called, from its resemblance to a door or shield. This foramen is somewhat wider above than below, and its greatest diameter is, from above downwards, and obliquely from within outwards. In the recent subject, it is almost completely closed by a strong fibrous membrane, called the *obturator* ligament. Upwards and outwards, where we observe a niche in the bone, the fibres of this ligament are separated, to allow a passage to the posterior crural nerve, an artery and vein. The great uses of this foramen seem to be to lighten the bones of the pelvis, and to afford a convenient lodgment to the obturator muscles. The three bones now described as constituting the os innominatum on each side, all concur to form the great *acetabulum*, or cotyloid cavity, which receives the head of the thigh-bone; the os ilium and os ischium making each about two-fifths, and the os pubis one-fifth, of the cavity. This acetabulum, which is of considerable depth, is of a spherical shape. Its brims are high, and, in the recent subject, it is tipped with cartilage. These brims, however, are higher above and externally, than they are internally and below, where we observe a niche in the bone (namely, the ischium), across which is stretched a ligament, forming a hole for the transmission of blood-vessels and nerves to the cavity of the joint. The cartilage which lines the acetabulum, is thickest at its circumference, and thinner within, where a little hole is to be observed, in which is placed the apparatus that serves to lubricate the joint, and facilitate its motions. We are likewise able to discover the impression made by the internal ligament of the os femoris, which, by being attached both to this cavity and to the head of the os femoris, helps to secure the latter in the acetabulum. The bones of the pelvis serve to support the spine and upper parts of the body, to lodge the intestines, urinary bladder, and other viscera; and likewise to unite the trunk to the lower extremities. But, besides these uses, they are destined, in the female subject, for other important purposes; and the accoucheur finds, in the study of these bones, the foundation of all midwifery knowledge. Several eminent writers are of opinion, that in difficult parturition, all the bones of the pelvis undergo a certain degree of separation. It has been observed, likewise, that the cartilage uniting the ossa pubis is thicker, and of a more spongy texture, in women than in men; and therefore more likely to swell and enlarge during pregnancy. That many instances of a partial separation of these bones, during labour, have happened, there can be no doubt; such a separation, however, ought by no means to be considered as a uniform and salutary work of nature, as some writers seem to think, but as the effect of disease. But there is another circumstance in regard to this part of osteology, which is well worthy of attention; and this is, the different capacities of the pelvis in the male and female subject. It has been observed that the os sacrum is shorter and broader in women than in men; the ossa ilia are also found more expanded; whence it happens, that in women the centre of gravity does not fall so directly on the upper part of the thigh as in men, and this seems to be the reason why, in general, they step with less firmness, and move their hips forward in walking. From these circumstances, also, the brim of the female pelvis is nearly of an oval shape, being considerably wider from side to side, than from the symphysis pubis to the os sacrum; whereas, in men, it is rounder, and everywhere of less diameter. The inferior opening of the pelvis is likewise proportionably larger in the female subject, the ossa ischia being more separated from each other, and the foramen ischii larger, so that, where the os ischium and os pubis are united together, they form a greater circle; the os sacrum is also more hollowed, though shorter, and the os coccygis more loosely connected, and, therefore, capable of a greater degree of motion than in men.

INOCULATION. *Inoculatio.* The insertion of a poison into any part of the body. It was mostly practised with that of the small-pox, because we had learned, from experience, that by so doing, we generally procured fewer pustules, and a much milder disease, than when the small-pox was taken in a natural way. Although the advantages were evident, yet objections were raised against inoculation, on the notion that it exposed the person to some risk, when he might have passed through life, without ever taking the disease naturally; but it is obvious that he was exposed to much greater danger, from the intercourse which he must have with his fellow-creatures, by taking the disorder in a natural way. It has also been adduced, that a person is liable to take the small-pox a second time, when produced at first by artificial means; but such instances are very rare, besides not being sufficiently authentic. We may conjecture that, in most of those cases, the matter used was not variolous, but that of some other eruptive disorder, such as the chicken-pox, which has often been mistaken for the small-pox. However, since the discovery of the preventive power of the cow-pox, small-pox inoculation has been rapidly falling into disuse. See *Variola vaccina.*

To illustrate the benefits arising from inoculation, it has been calculated that a third of the adults die who take the disease in a natural way, and about one-seventh of the children; whereas of those who are inoculated, and are properly treated afterward, the proportion is probably not greater than one in five or six hundred.

Inoculation is generally thought to have been introduced into Britain from Turkey, by Lady Mary Wortley Montague, about the year 1721, whose son had been inoculated at Constantinople, during her residence there, and whose infant daughter was the first that underwent the operation in this country. It appears, however, to have been well known before this period, both in the south of Wales and Highlands of Scotland. Mungo Park, in his travels into the interior of Africa, found that inoculation had been long practised by the Negroes on the Guinea coast; and nearly in the same manner, and at the same time of life, as in Europe. It is not clearly ascertained where inoculation really originated. It has been ascribed to the Circassians, who employed it as the means of preserving the beauty of their women. It appears more probable that accident first suggested the expedient among different nations, to whom the small-pox had long been known, independently of any intercourse with each other; and what adds to the probability of this conjecture is, that in most places where inoculation can be traced back, for a considerable length of time, it seems to have been practised chiefly by old women, before it was adopted by regular practitioners.

Many physicians held inoculation in the greatest contempt at first, from its supposed origin; others again discredited the fact of its utility; while others, on the testimony of the success in distant countries, believed in the advantages it afforded, but still did not think themselves warranted to recommend it to the families they attended; and it was not until the experiment of it had been made on six criminals (all of whom recovered from the disease and regained their liberty), that it was practised, in the year 1726, on the royal family, and afterward adopted as a general thing.

To ensure success from inoculation, the following precautions should strictly be attended to.

1. That the person should be of a good habit of body, and free from any disease, apparent or latent, in order that he may not have the disease and a bad constitution, or perhaps another disorder, to struggle with at the same time.

2. To enjoin a temperate diet and proper regimen; and, where the body is plethoric, or gross, to make use of gentle purges, together with mercurial and antimonial medicines.

3. That the age of the person be as little advanced as possible, but not younger if it can be avoided, than four months.

4. To choose a cool season of the year, and to avoid external heat, either by exposure to the sun, sitting by fires, or in warm chambers, or by going too warmly clothed, or being too much in bed.

5. To take the matter from a young subject, who has the small-pox in a favourable way, and who is otherwise healthy, and free from disease; and, when fresh matter can be procured, to give it the preference.

Where matter of a benign kind cannot be procured, and the patient is evidently in danger of the casual small-pox, we should not, however, hesitate a moment to inoculate from any kind of matter that can be procured; as what has been taken in malignant kinds of small-pox has been found to produce a very mild disease. The mildness or malignity of the disease appears, therefore, to depend little or not at all on the inoculating matter. Variolous matter, as well as the vaccine, by being kept for a length of time, particularly in a warm place, is apt, however, to undergo decomposition, by putrefaction; and then another kind of contagious material has been produced.

In inoculating, the operator is to make the slightest puncture or scratch imaginable in the arm of the person, rubbing that part of the lancet which is besmeared with matter repeatedly over it, by way of ensuring the absorption; and in order to prevent its being wiped off, the shirt sleeve ought not to be pulled down until the part is dry.

A singular circumstance attending inoculation is, that when this fails in producing the disease, the inoculated part nevertheless sometimes inflames and suppurates, as in cases where the complaint is about to follow; and the matter produced in those cases, is as fit for inoculation as that taken from a person actually labouring under the disease. The same happens very frequently in inoculation for the cow pox.

If, on the fourth or fifth day after the operation, no redness or inflammation is apparent on the edge of the wound, we ought then to inoculate in the other arm, in the same manner as before; or, for greater certainty, we may do it in both.

Some constitutions are incapable of having the disease in any form. Others do not receive the disease at one time, however freely exposed to its contagion, even though repeatedly inoculated, and yet receive it afterward by merely approaching those labouring under it.

On the coming on of the febrile symptoms, which is generally on the seventh day in the inoculated small-pox, the patient is not to be suffered to lie abed, but should be kept cool, and partake freely of antiseptic cooling drinks. See *Variola.*

INOSCULA'TION. (*Inosculatio;* from *in*, and *osculum*, a little mouth.) The running of the veins and arteries into one another, or the interunion of the extremities of the arteries and veins.

INSA'NIA. (From *in*, not, and *sanus*, sound.) Insanity, or deranged intellect. A genus of disease in the class *Neuroses*, and order *Vesaniæ*, characterized by erroneous judgment, from imaginary perceptions or recollections, attended with agreeable emotions in persons of a sanguine temperament. See *Mania.*

INSE'SSUS. (From *insideo*, to sit upon.) A hot-bath, simple or medicated, over which the patient sits.

INSIPIE'NTIA. (From *in*, and *sapientia*, wisdom.) A delirium without fever.

INSOLA'TIO. (From *in*, upon, and *sol*, the sun.) A disease which arises from a too great influence of the sun's heat upon the head, a coup de soleil.

INSPIRA'TION. (*Inspiratio;* from *in*, and *spiro*, to breathe.) The act of drawing the air into the lungs. See *Respiration.*

INSTINCT. (*Instinctus, ûs.* m.) Animals are not abandoned by nature to themselves: they are all employed in a series of actions; whence results that marvellous whole that is seen among organized beings. To incline animals to the punctual execution of those actions which are necessary for them, nature has provided them with *instinct;* that is, propensities, inclinations, wants, by which they are constantly excited, and forced to fulfil the intentions of nature.

Instinct may excite in two different modes, with or without knowledge of the end. The first is enlightened instinct, the second is blind instinct; the one is particularly the gift of man, the other belongs to animals.

In examining carefully the numerous phenomena which depend on instinct, we see that there is a double design in every animal:—1. The preservation of the individual. 2. The preservation of the species. Every animal fulfils this end in its own way, and according to its organization; there are therefore as many different instincts as there are different species; and as the organization varies in individuals, instinct presents individual differences sometimes strongly marked.

We recognise two sorts of instinct in man: the one depends more evidently on his organization, on his animal state; he presents it in whatever state he is found. This sort of instinct is nearly the same as that of animals. The other kind of instinct springs from the social state; and, without doubt, depends on organization: what vital phenomenon does not depend on it? But it does not display itself except when man lives in civilized society, and when he enjoys all the advantages of that state.

To the first, that may be called animal instinct, belong hunger, thirst, the necessity of clothing, of a covering from the weather; the desire of agreeable sensations; the fear of pain and of death; the desire to injure others, if there is any danger to be feared from them, or any advantage to arise from hurting them; the venereal inclinations; the interest inspired by children; inclination to imitation; to live in society, which leads man to pass through the different degrees of civilization, &c. These different instinctive feelings incline him to concur in the established order of organized beings. Man is, of all the animals, the one whose natural wants are most numerous, and of the greatest variety; which is in proportion to the extent of his intelligence: if he had only these wants, he would have always a marked superiority over the animals.

When man, living in society, can easily provide for all the wants which we have mentioned, he has then time and powers of action more than his original wants require: then new wants arise, that may be called social wants: such is that of a lively perception of existence; a want which, the more it is satisfied, the more difficult it becomes, because the sensations become blunted by habit.

This want of a vivid existence, added to the continually increasing feebleness of the sensations, causes a mechanical restlessness, vague desires, excited by the remembrance of vivid sensations formerly felt: in order to escape from this state, man is continually forced to change his object, or to overstrain sensations of the same kind. Thence arises an inconstancy which never permits our desires to rest, and a progression of desires, which, always annihilated by enjoyment, and irritated by remembrance, proceed forward without end; thence arises *ennui*, by which the civilized idler is incessantly tormented.

The want of vivid sensations is balanced by the love of repose and idleness in the opulent classes of society. These contradictory feelings modify each other, and from their reciprocal reaction results the love of power, of consideration, of fortune, &c. which gives us the means of satisfying both.

These two instinctive sensations are not the only ones which spring from the social state; a crowd of others arise from it, equally real, though less important; besides, the natural wants become so changed as no longer to be known; hunger is often replaced by a capricious taste; the venereal desires by a feeling of quite another nature, &c.

The natural wants have a considerable influence upon those which arise from society; these, in their turn, modify the former; and if we add age, temperament, sex, &c. which tend to change every sort of want, we will have an idea of the difficulty which the study of the instinct of man presents. This part of physiology is also scarcely begun. We remark, however, that the social wants necessarily carry along with them the enlargement of the understanding; there is no comparison in regard to the capacity of the mind, between a man in the higher class of society, and a man whose physical powers are scarcely sufficient to provide for his natural wants.

INTEGER. When applied to leaves, perianths, petals, &c. *folia integra*, means undivided; and is said of the simple leaves, as those of the orchises and grasses. The female flower of the oak affords an example of the *perianthium integrum*, and the petals of the *Nigella arvensis* and *Silene quinquevulnera* are described as *petala integra*.

INTEGERRIMUS. Most perfect or entire. Applied to leaves, the margin of which has no teeth, notches, or incisions. It regards solely the margin whereas the *folium integrum* respects the whole shape and has nothing to do with the margin.

INTERCO'STAL. (*Intercostalis;* from *inter*, between, and *costa*, a rib.) A name given to muscles, vessels, &c. which are between the ribs.

INTERCOSTAL ARTERIES. *Arteriæ intercostales.* The arteries which run between the ribs. The superior intercostal artery is a branch of the subclavian. The other intercostal arteries are given off from the aorta.

INTERCOSTAL MUSCLES. *Intercostales externi et interni.* Between the ribs on each side are eleven double rows of muscles. These are the *intercostales externi*, and *interni*. Galen has very properly observed, that they decussate each other like the strokes of the letter X. The *intercostales externi* arise from the lower edge of each superior rib, and, running obliquely downwards and forwards, are inserted into the upper edge of each inferior rib, so as to occupy the intervals of the ribs, from as far back as the spine to their cartilages; but from their cartilages to the sternum, there is only a thin aponeurosis covering the internal intercostales. The *intercostales interni* arise and are inserted in the same manner as the external. They begin at the sternum, and extend as far as the angles of the ribs, their fibres running obliquely backwards. These fibres are spread over a considerable part of the inner surface of the ribs, so as to be longer than those of the external intercostals. Some of the posterior portions of the internal intercostals pass over one rib, and are inserted into the rib below. Verheyen first described these portions as separate muscles, under the name of *infra costales*. Winslow has adopted the same name. Cowper, and after him Douglas, call them *costarum depressores proprii.* These distinctions, however, are altogether superfluous, as they are evidently nothing more than appendages of the intercostals. The number of these portions varies in different subjects. Most commonly there are only four, the first of which runs from the second rib to the fourth, the second from the third rib to the fifth, the third from the fourth rib to the sixth, and the fourth from the fifth rib to the seventh. The internal intercostals of the two inferior false ribs are frequently so thin, as to be with difficulty separated from the external; and, in some subjects, one or both of them seem to be altogether wanting. It was the opinion of the ancients, that the external intercostals serve to elevate, and the internal to depress the ribs. They were probably led to this opinion, by observing the different direction of their fibres; but it is now well known, that both have the same use, which is that of raising the ribs equally during inspiration. Fallopius was one of the first who ventured to call in question the opinion of Galen on this subject, by contending that both layers of the intercostals serve to elevate the ribs. In this opinion he was followed by Hieronymus Fabricius, our countryman Mayow, and Borelli. But, towards the close of the last century, Bayle, a writer of some eminence, and professor at Toulouse, revived the opinion of the ancients by the following arguments:—He observed, that the oblique direction of the fibres of the internal intercostals is such, that in each inferior rib, these fibres are nearer to the vertebræ than they are at their superior extremities, or in the rib immediately above; and that, of course, they must serve to draw the rib downwards, as towards the most fixed point. This plausible doctrine was adopted by several eminent writers, and among others, by Nicholls, Hoadley, and Schreiber; but above all, by Hamberger, who went so far as to assert, that not only the ribs, but even the sternum, are pulled down wards by these muscles, and constructed a particular instrument to illustrate this doctrine. He pretended likewise that the intervals of the ribs are increased by their elevation, and diminished by their depression; but he allowed that, while those parts of the internal intercostals that are placed between the bony part of the ribs pull them downwards, the anterior portions of the muscle, which are situated between the cartilages, concur with the external intercostals in raising them upwards. These opinions gave rise to a warm and interesting controversy, in which Hamberger and Haller were the principal disputants. The former argued chiefly from theory, and the latter from experiments on living animals, which demonstrate the fallacy of Hamberger's arguments, and prove, beyond a doubt, that the internal intercostals perform the same functions as the external.

INTERCOSTAL NERVE. *Nervus intercostalis.* Great intercostal nerve. Sympathetic nerve. The great intercostal nerve arises in the cavity of the cranium, from a branch of the sixth and one of the fifth pair, uniting into one trunk, which passes out of the cranium through the carotid canal, and descends by the sides of the bodies of the vertebræ of the neck, thorax, loins, and os sacrum: in its course, it receives the small accessory branches from all the thirty pair of spinal nerves. In the neck, it gives off three cervical ganglions, the upper, middle, and lower; from which the cardiac and pulmonary nerves arise. In the thorax, it gives off the splanchnic or anterior intercostal, which perforates the diaphragm, and forms the semilunar ganglions, from which nerves pass to all the abdominal viscera. They also form in the abdomen ten peculiar plexuses, distinguished by the name of the viscus, to which they belong, as the cœliac, splenic, hepatic, superior, middle, and lower mesenteric, two renal, and two spermatic plexuses. The posterior intercostal nerve gives accessory branches about the pelvis and ischiatic nerve, and at length terminates.

INTERCOSTAL VEINS. The intercostal veins empty their blood into the vena azygos.

INTERCU'RRENT. Those fevers which happen in certain seasons only, are called stationary: others are called, by Sydenham, intercurrents.

INTE'RCUS. (From *inter*, between, and *cutis*, the skin.) A dropsy between the skin and the flesh. See *Anasarca.*

INTERDE'NTIUM. (From *inter*, between, and *dens*, a tooth.) The intervals between teeth of the same order.

INTERDI'GITUM. (From *inter*, between, and *digitus*, a toe, or finger.) A corn between the toes, or wart between the fingers.

INTERFÆMI'NEUM. (From *inter*, between, and *fæmen*, the thigh.) The perinæum, or space between the anus and pudendum.

INTERLU'NIUS. (From *inter*, between, and *luna*, the moon; because it was supposed to affect those who were born in the wane of the moon.) The epilepsy.

Intermediate affinity. See *Affinity intermediate.*

INTERMITTENT. (*Intermittens*; from *inter*, between, and *mitto*, to send away.) A disease is so called which does not continue until it finishes one way or the other, as most diseases do, but ceases and returns again at regular or uncertain periods; as agues, &c.

Intermittent fever. See *Febris intermittens.*

INTERNODIS. Applied to a flowerstalk or peduncculus, when it proceeds from the intermediate part of a branch between two leaves; as in *Ehretia internodis.*

INTERNU'NTII DIES. (From *internuncio*, to go between.) Applied to critical days, or such as stand between the increase of a disorder and its decrease.

INTERO'SSEI MANUS. (*Interosseus*; from *inter*, between, and *os*, the bone.) These are small muscles situated between the metacarpal bones, and extending from the bones of the carpus to the fingers. They are divided into *internal* and *external*; the former are to be seen only on the palm of the hand, but the latter are conspicuous both on the palm and back of the hand. The *interossei interni* are three in number. The first, which Albinus names *posterior indicis*, arises tendinous and fleshy from the basis and inner part of the metacarpal bone of the forefinger, and likewise from the upper part of that which supports the middle finger. Its tendon passes over the articulation of this part of these bones with the forefinger, and, uniting with the tendinous expansion that is sent off from the extensor digitorum communis, is inserted into the posterior convex surface of the first phalanx of that finger. The second and third, to which Albinus gives the names of *prior annularis*, and *interrosseus auricularis*, arise, in the same manner, from the basis of the outsides of the metacarpal bones that sustain the ring-finger and the little finger, and are inserted into the outside of the tendinous expansion of the extensor digitorum communis that covers each of those fingers. These three muscles draw the fingers into which they are inserted, towards the thumb. The *interossei externi* are four in number; for among these is included the small muscle that is situated on the outside of the metacarpal bone that supports the forefinger. Douglas calls it *extensor tertii internodii indicis*, and Winslow *semi-interosseus indicis.* Albinus, who describes it among the interrossei, gives it the name of *prior indicis.* This first interosseus externus arises by two tendinous and fleshy portions. One of these springs from the upper half of the inner side of the first bone of the thumb, and the other from the ligaments that unite the os trapezoides to the metacarpal bone of the forefinger, and likewise from all the outside of this latter bone. These two portions unite as they descend, and terminate in a tendon, which is inserted into the outside of that part of the tendinous expansion from the extensor digitorum communis that is spread over the posterior convex surface of the forefinger. The second, to which Albinus gives the name of *prior medii*, is not quite so thick as the last described muscle. It arises by two heads, one of which springs from the inner side of the metacarpal bone of the forefinger, chiefly towards its convex surface, and the other arises from the adjacent ligaments, and from the whole outer side of the metacarpal bone that sustains the middle finger. These two portions unite as they descend, and terminate in a tendon, which is inserted, in the same manner, as the preceding muscle, into the outside of the tendinous expansion that covers the posterior part of the middle finger. The third belongs likewise to the middle finger, and is therefore named *posterior medii* by Albinus. It arises, like the last described muscle, by two origins, which spring from the roots of the metacarpal bones of the ring and middle fingers, and from the adjacent ligaments, and is inserted into the inside of the same tendinous expansion as the preceding muscle. The fourth, to which Albinus gives the name of *posterior annularis*, differs from the last two only in its situation, which is between the metacarpal bones of the ring and little fingers. It is inserted into the inside of the tendinous expansion of the extensor digitorum communis, that covers the posterior part of the ring-finger. All these four muscles serve to extend the fingers into which they are inserted, and likewise to draw them inwards, towards the thumb, except the third, or *posterii medii*, which, from its situation and insertion, is calculated to pull the middle finger outwards.

INTEROSSEI PEDIS. These small muscles, in their situation between the metatarsal bones, resemble the interossei of the hand, and, like them, are divided into *internal* and *external*. The *interossei pedis interni* are three in number. They arise tendinous and fleshy, from the basis and inside of the metatarsal bones of the middle, the third, and little toes, in the same manner as those of the hand, and they each terminate in a tendon that runs to the inside of the first joint of these toes, and from thence to their upper surface, where it loses itself in the tendinous expansion that is sent off from the extensors. Each of these three muscles serves to draw the toe into which it is inserted towards the great toe. The *interossei externi* are four in number. The first arises tendinous and fleshy from the outside of the root of the metatarsal bone of the great toe, from the os cuneiforme internum, and from the root of the inside of the metatarsal bone of the foretoe Its tendon is inserted into the inside of the tendinous expansion that covers the back part of the toes. The second is placed in a similar manner between the metatarsal bones of the fore and middle toes, and is inserted into the outside of the tendinous expansion on the back part of the foretoe. The third and fourth are placed between the two next metatarsal bones, and are inserted into the outside of the middle and third toes. The first of these muscles draws the foretoe inwards towards the great toe. The three others pull the toes, into which they are inserted, outwards. They all assist in extending the toes.

INTEROSSEOUS. (*Interosseus*; from *inter*, between, and *os*, a bone.) A name given to muscles ligaments, &c. which are between bones.

INTERPELLA'TUS. (From *interpello*, to interrupt.) A name given by Paracelsus to a disease attended with irregular or uncertain paroxysms.

INTERPOLA'TUS DIES. (From *interpolo*, to renew.) In Paracelsus, these are the days interpolated between two paroxysms.

INTERSCAPU'LIUM. (From *inter*, between, and *scapula*, the shoulder-blade.) That part of the spine which lies between the shoulders.

INTERSE'PTUM. (From *inter*, between, and *septum*, an enclosure.) The uvula and the septum narium.

INTERSPINA'LIS. (From *inter*, between, and *spina*, the spine.) Muscles, nerves, &c. are so named which are between the processes of the spine.

INTERSPINALES. The fleshy portions between the spinous processes of the neck, back, and loins, distinguished by the names of *interspinales colli, dorsi et lumborum.* Those which connect processes of the back and loins, are rather small tendons than muscles: they draw these processes nearer to each other.

INTERTRANSVERSA'LES. Four distinct small bundles of flesh, which fill up the spaces between the transverse processes of the vertebræ of the loins, and serve to draw them towards each other

INTERTRI'GO. (From *inter*, between, and *tero*, to rub.) An excoriation about the anus, groins, axilla, or other parts of the body, attended with inflammation and moisture. It is most commonly produced by the irritation of the urine, from riding, or some acrimony in children.

INTE'STINE. (*Intestinum;* from *intus*, within.) The convoluted membraneous tube that extends from the stomach to the anus, receives the ingested food, retains it a certain time, mixes with it the bile and pancreatic juice, propels the chyle into the lacteals, and covers the fæces with mucus, is so called. The intestines are situated in the cavity of the abdomen, and are divided into the small and large, which have, besides their size, other circumstances of distinction.

The *small* intestines are supplied internally with folds, called *valvulæ conniventes*, and have no bands on their external surface. The *large* intestines have no folds internally; are supplied externally with three strong muscular bands, which run parallel upon the surface, and give the intestines a saccated appearance; they have also small fatty appendages, called *appendiculæ epiploicæ.*

The first portion of the intestinal tube, for about the extent of twelve fingers' breadth, is called the *duodenum;* it lies in the epigastric region; makes three turnings, and between the first and second flexure receives by a common opening, the pancreatic duct, and the ductus communis choledochus. It is in this portion of the intestines that chylification is chiefly performed. The remaining portion of the small intestines is distinguished by an imaginary division into the jejunum and ileum.

The *jejunum*, which commences where the duodenum ends, is situated in the umbilical region, and is mostly found empty; hence its name: it is everywhere covered with red vessels, and, about an hour and a half after a meal, with destended lacteals.

The *ileum* occupies the hypogastric region and the pelvis, is of a more pallid colour than the former, and terminates by a transverse opening into the large intestines, which is called the *valve of the ileum, valve of the cæcum, or the valve of Tulpius.*

The beginning of the large intestines is firmly tied down in the right iliac region, and for the extent of about four fingers' breadth is called the *cæcum*, having adhering to it a worm-like process, called the *processus cæci vermiformis*, or *appendicula cæci vermiformis.* The great intestine then commences *colon*, ascends towards the liver, passes across the abdomen, under the stomach, to the left side, where it is contorted like the letter S, and descends to the pelvis: hence it is divided in this course into the *ascending portion, the transverse arch*, and the *sigmoid flexure.* When it has reached the pelvis, it is called the *rectum*, from whence it proceeds in a straight line to the anus.

The intestinal canal is composed of three membranes, or coats; a *common* one from the peritoneum, a *muscular coat*, and a *villous coat*, the villi being formed of the fine terminations of arteries and nerves, and the origins of lacteals and lymphatics. The intestines are connected to the body by the mesentery; the duodenum has also a peculiar collecting cellular substance, as have likewise the colon and rectum, by whose means the former is firmly accreted to the back, the colon to the kidneys, and the latter to the os coccygis, and, in women, to the vagina. The remaining portion of the tube is loose in the cavity of the abdomen. The arteries of this canal are branches of the *superior* and *inferior mesenteric*, and the *duodenal.* The veins evacuate their blood into the vena portæ. The nerves are branches of the eight pair and intercostals. The *lacteal vessels*, which originate principally from the jejunum, proceed to the glands in the mesentery.

INTRAFOLIACEUS. Applied to stipulæ, which are above the footstalk, and internal with respect to the leaf; as in *Ficus carica* and *Morus nigra.*

INTRICA'TUS. (From *intrico*, to entangle; so called from its intricate folds.) A muscle of the ear.

INTRI'NSECUS. (From *intra*, within, and *secus*, towards.) A painful disorder of an internal part

INTROCE'SSIO. (From *introcedo*, to go in.) *Depressio.* A depression or sinking of any part inwards.

INTUS-SUSCE'PTION. (*Intus-susceptio*, and *intro-susceptio;* from *intus*, within, and *suscipio*, to receive.) A disease of the intestinal tube, and most frequently of the small intestines; it consists in a portion of gut passing for some length within another portion.

I'NTYBUS. (From *in*, and *tuba*, a hollow instrument: so named from the hollowness of its stalk.) See *Cichorium endivia.*

I'NULA. (Contracted or corrupted from *helenium*, ηλενιον, fabled to have sprung from the tears of Helen.) 1. The name of a genus of plants in the Linnæan system. Class, *Syngenesia;* Order, *Polygamia superflua.*

2. The herb *inula*, or elecampane. See *Inula helenium.*

Inula, common. See *Inula helenium.*

INULA CRITHMOIDES. *Caaponga* of the Brazilians. *Trifolia spica; Crithmum marinum non spinosum.* The leaves and young stalks of this plant are pickled for the use of the table; they are gently diuretic.

INULA DYSENTERICA. The systematic name of the smaller inula, *Conyza media. Arnica Suedensis, Arnica spurio, Conyza: Inula—amplexicaulibus, cordato oblongis; caule villoso, paniculato; squamis calycinis, setaceis*, of Linnæus This indigenous plant was once considered as possessing great antidysenteric virtues. The whole herb is to the taste acrid, and at the same time rather aromatic. It is now fallen into disuse.

INULA HELENIUM. The systematic name of the common inula or elecampane. *Enula campana: Helenium. Inula—foliis amplexicaulibus ovatis rugosis subtus tomentosis, calycum squamis ovatis*, of Linnæus. This plant, though a native of Britain, is seldom met with in its wild state, but mostly cultivated. The root, which is the part employed medicinally, in its recent state, has a weaker and less grateful smell than when thoroughly dried, and kept for a length of time, by which it is greatly improved; its odour then approaching to that of Florentine orris-root. It was formerly in high estimation in dyspepsia, pulmonary affections, and uterine obstructions, but is now fallen into disuse. From the root of this plant, Rose first extracted the peculiar vegetable principle called *inulin.* Funke has since given the following as the analysis of elecampane root:—A crystallizable volatile oil; inulin; extractive; acetic acid; a crystallizable resin; gluten; a fibrous matter. See *Inulin.*

INULIN In examining the *Inula helenium*, or *Elecampane*, Rose imagined he discovered a new vegetable product, to which the name of *Inulin* has been given. It is white and pulverulent, like starch. When thrown on red-hot coals, it melts, diffusing a white smoke, with the smell of burning sugar. It yields, on distillation in a retort, all the products furnished by gum. It dissolves readily in hot water; and precipitates almost entirely on cooling, in the form of a white powder; but before falling down, it gives the liquid a mucilaginous consistence. It precipitates quickly on the addition of alkohol.

The above substance is obtained by boiling the root of this plant in four times its weight of water, and leaving the liquid in repose. Pelletier and Caventou have found the same starch-like matter in abundance in the root of colchicum: and Gautier in the root of pellitory.

INUSTION. (From *in*, and *uro*, to burn.) It is sometimes used for hot and dry seasons; and formerly by surgeons for the operation of the cautery.

INVERECU'NDUM OS. (From *in*, not, and *verecundus* modest.) An obsolete name of the frontal bones, from its being regarded as the seat of impudence.

INVERSION. *Inversio.* Turned inside outward

INVOLUCELLUM. A partial involucrum. See *Involucrum.*

INVOLU'CRUM. (From *in*, and *volvo*, to wrap up; because parts are enclosed by it.) In anatomy 1. A name of the pericardium.

2. A membrane which covers any part

n botany. A leafy calyx, remote from the flower, applied particularly to umbelliferous plants.

From the part of the umbel in which it is placed, it is called,

1. *Involucrum universale*, being at the base of the whole umbel; as in *Coriandrum sativum*, *Scandix cerefolium*, and *Cornus mascula*.

2. I. *partiale*, called *involucellum;* at the bottom of each umbellula, or partial stalk of the umbel; as in *Daucus carota*.

3. I. *dimidiatum*, surrounding the middle of the stalk at the base of the umbel, as in *Æthusa cynapium*.

From the number of the involucre leaves,

4. *Monophyllous;* as in *Coriander* and *Hermas*.

5. *Tryphillous;* as in *Bupleurum junceum*.

6. *Polyphillous;* as in *Bunium bulbocastanum*, and *Sium*.

7. *Pinnatifid;* as in *Daucus carota*, and *Sium angustifolium*.

8. *Reflex*, turned back; as in *Selinum monnieri*.

Solitary flowers rarely have an involucrum; yet it is found in the anemones.

INVOLUTUS. Involute. Rolled inwards. Applied to leaves, petals, &c. when their margins are turned inward; as in the leaves of *Pinguicula*, and petals of *Anethum*, *Pastinaca*, and *Bupleurum*.

IODATE. A compound of iodine with oxygen, and a metallic basis. The *oxiodes* of Davy.

IODES. (From ιος, verdigris.) Green matter thrown off by vomiting.

IODIC ACID. *Acidum iodicum*. Oxiodic acid. "When barytes water is made to act on iodine, a soluble hydriodate, and an insoluble iodate of barytes, are formed. On the latter, well washed, pour sulphuric acid, equivalent to the barytes present, diluted with twice its weight of water, and heat the mixture. The iodic acid quickly abandons a portion of its base, and combines with the water; but though even less than the equivalent proportion of sulphuric acid has been used, a little of it will be found mixed with the liquid acid. If we endeavour to separate this portion, by adding barytes water, the two acids precipitate together.

The above economical process is that of Gay Lussac; but Sir H. Davy, who is the first discoverer of this acid, invented one more elegant, and which yields a purer acid. Into a long glass tube, bent like the letter L inverted, (⅂) shut at one end, put 100 grains of chlorate of potassa, and pour over it 400 grains of muriatic acid, specific gravity 1.105. Put 40 grains of iodine into a thin long-necked receiver. Into the open end of the bent tube put some muriate of lime, and then connect it with the receiver. Apply a gentle heat to the sealed end of the former. Protoxide of chlorine is evolved, which, as it comes in contact with the iodine, produces combustion, and two new compounds, a compound of iodine and oxygen, and one of iodine and chlorine. The latter is easily separated by heat, while the former remains in a state of purity.

The iodic acid of Sir H. Davy is a white semitransparent solid. It has a strong acido-astringent taste, but no smell. Its density is considerably greater than that of sulphuric acid, in which it rapidly sinks. It melts, and is decomposed into iodine and oxygen, at a temperature of about 620°. A grain of iodic acid gives out 176.1, grain measure, of oxygen gas. It would appear from this, that iodic acid consists of 15.5 iodine, to 5 oxygen.

Iodic acid deliquesces in the air, and is, of course, very soluble in water. It first reddens and then destroys the blues of vegetable infusions. It blanches other vegetable colours. Between the acid prepared by Gay Lussac, and that of Sir H. Davy, there is one important difference. The latter, being dissolved, may, by evaporation of the water, pass not only to the inspissated syrup state, but can be made to assume a pasty consistence; and, finally, by a stronger heat, yields the solid substance unaltered. When a mixture of it, with charcoal, sulphur, resin, sugar, or the combustible metals, in a finely divided state, is heated, detonations are produced; and its solution rapidly corrodes all the metals to which Sir H. Davy exposed it, both gold and platinum, but much more intensely the first of these metals.

It appears to form combinations with all the fluid or solid acids which it does not decompose. When sulphuric acid is dropped into a concentrated solution of it in hot water, a solid substance is precipitated, which consists of the acid and the compound; for, on evaporating the solution by a gentle heat, nothing rises but water. On increasing the heat in an experiment of this kind, the solid substance formed fused; and on cooling the mixture, rhomboidal crystals formed of a pale yellow colour, which were very fusible, and which did not change at the heat at which the compound of oxygen and iodine decomposes, but sublimed unaltered. When urged by a much stronger heat, it partially sublimed, and partially decomposed, affording oxygen, iodine, and sulphuric acid.

With hydro-phosphoric, the compound presents phenomena precisely similar, and they form together a solid, yellow, crystalline combination.

With hydro-nitric acid, it yields white crystals in rhomboidal plates, which, at a lower heat than the preceding acid compounds, are resolved into hydronitric acid, oxygen, and iodine. By liquid muriatic acid, the substance is immediately decomposed, and the compound of chlorine and iodine is formed. All these acid compounds redden vegetable blues, taste sour, and dissolve gold and platinum. From these curious researches Sir H. Davy infers, that Gay Lussac's iodic acid is a sulpho-iodic acid, and probably a definite compound. However minute the quantity of sulphuric acid made to act on the iodide of barium may be, a part of it is always employed to form the compound acid; and the residual fluid contains both the compound acid and a certain quantity of the original salt."—*Ure*.

IODIDE. *Iode; Iodure*. A compound of iodine with a metal; as *Iodide of potassium*.

IODINE. (*Iodina;* from ιωδης, a violet colour, so termed from its beautiful colour.) A peculiar or un decompounded principle.

"Iodine was accidentally discovered, in 1812, by De Courtois, a manufacturer of saltpetre at Paris. In his processes for procuring soda from the ashes of seaweeds, he found the metallic vessels much corroded; and, in searching for the cause of the corrosion, he made this important discovery. But for this circumstance, nearly accidental, one of the most curious of substances might have remained for ages unknown, since nature has not distributed it, in either a simple or compound state, through her different kingdoms, but has confined it to what the Roman satirist considers as the most worthless of things, the vile seaweed.

Iodine derived its first illustration from Clement and Desormes. In their memoir, read at a meeting of the Institute, these able chemists described its principal properties. They stated its sp. gr. to be about 4; that it becomes a violet-coloured gas at a temperature below that of boiling water,—whence its name; that it combines with the metals, and with phosphorus and sulphur, and likewise with the alkalies and metallic oxides; that it forms a detonating compound with ammonia; that it is soluble in alkohol, and still more soluble in ether; and that, by its action upon phosphorus and upon hydrogen, a substance having the characters of muriatic acid is formed. In this communication they offered no decided opinion respecting its nature.

In 1813, Sir H. Davy happened to be on a visit to Paris, receiving, amid the political convulsions of France, the tranquil homage due to his genius. 'When Clement showed iodine to me,' says Sir H. Davy, 'he believed that the hydriodic acid was muriatic acid; and Gay Lussac, after his early experiments, made originally with Clement, formed the same opinion, and *maintained* it, when I *first* stated to him my belief, that it was a new and peculiar acid, and that iodine was a substance analogous in its chemical relations to chlorine.'

Iodine has been found in the following seaweeds, the *Algæ aquaticæ* of Linnæus:—

Fucus cartilagineus,	Fucus palmatus,
membranaceus,	filum,
filamentosus,	digitatus,
rubens,	saccharinus,
nodosus,	Ulva umbilicalis,
serratus,	pavonia,
siliquosus,	linza, and in sponge.

It is from the incinerated seaweed, or kelp, that iodine in quantities is to be obtained. Dr. Wollaston first communicated a precise formula for extracting it

Dissolve the soluble part of kelp in water. Concentrate the liquid by evaporation, and separate all the crystals that can be obtained. Pour the remaining liquid into a clean vessel, and mix with it an excess of sulphuric acid. Boil this liquid for some time. Sulphur is precipitated, and muriatic acid driven off. Decant off the clear liquid, and strain it through wool. Put it into a small flask, and mix it with as much black oxide of manganese as we used before of sulphuric acid. Apply to the top of the flask a glass tube, shut at one end. Then heat the mixture in the flask. The iodine sublimes into the glass tube. None can be obtained from sea-water.

Iodine is a solid, of a grayish-black colour and metallic lustre. It is often in scales similar to those of micaceous iron ore, sometimes in rhomboidal plates, very large and very brilliant. It has been obtained in elongated octohedrons, nearly half an inch in length; the axes of which were shown by Dr. Wollaston to be to each other, as the numbers 2, 3, and 4, at least so nearly, that in a body so volatile, it is scarcely possible to detect an error in this estimate, by the reflective goniometer. Its fracture is lamellated, and it is soft and friable to the touch. Its taste is very acrid, though it be very sparingly soluble in water. It is a deadly poison. It gives a deep brown stain to the skin, which soon vanishes by evaporation. In odour, and power of destroying vegetable colours, it resembles very dilute aqueous chlorine. The sp. gr. of iodine at 62½° is 4.948. It dissolves in 7000 parts of water. The solution is of an orange-yellow colour, and in small quantity tinges raw starch of a purple hue.

It melts, according to Gay Lussac, at 227° F., and is volatilized under the common pressure of the atmosphere, at the temperature of 350°. It evaporates pretty quickly at ordinary temperatures. Boiling water aids its sublimation, as is shown in the above process of extraction. The sp. gr. of its violet vapour is 8.678. It is a non-conductor of electricity. When the voltaic chain is interrupted by a small fragment of it, the decomposition of water instantly ceases.

Iodine is incombustible, but with azote it forms a curious detonating compound; and in combining with several bodies, the intensity of mutual action is such as to produce the phenomena of combustion. Its combinations with oxygen and chlorine are described, under iodic and chloriodic acids.

With a view of determining whether it was a simple or compound form of matter, Sir H. Davy exposed it to the action of the highly inflammable metals. When its vapour is passed over potassium heated in a glass tube, inflammation takes place, and the potassium burns slowly with a pale blue light. There was no gas disengaged when the experiment was repeated in a mercurial apparatus. The iodide of potassium is white, fusible at a red heat, and soluble in water. It has a peculiar acrid taste. When acted on by sulphuric acid, it effervesces, and iodine appears. It is evident that in this experiment there had been no decomposition; the result depending merely on the combination of iodine with potassium. By passing the vapour of iodide over dry red-hot potassa, formed from potassium, oxygen is expelled, and the above iodine results. Hence, we see, that at the temperature of ignition, the affinity between iodine and potassium is superior to that of the latter for oxygen. But iodine in its turn is displaced by chlorine, at a moderate heat, and if the latter be in excess, chloriodic acid is formed. Gay Lussac passed vapour of iodine in a red heat over melted subcarbonate of potassa; and he obtained carbonic acid and oxygen gases, in the proportions of two in volume of the first, and one of the second, precisely those which exist in the salt.

The oxide of sodium, and the subcarbonate of soda, are also completely decomposed by iodine. From these experiments it would seem, that this substance ought to disengage oxygen from most of the oxides; but this happens only in a small number of cases. The protoxides of lead and bismuth are the only oxides not reducible by mere heat, with which it exhibited that power. Barytes, strontian, and lime combine with iodine, without giving out oxygen gas, and the oxides of zinc and iron undergo no alteration in this respect. From these facts we must conclude, that the decomposition of the oxides by iodine depends less on the condensed state of the oxygen, than upon the affinity of the metal for iodine. Except barytes, strontian, and lime, no oxide can remain in combination with iodine at a red heat. For a more particular account of some iodides, see *Hydriodic acid;* the compounds of which, in the liquid or moist state, are *hydriodates*, but change, on drying, into *iodides*, in the same way as the muriates become chlorides.

From the proportion of the constituents in hydriodic acid, 15.5 has been deduced as the prime equivalent of iodine.

Iodine forms with sulphur a feeble compound, of a grayish-black colour, radiated like sulphuret of antimony. When it is distilled with water, iodine separates.

Iodine and phosphorus combine with great rapidity at common temperatures, producing heat without light. From the presence of a little moisture, small quantities of hydriodic acid gas are exhaled.

Oxygen expels iodine from both sulphur and phosphorus.

Hydrogen, whether dry or moist, did not seem to have any action on iodine at the ordinary temperature; but if we expose a mixture of hydrogen and iodine to a red heat in a tube, they unite together, and hydriodic acid is produced, which gives a reddish brown colour to water. Sir H. Davy threw the violet-coloured gas upon the flame of hydrogen, when it seemed to support its combustion. He also formed a compound of iodine with hydrogen, by heating to redness the two bodies in a glass tube.

Charcoal has no action upon iodine, either at a high or low temperature. Several of the common metals, on the contrary, as zinc, iron, tin, mercury, attack it readily, even at a low temperature, provided they be in a divided state. Though these combinations take place rapidly, they produce but little heat, and but rarely any light.

The compound of iodine and zinc, or iodide of zinc, is white. It melts readily, and is sublimed in the state of fine, acicular, four-sided prisms. It is very soluble in water, and rapidly deliquesces in the air. It dissolves in water without the evolution of any gas. The solution is slightly acid, and does not crystallize. The alkalies precipitate from it white oxide of zinc; while concentrated sulphuric acid disengages hydriodic acid and iodine, because sulphurous acid is produced. The solution is a hydriodate of oxide of zinc. When iodine and zinc are made to act on each other under water in vessels hermetically sealed, on the application of a slight heat, the water assumes a deep reddish-brown colour, because, as soon as hydriodic acid is produced, it dissolves iodine in abundance. But by degrees the zinc, supposed to be in excess, combines with the whole iodine, and the solution becomes colourless like water.

Iron is acted on by iodine in the same way as zinc; and a brown iodide results, which is fusible at a red heat. It dissolves in water, forming a light green solution, like that of muriate of iron. When the dry iodide was heated, by Sir H. Davy, in a small retort containing pure ammoniacal gas, it combined with the ammonia and formed a compound which volatilized without leaving any oxide.

The iodide of tin is very fusible. When in powder, its colour is a dirty orange-yellow, not unlike that of glass of antimony. When put into a considerable quantity of water, it is completely decomposed. Hydriodic acid is formed, which remains in solution in the water, and the oxide of tin precipitates in white flocculi. If the quantity of water be small, the acid, being more concentrated, retains a portion of oxide of tin and forms a silky orange-coloured salt, which may be almost entirely decomposed by water. Iodine and tin act very well on each other, in water of the temperature of 212°. By employing an excess of tin, we may obtain pure hydriodic acid, or at least an acid containing only traces of the metal. The tin must be in considerable quantity, because the oxide which precipitates on its surface, diminishes very much its action on iodine.

Antimony presents with iodine the same phenomena as tin; so that we might employ either for the preparation of hydriodic acid, if we were not acquainted with preferable methods.

The iodides of lead, copper, bismuth, silver, and mercury, are insoluble in water, while the iodides of the very oxidizable metals are soluble in that liquid. If we mix a hydriodate with the metallic solutions, all the metals which do not decompose water will give precipitates, while those which decompose that liquid will give none. This is at least the case with the above-mentioned metals

There are two iodides of mercury; the one yellow, the other red; both are fusible and volatile. The yellow or prot-iodide, contains one half less iodine than the deut-iodide. The latter when crystallized is a bright crimson. In general, there ought to be for each metal as many iodides as there are oxides and chlorides. All the iodides are decomposed by concentrated sulphuric and nitric acids. The metal is converted into an oxide, and iodine is disengaged. They are likewise decomposed by oxygen at a red heat, if we except the iodides of potassium, sodium, lead, and bismuth. Chlorine likewise separates iodine from all the iodides; but iodine, on the other hand, decomposes most of the sulphurets and phosphurets.

When iodine and oxides act upon each other in contact with water, very different results take place from those above described. The water is decomposed; its hydrogen unites with iodine, to form hydriodic acid; while its oxygen, on the other hand, produces with iodine, iodic acid. All the oxides, however, do not give the same results. We obtain them only with potassa, soda, barytes, strontian, lime, and magnesia. The oxide of zinc, precipitated by ammonia from its solution in sulphuric acid, and well washed, gives no trace of iodate and hydriodate.

From all the above-recited facts, we are warranted in concluding iodine to be *an undecompounded body*. In its specific gravity, lustre, and magnitude of its prime equivalent, it resembles the metals; but in all its chemical agencies, it is analagous to oxygen and chlorine. It is a non-conductor of electricity, and possesses, like these two bodies, the negative electrical energy with regard to metals, inflammable and alkaline substances; and hence, when combined with these substances in aqueous solution, and electrised in the voltaic circuit, it separates at the positive surface. But it has a positive energy with respect to chlorine: for when united to chlorine, in the chloriodic acid, it separates at the negative surface. This likewise corresponds with their relative attractive energy, since chlorine expels iodine from all its combinations. Iodine dissolves in carburet of sulphur, giving, in very minute quantities, a fine amethystine tint to the liquid.

Iodide of mercury has been proposed for a pigment. Orfila swallowed 6 grains of iodine; and was immediately affected with heat, constriction of the throat, nausea, eructation, salivation, and cardialgia. In ten minutes he had copious bilious vomitings, and slight colic pains. His pulse rose from 70 to about 90 beats in a minute. By swallowing large quantities of mucilage, and emollient clysters, he recovered, and felt nothing next day but slight fatigue. About 70 or 80 grains proved a fatal dose to dogs. They usually died on the fourth or fifth day.

Dr. Coindet of Geneva has recommended the use of iodine in the form of tincture, and also hydriodate of potassa or soda, as an efficacious remedy for the cure of glandular swellings, of the goitrous and scrofulous kind. I have found an ointment composed of 1 oz. hog's lard, and 1 drachm of iodide of zinc, a powerful external application in such cases. About a drachm of this ointment should be used in friction on the swelling once or twice a-day."—*Ure's Chem. Dict.*

[This powerful remedy, which has recently been introduced into practice, is obtained from the plants affording soda, or the vegetables called "Varecks," by the French, or from other species of the algæ or seaweeds. A species furnishing a more considerable portion of iodine than its congeners is the *Fucus saccharinus*, or *Sugar-seaweed*, belonging to the class *Cryptogamia*, order *Algæ*.

In the year 1815, Dr. Mitchill received from Mr. G. De Claubry, of Paris, his researches upon this subject. His particular objects were to find whether iodine existed in ocean-water, and the condition and manner of its evolution from the vegetables that furnished the soda or salt of Varecks. He ascribes the discovery of this substance to Messrs. Macquer and De La Salle, who, in their experiments upon the Varecks or seaweeds, discovered iodine in the mother-water of the soda they afforded. This fact he deemed sufficiently important to encourage chemists to look for it in the vegetables themselves, from which that kind of soda was obtained. He made a journey to the west of Normandy (in France) for the express purpose of examining upon the spot the different species of Fucus; and he obtained from the able botanist of Caen, various kinds of these marine plants, which he submitted to experiment. His analyses were chiefly made upon the following sorts, viz.

I. Of the Family of the Ulvæ.
- 1. The Ulva saccharina.
- 2. .. digitata.
- 3. The Fucus saccharinus, } of Linnæus
- 4. .. digitatus, } of Linnæus

II. Of the Family of the Varecks.
- 1. The Fucus vesiculosus.
- 2. .. serratus.
- 3. .. siliquosus.

III. Of the Family of the Ceramium.
- 1. The Ceramium filum, or the Fucus filum, of Linnæus.

Such and other seaweeds are gathered on the shores of the ocean, among other purposes, for that of being burned to ashes, for the preparation of the fixed alkali, called *the soda or salt of Varecks* by the French and Dutch, as distinguished from the soda or barilla, made by burning the maritime plant called salsola. The product of the above-mentioned seaweeds is a complicated mixture of things, such as,

1. A small quantity of the subcarbonate of soda.
2. A good deal of the hydro-chlorate of soda.
3. .. sulphate of soda.
4. Sulphate of magnesia.
5. Hydro-chlorate of potash and magnesia
6. Subcarbonate of potash.
7. A little sulphuretted sulphate of soda, and
8. A minute portion of the hydro-iodate of potash.

The poverty of this sort of soda gives it but little value in commerce, its chief consumption being in the glass manufactures. It is called *kelp*, and contains much less soda than *barilla*.

It was in the mother waters of the leys or lixiviums of kelp that iodine was first discovered, as is said by Mr. Courtois. All the foregoing products were consequent upon the preceding incineration of the fuci. As a number of these fuci are employed in their recent state as human food, (as is the fucus edulis) the several sorts acquired an interest corresponding to their usefulness, as applicable for manure, for making kelp or iodine, or for food.

On burning the fucus saccharinus, one of the results of a most elaborate and complicated analysis of the residue, was that potash was associated with *iodine* in the form of a *hydro-iodate*, the *hydro-iodate of potash*. As a general remark, he says, that the species of fuci which contain the most mucilage, contain more iodine than the others, by a large difference.

This analysis of ocean or sea-water, proved that it contained no iodine; therefore it may be fairly concluded, that the peculiar article under consideration, is prepared, or elaborated, by the living economy of these marine vegetables. Of the fuci he analyzed, the fucus saccharinus which contained more of it than the other species. This species, treated with sulphuric acid, yielded immediately the iodine it contained, without the process of burning to ashes. This saves the trouble of resorting to the *eau mere*, or mother water, to obtain it. The iodine has an affinity to oxygen, and under convenient circumstances, forms the *hydro-iodic acid*.

Iodine is particularly acted upon by starch, and other vegetable feculæ, whereby it acquires, in the cool and dry way by trituration, a violet colour, passing into blue and black, according to the relative proportions of the iodine and starch employed. The hue is *reddish* if the starch predominates; a *superb blue*, if the ingredients are duly apportioned; and *black*, if the iodine is in excess; as also *violets of different shades*, between the reds and blues. By a particular process, iodine may be obtained *white*. This is shown in the memoir of Messrs. Colin and Claubry, on the combination of iodine with vegetable and animal substances, as contained in the Annals of Chemistry for 1814.

It has lately been discovered, that *iodine existed in small quantity*, with a portion of carbon, and of the other muriate and carbonate of soda, in the officinal preparation called *burnt sponge*, or *pulvis spongiæ ustæ*.

The sponges are in modern zoology, classed among

the zoophytes. They are marine productions, of a fibrous and tough constitution, covered with a slimy matter, in which it has not yet been possible to discover either polypes, or other moveable parts, nor any decided proofs of animality. It seems, nevertheless, that living sponges evince a kind of shrinking, or contraction, on being touched, and that there is a sort of palpitation in the pores with which the body of the sponge is pierced.

From such feeble evidence of the animal nature of the sponge, it has been doubted by some naturalists, whether they ought to be referred to the animal kingdom. By others they have been roundly pronounced to be vegetables. Dr. Mitchill's opinion is, that from the analysis of sponge, the proximity of the results to those of varecks and other seaweeds, and more especially the detection and presence of iodine, is in favour of the vegetable character of sponge.

Burnt sponge was admitted into the Edinburgh New Dispensatory, for the first time, in 1786, by reason of the reputation it had acquired as a remedy for scrofulous and cutaneous diseases, for removing obstructions in the glands, and among others, for lessening and removing the bronchocele. There the process for reducing it to ashes is detailed. The dose is a scruple several times a-day.

Now, since the discovery of iodine in the ashes of sponge, modern physicians have ascribed the chief virtue, against the aforesaid disorders, to this ingredient. The conjecture is a rational one; for it is more probable its efficacy proceeds from the iodine than from the charcoal and neutral salts.

Upon the faith of this interpretation, it was conceived better to prescribe the iodine by itself, or in known and exact combination, than in form of burnt sponge, and as sponge contained this active principle, it was naturally concluded, that the iodine would be in all respects as good when prepared from the seawrecks as from sponges.

In that ugly and obstinate disorder, the goitre, Dr. Coindet, of Geneva, (in Switzerland,) has prescribed iodine with remarkable success. The preparation he employs requires explanation, by reason of its chemical intricacy. To understand the receipt we must recapitulate. The forms of iodine are,

1. Simple iodine. 2. Oxide of iodine, by starch or other feculæ. 3. Iodic-acid. 4. Hydro-iodic acid. 5. Hydro-iodate of potash, by burning, &c.

Dr. Coindet prescribes what is termed "*Ioduretted hydro-iodate of potash.*" To prepare this the hydro-iodic acid must first be procured, which is done thus: Take of alkoholic spirit, pure iodine, any quantities. Then pass sulphuretted hydrogen through the solution. This forms the *hydro-iodic acid.* The next process is, to take potash and hydro-iodic acid, and combine them to saturation. This forms Dr. Coindet's medicine. The *hydro-iodate of potash.*—To reduce this into a form for medicinal prescription, he proceeds as follows: Take of the hydro-iodate of potash, grs. 36. Pure iodine, grs. 10. Distilled water, ℥j. m.

This is the *ioduretted hydro-iodate of potash.* It is so active a preparation, that a full dose is from 5 to 10 drops three times a-day in syrup. The dose may be gradually increased, according to circumstances, but with great caution, to the extent of 20 drops. It must be remembered, whenever it is administered, an overdose must be avoided, as it acts with an extreme and dangerous effect upon the constitution.

They say, that after a few weeks' skilful administration, the external swelling will gradually disappear. Should the patient, while under a course of it, experience any considerable quickening of the pulse, a rapid loss of flesh, palpitation of the heart, a dry cough, restlessness, and want of sleep, and in certain cases with an increase of appetite for food, though the swelling shall undergo diminution, it will be necessary to intermit the medicine for some days; and afterward resume the use of it when the health and safety of the patient will permit.—*Notes from Mitchill's Lects. on Mat. Med.* A.]

IODO-SULPHURIC ACID. "When sulphuric acid is poured, drop by drop, into a concentrated and hot aqueous solution of iodic acid, there immediately results a precipitate of iodo-sulphuric acid, possessed of peculiar properties. Exposed gradually to the action of a gentle heat, the iodo-sulphuric acid melts, and crystallizes on cooling into rhomboids of a pale yellow colour. When strongly heated, it sublimes, and is partially decomposed; the latter portion being converted into oxygen, iodine, and sulphuric acid.

Phosphoric and nitric acids exhibit similar phenomena. These compound acids act with great energy on the metals. They dissolve gold and platinum."

IOLITE. Dichroite. Prismato-rhomboidal quartz of Mohs. This is of a colour intermediate between black, blue, and violet-blue. When viewed in the direction of the axis of the crystals, the colour is dark indigo-blue; but perpendicular to the axis of the crystals, pale brownish-yellow. It comes from Finland.

I'ONIS. (From ιον a violet.) A carbuncle of a violet colour.

IO'NTHUS. (From ιον, a violet, and ανθος, a flower.) A pimple in the face, of a violet colour.

IOTACI'SMUS. (From ιωτα, the Greek letter ι.) A defect in the tongue or organs of speech, which renders a person incapable of pronouncing his letters.

IPECACUA'NHA. (An Indian word.) See *Callicocca ipecacuanha.*

[IPECACUANHA SPURGE. See *Euphorbia ipecacuanha.* A.]

IPOMŒA. (So called by Linnæus from ιψ, which he unaccountably mistakes for the convolvulus plant, whereas it means a creeping sort of worm that infests and corrodes vines, and ομοιος, like. By this appellation he evidently intended to express the close resemblance of *Ipomœa* to the genus *Convolvulus,* with which it agrees in habit altogether.) The name of a genus of plants in the Linnæan system. Class, *Pentandria;* Order, *Monogynia.*

IPOMŒA QUAMOCLIT. *Batata peregrina.* The cathartic potato. If about two ounces are eaten at bedtime, they gently open the bowels by morning.

IQUETA'IA. The inhabitants of the Brazils give this name to the *Scrophularia aquatica,* which is there celebrated as a corrector of the ill flavour of senna.

IRACU'NDUS. (From *ira,* anger: so called because it forms the angry look.) A muscle of the eye.

IRIDIUM. A metal found with another, called osmium, in the black powder left after dissolving platinum. See *Platinum.*

I'RIS. (A rainbow: so called because of the variety of its colours.) 1. The anterior portion of the continuation of the choroid membrane of the eye, which is perforated in the middle by the pupil. It is of various colours. The posterior surface of the iris is termed the *uvea.* See *Choroid membrane.*

2. The *flower-de-luce,* from the resemblance of its flowers to the rainbow.

3. The name of a genus of plants in the Linnæan system. Class, *Triandria;* Order, *Monogynia.*

IRIS FLORENTINA. Florentine orris, or iris. The root of this plant, *Iris—corollis barbatis, caule foliis altiore subbifloro, floribus sessilibus,* of Linnæus, which is indigenous to Italy, in its recent state is extremely acrid, and, when chewed, excites a pungent heat in the mouth, that continues several hours: on being dried, this acrimony is almost wholly dissipated; the taste is slightly bitter, and the smell agreeable, and approaching to that of violets. The fresh root is cathartic, and for this purpose has been employed in dropsies. It is now chiefly used in its dried state, and ranked as a pectoral and expectorant; and hence has a place in the *trochisci amyli* of the pharmacopœias.

Iris, florentine. See *Iris florentina.*

IRIS GERMANICA. The systematic name of the common iris, or orris, or flower-de-luce. *Iris nostra.* The fresh roots of this plant, *Iris—corollis barbatis, caule foliis altiori multifloro, floribus inferioribus pedunculatis,* of Linnæus, have a strong, disagreeable smell, and an acrid, nauseous taste. They are powerfully cathartic, and are given in dropsical diseases, where such remedies are indicated.

IRIS NOSTRAS. See *Iris germanica.*

IRIS PALUSTRIS. See *Iris pseudacorus.*

IRIS PSEUDACORUS. The systematic name of the yellow water-flag. *Iris palustris; Gladiolus luteus; Acorus vulgaris.* This indigenous plant, *Iris—imberbis, foliis ensiformibus, petalis alternis, stigmatibus minoribus,* is common in marshes, and on the banks of rivers. It formerly had a place in the London Pharmacopœia, under the name of *Gladiolus luteus.* The root is without smell, but has an acrid styptic taste, and its juice, on being snuffed up the nostrils, produces a burning heat in the nose and mouth, accompanied by copious discharge from these organs: hence it is recommended both as an errhine and sialagogue. Given internally, when perfectly dry, its adstringent qualities are such as to cure diarrhœas. The expressed juice is likewise said to be a useful application to serpiginous eruptions and scrofulous tumours.

Irish Slate. See *Lapis Hybernicus.*

IRI'TIS. (*Iritis, idis.* f.; from *iris*, the name of the membrane.) Inflammation of the iris: it produces the symptoms of deep-seated or internal inflammation of the eye. See *Ophthalmia.*

IRON. *Ferrum.* Of all the metals, there is none which is so copiously and so variously dispersed through nature as iron. In animals, in vegetables, and in all parts of the mineral kingdom, we detect its presence. Mineralogists are not agreed with respect to the existence of native iron, though immense masses of it have been discovered, which could not have been the products of art; but there is much in favour of the notion that these specimens have been extracted by subterraneous fire. A mass of native iron, of 1600 pounds weight, was found by Pallas, on the river Denisei, in Siberia; and another mass of 300 pounds was found in Paraguay, of which specimens have been distributed everywhere. A piece of native iron, of two pounds weight, has been also met with at Kamsdorf, in the territories of Neustadt, which is still preserved there. These masses evidently did not originate in the places where they were found.

[Specimens of native iron have been found in several places in America, in situations which give rise to the conjecture, that they were of meteoric origin. One of the largest of these has been deposited by its owner, Colonel Gibs, in the Cabinet of the New-York Lyceum of Natural History. It is an irregular mass, weighing upwards of 3000 lbs. "Its surface, which is covered by a blackish crust, is greatly indented, from which it would appear that this mass had been in a soft state. On removing the crust, the iron, on exposure to moisture, soon becomes oxidated. Sp. gr. 7.400.

"It appears to consist entirely of iron, which possesses a high degree of malleability; experiments have been made without detecting nickel or any other metal. This enormous mass of iron is said to have been found near the Red river, in Louisiana."—*Bruce's Min. Journal.* A.]

There are a vast variety of iron ores: they may, however, be all arranged under the following genera; namely, sulphurets, carburets, oxides, and salts of iron. The sulphurets of iron form the ores called *Pyrites*, of which there are many varieties. Their colour is, in general, a straw-yellow, with a metallic lustre; sometimes brownish, which sort is attracted by the magnet. They are often amorphous, and often also crystallized. Iron, in the state of a carburet, forms the *graphite* of Werner (*plumbago*). This mineral occurs in kidney-form lumps of various sizes. Its colour is a dark iron-gray, or brownish-black; when cut, bluish-gray. It has a metallic lustre. Its texture is fine-grained. It is very brittle. The combination of iron with oxygen is very abundant. The common *magnetic iron-stone*, or *load-stone*, belongs to this class; as does *specular iron ore*, and all the different ores called *hæmatites*, or *blood-stone.* Iron, united to carbonic acid, exists in the *sparry iron ore.* Joined to arsenic acid, it exists in the ores called *arseniate of iron*, and *arseniate of iron and copper.*

[The different varieties of the ores of iron are arranged as follows in Cleaveland's Mineralogy, which is a standard work on the subject in the United States:—

Species 1. Native iron.
.. 2. Arsenical iron.
 a. Argentiferous arsenical iron.
.. 3. Sulphuret of iron. Iron Syrites.
 a. Common sulphuret of iron.
 b. Radiated .. ..
 c. Hepatic .. ..
 Sub-species 1. Magnetic sulphuret of iron.
 .. 2. Arsenical .. ..
.. 4. Magnetic oxide of iron
 a. Native magnet.
 b. Iron sand.
.. 5. Specular oxide of iron.
 Sub-species 1. Micaceous oxide of iron.
.. 6. Red oxide of iron.
 a. Scaly red oxide of iron.
 b. Red hematite.
 c. Compact red oxide of iron.
 d. Ochrey red oxide.
Species 7. Brown oxide of iron.
 a. Scaly red oxide of iron
 b. Hematitic .. ..
 c. Compact .. ..
 d. Ochrey .. ..
.. 8. Argillaceous oxide of iron.
 a. Columnar argillaceous oxide of iron.
 b. Granular .. .. ..
 c. Lenticular .. .. ..
 d. Nodular .. .. ..
 e. Common .. .. ..
 f. Bog ore.
.. 9. Carbonate of iron.
.. 10. Sulphate of iron.
.. 11. Phosphate of iron.
 a. Foliated phosphate of iron.
 b. Earthy .. ..
 c. Green iron earth.
.. 12. Arseniate of iron.
.. 13. Chromate of iron.
 a. Crystallized chromate of iron.
 b. Granular .. ..
 c. Amorphous .. .. A.]

Properties of iron.—Iron is distinguished from every other metal by its magnetical properties. It is attracted by the magnet, and acquires, under various conditions, the property of attracting other iron. Pure iron is of a whitish gray, or rather bluish colour very slightly livid; but when polished, it has a great deal of brilliancy. Its texture is either fibrous, fine-grained, or in dense plates. Its specific gravity varies from 7.6 to 7.8. It is the hardest and most elastic of all the metals. It is extremely ductile, and may therefore be drawn into wire as fine as a human hair; it is also more tenacious than any other metal; and yields with facility to pressure. It is extremely infusible, and when not in contact with the fuel, it cannot be melted by the heat which any furnace can excite; it is, however, softened by heat, still preserving its ductility; and when thus softened, different pieces may be united; this constitutes the valuable property of *welding.* It is very dilatable by heat. It is the only metal which takes fire by the collision of flint. Heated in contain with air it becomes oxidized. If intensely and briskly heated, it takes fire with scintillation, and becomes a black oxide. It combines with carbon, and forms what is called steel. It combines with phosphorus in a direct and an indirect manner, and unites with sulphur readily by fusion. It decomposes water in the cold slowly, but rapidly when ignited. It decomposes most of the metallic oxides. All acids act upon iron. Very concentrated sulphuric acid has little or no effect upon it, but when diluted it oxidizes it rapidly. The nitric acid oxidizes it with great vehemence. Muriate of ammonia is decomposed by it. Nitrate of potassa detonates very vigorously with it. Iron is likewise dissolved by alkaline sulphurets. It is capable of combining with a number of metals. It does not unite with lead or bismuth, and very feebly with mercury. It detonates by percussion with the oxygenated muriates.

Method of obtaining iron.—The general process by which iron is extracted from its ores, is first to roast them by a strong heat, to expel the sulphur, carbonic acid, and other mineralizers which can be separated by heat. The remaining ore, being reduced to small pieces, is mixed with charcoal, or coke; and is then exposed to an intense heat, in a close furnace, excited by bellows; the oxygen then combines with the carbon, forming carbonic acid gas during the process, and the oxide is reduced to its metallic state. There are likewise some fluxes necessary in order to facilitate the separation of the melted metal. The matrix of the iron ore is generally either argillaceous or calcareous, or sometimes a portion of siliceous earth; but whichever of these earths is present, the addition of one or both of the others makes a proper flux. These are therefore added in due proportion, according to the nature of the ores; and this mixture, *in contact with the fuel*, is exposed to a heat sufficient to reduce the oxide to its metallic state.

The metal thus obtained, and called smelted, pig, or cast iron, is far from being pure, always retaining a considerable quantity of carbon and oxygen, as well as several heterogeneous ingredients. According as one or other of these predominates, the property of the metal differs. Where the oxygen is present in a large proportion, the colour of the iron is whitish gray; it is extremely brittle, and its fracture exhibits an appearance of crystallization: where the carbon exceeds, it is of a dark gray, inclining to blue, or black, and is less brittle. The former is the *white*, the latter the *black crude iron of commerce*. The *gray* is intermediate to both. In many of these states, the iron is much more fusible than when pure; hence it can be fused and cast into any form; and when suffered to cool slowly, it crystallizes in octahedra: it is also much more brittle, and cannot therefore be either flattened under the hammer, or by the laminating rollers.

To obtain the iron more pure, or to free it from the carbon with which it is combined in this state, it must be refined by subjecting it to the operations of melting and forging. By the former, in which the metal is kept in fusion for some time, and constantly kneaded and stirred, the carbon and oxygen it contains are partly combined, and the produced carbonic acid gas is expelled: the metal at length becomes viscid and stiff; it is then subjected to the action of a very large hammer, or to the more equal, but less forcible pressure of large rollers, by which the remaining oxide of iron, and other impurities, not consumed by the fusion, are pressed out. The iron is now no longer granular nor crystallized in its texture; it is fibrous, soft, ductile, malleable, and totally infusible. It is termed forged, wrought, or bar iron, and is the metal in a purer state, though far from being absolutely pure.

The compounds of iron are the following:

1. *Oxides*; of which there are two, or perhaps three.

1*st*, The oxide, obtained either by digesting an excess of iron filings in water, by the combustion of iron wire in oxygen, or by adding pure ammonia to solution of green copperas, and drying the precipitate out of contact of air, is of a black colour, becoming white by its union with water, in the hydrate, attractible by the magnet, but more feebly than iron. By a mean of the experiments of several chemists, its composition seems to be,

Iron,	100	77.82	3.5
Oxygen,	28.5	22.18	1.0

2*d*, Deutoxide of Gay Lussac. He forms it by exposing a coil of fine iron wire, placed in an ignited porcelain tube, to a current of steam, as long as any hydrogen comes over. There is no danger, he says, of generating peroxide in this experiment, because iron, once in the state of deutoxide, has no such affinity for oxygen as to enable it to decompose water. It may also, he states, be procured by calcining strongly a mixture of 1 part of iron and 3 parts of the red oxide in a stoneware crucible, to the neck of which a tube is adapted to cut off the contact of air. But this process is less certain than the first, because a portion of peroxide may escape the reaction of the iron. But we may dispense with the trouble of making it, adds Thenard, because it is found abundantly in nature. He refers to this oxide, the crystallized specular iron ore of Elba, Corsica, Dalecarlia, and Sweden. He also classes under this oxide all the magnetic iron ores; and says, that the above-described protoxide does not exist in nature. From the synthesis of this oxide by steam, Gay Lussac has determined its composition to be,

Iron,	100	72.72
Oxygen,	37.5	27.28

3*d*, The red oxide. It may be obtained by igniting the nitrate, or carbonate; by calcining iron in open vessels; or simply by treating the metal with strong nitric acid, then washing and drying the residuum. Colcothar of vitriol, or thorough calcined copperas, may be considered as peroxide of iron. It exists abundantly native in the red iron ores. It seems to be a compound of,

Iron,	100	70 = 4 primes.
Oxygen,	43	30 = 3 primes.

2. *Chlorides* of iron; of which there are two, first examined in detail by Dr. John Davy.

The protochloride may be procured by heating to redness, in a glass tube with a very small orifice, the residue which is obtained by evaporating to dryness the green muriate of iron. It is a fixed substance, requiring a red heat for its fusion. It has a grayish, variegated colour, a metallic splendour, and a lamellar texture.

The deutochloride may be formed by the combustion of iron wire in chlorine gas, or by gently heating the green muriate in a glass tube. It is the volatile compound described by Sir H. Davy in his celebrated Bakerian lecture on oxymuriatic acid. It condenses after sublimation, in the form of small brilliant iridescent plates.

3. For the *iodide* of iron, see *Iodine*.

4. *Sulphurets* of iron; of which, according to Porrett, there are four, though only two are usually described, his protosulphuret and persulphuret.

5. *Carburets* of iron. These compounds form steel, and probably cast-iron; though the latter contains also some other ingredients. The latest practical researches on the constitution of these carburets, are those of Daniel.

6. *Salts of iron*.

1. *Protacetate of iron* forms small prismatic crystals, of a green colour, a sweetish styptic taste.

2. *Peracetate of iron* forms a reddish-brown, uncrystallizable solution, much used by the calico-printers, and prepared by keeping iron turnings, or pieces of old iron, for six months immersed in redistilled pyrolignous acid.

3. *Protarseniate of iron* exists native in crystals, and may be formed in a pulverulent state, by pouring arseniate of ammonia into sulphate of iron.

4. *Perarseniate of iron* may be formed by pouring arseniate of ammonia into peracetate of iron; or by boiling nitric acid on the protarseniate. It is insoluble.

5. *Antimoniate of iron* is white, becoming yellow insoluble.

6. *Borate*, pale yellow, insoluble.
7. *Benzoate*, yellow, do.
8. *Protocarbonate*, greenish, soluble
9. *Percarbonate*, brown, insoluble.
10. *Chromate*, blackish, do.
11. *Protocitrate*, brown crystals, soluble.
12. *Protoferroprussiate*, white, insoluble
13. *Perferroprussiate*, white, do.

This constitutes the beautiful pigment called Prussian blue.

14. *Protogallate*, colourless, soluble.
15. *Pergallate*, purple, insoluble.
16. *Protomuriate*, green crystals, very soluble.
17. *Permuriate*, brown, uncrystallizable, very soluble.
18. *Protonitrate*, pale green, soluble.
19. *Pernitrate*, brown, do.
20. *Protoxalate*, green prisms, do.
21. *Peroxalate*, yellow, scarcely soluble.
22. *Protophosphate*, blue, insoluble.
23. *Perphosphate*, white, do.
24. *Protosuccinate*, brown crystals, soluble.
25. *Persuccinate*, brownish-red, insoluble.
26. *Protosulphate*, green vitriol, or copperas. It is generally formed by exposing native pyrites to air and moisture, when the sulphur and iron both absorb oxygen, and form the salt.
27. *Persulphate*. Of this salt there seems to be four or more varieties, having a ferreous base, which consists, by Porrett, of 4 primes iron + 3 oxygen = 10 in weight, from which their constitution may be learned.

The tartrate and pertartrate of iron may also be formed; or by digesting cream of tartar with water or iron filings, a triple salt may be obtained, formerly called tartarized tincture of Mars.

These salts have the following general characters:—

1. Most of them are soluble in water; those with the protoxide for a base are generally crystallizable; those with the peroxide are generally not; the former are insoluble, the latter soluble in alkohol.

2. Ferroprussiate of potassa throws down a blue precipitate, or one becoming blue in the air.

3. Infusion of galls gives a dark purple precipitate, or one becoming so in the air.

4. Hydrosulphuret of potassa or ammonia gives a black precipitate; but sulphuretted hydrogen merely deprives the solutions of iron of their yellow-brown colour.

5. Phosphate of soda gives a whitish precipitate.

6. Benzoate of ammonia, yellow.

7. Succinate of ammonia, flesh-coloured with the peroxide.

The general medicinal virtues of iron, and the

several preparations of it, are to constringe the fibres, to quicken the circulation, to promote the different secretions in the remoter parts, and at the same time to repress inordinate discharges into the intestinal tube. By the use of chalybeates, the pulse is very sensibly raised, the colour of the face, though before pale, changes to a florid red; the alvine, urinary, and cuticular excretions, are increased.

When given improperly, or to excess, iron produces headache, anxiety, heats the body, and often causes hæmorrhages, or even vomiting, pains in the stomach, spasms, and pains of the bowels.

Iron is given in most cases of debility and relaxation; in passive hæmorrhages; in dyspepsia, hysteria, and chlorosis; in most of the cachexiæ; and it has lately been recommended as a specific in cancer. Where either a preternatural discharge, or suppression of natural secretions, proceeds from a languor, or sluggishness of the fluids, and weakness of the solids, this metal, by increasing the motion of the former and the strength of the latter, will suppress the flux, or remove the suppression; but where the circulation is already too quick, the solids too tense and rigid, where there is any stricture, or spasmodic contraction of the vessels, iron, and all the preparations of it, will aggravate both diseases. Iron probably has no action on the body when taken into the stomach, unless it be oxidized. But during its oxidizement, hydrogen gas is evolved, and accordingly we find that fœtid eructations and black fæces are considered as proofs of the medicine having taken effect. It can only be exhibited internally in the state of filings, which may be given in doses from five to twenty grains. Iron wire is to be preferred for pharmaceutical preparations, both because it is the most convenient form, and because it is the purest iron.

The medicinal preparations of iron now in use are:—

1. Subcarbonas ferri. See *Ferri subcarbonas.*
2. Sulphas ferri. See *Ferri sulphas.*
3. Ferrum tartarizatum. See *Ferrum tartarizatum.*
4. Liquor ferri alkalini. See *Ferri alkalini liquor.*
5. Tinctura acetatis ferri. See *Tinctura ferri acetatis.*
6. Tinctura muriatis ferri. See *Tinctura ferri muriatis.*
7. Tinctura ferri ammoniati. See *Tinctura ferri ammoniati.*
8. Vinum ferri. See *Vinum ferri.*
9. Ferrum ammoniatum. See *Ferrum ammoniatum.*
10. Oxidum ferri rubrum. See *Oxidum ferri rubrum.*
11. Oxidum ferri nigrum. See *Oxidum ferri nigrum.*

IRON-FLINT. This occurs in veins of ironstone, and in trap-rocks, near Bristol, and in many parts of Germany.

IRRITABILITY. (*Irritabilitas*; from *irrito*, to provoke.) *Vis insita* of Haller. *Vis vitalis* of Goerter. Oscillation of Boerhaave. Tonic power of Stahl. Muscular power of Bell. Inherent power of Cullen. The contractility of muscular fibres, or a property *peculiar* to muscles, by which they contract upon the application of certain stimuli, without a consciousness of action. This power may be seen in the tremulous contraction of muscles when lacerated, or when entirely separated from the body in operations. Even when the body is dead to all appearance, and the nervous power is gone, this contractile power remains till the organization yields, and begins to be dissolved. It is by this inherent power that a cut muscle contracts, and leaves a gap; that a cut artery shrinks and grows stiff after death. This irritability of muscles is so far independent of nerves, and so little connected with feeling, which is the province of the nerves, that, upon stimulating any muscle by touching it with caustic, or irritating it with a sharp point, or driving the electric spark through it, or exciting with the metallic conductors, as those of silver, or zinc, the muscle instantly contracts, although the nerve of that muscle be tied; although the nerve be cut so as to separate the muscle entirely from all connexion with the system; although the muscle be separated from the body; although the creature upon which the experiment is performed may have lost all sense of feeling, and have been long apparently dead. Thus a muscle, cut from the limb, trembles and palpitates a long time after; the heart, separated from the body, contracts when irritated; the bowels, when torn from the body, continue their peristaltic motion, so as to roll upon the table, ceasing to answer to stimuli only when they become stiff and cold; and too often, in the human body the vis insita loses the exciting power of the nerves, and then palsy ensues; or, losing all governance of the nerves, the vis insita, acting without the regulating power, falls into partial or general convulsions. Even in vegetables, as in the sensitive plant, this contractile power lives. Thence comes the distinction between the irritability of muscles and the sensibility of nerves: for the *irritability* of muscles survives the animals, as when it is active after death; survives the life of the part, or the feelings of the whole system, as in universal palsy, where the vital motions continue entire and perfect, and where the muscles, though not obedient to the will, are subject to irregular and violent actions; and it survives the connexion with the rest of the system, as when animals, very tenacious of life, are cut into parts: but *sensibility*, the property of the nerves, gives the various modifications of sense, as vision, hearing, and the rest; gives also the general sense of pleasure or pain, and makes the system, according to its various conditions, feel vigorous and healthy, or weary and low. And thus the eye feels, and the skin feels: but their appointed stimuli produce no emotions in these parts; they are sensible, but not irritable. The heart, the intestines, the urinary bladder, and all the muscles of voluntary motion, answer to stimuli with a quick and forcible contraction; and yet they hardly feel the stimuli by which these contractions are produced, or, at least, they do not convey that feeling to the brain. There is no consciousness of present stimulus in those parts which are called into action by the impulse of the nerves, and at the command of the will: so that muscular parts have all the irritability of the system, with but little feeling, and that little owing to the nerves which enter into their substance; while nerves have all the sensibility of the system, but no motion.

The discovery of this singular property belongs to our countryman Glisson; but Baron Haller must be considered as the first who clearly pointed out its existence, and proved it to be the cause of muscular motion.

The laws of irritability, according to Dr. Crichton, are, 1. After every action in an irritable part, a state of rest, or cessation from motion, must take place before the irritable part can be again incited to action. If, by an act of volition, we throw any of our muscles into action, that action can only be continued for a certain space of time; the muscle becomes relaxed, notwithstanding all our endeavours to the contrary, and remains a certain time in that relaxed state, before it can be again thrown into action. 2. Each irritable part has a certain portion or quantity of the principle of irritability which is natural to it, part of which it loses during action, or from the application of stimuli. 3. By a process wholly unknown to us, it regains this lost quantity, during its repose, or state of rest. In order to express the different quantities of irritability in any part, we say that it is either more or less redundant, or more or less defective. It becomes redundant in a part when the stimuli which are calculated to act on that part are withdrawn, or withheld for a certain length of time, because then no action can take place: while, on the other hand, the application of stimuli causes it to be exhausted, or to be deficient, not only by exciting action, but by some secret influence, the nature of which has not yet been detected; for it is a circumstance extremely deserving of attention, that an irritable part, or body, may be suddenly deprived of its irritability by powerful stimuli, and yet no apparent muscular or vascular action takes place at the time. A certain quantity of spirits, taken at once into the stomach, kills almost as instantaneously as lightning does: the same thing may be observed of some poisons, as opium, distilled laurel-water, the juice of the cerbera ahovai, &c. 4. Each irritable part has stimuli which are peculiar to it, and which are intended to support its natural action: thus, blood, which is the stimulus proper to the heart, and arteries, if, by any accident, it gets into the stomach, produces sickness, or vomiting. If the gall, which is the natural stimulus to the ducts of the liver, the gall-bladder, and the intestines, is by any accident effused into the ca-sity of the peritonæum, it excites too great action of the vessels of that part, and induces inflammation. The urine does not irritate the tender fabric of the kidneys, ureters, or bladder, except in such a degree as to preserve their healthy action; but if it be effused into the cellular membrane, it brings on such a violent action of the vessels of these parts, as to produce gangrene. Such stimuli are called *habitual* stimuli of parts 5. Each irritable part differs from the rest in regard to the quantity of irritability which it possesses. This law explains to us the reason of the great diversity which we observe in the action of various irritable parts; thus, the muscles of voluntary motion can remain a long time in a state of action, and if it be continued as long as possible, another considerable portion of time is required before they regain the irritability they lost; but the heart and arteries have a more short and sudden action, and their state of rest is equally so. The circular muscles of the intestines have also a quick action and short rest. The urinary bladder does not fully regain the irritability it loses during its contraction for a considerable space of time; the vessels which separate and throw out the menstrual discharge, act, in general, for three or four days, and do not regain the irritability they lose for a lunar month. 6. All stimuli produce action in proportion to their irritating powers. As a person approaches his hand to the fire, the action of all the vessels in the skin is increased, and it glows with heat; if the hand be approached still nearer, the action is increased to such an unusual degree as to occasion redness and pain; and if it be continued too long, real inflammation takes place; but if this heat be continued, the part at last loses its irritability, and a sphacelus or gangrene ensues. 7. The action of every stimulus is in an inverse ratio to the frequency of its application. A small quantity of spirits taken into the stomach, increases the action of its muscular coat, and also of its various vessels, so that digestion is thereby facilitated. If the same quantity, however, be taken frequently, it loses its effect. In order to produce the same effect as at first, a larger quantity is necessary; and hence the origin of dram-drinking. 8. The more the irritability of a part is accumulated, the more that part is disposed to be acted upon. It is on this account that the activity of all animals, while in perfect health, is much livelier in the morning than at any other part of the day; for, during the night, the irritability of the whole frame, and especially that of the muscles destined for labour, viz. the muscles for voluntary action, is reaccumulated. The same law explains why digestion goes on more rapidly the first hour after food is swallowed than at any other time; and it also accounts for the great danger that accrues to a famished person upon first taking in food. 9. If the stimuli which keep up the action of any irritable body be withdrawn for too great a length of time, that process on which the formation of the principle depends is gradually diminished, and at last entirely destroyed. When the irritability of the system is too quickly exhausted by heat, as is the case in certain warm climates, the application of cold invigorates the frame, because cold is a mere diminution of the overplus of that stimulus which was causing the rapid consumption of the principle. Under such or similar circumstances, therefore, cold is a tonic remedy; but if, in a climate naturally cold, a person were to go into a cold bath, and not soon return into a warmer atmosphere, it would destroy life just in the same manner as many poor people who have no comfortable dwellings are often destroyed, from being too long exposed to the cold in winter. Upon the first application of cold the irritability is accumulated, and the vascular system therefore is exposed to great action; but, after a certain time, all action is so much diminished, that the process, whatever it be, on which the formation of the irritable principle depends, is entirely lost. For further information on this interesting subject, see Dr. Crichton on Mental Derangement.

IRRITA'TION. *Irritatio.* The action produced by any stimulus.

ISA'TIS. (Ισατις of Dioscorides, and *Isatis* of Pliny, the derivation of which is unknown.) The name of a genus of plants in the Linnæan system. Class, *Tetradynamia;* Order, *Siliquosa.*

ISATIS TINCTORIA. *Glastum.* The systematic name of the plant used for dying called woad. It is said to be adstringent.

I'SCA. A sort of fungous excrescence of the oak, or of the hazel, &c. The ancients used it as the moderns used moxa.

ISCHÆ'MON. (From ισχω, to restrain, and αιμα, blood.) A name for any medicine which restrains or stops bleeding.

ISCHÆ'MUM. A species of *Andropogon.*

I'SCHIAS. (Ισχιας; from ισχιον, the hip.) A rheumatic affection of the hip-joint. See *Rheumatismus.*

ISCHIATOCE'LE. (From ισχιον, the hip, and κηλη, a rupture.) *Ischiocele.* An intestinal rupture, through the sciatic ligaments.

ISCHIO-CAVERNOSUS. See *Erector penis.*

ISCHIOCE'LE. See *Ischiatocele.*

I'SCHIUM. (From ισχις, the loin: so named because it is near the loin.) A bone of the pelvis of the fœtus, and a part of the os innominatum of the adult. See *Innominatum os.*

ISCHNOPHO'NIA. (From ισχνος, slender, and φωνη, the voice.) 1. A shrillness of the voice.

2. A hesitation of speech, or a stammering.

ISCHURE'TICA. (From ισχουρια, a suppression of the urine.) Medicines which relieve a suppression of the urine.

ISCHU'RIA. (From ισχω, to restrain, and ουρον, the urine.) A suppression of urine. A genus of disease in the class *Locales*, and order *Epischeses*, of Cullen. There are four species of ischuria:

1. *Ischuria renalis*, coming after a disease of the kidneys, with a troublesome sense of weight or pain in that part.

2. *Ischuria ureterica*, after a disease of the kidneys, with a sense of pain or uneasiness in the course of the ureters.

3. *Ischuria vesicalis*, marked by a frequent desire to make water, with a swelling of the hypogastrium, and pain at the neck of the bladder.

4. *Ischuria urethralis*, marked by a frequent desire to make water, with a swelling of the hypogastrium, and pain of some part of the urethra.

When there is a frequent desire of making water, attended with much difficulty in voiding it, the complaint is called a dysury, or strangury; and when there is a total suppression of urine, it is known by the name of an ischury. Both ischuria and dysuria are distinguished into acute, when arising in consequence of inflammation, and chronic, when proceeding from any other cause, such as calculus, &c.

The causes which give rise to these diseases, are an inflammation of the urethra, occasioned either by venereal sores or by a use of acrid injections, tumour or ulcer of the prostate gland, inflammation of the bladder or kidneys, considerable enlargements of the hæmorrhoidal veins, a lodgment of indurated fæces in the rectum, spasm at the neck of the bladder, the absorption of cantharides applied externally, or taken internally, and excess in drinking either spirituous or vinous liquors; but particles of gravel sticking at the neck of the bladder, or lodging in the urethra, and thereby producing irritation, prove the most frequent cause. Gouty matter falling on the neck of the bladder, will sometimes occasion these complaints.

In dysury there is a frequent inclination to make water, attended with a smarting pain, heat, and difficulty in voiding it, together with a sense of fulness in the region of the bladder. The symptoms often vary, however, according to the cause which has given rise to it. If it proceeds from a calculus in the kidney, or ureter, besides the affections mentioned, it will be accompanied with nausea, vomiting, and acute pains in the loins and regions of the ureter and kidney of the side affected. When a stone in the bladder, or gravel in the urethra, is the cause, an acute pain will be felt at the end of the penis, particularly on voiding the last drops of urine, and the stream of water will either be divided into two, or be discharged in a twisted manner, not unlike a cork-screw. If a scirrhus of the prostate gland has occasioned the suppression or difficulty of urine, a hard indolent tumour, unattended with any acute pain, may readily be felt in the perinæum, or by introducing the finger in ano.

Dysury is seldom attended with much danger, unless, by neglect, it should terminate in a total obstruction. Ischury may always be regarded as a dangerous complaint, when it continues for any length of time, from the great distention and often consequent inflammation which ensue. In those cases where neither a bougie nor a catheter can be introduced, the event in all probability, will be fatal, as few patients will submit to the only other means of drawing off the urine before a considerable degree of inflammation and tendency to gangrene have taken place.

ISERINE. (So called from the river Iser, near the origin of which it is found.) An iron black-coloured ore.

ISINGLASS. See *Ichthyocolla.*

ISO'CHRONOS. (From ισος, equal, and χρονος, time.) Preserving an equal distance of time between the beats; applied to the pulse.

ISO'CRATES. (From ισος, equal, and κεραννυμι, to mix.) Wine mixed with an equal quantity of water.

ISO'DROMUS. (From ισος, equal, and δρομος, a course.) The same as *Isochronos.*

ISOPY'RUM. (From ισος, equal, and πυρ, fire: so named from its flame-coloured flower.) The *Aquilegia vulgaris.*

ISO'TONUS. (From ισος, equal, and τονος, extension.) Applied to fevers which are of equal strength during the whole of the paroxysm.

I'SSUE. *Fonticulus.* An artificial ulcer made by cutting a portion of the skin, and burying a pea or some other substance in it, so as to produce a discharge of purulent matter.

I'STHMION. (From ισθμος, a narrow piece of land between two seas.) The fauces narrow passage between the mouth and gullet.

ISTHMUS VIEUSSENII. The ridge surrounding the remains of the foramen ovale, in the right auricle of the human heart.

ITHMOI'DES. See *Ethmoides.*

ITINERA'RIUM. (From *iter*, a way.) The catheter; also a staff used in cutting for the stone.

ITIS. From the time of Boerhaave, visceral inflammations have been generally distinguished by anatomical terms derived from the organ affected, with the Greek term *itis*, added as a suffix; as *cephalitis*, &c. *Itis* is sufficiently significant of its purpose; it is immediately derived from ιεμαι, which is itself a ramification from εω, and imports, not merely action, "putting or going forth," which is the strict and simple meaning of εω, but action in its fullest urgency, "violent or impetuous action." When this term then is added to the genitive case of the Greek name of an organ, it means inflammation of that viscus: hence, *hepatitis*, *nephritis*, *gastritis*, *carditis*, mean inflammation of the liver, kidney, stomach, heart.—*Good.*

I'VA PECANGA. See *Smilax sarsaparilla.*

IVORY. The tusk, or tooth of defence, of the male elephant. It is an intermediate substance between bone and horn. The dust is occasionally boiled to form jelly, instead of isinglass, for which it is a bad substitute. In 100 parts there are 24 gelatin, 64 phosphate of lime, and 0.1 carbonate of lime.

IVY. See *Hedera helix.*

Ivy, ground. See *Glecoma hederacea.*

Ivy-gum. See *Hedera helix.*

I'XIA. (From ιξος, glue.) 1. A name of the *Carina gummifera*, from its viscous juice.

2. (From ιξομαι, to proceed from.) A preternatural distention of the veins.

IXINE. See *Carlina gummifera.*

J

JA'CEA. (*Quia prodest hominibus tristitia jacentibus;* because it resists sorrow; or from ιαομαι, to heal.) The herb pansey, or heart's-ease. See *Viola tricolor.*

JACERANTA TINGA. See *Acorus calamus.*

JACI'NTHUS. See *Hyacinthus.*

Jack-by-the-hedge. See *Erysimum alliaria.*

JACOBÆ'A. (Named because it was dedicated to St. James, or because it was directed to be gathered about the feast of that saint.) See *Senecio Jacobœa.*

JADE. See *Nephrite.*

Jagged leaf. See *Erosus.*

JALAP. See *Convolvulus jalapa.*

JALA'PA. See *Convolvulus jalapa.*

JALA'PIUM. (From *Chalapa*, or *Xalapa*, in New Spain, whence it is brought.) See *Convolvulus jalapa.*

JALAPPA ALBA. White jalap. See *Convolvulus mecoacan.*

JAMAICA BARK. See *Cinchona caribœa.*

JAMAICA PEPPER. See *Myrtus pimenta.*

JA'MBLICHI SALES. A preparation with sal-ammoniac, some aromatic ingredients, &c. so called from Jamblichus, the inventor.

JA'NITOR. (From *janua*, a gate.) The pylorus, so called from its being, as it were, the door or entrance of the intestines.

Japan earth. See *Acacia catechu.*

JAPO'NICA TERRA. (So called from the place it came from.) See *Acacia catechu.*

JARGON. See *Zircon.*

JA'SMINUM. (*Jasminum;* from *jasmen*, Arab.; or from ιον, a violet, and οσμη, odour, on account of the fine odour of the flowers.) 1. The name of a genus of plants in the Linnæan system. Class, *Diandria;* Order, *Monogynia.*

2. The pharmacopœial name of the jessamine. See *Jasminum officinale.*

JASMINUM OFFICINALE. The systematic name of the jessamine-tree. The flowers of this beautiful plant have a very fragrant smell, and a bitter taste. They afford, by distillation, an essential oil, which is much esteemed in Italy to rub paralytic limbs, and in the cure of rheumatic pains.

JASPER. A sub-species of rhomboidal quartz, according to Jameson, who enumerates five kinds: Egyptian, striped, porcelain, common, agate jasper.

JA'TROPHA. (Most probably from ιατρος, a physician.) The name of a genus of plants in the Linnæan system. Class, *Monœcia;* Order, *Monadelphia.*

JATROPHA CURCAS. The systematic name of a p nt, the seeds of which resemble the castor-oil seeds. *Ricinus major; Ricinoides; Pineus purgans; Pinhones indici; Faba cathartica; Nux cathartica; Americana; Nux barbadensis.* The seed or nut so called in the pharmacopœias is oblong and black, the produce of the *Jatropha—foliis cordatis angulatis* of Linnæus. It affords a quantity of oil, which is given, in many places, as the castor-oil is in this country, to which it is very nearly allied. The seeds of the *Jatropha multifida* are of an oval and triangular shape, of a pale brown colour, are called purging-nuts, and give out a similar oil.

JATROPHA ELASTICA. The juice of this plant affords an elastic gum. See *Caoutchouc.*

JATROPHA MANIHOT. This is the plant which affords the Cassada root. *Cassada; Cacavi; Cassave; Cassava; Pain de Madagascar; Ricinus minor; Maniot; Yucca; Manibar; Aipi; Aipima coxera; Aipipoca; Janipha.* The leaves are boiled, and eaten as we do spinach. The root abounds with a milky juice, and every part, when raw, is a fatal poison. It is remarkable that the poisonous quality is destroyed by heat: hence the juice is boiled with meat, pepper, &c. into a wholesome soup, and what remains after expressing the juice, is formed into cakes or meal, the principal food of the inhabitants. This plant, which is a native of three quarters of the world, is one of the most advantageous gifts of Providence, entering into the composition of innumerable preparations of an economical nature.

Cassada roots yield a great quantity of starch, called tapioca, exported in little lumps by the Brazilians, and now well known to us as a diet for sick and weakly persons.

JEBB, JOHN, was born at London in 1736. He was originally devoted to the church, and after studying at Cambridge, entered into orders, and obtained a living in Norfolk in 1764. The year following, he published in conjunction with two friends, a selection from Newton's Principia, with notes, which was highly esteemed. He soon afterward returned to Cambridge, and engaged warmly as an advocate for a reform in church and state, as well as in the discipline of that university. At length, in 1775, he resigned all his offices in the church, the established doctrines of which he did not approve; and determined upon entering into the Medical profession He soon qualified himself for this, obtained a diploma from St. Andrews, and was admitted a licentiate of the London College of Physicians; and in the same year, 1778, he was elected a fellow of the Royal Society. In 1782 he published "Select Cases of Paralysis of the Lower Extremities;" which tend to support the practice of Pott, of applying caustics near the spine. To this work is added an interesting description of a very rare disease, catalepsy. The warmth of his political sentiments, however, obstructed his professional career; and the various fatigues and anxieties to which he exposed himself, in order to further his benevolent designs, exhausted his constitution so much, that he sunk a premature victim in 1786.

JECORA'RIA. (From *jecur*, the liver: so named from its supposed efficacy in diseases of the liver.) 1. The name of a plant. See *Marchantia polymorpha*.

2. A name given to a vein in the right hand, because it was usually opened in diseases of the liver.

JE'CUR. (*Jecur*, *oris.*, or *jecinoris*, neut.) The liver. See *Liver*.

JECUR UTERINUM. The placenta is, by some, thus called, from the supposed similitude of its office with that of the liver.

JEJU'NUM. (From *jejunus*, empty.) *Jejunum intestinum*. The second portion of the small intestines, so called because it is mostly found empty. See *Intestine*.

JELLY. See *Gelatin*.

JENITE. See *Lievrite*.

Jerusalem cowslips. See *Pulmonaria officinalis*.

Jerusalem oak. See *Chenopodium botrys*.

Jerusalem sage. See *Pulmonaria officinalis*.

JESSAMINE. See *Jasminum*.

JESUITA'NUS CORTEX. (From *jesuita*, a jesuit.) A name of the Peruvian bark, because it was first introduced into Europe by Father de Lugo, a jesuit. See *Cinchona*.

JESUI'TICUS CORTEX. See *Cinchona*.

Jesuit's bark. See *Cinchona*.

JET. (So called from the river *Gaza* in Lesser Asia, from whence it came.) A black bituminous coal, hard and compact, found in great abundance in various parts of France, Sweden, Germany, and Ireland. It is brilliant and vitreous in its fracture, and capable of taking a good polish by friction; it attracts light substances, and appears to be electric like amber; hence it has been called *black amber*. It has no smell, but when heated, it acquires one like bitumen judaicum.

Jew's Pitch. See *Bitumen judaicum*.

JOHN'S WORT. See *Hypericum*.

Jointed Leaf. See *Articulatus*.

["JONES, JOHN, M. D. The family of Dr. Jones was of Welsh extraction, and of the religious society of Friends. He was born in the town of Jamaica, (Long Island,) in Queen's county, New-York, in the year 1729; and received his education partly from his excellent parents, but chiefly at a private school in the city of New-York. He was early led, both by the advice of his father, and his own inclination, to the study of medicine.

Dr. Jones early indicated an attachment for that profession which, at a subsequent period, he cultivated with so much ardour, by his fondness for anatomical researches; and though, as it may be readily supposed, these could only be of the comparative kind, yet it is a remarkable fact, that this love for pursuits of the same nature has been noticed in the youth of some of the most distinguished anatomists that ever lived.

After completing his studies in this country, Dr. Jones visited Europe, in order to improve himself still farther in his profession.

Upon the return of Dr. Jones to this country, he settled in New-York, where his abilities soon procured him extensive practice. To the profession of surgery, in particular, he devoted much attention; he was the first who performed the operation of lithotomy in that city, and succeeded so well in several cases that offered shortly after his return, that his fame as an operator became generally known throughout the middle and eastern states of America.

Upon the institution of a medical school in the college of New-York, Dr. Jones was appointed professor of Surgery, upon which branch he gave several courses of lectures, and thereby diffused a taste for it among the students, and made known the improved methods of practice lately adopted in Europe, with which most of the practitioners in this country were entirely unacquainted.

For a considerable part of the previous life of Dr. Jones, he had been afflicted by the asthma, and for a long time had struggled to overcome that painful disease; but the exertions both of his own skill, and of the rest of his medical brethren in most parts of the continent, had hitherto proved ineffectual even to his relief. He determined, therefore, to take a voyage to Europe, and accordingly sailed for London Here, in a thick smoke and an impure atmosphere, where so many asthmatics have found such remarkable benefit, he also experienced a considerable alleviation of his complaint; and probably the permanent alteration in his health which he afterward enjoyed, may be in some measure attributed to the effects of his residence in London. He also employed himself during his continuance in the metropolis, in collecting subscriptions for an hospital in New-York, which he had been chiefly instrumental in establishing.

In London he again had an opportunity of seeing his friend, Mr. Pott, at the head of his profession, and of renewing that intercourse which had been previously commenced between them. He had now been for some years left to the guidance of his own judgment; but unlike many who suppose all knowledge to become stationary at the time of their leaving college, he was still willing to be taught by those who had formerly been his instructers, and who, from the great opportunities they enjoyed, would be enabled to afford him much information. Eager for the acquisition of knowledge, whenever and wherever it could be obtained, he again attended the lectures of his old master, Dr. Hunter, and those of his friend, Mr. Pott, who lost no opportunity of showing the consistency between his profession and proofs of respect: during his short stay there, he paid Dr. Jones the most particular attention, and presented him with a complete copy of his lectures, just before his departure from London. His kindness, however, did not end here; for in the frequent applications which he received for advice from all parts of this country, in difficult and important cases, he never failed to recommend his old pupil, as capable of affording any relief to be derived from surgical assistance. In consequence of this, his attendance was frequently desired in the different states; and while he showed, by his skill and success, that the opinion which had been formed of him was just, his fame became thereby diffused throughout the continent of America.

The following year he returned to his native country, the political situation of which, at that time, called loudly for the exertions of all her citizens. He again resumed his lectures, and delivered several courses, and in the autumn of the next year, 1775, published his "Plain Remarks upon Wounds and Fractures," which he inscribed to his old preceptor, Dr. Cadwallader, in a neat dedication. A work of this kind which would give the young practitioner clear notions of the improved mode of treating disease, without embarrassing him with refined speculations or useless disquisitions, was much wanted. He attempted no systematic arrangements, but simply treated of those subjects to which the attention of the surgeons of the army and navy would be most continually directed. No present could have been more acceptable to his country, and no gift more opportunely made; for in the situation of American affairs, many persons were chosen to act as surgeons, who, from their few opportunities, and their ignorance of the improvements that had lately been brought in practice, were but ill qualified for the office. His well-meant endeavours were not lost; for the improvements which he had made known, though new to most practitioners and surgeons, were readily adopted when recommended by such authority. This was the only work ever published by Dr. Jones; it might have, indeed, been readily supposed, that more would have come from his pen, considering how well qualified he was to make observations, and impart to others some portion of that knowledge of which he himself possessed so great a share. Such was actually his intention; and he had prepared another work for the press, but was prevented by the most base treachery from giving it to the world.

He died 1791, in the 63d year of his age. As a *Surgeon*, Dr. Jones stood at the head of the profession in this country; and he may be deservedly considered as the chief instrument in effecting the remarkable revolution in that branch of the healing art, which is now so apparent, by laying aside the former complicated modes of practice, and substituting those which are plain and simple. The operation to which he principally confined himself for many of the last years of his life, was lithotomy; and his success in this difficult and important object of a surgeon's duty, was great indeed. Even in the month before his death, in a most capital and nice operation, there did not appear to be any diminution of that dexterity and steadiness of hand, for which he had always been remarkable, and of which those not half his age might have boasted.

Connected with this part of his professional character, was his merit as an accoucheur; and in this difficult and important branch his success was great.

The merit of Dr. Jones as a physician was likewise considerable. Though educated in the school of Boerhaave, he never professed an implicit faith in that, or any other system. He was guided by just principles, and he varied his practice like every judicious physician, with the varying circumstances of the case. The success of his practice was the best proof of the truth of his principles, and of the judgment which directed their application."—*Thach. Med. Biog.* A.]

["JONES, WALTER, M. D., one of the most eminent physicians of our country, was born in Virginia, and received his medical education at the University of Edinburgh, where he was graduated about the year 1770. While at this institution he became a favourite of the school, and enjoyed the particular friendship and esteem of Cullen, and the other professors of that time.

On his return to his native country, he settled in Northumberland county, Virginia, where he acquired an extensive practice, and sustained throughout life the highest standing both as a scholar and physician. 'He was,' (says a distinguished gentleman, who for some time enjoyed his acquaintance,) 'for the variety and extent of his learning, the originality and strength of his mind, the sagacity of his observations, and the captivating powers of his conversation, one of the most extraordinary men I have ever known. He was an accurate observer of nature and of human character; and seemed to possess intuitively the faculty of discerning the hidden cause of disease, and of applying, with a promptness and decision peculiar to himself, the appropriate remedies.' For a few years he was returned a member of the national legislature; but he spent the most of his life in the practice of that profession of which he was a distinguished ornament."—*Thach. Med. Biog.* A.]

JUDGMENT. The judgment is the most important of the intellectual faculties. We acquire all our knowledge by this faculty; without it our life would be merely vegetative; we would have no idea either of the existence of other bodies, or of our own; for these two sorts of notions, like our knowledge, are the consequence of our faculty of judging.

To judge is to establish a relation between two ideas, or between two groups of ideas. When I judge of the goodness of a work, I feel that the idea of goodness belongs to the book which I have read; I establish a relation, I form to myself an idea of a different kind from that which arises from sensibility and memory.

A continuation of judgments linked together form an inference, or process of reasoning.

We see how important it is to judge justly, that is, to establish only those relations which really exist. If I judge that a poisonous substance is salutary, I am in danger of losing my life; my false judgment is therefore hurtful. It is the same with all those of the same kind. Almost all the misfortunes which oppress man in a moral sense, arise from errors of judgment; crimes, vices, bad conduct, spring from false judgment.

The science of logic has for its end the teaching of just reasoning: but pure judgment, or good sense, and false judgment, or *wrong-headedness*, depend on organization. We cannot change in this respect; we must remain as nature has made us. There are men endowed with the precious gift of finding relations of things which have never been perceived before. If these relations are very important, and beneficial to humanity, the authors are men of genius: if the relations are of less importance, they are considered men of wit, imagination. Men differ principally by their manner of feeling different relations, or of judging. The judgment seems to be injured by an extreme vivacity of sensations; hence we see that faculty become more perfect with age.—*Magendie's Physiology*

JUDICATO'RIUS. (From *judico*, to discern.) An obsolete term applied to a synocha of four days, because its termination may certainly be foreseen.

JUGA'LE OS. (*Jugalis*; from *jugum*, a yoke: from its resemblance, or because it is articulated, to the bone of the upper jaw, like a yoke.) *Os malæ; Os zygomaticum.* The ossa malarum are the prominent square bones which form the upper part of the cheeks. They are situated close under the eyes, and make part of the orbit. Each of these bones have three surfaces to be considered. One of these is exterior and somewhat convex. The second is superior and concave, serving to form the lower and lateral parts of the orbit. The third, which is posterior, is very unequal and concave, for the lodgment of the lower part of the temporal muscle. Each of these bones may be described as having four processes formed by their four angles. Two of these may be called *orbitar* processes. The superior one is connected with the orbitar process of the os frontis; and the inferior one with the malar process of the maxillary bone. The third is connected with the temporal process of the sphenoid bone; and the fourth forms a bony arch, by its connexion with the zygomatic process of the temporal bone. In infants, these bones are entire and completely ossified.

JU'GLANS. (*Quasi Jovis glans*, the royal fruit, from its magnitude.) 1. The name of a genus of plants in the Linnæan system. Class, *Monœcia;* Order, *Polyandria.* The walnut-tree.

2. The pharmacopœial name of the walnut. See *Juglans regia.*

JUGLANS REGIA. The systematic name of the walnut-tree. The tree which bears the walnut is the *Juglans—foliolis ovalibus glabris subserratis subæqualibus* of Linnæus. It is a native of Persia, but cultivated in this country. The unripe fruit, which has an astringent bitterish taste, and has been long employed as a pickle, is the part which was directed for medical use by the London College, on account of its athelmintic virtues. An extract of the green fruit is the most convenient preparation, as it may be kept for a sufficient length of time, and made agreeable to the stomach of the patient, by mixing it with cinnamon water.

The *putamen*, or green rind of the walnut, has been celebrated as a powerful anti-venereal remedy, for more than a century and a half; and Petrus Borellus has given directions for a decoction not unlike that which is commonly called the Lisbon diet-drink, in which the walnut, with its green bark, forms a principal ingredient. Ramazzini, whose works were published early in the present century, has likewise informed us, that in his time, the green rind of the walnut was esteemed a good anti-vinereal remedy in England. This part of the walnut has been much used in decoctions, during the last fifty years, both in the green and dried state; it has been greatly recommended by writers on the continent, as well as by those of our own country; and is, without doubt, a very useful addition to the decoction of the woods. Pearson has employed it during many years, in those cases where pains in the limbs and indurations of the membranes have remained, after the venereal disease has been cured by mercury; and he informs us that he has seldom directed it without manifest advantage.

Brambilla and Girtanner also contend for the anti venereal virtues of the green bark of the walnut: but the result of Pearson's experience will not permit him to add his testimony to theirs. I have given it, says he, in as large doses as the stomach could retain, and for as long a time as the strength of the patients, and the nature of their complaints would permit; but I have uniformly observed, that if they who take it be not previously cured of *lues venerea*, the peculiar symptoms will appear, and proceed in their usual course, in defiance of the powers of this medicine. The *Decoctum Lusitanicum* may be given with great advantage in many of those cutaneous diseases, which are attended with aridity of the skin; and I have had some opportunities of observing that when the putamen of the walnut has been omitted, either intentionally or by accident, the same good effects have not followed the taking of the decoction, as when it contained this ingredient. See *Juglans*.

JUGULAR. (*Jugularis;* from *jugulum*, the throat.) Belonging to the throat.

JUGULAR VEINS. The veins so called run from the head down the sides of the neck, and are divided, from their situation, into external and internal. The *external, or superficial jugular vein*, receives the blood from the frontal, angular, temporal, auricular, sublingual or ranine, and occipital veins. The *internal*, or *deep-seated jugular vein*, receives the blood from the lateral sinuses of the dura mater, the laryngeal and pharyngeal veins. Both jugulars unite, and form, with the subclavian vein, the superior vena cava, which terminates in the superior part of the right auricle of the heart.

JU'GULUM. (From *jugum*, a yoke; because the yoke is fastened to this part.) The throat or anterior part of the neck.

JUJUBA. (An Arabian word.) Jujube. See *Rhamnus zizyphus*.

JU'JUBE. See *Rhamnus zizyphus*.

JULY-FLOWER. See *Dianthus Caryophyllus*.

JUNCKER, GOTTLOB JOHN, was born in 1680 at Londorff, in Hesse. After the proper studies he graduated at Halle in 1718; and became afterward a distinguished professor there, as well as physician to the public hospital. His works, which are chiefly compilations, have been much esteemed, and are still occasionally referred to; especially as giving a compendious view of the doctrines of Stahl, which he espoused and taught. He has given a "Conspectus" of medicine, of surgery, of chemistry, and of several other departments of professional knowledge; also many academical theses on medical, chirurgical, and philosophical subjects. He died in 1752.

JU'NCUS. (An old Latin word, a *jungendo*, say the etymologists, from the use of the plants which bear this name in joining or binding things together.) The name of a genus of plants in the Linnæan system. Class, *Hexandria;* Order, *Monogynia*.

JUNCUS ODORATUS. See *Andropogon schænanthus*.

JUNIPER. See *Juniperus communis*.

Juniper gum. See *Juniperus communis*.

JUNI'PERUS. (From *juvenis*, young, and *pario*, to bring forth: so called because it produces its young berries while the old ones are ripening.) 1. The name of a genus of plants. Class, *Diœcia;* Order, *Monodelphia*.

2. The pharmacopœial name of the common juniper. See *Juniperus communis*.

JUNIPERUS COMMUNIS. The systematic name of the juniper-tree. *Juniperus—foliis ternis patentibus mucronatis, baccis longioribus*, of Linnæus. Both the tops and berries of this indigenous plant are directed in our pharmacopœias, but the latter are usually preferred, and are brought chiefly from Holland and Italy. Of their efficacy as a stomachic, carminative, diaphoretic, and diuretic, there are several relations by physicians of great authority: and medical writers have also spoken of the utility of the juniper in nephritic cases, uterine obstructions, scorbutic affections, and some cutaneous diseases. Our pharmacopœias direct the essential oil, and a spirituous distillation of the berries, to be kept in the shops. From this tree is also obtained a concrete resin, which has been called sandarach, or gum juniper. It exudes in white tears, more transparent than mastich. It is almost totally soluble in alkohol, with which it forms a white varnish that dries speedily. Reduced to powder it is called *pounce*, which prevents ink from sinking into paper from which the exterior coating of size has been scraped away.

JUNIPERUS LYCIA. The systematic name of the plant which affords the true frankincense. *Olibanum; Thus.* Frankincense has received different appellations, according to its different appearances; the single tears are called simply *olibanum*, or *thus;* when two are joined together, *thus masculum;* and when two are very large, *thus femininum;* if several adhere to the bark, *thus corticosum;* the fine powder which rubs off from the tears, *mica thuris*· and the coarser, *manna thuris.* The gum-resin, that is so called, is the juice of the *Juniperus—foliis ternis undique imbricatis ovatis obtusis*, and is brought from Turkey and the East Indies; but that which comes from India is less esteemed. It is said to ooze spontaneously from the bark of the tree, appearing in drops, or tears, of a pale yellowish, and sometimes of a reddish colour. Olibanum has a moderately strong and not very agreeable smell, and a bitterish, somewhat pungent taste: in chewing, it sticks to the teeth, becomes white, and renders the saliva milky. Laid on a red-hot iron, it readily catches flame, and burns with a strong diffusive and not unpleasant smell. On trituration with water, the greatest part dissolves into a milky liquor, which, on standing, deposites a portion of resinous matter. The gummy and resinous parts are nearly in equal proportions; and though rectified spirit dissolves less of the olibanum than water, it extracts nearly all its active matter. In ancient times, olibanum seems to have been in great repute in affections of the head and breast, coughs, hæmoptysis, and in various fluxes, both uterine and intestinal; it was also much employed externally. Recourse is now seldom had to this medicine, which is superseded by myrrh, and other articles of the resinous kind. It is, however, esteemed by many as an adstringent, and though not in general use, is considered as a valuable medicine in fluor albus, and debilities of the stomach and intestines: applied externally in the form of plaster, it is said to be corroborant, &c. and with this intention it forms the basis of the *emplastrum thuris*.

JUNIPERUS SABINA. The systematic name of the common or barren savin-tree. *Sabina; Savina; Sabina sterilis; Brathu. Juniperus—foliis oppositis erectis decurrentibus, oppositionibus pyxidatis*, of Linnæus. Savin is a native of the south of Europe and the Levant; it has long been cultivated in our gardens, and from producing male and female flowers on separate plants, it was formerly distinguished into the barren and berry-bearing savin. The leaves and tops of this plant have a moderately strong smell of the disagreeable kind, and a hot, bitterish, acrid taste. They give out great part of their active matter to watery liquors, and the whole to rectified spirit. Distilled with water they yield a large quantity of essential oil. Decoctions of the leaves, freed from the volatile principle by inspissation to the consistence of an extract, retain a considerable share of their pungency and warmth along with their bitterness, and have some degree of smell, but not resembling that of the plant itself. On inspissating the spirituous tincture, there remains an extract consisting of two distinct substances, of which one is yellow, unctuous, or oily, bitterish, and very pungent; the other black, resinous, less pungent, and sub-astringent. Savin is a powerful and active medicine, and has been long reputed the most efficacious in the materia medica, for producing a determination to the uterus, and thereby proving emmenagogue; it heats and stimulates the whole system very considerably, and is said to promote the fluid secretions. The power which this plant possesses (observes Dr. Woodville) in opening uterine obstructions, is considered to be so great, that we are told it has been frequently employed, and with too much success, for purposes the most infamous and unnatural. It seems probable, however, that its effects in this way have been somewhat overrated, as it is found, very frequently, to fail as an emmenagogue, though this, in some measure, may be ascribed to the smallness of the dose in which it has been usually prescribed by physicians; for Dr. Cullen observes, "that savin is a very acrid and heating substance, and I have been often, on account of these qualities, prevented from employing it in the quantity necessary to render it emmenagogue. I must own, however, that it shows a more powerful determination to the uterus than any other plant I have employed; but I have been frequently disappointed in this, and its heating qualities always require a great deal of caution." Dr. Home appears to have had very great success with this medicine, for in five cases of amenorrhœa, which occurred at the Royal Infirmary at Edinburgh, four were cured by the sabina, which he gave in powder from a scruple to a drachm twice a-day. He says it is well sui ed to the debile, but improper in plethoric habits, and therefore orders repeated bleedings before its exhibitions. Country people give the juice from the leaves and young tops of savin mixed with milk to their children, in order to destroy the worms; it generally operates by stool, and brings them away with it. The leaves cut small, and given to horses, mixed with their corn, destroy the bots. Externally, savin is recommended as an escharotic to foul ulcers, syphilitic warts, &c. A strong decoction of the plant in lard and wax forms a useful ointment to keep up a constant discharge from blisters. &c. See *Ceratum sabinæ*.

JU'PITER. The ancient chemical name of tin, because supposed under the government of that planet.

JURIN, James, was, during several years, an active member and Secretary of the Royal Society, and at his death in 1750, President of the College of Physicians. He distinguished himself by a series of seventeen dissertations, printed in the Philosophical Transactions, and afterward as a separate work, in which mathematical science was applied with considerable acuteness to physiological subjects. These papers, however, involved him in several philosophical controversies concerning the force of the heart, &c. He was a warm advocate for the practice of inoculation, which he proved greatly to lessen the violence of the small-pox: but he did not anticipate that it would increase the mortality upon the whole, by keeping up the infection, while many retained their prejudices against adopting it.

JUSTICIA. (So named in honour of Mr. Justice, who published the British Gardener's Director.) The name of a genus of plants. Class, *Diandria.* Order *Monogynia.*

JUVA'NTIA. (From *juvo*, to assist.) Whatever assists in relieving a disease.

JUVENTUS. See *Age.*

Juxtangi'na. (From *juxta*, near, and *angina*, a quinsy.) A disease resembling a quinsy

END OF VOL. I.

www.ingramcontent.com/pod-product-compliance
Lightning Source LLC
Chambersburg PA
CBHW071826270326
41929CB00013B/1905